Health Assessment in
Nursing

FOURTH EDITION

Janet Weber, RN, EdD
Professor
Department of Nursing
Southeast Missouri State University
Cape Girardeau, Missouri

Jane H. Kelley, RN, PhD
Adjunct Professor
School of Nursing
University of Mississippi Medical Center
Jackson, Mississippi

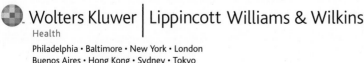
Wolters Kluwer | Lippincott Williams & Wilkins
Health

Philadelphia · Baltimore · New York · London
Buenos Aires · Hong Kong · Sydney · Tokyo

Acquisitions Editor: Elizabeth Nieginski
Project Manager: Katherine Burland
Editorial Assistant: Laura Scott
Director of Nursing Production: Helen Ewan
Art Director, Design: Joan Wendt
Art Director, Illustration: Brett MacNaughton
Manufacturing Coordinator: Karin Duffield
Vendor Manager: Beth Martz
Production Services: Macmillan Publishing Solutions

Fourth Edition

9 8 7 6 5 4 3

Library of Congress Cataloging-in-Publication Data

Weber, Janet.
  Health assessment in nursing / Janet Weber, Jane H. Kelley. — 4th ed.
      p. ; cm.
  Includes bibliographical references and index.
  ISBN 978-0-7817-8160-2 (alk. paper)
  1. Nursing assessment. I. Kelley, Jane, 1944– II. Title.
  [DNLM: 1. Nursing Assessment—methods. WY 100.4 W374h 2010]

  RT48.W43 2010
  610.73—dc22

                                                          2009028726

CCS0211

My husband, children, mother, father, and grandmothers who shared
their wisdom in special ways
Janet

My husband, mother, father, and grandmother, each of whom has helped me to
see the world through new eyes
Jane

But there's no vocabulary
For love within a family, love that's lived in
But not looked at, love within the light of which
All else is seen, the love within which
All other love finds speech.
This love is silent.
From **The Elder Statesman,** *T. S. Eliot (1888–1964)*

Contributors

Linda W. Bugle, PhD, RN
Professor of Nursing
Southeast Missouri State University
Anna, Illinois
CHAPTER 34: ASSESSING COMMUNITIES

Christina Byrd, MSN, ACNP-BC, ANP-BC, CNRN
Neurosciences Nurse Practitioner
Southeast Missouri Hospital
1701 Lacey Street
Cape Girardeau, Missouri
CHAPTER 27: NERVOUS SYSTEM

Jill C. Cash, MSN, APRN, CNP
Nurse Practitioner
Logan Primary Care
Marion, Illinois
CHAPTER 29: ASSESSING CHILDBEARING WOMEN
CHAPTER 30: ASSESSING NEWBORNS AND INFANTS
CHAPTER 31: ASSESSING CHILDREN AND ADOLESCENTS

Kathy Casteel, APRN, BC, FNP
Family Nurse Practitioner
Cape Girardeau Physician Associates
Cape Girardeau, Missouri
CHAPTER 26: MUSCULOSKELETAL SYSTEM

Nancy Collins, RN, MSN
Cardiology Nurse
DuPage Medical Group—Cardiology
Winfield, Illinois
CHAPTER 22: ABDOMEN

Rosie Danker, BSN, RN, CDE
Certified Diabetes Educator—Diabetes Rehab Nurse
St. Francis Medical Center
Cape Girardeau, Missouri
CHAPTER 28: PULLING IT ALL TOGETHER

Brenda Johnson, RN, PhD
Professor
Southeast Missouri State University
Cape Girardeau, MO
CHAPTER 32: ASSESSING FRAIL ELDERLY CLIENTS

Fleetwood Loustalot, PhD, FNP-BC, CDE
Adjunct Faculty
University of Mississippi Medical Center
School of Nursing
Jackson, Mississippi
CHAPTER 11: ASSESSING SPIRITUALITY AND RELIGIOUS
    PRACTICES

Bobbi Morris, APRN, FNP-BC
Instructor
Southeast Missouri State University
CHAPTER 28: PULLING IT ALL TOGETHER

Ann Sprengel, EdD, MSN, RN
Professor
Southeast Missouri State University
Cape Girardeau, Missouri
CHAPTER 12: ASSESSING NUTRITION
CHAPTER 21: PERIPHERAL VASCULAR SYSTEM

Cathy Young, DNSc, RN, FNP, BC
Associate Professor
Texas Tech University Health Science Center
Lubbock, Texas
CHAPTER 9: ASSESSING VICTIMS OF VIOLENCE
CHAPTER 23: FEMALE GENITALIA
CHAPTER 24: MALE GENITALIA

Maureen Anthony, PhD, RN, CDE
McAuley School of Nursing
University of Detroit
Detroit, Michigan

Maureen Belden, MS, RN
University of Michigan
Ann Arbor, Michigan

David Bennett, PhD
Kennesaw State University
Kennesaw, Georgia

Elizabeth Blunt, PhD, RN, CRNP
Drexel University
Philadelphia, Pennsylvania

Kathleen Bobay, PhD, RN, NEA-BC
College of Nursing
Marquette University
Milwaukee, Wisconsin

Cindy Bork, EdD, RN
Winona State University
Winona, Minnesota

Judy Ann Karpecki Bornais, RN, BA, BScN,
MSc, CDE
The University of Windsor
Windsor, Ontario

Linda A. Browne, MSN, BSN
Southwest Georgia Technical College
Thomasville, Georgia

Lorraine Cramp, RN, BA, BScN, MEd, PhD
Centennial College
Toronto, Ontario

Kathleen Curtis, BSN, RN
Mt. Carmel College of Nursing
Columbus, Ohio

Donna Davis, RN, NP-C, CNS, MSN
Imperial Valley College
Imperial, California

Julie Duff Cloutier, RN, BScN
Laurentian University
Sudbury, Ontario

Dana Edge, PhD, RN
University of Calgary
Calgary, Alberta

Brenda Eraut, RN, BSN
Douglas College
New Westminster, British Columbia

Sarah Evans, RN, MN
George Brown College
Toronto, Ontario

Helen Ewing
Centre for Nursing
Athabasca University
Athabasca, Alberta

Elizabeth Farren, PhD, MSN, BSN
Baylor University
Dallas, Texas

Cindy Fenske, MS, RN
University of Michigan
Ann Arbor, Michigan

Elizabeth Fornasier, RN, BScN, Med
George Brown College
Toronto, Ontario

Candace Ginsberg, MSN, RN, C-NP
College of St. Scholastica
Duluth, Minnesota

Lynne Harwood-Lunn, RN, BScN, MN
School of Nursing
York University
Toronto, Ontario

Anna Helewka, RPN, RN, BSN, MSN
Douglas College
New Westminster, British Columbia

Judy Hileman, ARNP, PhD
University of Missouri, Kansas City
Kansas City, Missouri

Karen Hoffman, ADAA
Indiana Wesleyan University
Marion, Indiana

Jane Kassens, MSN, CS, FNP
Georgia State University
Atlanta, Georgia

Kate Kniest, MSN
Harper College
Palatine, Illinois

Robin Eades Koch, RN, MSN, NNP
Piedmont Virginia Community College
Charlottesville, Virginia

Rhonda Lansdell, AND
Northeast Mississippi Community College
Booneville, Mississippi

Sandra Longman, BScN, MA
Seneca College
Toronto, Ontario

Noelle Lottes, RN, MS, CPNP, CFNP
Purdue University
West Lafayette, Indiana

Joanne Louis, BScN, RN, MSc
University of Toronto
Toronto, Ontario

Diana Mager, CRN, MSN
Fairfield University
Fairfield, Connecticut

Monique Mallet-Boucher, BScN, BEd, Med, MN
University of New Brunswick
Fredericton, New Brunswick

Shantia McCoy, MSN, CRNP
LaSalle University
Philadelphia, Pennsylvania

Sheila McKay, RN, MN
Red Deer College
Red Deer, Alberta

John McNulty, MS, RN
School of Nursing
University of Connecticut
Storrs, Connecticut

Wendy Mortimer, MSN, CRNP
Reading Hospital School of Allied Health
West Reading, Pennsylvania

Yvonne Nathan, EdD, RN
SUNY-Downstate Medical Center
Brooklyn, New York

Lynn Nichols, PhD, RN
St. John Fisher College
Rochester, New York

Laura Nicholson, RN, MN, ENC
Centennial College
Toronto, Ontario

Linda Nykolyn, RN, BScN
NorQuest College
Edmonton, Alberta

Pat O'Leary, DSN, RN, COI
Middle Tennessee State University
Murfreesboro, Tennessee

Pat Olsen, MN, RN
Shoreline Community College
Shoreline, Washington

Catherine Pagel, RN, MSN
Mercy College of Health Sciences
Des Moines, Iowa

Marilyn Pestano-Harte, RN, MSN
Florida International University
Miami, Florida

Karen Piotrowski, MSN, RNC
D'Youville College
Buffalo, New York

Nancy Prince, MSN, RN, FNP
Eastern Michigan University
Ypsilanti, Michigan

Jennifer Prinz
Spencerian College
Louisville, Kentucky

Mary Radford, RN, MSN
The University of Tennessee at Martin
Martin, Tennessee

Carol Reid
Century College
White Bear Lake, Minnesota

Lois Ripley, BSN, MS
West Virginia University, Parkersburg
Parkersburg, West Virginia

Margot Rykhoff, RN, BScN, MA(Ed)
Humber College Institute of Technology
and Advanced Learning
Toronto, Ontario

Mary Scott, RN, MSN, PhD
University of California, San Francisco
School of Nursing
San Francisco, California

Joyce Shanty, MS, RN
Indiana University of Pennsylvania
Indiana, Pennsylvania

Karen Smith, BN, PN
Centre for Nursing Studies
St. John's, Newfoundland

Judy Stauder, MSN, RN
Stark State College of Technology
Canton, Ohio

Audrey Steenbeek, PhD, MSN, BSN
Dalhousie University
Halifax, Nova Scotia

Lynne Thibeault, RN, BScN, NP-PHC, MEd
Confederation College
Thunder Bay, Ontario

Barbara Thompson, RN, BScN, MScN
Sault College
Sault Ste. Marie, Ontario

Valerie Trousdale, MSN, BSN
Baylor University
Dallas, Texas

Creina Twomey, C, BN, MN
Memorial University
St. John's, Newfoundland

Marsha Wamsley, RN, MS
Sinclair Community College
Dayton, Ohio

Ming Wang-Letzkus
California State University, Los Angeles
Los Angeles, California

Paige D. Wimberley, MSN, RN, CNS, CNE
Arkansas State University
Jonesboro, Arkansas

Sandra Wynn, MSN, BS, APRN, BC
Bluefield State College
Bluefield, West Virginia

Joanne Yastik, MSN, RN
University of Detroit Mercy
Detroit, Michigan

Patti Zuzelo, EdD, RN, CS
La Salle University
Philadelphia, Pennsylvania

Preface

With the fourth edition of *Health Assessment in Nursing,* our goal remains to help students acquire the skills they need to perform nursing assessments in today's ever changing health care environment. As nurses provide more care in a variety of settings—acute care agencies, clinics, family homes, rehabilitation centers, and long-term care facilities—they need to be more prepared than ever before to perform accurate, timely health assessments. No matter where a nurse practices, two components are essential for accurate collection of client data: a comprehensive knowledge base and expert nursing assessment skills. With that in mind, we have filled these pages with in-depth, accurate information; illustrations; and learning tools that help the student develop skills to collect both subjective and objective data. In addition to nursing assessment skills, today's nurses also need expert critical thinking skills to analyze the data they collect and to detect client problems—whether they are nursing problems that can be treated independently by nurses, collaborative problems that can be treated in conjunction with other health care practitioners, or medical problems that require referral to appropriate professionals. This textbook teaches students to use critical thinking skills to analyze the data they collect.

ORGANIZATION OF THE TEXT

This fourth edition of *Health Assessment in Nursing* has four units:

I.   Nursing Data Collection, Documentation, and Analysis
II. Integrative Holistic Nursing Assessment
III. Nursing Assessment of Physical Systems
IV. Nursing Assessment of Special Groups

Unit I describes the nurse's role in health assessment. It introduces the student to data collection and analysis as part of the nursing process. Separate chapters provide in-depth information about each step of the assessment process: collecting subjective data, collecting objective data, validating and documenting data, and analyzing the data. The process of using critical thinking skills to assess clients is discussed.

Unit II introduces the student to the unique perspective that the client should never be viewed as an isolated individual. Concepts covered in this unit are applicable throughout the entire client assessment. The unit begins by explaining how to obtain an overall view or general impression of the client. Assessment techniques to determine the client's mental status and comfort level are described; as are ways to determine if the client is a victim of violence; and ways that culture, spirituality, religion, and nutrition affect the client's holistic health.

Unit III immerses the student in actual assessment techniques for all body systems. Separate chapters cover techniques for each body system; and techniques to adapt for the older client are highlighted in each chapter. The unit concludes with a chapter on "Pulling It All Together," which shows the student how to integrate assessment of all body systems. Students can use the examples provided to model their own data collections,

analyses, and formulation of nursing diagnoses, collaborative problems, or referrals.

Unit IV reinforces the need to adapt assessment to the context of the client. Chapters provide specific information about ways to assess childbearing women, newborns and infants, children and adolescents, elderly clients, families, and communities. Separate chapters for each of these groups allow students easy access to the information they need when taking another course (i.e., pediatric nursing or community health nursing). For example, rather than look for toddler considerations in each body system chapter, the student can look to Chapter 31 to find head-to-toe information for the toddler. The chapter on assessing elderly clients provides an in-depth assessment of functional health of the frail elderly population.

ORGANIZATION OF THE ASSESSMENT CHAPTERS

Assessment chapters walk students through the entire assessment process from an anatomy and physiology review to data collection to analysis. Each assessment chapter includes the following organization:

• Structure and Function
• Health Assessment
• Collecting Subjective Data: The Nursing Health History
• Collecting Objective Data: Physical Examination
• Validating and Documenting Findings
• Analysis of Data
• Diagnostic Reasoning: Possible Conclusions
• Case Study

Structure and Function sections review key anatomy and physiology, which provide the knowledge base the nurse draws on to complete assessment. Health Assessment sections give in-depth assessment parameters, including nursing health history, physical assessment, and validation and documentation of the data. Nursing Health History information is presented in two columns; column one gives examples of questions to ask the client, and column two gives the rationale for asking the question. This approach helps students understand the "Whys" behind the "Whats," promoting critical thinking. Next, physical examination procedures are illustrated in a step-by-step fashion across three columns. Column one tells the student exactly how to perform specific aspects of the examination. Column two presents normal findings and normal variations, while column three presents a variety of abnormal findings. In addition, Abnormal Findings displays depict common abnormal findings, helping students to identify their findings. Sample documentation demonstrates proper documentation technique, a must for all students.

Analysis of the Data sections provide common nursing diagnoses (well, risk, and actual) and possible collaborative problems related to the specific body system. The case study uses a sample client to walk students through the diagnostic reasoning process.

THEMES OF THE TEXT

Health Promotion

Health promotion and client wellness are important baseline concepts in *Health Assessment in Nursing*. Asking the types of questions exemplified in the "Nursing History" sections of the chapters provides the nurse with an opportunity to promote health and healthful practices to clients—particularly in regard to nutrition, activity and exercise, sleep and rest, medication use and abuse, self care responsibilities, social activities, family relationships, education and careers, stress levels and coping strategies, and adaptation to the environment and community. Along these lines, the Promote Health displays contain "Risk Reduction Tips," which are an excellent resource for students to use to teach the client ways to reduce risk factors. Also, the text provides guidelines for how to perform self-examinations, including a skin self-examination, breast self-examination, and testicular self-examination.

Culture

In today's health care environment, both health care providers and health care recipients bring vast cultural variation to the marketplace, which in turn presents new ideas, practices, and challenges for nursing assessment. Consideration of culture is a high priority in *Health Assessment in Nursing*. It is not an aside to assessment—it is an integral part of it, which is why, in addition to a chapter introducing cultural concepts associated with assessment, normal and abnormal findings related to culture are integrated throughout the text exactly where the student would expect to find the information during an actual assessment. These considerations are highlighted by a special icon.

Lifespan

People today are living longer and healthier lives, making it more important than ever to meet the health needs of an aging population. Chapters in Unit III include information on how to adapt the assessment process to older clients, and describe how some physical changes are actually normal adaptations to aging rather than abnormal health findings. This information is also highlighted with an icon. Special individual chapters in Unit IV provide comprehensive discussions of the differences inherent in assessing very young and elderly clients, as well as child-bearing women. These chapters explain and illustrate the uniqueness of these differences in regard to body structures and functions, interview techniques, growth and development, and physical examination techniques.

Family and Community

Chapters devoted to assessing families and communities complete the text. The family chapter contains the theories of family function, family communication styles, nursing interview techniques for families, internal and external family structuring, and family development stages and tasks. A chapter on victims of violence assists the student in assessing the use of violence in families (see below). The community assessment chapter addresses the types of communities families and individuals live in and how the community enhances health or presents a barrier to effective, healthful functioning. How the physical environment of a community interacts with community health and social services is also explained and illustrated. This chapter is unique in that it assists the student with assessing the needs of a community in which a client lives. Again, this reinforces the concept of the client within the context of the community in which he or she lives.

MAJOR CHANGES TO THE FOURTH EDITION

This thoroughly updated edition includes several new features and chapters.

The chapters in **Unit II** emphasize the integrative holistic aspects of assessment, which are essential considerations with each client. Two **new chapters** have been added to this unit. **Assessing Mental Status and Psychosocial Developmental Level** has been created as a separate chapter from the neurological assessment chapter and placed at the beginning of the text to emphasize the importance of mental status and developmental level in obtaining a reliable client health history and clues to guide the nurse in the rest of the nursing assessment. **Assessing Culture,** another new chapter, has been added to cover cultural variations in communication and beliefs, and biological variations based on genetics and ethnicity. Chapter 9 on **Assessing Victims of Violence** has been reworked and moved from Unit IV, Assessment of Special Groups, to Unit II. Chapter 12 on **Assessing Nutrition** has expanded to include more variations of food recommendations including Canadian, Mediterranean, and vegetarian food guides. Finally, the **Pulling It All Together** chapter still focuses on assisting students to integrate all their knowledge into an organized, succinct format needed to perform a comprehensive "head-to-toe" physical examination. However, an addition to this chapter is a short **head-to-toe assessment format** that can be used on a daily basis to update ongoing client assessments. This format is commonly used in hospital settings by nurses who continually assess the client on an ongoing basis.

Features new to this edition include **COLDSPA Example,** which appears at the beginning of each chapter's Health History section; and **Applying COLDSPA,** which appears within each chapter's case study. These features provide samples of how the COLDSPA mnemonic can be applied to assessment of various body systems, and how nurses should follow up to client responses. **Spotlight** boxes highlight information about various assessment techniques and equipment; **Assessment Tool** boxes include process details and helpful questionnaires; and **Promote Health** boxes detail key information on a variety of health risks, including risk factors and risk reduction tips.

THE TEACHING-LEARNING PACKAGE

The fourth edition of *Health Assessment in Nursing* provides a robust teaching-learning package, including resources for both instructors and students.

Student Lab Manual to Accompany Health Assessment in Nursing

The combined study guide and lab manual is a significant resource that enhances learning and prepares the student for practice. It is designed to actively engage the learner. It offers self-test activities and interactive student group exercises that help students apply and retain the knowledge gained from the textbook. It also includes checklists to help the student capture important aspects of assessment.

Weber and Kelley's Interactive Nursing Assessment, Fourth Edition

Incorporating ten all new modules, the fourth edition of this engaging, interactive learning tool provides even more opportunity for students to refine their assessment skills. Structure and Function exercises test students' ability to correctly identify important anatomic structures and their function. Assessment exercises help students refine their data collection skills, and Analysis of the Data exercises provides students with an opportunity to practice diagnostic reasoning. The program also includes hundreds of NCLEX-style questions to test key concepts. It is available both for individual use on CD-ROM and for delivery via your institution's WebCT or Blackboard Learning Management System. This product also works in grade book software, allowing instructors to track students' progress.

Student Resource CD-ROM

The CD-ROM included with this text offers valuable resources for the student. A **Head-to-Toe Assessment Video,** created specifically for this text, walks the student through a comprehensive physical examination. This video takes a unique approach; a student nurse completes the examination under the supervision of an instructor. Students easily identify with the student nurse, and seeing a peer complete the examination helps build confidence. The CD-ROM also includes video demonstrating accurate collection of vital signs, illustrating and supporting the content from the general status chapter. In addition, the CD-ROM includes access to heart and breath sounds tutorials, giving students an opportunity to both hear the sounds and test their ability to identify normal and abnormal sounds. Additional exercises allow students to test their knowledge.

Instructor's Resource CD-ROM

The *Instructor's Resource CD-ROM to Accompany Health Assessment in Nursing* contains everything instructors need to bring health assessment to life for the student. The CD-ROM includes sample **Syllabi** for setting up your course and an integrated set of materials for every chapter:

- **Test Generator** featuring more than 900 questions
- Lively **PowerPoint slides** that include artwork and photographs from the text
- **Image Bank** featuring all the figures from each chapter
- **Assignments** for gauging student understanding
- **Discussion Topics** to encourage critical thinking
- **Case Studies** providing real life application of concepts
- **Lecture Outlines** for presenting key information to your students

The CD-ROM features these materials available for use in your institution's WebCT and Blackboard Learning Management System. It is available upon adoption of the text.

Janet Weber
Jane Kelley

Acknowledgements

With love, appreciation, and many thanks, we would like to acknowledge the following people for their help in making the fourth edition of *Health Assessment in Nursing* a reality.

JW:

- To Jane, my coauthor, for all your support in sharing your insights, research, and cultural expertise throughout the text
- To Bill, my husband, for your patience and encouragement on a long-term project
- To Joe and Wesley, my sons, for your humor and distractions to refresh my mind with what is really important in life
- To my mom, for your continued loving patience and support

JK:

- To Janet, precious friend, loyal colleague, and primary author, for encouraging my participation and for making the challenge a delightful experience
- To Arthur, my husband, for his sense of humor, creative outlook, and encouragement over the years
- To my mother, for inspiring me with an eagerness to learn

JW AND JK:

- To Elizabeth Nieginski, Executive Acquisitions Editor, for all your assistance and encouragement

- To Katherine Burland, Associate Development Editor, for your hard work, special insights, and creative ideas in making this fourth edition a pleasure to develop
- To all of our colleagues and contributors who have shared their expertise to make this book a reality
- To our students, who give us insight as to how one learns best
- To our friends, who give us endless hope and encouragement
- To Tom Mondeau, Mark Hill, Dr. Stanley Sides, Dr. Richard Martin, Dr. Michael Bennett, Curt Casteel, and Dr. Terri Woods for all your wonderful photography
- To Barbara Proud, for your excellent professional photography that is present throughout the text
- To Jill Cash and clients for your time, assessment, expertise, and participation in photo shoots—the beautiful photographs in "Assessing Newborns and Infants" and "Assessing Children and Adolescents" would not have been possible without you
- To ElderNet of Lower Merion—Narberth, Bryn Mawr, Pennsylvania, for your professionalism and kind assistance in eldercare
- To Amy Geller, Producer; Gus Freedman, photographer; Newton-Wellesley Hospital; and the kind nurses and patients for helping us update photographs throughout the book

Contents

1

Nurse's Role in Health Assessment: Collecting and Analyzing Data

Picture yourself in the following situations:

- You walk into Mrs. Smith's room for the first time. She is sitting on the edge of the bed crying and has not changed into a hospital gown. You introduce yourself and say, "You seem very upset." Mrs. Smith tells you that she is concerned about her husband being left at home alone while she is in the hospital for colon surgery.

- You make a follow-up visit to a new mother, Rebecca Brown, and her 3-day-old son. You arrive at the address provided to you and find Mrs. Brown and newborn living in a worn-down trailer. She appears very tired. When asked about this, she says that she has been unable to rest because of several visitors. "I don't mind the attention, but I'm sorta worried that my baby is gonna get sick because a lot of the people that have been coming over are sick with colds." Mrs. Brown also tells you that she has had trouble breast-feeding. You see the newborn in a crib and notice that his breathing is labored.

- While shopping in a grocery store, you notice a mother with three young children. The youngest, a boy, is in the grocery cart attempting to climb from the cart to the checkout counter. The child does not have on a safety belt; there is none available on the cart. The mother is gathering her coupons together and has her back to the boy to scold her two girls who are fighting with each other.

As a professional nurse, you will constantly observe situations and collect information to make nursing judgments. This occurs no matter what the setting: hospital, clinic, home, community, or long-term care. Each of the previous situations requires the collection of additional data before making a nursing judgment. For example, is Mr. Smith capable of caring for himself? What is the physical health status of the newborn in the trailer home? Does the community grocery store have any carts with child safety seat belts on them? Additional information may be gathered from further direct observations of the client and surroundings. In addition, you may also collect data by talking with the client, mother, or store manager.

You conduct many informal assessments every day. For example, when you get up in the morning, you check the weather and determine what would be the most appropriate clothing to wear. You assess whether you are hungry. Do you need a light or heavy breakfast? When will you be able to eat next? You may even assess the physical condition of your skin. Do you need moisturizing lotion? The assessments you make each day determine many of your actions and influence your comfort and success for the remainder of the day. Likewise, the professional nursing assessments you make on a client, family, or community determine nursing interventions that directly or indirectly influence the health status of your client.

INTRODUCTION TO HEALTH ASSESSMENT IN NURSING

Assessment: Step One of the Nursing Process

As you have learned, assessment is the first and most critical phase of the nursing process. If data collection is inadequate or inaccurate, incorrect nursing judgments may be made that adversely affect the remaining phases of the process: diagnosis, planning, implementation, and evaluation (Table 1-1). Although the assessment phase of the nursing process precedes the other phases in the formal nursing process, nurses are always aware that assessment is ongoing and continuous throughout all the phases of the nursing process. The nursing process should be thought of as circular, not linear (Fig. 1-1).

Focus of Health Assessment in Nursing

Virtually every health care professional performs assessments to make professional judgments related to clients. However, the purpose of a nursing health history and physical examination differs greatly from that of a medical or other type of health care examination (e.g., dietary assessment or examination for physical therapy).

Phase	Title	Description
Table 1-1	**Phases of the Nursing Process**	
I	Assessment	Collecting subjective and objective data
II	Diagnosis	Analyzing subjective and objective data to make a professional nursing judgment (nursing diagnosis, collaborative problem, or referral)
III	Planning	Determining outcome criteria and developing a plan
IV	Implementation	Carrying out the plan
V	Evaluation	Assessing whether outcome criteria have been met and revising the plan as necessary

The purpose of a nursing health assessment is to collect subjective and objective data to determine a client's overall level of functioning in order to make a professional clinical judgment. The nurse collects physiologic, psychological, sociocultural, developmental, and spiritual data *about* the client. Thus the nurse performs holistic data collection.

The mind, body, and spirit are considered to be interdependent factors that affect a person's level of health. The nurse, in particular, focuses on how the client's health status affects his activities of daily living and how the client's activities of daily living affect his health. For example, a client with asthma may have to avoid extreme temperatures and may not be able to enjoy recreational camping. If this client walks to work in a smoggy environment, it will adversely affect his asthma.

In addition, the nurse assesses how clients interact within their family, culture, and community and how the clients' health status affects the family and community. For example, a diabetic client may not be able to eat the same foods that the rest of the family enjoys. If this client develops complications of diabetes and has an amputation, the client may not be able to carry out his family responsibility of maintaining the yard. In addition, the client may no longer be able to work in the community as a bus driver. The nurse also assesses how family and community affect the individual client's health status. A supportive creative family may find alternative ways of cooking tasteful foods that are healthy for the entire family. The community may or may not have a diabetic support group for the client and the family.

In contrast, the physician performing a medical examination focuses primarily on the client's physiologic development status. Less focus may be placed on psychological, sociocultural, or spiritual well-being. Similarly, a physical therapist would focus more on the client's musculoskeletal system and ability to perform activities of daily living.

Framework for Health Assessment in Nursing

The framework used to collect nursing health assessment data differs from those used by other professionals. Using a nursing framework helps to organize information and promotes the collection of holistic data. This, in turn, provides clues that help to determine human responses.

Because there are so many nursing health assessment frameworks available for organizing data, using one assessment framework would limit the use of this text and ignore

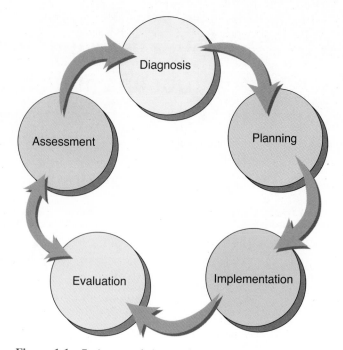

Figure 1-1 Each step of the nursing process depends on the accuracy of the preceding step. The steps are also overlapping because you may have to move more quickly for some problems than others. While *Evaluation* involves examining all the previous steps, it especially focuses on achieving desired outcomes. The arrow between *Assessment* and *Evaluation* goes in both directions because assessment and evaluation are ongoing processes as well as separate phases. When the outcomes are not as anticipated, the nurse needs to revisit (reassess) all the steps, collect new data, and formulate adjustments to the plan of care. (Adapted from Alfaro, R. (2006). *Applying nursing process: A tool for critical thinking* (6th ed.). Philadelphia: Lippincott Williams & Wilkins.)

many other valid nursing assessment framework methods. Therefore, the objective of this textbook is to provide the reader with the essential raw material necessary to perform a thorough health assessment without locking into one particular framework. Readers can take the information in this book and adapt it to the nursing assessment framework of their choice. The book is organized around a head-to-toe assessment of body parts and systems. In each chapter, the nursing health history is organized according to a "generic" nursing history framework, which is an abbreviated version of the complete nursing health history detailed in Chapter 3. The questions asked in each chapter concentrate on that particular body part or system and are broken down into four sections:

- History of Present Health Concern
- Past Health History
- Family History
- Lifestyle and Health Practices

After the health history, the physical assessment section provides the procedure, normal findings, and abnormal findings for each step of examination of a particular body part or system. The collected data based on the client's answers to the types of questions asked in the nursing history, along with the objective data gathered during the hands-on physical assessment, enable the nurse to make judgments concerning nursing diagnoses, collaborative problems, referral, and need for client teaching.

The end result of a nursing assessment is the formulation of nursing diagnoses (wellness, risk, or actual) that require nursing care, the identification of collaborative problems that require interdisciplinary care, and the identification of medical problems that require immediate referral.

Types of Assessment

The four basic types of assessment are

- Initial comprehensive assessment
- Ongoing or partial assessment
- Focused or problem-oriented assessment
- Emergency assessment

Each varies in the amount and type of data collected.

Initial Comprehensive Assessment

An initial comprehensive assessment involves collection of subjective data about the client's perception of her health of all body parts or systems, past health history, family history, and lifestyle and health practices (which includes information related to the client's overall function) as well as objective data gathered during a step-by-step physical examination.

The nurse typically collects the subjective data, especially those related to the client's overall function. However, depending on the setting (hospital, community, clinic, or home), other members of the health care team may participate in various parts of the objective data collection. For example, in a hospital setting the physician usually performs a total physical examination when the client is admitted (if this was not previously done in the physician's office). A physical therapist may perform a musculoskeletal examination, as in the case of a stroke patient, and a dietitian may take anthropometric measurements in addition to a subjective nutritional assessment. In a community clinic, a nurse practitioner may perform the entire physical examination. In the home setting, the nurse is usually responsible for performing most of the physical examination.

Regardless of who collects the data, a total health assessment (subjective and objective data regarding functional health and body systems) is needed when the client first enters a health care system and periodically thereafter to establish baseline data against which future health status changes can be measured and compared. Frequency of comprehensive assessments depends on the client's age, risk factors, health status, health promotion practices, and lifestyle.

Ongoing or Partial Assessment

An ongoing or partial assessment of the client consists of data collection that occurs after the comprehensive database is established. This consists of a mini-overview of the client's body systems and holistic health patterns as a follow-up on his health status. Any problems that were initially detected in the client's body system or holistic health patterns are reassessed in less depth to determine any major changes (deterioration or improvement) from the baseline data. In addition, a brief reassessment of the client's normal body system or holistic health patterns is performed to detect any new problems. This type of assessment is usually performed whenever the nurse or another health care professional has an encounter with the client. This type of assessment may be performed in the hospital, community, or home setting. For example, a client admitted to the hospital with lung cancer requires frequent assessment of lung sounds. A total assessment of skin would be performed less frequently, with the nurse focusing on the color and temperature of the extremities to determine level of oxygenation.

Focused or Problem-Oriented Assessment

A focused or problem-oriented assessment does not take the place of the comprehensive health assessment. It is performed when a comprehensive database exists for a client who comes to the health care agency with a specific health concern. A focused assessment consists of a thorough assessment of a particular client problem and does not cover areas not related to the problem. For example, if your client, John P., tells you that he has ear pain, you would ask him questions about the pain, possible hearing loss, dizziness, ringing in his ears, and personal ear care. Asking questions about his sexual functioning or his normal bowel habits would be unnecessary and inappropriate. The physical examination should focus on his ears, nose, mouth, and throat. At this time, it would not be appropriate to repeat all system examinations such as the heart and neck vessel or abdominal assessment.

Emergency Assessment

An emergency assessment is a very rapid assessment performed in life-threatening situations. In such situations (choking, cardiac arrest, drowning), an immediate diagnosis is needed to provide prompt treatment. An example of an emergency assessment is the evaluation of the client's airway, breathing, and circulation (known as the ABCs) when cardiac arrest is suspected. The major and only concern during this type of assessment is to determine the status of the client's life-sustaining physical functions.

STEPS OF HEALTH ASSESSMENT

The assessment phase of the nursing process has four major steps:

1. Collection of subjective data
2. Collection of objective data
3. Validation of data
4. Documentation of data

Although there are four steps, they tend to overlap and you may perform two or three steps concurrently. For example, you may ask your client, Jane Q., if she has dry skin while you are inspecting the condition of the skin. If she answers "no," but you notice that the skin on her hands is very dry, validation with the client may be performed at this point.

Each part of assessment is discussed briefly in the following sections. However, Chapters 2, 3, and 4 provide an in-depth explanation of each of the four assessment steps. In addition, the four steps of the assessment process format are carried throughout this text. All nursing assessment chapters contain the following sections: Collecting Subjective Data, Collecting Objective Data, and a combined Validation and Documentation section.

Preparing for the Assessment

Before actually meeting the client and beginning the nursing health assessment, there are several things you should do to prepare. It is helpful to review the client's record, if available.

Knowing the client's basic biographical data (age, sex, religion, and occupation) is useful. It provides background about chronic diseases and gives clues to how a present illness may impact the client's activities of daily living (ADL). Also useful is documented information regarding the client's medical diagnoses and progress notes. These give you an opportunity to verify what you read with what the client tells you and to ask further questions as needed. Reviewing the client's status with other health care team members who have taken care of or interacted with him is also helpful. Often a client may reveal and share important data with some team members and not others.

After reviewing the record or discussing the client's status with others, remember to keep an open mind and to avoid premature judgments that may alter your ability to collect accurate data. For example, do not assume a 30-year-old female client who happens to be a nurse knows everything regarding hospital routine and medical care or that a 60-year-old male client with diabetes mellitus needs client teaching regarding diet. Keep an open mind. Validate information with the client and be prepared to collect additional data.

Also use this time to educate yourself about the client's diagnoses or tests performed. The client may have a medical diagnosis that you have never heard of or that you have not dealt with in the past. You may review the record and find that the client had a special blood test and the results were abnormal and that you are not familiar with this test. At that time, you should consult the necessary resources (laboratory manual, textbook, or blood laboratory) to learn about the test and the implications of its findings.

Once you have gathered some basic data about the client, take a minute to reflect on your own feelings regarding your initial encounter with the client. For example, the client may be a 22-year-old with a drug addiction. If you are 22 years old and are a very health-conscious person who does not drink, smoke, take illegal drugs, or drink caffeine, you need to take time to examine your own feelings so you avoid biases, judgment, and the tendency to project your own feelings onto the client. You must be as objective and open as possible. Other client situations that may require more reflection time include those involving sexually transmitted diseases, terminal illnesses, amputation, paralysis, early teenage pregnancies, human immunodeficiency virus (HIV) infection or acquired immunodeficiency syndrome (AIDS), and abortion.

Finally, remember to obtain and organize materials that you will need for the assessment. The materials may be assessment tools such as a guide to interview questions or forms on which to record data collected during the health history interview and physical examination. Also gather any equipment (e.g., stethoscope, thermometer, otoscope) necessary to perform a nursing health assessment.

Collecting Subjective Data

Subjective data are sensations or symptoms (e.g., pain, hunger), feelings (e.g., happiness, sadness), perceptions, desires, preferences, beliefs, ideas, values, and personal information that can be elicited and verified only by the client. To elicit accurate subjective data, learn to use effective interviewing skills with a variety of clients in different settings. The major areas of subjective data include

- Biographical information (name, age, religion, occupation)
- Physical symptoms related to each body part or system (e.g., eyes and ears, abdomen)
- Past health history
- Family history
- Health and lifestyle practices (e.g., health practices that put the client at risk, nutrition, activity, relationships, cultural beliefs or practices, family structure and function, community environment)

The skills of interviewing and the complete health history are discussed in Chapter 3.

Collecting Objective Data

Objective data are directly observed by the examiner. These data include

- Physical characteristics (e.g., skin color, posture)
- Body functions (e.g., heart rate, respiratory rate)
- Appearance (e.g., dress and hygiene)
- Behavior (e.g., mood, affect)
- Measurements (e.g., blood pressure, temperature, height, weight)
- Results of laboratory testing (e.g., platelet count, x-ray findings)

This type of data is obtained by general observation and by using the four physical examination techniques: inspection, palpation, percussion, and auscultation. Another source of objective data is the client's medical/health record, which is the document that contains information about what other health care professionals (i.e., nurses, physicians, physical therapists, dietitians, social workers) observed about the client. Objective data may also be observations noted by the family or significant others about the client. See Table 1-2 for a comparison of objective and subjective data.

Validating Assessment Data

Validation of assessment data is a crucial part of assessment that often occurs along with collection of subjective and objective data. It serves to ensure that the assessment process is not ended before all relevant data have been collected, and it helps to prevent documentation of inaccurate data. What types of assessment data should be validated, the different ways to validate data, and identifying areas where data are missing are all parts of the process. Validation of data is discussed in detail in Chapter 4.

Documenting Data

Documentation of assessment data is an important step of assessment because it forms the database for the entire nursing process and provides data for all other members of the health care team. Thorough and accurate documentation is vital to ensure valid conclusions are made when the data are analyzed in the second step of the nursing process. Chapter 4 discusses the types of documentation, purpose of documentation, what to document, guidelines for documentation, and different types of documentation forms.

ANALYSIS OF ASSESSMENT DATA

Nursing Diagnosis: Step Two of the Nursing Process

Analysis of data (often called nursing diagnosis) is the second phase of the nursing process. Analysis of the collected data goes hand in hand with the rationale for performing a nursing

Table 1-2	Comparing Subjective and Objective Data	
	Subjective	**Objective**
Description	Data elicited and verified by the client	Data directly or indirectly observed through measurement
Sources	Client Family and significant others Client record Other health care professionals	Observations and physical assessment findings of the nurse or other health care professionals Documentation of assessments made in client record Observations made by the client's family or significant others
Methods used to obtain data	Client interview	Observation and physical examination
Skills needed to obtain data	Interview and therapeutic communication skills Caring ability and empathy Listening skills	Inspection Palpation Percussion Auscultation
Examples	"I have a headache." "It frightens me." "I am not hungry."	Respirations 16 per minute BP 180/100, apical pulse 80 and irregular X-ray film reveals fractured pelvis

assessment. The purpose of assessment is to arrive at conclusions about the client's health. To arrive at conclusions, the nurse must analyze the assessment data. Indeed, the nurse often begins to analyze the data in his mind while performing assessment. To achieve the goal or anticipated outcome of the assessment, the nurse makes sure that the data collected are as accurate and thorough as possible.

During this phase, you analyze and synthesize data to determine whether the data reveal a nursing concern (nursing diagnosis), a collaborative concern (collaborative problem), or a concern that needs to be referred to another discipline (referral).

A nursing diagnosis is defined by the North American Nursing Diagnosis Association (NANDA) as "a clinical judgment about individuals, family or community responses to actual and potential health problems and life processes. A nursing diagnosis provides the basis for selecting nursing interventions to achieve outcomes for which the nurse is accountable". Collaborative problems are defined as certain "physiological complications that nurses monitor to detect their onset or changes in status" (Carpenito, 2005). Nurses manage collaborative problems by implementing both physician- and nurse-prescribed interventions to reduce further complications. Referrals occur because nurses assess the "whole" (physical, psychological, social, cultural, and spiritual) client and, therefore, often identify problems that require the assistance of other health care professionals. Chapter 5 provides information about nursing diagnoses, collaborative problems, and referrals.

Process of Data Analysis

To arrive at nursing diagnoses, collaborative problems, or referral, you must go through the steps of data analysis. This process requires diagnostic reasoning skills, often called critical thinking. The process can be divided into seven major steps.

1. Identify abnormal data and strengths.
2. Cluster the data.
3. Draw inferences and identify problems.

4. Propose possible nursing diagnoses.
5. Check for defining characteristics of those diagnoses.
6. Confirm or rule out nursing diagnoses.
7. Document conclusions.

Each of these steps is explained in detail in Chapter 5. In addition, each assessment chapter in this text contains a section called "Analysis of Data," which uses these steps to analyze the assessment data presented in a specific client case study related to chapter content.

EVOLUTION OF THE NURSE'S ROLE IN HEALTH ASSESSMENT

The nurse's role in health assessment has changed significantly over the years. In the 21st century, the nurse's role in assessment continues to expand, becoming more crucial than ever before.

Past

Her long skirt swished with her stride and the flame of the oil lamp flickered as she approached the last bed in the dark and crowded infirmary. The tall, thin and frail man lay still on his back with his sunken eyes barely open. She spoke softly as she moved the light near him and gazed at his pale face. She placed the top of her hand over his fevered brow and felt the weak pulsation at his wrist. She wiped the beads of sweat from his temples, watched his heavy chest movements, and counted his loud breathing. She pressed a moist cloth to his dry lips, straightened his pillow, then moved to the window to write her notes.—N. Collins

As the previous passage indicates, physical assessment has been an integral part of nursing since the days of Florence Nightingale. Nurses relied on their natural senses; the client's face and body would be observed for "changes in color, temperature, muscle strength, use of limbs, body output, and degrees of nutrition, and hydration" (Nightingale, 1992). Palpation was used to measure pulse rate and quality and to locate the fundus of the puerperal woman (Fitzsimmons & Gallagher, 1978).

Examples of independent nursing practice using inspection, palpation, and auscultation have been recorded in nursing journals since 1901. Some examples reported in the *American Journal of Nursing* (1901–1938) include gastrointestinal palpation, testing eighth cranial nerve function, and examination of children in school systems. In addition, the *American Journal of Public Health* documents routine client and home inspection by public health nurses in the 1930s. This role of case finding, prevention of communicable diseases, and routine use of assessment skills in poor inner-city areas was performed through the Frontier Nursing Service and the Red Cross (Fitzsimmons & Gallagher, 1978). Nurses were also hired to conduct preemployment health stories and physical examinations for major companies, such as New York Telephone, from 1953 through 1960 (Bewes & Baillie, 1969; Cipolla & Collings, 1971).

Despite historical documentation of the use of assessment skills by nurses, it is generally recognized that the depth and scope of nursing assessment have expanded significantly over the past several decades because of rapid advances in biomedical knowledge and technology and through the promotion of primary health care. The early 1970s prompted nurses to develop an active role in the provision of primary health services and expanded the professional nurse role in conducting health histories and physical and psychological assessments (Holzemer, Barkauskas, & Ohlson, 1980; Lysaught, 1970).

Joint statements of the American Nurses Association and the American Academy of Pediatrics agreed that in-depth client assessments and on-the-spot diagnostic judgments would enhance the productivity of nurses and the health care of clients (Bullough, 1976; Fagin & Goodwin, 1972).

Acute care nurses in the 1980s employed the "primary care" method of delivery of care. Each nurse was autonomous in making comprehensive initial assessments from which individualized plans of care were established. In the 1990s, critical pathways or care maps guided the client's progression, with each stage based on specific protocols that the nurse was responsible for assessing and validating.

Over the last 20 years, the movement of health care from the acute care setting to the community and the proliferation of baccalaureate and graduate education solidified the nurses' role in holistic assessment. Advanced practice nurses have been increasingly used in the hospital as clinical nurse specialists and in the community as nurse practitioners. While state legislators and the American Medical Association struggled with issues of reimbursement and prescriptive services by nurses, government and societal recognition of the need for greater cost accountability in the health care industry brought the advent of diagnosis-related groups (DRGs) and promotion of health care coverage plans such as health maintenance organizations (HMOs) and preferred provider organizations (PPOs). Downsizing, budget cuts, and restructuring were the priorities of the 1990s. In turn, there was a demand for documentation of client assessments by all health care providers to justify health care services.

Present

The role of the nurse in assessment and diagnoses is more prevalent today than ever before in the history of nursing. Nurses from numerous international countries are expanding their assessment and nursing diagnosis skills (Baid, 2006;

Carroll-Johnson, 2004; Milligan & Neville, 2003). The rapidly evolving roles of nursing (e.g., forensic nursing) require extensive focused assessments and the development of related nursing diagnoses. Current focus on managed care and internal case management has had a dramatic impact on the assessment role of the nurse. The acute care nurse performs a focused assessment then incorporates assessment findings with a multidisciplinary team to develop a comprehensive plan of care. Critical care outreach nurses need enhanced assessment skills to safely assess critically ill clients who are outside the structured intensive care environment (Coombs & Moorse, 2002). Ambulatory care nurses assess and screen clients to determine the need for physician referrals. Home health nurses make independent diagnostic judgments. Public health nurses assess the needs of communities, school nurses monitor the growth and health of children, and hospice nurses assess the needs of the terminally ill clients and their families. In all settings, the nurse increasingly documents and retrieves assessment data through sophisticated computerized information systems (Lee, Delaney, & Moorhead, 2007). Nursing health assessment courses with informatics content are becoming the norm in baccalaureate programs. As the scope and environment for nursing assessment diversify, nurses must be prepared to assess populations of clients not only across the continuum of health but also by way of telecommunication systems with online data retrieval and documentation capabilities.

Future

Picture the nurse assessing a client who has "poor circulation." While in the client's home, the nurse can refresh his or her knowledge of the differences between arterial and venous occlusions, using a "point of need" learning file accessed over the Internet. Also immediately available are the agency's policies, procedures, and care maps. Digital pictures of the client's legs can be forwarded to the off-site nurse practitioner or physician for analysis. These networks have already been prototyped and will allow nurses to transmit and receive information by video cameras attached to portable computers or television sets in the client's home. The nurse can then discuss and demonstrate assessments with other health care professionals as clearly and quickly as if they were in the same room. Assessment data and findings can be documented over the Internet or in computerized medical records—some small enough to fit into a laboratory coat pocket and many activated by the nurse's voice.

The future will see increased specialization and diversity of assessment skills for nurses. While client acuity increases and technology advances, bedside nurses are challenged to make in-depth physiologic and psychosocial assessments while correlating clinical data from multiple technical monitoring devices. Bedside computers increasingly access individual client data as well as informational libraries and clinical resources (Graves, 2000). The communication of health assessment and clinical data will span a myriad of electronic interactivities and research possibilities. Health care networks already comprise a large hospital or medical center with referrals from smaller community hospitals; subacute, rehabilitation, and extended care units; HMOs; and home health services. These structures provide diverse settings and levels of care in which nurses will assess clients and facilitate their progress. New delivery systems such as "integrated clinical practice" for surgical care may require the nurse to assess and follow a client from the preoperative visit to a multidisciplinary outpatient clinic and even into the home by way of remote technology.

Nursing leaders envision tremendous growth of the nursing role in the managed care environment. The most marketable nurses will continue to be those with strong assessment and client teaching abilities and also those who are technologically savvy. The following factors will continue to promote opportunities for nurses with advanced assessment skills:

- Rising educational costs and focus on primary care that affect the numbers and availability of medical students
- Increasing complexity of acute care
- Growing aging population with complex comorbidities
- Expanding health care needs of single parents
- Increasing impact of children and the homeless on communities
- Intensifying mental health issues
- Expanding health service networks
- Increasing reimbursement for health promotion and preventive care services

Extensive research has resulted in several nursing languages to describe what nurses diagnose (Maas, 2004). This future development of nursing languages relies on the ability of practicing nurses to collect and analyze relevant client data to develop valid nursing diagnoses. Nurses will continue to be challenged to form client information and to move this information to knowledge through nursing informatics in order to improve health care. (Chastain, 2003).

CONTEXT AND HEALTH

In the past, health assessment has focused on the individual client. But there is a need to place individuals in the contexts that affect their health. The client's culture, family, and the community where the person lives may all affect his or her health status. When you look at a client, you need to perceive the person in these contexts and assess how they may be affecting the person's health. The person's family, community, and even spirituality are also affected by the individual's health status, even if only in subtle ways. Understanding or being aware of the client in context is essential to performing an effective health assessment. Remember, though, you must be aware of any perceived notions you have about the client's cultural, spiritual, community, or family context. Consider the following scenario to help illustrate the reason for seeing the client in context:

Mrs. Gutierrez, age 52, arrives at the clinic for diabetic teaching. She appears distracted and sad, uninterested in the teaching. The nurse suspects that Mrs. Gutierrez is upset by her diagnosis of diabetes. As the assessment progresses, the nurse learns that Mrs. Gutierrez has no appetite and no energy, wants to stay in bed all day, misses her sisters in Mexico, and cannot do her normal housekeeping or cooking. The nurse thinks that Mrs. Gutierrez is probably suffering from depression. But when the nurse asks Mrs. Gutierrez what she believes is causing her lack of appetite and low energy, Mrs. Gutierrez says she was shocked when her husband was hit by a car. He could not work for a month. She also says that she is suffering from *susto* and that a few days in bed will help her recover her soul and her health. The nurse decides to reschedule the diabetic teaching for a later time and just provide essential information to Mrs. Gutierrez at this visit.

What can be concluded from this scenario? Many systems are operating to create the context in which the client exists and functions. The nurse sees an individual client, but accurate interpretation of what the nurse sees depends on perceiving the client in context. Culture, family, and community operate as systems interacting to form the context.

A health assessment textbook for nurses focuses on providing a solid baseline for determining normal versus abnormal data gathered in a health history and physical assessment. This text must be supported by knowledge or concurrent instruction in medical–surgical and psychosocial nursing and, of course, anatomy and physiology. In this text, we can provide only a review of key concepts of these subjects.

As with anatomy and physiology, medical–surgical nursing, and psychosocial nursing content, a health assessment textbook can only provide key concepts related to culture, family, spirituality, and community. Many texts on transcultural nursing, family nursing, family therapy, social work, community nursing, and spiritual care exist to provide the knowledge base, concurrent instruction, or resources needed for exhaustive information. This assessment text emphasizes the need to consider the client in context for best practice in health assessment. For basic concepts of cultural, spiritual, family, and community assessment, see Chapters 10, 11, 33, and 34.

SUMMARY

Nursing health assessment differs in purpose, framework, and end result from all other types of professional health care assessment. Assessment is the first and most critical step of the nursing process and accuracy of assessment data affects all other phases of the nursing process. There are four types of nursing assessment: initial comprehensive, ongoing or partial, focused or problem-oriented, and emergency. Health assessment can be divided into four steps: collecting subjective data, collecting objective data, validation of data, and documentation of data.

It is difficult to discuss nursing assessment without taking the process one step further. Data analysis is the second step of the nursing process and the end result of nursing assessment. The purpose of data analysis is to reach conclusions concerning the client's health. These conclusions are in the form of nursing diagnoses, collaborative problems, or a need for referral. To arrive at conclusions, the nurse must go through seven steps of diagnostic reasoning or critical thinking.

The role of the nurse in health assessment has expanded drastically from the days of Florence Nightingale, when the nurse used the senses of sight, touch, and hearing to assess clients. Today communication and physical assessment techniques are used independently by nurses to arrive at professional clinical judgments concerning the client's health. In addition, advances in technology have expanded the role of assessment and the development of managed care has increased the necessity of assessment skills. Expert clinical assessment and informatics skills are absolute necessities for the future as nurses from all countries continue to expand their roles in all health care settings. Maintaining a focus on the clients in the contexts of their culture, family, and community is emphasized in this text.

References and Selected Readings

Alfaro-LeFevre, R. (2006). *Applying the nursing process: A tool for critical thinking* (6th ed.). Philadelphia: Lippincott Williams & Wilkins.

Anderson, M. C., Skillen, D. L., & Knight, C. L. (2001). Continuing care nurse's perception of need for physical assessment skills. *Journal of Gerontological Nursing, 27*(7), 23–29.

Baid, H. (2006). The process of conducting a physical assessment: A nursing perspective. *British Journal of Nursing, 15*(13), 710–714.

Bewes, D., & Baille, J. (1969). Pre-placement health screening by nurses. *Journal of Public Health, 12*(59), 2178–2184.

Bullough, B. (1976). Influences on role expansion. *American Journal of Nursing, 9*(76), 1476–1481.

Carpenito, L. J. (2005). *Nursing diagnosis: Application to clinical practice* (11th ed.). Philadelphia: Lippincott Williams & Wilkins.

Carroll-Johnson, R. M. (2004). Without borders. *International Journal of Nursing Terminologies and Classifications, 15*(1), 3–4.

Chastain, A. R. (2003). Nursing informatics: Past, present, and future. *Tennessee Nurse, 66*(1), 8–10.

Cipolla, J., & Collings, G. (1971). Nurse clinicians in industry. *American Journal of Nursing, 8*(71), 1530–1534.

Coombs, M. A., & Moorse, S. E. (2002). Physical assessment skills: A developing dimension of clinical nursing practice. *Intensive and Critical Care Nursing, 18*(4), 200–210.

Darbyshire, P. (2000). User-friendliness of computerized information systems. *Computers in Nursing, 18*(2), 93–99.

Fagin, C., & Goodwin, B. (1972). Baccalaureate preparation for primary care. *Nursing Outlook, 4*(20), 240–244.

Fitzsimmons, V., & Gallagher, L. (1978). Physical assessment skills: A historical perspective. *Nursing Forum, 4*(17), 345–355.

Holzemer, W., Barkauskas, V., & Ohlson, V. (1980). A program evaluation of four workshops designed to prepare nurse faculty in health assessment. *Journal of Nursing Education, 4*(19), 7–18.

Langer, S. (2000). Architecture of an image capable, web-based, electronic medical record. *Journal of Digital Imaging, 13*(2), 82–89.

Lee, M., Delaney, C., & Moorhead, S. (2007). Building a personal health record from: A nursing perspective. *International Journal of Medical Informatics, 4.* [Online version]. Available at https://www.researchgate.net/publication/6695832.

Lysaught, J. (1970). *An abstract for action.* New York: McGraw-Hill.

Maas, M. (2004). Nursing process outcome linkage research: Issues, current status, and health policy implications. *Medical Care, 42*(2), 11–40.

McManus, B. (2000). A move to electronic patient records in the community: A qualitative case study of a clinical data collection system. *Topics in Health Information Management, 20*(4), 23–37.

Milligan, K., & Neville, S. (2003). The contextualization of health assessment. *Nursing Praxis in New Zealand, 19*(1), 23–31.

Nightingale, F. (1992). Role expansion of role extension. *Nursing Forum, 4*(9), 380–399.

North American Nursing Diagnosis Association. (2009–2011). *Nursing diagnoses: Definitions and classification, 2009–2011* (6th ed.). Philadelphia: North American Nursing Diagnosis Association.

Purnell, L. D. & Paulanka, B. J. (Eds). (2003). *Transcultural health care: A culturally competent approach* (2nd ed.). Philadelphia: F.A. Davis.

Rushforth, H., Bliss, A., Burge, D., & Glasper, E. A. (2000). Nurse-led preoperative assessment: A study of appropriateness. *Pediatric Nursing, 12*(5), 15–20.

Simpson, R. (2004). Global informing: Impact and implications of technology in a global marketplace. *Nursing Informatics, 28*(2), 144–149.

Snyder-Halpern, R. (2000). Informatics nurse specialists: A role for the new century in health care. *Aspen's Advisor for Nurse Executives, 15*(4), 3–5.

Stricklin, M., Jones, S., & Niles, S. (2000). Home talk/healthy talk: Improving patients' health status with telephone technology. *Home Healthcare Nurse, 18*(1), 53–62.

Werfel, P. A. (2000). 20 Tips to perfect your assessment skills. *Journal of Emergency Medical Services, 25*(1), 68–70, 72–73.

2

Collecting Subjective Data

Collecting subjective data is an integral part of nursing health assessment. Subjective data consist of

- Sensations or symptoms
- Feelings
- Perceptions
- Desires
- Preferences
- Beliefs
- Ideas
- Values
- Personal information

These types of data can be elicited and verified only by the client. Subjective data provide clues to possible physiologic, psychological, and sociologic problems. They also provide the nurse with information that may reveal a client's risk for a problem as well as areas of strengths for the client.

The information is obtained through interviewing. Therefore, effective interviewing skills are vital to accurate and thorough collection of subjective data.

INTERVIEWING

Obtaining a valid nursing health history requires professional, interpersonal, and interviewing skills. The nursing interview is a communication process that has two focuses:

1. Establishing rapport and a trusting relationship with the client to elicit accurate and meaningful information and

2. Gathering information on the client's developmental, psychological, physiologic, sociocultural, and spiritual statuses to identify deviations that can be treated with nursing and collaborative interventions or strengths that can be enhanced through nurse–client collaboration.

Phases of the Interview

The nursing interview has three basic phases: introductory, working, and summary and closing phases. These phases are briefly explained by describing the roles of the nurse and client during each one.

Introductory Phase

After introducing himself to the client, the nurse explains the purpose of the interview, discusses the types of questions that will be asked, explains the reason for taking notes, and assures the client that confidential information will remain confidential. The nurse also makes sure that the client is comfortable (physically and emotionally) and has privacy. It is also essential for the nurse to develop trust and rapport at this point in the interview. This can begin by conveying a sense of priority and interest in the client. Developing rapport depends heavily on verbal and nonverbal communication on the part of the nurse. These types of communication are discussed later in the chapter.

Working Phase

During this phase, the nurse elicits the client's comments about major biographic data, reasons for seeking care, history of present health concern, past health history, family history, review of body systems for current health problems, lifestyle and health practices, and developmental level. The nurse then listens, observes cues, and uses critical thinking skills to interpret and validate information received from the client. The nurse and client collaborate to identify the client's problems and goals. The facilitating approach may be free-flowing or more structured with specific questions, depending on the time available and the type of data needed.

Summary and Closing Phase

During the summary and closing, the nurse summarizes information obtained during the working phase and validates problems and goals with the client (see Chapter 4). She also identifies and discusses possible plans to resolve the problem (nursing diagnoses and collaborative problems) with the client (see Chapter 5). Finally, the nurse makes sure to ask if anything else concerns the client and if there are any further questions.

Communication During the Interview

The client interview involves two types of communication—nonverbal and verbal. Several special techniques and certain general considerations will improve both types of communication and promote an effective and productive interview.

Nonverbal Communication

Nonverbal communication is as important as verbal communication. Your appearance, demeanor, posture, facial expressions, and attitude strongly influence how the client perceives the questions you ask. Never overlook this type of communication or take it for granted.

APPEARANCE

First take care to ensure that your appearance is professional. The client is expecting to see a health professional; therefore, you should look the part. Wear comfortable, neat clothes and a laboratory coat or a uniform. Be sure your name tag, including credentials, is clearly visible. Your hair should be neat and not in any extreme style; some nurses like to wear long hair pulled back. Fingernails should be short and neat; jewelry should be minimal.

DEMEANOR

Your demeanor should also be professional. When you enter a room to interview a client, display poise. Focus on the client and the upcoming interview and assessment. Do not enter the room laughing loudly, yelling to a coworker, or muttering under your breath. This appears unprofessional to the client and will have an effect on the entire interview process. Greet the client calmly and focus your full attention on her. Do not be overwhelmingly friendly or "touchy;" many clients are uncomfortable with this type of behavior. It is best to maintain a professional distance.

FACIAL EXPRESSION

Facial expressions are often an overlooked aspect of communication. Because facial expression often shows what you are truly thinking (regardless of what you are saying), keep a close check on your facial expression. No matter what you think about a client or what kind of day you are having, keep your expression neutral and friendly. If your face shows anger or anxiety, the client will sense it and may think it is directed toward him or her. If you cannot effectively hide your emotions, you may want to explain that you are angry or upset about a personal situation. Admitting this to the client may also help in developing a trusting relationship and genuine rapport.

Portraying a neutral expression does not mean that your face lacks expression. It means using the right expression at the right time. If the client looks upset, you should appear and be understanding and concerned. Conversely, smiling when the client is on the verge of tears will cause the client to believe that you do not care about his or her problem.

ATTITUDE

One of the most important nonverbal skills to develop as a health care professional is a nonjudgmental attitude. All clients should be accepted, regardless of beliefs, ethnicity, lifestyle, and health care practices. Do not act superior to the client or appear shocked, disgusted, or surprised at what you are told.

These attitudes will cause the client to feel uncomfortable opening up to you and important data concerning his or her health status could be withheld.

Being nonjudgmental involves not "preaching" to the client or imposing your own sense of ethics or morality on him. Focus on health care and how you can best help the client to achieve the highest possible level of health. For example, if you are interviewing a client who smokes, avoid lecturing condescendingly about the dangers of smoking. Also, avoid telling the client he or she is foolish or portraying an attitude of disgust. This will only harm the nurse–client relationship and will do nothing to improve the client's health. The client is, no doubt, already aware of the dangers of smoking. Forcing guilt on him is unhelpful. Accept the client, be understanding of the habit, and work together to improve the client's health. This does not mean you should not encourage the client to quit; it means that how you approach the situation makes a difference. Let the client know you understand that it is hard to quit smoking, support efforts to quit, and offer suggestions on the latest methods available to help kick the smoking habit.

SILENCE

Another nonverbal technique to use during the interview process is silence. Periods of silence allow you and the client to reflect and organize thoughts, which facilitates more accurate reporting and data collection.

LISTENING

Listening is the most important skill to learn and develop fully in order to collect complete and valid data from your client. To listen effectively, you need to maintain good eye contact, smile or display an open, appropriate facial expression, maintain an open body position (open arms and hands and lean forward). Avoid preconceived ideas or biases about your client. To listen effectively, you must keep an open mind. Avoid crossing your arms, sitting back, tilting your head away from the client, thinking about other things, or looking blank or inattentive. Becoming an effective listener takes concentration and practice.

In addition, several nonverbal affects or attitudes may hinder effective communication. They may promote discomfort or distrust. Display 2-1 describes communication to avoid.

Verbal Communication

Effective verbal communication is essential to a client interview. The goal of the interview process is to elicit as much data about the client's health status as possible. Several types of questions and techniques to use during the interview are discussed in the following sections.

OPEN-ENDED QUESTIONS

Open-ended questions are used to elicit the client's feelings and perceptions. They typically begin with the words "how" or "what." An example of this type of question is "How have you been feeling lately?" These types of questions are important because they require more than a one-word response from the client and, therefore, encourage description. Asking open-ended questions may help to reveal significant data about the client's health status.

DISPLAY 2-1	Communication to Avoid

Nonverbal Communication to Avoid

Excessive or Insufficient Eye Contact

Avoid extremes in eye contact. Some clients feel very uncomfortable with too much eye contact; others believe that you are hiding something from them if you do not look them in the eye. Therefore, it is best to use a moderate amount of eye contact. For example, establish eye contact when the client is speaking to you but look down at your notes from time to time. A client's cultural background often determines how he feels about eye contact (see Cultural Variations in Communication for more information).

Distraction and Distance

Avoid being occupied with something else while you are asking questions during the interview. This behavior makes the client believe that the interview may be unimportant to you. Avoid appearing mentally distant as well. The client will sense your distance and will be less likely to answer your questions thoroughly. Also try to avoid physical distance exceeding 2 to 3 feet during the interview. Rapport and trust are established when the client senses your focus and concern are solely on the client and the client's health. Physical distance may portray a noncaring attitude or a desire to avoid close contact with the client.

Standing

Avoid standing while the client is seated during the interview. Standing puts you and the client at different levels. You may be perceived as the superior, making the client feel inferior. Care of the client's health should be an equal partnership between the health care provider and the client. If the client is made to feel inferior, he or she will not feel empowered to be an equal partner and the potential for optimal health may be lost. In addition, vital information may not be revealed if the client believes that the interviewer is untrustworthy, judgmental, or disinterested.

Verbal Communication to Avoid

Biased or Leading Questions

Avoid using biased or leading questions. These cause the client to provide answers that may or may not be true. The way you phrase a question may actually lead the client to think you want her to answer in a certain way. For example, if you ask "You don't feel bad, do you?" the client may conclude that you do not think she should feel bad and will answer "no" even if this is not true.

Rushing Through the Interview

Avoid rushing the client. If you ask the client questions on top of questions, several things may occur. First, the client may answer "no" to a series of closed-ended questions when he or she would have answered "yes" to one of the questions if it was asked individually. This may occur because the client did not hear the individual question clearly or because the answers to most were "no" and the client forgot about the "yes" answer in the midst of the others. With this type of interview technique, the client may believe that his individual situation is of little concern to the nurse. Taking time with clients shows that you are concerned about their health and helps them to open up. Finally, rushing someone through the interview process undoubtedly causes important information to be left out of the health history. A client will usually sense that you are rushed and may try to help hurry the interview by providing abbreviated or incomplete answers to questions.

Reading the Questions

Avoid reading questions from the history form. This deflects attention from the client and results in an impersonal interview process. As a result, the client may feel ill at ease opening up to formatted questions.

The following example shows how open-ended questions work. Imagine yourself interviewing an elderly male client who is at the physician's office because of diabetic complications. He mentions casually to you, "Today is the two-month anniversary of my wife's death from cancer." Failure to follow up with an open-ended question such as "How does this make you feel?" may result in the loss of important data that could provide clues to the client's current state of health.

CLOSED-ENDED QUESTIONS

Use closed-ended questions to obtain facts and to focus on specific information. The client can respond with one or two words. The questions typically begin with the words "when" or "did." An example of this type of question is "When did your headache start?" Closed-ended questions are useful in keeping the interview on course. They can also be used to clarify or obtain more accurate information about issues disclosed in response to open-ended questions. For example, in response to the open-ended question "How have you been feeling lately?" the client says, "Well, I've been feeling really sick at my

stomach and I don't feel like eating because of it." You may be able to follow up and learn more about the client's symptom with a closed-ended question such as "When did the nausea start?"

LAUNDRY LIST

Another way to ask questions is to provide the client with a choice of words to choose from in describing symptoms, conditions, or feelings. This laundry list approach helps you to obtain specific answers and reduces the likelihood of the client's perceiving or providing an expected answer. For example, "Is the pain severe, dull, sharp, mild, cutting, or piercing?" "Does the pain occur once every year, day, month, or hour?" Repeat choices as necessary.

REPHRASING

Rephrasing information the client has provided is an effective way to communicate during the interview. This technique helps you to clarify information the client has stated; it also enables you and the client to reflect on what was said. For example, your client, Mr. G., tells you that he has been really tired and nauseated for 2 months and that he is scared because he fears that he has some horrible disease. You might rephrase the information by saying, "You are thinking that you have a serious illness?"

WELL-PLACED PHRASES

Client verbalization can be encouraged by well-placed phrases from the nurse. If the client is in the middle of explaining a symptom or feeling and believes that you are not paying attention, you may fail to get all the necessary information. Listen closely to the client during his or her description and use phrases such as "um-hum," "yes," or "I agree" to encourage the client to continue.

INFERRING

Inferring information from what the client tells you and what you observe in the client's behavior may elicit more data or verify existing data. Be careful not to lead the client to answers that are not true (see Verbal Communication to Avoid for more information). An example of inferring information follows: Your client, Mrs. J., tells you that she has bad pain. You ask where the pain is, and she says, "My stomach." You notice the client has a hand on the right side of her lower abdomen and seems to favor her entire right side. You say, "It seems you have more difficulty with the right side of your stomach" (use the word "stomach" because that is the term the client used to describe the abdomen). This technique, if used properly, helps to elicit the most accurate data possible from the client.

PROVIDING INFORMATION

Another important thing to consider throughout the interview is to provide the client with information as questions and concerns arise. Make sure you answer every question as well as you can. If you do not know the answer, explain that you will find out for the client. The more clients know about their own health, the more likely they are to become equal participants in caring for their health.

As with nonverbal communication, several verbal techniques may hinder effective communication (see Display 2-1).

Special Considerations during the Interview

Three variations in communication must be considered as you interview clients: gerontologic, cultural, and emotional. These variations affect the nonverbal and verbal techniques you use during the interview. Imagine, for example, that you are interviewing an 82-year-old woman and you ask her to describe how she has been feeling. She does not answer you and she looks confused. This older client may have some hearing loss. In such a case, you may need to modify the verbal technique of asking open-ended questions by following the guidelines provided.

Gerontologic Variations in Communication

Age affects and commonly slows all body systems to varying degrees. However, normal aspects of aging do not necessarily

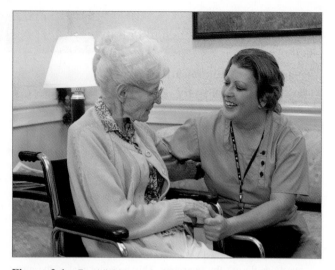

Figure 2-1 Establishing and maintaining trust, privacy, and partnership with older adults sets the tone for effectively collecting data and sharing concerns.

equate with a health problem, so it is important not to approach an interview with an elderly client assuming that there is a health problem. Older clients have the potential to be as healthy as younger clients.

When interviewing an elderly client, you must first assess hearing acuity. Hearing loss occurs normally with age, and undetected hearing loss is often misinterpreted as mental slowness or confusion. If you detect hearing loss, speak slowly, face the client at all times during the interview, and position yourself so that you are speaking on the side of the client that has the ear with better acuity. Do not yell at the client.

Older clients may have more health concerns than younger clients and may seek health care more often. Many times, older clients with health problems feel vulnerable and scared. They need to believe that they can trust you before they will open up to you about what is bothering them. Thus establishing and maintaining trust, privacy, and partnership with the older client is particularly important (Fig. 2-1). It is not unusual for elderly clients to be taken for granted and their health complaints ignored, causing them to become fearful of complaining. It is often disturbing to the older client that their health problems may be discussed openly among many health care providers and family members. Assure your elderly clients that you are concerned, that you see them as equal partners in health care, and that what is discussed will be between you, their health care provider, and them.

Speak clearly and use straightforward language during the interview with the elderly client. Ask questions in simple terms. Avoid medical jargon and modern slang. However, do not talk down to the client. Being older physically does not mean the client is slower mentally. Showing respect is very important. However, if the older client is mentally confused or forgetful, it is important to have a significant other (e.g., spouse, child, close friend) present during the interview to provide or clarify the data.

Cultural Variations in Communication

Ethnic/cultural variations in communication and self-disclosure styles may significantly affect the information obtained (Andrews & Boyle, 2002; Giger & Davidhizar, 2008;

Luckmann, 2000). Be aware of possible variations in the communication styles of yourself and the client. If misunderstanding or difficulty in communicating is evident, seek help from an expert, what some professionals call a "culture broker." This is someone who is thoroughly familiar not only with the client's language, culture, and related health care practices but also with the health care setting and system of the dominant culture. Frequently noted variations in communication styles include

- Reluctance to reveal personal information to strangers for various culturally-based reasons
- Variation in willingness to openly express emotional distress or pain
- Variation in ability to receive information (listen)
- Variation in meaning conveyed by language. For example, a client who does not speak the predominant language may not know what a certain medical term or phrase means and, therefore, will not know how to answer your question. Use of slang with non-native speakers is discouraged as well. Keep in mind that it is hard enough to learn proper language, let alone the idiom vernacular. The non-native speaker will likely have no idea what you are trying to convey.
- Variation in use and meaning of nonverbal communication: eye contact, stance, gestures, demeanor. For example, direct eye contact may be perceived as rude, aggressive, or immodest by some cultures but lack of eye contact may be perceived as evasive, insecure, or inattentive by other cultures. A slightly bowed stance may indicate respect in some groups; size of personal space affects one's comfortable interpersonal distance; touch may be perceived as comforting or threatening.
- Variation in disease/illness perception: Culture-specific syndromes or disorders are accepted by some groups

(e.g., in Latin America, *susto* is an illness caused by a sudden shock or fright).
- Variation in past, present, or future time orientation (e.g., the dominant U.S. culture is future oriented; other cultures may focus more on the past or present)
- Variation in the family's role in the decision-making process: A person other than the client or the client's parent may be the major decision maker about appointments, treatments, or follow-up care for the client.

You may have to interview a client who does not speak your language. To perform the best interview possible, it is necessary to use an interpreter. Possibly the best interpreter would be a culture expert (or culture broker). Consider the relationship of the interpreter to the client. If the interpreter is the client's child or a person of a different sex, age, or social status, interpretation may be impaired. Also keep in mind that communication through use of pictures may be helpful when working with some clients.

Emotional Variations in Communication

Not every client you encounter will be calm, friendly, and eager to participate in the interview process. Clients' emotions vary for a number of reasons. They may be scared or anxious about their health or about disclosing personal information, angry that they are sick or about having to have an examination, depressed about their health or other life events, or they may have an ulterior motive for having an assessment performed. Clients may also have some sensitive issues with which they are grappling and may turn to you for help. Some helpful ways to deal with various clients with various emotions are discussed in Display 2-2.

| DISPLAY 2-2 | **Interacting with Clients with Various Emotional States** |

When Interacting With an Anxious Client
- Provide the client with simple, organized information in a structured format.
- Explain who you are and your role and purpose.
- Ask simple, concise questions.
- Avoid becoming anxious like the client.
- Do not hurry and decrease any external stimuli.

When Interacting With an Angry Client
- Approach this client in a calm, reassuring, in-control manner.
- Allow him to ventilate feelings. However, if the client is out of control, do not argue with or touch the client.
- Obtain help from other health care professionals as needed.
- Avoid arguing and facilitate personal space so the client does not feel threatened or cornered.

When Interacting With a Depressed Client
- Express interest in and understanding of the client and respond in a neutral manner.
- Do not try to communicate in an upbeat, encouraging manner. This will not help the depressed client.

When Interacting With a Manipulative Client
- Provide structure and set limits.
- Differentiate between manipulation and a reasonable request.
- If you are not sure whether you are being manipulated, obtain an objective opinion from other nursing colleagues.

When Interacting With a Seductive Client
- Set firm limits on overt sexual client behavior and avoid responding to subtle seductive behaviors.
- Encourage client to use more appropriate methods of coping in relating to others.

When Discussing Sensitive Issues (for example, Sexuality, Dying, Spirituality)
- First be aware of your own thoughts and feelings regarding dying, spirituality, and sexuality; then recognize that these factors may affect the client's health and may need to be discussed with someone.
- Ask simple questions in a nonjudgmental manner.
- Allow time for ventilation of client's feelings as needed.
- If you do not feel comfortable or competent discussing personal, sensitive topics, you may make referrals as appropriate, for example, to a pastoral counselor for spiritual concerns or other specialists as needed.

COMPLETE HEALTH HISTORY

The health history is an excellent way to begin the assessment process because it lays the groundwork for identifying nursing problems and provides a focus for the physical examination. The importance of the health history lies in its ability to provide information that will assist the examiner in identifying areas of strength and limitation in the individual's lifestyle and current health status. Data from the health history also provide the examiner with specific cues to health problems that are most apparent to the client. Then these areas may be more intensely examined during the physical assessment. When a client is having a complete, head-to-toe physical assessment, collection of subjective data usually requires that the nurse take a complete health history. The complete health history is modified or shortened when necessary. For example, if the physical assessment will focus on the heart and neck vessels, the subjective data collection would be limited to the data relevant to the heart and neck vessels.

Taking a health history should begin with an explanation to the client of why the information is being requested, for example, "so that I will be able to plan individualized nursing care with you." This section of the chapter explains the rationale for collecting the data, discusses each portion of the health history, and provides sample questions. The health history has eight sections:

- Biographic data
- Reasons for seeking health care
- History of present health concern
- Past health history
- Family health history
- Review of body systems (ROS) for current health problems
- Lifestyle and health practices profile
- Developmental level

The organization for collecting data in this text is a generic nursing framework that the nurse can use as is or adapt to use with any nursing framework. See Assessment Tool 2-1 for a summary of the components of a complete client health history. This can be used as a guide for collecting subjective data from the client.

Biographic Data

Biographic data usually include information that identifies the client, such as name, address, phone number, gender, and who provided the information—the client or significant others. The client's birth date, Social Security number, medical record number, or similar identifying data may be included in the biographic data section.

When students are collecting the information and sharing it with instructors, addresses and phone numbers should be deleted and initials used to protect the client's privacy. The name of the person providing the information needs to be included, however, to assist in determining its accuracy. The client is considered the primary source and all others (including the client's medical record) are secondary sources. In some cases, the client's immediate family or caregiver may be a more accurate source of information than the client. An example would be an elderly client's wife who has kept the client's medical records for years or the legal guardian of a mentally compromised client. In any event, validation of the information by a secondary source may be helpful.

The client's culture, ethnicity, and subculture may begin to be determined by collecting data about date and place of birth, nationality or ethnicity, marital status, religious or spiritual practices, and primary and secondary languages spoken, written, and read. This information helps the nurse to examine special needs and beliefs that may affect the client or family's health care. A person's primary language is usually the one spoken in the family during early childhood and the one in which the person thinks. However, if the client was educated in another language from kindergarten on, that may be the primary language and the birth language would be secondary.

Gathering information about the client's educational level, occupation, and working status at this point in the health history assists the examiner to tailor questions to the client's level of understanding. In addition, this information can help to identify possible client strengths and limitations affecting health status. For example, if the client was recently downsized from a high-power, high-salary position, the effects of overwhelming stress may play a large part in his or her health status.

Finally, asking who lives with the client and identifying significant others indicates the availability of potential caregivers and support people for the client. Absence of support people would alert the examiner to the (possible) need for finding external sources of support.

Reason(s) for Seeking Health Care

This category includes two questions: "What is your major health problem or concerns at this time?" and "How do you feel about having to seek health care?" The first question assists the client to focus on his most significant health concern and answers the nurse's question, "Why are you here?" or "How can I help you?" Physicians call this the client's chief complaint (CC), but a more holistic approach for phrasing the question may draw out concerns that reach beyond just a physical complaint and may address stress or lifestyle changes.

The second question, "How do you feel about having to seek health care?" encourages the client to discuss fears or other feelings about having to see a health care provider. For example, a woman visiting a nurse practitioner states her major health concern: "I found a lump in my breast." This woman may be able to respond to the second question by voicing fears that she has been reluctant to share with her significant others. This question may also draw out descriptions of previous experiences—both positive and negative—with other health care providers.

History of Present Health Concern

This section of the health history takes into account several aspects of the health problem and asks questions whose answers can provide a detailed description of the concern. First, encourage the client to explain the health problem or symptom in as much detail as possible by focusing on the onset, progression, and duration of the problem; signs and symptoms and related problems; and what the client perceives as causing the problem. You may also ask the client to evaluate what makes the problem worse, what makes it better, which treatments have been tried, what effect the problem has had on daily life or lifestyle, what expectations are held about recovery, and what is the client's ability to provide self-care.

Because there are many characteristics to be explored for each symptom, a memory helper—known as a mnemonic—can help the nurse to complete the assessment of the sign,

ASSESSMENT TOOL 2-1 **Nursing Health History Format (Used for Client Care Plan)**

Biographical Data

Name
Address
Phone
Gender
Provider of history (patient or other)
Birth date
Place of birth
Race or ethnic background
Educational Level
Occupation
Significant others or support persons

Reasons for Seeking Health Care

Reason for seeking health care
Feelings about seeking health care

History of Present Health Concern

Character (How does it feel, look, smell, sound, etc.?)
Onset (When did it begin; is it better, worse, or the same since it began?)
Location (Where is it? Does it radiate?)
Duration (How long it lasts? Does it recur?)
Severity (How bad is it on a scale of 1 [barely noticeable] to 10 [worst pain ever experienced]?)
Pattern (What makes it better? What makes it worse?)
Associated factors (What other symptoms do you have with it? Will you be able to continue doing your work or other activities [leisure or exercise]?)

Past Health History

Problems at birth
Childhood Illnesses
Immunizations to date
Adult illnesses (physical, emotional, mental)
Surgeries
Accidents
Prolonged pain or pain patterns
Allergies

Family Health History

Age of parents (Living? Deceased date?)
Parent illnesses
Grandparents' Illnesses
Aunts' and uncles' age and illnesses
Children's ages and illnesses or handicaps

Review of Systems for Current Health Problems

Skin, Hair, and Nails: color, temperature, condition, rashes, lesions, sweating, hair loss dandruff
Head and Neck: headache, stiffness, difficulty swallowing, enlarged lymph nodes
Ears: pain, ringing, buzzing, drainage, difficulty hearing, exposure to loud noises, dizziness
Eyes: pain, infections, vision, redness, tearing, halos, blurring, black spots, flashes, double vision
Mouth, Throat, Nose, and Sinuses: mouth pain, sore throat, lesions, hoarseness, nasal obstruction, sneezing, coughing, snoring, nosebleeds

Thorax and Lungs: pain, difficulty breathing, shortness of breath with activities, orthopnea, cough, sputum, hemoptysis, respiratory infections
Breasts and Regional Lymphatics: pain, lumps, discharge from nipples, dimpling or changes in breast size, swollen tender lymph nodes in axilla
Heart and Neck Vessels: chest pain or pressure, palpitations, edema, last blood pressure, last ECG
Peripheral Vascular: leg or feet pain, swelling of feet or legs, sores on feet or legs, color of feet and legs
Abdomen: pain, indigestion, difficulty swallowing, nausea and vomiting. Gas, jaundice, hernias
Male Genitalia: painful urination, frequency or difficulty starting or maintaining urinary system, blood in urine, sexual problems, penile lesions, penile pain, scrotal swelling, difficulty with erection or ejaculation, exposure to sexually transmitted diseases
Female Genitalia: pelvic pain, voiding pain, sexual pain, voiding problems (dribbling, incontinence) age of menarche or menopause (date of last menstrual period), pregnancies and types of problems, abortions, sexually transmitted diseases, hormone replacement therapy, birth control methods
Anus, Rectum, and Prostate: pain, with refection, hemorrhoids, bowel habits, constipation, diarrhea, blood in stool
Musculoskeletal: pain, swelling, red, stiff joints, strength of extremities, abilities to care for self and work
Neurological: mood, behavior, depression, anger, headaches, concussions, loss of strength or sensation, coordination, difficulty with speech, memory problems, strange thoughts or actions, difficulty reading or learning

Lifestyle and Health Practices

Description of a typical day (AM to PM)
24-hour dietary intake (foods and fluids)
Who purchases and prepares meals
Activities on a typical day
Exercise habits and patterns
Sleep and rest habits and patterns
Use of medications and other substances (caffeine, nicotine, alcohol, recreational drugs)
Self concept
Self-care responsibilities
Social activities for fun and relaxation
Social activities contributing to society
Relationships with family, significant others, and pets
Values, religious affiliation, spirituality
Past, current, and future plans for education
Type of work, level of job satisfaction, work stressors
Finances
Stressors in life, coping strategies used
Residency, type of environment, neighborhood, environmental risks

Developmental Level

Young Adult: Intimacy versus Isolation
Middlescent: Generativity versus Stagnation
Older Adult: Ego Integrity versus Despair

DISPLAY 2-3	Components of the COLDSPA Symptom Analysis Mnemonic

Mnemonic	Question
Character	Describe the sign or symptom (feeling, appearance, sound, smell, or taste if applicable).
Onset	When did it begin?
Location	Where is it? Does it radiate? Does it occur anywhere else?
Duration	How long does it last? Does it recur?
Severity	How bad is it? How much does it bother you?
Pattern	What makes it better or worse?
Associated factors/How it **A**ffects the client	What other symptoms occur with it? How does it affect you?

symptom, or health concern. Many mnemonics have been developed for this purpose (e.g., PQRST, COLDSPAR, COLDSTER, LOCSTAAM). The mnemonic used in this text is COLDSPA, which is designed to help the nurse explore symptoms, signs, or health concerns (see Display 2-3). The COLDSPA Example provides a sample application of the COLDSPA mnemonic adapted to analyze back pain.

The client's answers to the questions provide the nurse with a great deal of information about the client's problem and especially how it affects lifestyle and activities of daily living. This helps the nurse to evaluate the client's insight into the problem and the client's plans for managing it. The nurse can also begin to postulate nursing diagnoses from this initial information.

Problems or symptoms particular to body parts or systems are covered in the Nursing History section under "History of Present Health Concern" in the physical assessment chapters.

Each identified symptom must be described for clear understanding of probable cause and significance.

Past Health History

This portion of the health history focuses on questions related to the client's past, from the earliest beginnings to the present. These questions elicit data related to the client's strengths and weaknesses in her health history. The client's strengths may be physical (e.g., optimal body weight), social (e.g., active in community services) emotional (e.g., expresses feeling openly), or spiritual (often turns to faith for support). The data may also point to trends of unhealthy behaviors such as smoking or lack of physical activity. The information gained from these questions assists the nurse to identify risk factors that stem from previous health problems. Risk factors may be to the client or to his significant others.

Sample Application of COLDSPA: Exploring the Symptoms of Back Pain

Mnemonic	General Question	Adapted Question
Character	Describe the sign or symptom (feeling, appearance, sound, smell, or taste if applicable).	"What does the pain feel like?"
Onset	When did it begin?	"When did this pain start?"
Location	Where is it? Does it radiate? Does it occur anywhere else?	"Where does it hurt the most? Does it radiate or go to any other part of your body?"
Duration	How long does it last? Does it recur?	"How long does the pain last? Does it come and go or is it constant?"
Severity	How bad is it? How much does it bother you?	"How intense is the pain? Rate it on a scale of 1 to 10."
Pattern	What makes it better or worse?	"What makes your back pain worse or better? Are there any treatments you've tried that relieve the pain?"
Associated factors/How it **A**ffects the client	What other symptoms occur with it? How does it affect you?	"What do you think caused it to start? Do you have any other problems that seem related to your back pain? How does this pain affect your life and daily activities?"

Information covered in this section includes questions about birth, growth, development, childhood diseases, immunizations, allergies, previous health problems, hospitalizations, surgeries, pregnancies, births, previous accidents, injuries, pain experiences, and emotional or psychiatric problems. Sample questions include

- "Can you tell me how your mother described your birth? Were there any problems? As far as you know, did you progress normally as you grew to adulthood? Were there any problems that your family told you about or that you experienced?"
- "What diseases did you have as a child such as measles or mumps? What immunizations did you get and are you up to date now?" (See Display 2-4 for recommended immunizations.)
- "Do you have any chronic illnesses? If so, when was it diagnosed? How is it treated? How satisfied have you been with the treatment?"

- "What illnesses or allergies have you had? How were the illnesses treated?"
- "Have you ever been pregnant and delivered a baby? How many times have you been pregnant/delivered?"
- "Have you ever been hospitalized or had surgery? If so, when? What were you hospitalized for or what type of surgery did you have? Were there any complications?"
- "Have you experienced any accidents or injuries? Please describe them."
- "Have you experienced pain in any part of your body? Please describe the pain."
- "Have you ever been diagnosed with/treated for emotional or mental problems? If so, please describe their nature and any treatment received. Describe your level of satisfaction with the treatment."

(text continues on page 21)

DISPLAY 2-4	**Recommended Adult Immunization Schedule (2007–2008)**

Note: These recommendations must be read with the footnotes that follow.

Recommended adult immunization schedule, by vaccine and age group United States, October 2007–September 2008

VACCINE ▼ AGE GROUP ►	19–49 years	50–64 years	≥ 65 years
Tetanus, diphtheria, pertussis (Td/Tdap)[1],*	1 dose Td booster every 10 yrs / Substitute 1 dose of Tdap for Td		
Human papillomavirus (HPV)[2],*	3 doses females (0, 2, 6 mos)		
Measles, mumps, rubella (MMR)[3],*	1 or 2 doses	1 dose	
Varicella[4],*	2 doses (0, 4–8 wks)		
Influenza[5],*		1 dose annually	
Pneumococcal (polysaccharide)[6,7]	1–2 doses		1 dose
Hepatitis A[8],*	2 doses (0, 6–12 mos or 0, 6–18 mos)		
Hepatitis B[9],*	3 doses (0, 1–2, 4–6 mos)		
Meningococcal[10],*	1 or more doses		
Zoster[11]			1 dose

*Covered by the Vaccine Injury Compensation Program.

For all persons in this category who meet the age requirements and who lack evidence of immunity (e.g., lack documentation of vaccination or have no evidence of prior infection)

Recommended if some other risk factor is present (e.g., on the basis of medical, occupational, lifestyle, or other indications)

Report all clinically significant postvaccination reactions to the Vaccine Adverse Event Reporting System (VAERS). Reporting forms and instructions on filing a VAERS report are available at www.vaers.hhs.gov or by telephone, 800-822-7967.

Information on how to file a Vaccine Injury Compensation Program claim is available at www.hrsa.gov/vaccinecompensation or by telephone, 800-338-2382. To file a claim for vaccine injury, contact the U.S. Court of Federal Claims, 717 Madison Place, N.W., Washington, D.C. 20005: telephone, 202-357-6400.

Additional information about the vaccines in this schedule, extent of available data, and contraindications for vaccination is also available at www.coc.gov/vaccines or from the CDC-INFO Contact Center at 800-CDC-INFO (800-232-4636) in English and Spanish, 24 hours a day, 7 days a week.

Use of trade names and commercial sources is for identification only and does not imply endorsement by the U.S. Department of Health and Human Services.

CS115143

continued on page 18

Vaccines that might be indicated for adults based on medical and other indications United States, October 2007–September 2008

INDICATION ▶ VACCINE ▼	Pregnancy	Immuno-compromising conditions (excluding human immunodeficiency virus [HIV]), medications, radiation[13]	HIV infection[3,12,13] CD4+ T lymphocyte count <200 cells/μL	HIV infection[3,12,13] CD4+ T lymphocyte count ≥200 cells/μL	Diabetes, heart disease, chronic pulmonary disease, chronic alcoholism	Asplenia[12] (including elective splenectomy and terminal complement component deficiencies)	Chronic liver disease	Kidney failure, end-stage renal disease, receipt of hemodialysis	Health-care personnel
Tetanus, diphtheria, pertussis (Td/Tdap)[1,*]	1 dose Td booster every 10 yrs				Substitute 1 dose of Tdap for Td				
Human papillomavirus (HPV)[2,*]		3 doses for females through age 26 yrs (0, 2, 6 mos)							
Measles, mumps, rubella (MMR)[3,*]	Contraindicated	Contraindicated	Contraindicated	1 or 2 doses					
Varicella[4,*]	Contraindicated	Contraindicated	Contraindicated	2 doses (0, 4–8 wks)					
Influenza[5,*]			1 dose TIV annually						1 dose TIV or LAIV annually
Pneumococcal (polysaccharide)[6,7]					1–2 doses				
Hepatitis A[8,*]		2 doses (0, 6–12 mos, or 0, 6–18 mos)							
Hepatitis B[9,*]		3 doses (0, 1–2, 4–6 mos)							
Meningococcal[10,*]		1 or more doses							
Zoster[11]	Contraindicated	Contraindicated					1 dose		

Recommended if some other risk factor is present (e.g., on the basis of medical, occupational, lifestyle, or other indications)

For all persons in this category who meet the age requirements and who lack evidence of immunity (e.g., lack documentation of vaccination or have no evidence of prior infection)

*Covered by the Vaccine Injury Compensation Program.

These schedules indicate the recommended age groups and medical indications for which administration of currently licensed vaccines is commonly indicated for adults ages 19 years and older, as of October 1, 2007. Licensed combination vaccines may be used whenever any components of the combination are indicated and when the vaccine's other components are not contraindicated. For detailed recommendations on all vaccines, including those used primarily for travelers or that are issued during the year, consult the manufacturers' package inserts and the complete statements from the Advisory Committee on Immunization Practices (www.cdc.gov/vaccines/pubs/acip-list.htm).

The recommendations in this schedule were approved by the Centers for Disease Control and Prevention's (CDC) Advisory Committee on Immunization Practices (ACIP), the American Academy of Family Physicians (AAFP), the American College of Obstetricians and Gynecologists (ACOG), and the American College of Physicians (ACP).

DEPARTMENT OF HEALTH AND HUMAN SERVICES
CENTERS FOR DISEASE CONTROL AND PREVENTION

CDC

continued

Footnotes
Recommended Adult Immunization Schedule • United States, October 2007–September 2008

For complete statements by the Advisory Committee on Immunization Practices (ACIP), visit www.cdc.gov/vaccines/pubs/ACIP-list.htm.

1. Tetanus, diphtheria, and acellular pertussis (Td/Tdap) vaccination

Tdap should replace a single dose of Td for adults aged <65 years who have not previously received a dose of Tdap. Only one of two Tdap products (Adacel® [sanofi pasteur]) is licensed for use in adults.

Adults with uncertain histories of a complete primary vaccination series with tetanus and diphtheria toxoid–containing vaccines should begin or complete a primary vaccination series. A primary series for adults is 3 doses of tetanus and diphtheria toxoid–containing vaccines; administer the first 2 doses at least 4 weeks apart and the third dose 6–12 months after the second. However, Tdap can substitute for any one of the doses of Td in the 3-dose primary series. The booster dose of tetanus and diphtheria toxoid–containing vaccine should be administered to adults who have completed a primary series and if the last vaccination was received ≥10 years previously. Tdap or Td vaccine may be used, as indicated.

If the person is pregnant and received the last Td vaccination ≥10 years previously, administer Td during the second or third trimester; if the person received the last Td vaccination in <10 years, administer Tdap during the immediate postpartum period. A one-time administration of 1 dose of Tdap with an interval as short as 2 years from a previous Td vaccination is recommended for postpartum women, close contacts of infants aged <12 months, and all health-care workers with direct patient contact. In certain situations, Td can be deferred during pregnancy and Tdap substituted in the immediate postpartum period, or Tdap can be administered instead of Td to a pregnant woman after an informed discussion with the woman.

Consult the ACIP statement for recommendations for administering Td as prophylaxis in wound management.

2. Human papillomavirus (HPV) vaccination

HPV vaccination is recommended for all females aged ≤26 years who have not completed the vaccine series. History of genital warts, abnormal Papanicolaou test, or positive HPV DNA test is not evidence of prior infection with all vaccine HPV types; HPV vaccination is still recommended for these persons.

Ideally, vaccine should be administered before potential exposure to HPV through sexual activity; however, females who are sexually active should still be vaccinated. Sexually active females who have not been infected with any of the HPV vaccine types receive the full benefit of the vaccination. Vaccination is less beneficial for females who have already been infected with one or more of the HPV vaccine types.

A complete series consists of 3 doses. The second dose should be administered 2 months after the first dose; the third dose should be administered 6 months after the first dose.

Although HPV vaccination is not specifically recommended for females with the medical indications described in Figure 2, "Vaccines that might be indicated for adults based on medical and other indications," it is not a live-virus vaccine and can be administered. However, immune response and vaccine efficacy might be less than in persons who do not have the medical indications described or who are immunocompetent.

3. Measles, mumps, rubella (MMR) vaccination

Measles component: Adults born before 1957 can be considered immune to measles. Adults born during or after 1957 should receive ≥1 dose of MMR unless they have a medical contraindication, documentation of ≥1 dose, history of measles based on health-care provider diagnosis, or laboratory evidence of immunity.

A second dose of MMR is recommended for adults who 1) have been recently exposed to measles or are in an outbreak setting; 2) have been previously vaccinated with killed measles vaccine; 3) have been vaccinated with an unknown type of measles vaccine during 1963–1967; 4) are students in postsecondary educational institutions; 5) work in a health-care facility; or 6) plan to travel internationally.

Mumps component: Adults born before 1957 can generally be considered immune to mumps. Adults born during or after 1957 should receive 1 dose of MMR unless they have a medical contraindication, history of mumps based on health-care provider diagnosis, or laboratory evidence of immunity.

A second dose of MMR is recommended for adults who 1) are in an age group that is affected during a mumps outbreak; 2) are students in postsecondary educational institutions; 3) work in a health-care facility; or 4) plan to travel internationally. For unvaccinated health-care workers born before 1957 who do not have other evidence of mumps immunity, consider administering 1 dose on a routine basis and strongly consider administering a second dose during an outbreak.

Rubella component: Administer 1 dose of MMR vaccine to women whose rubella vaccination history is unreliable or who lack laboratory evidence of immunity. For women of childbearing age, regardless of birth year, routinely determine rubella immunity and counsel women regarding congenital rubella syndrome. Women who do not have evidence of immunity should receive MMR vaccine upon completion or termination of pregnancy and before discharge from the health-care facility.

4. Varicella vaccination

All adults without evidence of immunity to varicella should receive 2 doses of single-antigen varicella vaccine unless they have a medical contraindication. Special consideration should be given to those who 1) have close contact with persons at high risk for severe disease (e.g., health-care personnel and family contacts of immunocompromised persons) or 2) are at high risk for exposure or transmission (e.g., teachers; child care employees; residents and staff members of institutional settings, including correctional institutions; college students; military personnel; adolescents and adults living in households with children; nonpregnant women of childbearing age; and international travelers).

Evidence of immunity to varicella in adults includes any of the following: 1) documentation of 2 doses of varicella vaccine at least 4 weeks apart; 2) U.S.-born before 1980 (although for health-care personnel and pregnant women, birth before 1980 should not be considered evidence of immunity); 3) history of varicella based on diagnosis or verification of varicella by a health-care provider (for a patient reporting a history of or presenting with an atypical case, a mild case, or both, health-care providers should seek either an epidemiologic link with a typical varicella case or to a laboratory-confirmed case or evidence of laboratory confirmation, if it was performed at the time of acute disease); 4) history of herpes zoster based on health-care provider diagnosis; or 5) laboratory evidence of immunity or laboratory confirmation of disease.

Assess pregnant women for evidence of varicella immunity. Women who do not have evidence of immunity should receive the first dose of varicella vaccine upon completion or termination of pregnancy and before discharge from the health-care facility. The second dose should be administered 4–8 weeks after the first dose.

5. Influenza vaccination

Medical indications: Chronic disorders of the cardiovascular or pulmonary systems, including asthma; chronic metabolic diseases, including diabetes mellitus, renal or hepatic dysfunction, hemoglobinopathies, or immunosuppression (including immunosuppression caused by medications

continued on page 20

or human immunodeficiency virus [HIV]); any condition that compromises respiratory function or the handling of respiratory secretions or that can increase the risk of aspiration (e.g., cognitive dysfunction, spinal cord injury, or seizure disorder or other neuromuscular disorder); and pregnancy during the influenza season. No data exist on the risk for severe or complicated influenza disease among persons with asplenia; however, influenza is a risk factor for secondary bacterial infections that can cause severe disease among persons with asplenia.

Occupational indications: Health-care personnel and employees of long-term care and assisted-living facilities.

Other indications: Residents of nursing homes and other long-term care and assisted-living facilities; persons likely to transmit influenza to persons at high risk (e.g., in-home household contacts and caregivers of children aged 0–59 months, or persons of all ages with high-risk conditions); and anyone who would like to be vaccinated. Healthy, nonpregnant adults aged ≤49 years without high-risk medical conditions who are not contacts of severely immunocompromised persons in special care units can receive either intranasally administered live, attenuated influenza vaccine (FluMist®) or inactivated vaccine. Other persons should receive the inactivated vaccine.

6. Pneumococcal polysaccharide vaccination

Medical indications: Chronic pulmonary disease (excluding asthma); chronic cardiovascular diseases; diabetes mellitus; chronic liver diseases, including liver disease as a result of alcohol abuse (e.g., cirrhosis); chronic alcoholism, chronic renal failure or nephrotic syndrome; functional or anatomic asplenia (e.g., sickle cell disease or splenectomy [if elective splenectomy is planned, vaccinate at least 2 weeks before surgery]); immunosuppressive conditions; and cochlear implants and cerebrospinal fluid leaks. Vaccinate as close to HIV diagnosis as possible.

Other indications: Alaska Natives and certain American Indian populations and residents of nursing homes or other long-term care facilities.

7. Revaccination with pneumococcal polysaccharide vaccine

One-time revaccination after 5 years for persons with chronic renal failure or nephrotic syndrome; functional or anatomic asplenia (e.g., sickle cell disease or splenectomy); or immunosuppressive conditions. For persons aged ≥65 years, one-time revaccination if they were vaccinated ≥5 years previously and were aged <65 years at the time of primary vaccination.

8. Hepatitis A vaccination

Medical indications: Persons with chronic liver disease and persons who receive clotting factor concentrates.

Behavioral indications: Men who have sex with men and persons who use illegal drugs.

Occupational indications: Persons working with hepatitis A virus (HAV)–infected primates or with HAV in a research laboratory setting.

Other indications: Persons traveling to or working in countries that have high or intermediate endemicity of hepatitis A (a list of countries is available at wwwn.cdc.gov/travel/contentdiseases.aspx) and any person seeking protection from HAV infection.

Single-antigen vaccine formulations should be administered in a 2-dose schedule at either 0 and 6–12 months (Havrix®), or 0 and 6–18 months (Vaqta®). If the combined hepatitis A and hepatitis B vaccine (Twinrix®) is used, administer 3 doses at 0, 1, and 6 months.

9. Hepatitis B vaccination

Medical indications: Persons with end-stage renal disease, including patients receiving hemodialysis; persons seeking evaluation or treatment for a sexually transmitted disease (STD); persons with HIV infection; and persons with chronic liver disease.

Occupational indications: Health-care personnel and public-safety workers who are exposed to blood or other potentially infectious body fluids.

Behavioral indications: Sexually active persons who are not in a long-term, mutually monogamous relationship (e.g., persons with more than 1 sex partner during the previous 6 months); current or recent injection-drug users; and men who have sex with men.

Other indications: Household contacts and sex partners of persons with chronic hepatitis B virus (HBV) infection; clients and staff members of institutions for persons with developmental disabilities; international travelers to countries with high or intermediate prevalence of chronic HBV infection (a list of countries is available at wwwn.cdc.gov/travel/contentdiseases.aspx); and any adult seeking protection from HBV infection.

Settings where hepatitis B vaccination is recommended for all adults: STD treatment facilities; HIV testing and treatment facilities; facilities providing drug-abuse treatment and prevention services; health-care settings targeting services to injection-drug users or men who have sex with men; correctional facilities; end-stage renal disease programs and facilities for chronic hemodialysis patients; and institutions and nonresidential day care facilities for persons with developmental disabilities.

Special formulation indications: For adult patients receiving hemodialysis and other immunocompromised adults, 1 dose of 40 μg/mL (Recombivax HB®) or 2 doses of 20 μg/mL (Engerix-B®), administered simultaneously.

10. Meningococcal vaccination

Medical indications: Adults with anatomic or functional asplenia, or terminal complement component deficiencies.

Other indications: First-year college students living in dormitories; microbiologists who are routinely exposed to isolates of *Neisseria meningitidis;* military recruits; and persons who travel to or live in countries in which meningococcal disease is hyperendemic or epidemic (e.g., the "meningitis belt" of sub-Saharan Africa during the dry season [December–June]), particularly if their contact with local populations will be prolonged. Vaccination is required by the government of Saudi Arabia for all travelers to Mecca during the annual Hajj.

Meningococcal conjugate vaccine is preferred for adults with any of the preceding indications who are aged ≤55 years, although meningococcal polysaccharide vaccine (MPSV4) is an acceptable alternative. Revaccination after 3–5 years might be indicated for adults previously vaccinated with MPSV4 who remain at increased risk for infection (e.g., persons residing in areas in which disease is epidemic).

11. Herpes zoster vaccination

A single dose of zoster vaccine is recommended for adults aged ≥60 years regardless of whether they report a prior episode of herpes zoster. Persons with chronic medical conditions may be vaccinated unless a contraindication or precaution exists for their condition.

12. Selected conditions for which *Haemophilus influenzae* type b (Hib) vaccine may be used

Hib conjugate vaccines are licensed for children aged 6 weeks–71 months. No efficacy data are available on which to base a recommendation concerning use of Hib vaccine for older children and adults with the chronic conditions associated with an increased risk for Hib disease. However, studies suggest good immunogenicity in patients who have sickle cell disease, leukemia, or HIV infection or who have had splenectomies; administering vaccine to these patients is not contraindicated.

13. Immunocompromising conditions

Inactivated vaccines are generally acceptable (e.g., pneumococcal, meningococcal, and influenza [trivalent inactivated influenza vaccine]), and live vaccines generally are avoided in persons with immune deficiencies or immune suppressive conditions. Information on specific conditions is available at www.cdc.gov/vaccines/pubs/acip-list.htm.

How clients frame their previous health concerns suggests how they feel about themselves and is an indication of their sense of responsibility for their own health. For example, a client who has been obese for years may blame himself for developing diabetes and fail to comply with his diet, whereas another client may be very willing to share the treatment of her diabetes and success with an insulin pump in a support group. Some clients are very forthcoming about their past health status; others are not. It is helpful to have a series of alternative questions for less responsive clients and for those who may not understand what is being asked.

Family Health History

As researchers discover more and more health problems that seem to run in families and that are genetically based, the family health history assumes greater importance. In addition to genetic predisposition, it is also helpful to see other health problems that may have affected the client by virtue of having grown up in the family and being exposed to these problems. For example, a gene predisposing a person to smoking has not yet been discovered but a family with smoking members can affect other members in at least two ways. First, the second-hand smoke can compromise the physical health of nonsmoking members; second, the smoker may serve as a negative role model for children, inducing them to take up the habit as well. Another example is obesity; recognizing it in the family history can alert the nurse to a potential risk factor.

The family history should include as many genetic relatives as the client can recall. Include maternal and paternal grandparents, aunts and uncles on both sides, parents, siblings, and the client's children. Such thoroughness usually identifies those diseases that may skip a generation such as autosomal recessive disorders. Include the client's spouse but indicate that there is no genetic link. Identifying the spouse's health problems could explain disorders in the client's children not indicated in the client's family history.

Drawing a genogram helps to organize and illustrate the client's family history. Use a standard format so others can easily understand the information. Also provide a key to the symbols used. Usually female relatives are indicated by a circle and male relatives by a square. A deceased relative is noted by marking an X in the circle or square and listing the age at death and the cause of death. Identify all relatives, living or dead, by age and provide a brief list of diseases or conditions. If the relative has no problems, the letters "A/W" (alive and well) should be placed next to the age. Straight vertical and horizontal lines are used to show relationships. A horizontal dotted line can be used to indicate the client's spouse; a vertical dotted line can be used to indicate adoption. A sample genogram is illustrated in Figure 2-2.

After the diagrammatic family history, prepare a brief summary of the kinds of health problems present in the family. For example, the client in the genogram depicted in the accompanying figure has longevity, obesity, heart disease, hypertension (HTN), arthritis, thyroid disorders, non–insulin-dependent diabetes mellitus (NIDDM, also known as type 2 diabetes), alcoholism, smoking, myopia, learning disability, hyperactivity disorder, and cancer (one relative) on his maternal side. On the client's paternal side are obesity, heart disease, hypercholesterolemia, back problems, arthritis, myopia, and cancer. The paternal history is not as extensive as the maternal history because the client's father was adopted. In addition, the client's sister is obese and has Graves' disease and hypercholesterolemia. His wife has arthritis; his children are both A/W.

Review of Systems (ROS) for Current Health Problems

In the review of systems (or review of body systems), each body system is addressed and the client is asked specific questions to draw out current health problems or problems from the recent past that may still affect the client or that are recurring. Care must be taken in this section to include only the client's subjective information and not the examiner's observations. There is a tendency, especially with more experienced nurses, to fill up the spaces with observations such as "erythema of the right eye" or "several vesicles on the client's upper extremities."

During the review of body systems, document the client's descriptions of her health status for each body system and note the client's denial of signs, symptoms, diseases, or problems that the nurse asks about but are not experienced by the client. For example, under the area "Head and Neck," the client may respond that there are no problems but on questioning from the nurse about headaches, stiffness, pain, or cracking in the neck with motion, swelling in the neck, difficulty swallowing, sore throat, enlarged lymph nodes, and so on, the client may suddenly remember that he did have a sore throat a week ago that he self-treated with zinc lozenges. This information might not have emerged without specific questions. Also, if the lone entry "no problems" is entered on the health history form, other health care professionals reviewing the history cannot even ascertain what specific questions had been asked, if any.

The questions about problems and signs or symptoms of disorders should be asked in terms that the client understands, but findings may be recorded in standard medical terminology. If the client appears to have a limited vocabulary, the nurse may need to ask questions in several different ways and use very basic lay terminology. If the client is well educated and seems familiar with medical terminology, the nurse should not insult her by talking at a much lower level. The most obvious information to collect for each body part or system is listed below. See the physical assessment chapters for in-depth questions and rationales for each particular body part or system.

- *Skin, hair, and nails:* Skin color, temperature, condition, excessive sweating, rashes, lesions, balding, dandruff, condition of nails
- *Head and neck:* Headache, swelling, stiffness of neck, difficulty swallowing, sore throat, enlarged lymph nodes
- *Eyes:* Vision, eye infections, redness, excessive tearing, halos around lights, blurring, loss of side vision, moving black spots/specks in visual fields, flashing lights, double vision, and eye pain
- *Ears:* Hearing, ringing or buzzing, earaches, drainage from ears, dizziness, exposure to loud noises
- *Mouth, throat, nose, and sinuses:* Condition of teeth and gums; sore throats; mouth lesions; hoarseness; rhinorrhea; nasal obstruction; frequent colds; sneezing or itching of eyes, ears, nose, or throat; nose bleeds; snoring
- *Thorax and lungs:* Difficulty breathing, wheezing, pain, shortness of breath during routine activity, orthopnea, cough or sputum, hemoptysis, respiratory infections

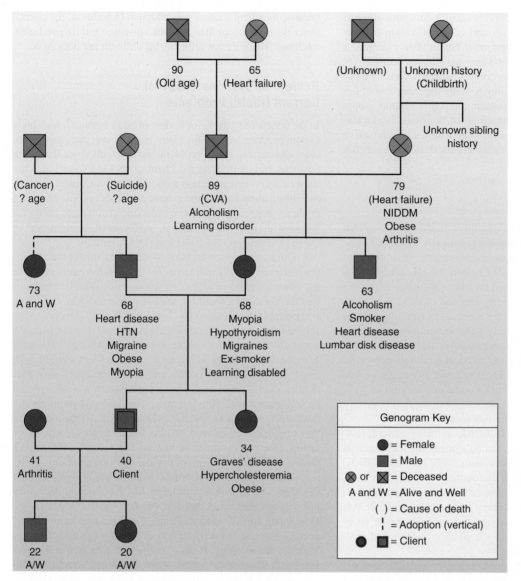

Genogram Key

● = Female
■ = Male
⊗ or ⊠ = Deceased
A and W = Alive and Well
( ) = Cause of death
┊ = Adoption (vertical)
● ■ = Client

Figure 2-2 Genogram of a 40-year-old male client.

- *Breasts and regional lymphatics:* Lumps or discharge from nipples, dimpling or changes in breast size, swollen or tender lymph nodes in axilla
- *Heart and neck vessels:* Last blood pressure, ECG tracing or findings, chest pain or pressure, palpitations, edema
- *Peripheral vascular:* Swelling, or edema, of legs and feet; pain; cramping; sores on legs; color or texture changes on the legs or feet
- *Abdomen:* Indigestion, difficulty swallowing, nausea, vomiting, abdominal pain, gas, jaundice, hernias
- *Male genitalia:* Excessive or painful urination, frequency or difficulty starting and maintaining urinary stream, leaking of urine, blood noted in urine, sexual problems, perineal lesions, penile drainage, pain or swelling in scrotum, difficulty achieving an erection and/or difficulty ejaculating, exposure to sexually transmitted infections
- *Female genitalia:* Sexual problems; sexually transmitted diseases; voiding problems (e.g., dribbling, incontinence); reproductive data such as age at menarche, menstruation (length and regularity of cycle), pregnancies, and type of or problems with delivery, abortions, pelvic pain, birth control, menopause (date or year of last menstrual period), and use of hormone replacement therapy

- *Anus, rectum, and prostate:* Bowel habits, pain with defecation, hemorrhoids, blood in stool, constipation, diarrhea
- *Musculoskeletal:* Swelling, redness, pain, stiffness of joints, ability to perform activities of daily living, muscle strength
- *Neurologic:* General mood, behavior, depression, anger, concussions, headaches, loss of strength or sensation, coordination, difficulty speaking, memory problems, strange thoughts and/or actions, difficulty learning

Lifestyle and Health Practices Profile

This is a very important section of the health history because it deals with the client's human responses, which include nutritional habits, activity and exercise patterns, sleep and rest patterns, use of medications and substances, self-concept and self-care activities, social and community activities, relationships, values and beliefs system, education and work, stress level and coping style, and environment.

Here clients describe how they are managing their lives, their awareness of healthy versus toxic living patterns, and the strengths and supports they have or use. When assessing this area, use open-ended questions to promote a dialogue with the client. Follow up with specific questions to guide the discussion and clarify the information as necessary. Be sure to pay special attention to the cues the client may provide that point to possibly more significant content. Take brief notes so that pertinent data are not lost and so there can be follow-up if some information needs clarification or expansion. If clients give permission and it does not seem to cause anxiety or inhibition, using an audiocassette recorder frees the nurse from the need to write while clients talk.

In this section, each area is discussed briefly then followed by a few sample questions.

Description of Typical Day

This information is necessary to elicit an overview of how the client sees his usual pattern of daily activity. The questions you ask should be vague enough to allow the client to provide the orientation from which the day is viewed, for example, "Please tell me what an average or typical day is for you. Start with awakening in the morning and continue until bedtime." Encourage the client to discuss a usual day, which, for most people, includes work or school. If the client gives minimal information, additional specific questions may be asked to draw out more details.

Nutrition and Weight Management

Ask the client to recall what consists of an average 24-hour intake for her with emphasis on what foods are eaten and in what amounts. Also ask about snacks, fluid intake, and other substances consumed. Depending on the client, you may want to ask who buys and prepares the food and when and where meals are eaten. These questions uncover food habits that are health promoting as well as those that are less desirable. The client's answers about food intake should be compared with the guidelines illustrated in the "food pyramid" (See Chapter 12). The food pyramid, developed by the U.S. Department of Agriculture, is designed to teach people what types and amounts of food to eat to ensure a balanced diet, to promote health, and to prevent disease. Consider reviewing the food pyramid with the client and explaining what a serving size is. The client's fluid intake should be compared with the general recommendation of six to eight glasses of water or noncaffeinated fluids daily. It is also important to ask about the client's bowel and bladder habits at this time (included in review of symptoms).

Sample questions include

- "What do you usually eat during a typical day? Please tell me the kinds of foods you prefer, how often you eat throughout the day, and how much you eat."
- "Do you eat out at restaurants frequently?"
- "Do you eat only when hungry? Do you eat because of boredom, habit, anxiety, depression?"
- "Who buys and prepares the food you eat?"
- "Where do you eat your meals?"
- "How much and what types of fluids do you drink?"

Activity Level and Exercise

Next, assess how active the client is during an average week either at work or at home. Inquire about regular exercise. Some clients believe that if they do heavy physical work at their job, they do not need additional exercise. Make it a point to distinguish between activity done when working, which may be stressful and fatiguing, and exercise, which is designed to reduce stress and strengthen the individual. Compare the client's answers with the recommended exercise regimen of regular aerobic exercise for 20 to 30 minutes at least three times a week. Explain to the client that regular exercise reduces the risk of heart disease, strengthens heart and lungs, reduces stress, and manages weight.

Sample questions include

- "What is your daily pattern of activity?"
- "Do you follow a regular exercise plan? What types of exercise do you do?"
- "Are there any reasons why you cannot follow a moderately strenuous exercise program?"
- "What do you do for leisure and recreation?"
- "Do your leisure and recreational activities include exercise?"

Sleep and Rest

Inquire whether the client feels he is getting enough sleep and rest. Questions should focus on specific sleep patterns such as how many hours a night the person sleeps, interruptions, whether the client feels rested, problems sleeping (e.g., insomnia), rituals the client uses to promote sleep, and concerns the client may have regarding sleep habits. Some of this information may have already been presented by the client, but it is useful to gather data in a more systematic and thorough manner at this time. Inquiries about sleep can bring out problems, such as anxiety, which manifests as sleeplessness, or inadequate sleep time, which can predispose the client to accidents. Compare the client's answers with the normal sleep requirement for adults, which is usually between 5 and 8 hours a night. Keep in mind sleep requirements vary depending on age, health, and stress levels.

Sample questions include

- "Tell me about your sleeping patterns."
- "Do you have trouble falling asleep or staying asleep?"
- "How much sleep do you get each night?"
- "Do you feel rested when you awaken?"
- "Do you nap during the day? How often and for how long?"
- "What do you do to help you fall asleep?"

See Promote Health—Insomnia and Display 2-5. For more detailed discussions of sleep and insomnia, see Cochran (2003), Turkoski (2006), and the National Sleep Foundation website.

Medication and Substance Use

The information gathered about medication and substance use provides the nurse with information concerning lifestyle and a client's self-care ability. Medication and substance use can affect the client's health and cause loss of function or impaired senses. In addition, certain medications and substances can increase the client's risk for disease. Because many people use vitamins or a variety of herbal supplements, it is important to ask which and how often. Prescription medications and these supplements may interact (e.g., garlic decreases coagulation and interacts with warfarin [Coumadin]).

Sample questions include

- "What medications have you used in the recent past and currently, both those that your doctor prescribed and those you can buy over the counter at a drug or grocery store? For what purpose did you take the medication? How much (dose) and how often did you take the medication?"
- "How much beer, wine, or other alcohol do you drink on the average?"

PROMOTE HEALTH
Insomnia

Overview

Many people experience occasional insomnia, but chronic insomnia can become a problem with daytime functioning. Insomnia occurs when one's normal sleep pattern is interrupted, resulting in less sleep or less satisfying sleep. More women than men report insomnia, especially those over 30 years of age. Also, persons of lower socioeconomic status or with chronic medical or psychiatric problems have higher rates of insomnia. Many physical, behavioral, or pharmacological factors can affect sleep. Common sleep disorders include obstructive sleep apnea, narcolepsy, restless leg syndrome, circadian rhythm disorders (causing inability to sleep at usual times), psychological disorders such as depression, and

psychiatric disorders. These disorders can be caused by intake of stimulant medications, consumption of substances such as caffeine, nicotine, and alcohol near bedtime, lighted and noisy environment, exercise close to bedtime or little exercise (sedentary).

Sleep is divided into various stages including rapid eye movement (REM) and non-rapid eye movement (NREM) sleep cycles. Brain waves and body functions correlate with the cycles, with slow brain waves and decreased body function rates during NREM. Both REM and NREM sleep are necessary for adequate rest, and disruption in any sleep stage can cause sleep disturbance. However, loss of total sleep time affects cognitive function the most.

Risk Factors

- Chronic medical, psychological, or psychiatric disorder
- Airway obstruction
- Narcolepsy
- Restless leg syndrome
- Stimulant medications intake
- Caffeine or alcohol consumption, or near bedtime smoking or heavy smoking
- Exercises, little or close to bedtime
- Lighted and noisy sleep environment, or an uncomfortable temperature
- Shift working or variable bedtimes
- Female over 30 years old
- Lower socioeconomic status

Teach Risk Reduction Tips

- Maintain a regular bedtime and wake time schedule, including weekends
- Establish a regular, relaxing bedtime routine, such as soaking in a hot bath or hot tub and then reading a book or listening to soothing music

- Create a sleep-conducive environment that is dark, quiet, comfortable, and cool
- Sleep on a comfortable mattress and pillows
- Use your bedroom only for sleep and sex
- Finish eating at least 2 to 3 hours before your regular bedtime
- Exercise regularly; it is best to complete your workout at least a few hours before bedtime
- Avoid caffeine (e.g., coffee, tea, soft drinks, chocolate) close to bedtime
- Avoid nicotine (e.g., cigarettes, tobacco products) close to bedtime
- Avoid alcohol close to bedtime
- Eat a light snack before bed if hungry
- Do not watch the clock
- Drink warm milk

(Risk Reduction Tips from National Sleep Foundation, 2007, and Cochran, 2003)

- "Do you drink coffee or other beverages containing caffeine (e.g., cola)?" If so, how much and how often?
- "Do you now or have you ever smoked cigarettes or used any other form of nicotine? How long have you been smoking/did you smoke? How many packs per week? Tell me about any efforts to quit."
- "Have you ever taken any medication not prescribed by your healthcare provider? If so, when, what type, how much, and why?"
- "Have you ever used, or do you now use, recreational drugs? Describe any usage."
- "Do you take vitamins or herbal supplements? If so, what?"

Self-Concept and Self-Care Responsibilities

This includes assessment of how the client views herself and investigation of all behaviors that a person does to promote her health. Examples of subjects to be addressed include sexual

responsibility; basic hygiene practices; regularity of health care checkups (i.e., dental, visual, medical); breast/testicular self-examination; and accident prevention and hazard protection (e.g., seat belts, smoke alarms, and sunscreen).

You can correlate answers to questions in this area with health-promotion activities discussed previously and with risk factors from the family history. This will help to point out client strengths and needs for health maintenance. Questions to the client can be open-ended but the client may need prompting to cover all areas.

Sample questions include

- "What do you see as your talents or special abilities?"
- "How do you feel about yourself? About your appearance?"
- "Can you tell me what activities you do to keep yourself safe, healthy, or to prevent disease?"
- "Do you practice safe sex?"
- "How do you keep your home safe?"
- "Do you drive safely?"

DISPLAY 2-5	Stanford Sleepiness Scale

This is a quick way to assess how alert you are feeling. During the day when you go about your business, ideally you would want a rating of "1." Take into account that most people have two peak times of alertness daily, at about 9 AM and 9 PM. Alertness wanes to its lowest point at around 3 PM and after that it begins to build again. Rate your alertness at different times during the day. If your score is greater than "3" during a time when you should feel alert, you may have a serious sleep debt and require more sleep.

Degree of Sleepiness	*Scale Rating*
Feeling active, vital, alert, or wide awake	1
Functioning at high levels, but not at peak; able to concentrate	2
Awake, but relaxed; responsive but not fully alert	3
Somewhat foggy, let down	4
Foggy; losing interest in remaining awake; slowed down	5
Sleepy, woozy, fighting sleep; prefer to lie down	6
No longer fighting sleep, sleep onset soon; having dream-like thoughts	7
Asleep	X

(Stanford Sleepiness Scale. Available at http://stanford.edu/~dement/sss.html)

- "How often do you have medical checkups or screenings?"
- "How often do you see the dentist or have your eyes (vision) examined?"

Social Activities

Questions about social activities help the nurse to discover what outlets the client has for support and relaxation and if the client is involved in the community beyond family and work. Information in this area also helps to determine the client's current level of social development. Sample questions include

- "What do you do for fun and relaxation?"
- "With whom do you socialize most frequently?"
- "Are you involved in any community activities?"
- "How do you feel about your community?"
- "Do you think that you have enough time to socialize?"
- "What do you see as your contribution to society?"

Relationships

Ask clients to describe the composition of the family into which they were born and about past and current relationships with these family members. In this way, you can assess problems and potential support from the client's family of origin. In addition, similar information should be sought about the client's current family (Fig. 2-3). If the client does not have any family by blood or marriage, then information should be gathered about any significant others (including pets) that may constitute the client's "family."

Sample questions include

- "Who is (are) the most important person(s) in your life? Describe your relationship with that person."
- "What was it like growing up in your family?"
- "What is your relationship like with your spouse?"
- "What is your relationship like with your children?"

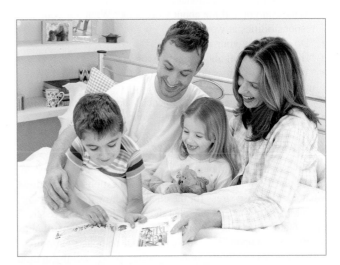

Figure 2-3 Discussing family relationships is a key way to assess support systems.

- "Describe any relationships you have with significant others."
- "Do you get along with your in-laws?"
- "Are you close to your extended family?"
- "Do you have any pets?"
- "What is your role in your family? Is it an important role?"
- "Are you satisfied with your current sexual relationships? Have there been any recent changes?"

Values and Belief System

Assess the client values. In addition, discuss the clients' philosophical, religious, and spiritual beliefs. Some clients may not be comfortable discussing values or beliefs. Their feelings should be respected. However, the data can help to identify important problems or strengths.

Sample questions include

- "What is most important to you in life?"
- "What do you hope to accomplish in your life?"
- "Do you have a religious affiliation? Is this important to you?"
- "Is a relationship with God (or another higher power) an important part of your life?"
- "What gives you strength and hope?"

Education and Work

Questions about education and work help to identify areas of stress and satisfaction in the client's life. If the client does not perceive that he has enough education or his work is not what he enjoys, he may need assistance or support to make changes. Sometimes discussing this area will help the client feel good about what he has accomplished and promote his sense of life satisfaction. Questions should bring out data about the kind and amount of education the client has, whether the client enjoyed school, whether he perceives his education as satisfactory or whether there were problems, and what plans the client may have for further education, either formal or informal. Similar questions should be asked about work history.

Sample questions include

- "Tell me about your experiences in school or about your education."
- "Are you satisfied with the level of education you have? Do you have future educational plans?"
- "What can you tell me about your work? What are your responsibilities at work?"
- "Do you enjoy your work?"
- "How do you feel about your coworkers?"
- "What kind of stress do you have that is work related? Any major problems?"
- "Who is the main provider of financial support in your family?"
- "Does your current income meet your needs?"

Stress Levels and Coping Styles

To investigate the amount of stress clients perceive they are under and how they cope with it, ask questions that address what events cause stress for the client and how they usually respond. In addition, find out what the client does to relieve stress and whether these behaviors or activities can be construed as adaptive or maladaptive. To avoid denial responses, nondirective questions or observations regarding previous information provided by the client may be an easy way to get the client to discuss this subject.

Sample questions include

- "What types of things make you angry?"
- "How would you describe your stress level?"
- "How do you manage anger or stress?"
- "What do you see as the greatest stressors in your life?"
- "Where do you usually turn for help in a time of crisis?"

Environment

Ask questions regarding the client's environment to assess health hazards unique to the client's living situation and lifestyle. Look for physical, chemical, or psychological situations that may put the client at risk. These may be found in the client's neighborhood, home, work, or recreational environment. They may be controllable or uncontrollable.

Sample questions include

- "What risks are you aware of in your environment such as in your home, neighborhood, on the job, or any other activities in which you participate?"
- "What types of precautions do you take, if any, when playing contact sports, using harsh chemicals or paint, or operating machinery?"
- "Do you believe you are ever in danger of becoming a victim of violence? Explain."

SUMMARY

Collecting subjective data is a key step of nursing health assessment. Subjective data consist of information elicited and verified only by the client. Interviewing is the means by which subjective data are gathered. Two types of communication are useful for interviewing: nonverbal and verbal. Variations in communication, such as gerontologic, cultural, and emotional variations, may be encountered during the client interview.

The complete health history is performed to collect as much subjective data about a client as possible. It consists of eight sections: biographic data, reasons for seeking health care, history of present health concern, past health history, family health history, review of body systems (ROS) for current health problems, lifestyle and health practices, and developmental level.

References and Selected Readings

Andrews, M., & Boyle, J. (2002). *Transcultural concepts in nursing care* (4th ed.). Philadelphia: Lippincott Williams & Wilkins.

Brush, B. L. (2000). Assessing spirituality in primary care practice: Is there time? *Clinical Excellence for Nurse Practitioners, 4*(2), 67–71.

Chambers, S. (2003). Use of non-verbal communication skills to improve nursing care. *British Journal of Nursing, 12*(14), 874–878.

Cochran, H. (2003). Diagnose and treat primary insomnia. *The Nurse Practitioner, 28*(9), 13–27.

DiMartino, G. (2000). Legal issues: The patient history. *Dynamic Chiropractic, 18*(14), 26.

Giger, J., & Davidhizar, R. (2008). *Transcultural nursing: Assessment and intervention* (5th ed.). St. Louis: Mosby-Year Book.

Heery, K. (2000). Straight talk about the patient intervention. *Nursing, 2000, 20*(6), 66–67.

Interview of older adult. (n.d.). Available at http://www.medicine.arizona.edu/aamc-hartford

Luckmann, J. (2000). *Transcultural communication in health care.* Albany, NY: Delmar.

National Sleep Foundation. (2007). Health sleep tips. Available at http://www.sleepfoundation.org

Piasecki, M. (2003). *Clinical communication handbook.* Maldon, MA: Blackwell Science.

Price, B. (2004). Conducting sensitive patient interviews. *Nursing Standard, 18*(38), 45–52.

Schuster, C. S., & Asburn, S. S. (1992). *The process of human development: A holistic life-span approach* (3rd ed.). Philadelphia: J. B. Lippincott.

Thompson, T. L. (2003). *Handbook of health communication.* Malwah, NJ: Lawrence Erlbaum Associates.

Turkoski, B. (2006). Pharmacology: Managing insomnia. *Orthopaedic Nursing, 25*(5), 339–345.

3

Collecting Objective Data

A complete nursing assessment includes both the collection of subjective data (discussed in Chapter 2) and the collection of objective data. Objective data include information about the client that the nurse directly observes during interaction with him and information elicited through physical assessment (examination) techniques.

To become proficient with physical assessment skills, the nurse must have basic knowledge in three areas:

- Types of and operation of equipment needed for the particular examination (e.g., penlight, sphygmomanometer, otoscope, tuning fork, stethoscope)
- Preparation of the setting, oneself, and the client for the physical assessment
- Performance of the four assessment techniques: inspection, palpation, percussion, and auscultation

EQUIPMENT

Each part of the physical examination requires specific pieces of equipment. Table 3-1 lists equipment necessary for each part of the examination and describes the general purpose of each piece of equipment. More detailed descriptions of each piece of equipment and the procedures for using them are provided in the chapters on the body systems where each piece is used, e.g., techniques for using an ophthalmoscope is included in the eye assessment chapter. However, because the stethoscope is used during the assessment of many body systems, this chapter includes a description of it and guidelines on how to use it.

Prior to the examination, collect the necessary equipment and place it in the area where the examination will be performed. This promotes organization and prevents the nurse from leaving the client to search for a piece of equipment.

PREPARING FOR THE EXAMINATION

How well you prepare the physical setting, yourself, and the client can affect the quality of the data you elicit. As an examiner, you must make sure that you have prepared for all three aspects before beginning an examination. Practicing with a friend, relative, or classmate will help you to achieve proficiency in all three aspects of preparation.

Preparing the Physical Setting

The physical examination may take place in a variety of physical settings such as a hospital room, outpatient clinic, physician's office, school health office, employee health office, or a client's home. It is important that the nurse strive to ensure that the examination setting meets the following conditions:

- Comfortable, warm room temperature—Provide a warm blanket if the room temperature cannot be adjusted.
- Private area free of interruptions from others—Close the door or pull the curtains if possible.
- Quiet area free of distractions—Turn off the radio, television, or other noisy equipment.
- Adequate lighting—It is best to use sunlight (when available). However, good overhead lighting is sufficient. A portable lamp is helpful for illuminating the skin and for viewing shadows or contours.
- Firm examination table or bed at a height that prevents stooping—A roll-up stool may be useful when it is necessary for the examiner to sit for parts of the assessment.
- A bedside table/tray to hold the equipment needed for the examination

Preparing Oneself

As a beginning examiner, it is helpful to assess your own feelings and anxieties before examining the client. Anxiety is easily conveyed to the client, who may already feel uneasy and self-conscious about the examination. Self-confidence in performing a physical assessment can be achieved by practicing the techniques on a classmate, friend, or relative. Your "pretend client" should be encouraged to simulate the client role as closely as possible. It is also important to perform some of your practice assessments with an experienced instructor or practitioner who can give you helpful hints and feedback on your technique.

Another important aspect of preparing yourself for the physical assessment examination is preventing the transmission of infectious agents. In 2007, the Centers for Disease Control and Prevention (CDC) and the Hospital Infection Control Practices Advisory Committee (HICPAC) updated Standard Precautions to be followed by all health care workers caring for clients (CDC & HICPAC, 2007). These Standard Precautions

Table 3-1	Equipment Needed for Physical Examinations

Equipment Needed	Purpose
For All Examinations	
Gloves	To protect examiner in any part of the examination when the examiner may have contact with blood, body fluids, secretions, excretions, and contaminated items or when disease-causing agents could be transmitted to or from the client
For Vital Signs	
Sphygmomanometer	To measure diastolic and systolic blood pressure
Stethoscope	To auscultate blood sounds when measuring blood pressure
Thermometer (oral, rectal, tympanic, electronic)	To measure body temperature
Watch with second hand	To time heart rate, pulse rate
Pain rating scale	To determine perceived pain level
For Anthropometric Measurements	
Skinfold calipers	To measure skinfold thickness of subcutaneous tissue
Flexible tape measure	To measure mid-arm circumference
Platform scale with height attachment	To measure height and weight
For Skin, Hair, and Nail Examination	
Ruler with centimeter markings	To measure size of skin lesions
Magnifying glass	To enlarge visibility of lesion
Wood's light	To test for fungus
For Head and Neck Examination	
Small cup of water	To help client swallow during examination of the thyroid gland
For Eye Examination	
Penlight	To test pupillary constriction
Snellen chart	To test distant vision
Ophthalmoscope	To view the red reflex and to examine the retina of the eye
Cover card	To test for strabismus
Newspaper or Rosenbaum Pocket Screener	To test near vision
For Ear Examination	
Otoscope	To view the ear canal and tympanic membrane
Tuning fork	To test for bone and air conduction of sound
For Mouth, Throat, Nose, and Sinus Examination	
Penlight	To provide light to view the mouth and throat and to transilluminate the sinuses
Tongue depressor	To depress tongue to view throat, check looseness of teeth, view cheeks, and check strength of tongue
Piece of small gauze	To grasp tongue to examine mouth
Otoscope with wide-tip attachment	To view the internal nose
For Thoracic and Lung Examination	
Stethoscope (diaphragm)	To auscultate breath sounds
Marking pencil and centimeter ruler	To measure diaphragmatic excursion
For Heart and Neck Vessel Examination	
Stethoscope (bell and diaphragm)	To auscultate heart sounds
Two centimeter rulers	To measure jugular venous pressure
For Abdominal Examination	
Stethoscope	To detect bowel sounds
Marking pencil and tape measure with centimeter markings	To mark area of percussion of organs to measure size
Two small pillows	To place under knees and head to promote relaxation of abdomen
For Female Genitalia Examination	
Vaginal speculum and lubricant	To inspect cervix through dilatation of the vaginal canal
Slides or specimen container, bifid spatula, and cotton-tipped applicator	To obtain endocervical swab and cervical scrape and vaginal pool sample
For Anus, Rectum, Prostate Examination	
Lubricating jelly	To promote comfort for client
Specimen container	To test for occult blood
For Peripheral Vascular Examination	
Stethoscope and sphygmomanometer	To auscultate vascular sounds and measure blood pressure
Flexible tape measure	To measure size of extremities for edema
Cotton ball and paper clip	To detect light, blunt, and sharp touch
Tuning fork	To detect vibratory sensation
Doppler ultrasound probe blood	To detect pressure and weak pulses not easily heard with a stethoscope
For Musculoskeletal Examination	
Tape measure	To measure size of extremities
Goniometer	To measure degree of flexion and extension of joints

continued

Table 3-1	Equipment Needed for Physical Examinations *Continued*

Equipment Needed	Purpose
For Neurologic Examination	
Tuning fork	To test for vibratory sensation
Cotton wisp, paper clip	To test for light, sharp, and dull touch and two-point discrimination
Soap, coffee	To test for smelling perception
Salt, sugar, lemon, pickle juice	To test for taste perception
Tongue depressor	To test for rise of uvula and gag reflex
Reflex hammer	To test deep tendon reflexes
Coin or key	To test for stereognosis (ability to recognize objects by touch)

appear in Display 3-1; they are a modified combination of the original Universal Precautions and Body Substance Isolation Guidelines and updated each year as necessary. The specific precaution or combination of precautions varies with the care to be provided. For example, performing venipuncture requires only gloves, but intubation requires gloves, gown, and face shield, mask, or goggles. General principles to keep in mind while performing a physical assessment include the following:

- Wash your hands before beginning the examination, immediately after accidental direct contact with blood or other body fluids (you should wear gloves if there is a chance that you will come in direct contact with blood or other body fluids), and after completing the physical examination or after removing gloves. If possible, wash your hands in the examining room in front of the client. This assures your client that you are concerned about his or her safety.
- Wear gloves if you have an open cut or skin abrasion, if the client has an open or weeping cut, if you are collecting body fluids (e.g., blood, sputum, wound drainage, urine, or stools) for a specimen, if you are handling contaminated surfaces (e.g., linen, tongue blades, vaginal speculum), and when you are performing an examination of the mouth, an open wound, genitalia, vagina, or rectum. Change gloves if moving from contaminated to clean body site, and between patients.
- If a pin or other sharp object is used to assess sensory perception, discard the pin and use a new one for your next client.
- Wear a mask and protective eye goggles if you are performing an examination in which you are likely to be splashed with blood or other body fluid droplets (e.g., if you are performing an oral examination on a client who has a chronic productive cough).

Approaching and Preparing the Client

The nurse–client relationship should be established during the client interview before the physical examination takes place. This is important because it helps to alleviate any tension or anxiety that the client is experiencing. At the end of the interview, explain to the client that the physical assessment will follow and describe what the examination will involve. For example, you might say to a client, "Mr. Smith, based on the information you have given me, I believe that a complete physical examination should be performed so I can better assess your health status. This will require you to remove your clothing and to put on this gown. You may leave on your underwear until it is time to perform the genital examination."

Respect the client's desires and requests related to the physical examination. Some client requests may be simple such as asking to have a family member or friend present during the examination. Another request may involve not wanting certain parts of the examination (e.g., breast, genitalia) to be performed. In this situation, you should explain to the client the importance of the examination and the risk of missing important information if any part of the examination is omitted. Ultimately, however, whether or not to have the examination is the client's decision. Some health care providers ask the client to sign a consent form before a physical examination, especially in situations where a vaginal or rectal examination will be performed.

If a urine specimen is necessary, explain to the client the purpose of a urine sample and the procedure for giving a sample; provide him or her with a container to use. If a urine sample is not necessary, ask the client to urinate before the examination to promote an easier and more comfortable examination of the abdomen and genital areas. Ask the client to undress and put on an examination gown. Allow him or her to keep on underwear until just before the genital examination to promote comfort and privacy. Leave the room while the client changes into the gown and knock before reentering the room to ensure the client's privacy.

Begin the examination with the less intrusive procedures such as measuring the client's temperature, pulse, blood pressure, height, and weight. These nonthreatening/nonintrusive procedures allow the client to feel more comfortable with you and help to ease client anxiety about the examination. Throughout the examination, continue to explain what procedure you are performing and why you are performing it. This helps to ease your client's anxiety. It is usually helpful to integrate health teaching and health promotion during the examination (e.g., breast self-examination technique during the breast examination).

Approach the client from the right-hand side of the examination table or bed because most examination techniques are performed with the examiner's right hand (even if the examiner is left-handed). You may ask the client to change positions frequently, depending on the part of the examination being performed. Prepare the client for these changes at the beginning of the examination by explaining that these position changes are necessary to ensure a thorough examination of each body part and system. Many clients need assistance getting into the required position. Display 3-2 illustrates various positions and provides guidelines for using them during the examination. Display 3-3 provides considerations for older adult clients.

(text continues on page 35)

DISPLAY 3-1	CDC* and HICPAC† Isolation Precaution Guidelines

Standard Precautions

Assume that every person is potentially infected or colonized with an organism that could be transmitted in the health care setting, and apply the following infection control practices during the delivery of health care.

Hand Hygiene

- During the delivery of health care, avoid unnecessary touching of surfaces in close proximity to the patient to prevent both contamination of clean hands from environmental surfaces and transmission of pathogens from contaminated hands to surfaces.
- When hands are visibly dirty, contaminated with proteinaceous material, or visibly soiled with blood or body fluids, wash hands with either a nonantimicrobial soap and water or an antimicrobial soap and water.
- If hands are not visibly soiled, or after removing visible material with nonantimicrobial soap and water, decontaminate hands in the clinical situations described later. The preferred method of hand decontamination is with an alcohol-based hand rub. Alternatively, hands may be washed with an antimicrobial soap and water. Frequent use of alcohol-based hand rub immediately following hand washing with nonantimicrobial soap may increase the frequency of dermatitis. Perform hand hygiene
  - Before having direct contact with patients
  - After contact with blood, body fluids or excretions, mucous membranes, nonintact skin, or wound dressings
  - After contact with a patient's intact skin (e.g., when taking a pulse or blood pressure or lifting a patient)
  - If hands will be moving from a contaminated body site to a clean body site during patient care
  - After contact with inanimate objects (including medical equipment) in the immediate vicinity of the patient
  - After removing gloves
- Wash hands with nonantimicrobial soap and water or with antimicrobial soap and water if contact with spores (e.g., *Clostridium difficile* or *Bacillus anthracis*) is likely to have occurred. The physical action of washing and rinsing hands under such circumstances is recommended because alcohols, chlorhexidine, iodophors, and other antiseptic agents have poor activity against spores.
- Do not wear artificial fingernails or extenders if duties include direct contact with patients at high risk for infection and associated adverse outcomes (e.g., those in ICUs or operating rooms).
  - Develop an organizational policy on the wearing of nonnatural nails by health care personnel who have direct contact with patients outside of the groups specified in the preceding text.

Personal Protective Equipment (PPE)

- Observe the following principles of use:
  - Wear PPE (gloves, gown, mouth/nose/eye protection) when the nature of the anticipated patient interaction indicates that contact with blood or body fluids may occur.
  - Prevent contamination of clothing and skin during the process of removing PPE.

  - Before leaving the patient's room or cubicle, remove and discard PPE.
- **Gloves**
  - Wear gloves when it can be reasonably anticipated that contact with blood or other potentially infectious materials, mucous membranes, nonintact skin, or potentially contaminated intact skin (e.g., of a patient incontinent of stool or urine) could occur.
  - Wear gloves with fit and durability appropriate to the task.
    - Wear disposable medical examination gloves for providing direct patient care.
    - Wear disposable medical examination gloves or reusable utility gloves for cleaning the environment or medical equipment.
  - Remove gloves after contact with a patient and/or the surrounding environment (including medical equipment) using proper technique to prevent hand contamination. Do not wear the same pair of gloves for the care of more than one patient. Do not wash gloves for the purpose of reuse since this practice has been associated with transmission of pathogens.
  - Change gloves during patient care if the hands will move from a contaminated body site (e.g., perineal area) to a clean body site (e.g., face).
- **Gowns**
  - Wear a gown that is appropriate to the task, to protect skin and prevent soiling or contamination of clothing during procedures and patient care activities when contact with blood, body fluids, secretions, or excretions is anticipated.
    - Wear a gown for direct patient contact if the patient has uncontained secretions or excretions.
    - Remove gown and perform hand hygiene before leaving the patient's environment.
  - Do not reuse gowns, even for repeated contacts with the same patient.
  - Routine donning of gowns upon entrance into a high-risk unit (e.g., ICU, NICU, or HSCT unit) is not indicated.
- **Mouth, nose, eye protection**
  - Use PPE to protect the mucous membranes of the eyes, nose, and mouth during procedures and patient care activities that are likely to generate splashes or sprays of blood, body fluids, secretions, and excretions. Select masks, goggles, face shields, and combinations of each according to the need anticipated by the task performed.
  - During aerosol-generating procedures (e.g., bronchoscopy, suctioning of the respiratory tract [if not using in-line suction catheters], endotracheal intubation) in patients who are not suspected of being infected with an agent for which respiratory protection is otherwise recommended (e.g., *Mycobacterium tuberculosis*, SARS‡, or hemorrhagic fever viruses), wear one of the following: a face shield that fully covers the front and sides of the face, a mask with attached shield, or a mask and goggles (in addition to gloves and gown).

*CDC: Center for Disease Control and Prevention
†HICPAC: Healthcare Infection Control Practices Advisory Committee.
‡SARS: Severe Acute Respiratory Syndrome

continued

DISPLAY 3-1   CDC and HICPAC Isolation Precaution Guidelines *Continued*

- **Respiratory hygiene/cough etiquette**
  - Educate health care personnel on the importance of source control measures to contain respiratory secretions to prevent droplet and fomite transmission of respiratory pathogens, especially during seasonal outbreaks of viral respiratory tract infections (e.g., influenza, RSV[§], adenovirus, parainfluenza virus) in communities.
  - Implement the following measures to contain respiratory secretions in patients and accompanying individuals who have signs and symptoms of a respiratory infection, beginning at the point of initial encounter in a health care setting (e.g., triage, reception and waiting areas in emergency departments, outpatient clinics, and physician offices).
    - Post signs at entrances and in strategic places (e.g., elevators, cafeterias) within ambulatory and inpatient settings with instructions to patients and other persons with symptoms of a respiratory infection to cover their mouths/noses when coughing or sneezing, to use and dispose of tissues, and to perform hand hygiene after hands have been in contact with respiratory secretions.
    - Provide tissues and no-touch receptacles (e.g., pedal-operated lid or open, plastic-lined waste basket) for disposal of tissues.
    - Provide resources and instructions for performing hand hygiene in or near waiting areas in ambulatory and inpatient settings; provide conveniently located dispensers of alcohol-based hand rubs and, where sinks are available, supplies for hand washing.
    - During periods of increased prevalence of respiratory infections in the community (e.g., as indicated by increased school absenteeism or increased number of patients seeking care for a respiratory infection), offer masks to coughing patients and other symptomatic persons (e.g., persons who accompany ill patients) upon entry into the facility or medical office and encourage them to maintain special separation, ideally a distance of at least 3 ft., from others in common waiting areas. Some facilities may find it logistically easier to institute this recommendation year-round as a standard of practice.
- **Patient placement**
  - Include the potential for transmission of infectious agents in patient placement decisions. Place patients who pose a risk for transmission to others (e.g., uncontained secretions, excretions, or wound drainage; infants with suspected viral respiratory or gastrointestinal infections) in a single-patient room when available.
  - Determine patient placement based on the following principles:
    - Route(s) of transmission of the known or suspected infectious agent
    - Risk factors for transmission in the infected patient
    - Risk factors for adverse outcomes resulting from an HAI[§§] in other patients in the area or room being considered for patient placement
    - Availability of single-patient rooms

    - Patient options for room sharing (e.g., cohorting patients with the same infection)
- **Patient care equipment and instruments/devices**
  - Establish policies and procedures for containing, transporting, and handling patient care equipment and instruments/devices that may be contaminated with blood or body fluids.
  - Remove organic material from critical and semicritical instrument/devices using recommended cleaning agents before high-level disinfection and sterilization to enable effective disinfection and sterilization processes.
  - Wear PPE (e.g., gloves, gown), according to the level of anticipated contamination, when handling patient care equipment and instruments/devices that are visibly soiled or may have been in contact with blood or body fluids.
- **Care of the environment**
  - Establish policies and procedures for routine and targeted cleaning of environmental surfaces as indicated by the level of patient contact and degree of soiling.
  - Clean and disinfect surfaces that are likely to be contaminated with pathogens, including those that are in close proximity to the patient (e.g., bed rails, overbed tables) and frequently touched surfaces in the patient care environment (e.g., door knobs, surfaces in and surrounding toilets in patients' rooms), on a more frequent schedule compared to that for other surfaces (e.g., horizontal surfaces in waiting rooms).
  - Use EPA-registered disinfectants that have microbiocidal (i.e., killing) activity against the pathogens most likely to contaminate the patient care environment, in accordance with the manufacturer's instructions.
    - Review the efficacy of in-use disinfectants when evidence of continuing transmission of an infectious agent (e.g., rotavirus, *C. difficile*, norovirus) may indicate resistance to the in-use product and change to a more effective disinfectant as indicated.
  - In facilities that provide health care to pediatric patients or have waiting areas with child's play toys (e.g., obstetric/gynecology offices and clinics), establish policies and procedures for cleaning and disinfecting toys at regular intervals. Use the following principles in developing this policy and procedures:
    - Select toys that can be easily cleaned and disinfected
    - Do not permit use of stuffed furry toys if they will be shared
    - Clean and disinfect large stationary toys (e.g., climbing equipment) at least weekly and whenever visibly soiled
    - If toys are likely to be mouthed, rinse with water after disinfection; alternatively, wash in a dishwasher
    - When a toy requires cleaning and disinfection, do so immediately or store in a designated labeled container separate from toys that are clean and ready for use
  - Include multiuse electronic equipment in policies and procedures for preventing contamination and for cleaning and disinfecting, especially those items that are used by patients, those used during delivery of patient care, and mobile devices that are moved in and out of patient rooms frequently (e.g., daily).

[§]RSV: Respiratory Syncytial Virus

[§§]HAI: Healthcare Associated Infections

continued on page 32

DISPLAY 3-1   **CDC and HICPAC Isolation Precaution Guidelines** *Continued*

- No recommendation for use of removable protective covers or washable keyboards. *Unresolved issue*
- **Textiles and laundry**
  - Handle used textiles and fabrics with minimum agitation to avoid contamination of air, surfaces, and persons.
  - If laundry chutes are used, ensure that they are properly designed, maintained, and used in a manner to minimize dispersion of aerosols from contaminated laundry.
- **Safe injection practices**
  The following recommendations apply to the use of needles, cannulas that replace needles, and, where applicable, intravenous delivery systems.
  - Use aseptic technique to avoid contamination of sterile injection equipment.
  - Do not administer medications from a syringe to multiple patients, even if the needle or cannula on the syringe is changed. Needles, cannulas, and syringes are sterile, single-use items; they should not be reused for another patient or used to access a medication or solution that might be intended for a subsequent patient.
  - Use fluid infusion and administration sets (i.e., intravenous bags, tubing, and connectors) for one patient only, and dispose appropriately after use. Consider a syringe or needle/cannula contaminated once it has been used to enter or connect to a patient's intravenous infusion bag or administration set.

- Use single-dose vials for parenteral medications whenever possible.
- Do not administer medications from single-dose vials or ampules to multiple patients or combine leftover contents for later use.
- If multidose vials must be used, both the needle or cannula and syringe used to access the multidose vial must be sterile.
- Do not keep multidose vials in the immediate patient treatment area and store in accordance with the manufacturer's recommendations; discard if sterility is compromised or questionable.
- Do not use bags or bottles of intravenous solution as a common source of supply for multiple patients.
- **Infection control practices for special lumbar puncture procedures**
  Wear a surgical mask when placing a catheter or injecting material into the spinal canal or subdural space (i.e., during myelograms, lumbar puncture, and spinal or epidural anesthesia).
- **Worker safety**
  Adhere to federal and state requirements for protection of health care personnel from exposure to bloodborne pathogens.

(From CDC and HICPAC. (2007). *Guidelines for isolation precautions: Preventing transmission of infectious agents in healthcare settings 2007. Part III.A. Standard precautions.* Atlanta: CDC.)

DISPLAY 3-2   **Positioning the Client**

Sitting Position

The client should sit upright on the side of the examination table. In the home or office setting, the client can sit on the edge of a chair or bed. This position is good for evaluating the head, neck, lungs, chest, back, breasts, axillae, heart, vital signs, and upper extremities. This position is also useful because it permits full expansion of the lungs and it allows the examiner to assess symmetry of upper body parts. Some clients may be too weak to sit up for the entire examination. They may need to lie down (supine position) and rest throughout the examination. Other clients may be unable to tolerate the position for any length of time. An alternative position is for the client to lie down with his or her head elevated.

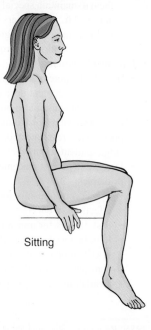

Sitting

continued

| DISPLAY 3-2 | **Positioning the Client** *Continued* |

Supine Position

Ask the client to lie down with the legs together on the examination table (or bed if in a home setting). A small pillow may be placed under the head to promote comfort. If the client has trouble breathing, the head of the bed may need to be raised. This position allows the abdominal muscles to relax and provides easy access to peripheral pulse sites. Areas assessed with the client in this position may include head, neck, chest, breasts, axillae, abdomen, heart, lungs, and all extremities.

Dorsal Recumbent Position

The client lies down on the examination table or bed with the knees bent, the legs separated, and the feet flat on the table or bed. This position may be more comfortable than the supine position for clients with pain in the back or abdomen. Areas that may be assessed with the client in this position include head, neck, chest, axillae, lungs, heart, extremities, breasts, and peripheral pulses. The abdomen should not be assessed because the abdominal muscles are contracted in this position.

SIMS' Position

The client lies on his or her right or left side with the lower arm placed behind the body and the upper arm flexed at the shoulder and elbow. The lower leg is slightly flexed at the knee while the upper leg is flexed at a sharper angle and pulled forward. This position is useful for assessing the rectal and vaginal areas. The client may need some assistance getting into this position. Clients with joint problems and elderly clients may have some difficulty assuming and maintaining this position.

Standing Position

The client stands still in a normal, comfortable, resting posture. This position allows the examiner to assess posture, balance, and gait. This position is also used for examining the male genitalia.

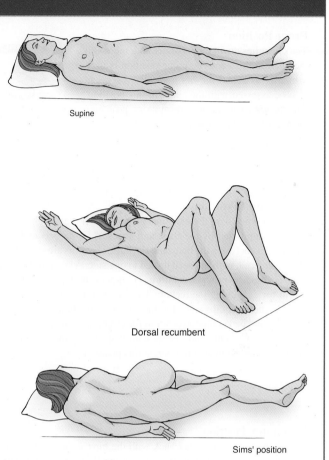

Supine

Dorsal recumbent

Sims' position

Standing

continued on page 34

DISPLAY 3-2	Positioning the Client *Continued*

Prone Position

The client lies down on his or her abdomen with the head to the side. The prone position is used primarily to assess the hip joint. The back can also be assessed with the client in this position. Clients with cardiac and respiratory problems cannot tolerate this position.

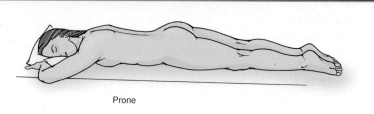

Prone

Knee–Chest Position

The client kneels on the examination table with the weight of the body supported by the chest and knees. A 90-degree angle should exist between the body and the hips. The arms are placed above the head, with the head turned to one side. A small pillow may be used to provide comfort. The knee–chest position is useful for examining the rectum. This position may be embarrassing and uncomfortable for the client, and, therefore, the client should be kept in the position for as limited a time as possible. Elderly clients and clients with respiratory and cardiac problems may be unable to tolerate this position.

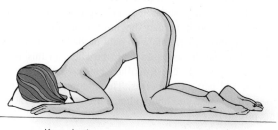

Knee-chest

Lithotomy Position

The client lies on his or her back with the hips at the edge of the examination table and the feet supported by stirrups. The lithotomy position is used to examine the female genitalia, reproductive tracts, and the rectum. The client may require assistance getting into this position. It is an exposed position, and clients may feel embarrassed. In addition, elderly clients may not be able to assume this position for very long or at all. Therefore, it is best to keep the client well draped during the examination and to perform the examination as quickly as possible.

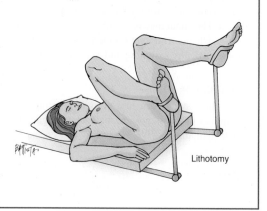

Lithotomy

DISPLAY 3-3	General Considerations for Examining Older Adults

- Some positions may be very difficult or impossible for the older client to assume or maintain because of decreased joint mobility and flexibility (see Display 3-2). Therefore, try to perform the examination in a manner that minimizes position changes.
- It is a good idea to allow rest periods for the older adult, if needed.

- Some older clients may process information at a slower rate. Therefore, explain the procedure and integrate teaching in a clear and slow manner.
- See Chapter 32 for physical examination of the frail elderly client.

PHYSICAL EXAMINATION TECHNIQUES

Four basic techniques must be mastered before you can perform a thorough and complete assessment of the client. These techniques are *inspection, palpation, percussion*, and *auscultation*. This chapter provides descriptions of each technique along with guidelines on how to perform the basic technique. Using each technique for assessing specific body systems is described in the appropriate chapter. After performing each of the four assessment techniques, the examiner should ask herself questions that will facilitate analysis of the data and determine areas in which more data may be needed. These questions include

- Did I inspect, palpate, percuss, or auscultate any deviations from the normal findings? (Normal findings are listed in the second column of the Physical Assessment sections in the body systems chapters.)
- If there is a deviation, is it a normal physical, gerontologic, or cultural finding; an abnormal adult finding; or an abnormal physical, gerontologic, or cultural finding? (Normal gerontologic and cultural findings are in the second column of the Physical Assessment sections in the body systems chapters. Abnormal adult, gerontologic, and cultural findings can be found in the third column of the Physical Assessment sections.)
- Based on my findings, do I need to ask the client more questions to validate or obtain more information about my inspection, palpation, percussion, or auscultation findings?
- Based on my observations and data, do I need to focus my physical assessment on other related body systems?
- Should I validate my inspection, palpation, percussion, or auscultation findings with my instructor or another practitioner?
- Should I refer the client and data findings to a primary care provider?

These questions help ensure that data is complete and accurate and facilitate analysis.

Inspection

Inspection involves using the senses of vision, smell, and hearing to observe and detect any normal or abnormal findings. This technique is used from the moment that you meet the client and continues throughout the examination. Inspection precedes palpation, percussion, and auscultation because the latter techniques can potentially alter the appearance of what is being inspected. Although most of the inspection involves the use of the senses only, a few body systems require the use of special equipment (e.g., ophthalmoscope for the eye inspection, otoscope for the ear inspection).

Use the following guidelines as you practice the technique of inspection:

- Make sure the room is a comfortable temperature. A too-cold or too-hot room can alter the normal behavior of the client and the appearance of the client's skin.
- Use good lighting, preferably sunlight. Fluorescent lights can alter the true color of the skin. In addition, abnormalities may be overlooked with dim lighting.
- Look and observe before touching. Touch can alter appearance and distract you from a complete, focused observation.
- Completely expose the body part you are inspecting while draping the rest of the client as appropriate.

Table 3-2	Parts of Hand to Use When Palpating	
Hand Part	**Sensitive To**	
Fingerpads	Fine discriminations: pulses, texture, size, consistency, shape, crepitus	
Ulnar or palmar surface	Vibrations, thrills, fremitus	
Dorsal (back) surface	Temperature	

- Note the following characteristics while inspecting the client: color, patterns, size, location, consistency, symmetry, movement, behavior, odors, or sounds.
- Compare the appearance of symmetric body parts (e.g., eyes, ears, arms, hands) or both sides of any individual body part.

Palpation

Palpation consists of using parts of the hand to touch and feel for the following characteristics: *texture* (rough/smooth), *temperature* (warm/cold), *moisture* (dry/wet), *mobility* (fixed/movable/still/vibrating), *consistency* (soft/hard/fluid filled), *strength of pulses* (strong/weak/thready/bounding), *size* (small/medium/large), *shape* (well defined/irregular), and *degree of tenderness*.

Three different parts of the hand—the fingerpads, ulnar/palmar surface, and dorsal surface—are used during palpation. Each part of the hand is particularly sensitive to certain characteristics. Determine which characteristic you are trying to palpate and refer to Table 3-2 to find which part of the hand is best to use. Several types of palpation can be used to perform an assessment; they include light, moderate, deep, or bimanual palpation. The depth of the structure being palpated and the thickness of the tissue overlying that structure determine whether you should use light, moderate, or deep palpation. Bimanual palpation is the use of both hands to hold and feel a body structure.

In general, the examiner's fingernails should be short and the hands should be a comfortable temperature. Standard precautions should be followed if applicable. Proceed from light palpation, which is safest and the most comfortable for the client, to moderate palpation and finally to deep palpation. Specific instructions on how to perform the four types of palpation follow:

- *Light palpation:* To perform light palpation (Fig. 3-1), place your dominant hand lightly on the surface of the structure.

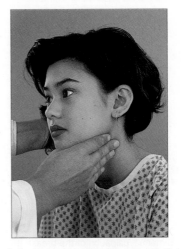

Figure 3-1 Light palpation. (Photo by B. Proud.)

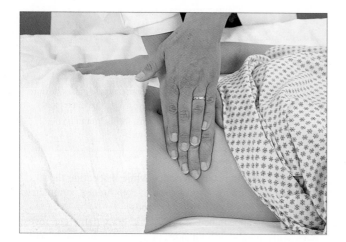

Figure 3-2 Deep palpation. (Photo by B. Proud.)

There should be very little or no depression (less than 1 cm). Feel the surface structure using a circular motion. Use this technique to feel for pulses, tenderness, surface skin texture, temperature, and moisture.

* *Moderate palpation:* Depress the skin surface 1 to 2 cm (0.5 to 0.75 inch) with your dominant hand, and use a circular motion to feel for easily palpable body organs and masses. Note the size, consistency, and mobility of structures you palpate.
* *Deep palpation:* Place your dominant hand on the skin surface and your nondominant hand on top of your dominant hand to apply pressure (Fig. 3-2). This should result in a surface depression between 2.5 and 5 cm (1 and 2 inches). This allows you to feel very deep organs or structures that are covered by thick muscle.
* *Bimanual palpation:* Use two hands, placing one on each side of the body part (e.g., uterus, breasts, spleen) being palpated (Fig. 3-3). Use one hand to apply pressure and the other hand to feel the structure. Note the size, shape, consistency, and mobility of the structures you palpate.

Percussion

Percussion involves tapping body parts to produce sound waves. These sound waves or vibrations enable the examiner to assess underlying structures. Percussion has several different assessment uses, including

* *Eliciting pain:* Percussion helps to detect inflamed underlying structures. If an inflamed area is percussed, the client's response may indicate or the client will report that the area feels tender, sore, or painful.
* *Determining location, size, and shape:* Percussion note changes between borders of an organ and its neighboring organ can elicit information about location, size, and shape.
* *Determining density:* Percussion helps to determine whether an underlying structure is filled with air or fluid or is a solid structure.
* *Detecting abnormal masses:* Percussion can detect superficial abnormal structures or masses. Percussion vibrations penetrate approximately 5 cm deep. Deep masses do not produce any change in the normal percussion vibrations.
* *Eliciting reflexes:* Deep tendon reflexes are elicited using the percussion hammer.

The three types of percussion are *direct, blunt,* and *indirect.* Direct percussion (Fig. 3-4) is the direct tapping of a body part with one or two fingertips to elicit possible tenderness (e.g., tenderness over the sinuses). Blunt percussion (Fig. 3-5) is used to detect tenderness over organs (e.g., kidneys) by placing one hand flat on the body surface and using the fist of the other hand to strike the back of the hand flat on the body surface. Indirect or mediate percussion (Fig. 3-6) is the most commonly used method of percussion. The tapping done with this type of percussion produces a sound or tone that varies

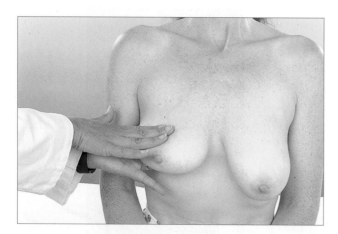

Figure 3-3 Bimanual palpation of the breast. (Photo by B. Proud.)

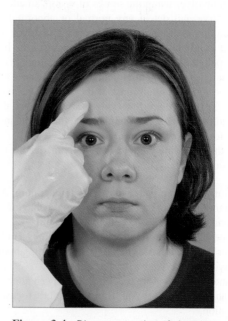

Figure 3-4 Direct percussion of sinuses.

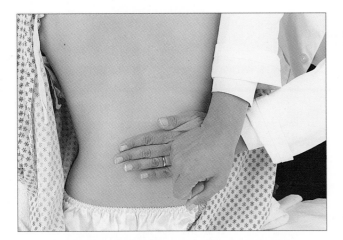

Figure 3-5 Blunt percussion of kidneys. (Photo by B. Proud.)

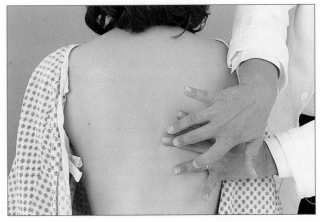

Figure 3-6 Indirect or mediate percussion of lungs. (Photo by B. Proud.)

with the density of underlying structures. As density increases, the sound of the tone becomes quieter. Solid tissue produces a soft tone, fluid produces a louder tone, and air produces an even louder tone. These tones are referred to as percussion notes and are classified according to origin, quality, intensity, and pitch (Table 3-3).

The following techniques help to develop proficiency in the technique of indirect percussion:

- Place the middle finger of your nondominant hand on the body part you are going to percuss.
- Keep your other fingers off the body part being percussed because they will damp the tone you elicit.
- Use the pad of your middle finger of the other hand (ensure that this fingernail is short) to strike the middle finger of your nondominant hand that is placed on the body part.
- Withdraw your finger immediately to avoid damping the tone.
- Deliver two quick taps and listen carefully to the tone.
- Use quick, sharp taps by quickly flexing your wrist, not your forearm.

Practice percussing by tapping your thigh to elicit a flat tone and your puffed-out cheek to elicit a tympanic tone. A good way to detect changes in tone is to fill a carton halfway with fluid and practice percussing on it. The tone will change from resonance over air to a duller tone over the fluid.

Auscultation

Auscultation is a type of assessment technique that requires the use of a stethoscope to listen for heart sounds, movement of blood through the cardiovascular system, movement of the bowel, and movement of air through the respiratory tract. A stethoscope is used because these body sounds are not audible to the human ear. The sounds detected using auscultation are classified according to the intensity (loud or soft), pitch (high or low), duration (length), and quality (musical, crackling, raspy) of the sound (see Equipment Spotlight 3–1).

The following guidelines should be followed as you practice the technique of auscultation:

- Eliminate distracting or competing noises from the environment (e.g., radio, television, machinery).
- Expose the body part you are going to auscultate. Do not auscultate through the client's clothing or gown. Rubbing against the clothing obscures the body sounds.
- Use the diaphragm of the stethoscope to listen for high-pitched sounds, such as normal heart sounds, breath sounds, and bowel sounds, and press the diaphragm firmly on the body part being auscultated.
- Use the bell of the stethoscope to listen for low-pitched sounds such as abnormal heart sounds and bruits (abnormal loud, blowing, or murmuring sounds heard during auscultation). Hold the bell lightly on the body part being auscultated.

Table 3-3 Sounds (Tones) Elicited by Percussion

Sound	Intensity	Pitch	Length	Quality	Example of Origin
Resonance (heard over part air and part solid)	Loud	Low	Long	Hollow	Normal lung
Hyper-resonance (heard over mostly air)	Very loud	Low	Long	Booming	Lung with emphysema
Tympany (heard over air)	Loud	High	Moderate	Drumlike	Puffed-out cheek, gastric bubble
Dullness (heard over more solid tissue)	Medium	Medium	Moderate	Thudlike	Diaphragm, pleural effusion, liver
Flatness (heard over very dense tissue)	Soft	High	Short	Flat	Muscle, bone, sternum, thigh

EQUIPMENT SPOTLIGHT 3–1   How to Use the Stethoscope

The stethoscope is used to listen for (auscultate) body sounds that cannot ordinarily be heard without amplification (eg, lung sounds, bruits, bowel sounds, and so forth). To use a stethoscope, follow these guidelines:

1. Place the earpieces into the outer ear canal. They should fit snugly but comfortably to promote effective sound transmission. The earpieces are connected to binaurals (metal tubing), which connect to rubber or plastic tubing. The rubber or plastic tubing should be flexible and no more than 12 inches long to prevent the sound from diminishing.
2. Angle the binaurals down toward your nose. This will ensure that sounds are transmitted to your eardrums.
3. Use the diaphragm of the stethoscope to detect high-pitched sounds. The diaphragm should be at least 1.5 inches wide for adults and smaller for children. Hold the diaphragm firmly against the body part being auscultated.
4. Use the bell of the stethoscope to detect low-pitched sounds. The bell should be at least 1 inch wide. Hold the bell lightly against the body part being auscultated.

Some Do's and Don'ts

• Warm the diaphragm or bell of the stethoscope before placing it on the client's skin.
• Explain what you are listening for and answer any questions the client has. This will help to alleviate anxiety.
• Do not apply too much pressure when using the bell—too much pressure will cause the bell to work like the diaphragm.
• Avoid listening through clothing, which may obscure or alter sounds.

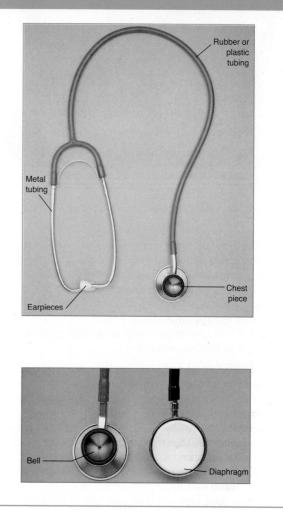

SUMMARY

Collecting objective data is essential for a complete nursing assessment. The nurse must have knowledge of and skill in three basic areas to become proficient in collecting objective data: necessary equipment and how to use it; preparing the setting, oneself, and the client for the examination; and how to perform the four basic assessment techniques. Collecting objective data requires a great deal of practice to become proficient. Proficiency is needed because how the data are collected can affect the accuracy of the information elicited.

References and Selected Readings

Anderson, I. (2007). Use of Doppler ultrasound in assessing big ulcers. *Nursing Standards, 21*(47), 50–56, 58.

Askin, D. F. (2007a). Physical assessment of the newborn. Part 1 of 2: Preparation through auscultation. *Nursing for Women's Health, 11*(3), 292–303.

Askin, D. F. (2007b). Physical assessment of the newborn. Part 2 of 2: Inspection through palpation. *Nursing for Women's Health, 11*(3), 304–315.

Centers for Disease Control and Prevention (CDC) and the Hospital Infection Control Practices Advisory Committee (HICPAC). (2007). *Guidelines for isolation precautions: Preventing transmission of infection agents in healthcare settings 2007. Part III. A. Standard precautions.* Atlanta: CDC.

Coombs, M. A., & Moorse, S. E. (2002). Physical assessment skills: A developing dimension of clinical nursing practice. *Intensive and Critical Care Nursing, 18,* 200–210.

Ferns, T. (2007). Respiratory auscultation: How to use a stethoscope. *Nursing Times, 103*(24), 28–29.

Fleury, J., & Keller, C. (2000). Assessment. Cardiovascular risk assessment in elderly individuals. *Journal of Gerontological Nursing, 26*(5), 30–37.

Gaskin, P. R. A., Owens, S. E., Tainer, N. S., Sanders, S. P., & Li, J. S. (2000). Clinical auscultation skills in pediatric residents. *Pediatrics, 105*(6), 1184–1186.

Jevon, P., & Cunnington, A. (2007a). Cardiovascular examination. Part one of the four part series: Measuring jugular venous pressure. *Nursing Times, 103*(25), 28–29.

Jevon, P., & Cunnington, A. (2007b). Cardiovascular examination: Part two: Inspection and palpation of the precordium. *Nursing Times, 103*(26), 26–27.

Jevon, P., & Cunnington, A. (2007c). Cardiovascular examination. Part three: Auscultation of the heart. *Nursing Times, 103*(27), 24–25.

Jevon, P., & Cunnington, A. (2007d). Cardiovascular examination. Part four: Auscultation of the heart. *Nursing Times, 103*(28), 26–27.

Mangione, S. (2000). *Physical diagnosis secrets.* Philadelphia: Hanley and Belfus Inc.

O'Keefe, M. (2001). Revitalizing the art of auscultation. *Journal of Emergency Medical Services, 26*(5), 79–80.

Schiff, L. (2000). Stethoscopes. *RN, 63*(7), 63–64.

Schindler, D. M. (2007). Practical cardiac auscultation. *Critical Care Nursing Quarterly, 30*(2), 166–180.

Smith, G. R. (2000). Devices for measuring blood pressure. *Professional Nurse, 15*(5), 337–340.

4

Validating and Documenting Data

Although validation and documentation of data often occur concurrently with collection of subjective and objective assessment data, looking at each step separately can help to emphasize each step's importance in nursing assessment.

VALIDATING DATA

Purpose of Validation

Validation of data is the process of confirming or verifying that the subjective and objective data you have collected are reliable and accurate. The steps of validation include deciding whether the data require validation, determining ways to validate the data, and identifying areas where data are missing. Failure to validate data may result in premature closure of the assessment or collection of inaccurate data. Errors during assessment cause judgments to be made on unreliable data, which result in diagnostic errors during the second part of the nursing process—analysis of data (determining nursing diagnoses). Thus validation of the data collected during assessment of the client is crucial to the first step of the nursing process.

Data Requiring Validation

Not every piece of data you collect must be verified. For example, you would not need to verify or repeat the client's pulse, temperature, or blood pressure unless certain conditions exist. Conditions that require data to be rechecked and validated include

- Discrepancies or gaps between the subjective and objective data. For example, a male client tells you that he is very happy despite learning that he has terminal cancer.
- Discrepancies or gaps between what the client says at one time then at another time. For example, your female patient says she has never had surgery but later in the interview she mentions that her appendix was removed at a military hospital when she was in the Navy.
- Findings that are very abnormal and/or inconsistent with other findings. For example, the following are inconsistent

with each other: the client has a temperature of 104°F, is resting comfortably, and her skin is warm to the touch and not flushed.

Methods of Validation

There are several ways to validate your data:

- Recheck your own data through a repeat assessment. For example, take the client's temperature again with a different thermometer.
- Clarify data with the client by asking additional questions. For example, if a client is holding his abdomen the nurse may assume he is having abdominal pain, when actually the client is very upset about his diagnosis and is feeling nauseated.
- Verify the data with another health care professional. For example, ask a more experienced nurse to listen to the abnormal heart sounds you think you have just heard.
- Compare your objective findings with your subjective findings to uncover discrepancies. For example, if the client states that she "never gets any time in the sun," yet has dark, wrinkled, suntanned skin, you need to validate the client's perception of never getting any time in the sun.

Identification of Areas Where Data Are Missing

Once you establish an initial database, you can identify areas where more data are needed. You may have overlooked certain questions. In addition, as data are examined in a grouped format, you may realize that additional information is needed. For example, if an adult client weighs only 98 lb, you would explore further to see if the client recently lost weight or this has been the usual weight for an extended time. If a client tells you he lives alone, you may need to identify the existence of a support system, his or her degree of social involvement with others, and his ability to function independently.

DOCUMENTING DATA

In addition to validation, documentation of assessment data is another crucial part of the first step in the nursing process. The significance of this aspect of assessment is addressed specifically by various state nurse practice acts, accreditation and/or reimbursement agencies (e.g., The Joint Commission on Accreditation of Healthcare Organizations [JCAHO], Medicare, Medicaid), professional organizations (local, state, and national), and institutional agencies (acute, transitional, long-term, and home care). JCAHO, for example, has specific standards that address documentation for assessments.

Health care institutions have developed assessment and documentation policies and procedures that provide not only the criteria for documenting but also assistance in completing the forms. The categories of information on the forms are designed to ensure that the nurse gathers pertinent information needed to meet the standards and guidelines of the specific institutions mentioned previously and to develop a plan of care for the client.

Purpose of Documentation

The primary reason for documenting the initial assessment is to provide the health care team with a database that becomes the foundation for care of the client. It helps to identify health problems, formulate nursing diagnoses, and plan immediate and ongoing interventions. If the nursing diagnosis is made without supporting assessment data, incorrect conclusions and interventions may result.

The initial and ongoing assessment documentation database also establishes a way to communicate with the multidisciplinary team members. With the advent of computer-based documentation systems, this database can link to other documents and health care departments, eliminating repetition of similar data collection by other health team members. Display 4-1 describes the many other purposes that assessment documentation serves.

Nurses use comprehensive and systematic nursing databases that streamline data collection and organization yet maintain a concise record that satisfies legal standards.

Information Requiring Documentation

Every institution is unique when it comes to documenting assessments. However, two key elements need to be included in every documentation: nursing history and physical assessment, also known as subjective and objective data. Most data collection starts with subjective data and ends with objective data.

As discussed in previous chapters, subjective data consist of the information that the client or significant others tell the nurse, and objective data are what the nurse observes through inspection, palpation, percussion, or auscultation. It is important to remember to document only what the client tells you and what you observe—not what you interpret or infer from the data. Interpretation or inference is performed during the analysis phase of the nursing process (see Chapter 5).

Subjective Data

Subjective data typically consist of biographic data, current health concern(s) and symptoms (or the client's chief complaint), past health history, family history, and lifestyle and health practices information:

- Biographic data typically consist of the client's name, age, occupation, ethnicity, and support systems or resources.
- The present health concern review is recorded in statements that reflect the client's current symptoms. Statements should begin, "Client (or significant other) states. . . ." Describe items as accurately and descriptively as possible. For example, if a client complains of difficult breathing, report how the client describes the problem, when the problem started, what started it, how long it occurred, and what makes the breathing better or worse. Use a memory tool, such as COLDSPA described in Chapter 2, to further explore every symptom reported by the client. This information provides the health care team members with details that help in diagnosis and clinical problem solving. Sometimes you may need to record the absence of specific signs and symptoms (e.g., no vomiting, diarrhea, or constipation).

DISPLAY 4-1	Purposes of Assessment Documentation

- Provides a chronologic source of client assessment data and a progressive record of assessment findings that outline the client's course of care.
- Ensures that information about the client and family is easily accessible to members of the health care team; provides a vehicle for communication; and prevents fragmentation, repetition, and delays in carrying out the plan of care.
- Establishes a basis for screening or validating proposed diagnoses.
- Acts as a source of information to help diagnose new problems.
- Offers a basis for determining the educational needs of the client, family, and significant others.

- Provides a basis for determining eligibility for care and reimbursement. Careful recording of data can support financial reimbursement or gain additional reimbursement for transitional or skilled care needed by the client.
- Constitutes a permanent legal record of the care that was or was not given to the client.
- Forms a component of client acuity system or client classification systems (Eggland & Heinemann, 1994). Numeric values may be assigned to various levels of care to help determine the staffing mix for the unit.
- Provides access to significant epidemiologic data for future investigations and research and educational endeavors.
- Promotes compliance with legal, accreditation, reimbursement, and professional standard requirements.

- Past health history data tell the nurse about events that happened before the client's admission to the health care facility or the current encounter with the client. The data may be about previous hospitalizations, surgeries, treatment programs, acute illness, chronic illnesses, and injuries. Be sure to include all pertinent information, e.g., dates of hospitalization. Also be sure to include all data, even negative history (e.g., "client denies prior surgeries.")
- Family history data include information about the client's biologic family (e.g., family history of diseases or behaviors that may be genetic or familial). A genogram may be helpful in recording family history (see Chapter 2).
- Lifestyle and health practices information typically details risk behaviors such as past or present smoking; alcohol use; medication (prescribed, over-the-counter, or illicit) use; environmental factors that may affect health; social and psychological factors that may affect the client's health; client and family health education needs; family and other relationships; and treatment and disease data. Be sure to be comprehensive, yet succinct.

Objective Data

After you complete the nursing history, the physical examination begins. This examination includes inspection, palpation, percussion, and auscultation. These data help to further define the client's problems, establish baseline data for ongoing assessments, and validate the subjective data obtained during the nursing history interview. A variety of systematic approaches may be used: namely, head-to-toe, major body systems, functional health patterns, or human response patterns.

No matter which approach is used, general rules apply:

- Make notes as you perform the assessments, and document as concisely as possible.
- Avoid documenting general non-descriptive or non-measurable terms such as normal, abnormal, good, fair, satisfactory, or poor.
- Instead, use specific descriptive and measurable terms (i.e., 3 inches in diameter, red excoriated edges, with purulent yellow drainage) about what you inspected, palpated, percussed, and auscultated.

Guidelines for Documentation

The way that the nursing assessments are recorded varies among practice settings. However, several general guidelines apply to all settings. They include

- *Document legibly or print neatly in nonerasable ink.* Errors in documentation are usually corrected by drawing one line through the entry, writing "error," and initialing the entry. Never obliterate the error with white paint or tape, an eraser, or a marking pen. Keep in mind that the health record is a legal document.
- *Use correct grammar and spelling.* **Use only abbreviations that are acceptable and approved by the institution.** Avoid slang, jargon, or labels unless they are direct quotes.
- *Avoid wordiness that creates redundancy.* For example, do not record: "Auscultated gurgly bowel sounds in right upper, right lower, left upper, and left lower abdominal quadrants. Heard 36 gurgles per minute." Instead record: "Bowel sounds present in all quadrants at 36/minute."
- *Use phrases instead of sentences to record data.* For example, avoid recording: "The client's lung sounds were clear both in the right and left lungs." Instead record: "Bilateral lung sounds clear."
- *Record data findings, not how they were obtained.* For example, do not record: "Client was interviewed for past history of high blood pressure, and blood pressure was taken." Instead record: "Has 3-year history of hypertension treated with medication. BP sitting right arm 140/86, left arm 136/86."
- *Write entries objectively without making premature judgments or diagnoses.* Use quotation marks to identify clearly the client's responses. For example, record: "Client crying in room, refuses to talk, husband has gone home" instead of "Client depressed due to fear of breast biopsy report and not getting along well with husband." Avoid making inferences and diagnostic statements until you have collected and validated all data with client and family.
- *Record the client's understanding and perception of problems.* For example, record: "Client expresses concern regarding being discharged soon after gallbladder surgery because of inability to rest at home with six children."
- *Avoid recording the word "normal" for normal findings.* For example, do not record: "Liver palpation normal." Instead record: "Liver span 10 cm in right MCL and 4 cm in MSL. No tenderness on palpation." In some health care settings, however, only abnormal findings are documented if the policy is to chart by exception only. In that case, no normal findings would be documented in any format.
- *Record complete information and details for all client symptoms or experiences.* For example, do not record: "Client has pain in lower back." Instead record: "Client reports aching-burning pain in lower back for 2 weeks. Pain worsens after standing for several hours. Rest and ibuprofen used to take edge off pain. No radiation of pain. Rates pain as 7 on scale of 1 to 10."
- *Include additional assessment content when applicable* (e.g., include information about the caregiver or last physician contact).
- *Support objective data with specific observations obtained during the physical examination.* For example, when describing the emotional status of the client as depressed, follow it with a description of the ways depression is demonstrated such as "dressed in dirty clothing, avoids eye contact, unkempt appearance, and slumped shoulders."

Assessment Forms Used for Documentation

Standardized assessment forms have been developed to ensure that content in documentation and assessment data meets regulatory requirements and provides a thorough database. The type of assessment form used for documentation varies according to the health care institution. In fact, a variety of assessment forms may even be used within an institution. Typically, however, three types of assessment forms are used to document data: an

---

DISPLAY 4-2 **Features of Types of Initial Assessment Documentation Forms**

Open-Ended Forms (Traditional form)
- Calls for narrative description of problem and listing of topics
- Provides lines for comments
- Individualizes information
- Provides "total picture," including specific complaints and symptoms in the client's own words
- Increases risk of failing to ask a pertinent question because questions are not standardized
- Requires a lot of time to complete the database

Cued or Checklist Forms
- Standardizes data collection
- Lists (categorizes) information that alerts the nurse to specific problems or symptoms assessed for each client (see Fig. 4-1)
- Usually includes a comment section after each category to allow for individualization
- Prevents missed questions
- Promotes easy, rapid documentation
- Makes documentation somewhat like data entry because it requires nurse to place checkmarks in boxes instead of writing narrative

- Poses chance that a significant piece of data may be missed because the checklist does not include the area of concern

Integrated Cued Checklist
- Combines assessment data with identified nursing diagnoses
- Helps cluster data, focuses on nursing diagnoses, assists in validating nursing diagnosis labels, and combines assessment with problem listing in one form
- Promotes use by different levels of caregivers, resulting in enhanced communication among the disciplines

Nursing Minimum Data Set
- Comprises format commonly used in long-term care facilities
- Has a cued format that prompts nurse for specific criteria; usually computerized
- Includes specialized information, such as cognitive patterns, communication (hearing and vision) patterns, physical function and structural patterns, activity patterns, restorative care, and the like
- Meets the needs of multiple data users in the health care system
- Establishes comparability of nursing data across clinical populations, settings, geographic areas, and time

---

initial assessment form, frequent or ongoing assessment forms, and focused or specialized assessment forms.

Initial Assessment Form

An initial assessment form is called a nursing admission or admission database. Four types of frequently used initial assessment documentation forms are known as open-ended, cued or checklist, integrated cued checklist, and nursing minimum data set (NMDS) forms. Display 4-2 describes each type of initial assessment form. In addition, Figure 4-1 is an example of the cued or checklist admission documentation form used in an acute care setting.

Frequent or Ongoing Assessment Form

Various institutions have created flow charts that help staff to record and retrieve data for frequent reassessments. Examples of two types of flow charts are the frequent vital signs sheet, which allows for vital signs to be recorded in a graphic format that promotes easy visualization of abnormalities, and the assessment flow chart, which allows for rapid comparison of recorded assessment data from one time period to the next (Fig. 4-2).

Progress notes (Fig. 4-3) may be used to document unusual events, responses, significant observations, or interactions because the data are inappropriate for flow records. Flow sheets streamline the documentation process and prevent needless repetition of data. Emphasis is placed on quality, not quantity, of documentation.

Focused or Specialty Area Assessment Form

Some institutions may use assessment forms that are focused on one major area of the body for clients who have a particular problem. Examples include cardiovascular or neurologic assessment documentation forms. In addition, forms may be customized. For example, a form may be used as a screening tool to assess specific concerns or risks such as falling or skin problems. These forms are usually abbreviated versions of admission data sheets with specific assessment data related to the purpose of the assessment (Fig. 4-4).

SUMMARY

Validation and documentation are two crucial aspects of nursing health assessment. Nurses need to concentrate on learning how to perform these two steps of assessment thoroughly and accurately.

Validation of data verifies the assessment data that you have gathered from the client. It consists of determining which data require validation, implementing techniques to validate, and identifying areas that require further assessment data.

Documentation of data is the act of recording the client assessment findings. Nurses first need to understand the purpose of documentation, next learn which information to document, then be aware of and follow the individual documentation guidelines of their particular health care facility. In addition, it is important for nurses to be familiar with the different documentation forms used in other health care institutions.

| SOUTHEAST MISSOURI HOSPITAL | ADULT ADMISSION HEALTH HISTORY | NAME:
SEX:
PHYS: | Account #:
Med Rec #:
DOB: AGE: |

Unless the nurse asks you to, you do NOT need to complete this again if the last admission was after Feb 1, 2001.

Unable to take history   ☐ Patient confused/unresponsive
☐ Patient not accompanied by family/significant other(s)   ☐ History taken from previous medical record

YES NO HEALTH MANAGEMENT   COMMENTS

Patient lives: ☐ Home   ☐ Other_____
☐ ☐ Live alone
      Primary support person:_____
☐ ☐ Receives home care services
☐ ☐ Metal or foreign objects in body
      (i.e., shrapnel, metal slivers)_____
☐ ☐ Mechanical devices on or implanted
      in the body_____
☐ ☐ Have you ever smoked?_____
      packs per day____#years____date quit_____
☐ ☐ Drink alcohol? Drinks per day_____
☐ ☐ Used/uses recreational drugs_____

NUTRITION/ METABOLIC
☐ ☐ Special diet/restrictions at home_____
☐ ☐ Undesired weight loss_____
☐ ☐ Undesired weight gain_____
☐ ☐ Recent loss of appetite_____
☐ ☐ Difficulty eating/swallowing_____
      ☐ onset during the last 7 days_____
☐ ☐ Recent vomiting (more than 3 days)_____
☐ ☐ Stomach/intestinal problems_____
      (i.e., hiatus hernia, severe heartburn, reflux, etc)
☐ ☐ Feeding tube   Company:_____

METABOLIC
☐ ☐ Have you ever had cancer_____
☐ ☐ Medication pump   Company:_____
☐ ☐ Diabetes—for how long:_____
☐ ☐ Thyroid problems_____

RESPIRATORY/ CIRCULATORY
☐ ☐ Recent cold, flu, sore throat_____
☐ ☐ Asthma or emphysema_____
☐ ☐ Pneumonia/bronchitis_____
☐ ☐ COPD_____
☐ ☐ Shortness of breath_____
☐ ☐ Taking breathing treatments_____
☐ ☐ Uses oxygen   Company:_____
☐ ☐ Sleep apnea_____
☐ ☐ Uses CPAP or other device   Company:_____

CARDIOVASCULAR
☐ ☐ CHF (congestive heart failure)_____
☐ ☐ Chest pain or heart attack_____
☐ ☐ Pacemaker_____
☐ ☐ Mitral valve prolapse_____
☐ ☐ Heart murmur_____
☐ ☐ Rheumatic fever_____
☐ ☐ High blood pressure_____
☐ ☐ Circulatory trouble_____

ELIMINATION
☐ ☐ Kidney or urinary problems_____
☐ ☐ Bladder/voiding problems_____
☐ ☐ Uses a catheter_____
☐ ☐ Has an ostomy_____

SEXUALITY/REPRODUCTIVE
Female:
Number of pregnancies_____
Number of live births_____
Date of last menstrual period_____
☐ ☐ Is there a chance you are_____
      pregnant

YES NO HEMATOLOGY
☐ ☐ Bleeding/bruising tendency_____
☐ ☐ Ever had blood transfusions_____
☐ ☐ Ever had severe anemia_____
☐ ☐ Ever had blood clots_____

ACTIVITY/EXERCISE
☐ ☐ Needs help with self care_____
      ☐ onset during last 7 days
☐ ☐ Problems with walking_____
      ☐ onset during last 7 days
☐ ☐ Arm/leg weakness/paralysis_____
      ☐ onset during last 7 days
☐ ☐ Bone/joint problems or arthritis_____
☐ ☐ Back or neck problems_____
☐ ☐ Recent fracture or surgical procedure_____
      involving the arms, legs or spine:
      Use of special equipment
☐ ☐ Walker   ☐ Brought with patient
                  Company obtained from:_____
☐ ☐ Wheelchair ☐ Brought with patient
                  Company obtained from:_____
☐ ☐ Cane   ☐ Brought with patient
                  Company obtained from:_____
☐ ☐ Crutches   ☐ Brought with patient
                  Company obtained from:_____
☐ ☐ Other   ☐ Brought with patient
                  Company obtained from:_____

COGNITIVE/PERCEPTUAL
☐ ☐ Stroke_____
☐ ☐ Memory loss or confusion_____
☐ ☐ Difficulty speaking or communicating_____
      ☐ onset during last 7 days
☐ ☐ Fainting spells or dizziness_____
☐ ☐ Convulsions, seizures, or epilepsy_____
☐ ☐ Nervous or mental disorders_____
☐ ☐ Eye problems or glaucoma_____
☐ ☐ Hearing problems_____
☐ ☐ Claustrophobia—If yes, how bad:_____

EDUCATION
☐ ☐ Is there anything you would like to learn about your
      condition? Explain:_____
Education needs for the following departments:
Patient educators   Receives ☐ Needs ☐ _____
Cardiac rehab   Receives ☐ Needs ☐ _____
Nutrition services   Receives ☐ Needs ☐ _____
Respiratory ther.   Receives ☐ Needs ☐ _____
Pulmonary rehab   Receives ☐ Needs ☐ _____

VALUE/BELIEF
☐ ☐ Is there anything in your religious or cultural belief
      that affects the care we provide or how we treat you?
      Explain:_____
      _____

☐ ☐ Would you like hospital chaplain to visit?

INFECTIOUS DISEASE
☐ ☐ Confirmed HIV positive
☐ ☐ Ever had hepatitis

      What type:_____   Year_____
☐ ☐ Ever had MRSA   Year_____
☐ ☐ Ever had VRE   Year_____
☐ ☐ Ever had tuberculosis (TB)   Year_____
☐ ☐ Ever had chicken pox   ☐ Vaccine
☐ ☐ Had contact with chicken pox 10–21 days ago?

Figure 4-1 Printout of computerized admission form. (Source: Used with permission from Southeast Missouri Hospital, Cape Girardeau, MO.)

SOUTHEAST MISSOURI HOSPITAL	ADULT ADMISSION HEALTH HISTORY	NAME: SEX: PHYS:		Account #: Med Rec #:
			DOB:	AGE:

Previous surgeries: (type, date, and facility)

Allergic to latex: ☐ Yes   ☐ No   Symptoms

Food allergies:	Symptoms

Medication allergies:	Symptoms

Other allergies:	Symptoms

Figure 4-1 *Continued*

PATIENT ASSESSMENT FLOWSHEET

INITIALS/SIGNATURE _____

_____

_____

_____

_____

Date _____

Addressograph

INITIAL ASSESSMENT	2300–0700 TIME/INITIALS _____	0700–1500 TIME/INITIALS _____	1500–2300 TIME/INITIALS _____
NUTRITION/ METABOLIC	SKIN: ☐ Dry ☐ Intact ☐ Warm ☐ Cold ☐ Other _____ Turgor: _____ ☐ N/V _____ TUBES: (feeding) _____ IV: Date Of Insertion: _____ SITE: _____ FLUIDS: _____ WOUNDS/DRSGS: _____	SKIN: ☐ Dry ☐ Intact ☐ Warm ☐ Cold ☐ Other _____ Turgor: _____ ☐ N/V _____ TUBES: (feeding) _____ IV: Date Of Insertion: _____ SITE: _____ FLUIDS: _____ WOUNDS/DRSGS: _____	SKIN: ☐ Dry ☐ Intact ☐ Warm ☐ Cold ☐ Other _____ Turgor: _____ ☐ N/V _____ TUBES: (feeding) _____ IV: Date Of Insertion: _____ SITE: _____ FLUIDS: _____ WOUNDS/DRSGS: _____
RESPIRATORY/ CIRCULATORY	BREATH SOUNDS: _____ RESPIRATIONS: _____ OXYGEN: _____ PULSE OX: _____ ☐ Cough _____ ☐ Sputum _____ APICAL PULSE: _____ ☐ Regular ☐ Irregular TELEMETRY: _____ NAILBED COLOR: ☐ Pink ☐ Pale ☐ Blue PEDAL PULSES: R ☐— ☐+ L ☐— ☐+ EDEMA: R ☐— ☐+ L ☐— ☐+ CALF R ☐— ☐+ TENDERNESS: L ☐— ☐+	BREATH SOUNDS: _____ RESPIRATIONS: _____ OXYGEN: _____ PULSE OX: _____ ☐ Cough _____ ☐ Sputum _____ APICAL PULSE: _____ ☐ Regular ☐ Irregular TELEMETRY: _____ NAILBED COLOR: ☐ Pink ☐ Pale ☐ Blue PEDAL PULSES: R ☐— ☐+ L ☐— ☐+ EDEMA: R ☐— ☐+ L ☐— ☐+ CALF R ☐— ☐+ TENDERNESS: L ☐— ☐+	BREATH SOUNDS: _____ RESPIRATIONS: _____ OXYGEN: _____ PULSE OX: _____ ☐ Cough _____ ☐ Sputum _____ APICAL PULSE: _____ ☐ Regular ☐ Irregular TELEMETRY: _____ NAILBED COLOR: ☐ Pink ☐ Pale ☐ Blue PEDAL PULSES: R ☐— ☐+ L ☐— ☐+ EDEMA: R ☐— ☐+ L ☐— ☐+ CALF R ☐— ☐+ TENDERNESS: L ☐— ☐+

Figure 4-2 Assessment flow sheet. Form is used when computerized form is unavailable. (Source: Used with permission from Southeast Missouri Hospital, Cape Girardeau, MO.)

PATIENT ASSESSMENT FLOWSHEET, Page 2

Addressograph   Date _____

INITIAL ASSESSMENT	2300-0700 TIME/INITIALS _____	0700-1500 TIME/INITIALS _____	1500-2300 TIME/INITIALS _____
ELIMINATION	ABDOMEN: ☐ Soft ☐ Firm ☐ Nondistended ☐ Distended BOWEL SOUNDS: ☐ Normoactive ☐ Hyperactive ☐ Hypoactive ☐ Absent LBM: _____ TUBES: _____ 	ABDOMEN: ☐ Soft ☐ Firm ☐ Nondistended ☐ Distended BOWEL SOUNDS: ☐ Normoactive ☐ Hyperactive ☐ Hypoactive ☐ Absent LBM: _____ TUBES: _____ 	ABDOMEN: ☐ Soft ☐ Firm ☐ Nondistended ☐ Distended BOWEL SOUNDS: ☐ Normoactive ☐ Hyperactive ☐ Hypoactive ☐ Absent LBM: _____ TUBES: _____
ACTIVITY/ EXERCISE	MAE: ☐ Full ☐ Impaired Fall Prevention _____	MAE: ☐ Full ☐ Impaired Fall Prevention _____	MAE: ☐ Full ☐ Impaired Fall Prevention _____
COGNITIVE/ PERCEPTUAL	LOC: ☐ Alert ☐ Lethargic ☐ Unresponsive ORIENTATION: ☐ Person ☐ Place ☐ Time ☐ Pain _____ 	LOC: ☐ Alert ☐ Lethargic ☐ Unresponsive ORIENTATION: ☐ Person ☐ Place ☐ Time ☐ Pain _____ 	LOC: ☐ Alert ☐ Lethargic ☐ Unresponsive ORIENTATION: ☐ Person ☐ Place ☐ Time ☐ Pain _____
PLAN OF CARE	Discussed Plan of Care with: ☐ Patient ☐ Family/Significant Other(s)	Discussed Plan of Care with: ☐ Patient ☐ Family/Significant Other(s)	Discussed Plan of Care with: ☐ Patient ☐ Family/Significant Other(s)
CARE PER STANDARD			
ONGOING PATIENT TEACHING (Time and Initial each entry)	☐ Video ☐ Handout/Booklet _____ ☐ Verbal - See Nurses Notes ☐ Pt/Family Response: _____	☐ Video ☐ Handout/Booklet _____ ☐ Verbal - See Nurses Notes ☐ Pt/Family Response: _____	☐ Video ☐ Handout/Booklet _____ ☐ Verbal - See Nurses Notes ☐ Pt/Family Response: _____
EDUCATIONAL (To be completed on Admission and PRN)	Motivation: ☐ Appears Interested ☐ Seems Uninterested ☐ Denies Need for Education Factors Affecting Teaching: _____	Motivation: ☐ Appears Interested ☐ Seems Uninterested ☐ Denies Need for Education Factors Affecting Teaching: _____	Motivation: ☐ Appears Interested ☐ Seems Uninterested ☐ Denies Need for Education Factors Affecting Teaching: _____

Figure 4-2   *Continued*

01/15/09 Client short of breath with labored respirations of 32/minute. Chest barrel shaped. Skin reddish. Decreased tactile fremitus percussed bilaterally. Bilateral hyperresonance. Respiratory and diaphragmatic excursion decreased. Has nonproductive cough, decreased breath sounds with wheezing and prolonged expirations. Client states, "I'm so short of breath."

Figure 4-3 Documentation of assessment findings on a narrative progress note.

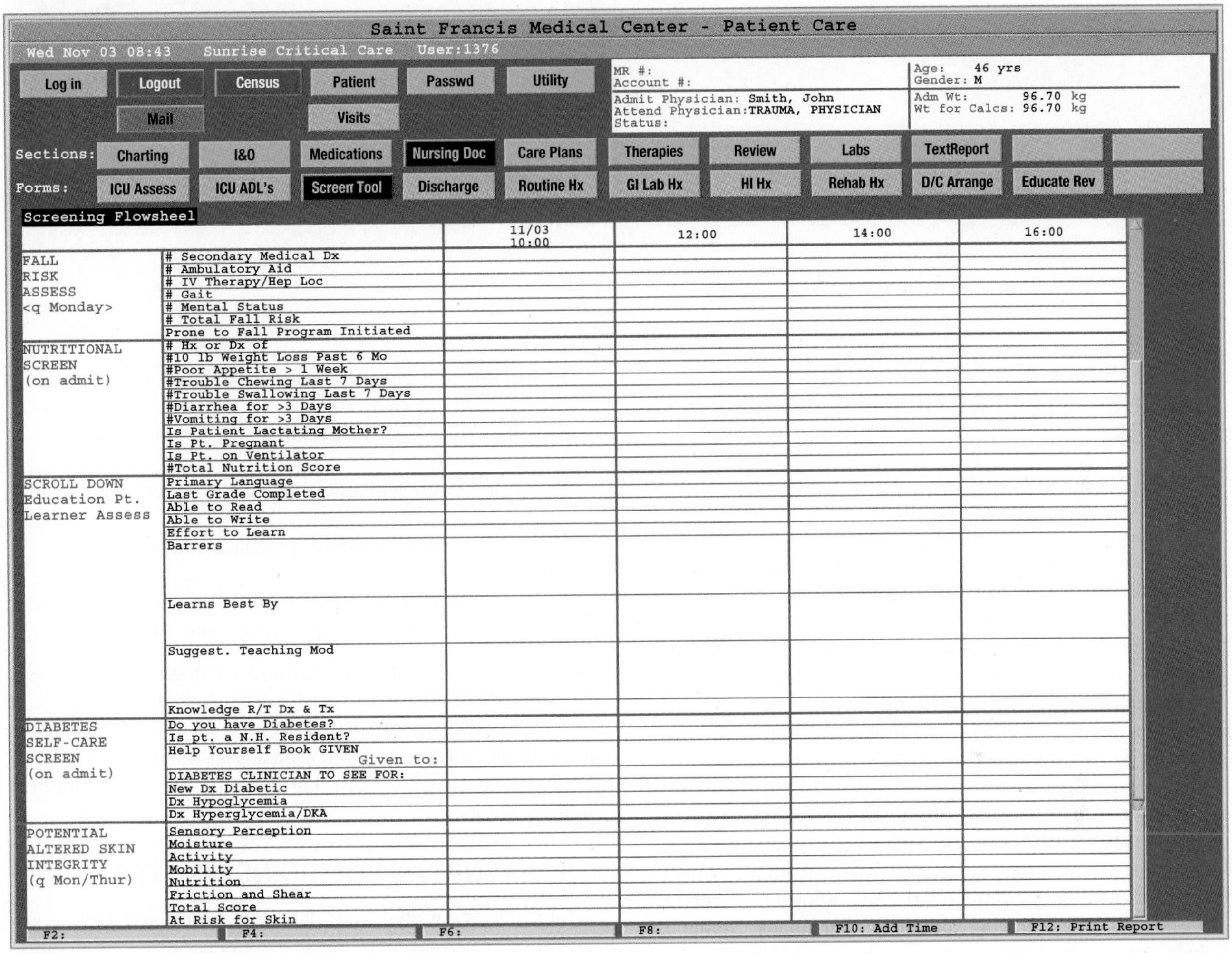

Saint Francis Medical Center - Patient Care

Wed Nov 03 08:43   Sunrise Critical Care   User:1376

| Log in | Logout | Census | Patient | Passwd | Utility |
| Mail | | | Visits | | |

MR #:
Account #:
Admit Physician: Smith, John
Attend Physician: TRAUMA, PHYSICIAN
Status:

Age: 46 yrs
Gender: M
Adm Wt: 96.70 kg
Wt for Calcs: 96.70 kg

Sections: | Charting | I&O | Medications | Nursing Doc | Care Plans | Therapies | Review | Labs | TextReport |
Forms: | ICU Assess | ICU ADL's | Screen Tool | Discharge | Routine Hx | GI Lab Hx | HI Hx | Rehab Hx | D/C Arrange | Educate Rev |

Screening Flowsheet

		11/03 10:00	12:00	14:00	16:00
FALL RISK ASSESS <q Monday>	# Secondary Medical Dx				
	# Ambulatory Aid				
	# IV Therapy/Hep Loc				
	# Gait				
	# Mental Status				
	# Total Fall Risk				
	Prone to Fall Program Initiated				
NUTRITIONAL SCREEN (on admit)	# Hx or Dx of				
	#10 lb Weight Loss Past 6 Mo				
	#Poor Appetite > 1 Week				
	#Trouble Chewing Last 7 Days				
	#Trouble Swallowing Last 7 Days				
	#Diarrhea for >3 Days				
	#Vomiting for >3 Days				
	Is Patient Lactating Mother?				
	Is Pt. Pregnant				
	Is Pt. on Ventilator				
	#Total Nutrition Score				
SCROLL DOWN Education Pt. Learner Assess	Primary Language				
	Last Grade Completed				
	Able to Read				
	Able to Write				
	Effort to Learn				
	Barrers				
	Learns Best By				
	Suggest. Teaching Mod				
	Knowledge R/T Dx & Tx				
DIABETES SELF-CARE SCREEN (on admit)	Do you have Diabetes?				
	Is pt. a N.H. Resident?				
	Help Yourself Book GIVEN Given to:				
	DIABETES CLINICIAN TO SEE FOR:				
	New Dx Diabetic				
	Dx Hypoglycemia				
	Dx Hyperglycemia/DKA				
POTENTIAL ALTERED SKIN INTEGRITY (q Mon/Thur)	Sensory Perception				
	Moisture				
	Activity				
	Mobility				
	Nutrition				
	Friction and Shear				
	Total Score				
	At Risk for Skin				

| F2: | F4: | F6: | F8: | F10: Add Time | F12: Print Report |

Figure 4-4 Portions of a computerized screening flow sheet. The full assessment document includes cells for systemic findings as well as functional data, such as nutrition, activities of daily living, and client education needs. (Source: Used with permission from Saint Francis Medical Center, Cape Girardeau, MO.)

References and Selected Readings

Allen, J., & Englebright, J. (2000). Patient-centered documentation: An effective and efficient use of clinical information system. *Journal of Nursing Administration, 30*(2), 90–95.

Brooke, P. S. (2000). Long-term care demands precise documentation. *Nursing Management, 31*(11), 23–24.

Clark, E. B., Luce, J. M., Curtis, J. R., Danis, M., Levy, M., Nelson, J., Solomo, M. Z., & Robert Wood Johnson Foundation Critical Care End-of-Life Person's Workgroup. (2004). A content analysis of forms, guidelines, and other materials documenting end-of-life care in intensive care units. *Journal of Critical Care, 19*(2), 108–117.

Complete guide to documentation (2nd ed.). (2007). Philadelphia: Lippincott Williams & Wilkins.

Häyrinen, K., Saranto, K., & Nykänen, P. (2007). Definition, structure content, use and impacts of electronic health records: A review of the research literature. *International Journal of Medical Informatics, 77*(5), 291–304.

Karkkainen, O., & Eriksson, K. (2004). A theoretical approach to documentation of care. *Nursing Science Quarterly, 17*(3), 268–272.

Kunihara, Y., Asai, N., Ishimoto, E., Kawamata, S., & Nakamura, S. (2007). A survey of the effects of the full computerized nursing records system on sharing nursing records among health professionals. *Medinfo, 12*(PTI), 360–363.

Marbut, M., & Dansby-Kelly, A. (2006). Great expectations: JCAHO-compliant nursing documentation. *Insight, 31*(4), 20–21.

Martin, R. H. (2004). Clearly, carefully, and completely. *Advanced Nursing Practitioner, 12*(6), 18.

McManus, B. (2000). A move to electronic patient records in the community: A qualitative case study of a clinical data collection system. *Topics in Health Information Management, 20*(4), 23–37.

Morris, K. (2002). Are there some general rules concerning documentation? *Ohio Nurses Review, 77*(2), 16.

Murphy, E. (2003). Charting by exception. *AORNJ, 78*(5), 821–823.

Platt, A., & Reed, B. (2001). Meet new pain standards with new technology. Documentation takes a leap into your hands. *Nursing Management, 32*(3), 40–43.

Plawecki, L. H., & Plawecki, H. M. (2007). Your choice: Documentation or litigation? *Journal of Gerontological Nursing, 33*(9), 3–4.

Smith, L. S. (2004). Documenting refusal of treatment. *Nursing, 34*(4), 79.

Stephens, S., & Mason, S. (2004). Putting it together: A documentation system that works. *Nursing Management, 30*(3), 43–47.

5

Analyzing Data Using Critical Thinking Skills

ANALYSIS OF DATA AND CRITICAL THINKING—STEP TWO OF THE NURSING PROCESS

Data analysis is often referred to as the diagnostic phase because the end result or purpose of this phase is the identification of a nursing diagnosis (wellness, actual, or risk), collaborative problem, or need for referral to another health care professional.

As the second step or phase of the nursing process, data analysis is a very difficult step because the nurse is required to use diagnostic reasoning skills to interpret data accurately. Diagnostic reasoning is a form of critical thinking. Because of the complex nature of nursing as both a science and an art, the nurse must think critically—in a rational, self-directed, intelligent, and purposeful manner.

Critical thinking is the way in which the nurse processes information using knowledge, past experiences, intuition, and cognitive abilities to formulate conclusions or diagnoses. The nurse must develop several characteristics to think critically (Display 5-1). An open mind and exploration of alternatives are essential when making judgments and plans. Sound rationale must support judgments and ideas; avoid hurried decisions. The critical thinker reflects on thoughts and gathers more information when necessary. Then, too, the critical thinker uses each clinical experience to learn new information and to add to the knowledge base. Another important aspect of critical thinking involves awareness of human interactions and the environment, which provide cues and directly influence decisions and judgments (see Display 5-1). Ask yourself the following questions to determine your critical thinking skills:

- Do you reserve your final opinion or judgment until you have collected more or all of the information?
- Do you support your opinion or comments with supporting data, sound rationale, and literature?
- Do you explore and consider other alternatives before making a decision?
- Can you distinguish between a fact, opinion, cue, or inference?

- Do you ask your client for more information or clarification when you do not understand?
- Do you validate your information and judgments with experts in the field?
- Do you use your past knowledge and experiences to analyze data?
- Do you try to avoid biases or preconceived ways of thinking?
- Do you try to learn from past mistakes in your judgments?
- Are you open to the fact that you may not always be right?

If you answered "yes" to most of these questions, you have already started to develop a critical thinking mindset. If you need practice, many books (some with practice exercises) are available on how to think critically as a nurse. Such books can help the nurse to learn and continue to develop, critical thinking skills.

THE DIAGNOSTIC REASONING PROCESS

Before you begin analyzing data, make sure you have accurately performed the steps of the assessment phase of the nursing process (collection and organization of assessment data, validation of data, and documentation of data). This information will have a profound effect on the conclusions you reach in the analysis step of the nursing process.

If you are confident of your work during the assessment phase, you are ready to analyze your data—the diagnostic phase of the nursing process. This phase consists of the following essential components: grouping and organizing data, validating data and comparing the data with norms, clustering data to make inferences, generating possible hypotheses regarding the client's problems, formulating a professional clinical judgment, and validating the judgment with the client. These basic components have been organized in various ways to break the process of diagnostic reasoning into easily understood steps. Regardless of how the information is organized or the title of the steps, diagnostic reasoning always consists of these components.

This text presents seven distinct steps to provide a clear, concise explanation of how to perform data analysis. Each step

DISPLAY 5-1	Essential Elements of Critical Thinking

- Keep an open mind.
- Use rationale to support opinions or decisions.
- Reflect on thoughts before reaching a conclusion.
- Use past clinical experiences to build knowledge.
- Acquire an adequate knowledge base that continues to build.
- Be aware of the interactions of others.
- Be aware of the environment.

is described in detail. In addition, these seven steps are used throughout the text in "Analysis of Data" sections of the assessment chapters. We will use the following case as an example of implementing diagnostic reasoning:

Mary Michaelson, a 29-year-old divorced woman, works as an office manager for a large, prestigious law firm. She reports she recently went to see a doctor because "my hair was falling out in chunks, and I have a red rash on my face and chest. It looks like a bad case of acne." After doing some blood work, her physician diagnosed her condition as discoid lupus erythematosus (DLE). She says she has come to see you, the occupational health nurse, because she feels "so ugly," and she is concerned that she may lose her job because of how she looks.

During the interview, she tells you that she is a surfer and is out in the sun all day nearly every weekend. She shares that she uses sunscreen but forgets to put it on at regular intervals during the day.

Your physical examination reveals an attractive, tanned, thin, anxious-appearing young woman. You note confluent and nonconfluent maculopapular lesions on her neck, chest above the nipple line, and over the shoulders and upper back to about the level of the T5 vertebra. Many of the lesions appear as red, scaling plaques with depressed, pale centers. A few of the lesions on her forehead and cheeks appear blistered. Patchy alopecia is also present. Her vital signs are within normal limits, and no other abnormalities are apparent at this time.

Step One—Identify Abnormal Data and Strengths

Identifying abnormal findings and client strengths requires the nurse to have and use a knowledge base of anatomy and physiology, psychology, and sociology. In addition, collected assessment data should be compared with findings in reliable charts and reference resources that provide standards and values for physical and psychological norms (i.e., height, nutritional requirements, growth and development). Additionally the nurse should have a basic knowledge of risk factors for the client. Risk factors are based on client data such as gender, age, ethnic background, and occupation. Therefore, the nurse needs to have access to both the data supplied by the client and the known risk factors for specific diseases or disorders.

The nurse's knowledge of anatomy and physiology, psychology, and sociology; use of reference materials; and attention to risk factors help to identify strengths, risks, and abnormal findings.

> **Clinical Tip** • *Identified strengths are used in formulating wellness diagnoses. Identified potential weaknesses are used in formulating risk diagnoses, and abnormal findings are used in formulating actual nursing diagnoses.*

Remember to analyze both subjective and objective data when identifying strengths and abnormal findings. Using Ms. Michaelson's case, you may identify the following:

Identified Abnormal Data and Strengths: Subjective

- "Hair falling out in chunks"
- Red rash on face and chest, "looks like a bad case of acne"
- "So ugly"
- Concerned that she may lose her job because of how she looks
- Surfer—out in the sun all day on weekends—minimal use of sunscreen
- Sought out occupational health nurse

Identified Abnormal Data and Strengths: Objective

- Anxious appearance
- Diagnosed with discoid lupus erythematosus
- Red, raised plaques on face, neck, shoulders, back, and chest
- Patchy alopecia

Step Two—Cluster Data

During step two, the nurse looks at the identified abnormal findings and strengths for cues that are related. Cluster both abnormal cues and strength cues; a particular nursing framework should be used as a guide when possible. Using the sample case, one identified cue cluster would be

- Rash on face, neck, chest, and back
- Patchy alopecia
- "So ugly"

While you are clustering the data during this step, you may find that certain cues are pointing toward a problem but that more data are needed to support the problem. For example, a client may have a nonproductive cough with labored respirations at a rate of 24/min. However, you have gathered no data on the status of breath sounds. In such a situation, you would need to assess the client's breath sounds to formulate an appropriate nursing diagnosis or collaborative problem.

Step Three—Draw Inferences

Step three requires the nurse to write down hunches about each cue cluster. For example, based on the cue cluster presented in step two—rash on face, neck, chest, and back; patchy alopecia; "so ugly"—you would write down what you think these data are saying and determine whether it is something that the nurse can treat independently. Your hunch about this data cluster might be "Changes in physical appearance are affecting self-perception." This is something for which the nurse would intervene and treat independently. Therefore, the nurse would move to step four: analysis of data to formulate a nursing diagnosis.

However, if the inference you draw from a cue cluster suggests the need for both medical and nursing interventions to resolve the problem, you would attempt to generate collaborative problems. Collaborative problems are defined as "certain physiological complications that nurses monitor to detect their onset or changes in status; nurses manage collaborative problems using physician-prescribed and nursing-prescribed interventions to minimize the complications of events" (Carpenito-Moyet, 2004).

Collaborative problems are equivalent in importance to nursing diagnoses but represent the interdependent or collaborative role of nursing. A list of collaborative problems is given in Appendix C.

Another purpose of step three is the referral of identified problems for which the nurse cannot prescribe definitive treatment. Referring can be defined as connecting clients with other professionals and resources. For example, if the collaborative problem for which the nurse is monitoring occurs, an immediate referral to the client's physician or nurse practitioner is necessary for implementing medical treatment. Another example may be a diabetic client who is having trouble understanding the exchange diet. Although the nurse has knowledge in this area, referral to a dietitian can provide the client with updated materials and allow the nurse more time to deal with client problems within the nursing domain. Another important reason for referral is the identification or suspicion of a medical problem based on the subjective and objective data collected. In such cases, referral to the client's physician, nurse practitioner, or another specialist is necessary.

The referral process differs from health care setting to health care setting. Sometimes the nurse makes a direct referral; other times it may be the policy to notify the nurse practitioner or physician who, if unable to intervene, will make the referral. To save time and to provide high-quality care for the client, make sure you are familiar with the referral process used in your health care setting.

Step Four—Propose Possible Nursing Diagnoses

If resolution of the situation requires primarily nursing interventions, you would hypothesize and generate possible nursing diagnoses. The nursing diagnoses may be wellness diagnoses, risk diagnoses, or actual diagnoses (Kelley, Frisch & Avant, 1995).

A wellness diagnosis indicates that the client has the opportunity for enhancement of a health state. There are occasions when clients are ready to improve an already healthy level of function. When such an opportunity exists, the nurse can support the client's movement toward greater health and wellness by identifying "opportunities for enhancement."

A risk diagnosis indicates the client does not currently have the problem but is at high risk for developing it (e.g., Risk for Impaired Skin Integrity related to immobility, poor nutrition, and incontinence).

An actual nursing diagnosis indicates the client is currently experiencing the stated problem or has a dysfunctional pattern (e.g., Impaired Skin Integrity: Reddened area on right buttocks). Table 5-1 provides a comparison of wellness, risk, and actual nursing diagnoses. Appendix B provides a list of common nursing diagnoses.

Using the sample case: The cue cluster from step two was determined to be something for which the nurse could intervene. Changes in physical appearance are affecting self-perception. One possible nursing diagnosis based on this inference is Body Image Disturbance related to changes in physical appearance.

Step Five—Check for Defining Characteristics

At this point in analyzing the data, the nurse must check for defining characteristics for the data clusters and hypothesized diagnoses in order to choose the most accurate diagnoses and delete those diagnoses that are not valid or accurate for the client. This step is often difficult because diagnostic labels overlap, making it hard to identify the most appropriate diagnosis. For example, the diagnostic categories of Impaired Gas Exchange, Ineffective Airway Clearance, and Ineffective Breathing Patterns all reflect respiratory problems but each is used to describe a very different human response pattern and set of defining characteristics.

Reference texts such as North American Nursing Diagnosis Association (NANDA) *Nursing Diagnoses: Definitions and Classifications 2009–2011* can assist the nurse to determine when and when not to use each nursing diagnostic category (NANDA, 2009–2011). It assists with ruling out invalid diagnoses and selecting valid diagnoses. Thus both the definition and defining characteristics should be compared with the client's set of data (cues) to make sure that the correct diagnoses are chosen for the client. For an example of how to check for defining characteristics, consider the nursing diagnosis hypothesized

Table 5-1	Comparison of Wellness, Risk, and Actual Nursing Diagnoses		
	Wellness Diagnoses	**Risk Diagnoses**	**Actual Diagnoses**
Client status	State of harmony and balance	State of risk for identified problem	State of health problems
Format for stating	Readiness for enhanced . . . or for enhanced	"Risk for . . ."	Nursing diagnoses and "related to" clause
Examples	Readiness for enhanced body image	Risk for Altered Body Image	Disturbed Body Image related to hand wound that is not healing
	Readiness for enhanced family processes	Risk for Altered Family Processes	Interrupted Family Processes related to hospitalization of patient
	Readiness for enhanced effective breast-feeding	Risk for Ineffective Breast-feeding	Ineffective Breast-feeding related to poor mother–infant attachment
	Readiness for enhanced skin integrity	Risk for Impaired Skin Integrity	Impaired Skin Integrity related to immobility

in step four. A major defining characteristic is "verbal negative response to actual change in structure." A minor defining characteristic is negative feelings.

Step Six—Confirm or Rule Out Diagnoses

If the cue cluster data do not meet the defining characteristics, you can rule out that particular diagnosis. If the cue cluster data do meet the defining characteristics, the diagnosis should be verified with the client and other health care professionals who are caring for the client. Tell the client what you perceive his diagnosis to be. Often nursing diagnosis terminology is difficult for the client to understand. For example, you would not tell the client that you believe that he has Impaired Nutrition: Less Than Body Requirements. Instead you might say that you believe that current nutritional intake is not adequate to promote healing of body tissues. Then you would ask the client if this seemed to be an accurate statement of the problem. It is essential that the client understand the problem so treatment can be properly implemented. If the client is not in a coherent state of mind to help validate the problem, consult with family members or significant others or even other health care professionals.

Validation is also important with the client who has a collaborative problem or who requires a referral. If the client has a collaborative problem, you need to inform her about which signs you are monitoring. For example, you might tell the client you will be monitoring blood pressure and level of consciousness every 30 minutes for the next several hours. It is also important to collaborate with the client regarding referrals to determine what is needed to resolve the problem and to discuss possible resources to help the client. When possible, provide the client with a list of possible resources (including availability and cost). Help the client to make the contact by phone or letter. Then follow up to determine if the referral was made and if the client was connected to the appropriate resources.

Using the sample case, we have identified the nursing diagnosis Body Image Disturbance related to changes in physical appearance. You may accept the diagnosis because it meets defining characteristics and is validated by the client.

Step Seven—Document Conclusions

Be sure to document all of your professional judgments and the data that support those judgments. Documentation of data collection before analysis is described in Chapter 4. Guidelines for correctly documenting nursing diagnoses, collaborative problems, and referrals are described in the sections that follow.

Nursing diagnoses are often documented and worded in different formats. The most useful formats for wellness, risk, and actual nursing diagnoses are described below. In addition, the major conclusions of a nursing assessment are compared in Table 5-2.

Wellness Nursing Diagnoses

Wellness diagnoses represent those situations in which the client does not have a problem but is at a point where he or she can attain a higher level of health. This type of diagnosis is worded *Readiness for enhanced.* . . . and indicates an opportunity to make greater, to increase quality of, or to attain the most desired level of function in the area of the diagnostic category.

When documenting these diagnoses, it is best to use the following format:

> Readiness to enhanced + diagnostic label + related to (r/t) + etiology + as manifested by (AMB) + symptoms (defining characteristics)
>
> *Example:* Readiness for Enhanced Effective Breast-feeding r/t confident mother, full-term healthy infant, and normal breast structure AMB infant contentment after feeding and mother's request to continue to breast-feed

Wellness diagnoses other than those for which NANDA has labels may be formulated by using the following format:

> Readiness for enhanced + NANDA problem-oriented diagnostic label minus the modifiers + r/t + etiology + AMB + symptoms (defining characteristics)
>
> *Example:* Readiness for Enhanced Parenting r/t effective bonding with children and effective basic parenting skills AMB parent's verbalized concern to continue effective parenting skills during child's illness

Risk Nursing Diagnoses

A risk diagnosis describes a situation in which an actual diagnosis will most likely occur if the nurse does not intervene. In this case, the client does not have any symptoms or defining characteristics that are manifested, and thus a shorter statement is sufficient:

> Risk for + diagnostic label + related to (r/t) + etiology
>
> *Example:* Risk for Infection r/t presence of dirty knife wound, leukopenia, and lack of client knowledge of how adequately to care for the wound

Actual Nursing Diagnoses

The most useful format for an actual nursing diagnosis is

> NANDA label (for problem) + r/t + etiology + AMB + defining characteristics
>
> *Example:* Fatigue r/t an increase in job demands and personal stress AMB client's statements of feeling exhausted all of the time and inability to perform usual work and home responsibilities (e.g., cooking, cleaning).

Shorter formats are often used to describe client problems. However, this format provides all of the necessary information and provides the reader with the clearest and most accurate description of the client's problem.

Collaborative Problems and Referrals

Collaborative problems should be documented as Risk for Complications (or RC): _____ (what the problem is). Nursing goals for the collaborative problem should be documented as well as which parameters the nurse must monitor and how often they should be monitored. The nurse also needs to indicate when the physician or nurse practitioner should be notified and to identify nursing interventions to help prevent the complication from occurring and nursing interventions to be initiated if a change occurs. If a referral is indicated, document the problem (or suspected problem), the need for immediate referral, and to whom the client is being referred.

Table 5-2	Major Conclusions of Assessment				
	Wellness Nursing Diagnosis	**Actual Problem Nursing Diagnosis**	**Potential Problem Nursing Diagnosis**	**Collaborative Problem**	**Problem for Referral**
Who identifies the concern?	Nurse	Nurse	Nurse	Nurse or other provider	Nurse or other provider
Who deals with the concern?	Nurse (independent practice)	Nurse (independent practice)	Nurse (independent practice)	Nurse (interdependent practice)	Other provider
What content knowledge is needed?	Nursing science Sciences Basic studies	Nursing science Sciences Basic studies	Nursing science Sciences Basic studies	Nursing science Sciences Basic studies Domain of other providers	Nursing science Sciences Basic studies Domain of other providers
What minimum work experience is needed?	Average	Average	Better than average	Average	Average
What does first part of conclusion statement look like?	Opportunity to enhance . . .	Taxonomy label or other descriptive label	Usually taxonomy label of "Risk for . . ."	Risk for Complication (RC)	N/A
Are related factors included?	Yes (but not mandatory)	Yes, unless unknown	Yes (mandatory)	Sometimes	N/A
What might complete statement look like?	Readiness for Enhanced Effective Breast-feeding r/t confident mother, full-term healthy infant, and normal breast structure	Disturbed Self-Esteem r/t knowledge deficit, ineffective coping as new mother, and loss of job	Risk for Impaired Skin Integrity r/t immobility, incontinence and fragile skin	RC: Rejection of kidney transplant	Unsafe housing (referral is necessary)

Using the sample case and cue cluster we have followed, the nurse would document the following conclusion:

"The following nursing diagnosis is appropriate for Ms. Michaelson at this time: Body Image Disturbance related to changes in physical appearance."

DEVELOPING DIAGNOSTIC REASONING EXPERTISE AND AVOIDING PITFALLS

A diagnosis or judgment is considered to be highly accurate if the diagnosis is consistent with all of the cues, supported by highly relevant cues, and as precise as possible (Lunney, 2003). Developing expertise with making professional judgments comes with accumulation of both knowledge and experience. One does not become an expert diagnostician overnight. It is a process that develops with time and practice. A beginning nurse attempts to make accurate diagnoses but, because of a lack of knowledge and experience, often finds that he or she has made diagnostic errors. Experts have an advantage because they know when exceptions can be applied to the rules that the novice is accustomed to using and applying. Beginning nurses tend to see things as right or wrong, whereas experts realize there are shades of gray or areas between right and wrong. Novices also tend to focus on details and may miss the big picture, whereas experts have a broader perspective in examining situations.

Although beginning nurses lack the depth of knowledge and expertise that expert nurses have, they can still learn to increase their diagnostic accuracy by becoming aware of, and avoiding, the several pitfalls of diagnosing. These pitfalls decrease the reliability of cues and decrease diagnostic accuracy. There are two

sets of pitfalls: those that occur during the assessment phase and those that occur during the analysis of data phase.

The first set of pitfalls is discussed in detail in Chapter 4. They include too many or too few data, unreliable or invalid data, and an insufficient number of cues available to support the diagnoses.

The second set of pitfalls occurs during the analysis phase. Cues may be clustered yet unrelated to each other. For example, the client may be very quiet and appear depressed. A nurse may assume the client is grieving because her husband died a year ago but the client may just be fatigued because of all the diagnostic tests she has just undergone.

Another common error is quickly diagnosing a client without hypothesizing several diagnoses. For example, a nurse may assume that a readmitted diabetic client with hyperglycemia has a knowledge deficit concerning the exchange diet. However, further exploration of data reveals that the client has low self-esteem and feelings of powerlessness and hopelessness in controlling a labile, fluctuating blood glucose level. The nurse's goal is to avoid making diagnoses too quickly without taking sufficient time to process the data.

Another pitfall to avoid is incorrectly wording the diagnostic statement. This leads to an inaccurate picture of the client for others caring for him. Finally, do not overlook consideration of the client's cultural background when analyzing data. Clients from other cultures may be misdiagnosed because the defining characteristics and labels for specific diagnoses do not accurately describe the human responses in their culture. Therefore, it is essential to look closely at cultural norms and responses for various clients.

ANALYSIS OF DATA THROUGHOUT HEALTH ASSESSMENT IN NURSING

The whole purpose of assessing a client's health status is to analyze the subjective and objective data collected. Therefore, because analysis of data is such a natural next step, the importance of illustrating the link between assessment and analysis for each body part or system assessment chapter is apparent. In the clinical assessment chapters of this textbook, *Analysis of Data* has been developed to help the reader visualize, understand, and practice analyzing data (diagnostic reasoning).

Analysis of Data consists of two sections. The first section, called Diagnostic Reasoning: Possible Conclusions, contains possible nursing diagnoses, collaborative problems, and referrals for the material covered in the particular chapter. This list is presented so that the reader becomes familiar with common possible conclusions seen with the particular body part or system. It also provides a convenient list for the reader to refer to while working through the case study in section three or completing the critical thinking exercise in the study guide/laboratory manual that is a companion piece for the textbook.

The second section is entitled Case Study. This section consists of a case study followed by the seven key steps of analysis and the accompanying data for each step based on the case study. This section illustrates exactly how to analyze data and which information to include in each of the seven key steps of diagnostic reasoning. It helps the reader grasp the concepts of critical thinking and data analysis.

A critical thinking exercise, based on an actual case, is presented in the study guide/laboratory manual. Blank spaces are provided under each key step. This exercise encourages the reader to build critical thinking and data analysis skills. The reader can do this by working through the seven key steps of diagnostic reasoning based on the information in the case study and by documenting data and conclusions in the space provided. In addition, Interactive Nursing Assessment provides further opportunity to practice both collecting and analyzing data.

SUMMARY

Analysis of data is the second step of the nursing process. It is the purpose and end result of assessment. It is often called the diagnostic phase because the purpose of this phase is identification of nursing diagnoses, collaborative problems, or need for referral to another health care professional. The thought process required for data analysis is called diagnostic reasoning—a form of critical thinking. Therefore, it is important to develop the characteristics of critical thinking in order to analyze the data as accurately as possible.

Seven key steps have been developed for this text that clearly explain how to analyze assessment data. These steps include

1. Identify abnormal data and strengths.

2. Cluster data.

3. Draw inferences.

4. Propose possible nursing diagnoses.

5. Check for presence of defining characteristics.

6. Confirm or rule out nursing diagnoses.

7. Document conclusions.

Keep in mind that developing expertise in formulating nursing diagnoses requires much knowledge and experience as a nurse. However, the novice nurse can learn to increase diagnostic accuracy by becoming aware of, and avoiding, the pitfalls of diagnosing.

Because analysis of data is so closely linked to assessment, a special part on analysis of data is included in each body part or system assessment chapter.

References and Selected Readings

Alfaro, R. (2002). *Applying nursing process: Promoting collaborative care*. Philadelphia: Lippincott Williams & Wilkins.

Aquilino, M. L., & Keenan, G. (2000). Having our say: Nursing's standardized nomenclatures. *American Journal of Nursing, 100*(7), 33–38.

Carpenito-Moyer, L. J. (2007). *Nursing diagnosis: Applications to clinical practice* (12th ed.). Philadelphia: Lippincott Williams & Wilkins.

Cholowski, K. M., & Chan, L. K. (2004). Cognitive factors in student nurses' clinical problem solving. *Journal of Evaluating Clinical Practice, 10*(1), 85–95.

Doenges, M. E., & Moorhouse, M. F. (2008). *Application of nursing process and nursing diagnoses: An interactive text of diagnostic reasoning* (5th ed.). Philadelphia: F. A. Davis.

Ferrario, C. G. (2003). Experienced and less-experienced nurses' diagnostic reasoning: Implications for fostering students' critical thinking. *International Journal of Nursing Terminologies and Classifications, 14*(2), 41–52.

Forneris, S. G. (2004). Exploring the attributes of critical thinking: A conceptual basis. *International Journal of Nursing Education and Scholarship, 1*(1), (Article 9).

Glaser, V. (2000). Five diagnostic controversies. *Patient Care, 34*(3), 179–182, 185–186, 191–194.

Green, C. (2000). *Critical thinking in nursing*. Upper Saddle River, NJ: Prentice Hall.

Hardiker, N. R., Bakken, S., & Hoy, D. (2002). Formal nursing terminology systems: A means to an end. *Journal of Biomedical Informatics, 35*(5–6), 298–305.

Johnson, M., Bulechek, G., McCloskey Docterman, J., Maas, M., Moorhead, S., & Swanson, E. (2005). *NANDA, NOC, and NIC linkages: Nursing diagnoses, outcomes, and interventions* (2nd ed.). St. Louis: Elsevier Mosby.

Lunney, M. (2003). Critical thinking and accuracy of nurses' diagnoses. *International Journal of Nursing Terminologies and Classifications, 14*(3), 96–107.

McCloskey, M. C., & Bulechek, G. M. (2003). *Nursing interventions classification (NIC)* (2nd ed.). St. Louis: C. V. Mosby.

North American Nursing Diagnosis Association. (2009–2011). *Nursing diagnoses: Definitions and classification, 2009–2011*. Philadelphia: NANDA.

Rubenfeld, G., & Scheffer, B. (2006). *Critical thinking TACTICS for nurses: Tracking, assessing, and cultivating thinking to improve competency-based strategies*. Sudbury, MA: Jones & Bartlett.

Scroggins, L., & Harris, M. (2003). Evaluating nursing diagnoses. *International Journal of Nursing Terminologies and Classifications, 14*(4, Suppl. 8).

6

Assessing Mental
Status & Psychosocial
Developmental Level

Structure and Function

Mental status refers to a client's level of cognitive and emotional functioning and stability. Mental status is reflected in one's speech, appearance, and thought patterns. The ability to think clearly and respond appropriately to daily stressors of life is necessary to function effectively in the activities of daily living. The *American Heritage Dictionary of the English Language* (4th edition) defines **mental health** as "a state of emotional and psychological well-being in which an individual is able to use his or her cognitive and emotional capabilities, function in society, and meet the ordinary demands of everyday life." The lack of mental health is prevalent in Western societies today and may affect other body systems when prompt assessment and intervention is delayed.

The term "psychosocial development" is frequently used in nursing and refers to the client's mental and emotional health in addition to one's self-concept, role development, relationships, coping stress patterns, and spiritual beliefs. You will learn to assess both the mental status and psychosocial developmental level of the client in this chapter.

The structure and function of the neurological system can affect one's mental and psychosocial status. Cerebral abnormalities disturb the client's intellectual ability, communication ability, or emotional behaviors. Refer to Chapter 27 for a review of the structure and function of the cerebral cortex. Psychosocial status is also influenced by the psychosocial development the client has had over time. Erikson's theory of psychosocial development will be used in this text to determine the client's psychosocial developmental level. Refer to a psychology text for an in-depth review of Erikson's theory of developmental tasks.

Health Assessment

COLLECTING SUBJECTIVE DATA: THE NURSING HEALTH HISTORY

Be alert for all clues that reflect the client's mental and psychosocial status from the very first interaction you have with the client. Before asking questions to determine the client's mental and psychosocial status, explain the purpose of this part of the examination. Explain that some questions you ask may sound silly or irrelevant, but that they will help to determine how certain thought processes and activities of daily living are affecting the client's current health status. For example, it is only through in-depth questioning that the examiner may be able to tell that the client is having difficulty with concentration, which may be due to excessively stressful life situations or a neurological problem. Tell clients that they may refuse to answer any questions with which they are uncomfortable. Ensure confidentiality and respect for all that the clients share with you.

Problems with other body systems may affect mental status. For example, a client with a low blood sugar may report anxiety and other mental status changes. Regardless of the source of the problem, the client's total lifestyle and level of functioning may be affected. Because of the subjective nature of mental status and psychosocial developmental level, an in-depth nursing history is necessary to detect problems in this area affecting the client's activities of daily living. For example, the nurse will be able to find out that the client is having difficulty concentrating or remembering only through precise questioning during the interview.

Clients who are experiencing symptoms such as memory loss or confusion may fear that they have a serious condition such as a brain tumor or Alzheimer's disease. They may also fear a loss of control, independence, and role performance. Be sensitive to these fears and concerns because the client may decline to share important information with you if these concerns are not addressed. Often clients prefer to have a physiological problem rather than a mental disorder because of prior cultural beliefs that mental health problems may signify weakness and lack of control of oneself. Mental health problems often affect the client's self-image and self-concept in a negative manner.

While interviewing the client, you may encounter a variety of emotions expressed by the client. For example, clients may be very anxious about their health problem or angry that they are having a health problem. In addition you may have to discuss sensitive issues such as sexuality, dying, or spirituality with your client. Therefore, there are many interviewing skills you will need to develop to effectively complete a psychosocial history. For guidelines, see Display 2-2 "Interacting with clients with various emotional states."

BIOGRAPHICAL DATA

Question	Rationale
What is your name, address, and telephone number?	These answers will provide baseline data about the client's level of consciousness, memory, speech patterns, articulation, or speech defects. Inability to answer these questions may indicate a cognitive/neurological defect.
How old are you? Note if the client is male or female.	This information helps determine a reference point for which the client's psychosocial developmental level and appearance can be compared. Women tend to have a higher incidence of depression and anxiety, whereas men tend to have a higher incidence of substance abuse and psychosocial disorders.
What is your marital status?	Married adults often report less stress than single or divorced adults.
What is your educational level and where are you employed?	Psychosocial problems appear more often in those with lower incomes and lower educational levels. Clients from higher educational and socioeconomic levels tend to participate in more healthy lifestyles.

HISTORY OF PRESENT HEALTH CONCERN

Question	Rationale
What is your most urgent health concern at this time? Why are you seeking health care?	This information will help the examiner determine the client's perspective and ability to prioritize the reality of symptoms related to their current health status.

COLDSPA Example for Memory Loss

Use the **COLDSPA** mnemonic as a guideline to collect needed information for each symptom the client shares. In addition, the following questions help elicit important information.

Mnemonic	Question	Client Response Example
Character	Describe the sign or symptom (feeling, appearance, sound, smell, or taste if applicable).	"Cannot remember names of friends. I should know and sometimes cannot remember where I put things or where I am going next."
Onset	When did it begin?	"Three months—I thought it was stress, but it is getting worse."
Location	Where is it? Does it radiate? Does it occur anywhere else?	"I forget people's names at work and at church. I misplace things at work and home all the time."

continued

Mnemonic	Question	Client Response Example
Duration	How long does it last? Does it recur?	"I often have to ask people their name because I just cannot recall it. Sometimes it takes me 5 to 10 minutes to remember what I started out to do next."
Severity	How bad is it? How much does it bother you?	"I cannot get things done as fast as I used to because I am always forgetting what I intended to do and where I put things."
Pattern	What makes it better or worse?	"Sometimes it is better in the morning after a good night's sleep but gets worse as the day goes on."
Associated factors/How it **A**ffects the client	What other symptoms occur with it? How does it affect you?	"I have trouble getting my secretarial work done on time and I am afraid I am going to overlook or lose something important and lose my job."

PAST HEALTH HISTORY

Question	Rationale
Have you ever received medical treatment for a mental health problem or received any type of counseling services? Explain.	Some clients may have had a negative past experience with mental health care services.
Have you ever had any type of head injury, meningitis, encephalitis, or a stroke? What changes in your health did you notice as a result of these?	These conditions can affect the developmental level and the mental status of the client.
Do you have headaches? Describe.	Tension headaches may be seen in clients experiencing stressful situations.
Have you ever served in active duty in the armed forces? Explain.	Posttraumatic syndrome may be seen in veterans who experienced traumatic conditions in military combat.
Do you ever have trouble breathing or heart palpitations?	Clients with anxiety disorders may hyperventilate or have palpitations.

FAMILY HISTORY

Question	Rationale
Is there a history of mental health problems or Alzheimer's disease in your family?	Some psychiatric disorders may have a genetic or familial connection such as anxiety, depression, bipolar disorder and/or schizophrenia, or Alzheimer's disease.

LIFESTYLE AND HEALTH PRACTICES

Question	Rationale
Can you perform your normal activities of daily living? Describe a typical day. Describe your energy level.	Neurological and mental illnesses can alter one's responses to activities of daily living (ADLs). Depression may be seen in those with sedentary lifestyles. Anxious clients may be restless, while depressed clients may feel fatigued. Clients with eating disorders may exercise excessively.

continued on page 58

LIFESTYLE AND HEALTH PRACTICES *Continued*

Question	Rationale
Describe your normal eating habits.	Poor appetite may be seen with depression, eating disorders, and substance abuse.
Describe your daily bowel elimination patterns.	Irritable bowel syndrome or peptic ulcer disease may be associated with psychological disorders.
Describe your sleep patterns.	Insomnia is often seen in depression, anxiety disorders, bipolar disorder, and substance abuse.
Do you take any prescribed or over-the-counter medications? How much alcohol do you drink? Do you use recreational drugs such as marijuana, tranquilizers, barbiturates, or cocaine?	Use of these substances may alter one's level of consciousness, decrease response times, and cause changes in moods and temperament. Inappropriate use of any of these substances may indicate alcoholism or drug abuse problems.
Have you been exposed to any environmental toxins?	Cognition may be altered with toxin exposure.
What religious affiliations do you have?	Certain religious beliefs can affect the client's ability to cope in a positive or negative manner.
How do you feel about yourself and your relationship with others?	Clients with a low self-concept may be depressed or suffer from eating disorders or have substance abuse problems. Clients with psychological problems often have difficulty maintaining effective meaningful relationships.
What do you perceive as your role in your family or relationship with your significant other?	Mental health problems often interfere with one's role in families and relationships. In turn, stressful relationships or roles may interfere with one's mental health.

COLLECTING OBJECTIVE DATA: PHYSICAL EXAMINATION

Sometimes the mental status examination may be performed with a complete neurological assessment, which also includes assessment of cranial nerves, motor and cerebellar function, sensory function, and reflexes. Among all of these neurological assessments, the mental status exam assesses the highest level of cerebral integration. The advantage of assessing mental status at the very beginning of the head-to-toe examination is that it provides clues regarding the validity of the subjective information provided by the client throughout the exam. Thus it is best to determine validity of client responses before completing the entire physical exam only to learn that the client's answers to questions may have been inaccurate. If the nurse finds out that the client's thought processes are impaired, another means of obtaining necessary subjective data must be identified.

A comprehensive mental status examination is quite lengthy and involves great care on the part of the examiner to put the client at ease. There are several parts of the examination which include assessment of the client's level of consciousness, posture, gait, body movements, dress, grooming, hygiene, facial expressions, behavior and affect, speech, mood, feelings, expressions, thought processes, perceptions, and cognitive abilities. Cognitive abilities include orientation, concentration, recent and remote memory, abstract reasoning, judgment, visual perception, and constructional ability.

If time is limited and a quick standard measure is needed to evaluate or reevaluate one's mental state, the mental status examinations found in Assessment Tool 6-1 may be used to obtain a score for the client's mental status. If depression is suspected, the Depression Questionnaire (Self-Assessment 6-1) may be completed by the client. In addition, The Alzheimer's Guide (Assessment Tool 6-2) may be used by the examiner to determine if the client may have any early warning signs of Alzheimer's disease.

Preparing the Client

Some of the questions you will be asking when collecting both subjective and objective data may seem silly or may embarrass the client. For example, the client will be asked to explain the meaning of a proverb, such as "a stitch in time saves nine." They will also be asked to name the day of the week and explain where they are at the time of the exam. With practice you will learn how to infer this information without direct questioning, just by observing the client's responses to other questions during the exam.

Equipment

- Pencil and paper
- Saint Louis University Mental Status (SLUMS) Examination Tool and The Confusion Assessment Method (CAM)
- Depression Questionnaire
- Alzheimer's Guide of Early Warning Signs

ASSESSMENT TOOL 6-1   Mental Status Examinations

Saint Louis University

Mental Status (SLUMS) Examination

Name _____   Age _____

Is patient alert? _____   Level of education _____

❶ 1. What day of the week is it?

❶ 2. What is the year?

❶ 3. What state are we in?

4. Please remember these five objects. I will ask you what they are later.
   Apple   Pen   Tie   House   Car

5. You have $100 and you go to the store and buy a dozen apples for $3 and a tricycle for $20.
❶ How much did you spend?
❷ How much do you have left?

6. Please name as many animals as you can in one minute.
❶ 0–5 animals   ❷ 5–10 animals   ❸ 10–15 animals   ❹ 15+ animals

❺ 7. What were the 5 objects I asked you to remember? 1 point for each one correct.

8. I am going to give you a series of numbers and I would like you to give them to me backwards.
   For example, if I say 42, you would say 24.
❶ 87   ❷ 649   ❸ 8537

9. This is a clock face. Please put in the hour markers and the time at ten minutes
   to eleven o'clock.
❷ Hour markers okay
❷ Time correct

❶ 10. Please place an X in the triangle.

❶ Which of the above figures is largest?

11. I am going to tell you a story. Please listen carefully because afterwards, I'm going to ask you some questions about
   it.

   Jill was a very successful stockbroker. She made a lot of money on the stock market. She then met Jack, a devastatingly
   handsome man. She married him and had three children. They lived in Chicago. She then stopped work and stayed at home
   to bring up her children. When they were teenagers, she went back to work. She and Jack lived happily ever after.

❷ What was the female's name?   ❷ What work did she do?
❷ When did she go back to work?   ❷ What state did she live in?

Scoring

High School Education		Less than High School Education
27–30	Normal	20–30
20–27	MCI	14–19
1–19	Dementia	1–14

continued on page 60

ASSESSMENT TOOL 6-1   **Mental Status Examinations** *Continued*

The Confusion Assessment Method (CAM) Instrument

1. [Acute Onset] Is there evidence of an acute change in mental status from the patient's baseline?

2A. [Inattention] Did the patient have difficulty focusing attention, for example, being easily distractable, or having difficulty keeping track of what was being said?

2B. [If present or abnormal] Did this behavior fluctuate during the interview, that is, tend to come and go or increase and decrease in severity?

3. [Disorganized thinking] Was the patient's thinking disorganized or incoherent, such as rambling or irrelevant conversation, unclear or illogical flow of ideas, or unpredictable switching from subject to subject?

4. [Altered level of consciousness] Overall, how would you rate this patient's level of consciousness? (Alert [normal]; Vigilant [hyperalert, overly sensitive to environmental stimuli, startled very easily]; Lethargic [drowsy, easily aroused]; Stupor [difficult to arouse]; Coma [unarousable]; Uncertain)

5. [Disorientation] Was the patient disoriented at any time during the interview, such as thinking that he or she was somewhere other than the hospital, using the wrong bed, or misjudging the time of day?

6. [Memory impairment] Did the patient demonstrate any memory problems during the interview, such as inability to remember events in the hospital or difficulty remembering instructions?

7. [Perceptual disturbances] Did the patient have any evidence of perceptual disturbances, for example, hallucinations, illusions, or misinterpretations (such as thinking something was moving when it was not)?

8A. [Psychomotor agitation] At any time during the interview did the patient have an unusually increased level of motor activity such as restlessness, picking at bedclothes, tapping fingers or making frequent sudden changes of position?

8B. [Psychomotor retardation] At any time during the interview did the patient have an unusually decreased level of motor activity such as sluggishness, staring into space, staying in one position for a long time or moving very slowly?

9. [Altered sleep-wake cycle] Did the patient have evidence of disturbance of the sleep-wake cycle, such as excessive daytime sleepiness with insomnia at night?

The Confusion Assessment Method (CAM) Diagnostic Algorithm

Feature 1: *Acute Onset or Fluctuating Course*

This feature is usually obtained from a family member or nurse and is shown by positive responses to the following questions: Is there evidence of an acute change in mental status from the patient's baseline? Did the (abnormal) behavior fluctuate during the day, that is, tend to come and go, or increase and decrease in severity?

Feature 2: *Inattention*

This feature is shown by a positive response to the following question: Did the patient have difficulty focusing attention, for example, being easily distractible, or having difficulty keeping track of what is being said?

Feature 3: *Disorganized thinking*

This feature is shown by a positive response to the following question: Was the patient's thinking disorganized or incoherent, such as rambling or irrelevant conversation, unclear or illogical flow of ideas, or unpredictable switching from subject to subject?

Feature 4: *Altered Level of consciousness*

This feature is shown by any answer other than "alert" to the followitn question: Overall, how would you rate this patient's level of consciousness? (Alert [normal]; Vigilant [hyperalert, overly sensitive to environmental stimuli, startled very easily]; Lethargic [drowsy, easily aroused]; Stupor [difficult to arouse]; Coma [unarousable])

The diagnosis of delirium by CAM requires the presence of features 1 and 2 and either 3 or 4.

The Confusion Assessment Method (CAM) Algorithm: Inouye SK, vanDyck CH, Alessi CA, Balkin S. Siegal AP, Horwitz RI. Clarifying Confusion: The Confusion Assessment Method: A New Method for Detection of Delirium. Ann Intern Med. 1990; 113:941–48. Used with Permission.

SELF-ASSESSMENT 6-1   Depression Questionnaire

The following DEPRESSION QUESTIONNAIRE has 16 simple questions that may help identify common symptoms of depression. The results can be a helpful way to discuss your condition with your healthcare provider and actually help him/her diagnose your condition. After answering the questions provided on the following pages, print the completed questionnaire and discuss any concerns with your doctor.

As with any medical illness or condition, only your doctor or other qualified healthcare professional can provide a diagnosis of depression. The following questionnaire is intended to help you discuss symptoms with a qualified healthcare professional. This questionnaire is not intended to serve as a substitute for a diagnosis of depression by a qualified healthcare professional. If you think you may have depression, you should visit your doctor or other qualified healthcare professional as soon as possible.

Complete the questionnaire below and take the results to your doctor.

Choose the items that best describe you over the last 7 days.

1. Falling Asleep
0   I never take longer than 30 minutes to fall asleep.
1   I take at least 30 minutes to fall asleep, less than half the time.
2   I take at least 30 minutes to fall asleep, more than half the time.
3   I take more than 60 minutes to fall asleep, more than half the time.

2. Sleep During the Night
0   I do not wake up at night.
1   I have a restless, light sleep with a few brief awakenings each night.
2   I wake up at least once a night, but I go back to sleep easily.
3   I awaken more than once a night and stay awake for 20 minutes or more, more than half the time.

3. Waking Up Too Early
0   Most of the time, I awaken no more than 30 minutes before I need to get up.
1   More than half the time I awaken more than 30 minutes before I need to get up.
2   I almost always awaken at least one hour or so before I need to, but I go back to sleep eventually.
3   I awaken at least one hour before I need to, and can't go back to sleep.

4. Sleeping Too Much
0   I sleep no longer than 7–8 hours/night, without napping during the day.
1   I sleep no longer than 10 hours in a 24-hour period including naps.
2   I sleep no longer than 12 hours in a 24-hour period including naps.
3   I sleep longer than 12 hours in a 24-hour period including naps.

5. Feeling Sad
0   I do not feel sad.
1   I feel sad less than half the time.
2   I feel sad more than half the time.
3   I feel sad nearly all of the time.

(Please complete either 6 or 7)

6. Decreased Appetite
0   There is no change in my usual appetite.
1   I eat somewhat less often or lesser amounts of food than usual.
2   I eat much less than usual and only with personal effort.
3   I rarely eat within a 24-hour period, and only with extreme personal effort or when others persuade me to eat.

7. Increased Appetite
0   There is no change from my usual appetite.
1   I feel a need to eat more frequently than usual.
2   I regularly eat more often and/or greater amounts of food than usual.
3   I feel driven to overeat both at mealtime and between meals.

(Please complete either 8 or 9)

8. Decreased Weight (Within the Last Two Weeks)
0   I have not had a change in my weight.
1   I feel as if I've had a slight weight loss.
2   I have lost 2 pounds or more.
3   I have lost 5 pounds or more.

9. Increased Weight (Within the Last Two Weeks)
0   I have not had a change in my weight.
1   I feel as if I've had a slight weight gain.
2   I have gained 2 pounds or more.
3   I have gained 5 pounds or more.

10. Concentration/Decision-Making
0   There is no change in my usual capacity to concentrate or make decisions.
1   I occasionally feel indecisive or find that my attention wanders.
2   Most of the time, I struggle to focus my attention or to make decisions.
3   I cannot concentrate well enough to read or cannot make even minor decisions.

11. View of Myself
0   I see myself as equally worthwhile and deserving as other people.
1   I am more self-blaming than usual.
2   I largely believe that I cause problems for others.
3   I think almost constantly about major and minor defects in myself.

12. Thoughts of Death or Suicide
0   I do not think of suicide or death.
1   I feel that life is empty or wonder if it's worth living.
2   I think of suicide or death several times a week for several minutes.
3   I think of suicide or death several times a day in some detail, or I have made specific plans for suicide or have actually tried to take my life.

continued on page 62

SELF ASSESSMENT 6-1 | **Depression Questionnaire** *Continued*

13. General Interest
0 There is no change from usual in how interested I am in other people or activities.
1 I notice that I am less interested in people or activities.
2 I find I have interest in only one or two of my formerly pursued activities.
3 I have virtually no interest in formerly pursued activities.

14. Energy Level
0 There is no change in my usual level of energy.
1 I get tired more easily than usual.
2 I have to make a big effort to start or finish my usual daily activities (for example, shopping, homework, cooking or going to work).
3 I really cannot carry out most of my usual daily activities because I just don't have the energy.

15. Feeling Slowed Down
0 I think, speak, and move at my usual rate of speed.
1 I find that my thinking is slowed down or my voice sounds dull or flat.
2 It takes me several seconds to respond to most questions and I'm sure my thinking is slowed.
3 I am often unable to respond to questions without extreme effort.

16. Feeling Restless
0 I do not feel restless.
1 I'm often fidgety, wringing my hands, or need to shift how I am sitting.
2 I have impulses to move about and am quite restless.
3 At times, I am unable to stay seated and need to pace around.

Depression Questionnaire Scoring

Each of the four possible answers to each quiz question is given an ascending numerical value from 0 to 3, and the total test score is calculated by using the following formula:

Enter the highest score on any 1 of the 4 sleep items, questions 1–4 _____

Enter the score from question 5 _____

Enter the highest score on any 1 appetite/weight item, questions 6–9 _____

Enter the score from question 10 _____

Enter the score from question 11 _____

Enter the score from question 12 _____

Enter the score from question 13 _____

Enter the score from question 14 _____

Enter the highest score on either of the 2 psychomotor items, questions 15 and 16 _____

TOTAL SCORE (Range 0–27) _____

Interpreting the scores

0–5	None
6–10	Mild
11–15	Moderate
16–20	Severe
21–27	Very Severe

© 2000, A. John Rush, M.D., Quick Inventory of Depressive Symptomatology (Self Report) (QIDS-SR).

ASSESSMENT TOOL 6-2 | **The Alzheimer's Guide**

Seven Alzheimer's Warning Signs

1. Asking the same question over and over again
2. Repeating the same story, word for word, again and again
3. Forgetting how to cook, or how to make repairs, or how to play cards—activities that were previously done with ease and regularity
4. Losing one's ability to pay bills or balance one's checkbook

5. Getting lost in familiar surroundings, or misplacing household objects
6. Neglecting to bathe, or wearing the same clothes over and over again, while insisting that they have taken a bath or that their clothes are still clean
7. Relying on someone else, such as a spouse, to make decisions or answer questions they previously would have handled themselves (WebMD, 2005–2007)

Used with permission of University of South Florida, Suncoast Gerontology Center.

PHYSICAL ASSESSMENT

Assessment Procedure	Normal Findings	Abnormal Findings

Mental Status and Level of Consciousness

Inspection

Observe the client's level of consciousness. Ask the client his or her name, address, and phone number (Fig. 6-1).

Client is alert and oriented to what is happening at the time of the interview and physical assessment. Client is alert to person, place, day, and time, and responds to your questions and interacts appropriately.

Although the older client's response and ability to process information may be slower, he or she is normally alert and oriented.

If the client does not respond appropriately, *call the client's name and note the response.* If the client does not respond, call the name louder. If necessary, shake the client gently. If the client still does not respond, apply a painful stimulus.

Client is alert and awake with eyes open and looking at examiner. Client responds appropriately.

The following levels of consciousness are abnormal:

Lethargy: Client opens eyes, answers questions, and falls back asleep.

Obtunded: Client opens eyes to loud voice, responds slowly with confusion, seems unaware of environment.

Stupor: Client awakens to vigorous shake or painful stimuli but returns to unresponsive sleep.

Coma: Client remains unresponsive to all stimuli; eyes stay closed. Client with lesions of the corticospinal tract draws hands up to chest (*decorticate* or abnormal flexor posture) when stimulated (Fig. 6-2).

Client with lesions of the diencephalon, midbrain, or pons extends arms and legs, arches neck and rotates hands and arms internally (*decerebrate* or abnormal extensor posture) when stimulated (Fig. 6-3).

> ➤ **Clinical Tip** • When assessing the level of consciousness, always begin with the least noxious stimulus: verbal, tactile, to painful.

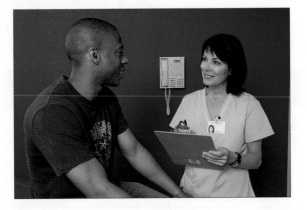

Figure 6-1   Assessing level of consciousness.

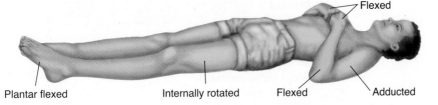

Flexed

Plantar flexed   Internally rotated   Flexed   Adducted

Figure 6-2   Decorticate posture.

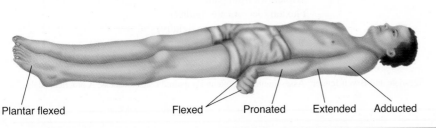

Plantar flexed   Flexed   Pronated   Extended   Adducted

Figure 6-3   Decerebrate posture.

continued

PHYSICAL ASSESSMENT *Continued*

Assessment Procedure	Normal Findings	Abnormal Findings
Use the Glasgow Coma Scale (GCS) for clients who are at high risk for rapid deterioration of the nervous system (Assessment Tool 6-3).	GCS score of 14 indicates an optimal level of consciousness.	GCS score of less than 14 indicates some impairment in the level of consciousness. A score of 3, the lowest possible score, indicates deep coma.
Observe posture, gait, and body movements. Be alert for tense, nervous, fidgety, and restless behavior, which may be seen in anxiety or may simply reflect the client's apprehension during a physical examination.	The client appears to be relaxed with shoulders and back erect when standing or sitting. Gait is rhythmic and coordinated with arms swinging at sides.	Slumped posture may reflect feelings of powerlessness or hopelessness characteristic of depression or organic brain disease. Bizarre body movements and behavior may be noted in schizophrenia or may be a side effect of drug therapy or other activity. Tense or anxious clients may elevate their shoulders toward their ears and hold the entire body stiffly.
Observe behavior and affect.	Client is cooperative and purposeful in his or her interactions with others. Mild to moderate anxiety may be normal in a client who is having a health assessment performed. Affect is appropriate for the client's situation.	Uncooperative, bizarre behavior may be seen in the angry, mentally ill, or violent client. Anxious clients are often fidgety and restless. Some degree of anxiety is often seen in ill clients. Apathy or crying may be seen with depression. Incongruent behavior may be seen in clients who are in denial of problems or illness. Prolonged, euphoric laughing is typical of mania.

In the older adult, purposeless movements, wandering, aggressiveness, or withdrawal may indicate neurological deficits. |

ASSESSMENT TOOL 6-3   Using the Glasgow Coma Scale

The Glasgow Coma Scale is useful for rating one's response to stimuli. The client who scores 10 or lower needs emergency attention. The client with a score of 7 or lower is generally considered to be in a coma.

		Score
Eye opening response	Spontaneous opening	4
	To verbal command	3
	To pain	2
	No response	1
Most appropriate verbal response	Oriented	5
	Confused	4
	Inappropriate words	3
	Incoherent	2
	No response	1
Most integral motor response (arm)	Obeys verbal commands	6
	Localizes pain	5
	Withdraws from pain	4
	Flexion (decorticate rigidity)	3
	Extension (decerebrate rigidity)	2
	No response	1
TOTAL SCORE		3 to 15

Reprinted from *The Lancet, 304/7872,* Graham Teasdale and Bryan Jennett, Assessment of coma and impaired consciousness: A practical scale, pg 4, © 1974, with permission from Elsevier.

continued

Assessment Procedure	Normal Findings	Abnormal Findings
Observe dress and grooming. Keep the examination setting and the reason for the assessment in mind as you note the client's degree of cleanliness and attire. For example, if the client arrives directly from home, he or she may be neater than if he or she comes to the assessment from the workplace. ➤ *Clinical Tip • Be careful not to make premature judgments regarding the client's dress. Styles and clothing fads (e.g., torn jeans, oversized clothing, baggy pants), developmental level, socioeconomic level, and culture, all influence a person's dress (e.g., Indian women wear saris; Hasidic Jewish men wear black suits and black skull caps).*	Dress is appropriate for occasion and weather. Dress varies considerably from person to person, depending on individual preference. There may be several normal dress variations depending on the client's developmental level, age, socioeconomic level, and culture or subculture. Some older adults may wear excess clothing because of slowed metabolism and loss of subcutaneous fat, resulting in cold intolerance.	Unusually meticulous grooming and finicky mannerisms may be seen in obsessive-compulsive disorder. Poor hygiene and inappropriate dress may be seen in depression, schizophrenia, dementia, and Alzheimer's disease. One-sided neglect may result from lesion in the opposite parietal cortex, usually the nondominant side. Uncoordinated clothing, extremely light clothing, or extremely warm clothing for the weather conditions may be seen on mentally ill, grieving, depressed, or poor clients. This may also be noted in clients with heat or cold intolerances. Extremely loose clothing held up by pins or a belt may suggest recent weight loss. Clients wearing long sleeves in warm weather may be protecting themselves from the sun or covering up needle marks secondary to drug abuse. Soiled clothing may indicate homelessness, elderly vision deficits, or mental illness.
Observe hygiene. Determine what the normal level of hygiene is for the client's developmental and socioeconomic level and cultural background.	The client is clean and groomed appropriately for occasion. Stains on hands and dirty nails may reflect certain occupations such as mechanic or gardener. Asians and Native Americans have fewer sweat glands and, therefore, less obvious body odor than most Caucasians and black Africans, who have more sweat glands. Additionally some cultures do not use deodorant products (see Chapter 13 for more information).	A dirty, unshaven, unkempt appearance with a foul body odor may reflect depression, drug abuse, or low socioeconomic level (i.e., homeless client). Poor hygiene may be seen in dementia or other conditions that indicate a self-care deficit. If the client is cared for by others, poor hygiene may reflect neglect by caregiver or caregiver role strain. Breath odors from smoking or from drinking alcoholic beverages may be noted as may diet-related odors such as garlic or soy products.
Observe facial expressions. Note particularly eye contact and affect.	Client maintains good eye contact, smiles, and frowns appropriately.	Poor eye contact is seen in depression or apathy. Extreme facial expressions of happiness, anger, or fright may be seen in anxious clients. Clients with Parkinson's disease may have a mask-like, expressionless face. Staring watchfulness appears in metabolic disorders and anxiety. Inappropriate facial expressions (e.g., smiling when expressing sad thoughts) may indicate mental illness. Drooping or gross asymmetry occurs with neurological disorder or injury (e.g., Bell's palsy or stroke).

continued

PHYSICAL ASSESSMENT *Continued*

Assessment Procedure	Normal Findings	Abnormal Findings
Observe speech. Observe and listen to tone, clarity, and pace of speech.	Speech is in a moderate tone, clear, with moderate pace, and culturally appropriate. Normally in older adults, responses may be slowed but speech should be clear and moderately paced.	Slow, repetitive speech is characteristic of depression or Parkinson's disease. Loud, rapid speech may occur in manic phases of bipolar disorder. Disorganized speech, consistent (nonstop) speech, or long periods of silence may indicate mental illness or a neurological disorder (e.g., dysarthria, dysphasia, speech defect, garbled speech). Table 6-1 provides further information about voice and speech problems.
If the client has difficulty with speech, perform additional tests: • Ask the client to name objects in the room. • Ask the client to read from printed material appropriate for his or her educational level. • Ask the client to write a sentence. ➤ *Clinical Tip* • *Speech is largely influenced by experience, level of education, and culture.*	Client names familiar objects without difficulty. Reads age-appropriate written print. Writes a coherent sentence with correct spelling and grammar.	Client cannot name objects correctly, read print correctly, or write a basic correct sentence. Deficits in this area require further neurologic assessment to identify any dysfunction of higher cortical levels.
Observe mood, feelings, and expressions. Ask client "How are you feeling today?" and "What are your plans for the future?" ➤ *Clinical Tip* • *Moods and feelings often vary from sadness to joy to anger, depending on the situation and circumstance.*	Cooperative or friendly, expresses feelings appropriate to situation, verbalizes positive feelings regarding others and the future, expresses positive coping mechanisms (support groups, exercise, sports, hobbies, counseling).	Expression of prolonged negative, gloomy, despairing feelings is noted in depression (see Self-Assessment 6-1). Expression of elation and grandiosity, high energy level, and engagement in high-risk but pleasurable activities is seen in manic phases. Excessive worry may be seen in anxiety or obsessive-compulsive disorders. Eccentric moods not appropriate to the situation are seen in schizophrenia.

Table 6-1   Sources of Voice and Speech Problems

Problem	Description	Source
Dysphonia	Voice volume disorder	Laryngeal disorders or impairment of cranial nerve X (vagus nerve)
Cerebellar dysarthria	Irregular, uncoordinated speech	Multiple sclerosis
Dysarthria	Defect in muscular control of speech (eg, slurring)	Lesions of the nervous system, Parkinson's disease, or cerebellar disease
Aphasia	Difficulty producing or understanding language	Motor lesions in the dominant cerebral hemisphere
Wernicke's aphasia	Rapid speech that lacks meaning	Lesion in the posterior superior temporal lobe
Broca's aphasia	Slowed speech with difficult articulation, but fairly clear meaning	Lesion in the posterior inferior frontal lobe

continued

Assessment Procedure	Normal Findings	Abnormal Findings
Observe thought processes and perceptions. Observe thought processes for clarity, content, and perception by inquiring about client's thoughts and perceptions expressed. Use statements such as "Tell me more about what you just said." or "Tell me what your understanding is of the current situation or your health." ➤ *Clinical Tip* • *When assessing the mental status of an older client, be sure first to check vision and hearing before assuming the client has a mental problem.*	Client expresses full, free-flowing thoughts; follows directions accurately; expresses realistic perceptions; is easy to understand and makes sense; does not voice suicidal thoughts.	Abnormal processes include persistent repetition of ideas, illogical thoughts, interruption of ideas, invention of words, or repetition of phrases as in schizophrenia; rapid flight of ideas, repetition of ideas, and use of rhymes and punning as in manic phases of bipolar disorder; continuous, irrational fears, and avoidance of an object or situation as in phobias; delusion, extreme apprehension; compulsions; obsessions; and illusions are also abnormal (see the glossary for definitions).
Identify possibly destructive or suicidal tendencies in client's thought processes and perceptions by asking, "How do you feel about the future?" or "Have you ever had thoughts of hurting yourself or doing away with yourself?" or "How do others feel about you?"	Verbalizes positive, healthy thoughts about the future and self.	Clients who are suicidal may share past attempts of suicide, give plan for suicide, verbalize worthlessness about self, joke about death frequently. Clients who are depressed or feel hopeless are at higher risk for suicide.
Use Geriatric Depression Scale if depression is suspected in the older client (see Chapter 32). Read the questions to the client if the client cannot read.	Scores 10 or less.	Scores between 10 and 30 may indicate depression.
Observe cognitive abilities. *Orientation:* Ask for the client's name and names of family members (person), the time such as hour, day, date, or season (time), and where the client lives or is now (place). ➤ *Clinical Tip* • *When assessing orientation to time, place, and person, remember that orientation to time is usually lost first and orientation to person is usually lost last.*	Client is aware of self, others, time, home address, and current location. Some older clients may seem confused, especially in a new or acute care setting, but most know who and where they are and the current month and year.	Reduced degree of orientation may be seen with organic brain disorders or psychiatric illness such as withdrawal from chronic alcohol use or schizophrenia. (*Note:* Schizophrenia may be marked by hallucinations—sensory perceptions that occur without external stimuli—as well as disorientation.)
Concentration: Note the client's ability to focus and stay attentive to you during the interview and examination. Give the client directions such as "Please pick up the pencil with your left hand, place it in your right hand, then hand it to me."	Client listens and can follow directions without difficulty. Some older clients may like to reminisce and tend to wander somewhat from the topic at hand.	Distraction and inability to focus on task at hand are noted in anxiety, fatigue, attention deficit disorders, and impaired states due to alcohol or drug intoxication.
Recent Memory: Ask the client "What did you have to eat today?" or "What is the weather like today?"	Recalls recent events without difficulty. Some older clients may exhibit hesitation with short-term memory.	Inability to recall recent events is seen in delirium, dementia, depression, and anxiety.
Remote Memory: Ask the client: "When did you get your first job?" or "When is your birthday?" Information on past health history also gives clues as to the client's ability to recall remote events.	Client correctly recalls past events.	Inability to recall past events is seen in cerebral cortex disorders.

continued

PHYSICAL ASSESSMENT *Continued*

Assessment Procedure	Normal Findings	Abnormal Findings
Use of Memory to Learn New Information: Ask the client to repeat four unrelated words. The words should not rhyme and they cannot have the same meaning (e.g., rose, hammer, automobile, brown). Have the client repeat these words in 5 minutes, again in 10 minutes, and again in 30 minutes.	Client is able to recall words correctly after a 5-, a 10-, and a 30-minute period. Clients older than 80 should recall two to four words after 5 minutes and possibly after 10 and 30 minutes with hints that prompt recall.	Inability to recall words after a delayed period is seen in anxiety, depression, or Alzheimer's disease. If Alzheimer's is a concern, use Assessment Tool 6-2 to determine with the client and family if early warning signs are present. Refer to Promote Health—Dementias for more information about Alzheimer's disease and other forms of dementia.
Abstract Reasoning: Ask the client to compare objects. For example, "How are an apple and orange the same? How are they different?" Also ask the client to explain a proverb. For example, "A rolling stone gathers no moss" or "A stitch in time saves nine." ➤ *Clinical Tip • If clients have limited education, note their ability to joke or use puns, which also requires abstract reasoning.*	Client explains similarities and differences between objects and proverbs correctly. The client with limited education can joke and use puns correctly.	Inability to compare and contrast objects correctly or interpret proverbs correctly is seen in schizophrenia, mental retardation, delirium, and dementia.
Judgment: Ask the client, "What do you do if you have pain?" or "What would you do if you were driving and a police car was behind you with its lights and siren turned on?"	Answers to questions are based on sound rationale.	Impaired judgment may be seen in organic brain syndrome, emotional disturbances, mental retardation, or schizophrenia.
Visual Perceptual and Constructional Ability: Ask the client to draw the face of a clock or copy simple figures (Fig. 6-4).	Draws the face of a clock fairly well. Can copy simple figures.	Inability to draw the face of a clock or copy simple figures correctly is seen with mental retardation, dementia, or parietal lobe dysfunction of the cerebral cortex.

Figure 6-4 Figures to be drawn by client.

Assessment Procedure	Normal Findings	Abnormal Findings
Use the Saint Louis University Mental Status (SLUMS) Examination if time is limited and a quick measure is needed to evaluate cognitive function. If further assessment is needed to distinguish delirium from other types of cognitive impairment use The Confusion Assessment Method (CAM) (See Assessment Tool 6-1). ➤ *Clinical Tip • This examination tests level of orientation, memory, speech, and cognitive functions but not mood, feelings, expressions, thought processes, or perceptions.*	A score between 27–30 for clients with a high school education and a score of 20–30 for clients with less than a high school education is considered normal.	For clients with a high school education a score of 20–27 indicates mild cognitive impairment (MCI) and for clients with less than high school education a score of 14–19 indicates MCI. For clients with a high school education a score of 1–19 indicates dementia and for clients with less than high school education a score of 1–14 indicates dementia. A diagnosis of delirium by CAM requires the presence of features 1 and 2 and either 3 or 4 under the CAM Diagnostic Algorithm (Assessment Tool 6-1). *Caution:* Note that potential harm from labeling or identifying clients with possible dementia must be weighed against benefits of assessment (Patterson, 2000).

PROMOTE HEALTH
Dementias

Overview

Dementia is the name given to loss of cognitive skills. These changes occur because of brain diseases or trauma. The cognitive changes can have a rapid or a gradual onset. Cognitive changes resulting from dementias include decision making/judgment, memory, spatial orientation, thinking/reasoning, verbal communication, personal safety, hygiene or nutrition neglect, and coordination and balance (Alzheimer's Association, 2007). Note that memory loss by itself is not necessarily a sign of dementia. It is predicted that about 33% of women and 20% of men over 65 years of age will develop dementia (Yaffe, 2007).

General symptoms of dementia (Alzheimer's Association, 2007):
- Repeatedly asking the same questions
- Becoming lost or disoriented in familiar places
- Being unable to follow directions
- Getting disoriented as to the date or time of day
- Not recognizing and being confused about familiar people
- Having difficulty with routine tasks such as paying the bills
- Neglecting personal safety, hygiene, and nutrition

Alzheimer's disease, the most common dementia of the elderly, results from gradual destruction of brain nerve cells and a shrinking brain. Symptoms resemble general dementia symptoms but include loss of recent memory, depression, anxiety, personality changes, unpredictable quirks or behaviors, and problems with language, calculation, and abstract thinking. Late in the disease, delusions and hallucinations can occur (Alzheimer's Association, 2007).

Vascular dementia (multi-infarct dementia) results from small strokes or brain blood supply changes usually caused by blood clots in small vessels. Brain location causes variation in symptoms and the symptoms may have a sudden onset. Wandering or getting lost in familiar surroundings; moving with rapid, shuffling steps; loss of bladder or bowel control; laughing or crying inappropriately; difficulty following instructions; and problems handling money are characteristic (Alzheimer's Association, 2007). This dementia has no cure and is not reversible.

A person can have mixed dementia. Other diseases that may have a dementia component or symptoms similar to dementia include Pick's disease, Creutzfeldt–Jakob disease, Huntington's disease, Parkinson's disease, and Lewy body disease, as well as other central nervous system conditions, systemic conditions (nutrition, fever, hormone, poisoning-related), substance abuse, and psychological stress and psychosis.

Aging has common forms of decline that are often *mistaken* for dementia or resemble dementia. These include slower thinking, problem solving, learning, and recall; decreased attention and concentration; more distractedness; and need for hints to jog memory.

Risk Factors
- Vascular, cerebrovascular, or cardiovascular disease (CVA, diabetes mellitus type II, cardiac disease, and hypertension), especially with the metabolic syndrome factors abdominal obesity, hypertriglyceridemia, low levels of high-density lipoproteins (HDL), hypertension, hyperglycemia
- Physical, intellectual, social, and nutritional habits
- Age; slightly higher in females over 80 years old
- Obesity (especially abdominal) and for obese cigarette smokers
- Genetics, but it is not well understood how diet and environment interact with genetics
- Gait disturbances may correlate with early dementia
- Diet, especially high cholesterol
- Environment, especially heavy metals
- Cigarette smoking
- Alcohol consumption

Teach Risk Reduction Tips
- Consult primary care provider to control vascular, cerebrovascular, cardiovascular diseases, especially including hypertension, diabetes mellitus II, and cardiac disease.
- Maintain active engagement in mental, physical, and social activities
- Eat a healthy diet avoiding high cholesterol and including a variety of fruits and vegetables
- Ask a primary health provider about the possible preventive effects and safety of nonsteroidal anti-inflammatory drugs (NSAIDs); hormonal therapy; antihypertensive medications, especially potassium-sparing diuretics; antioxidants. Ask about including about 2000 to 8000 mg per day of the spice curcumin in one's diet (Alzheimer's Disease Health Center, 2005).

DEVELOPMENTAL LEVEL: PSYCHOSOCIAL STATUS

Determining the client's developmental level is essential to complete the client's portrait. You do not need to ask the client additional questions unless major gaps in the data collection are found or clarification is needed. Instead, group and analyze the data obtained during the health history and compare them with normal developmental parameters (e.g., height, weight, Erikson's psychosocial developmental stages; see Learning theories, 2009). This requires integrating all that has been learned about the client by the health history and using critical thinking to determine any developmental impairments. Standard growth charts can be used to determine physical development.

However, when assessing adults, the area most likely to yield delays or unresolved problems occurs in the psychosocial domain of development. The theorist Erik H. Erikson developed a psychosocial theory that identifies a number of dichotomous concepts to describe growth from birth to death

Table 6-2	Erik H. Erikson's Psychosocial Developmental Levels		
Developmental Level	**Basic Task**	**Negative Counterpart**	**Basic Virtues**
1. Infant	Basic trust	Basic mistrust	Drive and hope
2. Toddler	Autonomy	Shame and doubt	Self-control and will power
3. Preschooler	Initiative	Guilt	Direction and purpose
4. Schoolager	Industry	Inferiority	Method and competence
5. Adolescent	Identity	Role confusion	Devotion and fidelity
6. Young adult	Intimacy	Isolation	Affiliation and love
7. Middlescent	Generativity	Stagnation	Production and care
8. Older adult	Ego-integrity	Despair	Renunciation and wisdom

Adapted from Erikson's Stages of Personality Development, from CHILDHOOD and SOCIETY by Erik H. Erikson. Copyright 1950, © 1963 by W.W. Norton & Company, Inc., renewed © 1978, 1991, by Erik H. Erikson. Used by permission of W.W. Norton & Company, Inc.

(Table 6-2). Although there are implied age ranges attached to these stages and it is hoped that a person might move through them in an orderly fashion, this does not always occur. Thus it is important to look at the client's behavior rather than age to identify the stage of development related to one's age.

Strong indicators that the client is functioning much below the usual behavior for her age range may specify areas for possible nursing diagnoses (developmental delay) and nursing intervention. Sometimes a person skips one or more developmental levels and, at a later stage of maturity, goes back and successfully works through the missed levels. A thorough knowledge of the behaviors and approximate age levels provides the nurse with a powerful tool for assessing and helping a client grow to his or her full potential. Although accomplishment of all of the tasks in the stage before moving on is ideal, it is believed that partial resolution is adequate for health, growth, and development.

The psychosocial developmental stages of the young adult, middle-aged adult, and older adult are discussed in detail in the following section. Each section includes important questions to ask yourself about the client to determine if he or she has accomplished all of the required tasks in a particular psychosocial developmental stage. If the adult client does not seem even to have advanced psychologically to the intimacy versus isolation stage, refer to the earlier stages seen in children and adolescents, which are discussed in Chapter 31.

ASSESSMENT OF ERIKSON'S STAGES (1991) OF PSYCHOSOCIAL DEVELOPMENT

Assessment Procedure	Normal Findings	Abnormal Findings
Determine the client's psychosocial developmental level by answering the following questions. If you do not have enough data to answer these questions, you may need to ask the client additional questions or make further observations.		

Does the Young Adult
- Accept self—physically, cognitively, and emotionally?
- Have independence from the parental home?
- Express love responsibly, emotionally, and sexually?
- Have close or intimate relationships with a partner?
- Have a social group of friends?
- Have a philosophy of living and life?
- Have a profession or a life's work that provides a means of contribution?
- Solve problems of life that accompany independence from the parental home?

Intimacy
The young adult should have achieved self-efficacy during adolescence and is now ready to open up and become intimate with others. Although this stage focuses on the desire for a special and permanent love relationship, it also includes the ability to have close, caring relationships with friends of both sexes and a variety of ages. Spiritual love also develops during this stage. Having established an identity apart from the childhood family, the young adult is now able to form adult friendships with his parents and siblings. However, the young adult will always be a son or daughter.

Isolation
If the young adult cannot express emotion and trust enough to open up to others, social and emotional isolation may occur. Loneliness may cause the young adult to turn to addictive behaviors such as alcoholism, drug abuse, or sexual promiscuity. Some people try to cope with this developmental stage by becoming very spiritual or social, playing an acceptable role, but never fully sharing who they are or becoming emotionally involved with others. When adults successfully navigate this stage, they have stable and satisfying relationships with important others.

continued

Assessment Procedure	Normal Findings	Abnormal Findings
Does the Middle-aged Adult • Have healthful life patterns? • Derive satisfaction from contributing to growth and development of others? • Have an abiding intimacy and long-term relationship with a partner? • Maintain a stable home? • Find pleasure in an established work or profession? • Take pride in self and family accomplishments and contributions? • Contribute to the community to support its growth and development?	**Generativity** During this stage, the middle-aged adult is able to share self with others and establish nurturing relationships. The adult will be able to extend self and possessions to others. Although traditionalists tend to think of generativity in terms of raising one's children and guiding their lives, generativity can be realized in several ways even without having children. Generativity implies mentoring and giving to future generations. This can be accomplished by producing ideas, products, inventions, paintings, writings, books, films, or any other creative endeavors that are then given to the world for the unrestricted use of its people. Generativity also includes teaching others, children or adults, mentoring young workers, or providing experience and wisdom to assist a new business to survive and grow. Also implied in this stage is the ability to guide, then let go of one's creations. Successful movement through this stage results in a fuller and more satisfying life and prepares the mature adult for the next stage.	**Stagnation** Without this important step, the gift is not given and the stage does not come to successful completion. Stagnation occurs when the middle-aged person has not accomplished one or more of the previous developmental tasks, and is unable to give to future generations. Sometimes severe losses may result in withdrawal and stagnation. In these cases, the person may have total dependency on work, a favorite child, or even a pet, and be incapable of giving to others. A project may never be finished or schooling completed because the person cannot let go and move on. Without a creative outlet, a paralyzing stagnation sets in.
Does the Older Adult • Adjust to the changing physical self? • Recognize changes present as a result of aging, in relationships and activities? • Maintain relationships with children, grandchildren, and other relatives? • Continue interests outside of self and home? • Complete transition from retirement at work to satisfying alternative activities? • Establish relationships with others who are his or her own age? • Adjust to deaths of relatives, spouse, and friends? • Maintain a maximum level of physical functioning through diet, exercise, and personal care? • Find meaning in past life and face inevitable mortality of self and significant others? • Integrate philosophical or religious values into self-understanding to promote comfort? • Review accomplishments and recognize meaningful contributions he or she has made to community and relatives?	**Integrity** According to Erikson (1950), a person in this stage looks back and either finds that life was good or despairs because goals were not accomplished. This stage can extend over a long time and include excursions into previous stages to complete unfinished business. Successful movement through this stage does not mean that one day a person wakes up and says, "My life has been good"; rather, it encompasses a series of reminiscences in which the person may be able to see past events in a new and more positive light. This can be a very rich and rewarding time in a person's life, especially if there are others with whom to share memories and who can assist with reframing life experiences (Fig. 6-5). For some people, resolution and acceptance do not come until the final weeks of life, but this still allows for a peaceful death.	**Despair** If the older person cannot feel grateful for his or her life, cannot accept those less desirable aspects as merely part of living, or cannot integrate all of the experiences of life, then the person will spend his or her last days in bitterness and regret and will ultimately die in despair.

continued

Assessment Procedure	Normal Findings	Abnormal Findings

> **Clinical Tip** • Erikson's Psychosocial Developmental Stages are based on ego development with distinct conflicts (indicated as "Normal and Abnormal Findings" in this section) across the lifespan. These stages are a lifelong process and may overlap each other.

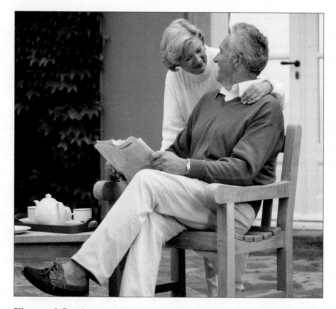

Figure 6-5 Older adulthood can be a rich and rewarding time to review life events.

VALIDATING AND DOCUMENTING FINDINGS

Validate the mental status and psychosocial assessment data you have collected. This is necessary to verify that the data are reliable and accurate. Document the data following the health care facility or agency policy.

> **Clinical Tip** • When documenting your assessment findings, it is better to describe the client's response than to label his or her behavior.

Sample of Subjective Data

Provided correct biographical information regarding: age (54 years), address, and marital status (married). Holds a master's degree in elementary education. Teaches sixth grade mathematics. Concerned about forgetting students' names in his class over the past semester. Also misplaces objects more frequently than in the past. Concerned that this will impair his abilities as a teacher. Memory and misplacing of things gets worse as the day progresses. No history of stroke, meningitis, or head injury. No family history of Alzheimer's disease. Brother had bipolar disorder. Is able to perform normal activities of daily living but is getting more difficult to concentrate on grading math papers at nighttime. Becomes tired quicker than in the past. Awakens two times a night but is able to go back to sleep within 30 minutes. Reports good appetite and normal bowel routine. Active in his church community. Positive about current activities of daily living, including work, exercise, and leisure. Expressed positive relationships with wife and children.

Sample of Objective Data

Mental status: Alert and oriented to person, place, day, and time. Clean and well-groomed appearance. Good eye contact, with pleasant, cooperative disposition. Speech clear with moderate tone. Somewhat anxious over forgetting names and location of objects. Looking forward to retirement in about 8 years. Able to name familiar objects in exam room. Expresses clear, realistic, logical thought processes about the past and future. Recalls what he ate for breakfast and past dates of family members' birthdays. Repeated four unrelated words after 5 minutes, repeated one after 10 minutes, unable to repeat after 10 minutes. Explained the meaning of common proverbs. Explained what to do in an emergency situation in the classroom. Correctly drew the face of a clock. Scored 28 on the Saint Louis University Mental Status (SLUMS) examination. Appears to have reached the psychosocial development level of "generativity." Expressed enjoyment and satisfaction in roles as husband, father, grandfather, teacher, and church member.

Analysis of Data

After collecting subjective and objective data pertaining to general survey and vital signs, identify abnormal findings and the client's strengths. Then cluster the data to reveal any significant patterns or abnormalities. These data may then be used to make clinical judgments about the client.

DIAGNOSTIC REASONING: POSSIBLE CONCLUSIONS

Some possible conclusions related to your mental status exam and assessment of the client's psychosocial developmental level are discussed in the following text.

Selected Nursing Diagnoses

After collecting subjective and objective data pertaining to the general survey, you will need to identify abnormals and cluster the data to reveal any significant patterns or abnormalities. These data will then be used to make clinical judgments (nursing diagnoses: wellness, risk, or actual) about the status of the client's general survey. Following is a list of selected nursing diagnoses that you may identify when analyzing data for this part of the assessment.

Wellness Diagnoses

- Health-Seeking Behaviors related to desire and request to learn more about health promotion
- Readiness for Enhanced Communication

Risk Diagnoses

- Risk for Self-Directed Violence related to depression, suicidal tendencies, developmental crisis, lack of support systems, loss of significant others, poor coping mechanisms and behaviors
- Risk for Developmental Delay related to lack of healthy environmental stimulation and activities

Actual Diagnoses

- Impaired Verbal Communication related to international language barrier (inability to speak English of accepted dominant language)
- Impaired Verbal Communication related to hearing loss
- Impaired Verbal Communication related to inability to clearly express self or understand others (aphasia)

- Impaired Verbal Communication related to aphasia, psychological impairment, or organic brain disorder
- Acute or Chronic Confusion related to dementia, head injury, stroke, alcohol or drug abuse
- Impaired Memory related to dementia, stroke, head injury, alcohol or drug abuse
- Dressing/Grooming Self-Care Deficit related to confusion and lack of resources/support from caregivers
- Disturbed Thought Processes related to alcohol or drug abuse, psychotic disorder, or organic brain dysfunction
- Social Isolation related to inability to relate/communicate effectively with others

Selected Collaborative Problems

After you group the data, it may become apparent that certain collaborative problems emerge. Remember that collaborative problems differ from nursing diagnoses in that they cannot be prevented by nursing interventions. However, these physiological complications of medical conditions can be detected and monitored by the nurse. In addition, the nurse can use physician- and nurse-prescribed interventions to minimize the complications of these problems. The nurse may also have to refer the client in such situations for further treatment of the problem. Following is a list of collaborative problems that may be identified when obtaining a general impression. These problems are worded as Risk for Complications (or RC), followed by the problem.

- RC: Stroke
- RC: Increased intracranial pressure
- RC: Seizures
- RC: Meningitis
- RC: Depression

Medical Problems

After you group the data, it may become apparent that the client has signs and symptoms that require psychiatric medical diagnosis and treatment. Refer to a primary care provider as necessary.

CASE STUDY

The case study demonstrates how to analyze assessment data for a specific client. The critical thinking exercises included in the study guide/lab manual and interactive product that complement this text also offer opportunities to analyze assessment data.

Mrs. Jane Wilson, a 61-year-old Caucasian female, has come to the local family clinic where you work. She is accompanied by her husband, Steve. When you ask her the reason for her visit, she states, "I'm very nervous and not thinking straight."

Mrs. Wilson reports sleep difficulties, loss of appetite, and a general feeling of anxiety. She says that she has excessively been "worrying over little things." She is fearful of someone breaking into her house and often checks and rechecks the locks despite her husband reassuring her the doors are locked. She states, "I'm afraid I am losing my mind."

When you ask her about her daily routine, she tells you she is unable to concentrate and has a hard time completing household chores. She reports feeling confused, tired, and depressed. She denies any plans to hurt herself.

Mrs. Wilson is appropriately dressed for the season and situation. She looks pale and thin but appears her stated age. Her hair is disheveled and she is not wearing any jewelry or makeup. Her husband informs you that she used to never leave the house without makeup and accessories, so he is worried

continued on page 74

about her. She sits quietly, slumped over in her chair and wrings her hands often. She has very brief eye contact and often stares at the floor. Her face is expressionless.

Mrs. Wilson appears alert and oriented to person, place, time, and situation. You, however, often have to repeat questions because she is having difficulty concentrating. Her speech is clear but low in volume; her responses are brief. She sometimes looks at her husband for reassurance. She is unable to recall some recent events including what she ate for dinner last night. She is unable to recall four objects 10 minutes after they were recited to her. Mrs. Wilson demonstrates the ability to answer remote memory questions accurately and displays appropriate decision-making skills.

Mrs. Wilson is 5 feet 5 inches tall and weighs 115 lbs. Her vital signs are tympanic temperature, 96.3°F; pulse, 82; respirations, 18; and blood pressure, 100/62. She does not appear to be in any physical distress. Her gait is steady and strong.

The following concept map illustrates the diagnostic reasoning process.

Applying COLDSPA

COLDSPA can be used to explore the client's symptoms of "anxiety and confusion" as illustrated below.

Mnemonic	Question	Data Provided	Missing Data
Character	Describe the sign or symptom (feeling, appearance, sound, smell, or taste if applicable).	"Very nervous and not thinking straight"	
Onset	When did it begin?		"When did these feelings first occur?"
Location	Where is it? Does it radiate? Does it occur anywhere else?		"Is there any place that you can feel calm or safe?"
Duration	How long does it last? Does it recur?		"Have these feelings been consistent since the onset?"
Severity	How bad is it? How much does it bother you?	Client fears someone is out to get her and that she is losing her mind. She leaves the house without makeup and accessories though she never did this in the past.	
Pattern	What makes it better or worse?	"I worry over little things."	"When do you feel most anxious? Is there anything that relieves or intensifies your feelings?"
Associated factors/How it **A**ffects the client	What other symptoms occur with it? How does it affect you?	Client is having difficulty sleeping, loss of appetite, and is confused, tired, and depressed.	

1) Identify abnormal findings and client strengths

Subjective Data

- "I'm very nervous and not thinking straight"
- Reports sleep difficulties, loss of appetite, and a general feeling of anxiety
- Says that she has excessively been "worrying over little things"
- Is fearful of someone breaking into her house and often checks and rechecks the locks, despite her husband reassuring her the doors are locked
- "I'm afraid I am losing my mind"
- Tells you she is unable to concentrate and has a hard time completing household chores
- Reports feeling confused, tired, and depressed
- Denies any plans to hurt herself
- Her husband informs you that she used to never leave the house without makeup and accessories, so he is worried about her

Objective Data

- 61-year-old Caucasian female
- Appropriately dressed for the season and situation
- Looks pale and thin, appears stated age, hair disheveled, not wearing jewelry or makeup
- Has very brief eye contact, often stares at the floor, face expressionless
- Wrings her hands often
- Appears alert and oriented to person, place, time, and situation
- You have to repeat questions because she is having difficulty concentrating
- Speech is clear, but low in volume, and her responses are brief
- Sometimes looks at her husband for reassurance
- Unable to recall some recent events, including what she ate for dinner last night
- Unable to recall four objects 10 minutes after they were recited to her
- Able to answer remote memory questions
- 5'5" tall and weighs 115 lbs
- Vital signs are tympanic temperature, 96.3F; pulse, 82; respirations, 18; and blood pressure, 100/62
- Does not appear to be in any physical distress
- Gait is steady and strong

2) Identify cue clusters

Cluster 1
- Reports sleep difficulties, loss of appetite, and a general feeling of anxiety
- Says that she has excessively been "worrying over little things"
- Is fearful of someone breaking into her house and often checks and rechecks the locks, despite her husband reassuring her the doors are locked
- Tells you she is unable to concentrate and has a hard time completing household chores
- You have to repeat questions because she is having difficulty concentrating
- Has very brief eye contact and often stares at the floor

Cluster 2
- Reports sleep difficulties, loss of appetite, and a general feeling of anxiety
- "I'm afraid I am losing my mind"
- Reports feeling confused, tired, and depressed
- Her husband informs you that she used to never leave the house without makeup and accessories, so he is worried about her
- Her hair is disheveled and she is not wearing any jewelry or makeup
- Her face is expressionless
- She sites quietly, slumped over in her chair

Cluster 3
- Reports loss of appetite
- Looks pale and thin
- 5'5" tall and weighs 115 lbs

3) Draw inferences

Client is nervous and experiencing anxiety r/t an unknown cause.

Client is possibly depressed. Refer to physician for evaluation.

Client may be undernourished.

4) List possible nursing diagnoses

Anxiety

Imbalanced Nutrition: Less than Body Requirements

5) Check for defining characteristics

Major: Diminished productivity, insomnia, extraneous movement, scared, worried, apprehensive, confusion, impaired attention
Minor: Poor eye contact

Major: None
Minor: Aversion to eating

6) Confirm or rule out diagnoses

Confirm diagnosis because it meets the major and minor defining characteristics

Rule out at this time, but monitor client's weight

7) Document conclusions

The following nursing diagnosis is appropriate:
- Anxiety

Potential collaborative problems include the following:
- RC: Depression

References and Selected Readings

Acorn, S. (1993). Use of the brief psychiatric scale by nurses. *Journal of Psychosocial Mental Health Services, 31*(5), 9–12.

Aird, T., & McIntosh, M. (2004). Nursing tools and strategies to assess cognition and confusion. *British Journal of Nursing, 13*(10), 621–626.

Brackley, M. H. (1997). Mental health assessment. *Nurse Practice Forum, 8*(3), 105–113.

Erikson, Erik H. (1991). Erikson's Stages of Personality Development. *Childhood and Society.* New York: W. W. Norton & Company, Inc.

Folstein, M., Anthony, J., Parhad, I., Duffy, B., & Gruenberg, E. (1985). The meaning of cognitive impairment in the elderly. *Journal of the American Geriatrics Society, 33*, 228–235.

Folstein, M. F., Folstein, S. E., & McHugh, P. R. (1975). Mini-mental state: A practical guide for grading the cognitive state of patients for the clinician. *Journal of Psychiatric Research, 12*(3), 89–198.

Learning theories. (2009). Available at http://www.learning-theories.com/eriksons-stages-of-development.

McConnell, E. A. (1997). Assessing altered mental states. *Nursing, 27*(4), 32d–32h.

Office of Disease Prevention and Health Promotion, US Department of Health and Human Services. (2000). *Healthy people 2010: Understanding and improving health* (2nd ed.). Washington, DC: Author.

Pangman, V. C., Sloan, J., & Guse, L. (2000). An examination of psychometric properties of the mini-mental state examination and the standardized mini-mental state examination: Implications for clinical practice. *Applied Nursing Research, 13*(4), 209–213.

Patterson, C. (2001). Screen for cognitive impairment and dementia in the elderly. Canadian Task Force on Preventive Health Care. Available at http://www.ctfphc.org.

Solomon, P. R., Hirschoff, A., Bridget, K., et al. (1998). A 7-minute neurocognitive screening battery highly sensitive to Alzheimer's disease. *Archives of Neurology, 55*, 349–355.

Solomon, P. R., & Pendelburry, W. W. (1998). Recognition of Alzheimer's disease: The 7-minute screen. *Family Medicine, 30*(4), 265–271.

Souder, E., & O'Sullivan, P. S. (2000). Nursing documentation versus standardized assessment of cognitive status in hospitalized mental patients. *Applied Nursing Research, 13*(1), 29–36.

Welch, D. C., & West, R. L. (1999). The short portable mental status questionnaire: Assessing cognitive ability in nursing home residents. *Nursing Research, 48*(6), 329–332.

Woods, P., Reed, V., & Collins, M. (2001). Measuring communication and social skills in high security forensic setting using the behavioral status index. *International Journal of Psychiatric Nursing Research, 7*(1), 761–777.

Yesevage, J. (1983). Development and validation of a geriatric depression screening scale: A preliminary report. *Journal of Psychiatric Research, 17*, 38–49.

Promote Health—Dementias

Alzheimer's Association. (2007a). Alzheimer's and other dementias: Understanding the differences. Available at http://www.helpguide.org/elder/alzheimers_dementias_types.

Alzheimer's Association. (2007b). International Conference on Prevention of Dementia session detail: Treating heart disease risk factors may slow Alzheimer's disease; Treating vascular risk factors may slow progression of Alzheimer's; Unexplained late-life weight loss may predict risk of dementia; "Motivational reserve" is a new concept complementing cognitive reserve. Available at http://alz.org/preventionconference/pc2007.

Alzheimer's Disease Health Center. (2005). Curry spice may fight Alzheimer's disease. *WebMD Medical News.* Available at http://www.webmd.com/alzheimers/news/20050105/curry-spice-may-fight-alzheimers-disease.

Berr, C., Akbaraly, T., Nourashemi, F., & Andrieu, S. (2007). [Epidemiology of dementia] (in French). *La Presse Medicale.* Available online through Entrez PubMed. Epub ahead of print.

Cereda, E., Sansone, V., Meola, G., & Malavazos, A. (2007). Increased visceral adipose tissue rather than BMI as a risk factor for dementia. *Age and Ageing.* Available online through Entrez PubMed. Epub ahead of print.

Chiang, C., Yip, P., Wu, S., Lu, C., Liou, C., Liu, H. (2007). Midlife risk factors for subtypes of dementia: A nested case–control study in Taiwan. *American Journal of Geriatric Psychiatry.* Available online through Entrez PubMed. Epub ahead of print.

Cole, A. R., Astell, A., Green, C., & Sutherland, C. (2007). Molecular connections between dementia and diabetes. *Neuroscience & Behavioral Review.* Available online through Entrez PubMed. Epub ahead of print.

Dosdunmu, R., Wu, J., Basha, M., & Zawia, N. (2007). Environmental and dietary risk factors in Alzheimer's disease. *Expert Review of Neurotherapeutics, 7*(7), 887–900.

Feldman, H. H., & Jacova, C. (2007). Primary prevention and delay of onset of AD/dementia. *Canadian Journal of Neurological Science, 34*(Suppl. 1), S84–S89.

Khachaturian, A., Zandi, P., Lyketsos, C., Hayden, K., Skoon, I., Norton, M., et al. (2006). Antihypertensive medication use and incident Alzheimer disease: the Cache County Study. *Archives of Neurology, 63*(5), 686–692.

Lahiri, D., Maloney, B., Basha, M., Ge, Y., & Zawia, N. (2007). How and when environmental agents and dietary factors affect the course of Alzheimer's disease: The "LEARn" model (latent early-life associate regulation) may explain the triggering of AD. *Current Alzheimer Research, 4*(2), 219–228.

Qiu, C., De Ronchi, D., & Fratiglioni, L. (2007). The epidemiology of the dementias: An update. *Current Opinion in Psychiatry, 20*(4), 380–385.

Ringman, J., Frautschy, S., Cole, G., Masterman, D., & Cummings, J. (2005). A potential role of the curry spice curcumin in Alzheimer's disease. *Current Alzheimer Research, 2.* Available online through PubMed.

Scherder, E., Eggermont, L., Swaab, D., van Heuvelen, M., Kamsma, Y., de Greef, M., et al. (2007). Gait in ageing and associated dementias; its relationship with cognition. *Neuroscience & Behavioral Review, 31*(4), 485–497.

WebMD. (2005–2007). Alzheimer's guide & Alzheimer's warning signs. Available at http://webmd.com/alzheimers/guide/7-alzheimers-warning-signs.

Yaffe, K. (2007a). Metabolic syndrome and cognitive decline. *Current Alzheimer Research, 4*(2), 123–136.

Yaffe, K. (2007b). Metabolic syndrome and cognitive disorders: Is the sum greater than its parts? *Alzheimer's Disease and Associated Disorders, 21*(2), 167–171.

7

Assessing General Status & Vital Signs

Structure and Function

The general survey is the first part of the physical exam that begins the moment the nurse meets the client. It requires the nurse to use all of her observational skills while interviewing and interacting with the client. These observations will lead to clues about the health status of the client. The outcome of the general survey provides the nurse with an overall impression of the client's whole being. The general survey includes observation of the client's

- Physical development and body build
- Gender and sexual development
- Apparent age as compared to reported age
- Skin condition and color
- Dress and hygiene
- Posture and gait
- Level of consciousness
- Behaviors, body movements, and affect
- Facial expression
- Speech
- Vital signs

The client's vital signs (pulse, respirations, blood pressure, temperature, and pain) are the body's indicators of health. Usually when a vital sign (or signs) is abnormal, something is wrong in at least one of the body systems. Traditionally, vital signs have included the client's pulse, respirations, blood pressure, and temperature. Today, "pain" is considered to be the "fifth vital sign" (Flaherty, 2001). Pain is inexpensive to assess and does not involve the use of fancy instruments, yet it can be an early predictor of impending disability. For example, early and correct assessment of a client's chest pain may promote early treatment and prevention of complications and the high cost of cardiovascular damage and/or failure.

OVERALL IMPRESSION OF THE CLIENT

The first time you meet a client, you tend to remember certain obvious characteristics. Forming an overall impression consists of a systematic examination and recording these general characteristics and impressions of the client. If possible, try to observe the client and environment quickly before interacting with the client. This gives you the opportunity to "see" the client before she assumes a social face or behavior and allows you to glimpse any distress, sadness, or pain before the client, knowingly or unknowingly, may mask it.

When you meet the client for the first time, observe any significant abnormalities in the client's skin color, dress, hygiene, posture and gait, physical development, body build, apparent age, and gender. If you observe abnormalities, you may need to perform an in-depth assessment of the body area that appears to be affected (e.g., an unusual gait may prompt you to perform a detailed musculoskeletal assessment). You should also generally assess the client's level of consciousness, level of comfort, behavior, body movements, affect, facial expression, speech and mental acuities. If you detect any abnormalities during your general impression examination, you will need to do an in-depth mental status examination. This examination is described in Chapter 6. Additional preparation involves creating a comfortable, non-threatening atmosphere to relieve anxiety in the client.

VITAL SIGNS

The nurse usually begins the "hands-on" physical examination by taking vital signs. This is a common, non-invasive physical assessment procedure that most clients are accustomed to. Vital signs provide data that reflect the status of several body systems including but not limited to the cardiovascular, neurological, peripheral vascular, and respiratory systems. Measure the client's temperature first, followed by pulse, respirations, and blood pressure. Measuring the temperature puts the client at ease and causes him or her to remain still for several minutes. This is important because pulse, respirations, and blood pressure are influenced by anxiety and activity. By easing the client's anxiety and keeping him or her still, you help to increase the accuracy of the data.

Temperature

For the body to function on a cellular level, a core body temperature between 36.5°C and 37.7°C (96.0°F and 99.9°F orally) must be maintained. An approximate reading of core body temperature can be taken at various anatomic sites. None of these is completely accurate; they are simply a good reflection of the core body temperature.

Several factors may cause normal variations in the core body temperature. Strenuous exercise, stress, and ovulation can raise temperature. Body temperature is lowest early in the morning (4 to 6 AM) and highest late in the evening (8 PM to midnight). Hypothermia (lower than 36.5°C or 96.0°F) may be seen in prolonged exposure to the cold, hypoglycemia, hypothyroidism, or starvation. Hyperthermia (higher than 38.0°C or 100°F) may be seen in viral or bacterial infections, malignancies, trauma, and various blood, endocrine, and immune disorders.

In the older adult, temperature may range from 95.0°F to 97.5°F. Therefore, the older client may not have an obviously elevated temperature with an infection or be considered hypothermic below 96°F.

Pulse

A shock wave is produced when the heart contracts and forcefully pumps blood out of the ventricles into the aorta. The shock wave travels along the fibers of the arteries and is commonly called the *arterial* or *peripheral pulse*. The body has many arterial pulse sites. One of them—the radial pulse—gives a good overall picture of the client's health status (see Chapter 21 for more information about additional pulse sites). Several characteristics should be assessed when measuring the radial pulse—rate, rhythm, amplitude and contour, and elasticity.

Amplitude can be quantified as follows:

1+ Thready or weak (easy to obliterate)

2+ Normal (obliterate with moderate pressure)

3+ Bounding (unable to obliterate or requires very firm pressure)

If abnormalities are noted during assessment of the radial pulse, further assessment should be performed. For more information on assessing pulses and abnormal pulse findings, refer to Chapters 20 and 21.

Respirations

The respiratory rate and character are additional clues to the client's overall health status. Respirations can be easily observed without alerting the client by watching chest movement before removing the stethoscope after you have completed counting the apical beat. Notable characteristics of respiration are rate, rhythm, and depth (see Chapter 18 for more information about respirations).

Blood Pressure

Blood pressure reflects the pressure exerted on the walls of the arteries. This pressure varies with the cardiac cycle, reaching a high point with systole and a low point with diastole (Fig. 7-1). Therefore, blood pressure is a measurement of the pressure of the blood in the arteries when the ventricles are contracted (systolic blood pressure) and when the ventricles are relaxed (diastolic blood pressure). Blood pressure is expressed as the ratio of the systolic pressure over the diastolic pressure. A client's blood pressure is affected by several factors:

• *Cardiac output*—Blood pressure increases with increased cardiac output and decreases with decreased cardiac output.

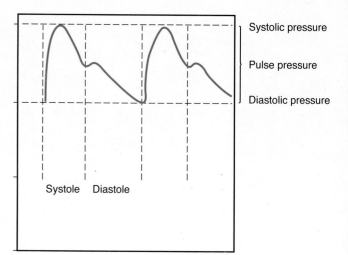

Figure 7-1 Blood pressure measurement identifies the amount of pressure in the arteries when the ventricles of the heart contract (systole) and when they relax (diastole).

• *Distensibility of the arteries*—Blood pressure increases when more effort is required to push blood through stiffened arteries.
• *Blood volume*—Blood pressure increases with increased volume and decreases with decreased volume.
• *Blood velocity*—Blood pressure increases when blood flow is slowed due to resistance and decreases when blood flow meets no resistance.
• *Blood viscosity (thickness)*—Blood pressure increases when the blood is thickened and decreases with thinning of the blood.

A client's blood pressure will normally vary throughout the day due to external influences. These include the time of day, caffeine or nicotine intake, exercise, emotions, pain, and temperature. The difference between systolic and diastolic pressure is termed the *pulse pressure*. The pulse pressure should be determined after the blood pressure is measured because it reflects the stroke volume—the volume of blood ejected with each heartbeat.

Blood pressure may also vary depending on the positions of the body and of the arm. Blood pressure in a normal person who is standing is usually slightly higher to compensate for the effects of gravity. Blood pressure in a normal reclining person is slightly lower because of decreased resistance.

Pain

Pain screening is very important in developing a comprehensive plan of care for the client. Therefore, it is essential to assess for pain at the initial assessment. When pain is present, it is important to identify the location, intensity, quality, duration, and any alleviating or aggravating factors to the client. Pain intensity measurement tools such as a 1 to 10 Likert scale (described in Chapter 8) may be used. Pain quality may be described as "dull," "sharp," "radiating," or "throbbing." The mnemonic device "COLDSPA" may help you to remember how to further assess pain if present. Chapter 8 provides in-depth information on the etiology of pain and pain assessment.

Health Assessment

COLLECTING SUBJECTIVE DATA: THE NURSING HEALTH HISTORY

COLDSPA Symptom Analysis Mnemonic

During the general survey, the **COLDSPA** mnemonic may be particularly helpful in exploring unusual signs and symptoms or problems reported, as you and the client ask and answer various questions during the health history interview.

Mnemonic	Question
Character	Describe the sign or symptom (feeling, appearance, sound, smell, or taste if applicable).
Onset	When did it begin?
Location	Where is it? Does it radiate? Does it occur anywhere else?
Duration	How long does it last? Does it recur?
Severity	How bad is it? How much does it bother you?
Pattern	What makes it better or worse?
Associated factors/How it **A**ffects the client	What other symptoms occur with it? How does it affect you?

Question	Rationale
General Survey Questions	
What are your name, address, and telephone number?	Answers to these questions provide verifiable and accurate identification data about the client. They also provide baseline information about level of consciousness, memory, speech patterns, articulation, or speech defects. For example, a client who is unable to answer these questions has cognitive/neurological deficits.
How old are you?	Establishes baseline for comparing appearance and development to chronologic age.
Do you know what your usual blood pressure is?	Knowing blood pressure indicates client is involved in own health care.
When and where did you last have your blood pressure checked?	Answer indicates if client consults professionals for health care, if client relies on possibly erroneous equipment in public places (e.g., drug stores), or if client has approved equipment at home that he is trained to use.
Have you had any high fevers that occur often or persistently?	A pattern of elevated temperatures may indicate a chronic infection or blood disorder such as leukemia.
Do you have any pain? If yes, describe the pain. How does it feel (dull, sharp, aching, throbbing)? How does area of pain look (shiny, bumpy, red, swollen, bruised)? When did it begin? Where is it? Does it radiate? How long does it last? Does it recur? How bad is it? What makes it better? What makes it worse? What other symptoms occur with it?	Exploring the pain in depth helps the nurse to understand the cause and significance of the pain.
Do you have any present health concerns?	This allows the client to voice her concerns and provides a focus for the examination.

COLLECTING OBJECTIVE DATA: PHYSICAL EXAMINATION

Preparing the Client

The general survey begins when the nurse first meets the client. During this time the nurse observes the client's posture, movements and overall appearance. To begin the interview for the mental status exam, the client should be in a comfortable sitting position in a chair, on the examination table, or on a bed in the home setting. Prepare the client for the mental status exam by explaining the purpose of the exam. Then explain that vital signs will be taken.

Equipment

- Thermometer: mercury-in-glass oral, axillary, or rectal thermometer; electronic thermometer; or tympanic thermometer
- Protective, disposable covers for type of thermometer used
- Aneroid or mercury sphygmomanometer or electronic blood pressure-measuring equipment
- Stethoscope
- Watch with a second hand

Physical Assessment

You may assess mental status effectively using the SLUMS or CAM tools found in Assessment Tools 6-1. Identify the equipment needed to measure vital signs and its proper use.

PHYSICAL ASSESSMENT

Assessment Procedure	Normal Findings	Abnormal Findings
General Impression		
Observe physical development, body build, and fat distribution.	A wide variety of body types fall within a normal range: from small amounts of fat and muscle to larger amounts of fat and muscle. See Chapter 12, "Assessing Nutrition," for more information. Body proportions are normal. Arm span (distance between finger tips with arms extended) is approximately equal. The distance from the head crown to the symphysis pubis is approximately equal to the distance from the symphysis pubis to the sole of the client's foot.	A lack of subcutaneous fat with prominent bones is a sign of malnutrition. Abundant fatty tissue is seen in obesity. Decreased height and delayed puberty, with chubbiness, are seen in hypopituitary dwarfism. Skeletal malformations with a decrease in height are seen in achondroplastic dwarfism. In gigantism, there is increased height and weight with delayed sexual development. Overgrowth of bones in the face, head, hands, and feet with normal height is seen in hyperpituitarism (acromegaly). Extreme weight loss is seen in anorexia nervosa. Arm span is greater than height, and pubis to sole measurement exceeds pubis to crown measurement in Marfan's syndrome. Excessive body fat that is evenly distributed is referred to as exogenous obesity. Central body weight gain with excessive cervical obesity (Buffalo's hump) is seen in Cushing's syndrome referred to as endogenous obesity. See Abnormal Findings 7.1.
Observe gender and sexual development.	Sexual development is appropriate for gender and age.	Abnormal findings include delayed puberty, male client with female characteristics, and female client with male characteristics.
Compare client's stated age with her apparent age and developmental stage.	Client appears to be her stated chronologic age.	Client appears older than actual chronologic age (e.g., due to hard life, manual labor, chronic illness, alcoholism, smoking).
Observe skin condition and color. ➤ *Clinical Tip* • *Keep in mind that underlying red tones from good circulation give a liveliness or healthy glow to all shades of skin color.*	Color is even without obvious lesions: light to dark beige-pink in light-skinned client; light tan to dark brown or olive in dark-skinned clients.	Abnormal findings include extreme pallor, flushed, or yellow in light-skinned client; loss of red tones and ashen gray cyanosis in dark-skinned client. See abnormal skin colors and their significance in Chapter 13.

continued

Assessment Procedure	Normal Findings	Abnormal Findings
Observe posture and gait.	Posture is erect and comfortable for age. Gait is rhythmic and coordinated with arms swinging at side.	Curvatures of the spine (lordosis, scoliosis, or kyphosis) may indicate a musculoskeletal disorder. Stiff, rigid movements are common in arthritis or Parkinson's disease (see Chapter 26). Slumped shoulders may signify depression. Clients with chronic pulmonary obstructive disease tend to lean forward, brace themselves with arms. In older adults, osteoporotic thinning and collapse of the vertebrae secondary to bone loss may result in kyphosis. In older men, gait may be wider based with arms held outward. Older women tend to have a narrow base and may waddle to compensate for a decreased sense of balance. Steps shorten with decreased speed and arm swing. Mobility may be decreased, and gait may be rigid.

Vital Signs

Temperature **To take oral temperature,** use an electronic thermometer with a disposable protective probe cover. Then place the thermometer under the client's tongue to the right or left of the frenulum deep in the posterior sublingual pocket. Ask the client to close his or her lips around the probe. Hold the probe until you hear a beep. Remove the probe and dispose of its cover by pressing the release button. Electronic thermometers give a digital reading in about 2 minutes.	Oral temperature is 36.5°C to 37.0°C (96.0°F to 99.9°F).	Oral temperature is below 36.5°C (96.0°F) or over 37.0°C (99.9°F).
To take axillary temperature, hold the glass or electronic thermometer under the axilla firmly by having the client hold the arm down and across the chest for 10 minutes.	The axillary temperature is 0.5°C (1°F) lower than the oral temperature.	
For rectal temperature, use this route only if other routes are not practical (e.g., client cannot cooperate, is comatose, cannot close mouth, or tympanic thermometer is unavailable). Cover the glass thermometer with a disposable, sterile sheath, and lubricate the thermometer. Wear gloves, and insert thermometer 1 inch into rectum. Hold a glass thermometer in place for 3 minutes; hold an electronic thermometer in place until the temperature appears in the display window.	The rectal temperature is between 0.4°C and 0.5°C (0.7°F and 1°F) higher than the normal oral temperature.	

continued

PHYSICAL ASSESSMENT *Continued*

Assessment Procedure	Normal Findings	Abnormal Findings
➤ *Clinical Tip* • *Never force the thermometer into the rectum or use a rectal thermometer for clients with severe coagulation disorders.*		
For tympanic temperature, an electronic tympanic thermometer measures the temperature of the tympanic membrane quickly and safely. It is also a good device for measuring core body temperature because the tympanic membrane is supplied by a tributary of the artery (internal carotid) that supplies the hypothalamus (the body's thermoregulatory center). Place the probe very gently at the opening of the ear canal for 2 to 3 seconds until the temperature appears in the digital display (Fig. 7-2).	The tympanic membrane temperature is about 0.8°C (1.4°F) higher than the normal oral temperature.	

Pulse

Assessment Procedure	Normal Findings	Abnormal Findings
Measure the radial pulse rate. Use the pads of your two middle fingers and lightly palpate the radial artery on the lateral aspect of the client's wrist (Fig. 7-3). Count the number of beats you feel for 30 seconds if the pulse rhythm is regular. Multiply by two to get the rate. Count for a full minute if the rhythm is irregular. Then, verify by taking an apical pulse as well.	A pulse rate ranging from 60 to 100 beats/min is normal for adults. Tachycardia may be normal in clients who have just finished strenuous exercise. Bradycardia may be normal in well-conditioned athletes.	*Tachycardia* is a rate greater than 100 beats/min. May occur with fever, certain medications, stress, and other abnormal states such as cardiac dysrhythmias. *Bradycardia* is a rate less than 60 beats/min. Sitting or standing for long periods may cause the blood to pool and decrease the pulse rate. Heart block or dropped beats can also manifest as bradycardia. Abnormal findings should be followed up with cardiac auscultation of the apical pulse (see Chapter 20 for more detail).

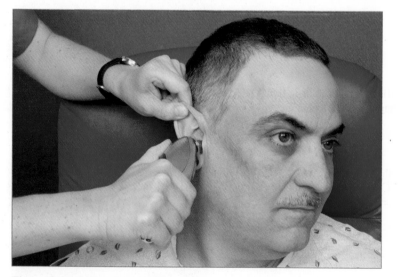

Figure 7-2 Taking a tympanic temperature.

continued

Assessment Procedure	Normal Findings	Abnormal Findings
Evaluate pulse rhythm.	There are regular intervals between beats.	Irregular intervals between beats should be followed up with auscultation of the apical pulse (see Chapter 20). When describing irregular beats, indicate whether they are regular irregular or irregular irregular.
Assess amplitude and contour.	Normally pulsation is equally strong in both wrists. Upstroke is smooth and rapid with a more gradual downstroke.	A bounding or weak and thready pulse is not normal. Delayed upstroke is also abnormal. Follow up on abnormal amplitude and contour findings by palpating the carotid arteries, which provides the best assessment of amplitude and contour (see Chapter 21).
Palpate arterial elasticity.	Artery feels straight, resilient, and springy. The older client's artery may feel more rigid, hard, and bent.	Artery feels rigid.

Respirations

Assessment Procedure	Normal Findings	Abnormal Findings
Monitor the respiratory rate. Observe the client's chest rise and fall with each breath. Count respirations for 30 seconds and multiply by 2 (refer to Chapter 16 for more information). ➤ *Clinical Tip* · *If you place the client's arm across the chest while palpating pulse, you can also count respirations. Do this by keeping your fingers on the client's pulse even after you have finished taking it.*	Between 12 and 20 breaths/min is normal. In the older adult, the respiratory rate may range from 15 to 22. The rate may increase with a shallower inspiratory phase because vital capacity and inspiratory reserve volume decrease with aging.	Fewer than 12 breaths/min or more than 20 breaths/min are abnormal.
Observe respiratory rhythm.	Rhythm is regular (if irregular, count for one full minute).	Rhythm is irregular (see Chapter 18 for more detail).

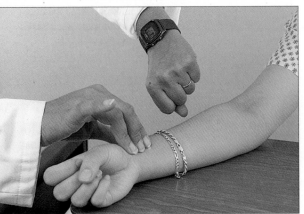

Figure 7-3 Timing the radial pulse rate. (© B. Proud.)

continued

PHYSICAL ASSESSMENT *Continued*

Assessment Procedure	Normal Findings	Abnormal Findings
Observe respiratory depth.	There is equal bilateral chest expansion of 1 to 2 inches.	There is unequal, shallow, or extremely deep chest expansion (see Chapter 18 for more detail) and labored or gasping breaths are abnormal.
Blood Pressure Measure blood pressure (Fig. 7-4). Spotlight Technique 7-1 and Display 7-1 provide guidelines.	Systolic pressure is <120 mmHg.	Tables 7-1 and 7-2 provide blood pressure classifications and recommended follow-up criteria. More than a 10 mmHg pressure difference between arms may indicate coarctation of the aorta or cardiac disease.
Measure on dominant arm first. Take blood pressure in both arms when recording it for the first time. Take subsequent readings in arm with highest measurement. ➤ **Clinical Tip** • *Advise client to avoid nicotine and caffeine for 30 minutes prior to measurement. Ask client to empty bladder before evaluating and avoid talking to the client while taking the reading. Each of these prevents elevating blood pressure prior to/during reading (Reeves, 1995; Mcalister & Strauss, 2001).*	Diastolic pressure is <80 mmHg; varies with individuals. A pressure difference of 10 mmHg between arms is normal.	More rigid, arteriosclerotic arteries account for higher systolic blood pressure in older adults. Systolic pressure over 140 but diastolic pressure under 90 is called isolated systolic hypertension.
If the client takes antihypertensives or has a history of fainting or dizziness, assess for possible orthostatic hypotension. Measure blood pressure with the client in a standing or sitting position after taking the pressure with the client in a supine position. ➤ **Clinical Tip** • *An ill client may not be able to stand; sitting is usually adequate to detect if the client truly has orthostatic hypotension.*	A drop of less than 20 mmHg from recorded sitting position is normal.	A drop of 20 mmHg or more from the recorded sitting blood pressure may indicate orthostatic (postural) hypotension. Orthostatic hypotension may be related to a decreased baroreceptor sensitivity, fluid volume deficit (e.g., dehydration), or certain medications (i.e., diuretics, antihypertensives). Symptoms of orthostatic hypotension include dizziness, lightheadedness, and falling. Further evaluation and referral to the client's primary care provider are necessary.

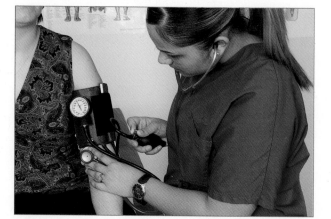

Figure 7-4   Measuring blood pressure.

continued on page 87

SPOTLIGHT TECHNIQUE 7-1 Measuring Blood Pressure

Preparation

Before measuring the blood pressure, consider the following behavioral and environmental conditions that can affect the reading:

- Room temperature too hot or cold
- Recent exercise
- Alcohol intake
- Nicotine use
- Muscle tension
- Bladder distension
- Background noise
- Talking (either patient or nurse)
- Arm position

Steps for Measuring Blood Pressure

1. Assemble your equipment so that the sphygmomanometer, stethoscope, and your pen and recording sheet are within easy reach.
2. Assist the client into a comfortable, quiet, restful position for 5 to 10 minutes. Client may lie down or sit.
3. Remove client's clothing from the arm and palpate the pulsations of the brachial artery. (If the client's sleeve can be pushed up to make room for the cuff, make sure that the clothing is not so constrictive that it would alter a correct pressure reading.)
4. Place the blood pressure cuff so that the midline of the bladder is over the arterial pulsation, and wrap the appropriate-sized cuff smoothly and snugly around the upper arm, 1 in. above the antecubital area so that there is enough room to place the bell of the stethoscope. The bladder inside the cuff should encircle 80% of the arm circumference in adults and 100% of the arm circumference in children younger than age 13. A cuff that is too small may give a false or abnormally high blood pressure reading. A mercury phygmomanometer is more reliable than an aneroid sphygmomanometer (Beevers, Lip, & O'Brien, 2001).
5. Support the client's arm slightly flexed at heart level with the palm up.
6. Put the earpieces of the stethoscope in your ears, then palpate the brachial pulse again and place the stethoscope lightly over this area. Position the mercury gauge on the manometer at eye level.
7. Adjust the screw above the bulb to tighten the valve on the air pump, and make sure that the tubing is not kinked or obstructed.
8. Inflate the cuff by pumping the bulb to about 30 mmHg above the point at which the radial pulse disappears. This will help you avoid missing an auscultatory gap.
9. Deflate the cuff slowly—about 2 mm per second—by turning the valve in the opposite direction while listening for the first of Korotkoff's sounds.
10. Read the point, closest to an even number, on the mercury gauge at which you hear the first faint but clear sound. Record this number as the systolic blood pressure. This is phase I of Korotkoff's sounds.
11. Next, note the point, closest to an even number, on the mercury gauge at which the sound becomes muffled (phase IV of the Korotkoff's sounds). Finally, note the point where the sound subsides completely (phase V of the Korotkoff's sounds). When both a change in sounds and a cessation of the sounds are heard, record the numbers at which you hear phase I, IV, and V sounds. Otherwise, record the first and last sounds.
12. Deflate the cuff at least another 10 mmHg to make sure you hear no more sounds. Then deflate completely and remove.
13. Record readings to the nearest 2 mmHg.

Cuff Selection Guidelines

The "ideal" cuff should have a bladder length that is 80% and a width that is at least 40% of the arm circumference (a length-to-width ratio of 2:1). A recent study comparing intra-arterial and auscultatory blood pressure concluded that the error is minimized with a cuff of 46% of the arm circumference. The recommended cuff sizes are

- 12×22 cm for arm circumference of 22 to 26 cm, which is the "small adult" size
- 16×30 cm for arm circumference of 27 to 34 cm, which is the "adult" size
- 16×36 cm for arm circumference of 35 to 44 cm, which is the "large adult" size
- 16×42 cm for arm circumference of 45 to 52 cm, which is the "adult thigh" size

Summary Points for Clinical Blood Pressure Measurement

- The patient should be seated comfortably with the back supported and the upper arm bared without constrictive clothing. The legs should not be crossed.
- The arm should be supported at heart level, and the bladder of the cuff should encircle at least 80% of the arm circumference.
- The mercury column should be deflated at 2 to 3 mm per second, and the first and last audible sounds should be taken as systolic and diastolic pressure. The column should be read to the nearest 2 mmHg.
- Neither the patient nor the observer should talk during the measurement.

(Based on information from American Heart Association. (2005). Recommendations for blood pressure measurement in humans and experimental animals. *Hypertension*, 45(1), 142–161. Available at http://hyper.ahajournals.org/cgi/content/full/45/1/142)

DISPLAY 7-1   **Identifying Korotkoff's Sounds**

Phase I

It is characterized by the first appearance of faint, clear, repetitive, tapping sounds that gradually intensify for at least two consecutive beats. This coincides approximately with the resumption of a palpable pulse. The number on the pressure gauge at which you hear the first tapping sound is the systolic pressure.

Phase II

It is characterized as muffled or swishing; these sounds are softer and longer than phase I sounds. They also have the quality of an intermittent murmur. They may temporarily subside, especially in hypertensive people. The loss of the sound during the latter part of phase I and during phase II is called the auscultatory gap. The gap may cover a range of as much as 40 mmHg; failing to recognize this gap may cause serious errors of underestimating systolic pressure or overestimating diastolic pressure.

Phase III

It is characterized by a return of distinct, crisp, and louder sounds as the blood flows relatively freely through an increasingly open artery.

Phase IV

It is characterized by sounds that are muffled, less distinct, and softer (with a blowing quality).

Phase V

It is characterized by all sounds disappearing completely. The last sound heard before this period of continuous silence is the onset of phase V and is the pressure commonly considered to define the diastolic measurement. (Some clinicians still consider the last sounds of phase IV the first diastolic value.)

Note: The American Heart Association recommends that values in phase IV and phase V be recorded when both a change in the sounds and a cessation in the sounds occur.

These recommendations apply particularly to children under age 13, pregnant women, and clients with high cardiac output or peripheral vasodilation. For example, such a blood pressure would be recorded as 120/80/64.

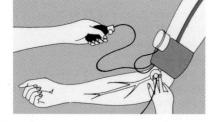

Initial silence.

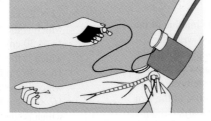

Turbulence.

Final silence.

(Adapted from American Heart Association [2005]. Recommendations for blood pressure measurement in humans and experimental animals. *Hypertension*, 45(1), 142–161. Available at http://hyper.ahajournals.org)

Table 7-1   **Categories for Blood Pressure Levels in Adults (Ages 18 and Older)**

Category	Blood Pressure Level (mmHg)	
	Systolic	Diastolic
Normal	<120	<80
Prehypertension	120–139	80–89
Stage 1 hypertension	140–159	90–99
Stage 2 hypertension	≥160	≥100

Source: These categories are from the National High Blood Pressure Education Program; National Heart, Lung, and Blood Institute; National Institutes of Health. Available at www.nhlbi.nih.gov/hbp/detect/categ/htm.

Assessment Procedure	Normal Findings	Abnormal Findings

Table 7-2 — Recommendations for Follow-Up Based on Initial Blood Pressure Measurements for Adults Without Acute End-Organ Damage

Initial Blood Pressure, mmHg*	Follow-Up Recommended[†]
Normal	Recheck in 2 years
Prehypertension	Recheck in 1 year[‡]
Stage 1 hypertension	Confirm within 2 months[‡]
Stage 2 hypertension	Evaluate or refer to source of care within 1 month. For those with higher pressures (e.g., >180/110 mmHg), evaluate and treat immediately or within 1 week depending on clinical situation and complications.

*If systolic and diastolic categories are different, follow recommendations for shorter time follow-up (e.g., 160/86 mmHg should be evaluated or referred to source of care within 1 month).

[†]Modify the scheduling of follow-up according to reliable information about past BP measurements, other cardiovascular risk factors, or target organ disease.

[‡]Provide advice about lifestyle modifications.

American Heart Association. (2008). Tenth Report of the Joint National Committee on Prevention, Detection, Evaluation, and Treatment of High Blood Pressure. Available at AHA website.

Assessment Procedure	Normal Findings	Abnormal Findings
Assess the pulse pressure—the difference between the systolic and diastolic blood pressure levels. Record in mmHg. For example, if the blood pressure was 120/80, then the pulse pressure would be 120 minus 80 or 40 mmHg.	Pulse pressure is 30 to 50 mmHg. Widening of the pulse pressure is seen with aging due to less elastic peripheral arteries.	A pulse pressure lower than 30 mmHg or higher than 50 mmHg may indicate cardiovascular disease.

Pain

Observe comfort level.	Client assumes a relatively relaxed posture without excessive position shifting. Facial expression is alert and pleasant.	Facial expression indicates discomfort (grimacing, frowning). Client may brace or holds body part that is painful. Breathing pattern indicates distress (shortness of breath, shallow, rapid breathing).
Ask the client if he or she has any pain.	No subjective report of pain	Any subjective report of pain should be further explored using the mnemonic COLDSPA. **Refer to Chapter 8 for further assessment of pain.**

Abnormal Findings 7-1   **Deviations Related to Physical Development, Body Build, and Fat Distribution**

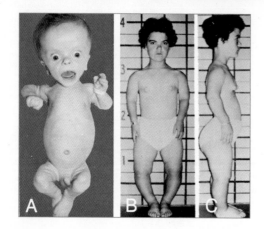

Dwarfism
These images show the associated decreased height and skeletal malformations.

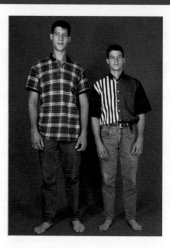

Gigantism
Note the disparity in height between the affected person and a person of the same age.

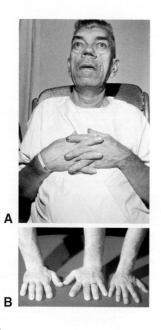

Acromegaly
The affected client shows the characteristic overgrowth of bones in the face, head, and hands.

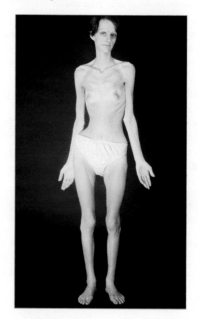

Anorexia nervosa
The client shows the emaciated appearance that follows self-starvation and accompanying extreme weight loss.

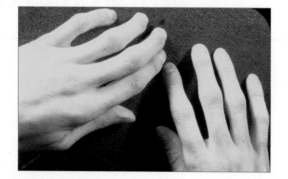

Marfan's syndrome
The elongated fingers are characteristic of this condition.

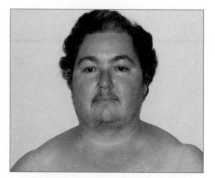

Cushing's syndrome
The affected client reflects the centralized weight gain.

VALIDATING AND DOCUMENTING FINDINGS

Validate the assessment data you have collected. This is necessary to verify that the data are reliable and accurate. Document the assessment data following the health care facility or agency policy.

Sample of Subjective Data

Mary Wright states age is 49 years, weight is 136 lbs. and height is 5 feet 4 inches. Has blood pressure checked with yearly physical exams. Usually 128/80. Does not run a fever but reports hot flashes on occasion. Does not have any pain or pain concerns. Voices happiness with family life and job as teacher. Just completed a master's degree in education and expresses interest in continuing her career teaching high school English.

Sample of Objective Data

Posture is erect and gait is smooth. Attractive female, neatly dressed in light weight clothes appropriate for summer season. Clean; nails well-groomed. Well-developed body build for age with even distribution of fat and firm muscle. Client is alert, friendly, cooperative, and answers questions with good eye contact. Smiles and laughs appropriately. Speech is fluent, clear, and moderately paced. Thoughts are free flowing. Able to recall recent events earlier in day (e.g., what she had for breakfast) without difficulty.

Oral temperature: 98.6°F; radial pulse: 84/min regular, bilateral, equally strong, and resilient; respirations: 16/min regular, equal bilateral chest expansion; blood pressure: sitting position—120/78 right arm, 124/80 left arm; standing position—124/80, RA; 126/82, LA.

Analysis of Data

After collecting subjective and objective data pertaining to general survey and vital signs, identify abnormal findings and client strengths. Then cluster the data to reveal any significant patterns or abnormalities. These data may then be used to make clinical judgments about the client.

DIAGNOSTIC REASONING: POSSIBLE CONCLUSIONS

Below are some possible conclusions related to your general survey, mental status exam, and vital signs.

Selected Nursing Diagnoses

After collecting subjective and objective data pertaining to the general survey, you will need to identify abnormals and cluster the data to reveal any significant patterns or abnormalities. These data will then be used to make clinical judgments (nursing diagnoses: wellness, risk, or actual) about the status of the client's general survey. Following is a list of selected nursing diagnoses that you may identify when analyzing data for this part of the assessment.

Wellness Diagnoses

- Health-Seeking Behaviors related to desire and request to learn more about health promotion

Risk Diagnoses

- Risk for Activity Intolerance related to deconditioned status
- Risk for Self-Directed Violence, related to depression, suicidal tendencies, developmental crisis, lack of support systems, loss of significant others, poor coping mechanisms and behaviors.

Actual Diagnoses

- Impaired Verbal Communication related to international language barrier (inability to speak English or accepted dominant language)
- Impaired Verbal Communication related to hearing loss
- Impaired Verbal Communication related to inability to clearly express self or understand others (aphasia)
- Impaired Verbal Communication related to aphasia, psychological impairment, or organic brain disorder
- Acute or Chronic Confusion related to dementia, head injury, stroke, alcohol or drug abuse.
- Impaired Memory related to dementia, stroke, head injury, alcohol or drug abuse
- Dressing/Grooming Self-Care Deficit related to impaired upper-extremity mobility and lack of resources
- Bathing/Hygiene Self-Care Deficit related to inability to wash body parts or inability to obtain water
- Disturbed Thought Processes related to alcohol or drug abuse, psychotic disorder, or organic brain dysfunction.
- Pain

Selected Collaborative Problems

After you group the data, it may become apparent that certain collaborative problems emerge. Remember that collaborative problems differ from nursing diagnoses in that they cannot be prevented by nursing interventions. However, these physiologic complications of medical conditions can be detected and monitored by the nurse. In addition, the nurse can use physician- and nurse-prescribed interventions to minimize the complications of these problems. The nurse may also have to refer the client in such situations for further treatment of the problem. Following is a list of collaborative problems that may be identified when obtaining a general impression. These problems are worded as Risk for Complications (or RC), followed by the problem.

- RC: Hypertension
- RC: Hypotension
- RC: Dysrhythmias
- RC: Hyperthermia
- RC: Hypothermia
- RC: Tachycardia

- RC: Bradycardia
- RC: Dyspnea
- RC: Hypoxemia

Medical Problems

After you group the data, it may become apparent that the client has signs and symptoms that require medical diagnosis and treatment. Refer to a primary care provider as necessary.

References and Selected Readings

Acromegaly.org. (n.d.). What is acromegaly? Available at http://www.acromegaly.org

Aird, T., & McIntosh, M. (2004). Nursing tools and strategies to assess cognition and confusion. *British Journal of Nursing, 13*(10), 621–626.

Alcenius, M. (2004). Successfully meet pain assessment standards. *Nursing Management, 35*(3), 12.

American Heart Association. (2005). Recommendations for blood pressure measurement in humans and experimental animals. *Hypertension, 45*(1), 142–161. Available at http://hyper.ahajournals.org/cgi/content/full/45/1/142

American Heart Association. (2008). Tenth Report of the Joint National Committee on Prevention, Detection, Evaluation, and Treatment of High Blood Pressure. Available at AHA website.

Artinian, N. T. (2004). Innovations in blood pressure monitoring: New, automated devices provide in-home or around-the-clock readings. *American Journal of Nursing, 104*(8), 52–59.

Baker, R. L. (2001). Pain assessment—the 5th vital sign. *Science of Psychosocial Processes, 14*(3), 152–154, 160.

Beevers, G., Lip, G., & O'Brien, E. (2001). *British Medical Journal, 322*(7295), 1167–1170.

Bern, L., Brandt, M., Nwanneka, M., Uzunma, A., Fisher, T., Shaver, Y., et al. (2007). Differences in blood pressure values obtained with automated and manual methods in medical inpatients. *MEDSURG Nursing, 6*(16), 356–362.

Body shape may be a reliable predictor of death in postmenopausal women with estrogen-dependent breast cancer. (2004, February). *Environmental Nutrition.* Available at http://www.highbeam.com/Environmental+Nutrition/publications.aspx (Accessed on February 01, 2004).

Braam, R., & Thien, T. (2005). Is the accuracy of blood pressure measuring devices underestimated at increasing blood pressure levels? *Blood Pressure Monitoring, 10*, 283–289.

Colin Bell, A., Adair, L., & Popkin, B. (2002). Ethnic differences in the association between body mass index and hypertension. *American Journal of Epidemiology, 155*(4), 346–353.

DeGowin, R., LeBlond, R., & Brown, D. (2004). *DeGowin's diagnostic examination.* Chicago: McGraw-Hill Professional.

Doerr, S. (2008). Hyperthermia and heat-related illness. Available at http://www.medicinenet.com

Erickson, R. (1976). Thermometer placement for oral temperature measurement in febrile adults. *International Journal of Nursing Studies, 38*, 671–675.

Flaherty, J. H. (2001). Guest editorial: "Who's taking your 5th vital sign?". *Journal of Gerontology: Medical Sciences, 56a*(7), M397–M399.

Folstein, M. F., Folstein, S. E., & McHugh, P. R. (1975). Mini-mental state: A practical guide for grading the cognitive state of patients for the clinician. *Journal of Psychiatric Research, 12*(3), 189–198.

Fothergill Bourbainnais, F., Perrefault, A., & Bouvette, M. (2004). Introduction of a pain and symptom assessment tool in the clinical setting—lessons learned. *Journal of Nursing Management, 12*, 194–200.

Gilbert, M., Barton, A. J., & Counsel, C. M. (2002). Comparison of oral and tympanic temperature in adult surgical patients. *Applied Nursing Research, 15*(1), 42–47.

Giuliano, K. (2005). Non-invasive blood pressure monitoring. In S. M. Burns (Ed.), *AACN protocols for practice: Non-invasive monitoring* (2nd ed., pp. 83–97). Sudbury, MA: Jones & Bartlett Publishers.

Introduction: Tachypnea. (2008). Available at http://cureresearch.com/t/tachypnea/into

Konopad, E., Kerr, J. R., Noseworthy, T., & Grace, H. (1994). A comparison of oral, axillary, rectal, and tympanic membrane temperatures of intensive care patients with and without an oral endotracheal tube. *Journal of Advanced Nursing, 20*(1), 77–84.

Layman, D. (2004). Stressors or stimula: Disturbers of body parameters. In *Physiology demystified: A self-teaching guide* (p. 41). Chicago: McGraw-Hill Professional.

Livingston, M. (2007). Sinus bradycardia. Available at http://www.emedicine.medscape.com [search emergency medicine and sinus bradycardia]

Mayo Clinic. (2007a). Anorexia nervosa. Available at http://www.mayoclinic.com [search by subject]

Mayo Clinic. (2007b). Dwarfism. Available at http://www.mayoclinic.com [search by subject]

Mayo Clinic. (2007c). Hypothermia. Available at http://www.mayoclinic.com [search by subject]

Mayo Clinic. (2007d). Low blood pressure (hypotension). Available at http://www.mayoclinic.com [search by subject]

Mayo Clinic. (2007e). Tachycardia. Available http://http://www.mayoclinic.com [search by subject]

McCallister, F. A., & Straus, S. E. (2001). Evidence-based treatment of hypertension. Measurement of blood pressure, and evidence-based review. *BMJ, 322*, 908–911.

Murphy, A. (2005). Links between body shape and heart disease: Are you an apple or a pear? Available at http://www.medicalnewstoday.com [search heart disease news body shape 2005]

Neuroexam.com. (n.d.). Gait. Available at http://www.neuroexam.com

Office of Disease Prevention and Health Promotion, U.S. Department of Health and Human Services. (2000). *Healthy people 2010: Understanding and improving health* (2nd ed.). Washington, DC: Author.

Pickering, T., Hall, J., Appel, L., Falkner, B., Graves, J., Hill, M., et al. (2005). Recommendations for blood pressure measurement in humans and experimental animals. Part 1: Blood pressure measurements in humans: A statement for professions from the subcommittee of professional and public education of the American Heart Association Council of High Blood Pressure Research. *Hypertension, 45*, 142–161.

Schubbe, J. (2004). Good posture helps reduce back pain. Available at http://www.spine-health.com/wellness/ergonomics/good-posture-helps-reduce-back-pain

Science Museums of Minnesota. (2000). Habits of the heart. Available at http://www.smm.org/heart/lessons

Smith, L. S. (2004). Using low-tech thermometers to measure body temperatures in older adults: A pilot study. *Journal of Gerontological Nursing, 29*(11), 26–33.

Souder, E., & O'Sullivan, P. S. (2000). Nursing documentation versus standardized assessment of cognitive status in hospitalized medical patients. *Applied Nursing Research, 13*(1), 29–36.

8

Assessing Pain: The 5th Vital Sign

Structure and Function

DEFINITION

The International Association for the Study of Pain (IASP) defines pain as "an unpleasant sensory and emotional experience, which we primarily associate with tissue damage or describe in terms of such damage, or both (IASP, 1994; Ranney," 2008). Recent literature has emphasized the importance and undertreatment of pain and has recommended that pain be the fifth vital sign. Some states in the United States have passed laws necessitating the adoption of an assessment tool and documenting pain assessment in patient charts along with temperature, pulse, heart rate, and blood pressure (see Chapter 7). Inadequate treatment of acute pain has been shown to result in physiological, psychological, and emotional distress that can lead to chronic pain (Dunwoody, Krenzischek, Pasero, Rathmell, & Polomano, 2008).

Pain is explained as a combination of physiological phenomena but with psychosocial aspects that influence perception of the pain. The most important definition of pain as it is experienced is that by McCaffery and Pasero (1999): "Pain is whatever the person says it is." This is an important concept for nurses to remember when assessing and treating pain.

PATHOPHYSIOLOGY

Several theories have tried to explain the concept of pain. Melzack and Wall in 1965 proposed the gate control model that emphasizes the importance of the central nervous system mechanisms of pain (see Fig. 8-1) (Wall & Melzack, 1994).

The pathophysiological phenomena of pain are associated with the central and peripheral nervous systems. The source of pain stimulates peripheral nerve endings (**nociceptors**), which transmit the sensations to the central nervous system. Various types of stimuli excite the nociceptors: mechanical, thermal, chemical (including chemical reactions in tissues causing ischemia or spasm). Nociceptors are distributed in the body, in the skin, subcutaneous tissue, skeletal muscle, joints, peritoneal surfaces, pleural membranes, dura mater, and blood vessel walls. Note that they are not located in the parenchyma of visceral organs. Physiological processes involved in pain perception (or nociception) include transduction, transmission, modulation, and perception.

Transduction of pain begins when a mechanical, thermal, or chemical stimulus results in tissue injury or damage stimulating the nociceptors, which are the primary afferent nerves for receiving painful stimuli. Noxious stimuli initiate a painful stimulus resulting in an inflammatory process that leads to release of cytokines and neuropeptides from circulating leukocytes, platelets, vascular endothelial cells, immune cells, and cells from within the peripheral nervous system. This results in the activation of the primary afferent nociceptors (A-delta and C-fibers). Furthermore, the nociceptors themselves release a substance P that enhances nociception, causing vasodilation, increased blood flow, and edema with further release of bradykinin, serotonin from platelets, and histamine from mast cells.

A-delta primary afferent fibers (small-diameter, lightly myelinated fibers) and C-fibers (unmyelinated, primary afferent fibers) are classified as nociceptors because they are stimulated by noxious stimuli. A-delta primary afferent fibers transmit fast pain to the spinal cord within 0.1 second, which is felt as pricking, sharp, or electric quality sensation and usually is caused by mechanical or thermal stimuli. C-fibers transmit slow pain within 1 second, which is felt as burning, throbbing, or aching and is caused by mechanical, thermal, or chemical stimuli usually resulting in tissue damage. By the direct excitation of the primary afferent fibers, the stimulus leads to the activation of the fiber terminals.

The transmission process is initiated by this inflammatory process, resulting in the conduction of an impulse in the primary afferent neurons to the dorsal horn of the spinal cord. There, neurotransmitters are released and concentrated in the substantia gelatinosa (which is thought to host the gating mechanism described in the gate control theory) and bind to specific receptors. The output neurons from the dorsal horn cross the anterior white commissure and ascend the spinal cord in the anterolateral quadrant in two ascending pathways (Fig. 8-2):

1. Spinothalamic tract (STT): ascends through the lateral edge of the medulla, lateral pons, and midbrain to the thalamus, then to the somatosensory cortex. It transmits location, quality, and intensity of acute pain and threatening events.

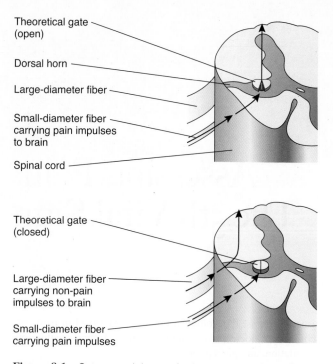

Theoretical gate (open)
Dorsal horn
Large-diameter fiber
Small-diameter fiber carrying pain impulses to brain
Spinal cord

Theoretical gate (closed)
Large-diameter fiber carrying non-pain impulses to brain
Small-diameter fiber carrying pain impulses

Figure 8-1 Gate control theory of pain

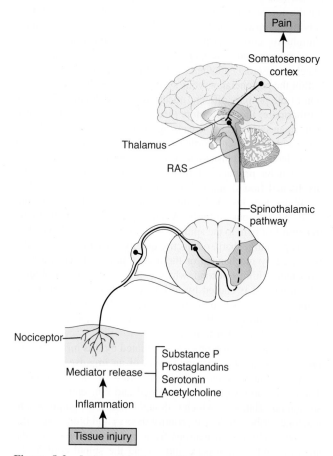

Pain
Somatosensory cortex
Thalamus
RAS
Spinothalamic pathway
Nociceptor
Substance P
Prostaglandins
Serotonin
Acetylcholine
Mediator release
Inflammation
Tissue injury

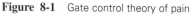

Figure 8-2 Pathways for transmitting pain.

2. Spinoreticular tract (SRT): ascends to the reticular formation, the pontine, medullary areas, and medial thalamic nuclei. It transmits pain information from the brainstem to the limbic area through noradrenergic bundles.

Modulation of pain is a difficult phenomenon. Modulation inhibits the pain message and involves the body's own endogenous neurotransmitters (endorphins, enkephalins, and serotonin) in the course of processing the pain stimuli.

The process of pain **perception** is still poorly understood. Studies have shown that the emotional status (depression and anxiety) affects directly the level of pain perceived and thus reported by patients. The hypothalamus and limbic system are responsible for the emotional aspect of the pain perception while the frontal cortex is responsible for the rational interpretation and response to pain.

PHYSIOLOGICAL RESPONSES TO PAIN

Pain elicits a stress response in the human body triggering the sympathetic nervous system, resulting in physiological responses such as the following:

- Anxiety, fear, hopelessness, sleeplessness, thoughts of suicide
- Focus on pain, reports of pain, cries and moans, frowns and facial grimaces
- Decrease in cognitive function, mental confusion, altered temperament, high somatization, and dilated pupils
- Increased heart rate, peripheral, systemic, and coronary vascular resistance, blood pressure
- Increased respiratory rate and sputum retention resulting in infection and atelectasis
- Decreased gastric and intestinal motility
- Decreased urinary output resulting in urinary retention, fluid overload, depression of all immune responses
- Increased antidiuretic hormone, epinephrine, norepinephrine, aldosterone, glucagons, decreased insulin, testosterone
- Hyperglycemia, glucose intolerance, insulin resistance, protein catabolism
- Muscle spasm resulting in impaired muscle function and immobility, perspiration

CLASSIFICATION

Pain is classified in several ways. Duration, location, etiology, and severity are four of these. Duration and etiology are often classified together to differentiate **acute pain**, **chronic nonmalignant pain**, and **cancer pain**.

- **Acute pain:** usually associated with a recent injury
- **Chronic nonmalignant pain:** usually associated with a specific cause or injury and described as a constant pain that persists for more than 6 months
- **Cancer pain:** often due to the compression of peripheral nerves or meninges or from the damage to these structures following surgery, chemotherapy, radiation, or tumor growth and infiltration.

Pain location classifications include

- **Cutaneous pain** (skin or subcutaneous tissue)
- **Visceral pain** (abdominal cavity, thorax, cranium)
- **Deep somatic pain** (ligaments, tendons, bones, blood vessels, nerves)

Another aspect of pain location is whether it is perceived at the site of the pain stimuli if it is **radiating** (perceived both at the source and extending to other tissues) or **referred** (perceived in body areas away from the pain source; see Fig. 8-3).

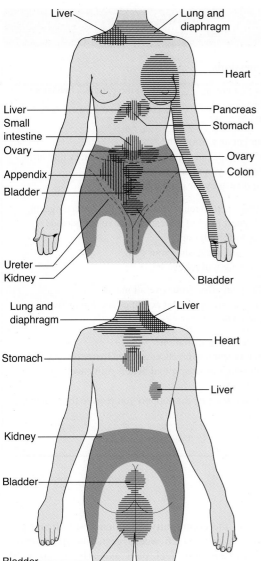

Figure 8-3 Areas of referred pain. (*Top*) Anterior view. (*Bottom*) Posterior view.

Phantom pain can be perceived in nerves left by a missing, amputated, or paralyzed body part.

Other types of pain not easily classified in the categories mentioned are **neuropathic pain** and **intractable pain**. Neuropathic pain causes an abnormal processing of pain messages and results from past damage to peripheral or central nerves due to sustained neurochemical levels, but exact mechanisms for the perception of neuropathic pain are unclear. Intractable pain is defined by its high resistance to pain relief.

THE SEVEN DIMENSIONS OF PAIN

The experience of pain is quite complex. It is more than the physiological and neurochemical responses. Silkman (2008) describes the multidimensional complexity of pain in seven dimensions: physical, sensory, behavioral, sociocultural, cognitive, affective, and spiritual. The **physical dimension** refers to the physiological effects just described. This dimension includes the patient's perception of the pain and the body's reaction to the stimulus. The **sensory dimension** concerns the quality of the pain and how severe the pain is perceived to be. This dimension includes the patient's perception of the pain's location, intensity, and quality. The **behavioral dimension** refers to the verbal and nonverbal behaviors that the patient demonstrates in response to the pain. The **sociocultural dimension** concerns the influences of the patient's social context and cultural background on the patient's pain experience. The **cognitive dimension** concerns "beliefs, attitudes, intentions, and motivations related to the pain and its management" (p. 14). Of course, beliefs, attitudes, intentions, and motivations are affected by all of the dimensions mentioned, but can be associated with the management part of the pain experience, which is dependent on cognition. The **affective dimension** concerns feelings, sentiments, and emotions related to the pain experience. The pain can affect the emotions and the emotions can affect the perception of pain. And finally, the **spiritual dimension** refers to the meaning and purpose that the person "attributes to the pain, self, others, and the divine" (p. 15). For some suggested questions to assess each dimension, see Assessment Tool 8-1.

ASSESSMENT TOOL 8-1	*Pain Dimensions: Sample Assessment Questions*

Here are examples of questions to ask your patient when assessing the seven dimensions of pain.

Dimension	**Sample Questions**
Physical: effect of anatomic structure and physiological functioning on the experience of pain	What surgeries or other medical procedures have you had? What medical conditions do you have? What conditions brought you to the hospital or doctor's office in the past?
Sensory: qualitative and quantitative descriptions of pain	Where is the pain located? What does the pain feel like? How would you rate the pain on a scale of 1 to 10, with 10 being the worst pain imaginable? When did the pain begin? How long does the pain usually last?

continued on page 94

ASSESSMENT TOOL 8-1	Pain Dimensions: Sample Assessment Questions *Continued*

Dimension	Sample Questions
Behavioral: verbal and nonverbal behaviors associated with pain	I notice that you are _____(fill in the patient's behavior, such as grimacing). Are you having pain?
Sociocultural: effect of social and cultural backgrounds on the experience of pain	What is your country of origin? Do you have any special cultural or social practices that influence the decisions you make about health care? How do you manage your pain at home?
Cognitive: thoughts, beliefs, attitudes, intentions, and motivations related to the experience of pain	How effective is the pain relief treatment you're currently getting? What's the highest level of education you've completed? What do you do for a living? What do you think is causing your pain? What do you think will relieve it?
Affective: feelings and emotions that result from pain	How does the pain affect your overall mood? Daily life and activities? Social activities and interactions? Personal relationships?
Spiritual: ultimate meaning and purpose attributed to pain, self, others, and the divine	What's your religious affiliation? What religious or spiritual practices and preferences do you have? How do your religious or spiritual beliefs influence your health care decisions? How would you describe the support you receive from friends and loved ones?

(From Silkman, C. (2008). Assessing the seven dimensions of pain. *American Nurse Today, 3*(2), 13–15. Used with permission.)

PAIN ASSESSMENT

Before beginning to collect data from the patient, there are several more elements of pain history that must be considered. The **developmental level** or **age** of the person makes a difference in assessment approach. Also, **culture** must be considered as cultural beliefs about pain and its treatment vary widely. **Cancer pain** is often considered separately because it can be caused by many elements of the disease or treatment, or by other sources of pain not related to the disease. A thorough pain assessment includes questions about **location, intensity, quality, pattern, precipitating factors**, and **pain relief**, as well as the effect of the pain on **daily activities**, what **coping strategies** have been used, and **emotional responses** to the pain. Note that pain assessment lends itself well to the COLDSPA mnemonic.

Developmental Level

The two extremes of development, pediatric (neonate to later childhood) and geriatric age groups, have characteristics that make pain assessment more difficult. Because pain has both sensory and emotional components, assessment strategies usually use quantitative and qualitative information. The American Pain Society (2008a) reports that chronic pain affects 15% to 20% of children, and Binasco (2003) noted studies that have shown that 33 million people aged 65 or older, 62% of nursing home residents and 25% to 50% of elders living in the community, experience significant pain. Even fetuses at least by 26 weeks gestation are known to perceive pain, and may feel pain as early as 20 weeks (Mahieu-Caputo, Dommergues, Muller, & Dumez, 2000). Obviously, then, even extremely premature infants and full-term neonates feel pain.

Not knowing whether fetuses, premature infants, neonates, young children, the elderly, and the cognitively impaired (elderly or others) are feeling pain can lead to gross undertreatment of pain in these people. The results of under-treated pain in any patient can be profound, resulting in both physical and psychological problems that can be avoided if pain is assessed and treated properly. Undertreated pain in children can lead to chronic pain conditions when they become adults.

Even cognitively intact elders, parents of children, and persons from certain cultures (see the following text) hold beliefs that may prevent the patient's pain from being assessed and treated correctly. Some people believe that pain is a punishment for past sins or behaviors, some believe it is a natural part of the aging process, and some believe that having pain indicates that a disease is getting worse or that death is near. For such reasons, patients or their families may give untrue answers to questions about pain. Some patients and health care providers also fear addiction from narcotics or opioids. Learning how to assess pain and teaching patients, families, and other health care providers about pain care are essential for nurses who provide high-quality care.

Pain in Persons Unable to Provide a Self-Report (Unconscious, Cognitively Impaired, Elders with Dementia, Intubated Patients, Infants, and Preverbal Toddlers)

For nonverbal persons or those with cognitive impairment, it has been recommended that the Hierarchy of Pain Assessment Techniques (McCaffery & Pasero, 1999) be used (Herr et al., 2006). The Hierarchy includes five items:

1. Self-report—always try to get a self-report, but note if unable and go on to the other items

2. Search for potential causes of pain—pathological conditions, procedures such as surgery, wound care, positioning, skin invasion by needle or catheter, or other known pain producers or diseases

3. Observe patient behaviors—many scales reflect pain-related behaviors of different patient types. See Pain Scales listed by Herr et al. and selected ones later in this chapter. Note: Patient behaviors may not accurately reflect pain intensity

4. Surrogate reporting (family members, parents, caregivers) of pain and behavior/activity changes—Note: Discrepancies may exist between self-report of pain and surrogate reports, and between surrogates and health care providers on judgments of pain and its intensity

5. Attempt an analgesic trial—a full protocol is recommended. After an analgesic is ordered, the nurse needs to observe for changes in self-report, if any, or in any behaviors

QUESTT Principles for Pain in Children

The mnemonic QUESTT was developed by Baker and Wong (1987) and described by the Texas Cancer Council's Cancer Pain Management in Children website (1999). Main points that underlie the mnemonic are that in clinical assessment of pain, regular and systematic assessment is essential; the health care provider should believe the patient's or family's report of the pain and should empower them by involving them in decision making. The mnemonic is

Question the child

Use pain-rating scales

Evaluate behavior and physiological changes

Secure parents' involvement

Take cause of pain into account

Take action and evaluate results

Cancer Pain

Cancer pain is a special category of pain because it may reflect all of the pain types at the same time or at different times during the course of the disease. Cancer pain may be caused by the cancer, its treatment, or its metastasis. Some important facts about cancer pain are as follows:

- It can be acute (sudden and severe) or chronic (lasting more than 3 months)
- Its types include somatic pain, visceral pain, and neuropathic pain
- It causes breakthrough pain (brief, severe pain that occurs in spite of pain medication) in many patients
- It depends on many factors, including the type and stage of the cancer
- It may be triggered by blocked blood vessels or pressure on a nerve from a tumor
- Side effects of cancer treatments, such as surgery, radiation, and chemotherapy, may include pain
- About 90% of patients with advanced cancer experience severe pain, which often is undertreated
- Cancer pain can result from
  - Blocked blood vessels causing poor circulation
  - Bone fracture from metastasis
  - Infection
  - Inflammation
  - Psychological or emotional problems
  - Side effects from cancer treatments (e.g., chemotherapy, radiation)
  - Tumor exerting pressure on a nerve (Healthcommunities .com, 1998–2008)

Cultural Expressions of Pain

Pain is a universal human experience, but how people respond to pain varies with the meaning placed on pain and the response expected from pain in the culture in which the person is raised. There are certain patterns of pain expression that vary across cultures. Pain can have several meanings that lead to these different response patterns. Refer to the examples shown in Display 8-1, "Cultural Expressions of Pain." Although these examples of differences in meaning and expression of pain show some of the cultural variations that are important for the nurse assessing for pain, the most important factor is this: Do Not Stereotype! This means that even though there are tendencies for people from a particular cultural background to exhibit

DISPLAY 8-1	Cultural Expressions of Pain

Cultural Group	Pain Expression/Beliefs
Asian and Asian-American	• Pain is natural • Use mind over body; positive thinking • Pain is honorable • Pain may be caused by past transgressions and helps to atone and achieve higher spirituality • Stigma against narcotic use may result in underreporting of pain
African-American	• Pain is a challenge to be fought • Pain is inevitable and is to be endured • Pain is stigmatized resulting in inhibition in expressing pain or seeking help • Pain may be a punishment from God • God and prayer will help more than medicine

continued on page 96

DISPLAY 8-1	**Cultural Expressions of Pain** *Continued*
Hindu	• Pain must be endured as part of preparing for the next life in the cycle of reincarnation • Must remain conscious when nearing death to experience the events of dying and perhaps rebirth
Native American	• Pain is to be endured • May not ask for medication due to respect for caregivers who should know their needs • Metaphors and images from nature are used to describe pain (Kaegi, 2004)
Hispanic	• Pain response is often very expressive, though pain must be endured to perform gender role duties • Pain is natural, but may be the result of sinful or immoral behavior
Jewish	• Pain is expressed openly with much complaining • Pain must be shared, recognized, and validated by others so that the experience is affirmed (Steele, 2002)

Before looking at how patients from cultures different from your own express their pain and the meaning pain has for them, it is very important for you, the caregiver, to recognize your own response to pain. How did you respond to pain in your family? What did you think about pain when you were a child? Did your parents respond the same way? What did they teach you about pain? Some are raised to deny pain, since it is just a normal part of life. Others are raised to respond verbally and loudly to pain, since it indicates an invasion of the body and is a sign that something bad has happened or will happen. Are you stoic? Are you vocal and loud, moaning or crying, if pain is intense?

Knowing your own response to pain lets you know a little about what you believe about pain. A perception that our responses and beliefs are "normal" and those of others are not can lead to miscommunications between nurses and patients.

To be a **culturally competent nurse** caring for patients in pain:

- Be aware of your own cultural and family values
- Be aware of your personal biases and assumptions about people with different values than yours
- Be aware and accept cultural differences between yourself and individual patients
- Be capable of understanding the dynamics of the difference
- Be able to adapt to diversity (Weissman, Gordon, & Bidar-Sielaff, 2002)

certain characteristics, many people of that culture will not. The nurse must assess what the person says about pain, what the person says about asking for pain medication, what the person says about the meaning pain has, how the person behaves when undergoing known-to-be painful procedures, and how the person behaves when others are present or absent. In other words, treat each patient as a unique individual, assess each patient, respect each patient's responses to pain, and treat each patient with dignity and consideration.

A variety of issues can create barriers to pain assessment (see Display 8-2). For an excellent source for interventions to overcome cultural and communication barriers when caring for patients in pain, see *What Color Is My Pain?* by Louise Kaegi (2004).

DISPLAY 8-2	**Barriers to Pain Assessment**

Barriers to correct pain assessment may be present and must be assessed as well. Cultural differences and physiological differences account for most of these. Consider cultural variation to exist in all patient populations and not just among persons from other countries. Also, gender differences are expressed differently in different cultures. Nurses' and other health care providers' beliefs about pain can also affect the assessment.

Barriers Based on Beliefs
- Acknowledging pain is not manly; it is a sign of weakness
- Pain is a punishment (often thought to be from God) for past mistakes, sins, or behaviors, and must be tolerated
- Pain indicates that my condition/disease is getting worse, and that I am going to die soon. If I don't acknowledge it, it won't be so bad.

- Pain medications are addictive; cause awful side effects; and make me "dopey," confused, and sleepy or unconscious
- All people have pain, especially as they age. This is just normal pain and I should not say anything about it.

Barriers Based on Physical Conditions
- The disease/illness/injury for which the patient is being treated is not the source of the pain
- Both the current disease and another disease are causing pain
- The patient expresses few, if any, pain-related behaviors once accommodated to prolonged chronic pain conditions

continued

DISPLAY 8-2	**Barriers to Pain Assessment** *Continued*

Barriers Based on Health Care Providers' Beliefs
- Patients who complain of pain frequently are just trying to get more pain medicine or are addicts wanting more narcotics, etc.
- Patients who complain of pain but don't show physical and behavioral signs of pain don't need more pain medication, whether they are chronic pain patients or acute pain patients

- Old people just have more pain
- Confused or demented patients, or very young patients, neonates, and fetuses don't feel pain
- Patients who are sleeping don't have pain
- Pain medication causes addiction/respiratory depression/too many side effects
- Giving as much pain medication as possible at night will make the patients sleep and not disturb the nurses

Health Assessment

COLLECTING SUBJECTIVE DATA: THE NURSING HEALTH HISTORY

There are few objective findings on which the assessment of pain can rely. Pain is a subjective phenomenon and thus the main assessment lies in the client's reporting. The client's description of pain is quoted. The exact words used to describe the experienced of pain are used to help in the diagnosis and management. Pain, its onset, duration, causes, alleviating and aggravating factors are assessed. Then the quality, intensity and the effects of pain on the physical, psychosocial, and spiritual aspects are questioned. Past experience with pain in addition to past and current therapies are explored.

(text continues on page 100)

HISTORY OF PRESENT HEALTH CONCERN

Review JCAHO standards (Display 8-3) and tips for collecting subjective data (Display 8-4) before assessing the client's subjective experience of pain.

Following Joint Commission standards and tips for collecting subjective data will enhance evaluation of the client's personal experience of pain.

continued on page 98

DISPLAY 8-3	**Joint Commission Standards for Pain Management**

Joint Commission Standards for Pain Management were revised and published in 2000–2001. The standards require healthcare providers and organizations to improve pain assessment and management for all patients.

- Recognize the right of patients to appropriate assessment and management of pain
- Screen for the existence and assess the nature and intensity of pain in all patients
- Record the results of the assessment in a way that facilitates regular reassessment and follow-up
- Determine and ensure staff competency in pain assessment and management, and address pain assessment and management in the orientation of all new staff
- Establish policies and procedures that support the appropriate prescription or ordering of effective pain medications
- Educate patients and their families about effective pain management
- Address patient needs for symptom management in the discharge planning process
- Maintain a pain control performance improvement plan

(From Chapman, C. R. (2000). New JCAHO standards for pain management: carpe diem! *APS Bulletin, 10*(4). Available at http://www.ampainsoc.org/pub/bulletin/jul00)

| DISPLAY 8-4 | **Tips for Collecting Subjective Data** |

- Maintain a quiet and calm environment that is comfortable for the patient being interviewed
- Maintain the client's privacy and ensure confidentiality
- Ask the questions in an open-ended format
- Listen carefully to the client's verbal descriptions and quote the terms used
- Watch for the client's facial expressions and grimaces during the interview
- DO NOT put words in the client's mouth
- Ask the client about past experiences with pain
- Believe the client's expression of pain

HISTORY OF PRESENT HEALTH CONCERN *Continued*

Question	Rationale
Are you experiencing pain now or have you in the past 24 hours?	To establish the presence or absence of perceived pain.
Where is the pain located?	The location of pain helps to identify the underlying cause.
Does it radiate or spread?	Radiating or spreading pain helps to identify the source. For example, chest pain radiating to the left arm is most probably of cardiac origin while the pain that is pricking and spreading in the chest muscle area is probably musculoskeletal in origin.
Are there any other concurrent symptoms accompanying the pain?	Accompanying symptoms also help to identify the possible source. For example, right lower quadrant pain associated with nausea, vomiting, and the inability to stand up straight is possibly associated with appendicitis.
When did the pain start?	The onset of pain is an essential indicator for the severity of the situation and suggests a source.
What were you doing when the pain first started?	This helps to identify the precipitating factors and what might have exacerbated the pain.
Is the pain continuous or intermittent?	This is also to help identify the nature of the pain.
If intermittent pain, how often do the episodes occur and for how long do they last?	Understanding the course of the pain provides a pattern that may help to determine the source.
Describe the pain in your own words.	Clients are quoted so that terms used to describe their pain may indicate the type and source. The most common terms used are: throbbing, shooting, stabbing, sharp, cramping, gnawing, hot-burning, aching, heavy, tender, splitting, tiring-exhausting, sickening, fearful, punishing.
What factors relieve your pain?	Relieving factors help to determine the source and the plan of care.
What factors increase your pain?	Identifying factors that increase pain helps to determine the source and helps in planning to avoid aggravating factors.
Are you on any therapy to manage your pain?	This question establishes any current treatment modalities and their effect on the pain. This helps in planning the future plan of care.
Is there anything you would like to add?	An open-ended question allows the client to mention anything that has been missed or the issues that were not fully addressed by the above questions.

continued

COLDSPA Example for Pain

Use the **COLDSPA** mnemonic as a guideline to collect needed information for each symptom the client shares. In addition, the following questions help elicit important information.

Mnemonic	Question	Client Response Example
Character	Describe the sign or symptom (feeling, appearance, sound, smell, or taste if applicable).	"My right lower side hurts. It is a steady aching that is getting worse."
Onset	When did it begin?	"Late last night."
Location	Where is it? Does it radiate? Does it occur anywhere else?	"It started in the middle of my stomach and now it is worse on my right side. It does not hurt anywhere else."
Duration	How long does it last? Does it recur?	"It has been ongoing since last night around 3 AM and is getting worse."
Severity	How bad is it? How much does it bother you?	"It hurts to walk or even move. I would rate it 8 on a scale of 10 (with 10 being the worst)."
Pattern	What makes it better or worse?	"It hurts constantly and gets worse if I move."
Associated factors/How it **A**ffects the client	What other symptoms occur with it? How does it affect you?	"I feel nauseated and like I may vomit. I cannot do anything except stay still or it gets worse."

PAST HEALTH HISTORY

Question	Rationale
Have you had any previous experience with pain?	Past experiences of pain may shed light on the previous history of the client in addition to possible positive or negative expectations of pain therapies.
Does this pain have any special meaning to you?	Some cultures view pain as a punishment or view pain as the main symptom to be treated as opposed to treating the underlying disease.

FAMILY HISTORY

Question	Rationale
Does any one in your family experience pain?	To assess possible family-related perceptions or any past experiences with persons in pain.
How does pain affect your family?	To assess how much the pain is interfering with the client's family relations.

LIFESTYLE AND HEALTH PRACTICES

Question	Rationale
What are your concerns about pain?	Identifying the client's fears and worries helps in prioritizing the plan of care and providing adequate psychological support.

continued on page 100

COLLECTING OBJECTIVE DATA: PHYSICAL EXAMINATION

Objective data are collected by using one of the pain assessment tools. There are many assessment tools, some of which are specific to special types of pain. The main issues in choosing the tool are its reliability and its validity. Moreover, the tool must be clear and, therefore, easily understood by the client, and require little effort from the client and the nurse.

Preparing the Client

In preparation for the interview, clients are seated in a quiet, comfortable and calm environment with minimal interruption. Explain to the client that the interview will entail questions to clarify the picture of the pain experienced in order to develop the plan of care.

Pain Assessment Scales

Select one or more pain assessment tools appropriate for the client. There are many pain assessment scales; for example, Visual Analog Scale (VAS), Numeric Pain Intensity Scale (NPI), Simple Descriptive Pain Intensity Scale, Graphic Rating Scale, Verbal Rating Scale, and Faces Pain Scales (FPS, FPS-R; see

Chapter 31). You can look at all of these and other scales at http://www.partnersagainstpain.com/professional-assessment/professional-assessment.aspx?id=2. Most of these scales have been shown to be reliable measures of patient pain. The three most popular scales are the Numeric Rating Scale (NRS), the Verbal Descriptor Scale, and the FPS, although VASs are often mentioned as very simple (see Figs. 8-4, 8-5, and 8-6). A pain assessment tool integrating several assessment tools and verbal translation to several languages has been developed (UCLA, n.d.). See the Universal Pain Assessment Tool (Fig. 8-7).

Assessing Pain in Older Adults

The NRS has been shown to be best for older adults with no cognitive impairment, and the Faces Pain Scale—Revised (FPS-R) for cognitively impaired adults (Flaherty, 2008).

Assessing Pain in Infants and Children

It is hard to evaluate pain in neonates and infants. Behaviors that indicate pain are used to assess their pain. One tool for such assessment is the N-PASS: Neonatal Pain, Agitation, & Sedation Scale (Hummel & Puchalski, 2000). Another popular tool for assessing pediatric pain is the FLACC Scale (Face, Legs, Activity, Cry, and Consolability; see Assessment Tool 8-2).

(text continues on page 102)

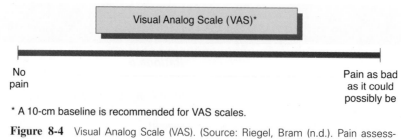

Figure 8-4 Visual Analog Scale (VAS). (Source: Riegel, Bram (n.d.). Pain assessment. Available at http://www.burnsurvivorsttw.org Burn Survivors Throughout The World, Inc. is an international nonprofit organization offering a support team, advocacy, medical referrals, email, chat room for burn survivors.)

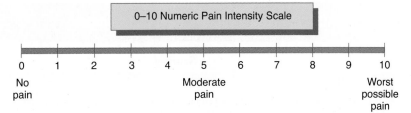

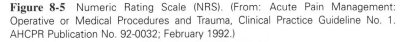

Figure 8-5 Numeric Rating Scale (NRS). (From: Acute Pain Management: Operative or Medical Procedures and Trauma, Clinical Practice Guideline No. 1. AHCPR Publication No. 92-0032; February 1992.)

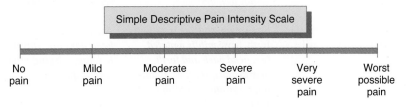

Figure 8-6 Verbal Descriptor Scale (VDS). (From: Acute Pain Management: Operative or Medical Procedures and Trauma, Clinical Practice Guidelline No. 1. AHCPR Publication No. 92-0032; February 1992.)

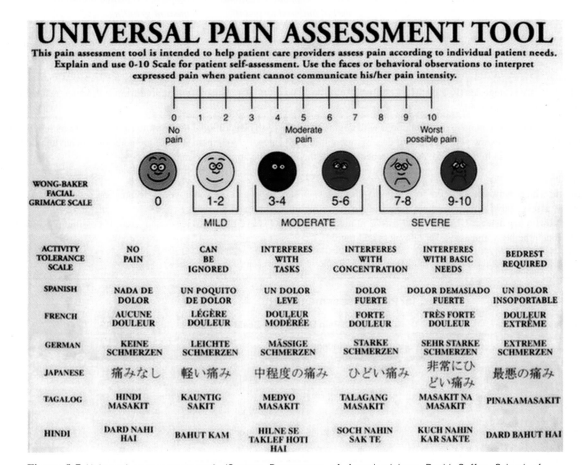

Figure 8-7 Universal assessment tool. (Source: Department of Anesthesiology, David Geffen School of Medicine at UCLA. Available at http://www.anes.ucla.edu/ pain/index.htm)

Assessing Cancer Pain

Memorial Sloan-Kettering Cancer Center has developed a cancer pain assessment tool that has four parts. This tool provides feedback on the type and level of pain as well as the patient's mood and pain relief from pain treatment (see Figure 8-8).

Three Initial Pain Assessment Tools

Three pain assessment tools that serve well for the patient's initial assessment are the Initial Pain Assessment Tool (McCaffery & Pasero, 1999), (see Figure 8-9) the Brief Pain Inventory (Short Form) (Cleeland, 1992), and for pediatric pain assessment, the Initial Pain Assessment for Pediatric Use Only (Otto, Duncan, & Baker, 1996).

ASSESSMENT TOOL 8-2   FLACC Scale for Pediatric Pain Assessment

Categories	Scoring		
	0	**1**	**2**
FACE	No particular expression or smile	Occasional grimace or frown, withdrawn, disinterested *appears sad or worried*	Frequent to constant frown, clenched jaw, quivering chin *distress-looking face: expression of fright or panic*
LEGS	Normal position or relaxed	Uneasy, restless, tense *occasional tremors*	Kicking, or legs drawn up *marked increase in spasticity, constant tremors or jerking*
ACTIVITY	Lying quietly, normal position moves easily	Squirming, shifting back and forth, tense *mildly agitated (eg. head back and forth, aggression); shallow, splinting respirations,intermittent sighs*	Arched, rigid, or jerking *severe agitation, head banging, shivering (not rigors); breath-holding, gasping or sharp intake of breath; severe splinting*
CRY	No cry (awake or asleep)	Moans or whimpers, occasional complaint *occasional verbal outburst or grunt*	Crying steadily, screams or sobs, frequent complaints *repeated outbursts, constant grunting*
CONSOLABILITY	Content, relaxed	Reassured by occasional touching, hugging,or being talked to, distractable	Difficult to console or comfort *pushing away caregiver, resisting care or comfort measures*

Each of the five categories (F) Face; (L) Legs; (A) Activity; (C) Cry; (C) Consolability is scored from 0-2, which results in a total score between zero and ten.

The revised FLACC can be used for children with cognitive disability. The additional descriptors (in italics) are included with the original FLACC. Review with parents the descriptors within each category. Ask them if there are additional behaviors that are better indicators of pain in their child. Add these behaviors to the tool in the appropriate category.

Procedure:
Patients who are awake: Observe for at least 1-2 minutes. Observe legs and body uncovered. Reposition patient or observe activity, assess body for tenseness and tone. Initiate consoling interventions if needed
Patients who are asleep: Observe for at least 2 minutes or longer. Observe body and legs uncovered. If possible reposition the patient. Touch the body and assess for tenseness and tone.

© 2002, The Regents of the University of Michigan. All Rights Reserved. Revision 2007: Voepel-Lewis

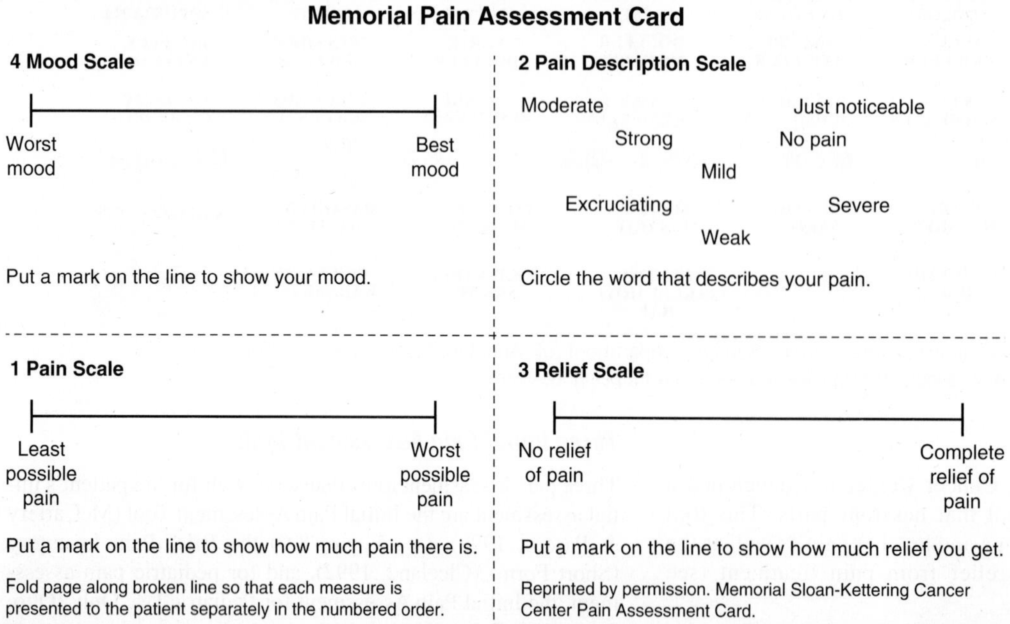

Memorial Pain Assessment Card

4 Mood Scale

Worst   Best
mood   mood

Put a mark on the line to show your mood.

2 Pain Description Scale

Moderate   Just noticeable
      Strong   No pain
              Mild
Excruciating   Severe
          Weak

Circle the word that describes your pain.

1 Pain Scale

Least   Worst
possible   possible
pain   pain

Put a mark on the line to show how much pain there is.

Fold page along broken line so that each measure is presented to the patient separately in the numbered order.

3 Relief Scale

No relief   Complete
of pain   relief of
                              pain

Put a mark on the line to show how much relief you get.

Reprinted by permission. Memorial Sloan-Kettering Cancer Center Pain Assessment Card.

A7012-AS-9

Figure 8-8 Memorial pain assessment card.

McCaffrey Initial Pain Assessment Tool

Date _____

Patient's Name _____ Age _____ Room _____

Diagnosis _____ Physician _____

Nurse _____

1. LOCATION: Patient or nurse marks drawing.

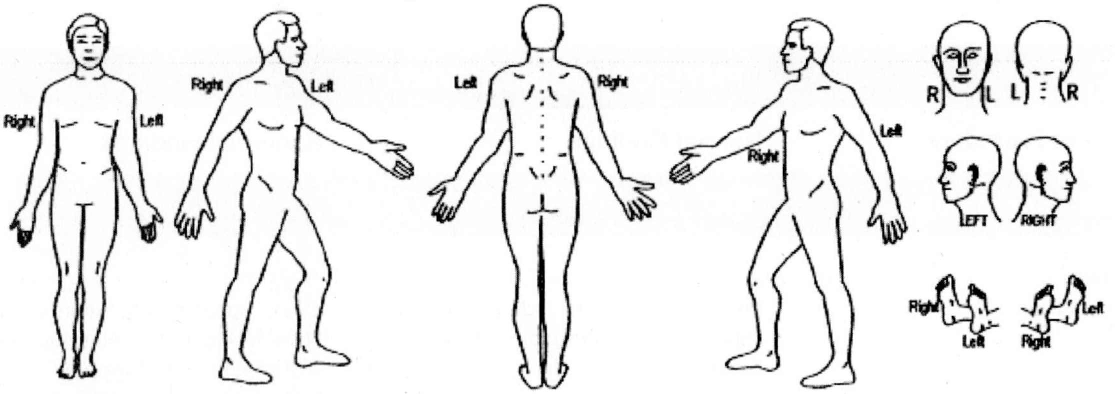

2. INTENSITY: Patient rates the pain. Scale used _____

    Present: _____

    Worst pain gets: _____

    Best pain gets: _____

    Acceptable level of pain: _____

3. QUALITY: (Use patient's own words, e.g., prick, ache, burn, throb, pull sharp) _____

    _____

4. ONSET, DURATION, VARIATIONS, RHYTHMS: _____

    _____

5. MANNER OF EXPRESSING PAIN? _____

    _____

    _____

6. WHAT RELIEVES THE PAIN? _____

    _____

    _____

7. WHAT CAUSES OR INCREASES THE PAIN? _____

    _____

    _____

8. EFFECTS OF PAIN: (Note decreased function, decreased quality of life.)

    Accompanying symptoms (e.g., nausea) _____

    Sleep _____

    Appetite _____

    Physical activity _____

    Relationship with others (e.g., irritability) _____

    Emotions (e.g., anger, suicidal, crying) _____

    Concentration _____

    Other _____

9. OTHER COMMENTS: _____

10. PLAN: _____

May be duplicated for use in clinical practice. From McCaffery M, Pasero C: Pain: Clinical manual, p. 60. Copyright ©1999, Mosby, Inc.

Figure 8-9 McCaffrey et al Initial Pain Assessment Tool.

Physical Assessment

During examination of the client, remember these key points:

- Choose an assessment tool reliable and valid to your culture.
- Explain to the client the purpose of rating the intensity of pain.
- Ensure the client's privacy and confidentiality.
- Respect the client's behavior towards pain and the terms used to express it.

Understand that different cultures express pain differently and maintain different pain thresholds and expectations.

PHYSICAL ASSESSMENT

Assessment Procedure	Normal Findings	Abnormal Findings
General Impression		
Inspection **Observe posture.**	Posture is upright when the client appears to be comfortable, attentive, and without excessive changes in position and posture.	Client appears to be slumped with the shoulders not straight (indicates being disturbed/uncomfortable). Client is inattentive and agitated. Client might be guarding affected area and have breathing patterns reflecting distress.
Inspection **Observe facial expression.**	Client smiles with appropriate facial expressions and maintains adequate eye contact.	Client's facial expressions indicate distress and discomfort, including frowning, moans, cries, and grimacing. Eye contact is not maintained, indicating discomfort. Nodding up and down or saying, "yeah, yeah," may not indicate a client's positive response to questions, but just listening or not wanting to be negative.
Inspect joints and muscles.	Joints appear normal (no edema); muscles appear relaxed.	Edema of a joint may indicate injury. Pain may result in muscle tension.
Observe skin for scars, lesions, rashes, changes or discoloration.	No inconsistency, wounds, or bruising is noted.	Bruising, wounds, or edema may be the result of injuries or infections, which may cause pain.
Vital Signs		
Inspection **Measure heart rate.**	Heart rate ranges from 60 to 100 beats per minute.	Increased heart rate may indicate discomfort or pain.
Measure respiratory rate.	Respiratory rate ranges from 12 to 20 breaths per minute.	Respiratory rate may be increased, and breathing may be irregular and shallow.
Measure blood pressure.	Blood pressure ranges from: Systolic: 100 to 130 mmHg Diastolic: 60 to 80 mmHg.	Increased blood pressure often occurs in severe pain.

Note: Refer to physical assessment chapter appropriate to affected body area. Body system assessment will include techniques for assessing for pain, e.g., palpating the abdomen for tenderness and performing range of motion test on the joints.

VALIDATING AND DOCUMENTING FINDINGS

Validate the pain assessment data you have collected. This is necessary to verify that the data are reliable and accurate. Document the assessment data following the health care facility or agency policy.

Sample Documentation of Subjective Data

Ms. S.B. is a 68-year-old female patient known previously as having osteoporosis. This visit she presents with low back pain, burning in nature, radiating to the left lower extremity associated with tingling and numbness sensation of the lower extremity. The pain is continuous and exacerbates mostly in the morning and after any movement. Pain is moderately relieved by pain medications and rest. "Pain is interfering with my activities of daily life. I am not able to bathe, dress, and perform the daily household chores. Also, I am not able to concentrate on my work anymore. I cannot sleep at night and I seem not to enjoy anything lately." Using the Visual Analog Scale (VAS), Ms. S.B. rates her pain to be 8/10.

Sample Documentation of Objective Data

Client comes in leaning on her daughter and has difficulty sitting down on the chair. Her posture is not upright and she seems to be agitated. She is frowning and grimacing most of the time. She is unable to concentrate and continue an idea. Her HR = 108 beats/min, RR = 22 breaths/min, BP = 135/80 mmHg.

Analysis of Data

DIAGNOSTIC REASONING: POSSIBLE CONCLUSIONS

After collecting subjective and objective data pertaining to the pain assessment, identify abnormal findings and client strengths. Then, cluster the data to reveal any significant patterns or abnormalities. These data may then be used to make clinical judgments about the status of the client's pain.

Selected Nursing Diagnoses

Following is a listing of selected nursing diagnoses (wellness, risk, or actual) that you may identify when analyzing the cue clusters.

Wellness Diagnoses

- Readiness for enhanced spiritual well-being related to coping with prolonged physical pain
- Readiness for enhanced comfort level

Risk Diagnoses

- Risk for activity intolerance related to chronic pain and immobility
- Risk for constipation related to nonsteroidal anti-inflammatory agents or opiates intake or poor eating habits
- Risk for spiritual distress related to anxiety, pain, life change, and chronic illness
- Risk for powerlessness related to chronic pain, healthcare environment, pain treatment-related regimen

Actual Diagnoses

- Acute pain related to injury agents (biological, chemical, physical, or psychological)
- Chronic pain related to chronic inflammatory process of rheumatoid arthritis
- Ineffective breathing pattern related to abdominal pain and anxiety
- Disturbed energy field related to pain and anxiety
- Fatigue related to stress of handling chronic pain
- Impaired physical mobility related to chronic pain
- Bathing/hygiene self-care deficit related to severe pain (specify)

Selected Collaborative Problems

After grouping the data, certain collaborative problems may become apparent. Remember that collaborative problems differ from nursing diagnoses in that they cannot be prevented by nursing intervention. However, these physiological complications of medical conditions can be detected and monitored by the nurse. In addition, the nurse can use physician- and nurse-prescribed interventions to minimize the complications of these problems. The nurse may also have to refer the client in such situations for further treatment of the problem. Following is a list of collaborative problems that may be identified when obtaining a general impression. These problems are worded as Risk for Complications (or RC), followed by the problem.

- RC: Angina
- RC: Decreased cardiac output
- RC: Endocarditis
- RC: Peripheral vascular insufficiency
- RC: Paralytic ileus/small bowel obstruction
- RC: Sickling crisis
- RC: Peripheral nerve compression
- RC: Corneal ulceration
- RC: Osteoarthritis
- RC: Joint dislocation
- RC: Pathologic fractures
- RC: Renal calculi

Medical Problems

After grouping the data, the client's signs and symptoms may clearly require medical diagnosis and treatment. Referral to a primary care provider is necessary.

CASE STUDY

The case study demonstrates how to analyze pain assessment data for a specific client. The critical thinking exercises included in the study guide/lab manual and interactive product that complement this text also offer opportunities to analyze assessment data.

L.B. is a 55-year-old male divorced with two children who works as a financial manager at a company. Two years ago, he experienced difficulty urinating and burning upon urination. Tests revealed prostate cancer. Mr. L.B. underwent prostatectomy followed by cycles of chemotherapy 1 year ago. For the past 8 to 10 months, he has complained of continuous low back pain and leg pain that exacerbates at night and while walking. "I sometimes feel that I will fall down while walking and at night I am awakened by stabbing deep dull pain in my legs. I am not able to sleep at night and during the day I feel tired and unable to proceed with my work, especially meeting my clients." Mr. L.B. also reports decreased appetite and weight loss of around 6 kg in the past 3 months.

During the physical exam, Mr. L.B. entered the room limping and sat on the chair with his shoulders slumped. He changes his position every 2 to 3 minutes looking anxious and uncomfortable with frowns and grimaces as facial expressions. He rates his pain on average on the Visual Analog Scale (VAS) to be 7/10. Vital signs: HR=110 beats/min, RR=22 breaths/min, BP=135/85 mmHg.

The following concept map illustrates the diagnostic reasoning process.

Applying COLDSPA

Applying **COLDSPA** for client symptoms: "back and leg pain."

Mnemonic	Question	Data Provided	Missing Data
Character	Describe the sign or symptom (feeling, appearance, sound, smell, or taste if applicable).	Low back and stabbing, deep, dull pain in legs	
Onset	When did it begin?	8 to 10 months ago	
Location	Where is it? Does it radiate? Does it occur anywhere else?	Lower back and legs	
Duration	How long does it last? Does it recur?	Continuous, gets worse at night and when walking	
Severity	How bad is it? How much does it bother you?	Client rates pain on the VAS to be 7/10. Limps when walking and changes position every 2 to 3 minutes to try to get comfortable. Makes facial grimaces and frowns. Sits with slumped shoulders.	
Pattern	What makes it better or worse?		"What makes the leg and back pain worse or better?"
Associated factors/How it **A**ffects the client	What other symptoms occur with it? How does it affect you?	Feels like he may fall when walking. Is tired and has trouble working during the day because he cannot sleep at night; the pain wakes him up. Decreased appetite and weight loss of 6 kg in the past 3 months.	

1) Identify abnormal findings and client strengths

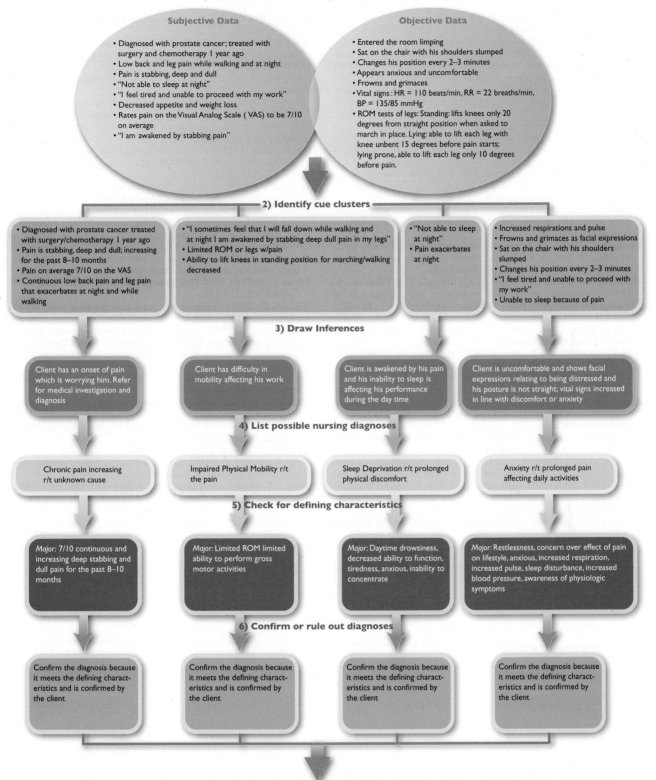

Subjective Data

- Diagnosed with prostate cancer; treated with surgery and chemotherapy 1 year ago
- Low back and leg pain while walking and at night
- Pain is stabbing, deep and dull
- "Not able to sleep at night"
- "I feel tired and unable to proceed with my work"
- Decreased appetite and weight loss
- Rates pain on the Visual Analog Scale (VAS) to be 7/10 on average
- "I am awakened by stabbing pain"

Objective Data

- Entered the room limping
- Sat on the chair with his shoulders slumped
- Changes his position every 2–3 minutes
- Appears anxious and uncomfortable
- Frowns and grimaces
- Vital signs: HR = 110 beats/min, RR = 22 breaths/min, BP = 135/85 mmHg
- ROM tests of legs: Standing: lifts knees only 20 degrees from straight position when asked to march in place. Lying: able to lift each leg with knee unbent 15 degrees before pain starts; lying prone, able to lift each leg only 10 degrees before pain.

2) Identify cue clusters

- Diagnosed with prostate cancer treated with surgery/chemotherapy 1 year ago
- Pain is stabbing, deep and dull; increasing for the past 8–10 months
- Pain on average 7/10 on the VAS
- Continuous low back pain and leg pain that exacerbates at night and while walking

- "I sometimes feel that I will fall down while walking and at night I am awakened by stabbing deep dull pain in my legs"
- Limited ROM or legs w/pain
- Ability to lift knees in standing position for marching/walking decreased

- "Not able to sleep at night"
- Pain exacerbates at night

- Increased respirations and pulse
- Frowns and grimaces as facial expressions
- Sat on the chair with his shoulders slumped
- Changes his position every 2–3 minutes
- "I feel tired and unable to proceed with my work"
- Unable to sleep because of pain

3) Draw Inferences

Client has an onset of pain which is worrying him. Refer for medical investigation and diagnosis

Client has difficulty in mobility affecting his work

Client is awakened by his pain and his inability to sleep is affecting his performance during the day time

Client is uncomfortable and shows facial expressions relating to being distressed and his posture is not straight; vital signs increased in line with discomfort or anxiety

4) List possible nursing diagnoses

Chronic pain increasing r/t unknown cause

Impaired Physical Mobility r/t the pain

Sleep Deprivation r/t prolonged physical discomfort

Anxiety r/t prolonged pain affecting daily activities

5) Check for defining characteristics

Major: 7/10 continuous and increasing deep stabbing and dull pain for the past 8–10 months

Major: Limited ROM limited ability to perform gross motor activities

Major: Daytime drowsiness, decreased ability to function, tiredness, anxious, inability to concentrate

Major: Restlessness, concern over effect of pain on lifestyle, anxious, increased respiration, increased pulse, sleep disturbance, increased blood pressure, awareness of physiologic symptoms

6) Confirm or rule out diagnoses

Confirm the diagnosis because it meets the defining characteristics and is confirmed by the client

Confirm the diagnosis because it meets the defining characteristics and is confirmed by the client

Confirm the diagnosis because it meets the defining characteristics and is confirmed by the client

Confirm the diagnosis because it meets the defining characteristics and is confirmed by the client

7) Document conclusions

Nursing diagnoses that are appropriate for this client include:
- Chronic Pain (increasing) r/t unknown cause
- Impaired Physical mobility r/t the pain
- Sleep Deprivation r/t prolonged physical discomfort
- Anxiety r/t prolonged pain affecting daily activities

Potential collaborative problems include the following:
RC: Prostate cancer metastasis

References and Selected Readings

Acute pain management: Operative or medical procedures and trauma. (1992, February). Clinical Practice Guidelines No. 1 (AHCPR Publication No. 92-0032). Rockville, MD: Agency for Healthcare Research and Quality.

American Pain Society. (2008a). Advocacy. Pediatric chronic pain: A position statement from the American Pain Society. Available at http://www.ampainsoc.org/advocacy/pediatric

American Pain Society. (2008b). Membership. Special interest groups: Geriatric pain. Available at http://www.ampainsoc.org/member/sigsites/geriatric

Binasco, K. (2003). Pain management for the geriatric patient. Available at http://www.medscape.com/viewarticle/44839

Cancer Pain Management in Children. (1999). Available at http://www.childcancerpain.org

Carrier-Kohlman, V., Lindsey, A., & West, C. (2003). Pathophysiologic phenomena in nursing: Human response to illness (3rd ed., pp. 235–254). St. Louis: Saunders.

Chapman, C. R. (2000). New JCAHO standards for pain management: carpe diem! APS Bulletin, 10(4). Available at http://www.ampainsoc.org/pub/bulletin/jul00

Cleeland, C. (1992). Brief pain inventory short form [BPI SF]. In C. Cleeland, D. Turk, & R. Melzack, Handbook of pain assessment (pp. 367–370, 383–384). New York: Guildford Press.

Dunwoody, C., Krenzischek, D., Pasero, C., Rathmell, J., & Polomano, R. (2008). Assessment, physiological monitoring, and consequences of inadequately treated acute pain. Pain Management Nursing, 9(1), S11–S21.

Flaherty, E. (2008). Pain assessment for older adults. AJN, 108(6), 45–47.

Healthcommunities.com. (1998–2008). Cancer pain. Available at http://www.oncologychannel.com/pain

Herr, K., Coyne, P., Key, T., Manworren, R., McCaffery, M., Merkel, S., et al. (2006). Pain assessment in the nonverbal patient: Position statement with clinical practice recommendations. Pain Management Nursing, 7(2), 44–52.

Hummel, P., & Puchalski, M. (2000). N-Pass: Neonatal pain, agitation, & sedation scale. Chicago: Loyola University Health System. Available at http://www.n-pass.com

International Association for the Study of Pain. (1994). Definition of pain. Available at http://www.iasp-pain.org

Jacox, A., Carr, D., Payne, R, et al. (1994, March).Management of cancer pain. Clinical Practice Guidelines No. 9 (AHCPR Publication No. 94-0592). Rockville, MD: Agency for Health Care Policy and Research, USDHHS.

Mahieu-Caputo, D., Dommergues, M., Muller, F., & Dumez, Y. (2000). Fetal pain. Presse Med, 29(12), 663–669. Available at http://opoids.com/endormorphins/foetpain

McCaffery, M., & Pasero, C. (1999). Pain: Clinical manual (2nd ed.). St. Louis: Mosby.

Memorial Pain Assessment Card. (n.d.). Available at http://www.partners-againstpain.com

NANDA International. (2007). Nursing diagnoses: Definitions & classification 2007–2008. Philadelphia: NANDA International.

Oncology Nursing Society. (2006). Cancer pain management. Available at http://www.ons.org/publication/positions/CancerPainManagement.shtml

Otto, S., Duncan, S., & Baker, L. (1996). Initial pain assessment for pediatric use only. Distributed by the City of Hope Pain/Palliative Care Resource Center. Available at http://www.cityofhope.org/prc/pain_assessment.asp

Phillips, D. M. (2000). JCAHO pain management standards are unveiled. Joint Commission on Accreditation of Healthcare Organizations. JAMA, 284(18), 2317–2318.

Price, S., & Wilson, L., (1997). Pathophysiology, clinical concepts of disease process (5th ed.). St. Louis: Mosby-Year Book.

Rankin, E., & Mitchel, M. (2000). Creating a pain management educational module for hospice nurses: Integrating the new JCAHO standards and the AHCPR pain management guidelines. Journal of Hospice and Palliative Nursing, 2(3), 91–100.

Ranney, D. (2008). Pain is a subjective experience. Available at http://www.ahs.uwaterloo.ca/~ranney/pain.html

Regan, J., & Peng, P. (2000). Neurophysiology of cancer pain. Cancer Control, 7(2), 111–119.

Silkman, C. (2008). Assessing the seven dimensions of pain. American Nurse Today, 3(2), 12–15.

Stratton Hill, C. (1997). Guidelines for treatment of cancer pain: The revised pocket edition of the final report of the Texas Cancer Council's Workgroup on Pain Control in Cancer Patients (2nd ed.). Austin, TX: Texas Cancer Council.

Universal Pain Assessment Tool (UCLA). (n.d.). Available at http://www.anes.ucla.edu/pain

VonBaeyer, C. (2007). Faces Pain Scale-Revised (FPS-R). Available at http://www.painsourcebook.ca

Wall, P., & Melzack, R. (1994). Textbook of pain (3rd ed.). London: Longman Group UK Ltd.

Weissman, Gordon, & Bidar-sielaff. (2002).

Wong, D., & Hess, C. (2000). Wong and Whaley's clinical manual of pediatric nursing (5th ed.). St. Louis: Mosby.

Wong, D., Hockenberry-Eatopn, M., Wilson, D., Windelstein, M., & Schwartz, P. (2001). Wong's essential of pediatric nursing (6th ed.). St. Louis: Mosby.

9

Assessing Victims of Violence

Structure and Function

"In this country, domestic violence is just about as common as giving birth—about four million instances of each. Think about that—hopelessness and hope, equally weighted in our society—and all too often, intermingled in the same woman's life . . . domestic violence is an unacknowledged epidemic in our country. And yet we're still shocked when the 'life of the party,' an expert in his field, a pillar of the community, turns out to be a wife-beater." Donna E. Shalala, former U.S. Secretary of Health and Human Services (March 1994).

WHAT IS FAMILY VIOLENCE?

Family violence can be defined as the controlling, coercive behaviors seen through the intentional acts of violence inflicted on those in familial or intimate relationships and includes intimate partner violence, child abuse, and elder mistreatment. Family violence affects people of all ages, sexes, religions, ethnicities and socioeconomic levels.

Categories of Family Violence

Categories of family violence include intimate partner violence, child abuse, and elder mistreatment.

Intimate partner violence (IPV) includes a range of behaviors including physical abuse, emotional abuse, economic abuse, psychological abuse, and sexual assault. Over time, IPV escalates in both severity and frequency unless intervention occurs.

The Child Abuse Prevention and Treatment Act (CAPTA) defines *child abuse* as

> any recent act or failure to act, resulting in imminent risk of serious harm, death, serious physical or emotional harm, sexual abuse, or exploitation of a child (a person under the age of 18, unless the child protection law of the State in which the child resides specifies a younger age for cases not involving sexual abuse) by a parent or caretaker (including any employee of a residential facility or any staff person providing out-of-home care) who is responsible for the child's welfare (Child Abuse Prevention and Treatment Act, Public Law 104–235, §111; 42 U.S.C. 510g, 2003).

The Child Welfare Information Gateway (2008) defines child abuse as: "physical or mental injury, sexual abuse, negligent treatment or maltreatment of a child under the age of 18 by a person who is responsible for the child's welfare under circumstances that indicate that the child's health or welfare is harmed." Child abuse may be either by commission or by omission and is rarely an isolated incident. There are four broad categories of child abuse: neglect, emotional abuse, sexual abuse, and physical abuse.

Elder mistreatment, formerly known as elder abuse includes physical abuse, neglect, exploitation, abandonment or prejudicial attitudes that decreases one's quality of life and is demeaning to those over the age of 65 years. The American Medical Association estimates that only one out of every 14 cases is reported (1993). Elder abuse is often difficult to assess because of isolation from the community, immobility of the older person, and inability to report because of cognitive impairments.

Elders are often unwilling to report their abuser, due to mistrust of law enforcement or due to a relationship with the abuser (i.e., son or daughter) that may create feelings of guilt, burden, dependence, or fear of abandonment. They may be unsure who to report the abuse to, doubt authorities' willingness to become involved, or fear that without their caregiver they will end up in an institution. Many elders prefer to stay in their own home even if it means suffering abuse at the hands of a caregiver.

Types of Violence

Types of family violence include physical abuse, psychological abuse, economic abuse, and sexual abuse.

Physical abuse includes pushing, shoving, slapping, kicking, choking, punching and burning. It may also involve holding, tying or other methods of restraint. The victim may be left in a dangerous place without resources. The abuser may refuse to help the victim when sick, injured or in need. Physical abuse may also involve attacking the victim with household items (lamps, radios, ashtrays, irons, etc.) or with common weapons (knives or guns).

Psychological abuse involves the use of constant insults or criticism, blaming the victim for things that are not the victim's fault, threats to hurt children or pets, isolation from supporters (family, friends or coworkers), deprivation, humiliation, and intimidation.

Economic abuse may be evidenced by preventing the victim from getting or from keeping a job, controlling money and limiting access to funds, and controlling knowledge of family finances.

Sexual abuse involves forcing the victim to perform sexual acts against her or his will, pursuing sexual activity after victim has said no, using violence during sex, and using weapons vaginally, orally, or anally.

Types of elder mistreatment include neglect, physical abuse, financial abuse, and psychological abuse, including humiliation, intimidation, and threats. The abuse may be from commission, but is frequently from omission.

WHY ASSESS FAMILY VIOLENCE?

It is estimated that more than one million women seek medical care for injuries related to abuse, resulting in 100,000 days of hospitalization, 30,000 emergency room visits, and 40,000 primary care visits a year. One out of four women treated for serious injuries are victims of IPV. Thirty percent of all murdered women are victims of IPV. IPV is the single major cause of injury to women, surpassing accidents, stranger rapes and stranger muggings (Datner & Ferrogiaro, 1999). In addition, children raised in homes with IPV are more likely to use violence as adults (Lamberg, 2000).

Today more than 3,000,000 children are referred to child protective services yearly. Forty-six out of every 1000 child abuse cases are substantiated. Four children die daily as a result of child abuse (Peddle, Wang, Diaz, & Reid, 2002).

The rate of violence against the aged by family members is 6.772 per 1000 older adults. The medical consequences of elder mistreatment include (1) inability of the frail elderly to handle the trauma, (2) inability to get food or medication because of neglect, (3) inability to pay for food or medication because of financial abuse, and (4) inability to deal with illness/malnutrition/problems because of depression associated with abuse.

The World Health Organization estimates that the cost of violence is greater than 4% of the gross domestic products of many countries. Abuse is not limited to one economic level, gender, age, or educational level, but can occur in any population. Historically, family violence was viewed as a private matter, but in reality it is a public health problem with a significant impact on health care systems.

HISTORICAL BACKGROUND

The prevalence of violence is not certain in early civilization, but Kolb (1971) observed that in recorded history only ten generations of humans have avoided war. This gives credence to those who argue the inevitability of violent behaviors.

Historical examination shows a propensity for violence since recorded history. It does indicate violence was present, but does not explain the cause. Beginning late in the twentieth century, more research and attention have been paid to violence.

History of Nursing and Domestic Violence

The battered women's movement began in the mid-1970s to meet the immediate needs of victims for safety and housing. Victims' advocates began to lobby the justice system about the bias against victims of domestic violence. Health care or what victims faced when they sought health care was not an initial focus; however, the nursing profession was involved with victims from the beginning.

In addition, several examples of nurses individually and collectively addressing the issue of domestic violence include

- In 1977, Barbara Parker, a nurse, published an article on the health-care concern of domestic violence. She was a founder of the House of Ruth shelter in Baltimore.
- The Ambulatory Nursing department of Brigham and Women's Hospital in Boston worked with the social work department and developed one of the first emergency department domestic violence protocols.
- In 1981, Jacqueline Campbell published a study showing that one of the major risk factors for homicide among women was domestic violence. Campbell later developed a Danger Assessment Screening Tool to identify risk factors of homicide in an abusive relationship (1981, 1988).
- In 1991, the American Nurses Association passed a resolution encouraging that topics related to domestic violence be included in nursing education.

In addition, nurses have been involved in addressing a number of domestic violence issues and the impact on health including sexually transmitted disease (STD), human immunodeficiency virus (HIV), unintentional pregnancy, injuries to the vaginal area, urinary tract infections, and battering during pregnancy.

History of Intimate Partner Violence

IPV has a long historical background. Historically, many societies were patriarchal. The patriarchal society supported domination, subordination, and control. Many aspects of many cultures still reflect these values, and IPV continues to be condoned in most societies. Historical examples of condoning and perpetuating IPV include

- The Bible provides early evidence of beatings, stonings, and even deaths of women when infidelity was suspected.
- The Declaration of Independence asserts all men are created equal, but does not mention women.
- Mississippi legalized wife beating in 1824.
- The first law to punish wife beaters was passed by North Carolina in 1874 but the courts indicated they would not hear cases unless there was evidence of damage or danger to life (Davidson, 1977).
- In 1915, a magistrate ruled that men could legally beat their wives at home as long as the stick used was not thicker than a man's thumb (Campbell & Humphreys, 1993).

When examining the problem of IPV, it is common to focus on the woman as the victim. Males also suffer from victimization, though this is commonly perceived as a rarity. Male victims report that if they inform about an incident to the police, it may not be filed and they are often ridiculed. Male victims suffer effects of trauma similar to those experienced by female victims (Huckle, 1995); when men attempt to leave their abuser, they face many of the same problems as female victims. However, they may have fewer options for assistance, as there are few if any facilities that offer shelter to male victims.

History of Child Abuse

There is also a long history of child abuse. Historical examples of violence against children include

- In early cultures, children were sacrificed to please the god of their parents. This sacrifice was viewed as a desirable act and indicated that the parents loved their god above their children.

- Children with birth defects were killed because of the belief that they had been possessed or had contact with demons. Children with seizure disorders, mental retardation, or mental illness were often exposed to torture to drive out the demons that possessed them.
- The clichés "spare the rod and spoil the child" and "just beat some sense into them" were used to indicate that beatings are necessary for the child to learn and to follow rules.
- In *Ingram versus Wright* (1977), the Supreme Court ruled in favor of the schools in a case that questioned the use of corporal punishment to discipline students in schools (Knitzer, 1977).

All 50 states now mandate child abuse reporting. Guidelines have been developed to aid clinicians in recognizing child abuse injuries, performing comprehensive examinations, recommending tests, documenting injuries, and reporting and testifying in child abuse cases.

- The long-term impact of child sexual abuse results in 6% of cases of alcohol abuse, illicit drug abuse, and depression (Barclay & Lie, 2007).
- In 2004, 152,250 children/adolescents were confirmed victims of physical abuse in the United States (Barclay & Lie, 2007).

THEORETICAL BACKGROUND

To discuss the theory of family violence, the concepts of violence and aggression need to be defined. *Violence* is an "execution of force used so as to injure or abuse" (Merriam-Webster, 2005). Violence tends to have a negative connotation when thought of as murder, torture, or hate but has more of a positive connotation if associated with self-defense or acts of war. The American culture condemns it; however, some movies, television programs, and literature glorify it. *Aggression* is defined as an unprovoked attack or warlike action (Merriam-Webster Online, 2005). Aggression also has both positive and negative connotations. The positive connotation is associated with the drive for success, as in aggressive men. The negative connotation is often associated with the notion of aggressive women, which often violates what is considered appropriate for gender norms.

This chapter briefly discusses five theories related to domestic violence: biological, psychoanalytical, social learning, cultural attitudes, and Walker's Cycle of Violence theory. The first four focus on basis of violence, whereas Walker's Cycle discusses the cyclic nature of violence. *Biological theory* asserts that violence is an innate characteristic of humans, based on neurophysiological states. Instinct has served to preserve the species so that those men who were more violent survived. *Psychoanalytical theory* states that violence results from the need to discharge hostility. In addition, frustration is the stimulus that leads to violence or aggression. *Social learning theory* describes both aggression and violence as learned responses that may be considered positive or as negative response depending on the situation. These behaviors are learned from not only the family, but also from the community and society. Some experts purport that *cultural attitudes* influence violence. For example, the acceptance of war as a justified means of resolving a conflict and corporal punishment as a method of discipline both developed from various cultural attitudes.

Walker (1979, 1984) describes the *Cycle of Violence theory*. He explains that abuse occurs in a predictable pattern.

During the beginning of a relationship, couples are rarely apart and the relationship is very intense. The abuser displays possessiveness and jealousy and starts to separate the victim from supportive relationships. Criticism is the herald of Phase 1, the tension-building phase. The abuser makes unrealistic demands. When the expectations are not satisfied, the criticism and/or ridicule escalates into shoving or slapping. The victims often blame themselves for failing to satisfy the unrealistic demands of the abuser. Phase 2, the acute battering stage, may be triggered by something minor but results in violence lasting up to 24 hours. The victim is rarely able to stop the abuse. Phase 3, the honeymoon phase, is described as a period of reconciliation. This phase begins after an incident of battery. The abuser is loving, promises never to abuse the victim again, and is very attentive to the victim. Then the cycle begins again (Frank & Roddowski, 1999).

Culture, race and ethnicity must also be considered in the theory of family violence. One needs to conduct a cultural assessment (using assessment guidelines) before attempting to understand family violence. Health-care providers are more likely to report child abuse in minority populations or in lower socioeconomic levels (ANA, 1998). Studies show little difference in rates of abuse in racial groups when income levels are included (Hawkins, 1993).

Violence in the Workplace

Nurses may also find themselves victims of violence in the workplace. Because of the nature of emergency departments, there are increased risks for staff, patients, and visitors. Patients with psychiatric illness, abusers of alcohol or drugs, patients in pain who have had to wait, and individuals who have been involved in gang violence are often seen in the emergency department. Staffing is often inadequate, fatigue is common, and tempers may not be controlled. Nurses may encounter the fears, frustration, and harassment of patients. Emergency department (ED) nurses surveyed reported that 36% had experienced violence in the past year while at work and 63% related an assault during their careers (Saxton Mahoney, 1990). Even with all the factors contributing to the potential for serious incidents, one of the greatest risks continues to be in caring for victims of IPV. Injured victims are often accompanied to the ED by the batterer. As the batterer has already shown the ability to inflict injury, he or she should be considered dangerous. By accompanying the victim, the batterer is attempting to maintain control of the victim and prevent reports from being filed.

Because of the potential for violence, health care facilities should have a safety plan to control potential violence and to ensure safety of the staff, patients, and visitors.

Assessing Victims of Violence

Screening for a history of current and past abuse is essential at the initial and annual visits regardless of the presence or absence of abuse indicators, and helps to identify mothers affected by IPV (Barclay, 2007). Screen at each visit if there is a history of abuse. Screen all pregnant women at least once per trimester and once postpartum (Washington State Department of Health, April 2004). Screen mothers during well child visits to the pediatrician. Also screen for abuse if the client is in a new relationship or if there are signs or symptoms indicating the presence of abuse.

As mentioned before, there are four areas to assess to determine the presence of family violence: physical abuse, psychological abuse, economic abuse, and sexual abuse.

With physical abuse, it is important to remember that physical abuse may start at any time during a relationship. The abuse may not be part of the presenting problem for which the client is being seen but may be the cause or etiology of the presenting problem. Consistent risk factors for women at risk have not been identified. Therefore, both abused and non-abused women require routine screening by health-care providers. The Family Violence Prevention Fund (1999) recommends that all female clients, age 14 and older, be screened for abuse when seen in emergency departments, urgent care centers, or primary health-care clinics.

Psychological abuse, also known as emotional abuse, has very great consequences—some believe even more than the effects of physical abuse (Strauss & Sweet, 1992). Examples of psychological abuse include threats of harm and intimidation. This type of abuse is difficult to assess because of the lack of a clearly defined diagnosis. Legal definitions of psychological abuse differ from state to state, which results in an underestimated number of cases reported. The majority of children who suffer from psychological abuse often use effective coping mechanisms and will not exhibit any pathologic behaviors.

Economic abuse, also known as financial abuse, is the improper exploitation of another person's personal assets, properties, or funds. Examples of this type of abuse include the cashing of another person's checks without authorization or permission, forging signatures, and misusing or stealing money or possessions. Economic abuse may also occur if someone deceives another into signing a will or contract, coerces a person into signing a will or contract, or controls another person's money and demands a detailed accounting of the funds. Statistics of economic abuse are difficult to find due to the under reporting by abused elders.

When sexual abuse is suspected, a complete physical examination is required. Disclosure of the incident may not occur for months or years after the sexual abuse event. Often sexual abuse, such as fondling, oral sex, or activity without penetration, does not involve physical injury. If sexual abuse is suspected, a trained interviewer should conduct a forensic interview. Both the interview and physical examination are part of the actual nursing interventions that assist the client to recover from the sexual abuse.

PREPARING YOURSELF FOR THE EXAMINATION

Before you can begin to effectively assess for the presence of family violence, you must first examine your feelings, beliefs, and biases regarding violence. Violence is a prevalent family and community health problem that needs to be confronted by society today. No one under any circumstances should be physically, sexually, or emotionally abused. As a nurse, it is imperative that you become active in interrupting or ending cycles of violence. During your assessment, be aware of "red flags" that may indicate the presence of family violence; these "red flags" are often hidden from others.

INTERVIEW TECHNIQUES

Creating a safe and confidential environment is essential to obtain concise and valid subjective data from the clients who have experienced domestic violence. For any client over the age of 3 years, ask any screening questions in a secure, private setting with no one else present in the room. Do not screen if there are any safety concerns for the client or for yourself.

Prior to screening, discuss any legal, mandatory reporting requirements or other limits to confidentiality. Screening may be done orally and in a written format or through computer-generated questions. Find a reliable interpreter if the client is non-English speaking.

Remember to ask questions and allow the client to answer completely. Do not interrupt the client. Convey a concerned and nonjudgmental attitude. Show appropriate empathy.

(text continues on page 118)

ASSESSMENT PROCEDURE

Assessment Procedure	Normal Findings	Abnormal Findings (Indicators of Violence or Potential Violence)
Family Violence Assessment		
Review the client's past health history and physical examination records if available.	No indicators of abuse are present.	Records include documentation of past assaults; unexplained injuries; unexplained symptoms of pain, nausea and vomiting or choking feeling; repeated visits to emergency department or clinic for injuries; signs and symptoms of anxiety; use of sedatives or tranquilizers; injuries during pregnancy; history of drug or alcohol abuse; history of depression and/or suicide attempts.

Assessment Procedure	Normal Findings	Abnormal Findings (Indicators of Violence or Potential Violence)
If partner/parent/caregiver is present at the visit, observe client's interactions with partner.	Client does not seem afraid of partner and answers questions independently. Partner appears supportive.	Partner criticizes client about appearance, feelings, and/or actions. Partner is not sensitive to client's needs. Partner refuses to leave client's presence. Partner attempts to speak for and answer questions for client. Client appears anxious and afraid of partner; is submissive or passive to negative comments from partner.
Interview **Perform the rest of the examination without the partner, parent, or caregiver present.** **Ask all clients:** Has anyone in your home ever hurt you? Do you feel safe in your home? Are you afraid of anyone in your home? Has anyone made you do anything you didn't want to do? Has anyone ever touched you without you telling them it was OK for them to do so? Has anyone ever threatened you?	Client answers no to all questions.	"Yes" to any of the questions indicates abuse.
For intimate partner violence, begin the screening by telling the client that it is important to routinely screen all clients for intimate partner violence because it affects so many women and men in our society. **Ask the client to fill out or help the client fill out the Abuse assessment screen in Assessment Tool 9-1.**	Client responds no to all three questions. If the client replies "no" to screening questions and is not being abused, it is important for the client to know that you are available if she ever experiences abuse in the future. Make statements that build trust such as: If your situation ever changes, please call me to talk about it. I am happy to hear that you are not being abused. If that should ever change, this is a safe place to talk. ➤ *Clinical Tip • Sometimes no matter how carefully you prepare the client and ask the questions she may not disclose abuse.*	"Yes" to any of the questions strongly indicates initial disclosure of abuse. You should do the following: • Acknowledge the abuse and her courage. • Use supportive statements such as "I'm sorry this is happening to you. This is not your fault. You are not responsible for his behavior. You are not alone. You don't deserve to be treated this way. Help is available to you." • Acknowledge her autonomy and right to self-determination. Reiterate confidentiality of disclosure.
For child abuse, use the guidelines in Display 9-1. Question the child about safety including physical abuse, sexual abuse, emotional abuse, and neglect.	Client shows no signs of abuse.	Client indicates someone has hurt them (physically, sexually, or emotionally). Child appears neglected.

continued on page 115

ASSESSMENT TOOL 9-1   Abuse Assessment Screen

1. WITHIN THE LAST YEAR, have you been hit, slapped, kicked, or otherwise physically hurt by someone?   YES   NO

   If YES, by whom? _____

   Total number of times _____

2. SINCE YOU'VE BEEN PREGNANT, have you been hit, slapped, kicked, or otherwise physically hurt by someone?   YES   NO

   If YES, by whom? _____

   Total number of times _____

MARK THE AREA OF INJURY ON THE BODY MAP. SCORE EACH
INCIDENT ACCORDING TO THE FOLLOWING SCALE:

SCORE

1 = Threats of abuse including use of a weapon   _____

2 = Slapping, pushing: no injuries and/or lasting pain   _____

3 = Punching, kicking, bruises, cuts and/or continuing pain   _____

4 = Beating up, severe contusions, burns, broken bones   _____

5 = Head injury, internal injury, permanent injury   _____

6 = Use of weapon; wound from weapon   _____

If any of the descriptions for the higher number apply, use the higher number.

3. WITHIN THE LAST YEAR, has anyone forced you to have sexual activities?   YES   NO

   If YES, who? _____

   Total number of times _____

   _____

Developed by the Nursing Research Consortium on Violence and Abuse. Readers are encouraged to reproduce and use this assessment tool.

DISPLAY 9-1   Considerations for Interviewing Children

- It is important to establish a reassuring environment for the interview.
- Although you may be uncomfortable questioning the child about abuse, do not convey this in the interactions with the child.
- It is important that you receive any information the child may disclose to you with interest. Be calm and accepting without showing surprise or distaste.
- Do not coerce the child to answer questions by offering a reward to answer your questions.
- Establish the child's understanding or developmental stage by asking simple questions (Name, how to spell name, age, birth date, how many eyes do you have, etc.). Then formulate questions keeping in mind child's ability to comprehend or language limitations. Use the child's comprehensive abilities and any language limitations to structure your interview/questions. Use terms for body parts or acts that the child uses.
- Questions must be direct to extract information without being leading. Children will answer questions. The majority disclose to questions specific to direct inquiry about the person suspected of abuse or related to type of abuse (Heger, et al., 2000).
- Avoid questions that can be answered with a yes or no. Give the child as many choices during the interview as possible. Use multiple choice or open-ended questions.
- The less information you supply in your questions and the more information the child gives answering the questions increases the credibility of the information gathered during the interview.

Assessment Procedure	Normal Findings	Abnormal Findings (Indicators of Violence or Potential Violence)
For elder mistreatment, start out by asking the elder to tell you about a typical day in their life. Be alert for indicators placing the elder at a high risk for abuse or neglect. Then ask Has anyone ever made you sign papers that you did not understand? Are you alone often? Has anyone refused to help you when you needed help? Has anyone ever refused to give you or let you take your medications?	Client answers no to all questions.	"Yes" to any of the questions indicates abuse.
Physical Examination **Perform a general survey.** Observe general appearance and body build.	Client appears stated age and well-developed.	Abused children may appear younger than stated age due to developmental delays or malnourishment. Older clients may appear thin and frail due to malnourishment.
Note dress and hygiene.	Client is well-groomed and dressed appropriately for season and occasion.	Poor hygiene and soiled clothing may indicate neglect. Long sleeves and pants in warm weather may be an attempt to cover bruising or other injuries. Victims of sexual abuse may dress provocatively.
Assess mental status.	Client is coherent and relaxed. A child shows proper developmental level for age.	Client is anxious, depressed, suicidal, withdrawn, or has difficulty concentrating. Client has poor eye contact or soft passive speech. Client is unable to recall recent or past events. Child does not meet developmental expectations.
Evaluate vital signs.	Vital signs are within normal limits.	Hypertension may be seen in victims of abuse.
Inspect skin.	Skin is clean, dry, and free of lesions or bruises. Skin fragility increases with age, bruising may occur with pressure and may mimic bruising associated with abuse. Be careful to distinguish between normal and abnormal findings.	Client has scars, bruises, burns, welts or swelling on face, breasts, arms, chest, abdomen, or genitalia.
Inspect the head and neck.	Head and neck are free of injuries.	Client has hair missing in clumps, subdural hematomas, or rope marks or finger/hand strangulation marks on neck.

continued

ASSESSMENT PROCEDURE *Continued*

Assessment Procedure	Normal Findings	Abnormal Findings (Indicators of Violence or Potential Violence)
Inspect the eyes.	Eyes are free of injury.	Client has bruising or swelling around eyes, unilateral ptosis of upper eyelids (due to repeated blows causing nerve damage to eyelids), or a subconjunctival hemorrhage.
Assess the ears.	Ears are clean and free of injuries.	Client has external or internal ear injuries.
Assess the abdomen.	Abdomen is free of bruises and other injuries and is nontender.	Client has bruising in various stages of healing. Assessment reveals intra-abdominal injuries. A pregnant client has received blows to abdomen.
Assess genitalia and rectal area.	Client is free of injury.	Client has irritation, tenderness, bruising, bleeding, or swelling of genitals or rectal area. Discharge, redness, or lacerations may indicate abuse in young children. Hemorrhoids are unusual in children and may be caused by sexual abuse. Extreme apprehension during examination may indicate physical or sexual abuse
Assess the musculoskeletal system.	Client shows full range of motion and has no evidence of injuries.	Dislocation of shoulder; old or new fractures of face, arms, or ribs; and poor ROM of joints are indicators of abuse.
Assess the neurologic system.	Client demonstrates normal neurologic function.	Abnormal findings include tremors, hyperactive reflexes, and decreased sensations to areas of old injuries secondary to neurological damage.

Additional Tools for Victims of IPV

If screening for IPV is positive, ask the client if she has a safety plan and where she would like to go when she leaves your agency.	Client has a plan.	If the client says she prefers to return home, ask her if it is safe for her to do so and have her complete the Danger Assessment Tool in Assessment Tool 9-3. Provide the client with contact information for shelters and groups. Encourage her to call with any concerns.
Assess her for safety issues in her home using Assessment Tool 9-2.		
Make a follow-up appointment and or referral as appropriate.		

ASSESSMENT TOOL 9-2 | Assessing a Safety Plan

Ask the client, do you
- Have a packed bag ready? Keep it hidden but make it easy to grab quickly?
- Tell your neighbors about your abuse and ask them to call the police when they hear a disturbance?
- Have a code word to use with your kids, family and friends. They will know to call the police and get you help?
- Know where you are going to go, if you ever have to leave?
- Remove weapons from the home?
- Have the following gathered:
  - Cash
  - Social Security cards/numbers for you and your children
  - Birth certificates for you and your children
  - Driver's license
  - Rent and utility receipts
  - Bank account numbers
  - Insurance policies and numbers
  - Marriage license
  - Jewelry
  - Important phone numbers
  - Copy of protection order

Ask children, do you:
- Know a safe place to go?
- Know who is safe to tell you are unsafe?
- Know how and when to call 911? Know how to make a collect call?

Inform children that it is their job to keep themselves safe; they should not interject themselves into adult conflict.

If the client is planning to leave
- Remind the client this is a dangerous time that requires awareness and planning.
- Review where the client is planning to go, shelter options, and the need to be around others to curtail violence.
- Review the client's right to possessions and list of possessions to take.

Adapted from material by Jacquelyn C. Campbell.

ASSESSMENT TOOL 9-3 | Danger Assessment

Several risk factors have been associated with increased risk of homicides (murders) of women and men in violent relationships. We cannot predict what will happen in your case, but we would like you to be aware of the danger of homicide in situations of abuse and for you to see how many of the risk factors apply to your situation.

Using the calendar, please mark the approximate dates during the past year when you were abused by your partner or ex partner. Write on that date how bad the incident was according to the following scale:

1. Slapping, pushing; no injuries and/or lasting pain
2. Punching, kicking; bruises, cuts, and/or continuing pain
3. "Beating up"; severe contusions, burns, broken bones, miscarriage
4. Threat to use weapon; head injury, internal injury, permanent injury, miscarriage
5. Use of weapon; wounds from weapon
(If **any** of the descriptions for the higher number apply, use the higher number.)

Mark **Yes** or **No** for each of the following.
("He" refers to your husband, partner, ex-husband, ex-partner, or whoever is currently physically hurting you.)

Yes	No	
_____	_____	1. Has the physical violence increased in severity or frequency over the past year?
_____	_____	2. Does he own a gun?
_____	_____	3. Have you left him after living together during the past year?
		3a. (If you have *never* lived with him, check here ___)
_____	_____	4. Is he unemployed?
_____	_____	5. Has he ever used a weapon against you or threatened you with a lethal weapon?
		5a. (If yes, was the weapon a gun? _____)
_____	_____	6. Does he threaten to kill you?
_____	_____	7. Has he avoided being arrested for domestic violence?
_____	_____	8. Do you have a child that is not his?
_____	_____	9. Has he ever forced you to have sex when you did not wish to do so?
_____	_____	10. Does he ever try to choke you?
_____	_____	11. Does he use illegal drugs? By drugs, I mean "uppers" or amphetamines, speed, angel dust, cocaine, "crack", street drugs or mixtures.
_____	_____	12. Is he an alcoholic or problem drinker?

continued on page 118

ASSESSMENT TOOL 9-3	Danger Assessment *Continued*

Yes	**No**	
_____	_____	13. Does he control most or all of your daily activities? (For instance: does he tell you who you can be friends with, when you can see your family, how much money you can use, or when you can take the car)? (If he tries, but you do not let him, check here: _____)
_____	_____	14. Is he violently and constantly jealous of you? (For instance, does he say "If I can't have you, no one can.")
_____	_____	15. Have you ever been beaten by him while you were pregnant? (If you have never been pregnant by him, check here: _____)
_____	_____	16. Has he ever threatened or tried to commit suicide?
_____	_____	17. Does he threaten to harm your children?
_____	_____	18. Do you believe he is capable of killing you?
_____	_____	19. Does he follow or spy on you, leave threatening notes or messages on answering machine, destroy your property, or call you when you don't want him to?
_____	_____	20. Have you ever threatened or tried to commit suicide?
_____	_____	Total "Yes" Answers

Thank you. Please talk to your nurse, advocate or counselor about what the Danger Assessment means in terms of your situation.
_____

Jacquelyn C. Campbell, Ph.D., R.N. Copyright, 2004.

VALIDATING AND DOCUMENTING FINDINGS

Validate any family violence data you have collected. This is necessary to verify that the data are reliable and accurate. Document your assessment data following the health-care facility or agency policy.

Sample Subjective Data

Client reports injuries to head, neck, and breasts. States, "I am having difficulty talking." Shares that she was beaten with a plastic ball bat on her head; denies any loss of consciousness. Reports pain and soreness of her neck and pain when speaking after being choked with a cord. Also reports multiple bites and bruising on both breasts. States, "This has happened on a number of occasions for the past 3 years." Denies any witnesses for any of the events.

Sample Objective Data

Ears: right tympanic membrane scar noted at 3 o'clock position; Eyes: conjunctival hemorrhage bilaterally; Neck: circular pattern of bruising and abrasions noted around the neck

Chest: respiration regular, 20 per minute; Breasts: right nipple, red, swollen with multiple abrasions noted around the areola; Abdomen: multiple bruises noted at various stages of healing

Analysis of Data

After you have collected your assessment data, you will need to analyze the data using diagnostic reasoning skills. Use the case study on the following pages as a guide to analyzing the assessment data for a specific client. In the same way, practice diagnostic reasoning skill in the critical thinking exercise included in the lab manual/study guide available for this textbook.

DIAGNOSTIC REASONING: POSSIBLE CONCLUSIONS

Listed below are some possible conclusions that may be drawn from assessment of family violence.

Selected Nursing Diagnoses

After collecting subjective and objective data pertaining to domestic violence, you will need to identify abnormals and cluster the data to reveal any significant patterns or abnormalities. These data will then be used to make clinical judgments (nursing diagnoses, wellness, risk, or actual) about the status of domestic violence in your client's life. The following is a listing of selected nursing diagnoses that you may identify when analyzing data for assessment of domestic violence in the family.

Wellness Diagnoses

- Readiness for Enhanced Family Processes
- Health-Seeking Behavior: requests information related to safety from domestic violence

Risk Diagnoses

- Risk for Impaired Parent/Infant/Child Family Processes related to the presence of domestic violence

- Risk for Violence (other directed) related to the presence of poor coping mechanisms and the misuse of alcohol and illegal drugs
- Risk for STDs and HIV related to participation in forced sexual relationships
- Risk for Powerlessness related to control of relationships, control of children and finances by abusive significant other
- Risk for Post-Trauma Syndrome related to the inability to remove self from abusive intimate relationships

Actual Diagnoses

- Dysfunctional Grieving related to loss of ideal relationship as evidenced by refusal to discuss feelings and prolonged denial
- Impaired Parenting related to choosing to remain living in the presence of an abusive marriage or intimate relationship
- Disturbed Personal Identity related to inability to function effectively outside of a victimized abusive role
- Rape-Trauma Syndrome related to the forced violent penetration against the client's will secondary to the lack of a safety plan for the victim
- Rape-Trauma Syndrome: Silent Reaction related to inability to discuss occurrences of a victim of rape
- Rape-Trauma Syndrome: Compound Reaction related to inability to function effectively in everyday activities after being a victim of rape
- Fear of losing an ineffective abusive intimate relationship related to unrealistic expectations of self and others
- Hopelessness related to remaining in a prolonged abusive relationship and inability to seek counseling and healthy supportive relationships
- Anxiety related to inconsistency of behaviors and instability of abusive spouse or parent

- Low Self-Esteem related to lack of confidence related to presence of prolonged physical, sexual, and emotional abuse

Selected Collaborative Problems

After grouping the data, you may see various collaborative problems emerge. Remember that collaborative problems differ from nursing diagnoses in that they cannot be prevented by nursing interventions. However, these physiologic complications of medical conditions can be detected and monitored by the nurse. In addition, the nurse can use physician- and nurse-prescribed interventions to minimize the complications of these problems. The nurse may also have to refer the client in such situations for further treatment of the problem. Following is a list of collaborative problems that may be identified when assessing a victim of family violence.

- RC: Fractures
- RC: Bruises
- RC: Concussion
- RC: Subdural hematoma
- RC: Subconjunctival hemorrhage
- RC: Intra-abdominal injury
- RC: Depression
- RC: Suicide
- RC: Death

Medical Problems

Once the data are grouped, certain signs and symptoms may become evident and may require medical diagnoses and treatment. Referral to primary health-care provider is necessary.

CASE STUDY

The case study presents assessment data for a specific client followed by an analysis of the data, working out the key steps and arriving at conclusions.

Clara Doubtfree, a 32-year-old, timid, and passive female, comes to the outpatient clinic accompanied by her husband and two small children, ages 6 years and 8 years. The family displays good hygiene and dress. Her husband assists her as she walked into the reception area. Ms. Doubtfree denied falling or being involved in an accident. She reports being hospitalized 6 months ago in another state with similar symptoms. She states, "My chest hurts and I cannot breathe easily." When asked about her injuries, she has poor eye contact and looks away or towards husband. Husband interrupts client frequently preventing from answering interview questions. The children cling to their mother.

You bring the client to the restroom to assist her to obtain a urine specimen. She begins to cry and discloses that her husband has been choking her, hitting her, and kicking her in the chest and stomach several times today and in the past. She states, " I know he is going to kill me; I just don't know when. I will not be able to stop him. He has been threatening to kill me

for the last 6 months. Now I'm afraid he will hurt my 8 year old, who he choked and then locked outside in the middle of the night."

Ms. Doubtfree appears frail and thin. Upon physical examination, you note a large area of discoloration and swelling noted on the right chest wall, bruising on right side of the abdomen and right hip, and decreased breath sounds over right lung. The client has rope burn and abrasions all around circumference of neck; her son also has abrasions around his neck. She has full range of motion but complains of pain with motion. Other than her injuries, her other body systems are intact. A radiograph reveals two fractured ribs and old healed fracture of left arm.

When questioned about old healed fracture on x-rays, the client states "I did not come to the doctor when he broke that arm because he threatened to kill me if I did."

The following concept map illustrates the diagnostic reasoning process.

continued on page 120

Applying COLDSPA

Applying **COLDSPA** for client symptoms: "chest pain."

Mnemonic	Question	Data Provided	Missing Data
Character	Describe the sign or symptom (feeling, appearance, sound, smell, or taste if applicable).	"My chest hurts and I cannot breathe easily"	
Onset	When did it begin?	"I had the same symptoms 6 months ago." In private, the client states, "My husband has been choking, hitting, and kicking me in the chest and stomach." She indicates this has occurred "several times today and in the past," and indicates fear for the safety of her children and for her own life.	
Location	Where is it? Does it radiate? Does it occur anywhere else?		Does your chest pain radiate? Do you have pain anywhere else?
Duration	How long does it last? Does it recur?		How long does this pain last? Does it recur?
Severity	How bad is it? How much does it bother you?		How bad is this chest pain? Does it limit your ability to move or go about your normal activites?
Pattern	What makes it better or worse?		Does this chest pain occur only when your husband physically hurts you?
Associated factors/ How it **A**ffects the client	What other symptoms occur with it? How does it affect you?	The client makes poor eye contact and looks at her husband frequently for answering questions. Children are clinging to their mother. The client is frail and thin, with bruising and swelling over the right chest wall.	How has this abusive situation affected your activities of daily living?

1) Identify abnormal findings and client strengths

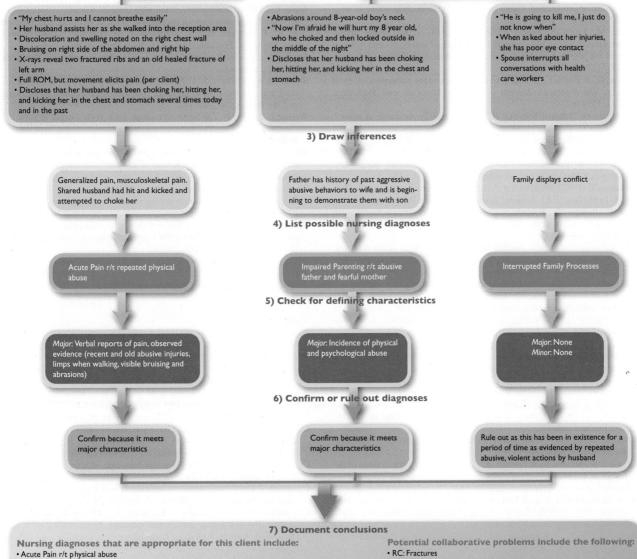

Subjective Data

- "My chest hurts and I cannot breathe easily"
- Discloses that her husband has been choking her, hitting her, and kicking her in the chest and stomach
- "I know he is going to kill me; I just don't know when. He has been threatening to kill me for the last 6 months"
- "Now I'm afraid he will hurt my 8 year old, who he choked and then locked outside in the middle of the night"
- When questioned about old healed fracture, client states "I did not come to the doctor when he broke that arm because he threatened to kill me if I did"

Objective Data

- Frail, thin, 32-year-old female
- Family displays good hygiene and dress
- Her husband assists her as she walked into the reception area
- When asked about her injuries, she has poor eye contact
- Spouse interrupts all conversations with health care workers
- Decreased breath sounds over right lung
- Large area of discoloration and swelling noted on the right chest wall
- Bruising on right side of the abdomen and right hip
- Rope burn and abrasions all around circumference of neck
- Abrasions around 8-year-old's neck
- Full ROM, but movement elicits pain (per client)
- X-rays reveal two fractured ribs and an old healed fracture of left arm

2) Identify cue clusters

- "My chest hurts and I cannot breathe easily"
- Her husband assists her as she walked into the reception area
- Discoloration and swelling noted on the right chest wall
- Bruising on right side of the abdomen and right hip
- X-rays reveal two fractured ribs and an old healed fracture of left arm
- Full ROM, but movement elicits pain (per client)
- Discloses that her husband has been choking her, hitting her, and kicking her in the chest and stomach several times today and in the past

---

- Abrasions around 8-year-old boy's neck
- "Now I'm afraid he will hurt my 8 year old, who he choked and then locked outside in the middle of the night"
- Discloses that her husband has been choking her, hitting her, and kicking her in the chest and stomach

---

- "He is going to kill me, I just do not know when"
- When asked about her injuries, she has poor eye contact
- Spouse interrupts all conversations with health care workers

3) Draw inferences

Generalized pain, musculoskeletal pain. Shared husband had hit and kicked and attempted to choke her

---

Father has history of past aggressive abusive behaviors to wife and is beginning to demonstrate them with son

---

Family displays conflict

4) List possible nursing diagnoses

Acute Pain r/t repeated physical abuse

Impaired Parenting r/t abusive father and fearful mother

Interrupted Family Processes

5) Check for defining characteristics

Major: Verbal reports of pain, observed evidence (recent and old abusive injuries, limps when walking, visible bruising and abrasions)

Major: Incidence of physical and psychological abuse

Major: None
Minor: None

6) Confirm or rule out diagnoses

Confirm because it meets major characteristics

Confirm because it meets major characteristics

Rule out as this has been in existence for a period of time as evidenced by repeated abusive, violent actions by husband

7) Document conclusions

Nursing diagnoses that are appropriate for this client include:
- Acute Pain r/t physical abuse
- Impaired Parenting r/t abusive father and fearful mother

Potential collaborative problems include the following:
- RC: Fractures
- RC: Hemorrhage
- RC: Intra-abdominal hemorrhages
- RC: Death

References and Selected Readings

American Medical Association. (1993). *Diagnostic and treatment guidelines on elder abuse.* Chicago, IL: American Medical Association.

American Nurses Association. (1998). *Culturally competent assessment for family violence.* Washington, DC: Author.

Barclay, L. (2007). Screening tool helps to identify mothers affected by intimate partner violence. Retrieved August 1, 2008 from http://www.medscape.com/viewarticle/568324

Barclay, L., & Lie, D. (2007). New guidelines issued for evaluating physical abuse in children. *Medscape Medical News.* Retrieved June 7, 2007 from http://cme.medscape.com/viewarticle/557883

Biller, H. (1995). The battered spouse made male. *Brown University Child Adolescent Behavior Letter, March 3,* 1–3.

Burgess, A., Brown, K., Bell, K., Ledray, L., & Poarch, J. (2005). Sexual abuse of older adults: Assessing for signs of a serious crime—and reporting it. *American Journal of Nursing, 105*(10), 66–71.

Campbell, J., & Humphreys, J. (1993). *Nursing care of survivors of family violence.* St. Louis: Mosby.

Child Abuse Prevention and Treatment Act. (2003). Public Law 104–235, 111; 42 U.S.C 510g.

Child Welfare Information Gateway. (2008). What is child abuse of neglect? Available at www.hhs.gov

Cohen, M., Levin, S., Gagin, R., & Friedman, G. (2007). Elder abuse: Disparities between older people's disclosure of abuse, evident signs of abuse and high risk of abuse. *Journal of the American Geriatrics Society, 55*(8), 1224–1450.

Collins, K., & Presnell, S. (2007). Elder neglect and the pathophysiology of aging. *The American Journal of Forensic Medicine and Pathology, 28*(2), 157–162.

Committee on National Statistics (CNSTAT). (2002). Available at www7.nationalacademies.org/cnstat

Cronin, G. (2007). Elder abuse: The same old story? *Emergency Nurse, 15*(3), 11–13.

Datner, E., & Ferroggiaro, A. (1999). Violence during pregnancy. *Emergency Medical Clinics of North America, 17*(3), 645.

Davidson, T. (1977). Wifebeating: A recurring phenomenon throughout history. In M. Roy (Ed.), *Battered Women.* New York: Van Nostrand.

Dyer, C., Pickens, S., Burnett, J. (2007). Vulnerable elders when it is no longer safe to live alone. *Journal of the American Medical Association, 298*(12), 1448–1450.

Elder mistreatment: Abuse, neglect and exploitation in an aging America. Available at http://www.nap.edu/books/0309084342/html/238.html

Ewen, B. (2007). Failure to protect laws: Protecting children or punishing mothers? *Journal of Forensic Nursing, 3*(2), 84–86.

Fagan, J. A., Steward, D. W., & Hansen, K. V. (1983). Violent men or violent husband? Background factors and situational correlates. In R. J. Gelles, G. T. Hotaling, M. A. Straus, & D. Finkelhor (Eds.), *The dark side of families.* Beverly Hills, CA: Sage.

Family Violence Prevention Fund. (1999). Preventing domestic violence: Clinical guidelines on routine screening. San Francisco: Family Violence Prevention Fund. Available at www.fvpf.org.

Frank, J., & Roddowski, M. (1999). Review of psychological issues in victims of domestic violence seen in emergency settings. *Emergency Medicine Clinics of North America, 17*(3), 657–677.

Gelles, R. J. (1997). *Intimate violence in families.* Thousand Oaks, CA: Sage Publications.

Hawkins, D. F. (1993). Inequality, culture, and interpersonal violence. *Health Affairs, 12*(4), 80–95.

Hayward, K., Steiner, S., & Sproule, K. (2007). Women's perceptions of the impact of a domestic violence treatment program for male perpetrators. *Journal of Forensic Nursing, 3*(2), 77–83.

Hegar, A. H., Emans, S. J., & Muram, D. (2000). *Evaluation of the sexually abused child: A medical textbook and photographic atlas.* New York: Oxford University Press.

Huckle, P. (1995). Male rape victims referred to a forensic psychiatric service. *Medical Sciences Law, 35,* 187–192.

Humphrey, J., & Campbell, J. C. (2009). *Family violence and nursing practice.* Philadelphia: Lippincott Williams & Wilkins.

Kingsnorth, R. (2006). Intimate partner violence: Predictors of recidivism in a sample of arrestees. *Violence Against Women, 12*(10), 917–935.

Knitzer, J. (1977). Spare the rod and spoil the child revisited. *American Journal of Orthopsychiatry, 47,* 372–373.

Kold, L. (1971). Violence and aggression: An overview. In J. Fawcett (Ed.), *Dynamics of violence* (pp. 40–50). Chicago: American Medical Association.

Lamberg, L. (2000). Domestic violence: What to ask, what to do. *Journal of the American Medical Association, 284*(5), 554.

Merriam-Webster Online. (2005). Available at http://www.m-w.com/.

Miller, S., & Meloy, M. (2006). Women's use of force: Voices of women arrested for domestic violence. *Violence Against Women, 12*(1), 89–115.

Nuddelman, J., Durborow, N., Grambs, M., & Letellier, P. (1997). *Best practices: Innovation domestic violence programs in health care settings.* San Francisco: Family Violence Prevention Fund.

Nursing Network on Violence Against Women International. (2004). Assessment tools. Available at www.nnvawi.org

Peddle, N., Wang, C. T., Diaz, J., & Reid, R. (2002). Current trends in child abuse prevention and fatalities—the 2000 fifty state survey. Available at http://member.preventchildabuse.org/site/DocServer/2000_50_survey.pdf?docID=143

Pillemer, K., & Finkelhor, D. (1988). The prevalence of elder abuse: a random sample survey. *The Gerontologist, 28,* 51–57.

Saxton Mahoney, B. (1990). The extent and response to victimization of emergency nurses in Pennsylvania. *Journal of Emergency Nursing, 17,* 282–294.

Schornstein, S. L. (1997). *Domestic violence and health care: What every professional needs to know.* Thousand Oaks, CA: Sage Publications.

Stark, E. (2001). Health intervention with battered women: From crisis intervention to complex social prevention. In C. M. Renzetti, J. L. Edleson, & R. K. Bergen (Eds.), *Sourcebook on violence against women* (pp. 345–370). Thousand Oaks, CA: Sage Publications.

Straus, M. & Gelles, R. (1990). *Violence in the American family.* New York: Transaction Press.

Straus, M. A., & Sweet, S. (1992). Verbal aggression in couples: Incidence rates and relationships to personal characteristics. *Journal of Marriage and the Family, 54,* 346–357.

Walker, L. E. (1979). *The battered woman.* New York: Harper & Row.

Walker, L. E. (1984). *The battered woman syndrome.* New York: Harper & Row.

Wang, J., Tseng, H., & Cheng, K. (2007). Development and testing of screening indicators for psychological abuse of older people. *Archives of Psychiatric Nursing, 21*(1), 40–47.

Washington State Department of Health. (2004). *Domestic violence and pregnancy: Guidelines for screening and referral* (Publication No. 950-143). Olympia, WA: Author.

Weise, D., & Daro, D. (1995). *Current trends on child abuse reporting and fatalities: The results of the 1994 Fifty State Survey.* Chicago: National Committee to Prevent Child Abuse.

Wolf, R. (1995). Abuse of the elderly. In R. Gelles (Ed.), *Visions 2010: Families and violence, abuse, and neglect* (pp. 8–10). Minneapolis: National Council on Family Relations.

Danger Assessment

Block, C. R., Engel, B., Naureckas, S. M., & Riordan, K. A. (1999). The Chicago women's health risk study: Lessons in collaboration. *Violence Against Women, 5,* 1158–1177.

Browne, A. (1987). *Battered women who kill.* New York: Free Press.

Browne, A. Williams, K., and Dutton, D. (1998). Homicide between intimate partners. In M. D. Smith & M. Zahn (Eds.), *Homicide: A sourcebook of social research* (pp. 149–164). Thousand Oaks, CA: Sage.

Campbell, J. C. (1995). *Assessing Dangerousness.* Newbury Park: Sage.

Campbell, J. C. (1992). "If I can't have you, no one can": Power and control in homicide of female partners. In J. Radford & D. E. H. Russell (Eds.), *Femicide: The politics of woman killing* (pp. 99–113). New York: Twayne.

Campbell, J. C. (1981). Misogyny and homicide of women. *Advances in Nursing Science, 3,* 67–85.

Campbell, J. C. (1986). Nursing assessment for risk of homicide with battered women. *Advances in Nursing Science, 8,* 36–51.

Campbell, D. W., Campbell, J. C., King, C., Parker, B., & Ryan, J. (1994). The reliability and factor structure of the index of spouse abuse with African-American battered women. *Violence and Victims, 9,* 259–274.

Campbell, J. C., Sharps, P., and Glass, N. (2000). Risk Assessment for Intimate Partner Homicide. In G. F. Pinard & L. Pagani (Eds.), *Clinical Assessment of Dangerousness: Empirical Contributions.* New York: Cambridge University Press.

Campbell, J. C., Soeken, K., McFarlane, J., & Parker, B (1998). Risk factors for femicide among pregnant and nonpregnant battered women. In J. C. Campbell (Ed.), *Empowering survivors of abuse: Health care for battered women and their children* (pp. 90–97). Thousand Oaks, CA: Sage.

Campbell, J. C., and Webster, D. (submitted). The Danger Assessment: Psychometric support from a case control study of intimate partner homicide.

Campbell, J. C., Webster, D., Koziol-McLain, J., et. al. (2003). Assessing risk factors for intimate partner homicide. *National Institute of Justice Journal* (250):14–19. (Full Text: http://ncjrs.org/pdffiles1/jr000250e.pdf)

Campbell, J. C. Webster, D., Koziol-McLain, J. et. al. (2003). Risk Factors for Femicide in Abusive Relationships: Results from a Multi-Site Case Control Study. *American Journal of Public Health, 93*(7): 1089–1097.

Diaz-Olavarrieta, C., Campbell, J. C., Garcia de la Cadena, C., Paz, F., & Villa, A. (1999). Domestic violence against patients with chronic neurologic disorders. *Archives of Neurology, 56,* 681–685.

Fagan, J. A., Stewart, D. E., & Hansen, K. (1983). Violent men or violent husbands? Background factors and situational correlates. In R. J. Gelles, G. Hotaling, M. A. Straus, & D. Finkelhor (Eds.), *The dark side of families* (pp. 49–68). Beverly Hills: Sage.

Ferraro, K. J. & Johnson, J. M. (1983). How women experience battering: The process of victimization. *Social Problems, 30,* 325–339.

Goodman, L., Dutton, M. and Bennett, M. (1999). Predicting repeat abuse among arrested batterers: Use of the danger assessment scale in the criminal justice system. *J. Interpers. Violence, 15,* 63–74.

Heckert, D. A., & Gondolf, E. W. (2004). Battered women's perceptions of risk versus risk factors and instruments in predicting repeat reassault. *J. Interpers. Violence 19*(7): 778–800.

Heckert, D. A., & Gondolf, E. W. (2001). Predicting levels of abuse and reassault among batterer program participants. Paper presented at the American Society of Criminology, Atlanta, GA.

McFarlane, J., Campbell, J. C., Sharps, P., & Watson, K. (2002). Abuse during pregnancy and femicide: urgent implications for women's health. *Obstet. Gynecol., 100,* 27–36.

McFarlane, J., Campbell, J. C., & Watson, K. (2002). Intimate Partner Stalking and Femicide: Urgent implications for women's safety. *Behavioral Sciences and the Law, 20,* 51–68.

McFarlane, J., Campbell, J. C., and Wilt, S., et al. (1999). Stalking and intimate partner femicide. *Homicide Studies* 3 (4): 300–316.

McFarlane, J., Parker, B., Soeken, K., & Bullock, L. (1992). Assessing for abuse during pregnancy: Severity and frequency of injuries and associated entry into prenatal care. *JAMA, 267,* 3176–3178.

McFarlane, J., Parker, B., & Soeken, K. (1996). Abuse during pregnancy: Associations with maternal health and infant birth weight. *Nursing Research, 45,* 37–42.

McFarlane, J, Soeken, K., Campbell, J. C, Parker, B., Reel, S., and Silva, C. (1998). Severity of abuse to pregnant women and associated gun access of the perpetrator. *Public Health Nurs. 15*(3): 201–206.

McFarlane, J., Soeken, K., Reel, S., Parker, B., & Siiva, C. (1997). Resource use by abused women following an intervention program: Associated severity of abuse and reports of abuse ending. *Public Health Nursing, 14,* 244–250.

Parker, B., McFarlane, J., & Soeken, K. (1994). Abuse during pregnancy: Effects on maternal complications and birth weight in adult and teenage women. *Obstetrics & Gynecology, 84,* 323–328.

Roehl, J. & Guertin, K. (1998). Current use of dangerousness assessments I sentencing domestic violence offenders Pacific Grove, CA: State Justice Institute.

Sharps, P. W., Koziol-McLain, J., and Campbell, J. C., et. al. (2001). Health Care Provider's Missed Opportunities for Preventing Femicide. *Prev. Med., 33,* 373–380.

Silva, C. McFarlane, J., and Soeken, K, et. al. (1997). Symptoms of posttraumatic stress disorder in abused women in a primary care setting. *Journal of Women's Health.* 6, 543–552.

Stuart, E. P. & Campbell, J. C. (1989). Assessment of patterns of dangerousness with battered women. *Issues Mental Health Nursing. 10,* 245–260.

Weisz, A., Tolman, R., & Saunders, D. G. (2000). Assessing the risk of severe domestic violence: The importance of survivor's predictions. *Journal of Interpersonal Violence, 15,* 75–90.

Williams, K. and Conniff, E. (2001). Legal Sanctions and the Violent Victimization of Women. Paper presented at the American Society of Criminology, Atlanta, GA.

CONTEXTS FOR ASSESSMENT

Culture includes among its elements family structure and function, spirituality and religion, and community. Together these form the major contexts for seeing a client as an individual or group but inseparable from the background contexts. The influence of culture, family, spirituality, and community on the health status of the client cannot be emphasized enough. The nurse must perceive the client within these contexts and be able to assess aspects of these contexts as necessary when performing a health assessment.

CULTURE: WHAT IS IT?

Nurses often ask "What is culture and why do we need to know something about it?" Other questions are as follows: How do culture and race differ? What about ethnicity? Minority? Do I have a culture? To answer these questions, it will first help to define the terms.

Culture may be defined as a shared system of values, beliefs, and learned patterns of behavior. Purnell and Paulanka (2003, p. 3) provide the following useful definition: "the totality of socially transmitted behavioral patterns, arts, beliefs, values, customs, lifeways, and all other products of human work and thought characteristic of a population or people that guide their worldview and decision making." The particular culture defines values (learned beliefs about what is held to be good or bad) and norms (learned behaviors that are perceived to be appropriate or inappropriate). So culture is learned, shared, associated with adaptation to the environment, and it is universal. All people have a socially transmitted culture. Our own culture forms our worldview based on the values, beliefs, and behaviors sanctioned by it. That worldview becomes, for us, reality.

If an individual has limited interaction with other cultural groups, his or her cultural worldview is the limit of his or her experience. The perception that one's worldview is the only acceptable truth and that one's beliefs, values, and sanctioned behaviors are superior to all others is called *ethnocentrism.*

Many people are aware of other cultures and their different beliefs, values, and accepted behaviors but do not recognize the great variation that can exist within any cultural group. Not recognizing this variation tends to lead to *stereotyping* all members of a particular culture, expecting group members to hold the same beliefs and behave in the same way.

Ethnicity, or a person's ethnic identity, exists when the person identifies with a "socially, culturally, and politically constructed group of individuals that holds a common set of characteristics not shared by others with whom its members come in contact" (Lipson, 1996, p. 8). Put another way, ethnicity describes subgroups that have a common history, ancestry, or other cultural identity and may relate to geographical origin, such as Southerners, Navajos, or Mexican Americans.

Race, in humans, is not a physical characteristic but a socially constructed concept that has meaning to a larger group. The concept of race "originates from societal desire to separate people based on their looks and culture . . . [it is] a vague, unscientific term referring to a group of genetically related individuals who share certain physical characteristics" (Bigby, 2003), but actually the genetic distinctiveness may not exist. Bigby argues that race "is reflected in American society in a way that ethnicity, culture, and class are not" (p. 2) because access to resources is often based on race categories. The primary race categories used by the U.S. government are American Indian/Alaska Native, Asian American, African American or black, Native Hawaiian/Pacific Islander, and white. Often the categories of non-Hispanic white or black are added along with Hispanic. You can see how genetics cannot serve as a basis for separating the groups.

Minority refers to a group who has less power or prestige within the society, but actually means a group with smaller population numbers. Since Caucasian Americans, or whites, are the majority in the United States and are expected to remain so for the next 30 or 40 years, all other groups would be minorities. But the term has a negative meaning in most uses, indicating a group that does not hold the "majority" values or does not behave in "appropriate" ways.

There are several reasons why nurses need to know about culture, including the long history of disparity in the level of health care received by persons from certain racial groups or minorities, and the problems of ethnocentrism and stereotyping mentioned earlier. To provide high-quality health care, nurses must know how to assess what is normal or abnormal for all persons who seek care. This necessitates cultural competence.

CULTURAL COMPETENCE

Cultural competence has a number of components and allows a nurse to integrate a cultural assessment into the health assessment of each client.

According to Campinha-Bacote (2007), there are five constructs in the cultural competence process: cultural awareness, cultural knowledge, cultural skill, cultural encounters, and cultural desire (For a model and description of Campinha-Bacote's "The Process of Cultural Competence in the Delivery of Healthcare Services," go to her website at www.transculturalcare.net).

Cultural Desire

The motivation to engage in intercultural encounters and acquire cultural competence is known as *cultural desire.* Campinha-Bacote's revised model is based on the assumption that the starting point of cultural competence is cultural desire. In other words, to be a culturally competent health care provider, the nurse must sincerely desire to acquire the cultural knowledge and skill necessary for effectively assessing the client. The nurse must also seek repeated encounters with people of the culture so that awareness, knowledge, and skill continually increase.

Cultural Awareness

Cultural awareness is the "deliberate, cognitive process in which the healthcare provider becomes appreciative and sensitive to the values, beliefs, life ways, practices and problem-solving strategies of a client's culture" (Campinha-Bacote, 1998). But first, cultural awareness involves "self-examination and in-depth exploration of one's own cultural background" (Campinha-Bacote, 2003). Health care providers need to examine their own prejudices and biases toward other cultures and explore how their own cultural beliefs and background may affect views of and interactions with clients of different cultures. The stages of cultural awareness are

- **Unconscious incompetence:** not aware that one lacks cultural knowledge; not aware that cultural differences exist
- **Conscious incompetence:** aware that one lacks knowledge about another culture; aware that cultural differences exist but not knowing what they are or how to communicate effectively with clients from different cultures
- **Conscious competence:** consciously learning about the client's culture and providing culturally relevant interventions; aware of differences; able to have effective transcultural interactions
- **Unconscious competence:** able to automatically provide culturally congruent care to clients from a different culture; having much experience with a variety of cultural groups and having an intuitive grasp of how to communicate effectively in transcultural encounters

Cultural Knowledge

Cultural knowledge is "the process of seeking and obtaining a sound educational foundation concerning the various world views of different cultures" (Campinha-Bacote, 1998). The client's worldview is the basis for his or her behaviors and interpretations of the world. For instance, the client's worldview will help to clarify his or her belief about what causes illness, what symptoms are defined as illness, and what are considered appropriate interactions within cultural groups. These characteristics based on worldview, along with biological (physical and pharmacological) variations, comprise the content of cultural knowledge useful for the nurse assessing a client from a different culture.

Cultural Skill

Cultural skill is "the ability to collect relevant cultural data regarding the client's health history and presenting problem as well as accurately performing a physical assessment" (Campinha-Bacote, 1998). Cultural skill involves learning how to complete cultural assessments and culturally based physical assessments and to interpret the data accurately.

Cultural Encounters

A *cultural encounter* is "the process that allows the healthcare provider to engage directly in face-to-face interactions with clients from culturally diverse backgrounds" (Campinha-Bacote, 1998). This process requires going beyond the study of a culture and limited interaction with three or four members of the culture. Repeated face-to-face encounters help to refine or modify the nurse's knowledge of the culture. The nurse must seek out many such encounters with the desire to understand more and more about the culture. Use the ASKED mnemonic to examine your cultural competence (The ASKED mnemonic is found on Campinha-Bacote's website www.transculturalcare.net and click on the Process of Cultural Competence Model).

Ask yourself about the level of your awareness, skill, knowledge, and desire for cultural competence, and the number of encounters you have had or desire to have with persons of cultures different from your own. Together and in different order, these make the word ASKED, to help you to remember to check up on your growing cultural competence as you seek opportunities to increase your competence. Ask yourself how aware you are of your own biases and prejudices toward people different from yourself. Ask yourself if you can complete a cultural assessment being sensitive to cultural differences and sensitivities. Ask yourself how much know about different cultures and ethnic groups, about their beliefs, customs, and biological variations. Ask yourself what level of interest you have in interacting with people from different cultures or ethnicities. And ask yourself is you really have interest in becoming culturally competent. [Based on Campinha-Bacote, J. (2007). The process of cultural competence in the delivery of healthcare services (5th ed.). Cincinnati, OH: Transcultural C.A.R.E. Associates.]

CULTURAL ASSESSMENT
Overview

Cultural assessment can mean adding elements of cultural assessment to the health assessment, or it can mean completing an entire cultural assessment. To know what and when to include cultural components in a health assessment, the nurse has to know how to complete an entire cultural assessment. For this reason, many categories that may vary across cultures will be described. The nurse can then be aware of the possibilities for variation and select those that are most important for assessing each client. Many of these cultural variation categories are covered in transcultural nursing and cultural anthropology texts, or can be found on the Internet. The more common cultural and biological variations that we encounter in the clinical setting will be described here.

Two main belief categories are included in a cultural assessment: those that affect the client approaching the health care system and provider and those that affect the disease, illness, or health state. Of course there is some overlap between them.

Cultural Beliefs and Values

- Dominant value orientation
  - Beliefs about human nature
  - Beliefs about relationship with nature
  - Beliefs about purpose of life
- Beliefs about health, illness, and healing
  - Beliefs about what causes disease
  - Beliefs about health
  - Beliefs about who serves in the role of healer or what practices bring about healing

Assessing these beliefs will help the nurse to understand the client's approach to health care providers and to illness and healing. For instance, if an individual believes that diseases are punishment from God or gods, then he or she may not seek help quickly or even at all. If an individual believes that evil spirits cause disease, he or she will seek out a person who can cast out evil spirits to heal him or her. If the individual believes that health is something that can be improved with exercise, eating the right foods, and other "healthy" behaviors, then seeking health care for early symptoms is usual. If the group's cultural healers play an important role, then an individual may not accept Western style health care without the involvement of the healer as well.

Factors Affecting Approach to Providers

- Ethnicity (assimilation or acculturation): How close to the primary culture does the person feel? To the ethnic group? Country of origin? Age at immigration (if applicable)? Frequency of travel to and from country of origin?
- Generational status: Age? Child, or parent, or grandparent? Family member or patient?
- Education level: Ability to understand spoken and written English? Ability to speak or write English? Acceptance of interpreter? Of interpreter of different age or gender?
- Religion: Acceptance of care by provider of different gender, age, or ethnic group? Level of modesty during care? Need for culturally specific healer to participate in care?
- Previous experience of care by primary health care system? Positive or negative experience?
- Occupation and income level: Ability to pay or use insurance? Embarrassment or fear due to inability to pay? Ability to follow prescribed care?
- Time dimensions: Focus on past, present, or future? Orientation to time (importance of time vs. immediate needs [arrives on time; arrives when convenient for self])?
- Space: Personal space distance? Comfortable with touch?
- Communication: Verbal, written language? Verbal and nonverbal language patterns? Eye contact? Who speaks to whom?

If the person seeking care is from a cultural group but is well acculturated to Western values, assuming that he or she follows practices of the culture group is stereotyping and will lead to conflict with the person. In some cultures, it still may be the practice that older family members have more say in health care and treatment than the patient himself or herself,

even if the patient is an adult (this is especially true for females). Education level plays an important role in health care but it is essential to assess language proficiency and the acceptance of an interpreter with specific characteristics. For instance, some cultures do not allow a young person or a person of different gender to hear personal details. Religious rules and norms may affect who can assess, who can treat, and what treatments are acceptable, among many other aspects of health care. Time, space, and communication will be discussed in the in the following section.

Factors Affecting Disease, Illness, Health State

- Biomedical variations
- Nutrition/dietary habits
- Family roles and organization, patterns
- Workforce issues
- High-risk behaviors
- Pregnancy and childbirth practices
- Death rituals
- Religious and spiritual beliefs and practices
- Health care practices
- Health care practitioners
- Environment

Biomedical variations will be covered in the following section, as will a brief discussion of nutrition/dietary habits. Family content is addressed in Chapter 33, and religious and spiritual content in Chapter 11. Knowing what issues the culturally different client may have at work and what high-risk behaviors are common to the cultural group, as well as the environment from which the client comes, can give clues to the current health status. Assessing health care practices will be discussed in the following section. As this is an assessment text, only the most common cultural and biological variations are covered here. Thorough content is available in transcultural nursing and cultural anthropology texts.

Communication and the Culturally Competent Interview

The first phase of assessment begins with meeting the client. This involves observation and communication. The meeting itself, nurse–client communication, and observation include many of the transcultural variations of time, space, and communication, and biomedical variations.

All communication is culturally based. Verbal communication can have many variations based on both language differences and usual tone of voice. For instance, a harsh tone of voice may be normal in some cultures and thought to be rude in others. Nonverbal communication has the most often misinterpreted variations. These variations include patterns of space, eye contact, body language and hand gestures, silence, and touch. Time is also interpreted to be a form of communication when two people from different cultures perceive time differently.

Time

Time is perceived to be measurable (Western) or fluid and flowing (Eastern cultures). Cultural groups tend to value time in the past, present, or future. Those focused on past value practices that are unchanged from ancestors and are often resistant to new ways. Those focused on the present put what is going on in the present above what will occur in the future. For instance, if a person has an appointment with you but is involved in a pleasurable activity at the time, then either the appointment will be missed or the person will arrive late. Those who are future oriented place value on deferring pleasure for a later gain. They are the ones who will value the care and treatment in expectation of improvement (this reflects Western values).

Space

As noted by Davis' 1990 classic article on cultural differences in personal space, "everyone who's ever felt cramped in a crowd knows that the skin is not the body's only boundary. We each wear a zone of privacy like a hoop skirt, inviting others in or keeping them out with body language—by how closely we approach, the angle at which we face them, and speed with which we break a gaze" (p. 4). Studies show that Asians and Americans tend to keep more space between themselves when speaking. Latins, both Mediterranean and Latin American, stay closer to each other; and Middle Easterners move in the closest.

Eye Contact and Face Positioning

Americans expect people talking to each other to maintain a fairly high level of eye contact. Those looking away and not giving "good eye contact" are thought to be rude or inattentive. But people from Eastern countries and Native Americans tend to look down to show respect to the person talking. Also, some African Americans look away when being talked to, but give a very high level of eye contact when speaking. An Anglo American unfamiliar with this pattern can get the impression that the person does not care what the caregiver is saying and is aggressive when talking. However, it is just a normal cultural variation in communication pattern.

Another variation is whether the persons face each other or stand with the face slightly to the side. American females (both Anglo and Hispanic American) tend to face each other, but males, and people of some other cultures, tend to stand with the face slightly away from the other speaker.

Body Language and Hand Gestures

There are too many elements of body language and hand gestures to cover them all; however, two major hand gestures of note are those for indicating height and those for indicating OK. Latins and others indicate height of an animal the way Americans indicate height of people—by putting the hand level at the indicated height. Latins indicate height for humans by bending the fingers up and putting the back of the hand at the height level. The Latin way is not noticed much by Anglo Americans, but the American way is an insult to Latins. The way Americans sign OK by making a circle with the thumb and forefinger is a definite and serious insult in many cultures around the world. So if any hand gesture is used, be sure to clarify if there seems to be a strange or unexpected reaction on the other person's part.

Silence

There are two types of silence. One is simply remaining silent for long periods; the other is used to space talking between two people carrying on a conversation. There are three patterns of the latter. In Eastern cultures there is a pause after each person speaks before the other does. The pause is thought to show respect and to allow for consideration of what has been said.

Westerners, including English speakers in the United States, tend to interrupt this silence leaving no pause between speakers; Americans tend to be uncomfortable with silence. In yet other cultures, such as Latin cultures, it is common for speakers to interrupt one another in conversation. This provides for overlap in speech. Within the culture, this indicates that the persons are deeply engaged in the conversation, but it is perceived to be rude by other cultures.

Touch

Touch is very culturally based. How much touch is comfortable and allowable, and by whom are all based on culture. The most modest and conservative cultures usually have religious rules about this. Touch of females by males in many of these cultures is restricted to male family members and may also be restricted among them. Even male physicians are not allowed to treat a female patient. In some religions, there are prohibitions on touching people considered to be unclean. There are prohibitions about touching parts of the body, especially the head, or touching children in some cultures because touch is a way to "give the evil eye" to another. In light of these cultural variations, a health care provider should always ask permission before touching anyone.

Autonomy

Autonomy is assumed to be a right of all health care consumers in the United States, meaning that an individual has the right to know about the diagnosis and treatment plans and to make decisions for himself or herself. However, autonomy is not an accepted value in many societies. In paternalistic or patriarchal societies, the father or the family is expected to be told of diagnoses and to make decisions about treatment. In many societies, women are not decision makers. Do not assume that the client expects autonomy; clarify with the client and family. Client autonomy is a legal issue in U.S. health care, so the family and client will need to have a clear explanation of this. The information should be presented in such a way as to avoid a hostile response or the withdrawal of the client from Western health care.

Diet and Nutrition

What we eat, how we eat it, and even when we eat are all culturally based. Dietary considerations in cultural assessment include the meaning of food to the individual, common foods eaten and rituals surrounding the eating, the distribution of food throughout a 24-hour day, religious beliefs about foods, beliefs about food and health promotion, and nutritional deficiencies associated with the ethnic group.

If possible, compare the nutrients of foods not usual in the United States with nutrition charts to understand how healthy a diet is, especially with regard to diseases such as diabetes mellitus. It is very difficult to get a client to change usual dietary habits drastically, even with knowledge of the interaction of diet and disease. What food means to the individual can also be very important. It may serve as a comfort, as closeness to ethnic roots or family. Providing food may be considered to reflect caring, love, and withdrawing food may be considered akin to torture. When the meal is served can seriously affect appetite. For those who usually eat a midday meal at 2 or 3 PM, it is unappetizing to see lunch served at 11 or 12 noon, and a 5 or 6 PM dinner is considered a late lunch rather than an evening meal. Religious beliefs affect what can and cannot be eaten, such as the prohibition of pork or pork products for Jews and Muslims. Asking about specific diet requirements or preferences is part of cultural assessment.

Spirituality

Spirituality is closely associated with culture and includes religious practices, faith, and a relationship with God or a higher being, and those things which bring meaning to life. See Chapter 11 for a detailed discussion of assessing spirituality.

Death Rituals

As noted by Purnell and Paulanka (2003), death rituals include views of death, euthanasia, and rituals for dying, burial, and bereavement, and are unlikely to vary from the original ethnic group's practices.

Practices that affect health care include such customs as ritual washing of the body, the number of family members present at the death of a family member, religious practices required during or after dying, acceptance of life- or death-prolonging treatments, beliefs about withdrawing life support, and beliefs about autopsy. Responses to death and grief vary. Some cultures expect loud wailing in grief with death (e.g., Latins, African Americans), while others expect solemn, quiet grief (e.g., Hindus). In addition, the expected duration of grief varies with culture.

Pregnancy and Childbearing

Accepted practices for getting pregnant, delivery, and child care vary across cultures. As Purnell and Paulanka (2003) noted, "More traditional, folk, and magicoreligious beliefs surround fertility control, pregnancy, childbearing, and postpartum practices in this cultural domain than in any other" (p. 30). Beliefs about conception, pregnancy, and childbearing are passed from generation to generation.

Fertility control varies by culture and religion. Use of sterilization is accepted by some, rejected by others, and forcibly used in other cultures. Rituals to restrict sexuality are used in some cultures, including female circumcision (removal of the clitoris or the vulva, with sewing together of the surrounding skin leaving only a small hole for urination and menstruation). Stoning or other forms of killing women who become pregnant out of wedlock is common in some Islamic cultures.

U.S. culture has pregnancy taboos just as others do. Pregnant women are expected to avoid environments with very loud noises, avoid smoking and alcohol, avoid high caffeine and drug intake, and be cautious about taking prescription and over-the-counter medications. Other cultures have pregnancy taboos such as having the mother avoid reaching over her head to prevent the umbilical cord from going around the baby's neck, not buying baby clothes before birth (Navajo), not permitting the father to see the mother or baby until the baby is cleaned (Belize and Panama), and many other beliefs (Purnell & Paulanka, 2003, p. 31).

Culture-Based Treatments

Culture-based treatments are often misinterpreted in Western health care settings, as they often produce marks on the skin that are interpreted as evidence of abuse. Assuming abuse can create a very bad nurse–client interaction and can cause the culturally different client to reject Western style health care in the future.

Some of the more common Asian treatments are cupping, coining, and moxibustion. *Cupping*, often used to treat back pain, involves placing heated glass jars on the skin. Cooling causes suction that leaves redness and bruising. *Coining* involves rubbing ointment into the skin with a spoon or coin. It leaves bruises or red marks but does not cause pain. It is used for "wind illness" (a fear of being cold or of wind, which causes loss of *yang*), fever, and stress-related illnesses such as headache. *Moxibustion* is the attachment of smoldering herbs to the end of acupuncture needles or placing the herbs on the skin; this causes scars that look like cigarette burns. It is used to strengthen one's blood and the flow of energy, and generally to maintain good health.

Other treatments are related to different beliefs about what causes disease. In many cultures an imbalance in *hot/cold* is believed to cause disease, so treatment would be to take foods, drinks, or medication of the opposite type (hot for a cold condition and cold for a hot condition). What is thought to be hot or cold has no relation to temperature. Cancer, headache, and pneumonia are described as cold, while diabetes mellitus, hypertension, and sore throat or infection are hot. One example of a Western versus Latino treatment belief difference is pregnancy. Pregnancy is a hot condition; iron-containing foods are also hot. So a pregnant female does not eat iron-containing foods. In Asian societies, hot/cold is also associated with the body's energy of *yin/yang*, which must remain in balance for health. These are balanced through diet, lifestyle, acupuncture, and herbs.

Some standard Western treatments are unacceptable in other cultures. Counseling or psychiatric treatments are resisted by Asians and many others because psychological or psychiatric illness is considered shameful.

Culture-Bound Syndromes

Culture-bound syndromes are conditions that are specific to various cultures and occur as a combination of psychiatric or psychological and physical symptoms. There is much debate about whether these syndromes are folk illnesses with behavior changes, local variations of Western psychiatric disorders, or whether they are not syndromes at all but locally accepted ways of explaining negative events in life.

Because clients perceive the syndromes to be conditions with specific symptoms, it is necessary to be familiar with them. It is important to acknowledge the client's belief that the symptoms form a disorder even if Western medicine calls it something else or does not see it as a specific disease. See Display 10-1 for a list and description of some of the more common culture-bound syndromes.

Many of the culture-bound syndromes are based on different beliefs in what causes disease. Some of the culturally based beliefs about disease causation include yin/yang out of balance, hot/cold imbalanced, and spirit possession. Such beliefs in these as causes of disease may form the bases of culturally-based syndromes. The symptoms related to the conditions are often specific to a particular culture.

Health Care Practices

Purnell and Paulanka (2003) divide the assessment of health care practices into six categories: Health-Seeking Beliefs and Behaviors, Responsibility for Health Care, Folklore Practices, Barriers to Health Care, Cultural Responses to Health and

(text continues on page 130)

DISPLAY 10-1	Culture-Bound Syndromes

Common culture-bound syndromes by geographical area are listed below along with brief descriptions of each.

Latin (American or Mediterranean)

Ataque de nervios	Results from stressful event and build up of anger over time. Shouting, crying, trembling, verbal or physical aggression, sense of heat in chest rising to head.
Empacho	Especially in young children, soft foods believed to adhere to stomach wall. Abdominal fullness, stomach ache, diarrhea with pain, vomiting. Confirmed by rolling egg over stomach and egg appears to stick to an area.
Mal de ojo (evil eye)	Children, infants at greatest risk; women more at risk than men. Cause often thought to be stranger's touch or attention. Sudden onset of fitful sleep, crying without apparent cause, diarrhea, vomiting, and fever.
Mal puesto or *brujeria*	See rootwork, Africa and African Origin in Americas.
Susto	Spanish word for "fright," caused by natural (cultural stressors) or supernatural (sorcery or witnessing supernatural phenomenon) means. Nervousness, anorexia, insomnia, listlessness, fatigue, muscle tics, diarrhea.

Africa and Africa Origin in Americas

Falling out or blacking out	Sudden collapse preceded by dizziness, spinning sensation. Eyes may remain open but unable to see. May hear and understand what is happening around them but unable to interact.
Rootwork	Belief that illnesses are supernatural in origin (witchcraft, voodoo, evil spirits, or evil person). Anxiety, gastrointestinal complaints, fear of being poisoned or killed.
Spell	Communicates with dead relatives or spirits, often with distinct personality changes (not considered pathological in culture of origin).
High blood	A slang term for high blood pressure, but also for thick or excessive blood that rises in the body. Often believed to be caused by overly rich foods.
Low blood	Not enough or weak blood caused by diet.
Bad blood	Blood contaminated, often refers to sexually transmitted diseases.
Boufee deliriante (Haiti)	A panic disorder with sudden agitated outbursts, aggressive behavior, confusion, excitement. May have hallucinations or paranoia.

Native American

Ghost sickness (Navajo)	Feelings of danger, confusion, futility, suffocation, bad dreams, fainting, dizziness, hallucinations, loss of consciousness. Possible preoccupation with death or someone who died.
Hi-Wa itck (Mohave)	Unwanted separation from a loved one. Insomnia, depression, loss of appetite, and sometimes suicide.
Pibloktoq or Arctic hysteria (Greenland Eskimos)	An abrupt onset, extreme excitement of up to 30 minutes often followed by convulsive seizures and coma lasting up to 12 hours, with amnesia of the event. Withdrawn or mildly irritable for hours or days before attack. During the attack, may tear off clothing, break furniture, shout obscenities, eat feces, run out into snow, do other irrational or dangerous acts.
Wacinko (Oglala Sioux)	Often reaction to disappointment or interpersonal problems. Anger, withdrawal, mutism, immobility, often leads to attempted suicide.

Middle East

Zar	Experience of spirit possession. Laugh, shout, weep, sing, hit head against wall. May be apathetic, withdrawn, refuse food, unable to carry out daily tasks. May develop long-term relationship with possessing spirit (not considered pathological in the culture).

Asian (South or East)

Amok (Malaysia)	Occurs among male (20–45 years old) after perceived slight or insult. Aggressive outbursts, violent or homicidal, aimed at people or objects, often with ideas of persecution. Amnesia, exhaustion, final return to previous state.
Koro (Malaysia, Southeast Asia)	Similar to conditions in China, Thailand, and other areas. Fear that genitalia will retract into the body, possibly leading to death. Causes vary, including inappropriate sex, mass cases from belief that eating swine flu–vaccinated pork is a cause.
Latah (Malaysia)	Occurs after traumatic episode or surprise. Exaggerated startle response (usually in women). Screaming, cursing, dancing, hysterical laughter, may imitate people, hypersuggestibility.

continued on page 130

DISPLAY 10-1   **Culture-Bound Syndromes** *Continued*

Shen kui (China)   Similar conditions that result from the belief that semen (or "vital essence") is being lost. Anxiety,
Dhat (India)   panic, sexual complaints, fatigue, weakness, loss of appetite, guilt, sexual dysfunction with no phys-
                        ical findings.

Taijin kyofusho (Japan)   Dread of offending or hurting others by behavior or physical condition such as body odor. Social phobia.
Wind illness (Asia)   Fear of wind, cold exposure causing loss of *yang* energy.

North America, Western Europe
Anorexia nervosa   Associated with intense fear of obesity. Severely restricted food and calorie intake.
Bulimia nervosa   Associated with intense fear of obesity. Binge eating and self-induced vomiting, laxative or diuretic use.

Modified from the following sources:

Baylor College of Medicine. (2005). Multicultural patient care: Special populations: African Americans. Available at
http://www.bcm.edu/mpc/special-af.html.

Bigby, J. (Ed.). (2003). *Cross-cultural medicine*. Philadelphia: American Academy of Physicians.

Culture-bound syndromes. Available at http://rjg42.tripod.com/culturebound_syndromes.htm.

Glossary of culture bound syndromes. (2001). Available at http://homepage.mac.com/mccajor/cbs_glos/html.

Juckett, G. (2005). Cross-cultural medicine. *American Family Physician, 72*(11). Available at http://www.aafp.org/afp/20051201/2267.html.

O'Neill, D. (2002–2006). Culture specific diseases. Available at http://anthro.palomar.edu/medical/med_4.htm.

DISPLAY 10-2   **Healthcare Practices**

Health-Seeking Beliefs and Behaviors
1. Identify predominant beliefs that influence healthcare practices.
2. Describe health promotion and prevention practices.

Responsibility for Healthcare
3. Describe the focus of acute-care practice (curative or fatalistic).
4. Explore who assumes responsibility for health care in this culture.
5. Describe the role of health insurance in this culture.
6. Explore practices associated with the use of over-the-counter medications.

Folklore Practices
7. Explore combinations of magicoreligious beliefs, folk, and traditional beliefs that influence healthcare behaviors.

Barriers to Healthcare
8. Identify barriers to health care such as language, economics, accessibility, and geography for this group.

Cultural Responses to Health and Illness
9. Explore cultural beliefs and responses to pain that influence interventions. Does pain have a special meaning?
10. Describe beliefs and views about mental illness in this culture.
11. Differentiate between the perceptions of mentally and physically handicapped in this culture.
12. Describe cultural beliefs and practices related to chronicity and rehabilitation.
13. Identify cultural perceptions of the sick role in this group.

Blood Transfusion and Organ Donation
14. Describe the acceptance of blood and blood products, organ donation, and organ transplantation among this group.

(Purnell, L., & Paulanka, B. [2003]. *Transcultural health care: A culturally competent approach*. Philadelphia: F.A. Davis.)

Illness, and Blood Transfusion and Organ Donation (see Display 10-2). The 14 items are easily understood as stated. Two, pain and blood, need a clearer explanation.

Pain

Pain is now the 5th vital sign in U.S. health care. Assessing pain is necessary for each client; however, the experience of pain may vary by cultural conditioning. Some believe that pain is punishment for wrongdoing; others believe it is atonement for wrongdoing. The response to pain is based on cultural values.

Some cultures, such as Asians, value controlling the response to pain, while others, such as Latins and Southern Europeans, value openly expressing pain. When the caregiver and the client come from different cultures, interpreting the actual level of pain being felt is difficult. It is necessary to explain the therapeutic reasons for treating pain so that a person from a stoic culture may become less reluctant to express or describe pain.

Blood

Use of blood products and blood transfusions is accepted by most religions except for Jehovah's Witnesses. Organ donation and autopsy are not accepted by certain cultural groups, including Christian Scientists, Orthodox Jews, Greeks, and some Spanish-speaking groups (because of the belief that the person will suffer in the after life if organs are removed or autopsy is done); African Americans are often suspicious of organ donation believing that the person will receive inadequate care so that organs can be harvested (Purnell & Paulanka, 2003).

Biological Variations

Genetics and environment, and their interaction, cause humans to vary biologically. Gene variations cause obvious differences like eye color and genetic diseases, such as trisomy 21. Genes are identified increasingly as playing a role in most diseases, even if only to increase or decrease a person's susceptibility to infectious or chronic diseases. Environment has also been proved to cause disease, but modern Western thought on disease causation leans toward a mingling of genetics and environment. If, for example, a person has lungs that are genetically "hardy," then exposure to smoking may not cause lung cancer or chronic lung disease.

Physical variations (resulting from genetics or cultural behaviors) are included directly in the normal and abnormal findings in the physical assessment chapters throughout the book. Integrating the information helps the nurse to attend to the possible variations during all assessments rather than having to seek the information elsewhere if the client appears to be from a different culture.

One limitation of this approach has to be acknowledged. Because characteristics vary along a continuum with many possible points of reference, it would be cumbersome to include every possible variation as the point from which a characteristic varies. Acknowledging that this is an imperfect approach, the authors have used the U.S. population majority group as the point from which variation is assessed. As U.S. population demographics change, the baseline point will have to change in future texts.

In his model of cultural competence, Purnell (Purnell & Paulanka, 2003) includes a category called biocultural ecology. This category refers to the client's physical, biological, and physiological variations such as variations in drug metabolism, disease, and health conditions. The term biocultural ecology presents an interesting perspective. However, this text uses the term biological variation to include human variation of a biological and physiological nature. Overfield (1995) divides the discussion of biological variation into sections as follows:

I.   Surface variations and anatomical differences
   A. Surface variation
     1. Color
     2. Secretions
     3. Surface anatomy
   B. Anatomical variation
     1. Body proportions
     2. Bones
     3. Pelvic measurements and newborn size
     4. Pulmonary function
     5. Teeth
     6. Soft tissue

II. Developmental variation in childhood
   A. Body size and proportion differences
   B. Developmental maturity differences
   C. Environmental effects
   D. Surface features
   E. Common clinical measurements
   F. Disease differential
   G. Other variations

III. Developmental variation in adulthood
   A. Body size, shape, and composition
   B. Surface manifestations
   C. Developmental changes
   D. Disease susceptibility

IV. Biochemical variation and differential disease susceptibility includes drug metabolism

V.   Environmentally related variation
   A. Climate
   B. Altitude
   C. Diet

VI. Sexual variation

Additionally, there are culturally based syndromes of diseases that are perceived to exist in some cultures but not perceived to exist in other cultures nor by the healthcare providers of other cultures.

Obviously, an assessment text cannot discuss all of the topics in biological variation. Only a sampling is included in this text. The variations selected for inclusion are among the most often seen or most likely to be interpreted incorrectly as normal or abnormal.

Surface Variation

Secretions as an example of a surface variation refer to the variation in apocrine and eccrine sweat secretions and the apocrine secretion of earwax. Sebaceous gland activity and secretion composition do not show significant variation.

Eccrine glands, distributed over the entire body, show no variation in number or distribution but do vary in activity based on environmental and individual adaptations (not by race). Persons born in the tropics have more functioning glands than those born in other areas and than those who move to the tropics later in life. Studies of Japanese and Solomon Islanders have noted this pattern (Overfield, 1995, p. 16). Eskimos have been noted to sweat less on their trunks and extremities but more on their faces than do Caucasians; this is believed to be an adaptation to allow thermoregulation without dampening clothes (Overfield, 1995, p. 16).

The amount of chloride excreted by sweat glands differs by ethnic or racial group and by environment. The sweat of people of black African origin has a low salt concentration, but the sweat of Caucasians acclimatized to the tropics also has a lower salt–chloride concentration than does the sweat of nonacclimatized Caucasians (Overfield, 1995, p. 16).

Apocrine glands, opening into the hair follicles in the axilla, groin, and pubic regions, around the anus, umbilicus, and breast areola, and in the external auditory canal, vary much in the number of functioning glands. Asians and Native Americans have fewer functioning apocrine glands than do most Caucasians and blacks (Overfield, 1995, p. 16). The amount of sweating and body odor is directly related to the function of apocrine glands, although the odor is probably related to the decomposition of lipids in the secretions. Prepubescent children, Asians, and Native Americans have no or limited underarm sweat and body odor.

Earwax, produced by the apocrine glands in the external ear, varies between dry and wet wax based on a genetic trait.

About 85% of Asians and Native Americans have dry earwax; about 97% of Caucasians and 99% of blacks have wet earwax (Overfield, 1995, p. 17). Reasons for the genetic variation are thought to include climate and disease susceptibility. For instance, women with dry earwax have a lower incidence of breast cancer.

Anatomical Variation

Lower extremity venous valves vary between Caucasians and black Africans. Black Africans have been noted to have fewer valves in the external iliac veins but many more valves lower in the leg than do Caucasians. The additional valves may account for the lower prevalence of varicose veins in blacks (Overfield, 1995, p. 28).

Developmental Variation

Maturity differences appear to be related to both genetics and environment. African American infants and children tend to be ahead of other American groups in motor development. However, studies of the effect of socioeconomic status indicate that lower-status children show earlier motor development than do higher-status children, irrespective of racial group (Overfield, 1995, p. 45). Overfield cautions those using the Denver Developmental Screening Test (DDST) because its development was based primarily on Caucasian American children. She suggests that any African American child who lags below the 50th percentile on motor development items should have further diagnostic procedures.

Biochemical Variation and Differential Disease Susceptibility

Drug metabolism differences, lactose intolerance, and malaria-related conditions, such as sickle cell disease, thalassemia, glucose-6-phosphate dehydrogenase (G6PD) deficiency, and Duffy blood group, are considered biochemical variations. Overfield (1995), Campinha-Bacote (1998), and Purnell and Paulanka (2003) provide extensive reviews of ethnic–racial group differences in drug metabolism. As far as lactose intolerance is concerned, most of the world's population is lactose intolerant. The ability to digest lactose after childhood relates to a mutation that occurs mainly in those of North and Central European ancestry and in some Middle Eastern populations (Overfield, 1995, p. 104). The malaria-related conditions would obviously occur in populations living in or originating from mosquito-infested locales such as the Mediterranean and Africa. These brief examples show that health status and health assessment are greatly influenced by biological variations. Many of the chapters in this text include physical characteristics to be assessed that have normal variations or that vary in the way abnormalities are expressed. These variations are inserted into the physical assessment discussions. Also, many of the chapters include risk factor discussions addressing common illnesses associated with the content of the chapter.

Drug Metabolism

There have been many studies on ethnic, racial, or biological variations in drug metabolism. As Purnell and Paulanka (2003) noted, Chinese are more sensitive to cardiovascular effects of some drugs and have increased absorption of antipsychotics, some narcotics, and antihypertensives. Eskimos, Native Americans, and Hispanics have increased risks for peripheral neuropathy with isoniazid. African Americans have a better response to diuretics than do whites.

Many conditions can alter drug metabolism as well; for instance, smoking accelerates it, malnutrition affects it, stress affects it, and diets such as low fat decrease absorption of some drugs. Cultural beliefs about taking medication affect their use.

Geographical and Ethnic Disease Variation

In general, chronic diseases predominate in developed countries and infectious diseases predominate in third world countries. However, there is some genetic and ethnic variation in addition to the chronic versus infection pattern. Often the studies in developing countries and on immigrants from these countries to the United States are limited. Patterns are known, however, and are often based on body size, lifestyle, and genetics. For instance, vascular diseases tend to be higher in African Americans and populations with larger body size and lifestyle habits such as smoking. Osteoporosis is more prevalent in small-framed people such as Asians. Knowing that some groups will be more prone to a disease or condition can help the nurse to more carefully assess each client. Following are examples of geographical or ethnic disease variations for the physical systems.

Skin, Hair, Nails

Skin cancer is highly feared among skin diseases. Fair-skinned people, especially those with light eyes and freckles, are at highest risk for developing skin cancers, although all people who are exposed to high levels of intense sunlight are at risk. Because ozone depletion is a factor in skin cancer risk, people living in Australia and southern Africa are at greater risk. Worldwide, 2 to 3 million nonmelanoma and 132,000 melanoma skin cancers occur each year (WHO, 2007).

Although darker skin is not as susceptible to skin cancers, some other skin conditions occur more frequently in darker-pigmented people (Skin of color, 2006). Darker-skinned people come from many ethnic and geographical groups including African Americans, Native Americans, Asians, and Latino or Hispanics. The conditions that are more common in darker skin are postinflammatory hyperpigmentation, vitiligo, pityriasis alba, dry or "ashy" skin, dermatosis papulosa nigra (flesh moles), keloids, keloid-like acne from shaving neck, and hair loss (if tightly curled and fragile hair and use of relaxers or tight rollers).

Head and Neck

The few cultural considerations that come into play are related to dependence on poorly maintained automobiles or bicycles, lack of use of protective gear, inadequate and unsafe housing, and unsafe celebratory practices (such as shooting guns to welcome the new year). In the United States, traumatic brain injury is especially prevalent among adolescents, young adults, and persons over 75 years of age, with males more than twice as much at risk than females. The CDC (2007) reported that TBI varies by cause and by age: for age 0 to 4 and 75 or above, falls; for other ages, especially 15 to 19, motor vehicle, bicycle, and other transportation accidents; struck by or against objects; and assaults, especially with firearms (including suicide attempts), particularly high in young males.

Eye

Visual impairment varies across age (greater after 50), gender (more in females), and geography (higher in Southeast Asia, Western Pacific, and Africa) (WHO, 2004). In all but highly developed countries, cataract is the leading cause of visual disease and blindness, followed by glaucoma and age-related macular degeneration (which is the leading cause in developed countries). Other diseases include trachoma, other corneal diseases, diabetic retinopathy, and diseases of children, such as cataract, prematurity retinopathy, and vitamin A deficiency (WHO, 2004).

Ear and Hearing Loss

The WHO (2005) recorded that of the 278 million people across the world with hearing loss in both ears, 80% live in low- to middle-income countries. The number is rising as the populations age. The main cause of hearing loss in children is chronic middle ear infection. At least 50% of hearing impairment is avoidable if diagnosed early and well managed, according to WHO. There have been reports that populations with shorter, wider, and more horizontal eustachian tubes (Native Americans, Eskimos, New Zealand Maoris, one Nigerian population, and some aborigines) have higher rates of otitis media (Casselbrant, Mandel, Kurs-Lasky, Rockette, & Bluestone, 1995). Overfield (1995) reported that African Americans have lower rates of both otitis media and noise-induced or other forms of hearing loss.

According to WHO, causes of hearing loss at or before birth are genetic (through one or both parents) and include birth complications such as prematurity, reduced oxygen for the baby, or mother's infections (e.g., rubella, syphilis); use of drugs affecting the baby's hearing (more than 130 drugs including gentamicin); and severe jaundice which can damage the baby's hearing nerve. After birth, infectious diseases, ototoxic drugs, head or ear injury, wax or foreign body blockage, excessive noise, and age can lead to hearing loss.

Mouth, Nose, Sinus

Oral diseases are prevalent in poorer populations in developed and developing countries. They include dental caries, periodontal disease, tooth loss, oral mucosal and oropharyngeal lesions and cancers, HIV-related diseases, and trauma. Poor living conditions including diet, nutrition, hygiene, and the use of alcohol, tobacco and tobacco-related products, and limited oral health care contribute to developing oral disease.

The incidence of oral cancer is different for different countries. This is attributed to environment rather than genetics. The use of smoking and smokeless tobacco and excessive alcohol are the main risk factors for oral cancer. Rates are higher in men than in women (ACS, 2007b). Very high rates (five to six times higher than in the United States) are reported for South Asia where tobacco mixed with betel nut, lime, spices, perfumes, and other substances is used for smoking and chewing (Mukherjea, 2004–2006). This practice is also used in South Asian rituals.

Sinusitis is widespread. However, the prevalence is higher in whites and African Americans than in Hispanics (Brigham & Women's Hospital, 2007).

Thorax and Lungs

Lung cancer is directly related to smoking and to the quantity of cigarettes smoked. However, according to an article on Medscape (Ethnic differences, 2006), African Americans and Native Hawaiians who smoke are more susceptible to lung cancer than are whites, Japanese Americans, or Latinos.

The *African Americans and Lung Disease Fact Sheet* (2007) provides an overview of various nonmalignant lung diseases. African Americans have the highest prevalence rate of asthma and are more likely to die from the disease than members of other U.S. racial or ethnic groups. Although African Americans smoke at rates similar to those of whites, they are less likely to have or die from chronic obstructive pulmonary disease (COPD). African Americans are less likely to take vaccines for flu and pneumonia and are more likely to work in occupations with risks for lung diseases. Sarcoidosis occurs more often in African Americans, Swedes, and Danes, and due to its reduction in reactivity of tuberculin makes it more difficult to detect tuberculosis. The higher rate of AIDS in African Americans predisposes them to immune suppression and related lung diseases. Infants and children of African Americans and non-Hispanic blacks have higher rates of sleep apnea and sudden infant death syndrome (SIDS) death. Somalis and other foreign born immigrants to the United States account for an increase in the incidence of tuberculosis (CDC, 2006).

Breasts and Lymphatic System

Both in situ and invasive breast cancer rates are similar across U.S. ethnic groups (National Cancer Institute, 2007a). White, Hawaiian, and black women have the highest rates; Korean, American Indian, and Vietnamese women have the lowest rates. Men can also have breast cancer, but the incidence is so low that widespread studies for ethnic differences have not been done.

Cultural beliefs about the causes of breast cancer, the meaning of breast cancer to the client and partner, the availability of or knowledge of services, fear due to illegal status of some immigrants, and other barriers affect the lower use of screening methods for breast cancer (Kaiser Health, 2007).

Heart and Neck Vessels

Heart disease and all cardiovascular diseases are higher in the southern states of the United States, known as the "Stroke Belt" (Howard, 2007). African American ethnicity and socioeconomic status are factors, along with obesity, diabetes mellitus, smoking, and high alcohol consumption rates. Other ethnic groups shown to have high rates of risk factors and cardiovascular disease are South Asians (Indians, Pakistanis, Bangladeshis, Sri Lankans) (BBC, 2000).

Peripheral Vascular System

A higher risk of peripheral artery disease has been found for black Americans even when controlling for risk factors of diabetes, hypertension, and obesity (body mass index) (Criqui et al., 2005). Varicose veins, on the other hand, are found in equal numbers and vary only by lifestyle (Epidemiology, n.d.).

Abdomen

Gallbladder disease and cancer vary by ethnic group in the United States. Native Americans and Mexican Americans have higher rates of disease and cancer (ACS, 2007a). Stomach cancer has an association with the prevalence of *Helicobacter pylori* (which also causes ulcers) and is highest in Korea and Japan, intermediate in Italy, and lowest in the United States (The Helicobacter Foundation, 2007).

Ashkenazi Jews have been found to have the highest lifetime risk for developing colorectal cancer (Hereditary cancer, 2005).

Cancer in general has a different pattern for Asian Americans than for those remaining in Asia. The rate of cancer is low for Asian Americans but the death rate from cancer is higher. There is a variable pattern of specific cancers across Asian groups (ACS, 2007b).

Female and Male Genitalia, Anus, Rectum, Prostate

Sexually transmitted diseases (chlamydia, herpes, human papilloma virus [HPV], syphilis, gonorrhea, and HIV/AIDS) vary across U.S. populations. Ethnic variation is thought to be due to rates of poverty, use of drugs, hygiene, and greater reporting in poorer community clinics (CDC, 2001). HIV/AIDS infection in parts of Southern Africa is higher than that in any other area of the world.

National Cancer Institute data for 1975 to 2000 show that the highest incidence of cervical cancer in the United States is among Hispanics and African Americans, and the lowest is among Native Americans and Alaskans. Related deaths occur more frequently among African Americans, Hispanics, and Native Americans.

In U.S. populations, incidence of prostate cancer is highest among African Americans and lowest among Native Americans and Alaska Natives, while deaths from prostate cancer are highest in African Americans and lowest in Asian/Pacific Islanders (National Cancer Institute, 2007b). Both prostate and cervical cancer rates reflect lower Asian incidence.

Musculoskeletal System

Bone mass density (BMD) peaks around 40 years of age in females and males, and then begins to decrease in both sexes and in all ethnic or racial groups (Overfield, 1995). BMD is higher in men and blacks and lowest in Asians except for Polynesians. Weight is associated with BMD (Barret-Connor et al., 2005). Osteoporosis and bone fractures are related to BMD and the Middle East, Latin America, and Asia are expecting dramatic increases in the next 20 years (IOF, 2001).

Ethnic variation in arthritis in the United States indicates that African Americans and whites have similar rates, while Hispanics have lower rates diagnosed by physicians, but higher work-related limitations and severe joint pain on diagnosis (Racial/ethnic differences, 2005). Regarding rheumatoid arthritis, African Americans have a lower genetic predisposition (10% carry the genetic marker) compared to Caucasians (25%) (The Scripps Research Institute, n.d.).

Nervous System

Cerebrovascular disease (CVA) has neurological effects but the cause is vascular. The same patterns of ethnic variation that occur in cardiovascular disease (see Chapters 20 and 21) occur with stroke. In the United States, the "stroke belt" (North Carolina, South Carolina, Georgia, Alabama, Mississippi, Louisiana, Arkansas, Tennessee) has greater occurrence of stroke and vascular disease, which may be due to high percentages of older adult and African American dietary factors. Children born and living in these states during childhood show greater risk for stroke in adulthood (Glymour, Avendano, & Berkman, 2007).

Occurrence of dementia, including Alzheimer's disease, is rising rapidly, especially in developing countries where the number of elderly is increasing (China, India, other South Asian and Pacific Island countries) (Alzheimer's Disease International, 2007). Over 50% of dementia cases in Caucasians are Alzheimer's, but the rate in developing countries and other ethnic groups has not been well studied.

SUMMARY OF DISEASE VARIATION

In general, chronic diseases predominate in the developed countries and infectious diseases predominate in third world countries. However, there is some genetic and ethnic variation in addition to the chronic versus infection pattern. Often the studies in developing countries are limited and the studies on immigrants from these countries to the US are also limited. Patterns are known, however, and are often based on body size, lifestyle and genetics. For instance, vascular diseases tend to be higher in African Americans and populations with larger body size and lifestyle habits such as smoking. Osteoporosis is more prevalent in small framed people such as Asians. Knowing that some groups will be more prone to a disease or condition can help the nurse to more carefully assess each client.

SUMMARY

To complete a culturally competent assessment, it is essential to interact with the client showing respect for the person, the family, and their beliefs. Challenge yourself to learn about many of the cultural groups in your geographical area and interact with them enough to gain some understanding and appreciation for their worldviews. Use your knowledge when meeting and assessing your clients, but be alert for behaviors, descriptions, or physical variations that need to be clarified as normal for their culture or abnormal and needing further assessment.

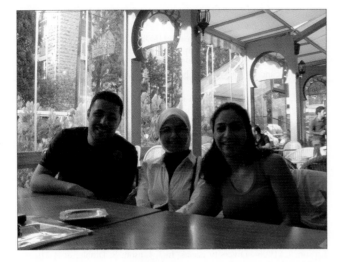

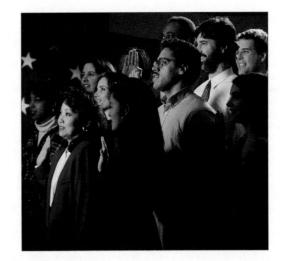

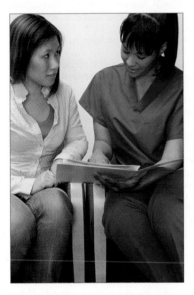

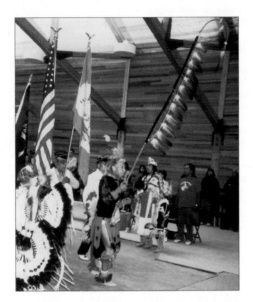

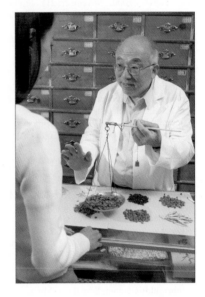

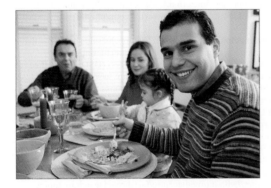

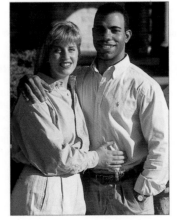

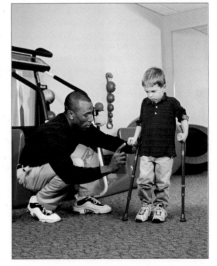

References and Selected Readings

African Americans and Lung Disease Fact Sheet. (2007). Available at http://www.lungusa.org.

Alzheimer's Disease International. (2007). Statistics. Available at http://www.alz.co.uk/research/statistics.html.

American Cancer Society (ACS). (2007a). What are the risk factors for gallbladder cancer? Available at http://www.cancer.org/docroot/CRI/content/CRI_2_4_2X_What_are_the_risk_factors_for_gall_bladder_cancer_68.asp.

American Cancer Society (ACS). (2007b). Cancer hits US Asian groups differently. Available at http://www.cancer.org/docroot/NWS/content/NWS_1_1x_Cancer_Hits_US_Asian_Groups_Differently.asp.

American Translators Association. Available at http://www.atanet.org

Andrews, M., & Boyle, J. (2002). Transcultural concepts in nursing care (2nd ed.). Philadelphia: Lippincott Williams & Wilkins.

Barret-Connor, E., Siris, E., Wehren, L., Miller, P., Abbott, T., et al. (2005). Osteoporosis and fracture risk in women of different ethnic groups. Journal of Bone and Mineral Research, 20(2), 185–194. Available at http://www.cababstractsplus.org/google/abstract.asp?AcNo=20053042047.

Baylor College of Medicine. (2005). Multicultural patient care: Special populations: African Americans. Available at http://www.bcm.edu/mpc/special-af.html.

BBC News. (2000, November 21). Ethnic heart disease gulf widens. Available at http://news.bbc.co.uk/2/hi/health/1032168.stm. [available on google.com by title]

Bigby, J. (Ed.). (2003). Cross-cultural medicine. Philadelphia: American College of Physicians.

Brigham and Women's Hospital. (2007). Risk factors for sinusitis. Available at http://healthgate.partners.org.

Campinha-Bacote, J. (1998). The process of cultural competence in the delivery of healthcare services (3rd ed.). Cincinnati, OH: Transcultural C.A.R.E. Associates.

Campinha-Bacote, J. (2003). The process of cultural competence in the delivery of healthcare services (4th ed.). Cincinnati, OH: Transcultural C.A.R.E. Associates.

Campinha-Bacote, J. (2007). The process of cultural competence in the delivery of healthcare services (5th ed.). Cincinnati, OH: Transcultural C.A.R.E. Associates.

Casselbrant, M., Mandel, E., Kurs-Lasky, M., Rockette, H., & Bluestone, C. (1995). Otitis media in a population of black American and while American infants, 0–2 years of age. International Journal of Pediatric Otorhinolaryngology, 33, 1–16.

Centers for Disease Control and Prevention (CDC). (2001). Tracking the hidden epidemics: Trends in STDs in the United States 2000. Available at http://www.cdc.gov/std/Trends2000/faq.htm#morecommon.

Centers for Disease Control and Prevention (CDC). (2006). Extrapulmonary tuberculosis among Somalis in Minnesota. Available at http://www.cdc.gov/ncidod/eid/vol12no09/05-0295.htm.

Centers for Disease Control and Prevention (CDC). (2007). Available at http://cdc.gov.

Criqui, M., Vargas, V., Denenberg, J., Ho, E., Allison, M., et al. (2005). Ethnicity and peripheral artery disease. Circulation, 112, 2703–2707. Available at http://circ.ahajournals.org/cgi/content/abstract/112/17/2703.

Culture-bound syndromes. Available at http://rjg42.tripod.com/culturebound_syndromes.htm.

Davis, L. (1990). Where do we stand? Health, 4–5.

Epidemiology. (n.d.). Available at http://www.medivein.com/siteuk/varicose/comprendre.html.

Ethnic and racial differences may affect lung cancer rates. (2006). Available at http://medscape.com.

Galanti, G. (2004). Caring for patients from different cultures. Philadelphia: University of Pennsylvania Press.

Giger, J., & Davidhizar, R. (2008). Transcultural nursing: Assessment and intervention (5th ed.). St. Louis: Mosby.

Glossary of culture bound syndromes. (2001). Available at http://homepage.mac.com/mccajor

Glymour, M., Avendano, M., & Berkman, L. (2007). Is the stroke belt worn from childhood? Stroke, 38(9), 2415–2421. Available at http://pt.wkhealth.com/pt/re/stroke/abstract.00007670-200709000-00007.htm;jsessionid=HDyXhs7zjhycds3p5H9ZqNJYh8LZJqLx00xGS8MXx2RS6sX2LfvM!1105064230!181195628!8091!-1.

Hereditary cancer. (2005). Available at http://www.medicalnewstoday.com/articles/21151.php.

Howard, V. (2007). From sea to shining sea: What is it about where you live and your stroke risk? Stroke, 38, 2210. Available at http://stroke.ahajournals.org/cgi/content/full/38/8/2210.

International Osteoporosis Foundation (IOF). (2001). Osteoporosis. Available at http://www.osteofound.org.

Juckett, G. (2005). Cross-cultural medicine. American Family Physician, 72(11). Available at http://www.aafp.org/afp/20051201/2267.html.

Kaiser health disparities report: A weekly look at race, ethnicity and health. (2007). Available at http://www.kaisernetwork.org/daily_reports/rep_index.cfm?DR_ID=44602.

Language Line Available at http://www.languageline.com

Leininger, M., & McFarland, M. (2002). Transcultural nursing: Concepts, theories, research & practice. New York: McGraw-Hill.

Lipson, J. (1996). Diversity issues. In J. Lipson, S. Dibble, & P. Minarik (Eds.), Culture and nursing care: A pocket guide (pp. 7–10). San Francisco: UCSF Nursing Press.

Louis Calder Memorial Library. (2005). Internet listings for cross cultural medicine. Available at http://calder.med.miami.edu/catalog/subject/cross_cultural_medicine.html.

Mukherjee, A. (2004–2006). Cultural influences on South Asian oral health disparities. Available at http://www.umdnj.edu

National Cancer Institute. (2007a). Breast: US racial/ethnic cancer patterns. Available at http://www.cancer.gov/statistics/cancertype/breast-racial-ethnic.

National Cancer Institute. (2007b). Cancer of the prostate. Available at http://seer.cancer.gov/statfacts/html/prost.html.

O'Neill, D. (2002–2006). Culture specific diseases. Available at http://anthro.palomar.edu/medical/med_4.htm.

Overfield, T. (1995). Biological variation in health and illness: Race, age, and sex differences. Menlo Park, CA: Addison-Wesley.

Petersen, P., Bourgeois, D., Ogawa, H., Estupinan-Day, S., & Ndiaye, C. (2005). The global burden of oral diseases and risk to oral health. Bulletin of the World Health Organization, 83(9), 641–720.

Purnell, L., & Paulanka, B. (2003). Transcultural health care: A culturally competent approach (2nd ed.). Philadelphia: F.A. Davis.

Racial/ethnic differences in the prevalence and impact of doctor-diagnosed arthritis—United States, 2002. (2005). MMWR, 54(5), 119–123. Available at http://www.cdc.gov/mmwR/preview/mmwrhtml/mm5405a3.htm.

Skin of color. (2006). Available at http://aad.org [insert Skin of Color into search box]

Spector, R. (2003). Cultural diversity in health and illness (6th ed.). Upper Saddle River, NJ: Prentice-Hall.

The Helicobacter Foundation. (2007). Stomach cancer. Available at http://www.helico.com/disease_stomach.html.

The Scripps Research Institute. (n.d.). Philanthropy. Research advances. Arthritis. Available at http://www.scripps.edu/philanthropy/arthritis.html.

University of Washington Medical Center. Culture clues tip sheets. Available at http://www.depts.washington.edu/pfes/cultureclues.html

U.S. Department of Health and Human Services (USDHHS) office of Minority Health Resource center. Available at http://www.omhrc.gov/CLAS

Wood, A. J. (2001). Racial differences in the response to drugs: Pointers to genetic differences. New England Journal of Medicine, 344, 1392–1396.

World Health Organization (WHO). (2004). Magnitude and causes of visual impairment. Available at http://who.int/mediacentre/factsheets [search by topic]

WHO. (2005). Deafness and hearing impairment. Available at http://who.int/mediacentre/factsheets [search by topic]

WHO. (2007). Ultraviolet radiation and the INTERSUN programme. Available at http://who.int/mediacentre/factsheets [search by topic]

11

Assessing Spirituality and Religious Practices

Structure and Function

INTRODUCTION TO SPIRITUAL ASSESSMENT

What Is Spirituality?

Spirituality and religion are important factors in health and can influence health decisions and outcomes. Recent polls suggest that more than 95% of Americans believe in God or a universal spirit or power, more than 50% of them pray on a daily basis, and an estimated one-third of them use complementary and alternative medical practices that include religious and/or spiritual practices (Barnes, Powell-Griner, McFann, & Nahin 2004; Gallup, 2006). Religious and spiritual conversation, debate, and lifestyles are frequently proclaimed and criticized through the media, peers, and everyday acquaintances. But what is religion? What is spirituality? People are often confused about religion and spirituality. The concepts are separate and distinct; different people use them in different ways (Display 11-1). Religion is defined as the rituals, practices, and experiences shared within a group that involve a search for the sacred (i.e., God, Allah, etc.). For some faiths, this idea of religion encompasses the concept of spirituality and is a natural outflow of that idea. Others may view spirituality as a separate concept, possibly disconnected from any religious institution. In fact, the number of persons describing themselves as "spiritual but not religious" has risen substantially over the past decade (Gallup, 2006). Spirituality is defined as a search for meaning and purpose in life; it seeks to understand life's ultimate questions in relation to the sacred. Spirituality has undergone tremendous growth in its conceptual understanding during the past 20 years. Thoughts about spirituality and religion may vary immensely from one client to the next. During a **spiritual assessment,** the healthcare professional should keep an objective perspective with the goal of meeting the client where she or he is. Knowing how spirituality can vary will help the nurse to identify possible coping responses; otherwise these resources might have gone unnoticed.

Why Assess Spirituality?

Public opinion and health care research give credence to the importance of the relationship of religion, spirituality, and health.

A large number of patients use spiritual resources during times of high stress (i.e., hospitalizations). Religion and spirituality have been related to a person's greater well-being in the face of chronic disease management and assistance adhering to medical regimens. Religion and spirituality can be powerful coping mechanisms when a person faces end-of-life issues. There is a wealth of information regarding religion, spirituality, and health. Among certain populations, religion and spirituality have been related to lower levels of mortality, less heart disease, lower blood pressure, less depression, lower levels of stress, less alcohol and tobacco abuse, greater well-being and optimism, and positive health habits (Koenig, McCullough, & Larson, 2001; Loustalot, Wyatt, May, et al., 2006). Clients have also called for medical providers to address spiritual issues during client-provider interactions. Nurses generally have more opportunities to address spiritual concerns with clients because nurses are the primary points of contact for most clients.

Nursing has a long history of incorporating spirituality into client care. Florence Nightingale wrote at length about a spiritual dimension that provided an inner strength. More recently modern nursing theorists have used spirituality as a major determinant in the grand theories that guide nursing practice. NANDA-approved nursing diagnoses have also been formulated to assist nurses in identifying and addressing the client's spiritual dimension. These references underlie a primary idea in nursing: clients are seen as **holistic** beings in body, mind, and spirit.

Some religions encourage positive health behaviors, greater mental health, and provide a strong social support network.

> **Clinical Tip •** *Plans for referral or intervention will develop out of the ongoing dialogue between the nurse and the client.*

For example, a client newly diagnosed with diabetes may be encouraged to join his local congregation's exercise program for support and accountability. The church-based program may provide support dimensions that are absent in a similar secular program. Or a nurse may facilitate a referral to an appropriate clergy member or hospital chaplain. In whatever form spirituality is incorporated into client care, the nurse should be respectful, open, and willing to discuss spiritual issues if seen as appropriate.

DISPLAY 11-1 | **Foundational Knowledge for Spiritual Assessment**

Religion

Definition: Rituals, practices, and experiences involving a search for the sacred (i.e., God, Allah, etc.)* that are shared within a group.

Defining Characteristics

- Formal
- Organized
- Group-oriented
- Ritualistic
- Objective, as in easily measurable (e.g., church attendance)

Spirituality

Definition: A search for meaning and purpose in life, which seeks to understand life's ultimate questions in relation to the sacred.

Defining Characteristics

- Informal
- Non-organized
- Self-reflection
- Experience

- Subjective, as in difficult to consistently measure (e.g., daily spiritual experiences, spiritual well-being, etc.)

Spiritual Assessment

Definition: Active and ongoing conversation that assesses the spiritual needs of the client.

Defining Characteristics

- Formal or informal
- Respectful
- Non-biased

Spiritual Care

Definition: Addressing the spiritual needs of the client as they unfold through spiritual assessment.

Defining Characteristics

- Individualistic
- Client oriented
- Collaborative

Note: God or Allah can be interchanged with universal spirit of higher power throughout this chapter as necessary to support the individual needs of the patient.

OVERVIEW OF SPIRITUAL ASSESSMENT AND NURSING CARE

Spiritual assessment does not begin at the bedside. The nurse's knowledge of the spiritual temperament of the community and his or her own spirituality will lead to greater ease when discussing the client's spirituality. To assist in assessing religion and spirituality, it would be useful to define the concepts as interconnected but separate ideas (see Fig. 11-1). With a growing proportion of the population identifying themselves as "spiritual but not religious," the use of the correct instrument or framework will determine the accuracy of the assessment.

Spirituality can be practiced through a wide variety of avenues. A limited list of spiritual activities may include prayer, meditation, yoga, *tai chi*, dietary restrictions, pilgrimage, confessions, reflection, forgiveness, and any other activity that includes a search for meaning and purpose in life. If a patient identifies spiritual activities, they should be encouraged if found beneficial to the overall health. Reconnecting with a previous spiritual activity may assist the patient in asserting a positive view of his or her situation. In addition, a working knowledge of the majority faiths' ideals, beliefs, and practices in the nurse's community would provide a useful foundation for spiritual care. When conducting any type of review of the denominations or faiths in a particular community, be aware that a client's spiritual dimension is subjective and may vary greatly between persons, even persons of the same denomination or faith. However, a general knowledge of the faiths may give context to some issues that certain religious groups face and provide time to develop appropriate interventions to meet those needs. A discussion with a hospital chaplain or clergy regarding the views of religious faiths in the nurse's community would also provide a greater understanding about the particular faith's views of health and give the nurse a resource for future referral or collaboration.

Collaboration and referral with pastoral chaplains or clergy are extremely important when dealing with religious issues in a health care setting. Many hospitals have staff pastoral chaplains, and community resources of different faiths are usually available through social work professionals. While nurses can assess and support many clients' spiritual needs, some situations are beyond the scope of nursing practice and require someone with more experience and knowledge about a particular faith. For example, a nurse from a Protestant faith faced with a Muslim client who has just been diagnosed with terminal cancer may not be able to speak to the client's end of life issues and may require referral to the appropriate professional.

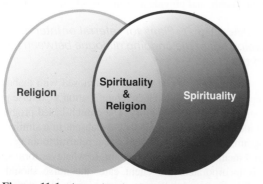

Figure 11-1 ▌ Interrelated yet separate concepts of religion and spirituality.

The Role of Religion and Spirituality in Health and Health Care Choices

A substantial amount of evidence shows the positive effects of spirituality on health. The global domains of practice, beliefs, and experiences cover religious or spiritual traditions and can be used to highlight the positive effects. Spiritual practices, which may include meditation or yoga, have the potential to encourage greater mental and physical health. Religious groups frequently view the body as a gift and encourage a lifestyle to mirror that belief. Avoidance of promiscuous sexual activity, shunning alcohol and tobacco use, and dietary guidelines each promote a healthy lifestyle. If discovered in discussion with the client, these positive health behaviors can be encouraged and supported. Religious beliefs can express a wide variety of values and practices and can have rituals (i.e., birth, death, illness) and end-of-life issues that may significantly affect the religion-health relationship. Table 11-1 provides a general review of the major religions and how their beliefs affect their healthcare decisions. Remember, as with culture, never make assumptions that all members of one group adopt all aspects. The client's spiritual experiences or spiritual history are subjective and may be the most relevant factor that guides conversation and decisions about referral or collaboration. Providing a time of silence for the client may encourage spiritual practices such as meditation, or the nurse may gather family member or clergy to participate in a prayer ritual.

Table 11-1 — Major World Religions and Common Health Beliefs

	Overview	Illness	End of Life	Nutrition
Buddhism Global: ±6% US: <1%	Suffering is a part of human existence, but the inward death of the self and senses leads to a state beyond suffering and existence.	Prayer and meditation are used for cleansing and healing. Terminal illness may be seen as a unique opportunity to reflect on life's ultimate meaning and the meaning of one's relation with the world. Therefore, it is important that medication does not interfere with consciousness.	Life is the opportunity to cultivate understanding, compassion, and joy for self and others. Death is associated with rebirth. Serene surroundings are important to the dignity of dying.	Many are strict vegetarians. Some holy days include fasting from dawn to dusk but considerations are allowed for the frail and elderly for whom fasting could create problems.
Hinduism Global: ±15% US: <1%	Nirvana (oneness with God) is the primary purpose of the religion. Many have an altar in their home for worship.	Illness is the result of past and current life actions (Karma). The right hand is seen as holy, and eating and intervention (IV) needs to be with the right hand to promote clean healing.	Death marks a passage because the soul has no beginning or end. At death the soul may be reborn as another person and one's Karma is carried forward. It is important for Karma to leave this life with as little negativity as possible to insure a better life next birth. Holy water and basil leaves may be placed on the body; sacred threads may be tied around wrists or neck. The deceased arms should be straightened.	Many but not all are vegetarians. Many holy days include fasting.
Islam Global: ±22% US: ±1.5%	Mohammed is believed to be the greatest of all prophets. Worship occurs in a mosque. Prayer occurs five times a day: dawn, sunrise, noon, afternoon, sunset, and evening. Prayers are done facing east toward the sacred place in Mecca and often occur on a prayer rug with ritual washing of hands, face and feet prior to prayer. Women are to be "modest" and are not to view men, other than their husbands, naked. The Islamic faith is presently one of the fastest growing religious groups in the United States.	Allah is in control of the beginning and end of life, and expressions of powerlessness are rare. To question or ask questions of healthcare providers is considered a sign of mistrust so clients and family are less likely to ask questions.	All outcomes, whether death or healing, are seen as predetermined by Allah. It is important for dying clients to face east and to die facing east. Prayer is offered but need not be done by an Imam (religious leader).	Consumption of pork or alcohol is prohibited. Other meats must meet ritual requirements and many use Kosher (Jewish ritual) foods because these meet the requirements of Islamic believers as well. During the holy days of Ramadan (29 days in December and/or January), neither food nor drink is taken between sunrise and sunset, though frail, ill and young children are exempt.

continued on page 140

Table 11-1	Major World Religions and Common Health Beliefs *Continued*

	Overview	Illness	End of Life	Nutrition
Christianity Global: ±33% US: ±85%	Beliefs focus around the Old and New Testaments of the Bible and view Jesus Christ as the Savior. Prayers may be directed to one or all of the Holy Trinity (God, Holy Spirit, and Jesus Christ). Beliefs usually culturally developed vary within denominations.	Most view illness as a natural process for the body and even as a testing of faith. Others may see illness as a curse brought on by living outside the laws of God and, therefore, retribution for personal evil.	There is belief in miracles, especially through prayer. Western medicine is usually held in high regard. Memorial services rather than funerals and cremation rather than burial are more common in Christian religions than in other sects.	No special or universal food beliefs are common to Christian religions, although there may be regional or cultural beliefs.
Judaism Global: <5% US: ±2%	Judaism includes religious beliefs and a philosophy for a code of ethics with four major groupings of Jewish beliefs: Reform, Reconstructionist, Conservative, and Orthodox. Prayer shawls are common and are often passed between generations of family. The clergy are known as Rabbi.	Restrictions related to work on holy days are removed to save a life. However, tests, signatures, and assessments for medical needs that can be scheduled to avoid holy days are appreciated.	Psalms and the last prayer of confession (vidui) are held at bedside. At death, arms are not crossed; any clothing or bandages with client's blood should be prepared for burial with the person. It is important that the whole person be buried together.	Orthodox or Kosher involves no mixing of meat with dairy; separate cooking and eating utensils are used for food preparation and consumption. Kosher laws include special slaughter and food handling. "Keeping Kosher" is predominantly an Orthodox practice. When food has passed Kosher laws of preparation, a symbol (K) appears on the label. Many holy days include a fasting period.

Adapted with permission from Napier-Tibere, B. (2002). *Diversity, healing and health care* [On-line]. Retrieved September 1, 2004, from the World Wide Web: http://www.gasi.org/diversity.htm. A website supported through grant funding from On Lok SeniorHealth, Inc., and Stanford University School of Medicine: Stanford Geriatric Education Center.

Barrett, D., Kurlan, G., & Johnson, T. (2001). *World Christian encyclopedia: A comparative survey of churches and religions in the modern world* (2nd ed.). New York: Oxford.

Particular religious views may negatively impact health. Failure to seek timely medical care and withholding "proper" medical care based on religious dogma are usually the most prominent ethical dilemmas faced by healthcare providers. Christian Scientists frequently rely on prayer alone to heal illnesses, rarely seek mainstream medical care, and have higher rates of mortality than the general population. Jehovah's Witnesses refuse blood transfusions due to their belief that the body cannot be sustained by another's blood and accepting a transfusion will bar the recipient from eternal salvation. Controversy has erupted when a child of a Jehovah's Witness is in need of a blood transfusion and the parents wish to withhold a possible lifesaving therapy. The U.S. Supreme Court has generally sided against parents' withholding medical therapies for religious reasons; the hospital's ethics committee should be consulted immediately to assist in this complex decision. Members of the Faith Assembly of Indiana have a negative view of modern health care and have an especially high rate of infant mortality due to limited prenatal care. While these are only specific denominational examples of the negative impact of religion on health, there are also generalized manifestations of religion's negative effects. Religion may lead to depression or anxiety over not meeting group expectations, and certain spiritual practices or participation in complementary and alternative medical practices may delay needed medical care. (Koenig, McCullough, & Larson, 2001; Barrett, Kurlan, & Johnson, 2001).

If a nurse is presented with a situation where religious or spiritual views have the potential to compromise adequate nursing care, the situation should be presented to a supervising staff member immediately. For complex cases, the situation may also be presented to the ethics committee of the institution or organization to assure appropriate measures are followed. Refer to the institutional or organizational handbook for specific instructions regarding individual cases.

Self-Understanding of Spirituality

Consistently nurses who are more aware of their spirituality are more comfortable discussing the potential spiritual needs of the client. Introspective reflection on one's own beliefs and biases about the relationship between spirituality and health can be undertaken through journaling, meditation, or discussions with interested persons. The nurse needs to ask

1. What are my/your views on the interaction between spirituality and health?

2. How would I/you respond to someone in spiritual distress or to someone requesting an intervention relating to spirituality?

3. How can I/you provide spiritual care?

These reflections help to provide a deeper understanding of the nurses' spiritual dimension and build confidence for future discussions on spirituality. While many nurses view spiritual assessment and care as an important part of nursing practice, training levels vary from institution to institution. However, nurses can train themselves to meet this vital need of the client. The nurse who understands the content of a spiritual assessment can use this knowledge also to increase self-understanding.

Approach to Spiritual Assessment

A spiritual assessment is similar to the many other assessments nurses perform on a daily basis. Gaining relevant information about the client's spirituality helps to identify related nursing diagnoses and needed interventions and can improve client care. Examples of spiritual assessment tools and general, appropriate open-ended questions will be provided later in the chapter.

There is no absolute in the timing of a spiritual assessment. Some professionals recommend inclusion with the initial assessment, while others argue for a delayed assessment after the nurse-client relationship has been established. The integration of both techniques may be the most useful because the spiritual assessment should not be viewed as static but rather an ongoing conversation between the nurse and client. If the nurse were proceeding through an initial assessment with relevant past medical history, it would be very appropriate to include general 'screening questions' related to clients' integration of spirituality into their personal health. (e.g., Do you consider yourself to be a religious or spiritual person? If so, how is this related to your health or healthcare decisions?)

➤ **Clinical Tip** • *Briefly addressing a client's spirituality will establish an open dialogue, and provide a foundation for any intervention or care that may be needed in the future.*

The client is focus of the spiritual assessment. Therefore, the nurse does not have to be spiritual to take a spiritual assessment. Objectivity is a key component in a high quality spiritual assessment. The questions in a spiritual assessment probe for beliefs that could affect client care. Divulged information is then utilized to support, encourage, or lead clients in harmonizing their personal relationships to spirituality and health. Some clients may not be connected to any religious group or have any interest in spirituality. These clients should be encouraged in whatever provides them strength in dealing with health care issues (i.e., family, friends, nature, etc.). If a client responds negatively to any aspect of the discussion of religion or spirituality, the nurse may collaborate with the hospital clergy or pastoral care department to further assess the situation and patient responses.

Spiritual Assessment

SPIRITUAL ASSESSMENT TECHNIQUES

Spirituality is multidimensional. It is also unique to each individual. These characteristics of spirituality can present difficulties in proper assessment. Many instruments to assess spirituality were derived within a particular faith background and may have little cross-cultural relevance. The most useful spiritual assessment techniques should have general introductory questions and not be specific to any religious denomination that would guide precise questions related to the client's specific spiritual needs.

Nonformal

There are numerous ways to perform a spiritual assessment. Many times it is helpful to have a quick reference to guide assessment. Acronyms related to the assessment of spirituality have been published (e.g., FICA–Assessment Tool 11-1) and can serve as excellent reminders when assessing a concept with many attributes. Techniques such as these are nonformal yet have somewhat systematic approaches. They are nonformal in the sense of asking open-ended questions and allowing the client to disclose pertinent information. They are systematic to the extent that the client's responses guide future choices of questions, and they may cover numerous practices in which the client may or may not be involved (e.g., prayer, organized religion, etc.).

ASSESSMENT TOOL 11-1	FICA Spiritual Assessment Tool

F: Faith and Beliefs
I: Importance and influence
C: Community
A: Address

Detailed questions relating to acronym:

F: What is your faith or belief?
Do you consider yourself spiritual or religious?
What things do you believe in that give meaning to your life?

I: Is it important in your life?
What influence does it have on how you take care of yourself?
How have your beliefs influenced your behavior during this illness?
What role do your beliefs play in regaining your health?

C: Are you part of a spiritual or religious community?
Is this of a support to you?
Is there a person or group of people who you really love or who are really important to you?

A: How would you like me, your [nurse], to address these issues in your health care?

General recommendations when taking a spiritual history:

1. Consider spirituality as a potentially important component of every client's physical well-being and mental health.
2. Address spirituality at each complete physical examination and continue addressing it at follow-up visits if appropriate. In patient care, spirituality is an ongoing issue.
3. Respect a client's privacy regarding spiritual beliefs; do not impose your beliefs on others.
4. Make referrals to chaplains, spiritual directors, or community resources as appropriate.
5. Be aware that your own spiritual beliefs will help you personally and will overflow in your encounters with those for whom you are to make the [nurse]-patient encounter a more humanistic one.

Adapted from Puchalski, C. (2001). Taking a spiritual history allows clinicians to understand patients more fully. In M. Solomon, A. Romer, K. Heller, & D. Weissman (Eds.), *Innovations in end-of-life care: Practical strategies & international perspectives* (Vol. II). Larchmont, NY: Mary Ann Liebert.

Formal

The client's spirituality and religiosity can also be assessed with formal instruments (Assessment Tools 11-2 and 11-3). While many of these measures are paper-and-pencil self-response, they begin a dialogue and could be employed as important screening tools. Completion of a self-response spiritual or religious assessment instrument in conjunction with other past medical history could uncover strengths or deficiencies that may have initially gone unnoticed. For example, a client responds negatively to the question, "I find comfort in my religion or spirituality" during the initial history taking. During future conversations, the nurse could incorporate this into conversation and possibly reconnect the distressed client to an effective source of spiritual support.

The following information provides examples for spiritual assessment. The normal and abnormal findings in no way encompass all of the appropriate responses from the client. Use the informal in the normal and abnormal sections as a guide only.

(text continues on page 145)

SPIRITUAL ASSESSMENT

Assessment Procedure	Normal Findings	Abnormal Findings
Listen to client's story and seek clarification where needed. Support client to develop trust. Ask client: Do you consider yourself to be a religious or spiritual person? If so, how is this related to your health or healthcare decisions?	Client makes reference to involvement in religious groups and/or spiritual practices that have provided comfort and social support. Describes belief that prayer reduces stress and heals disease.	Reports lost connections to his religious group, while continuing to focus on the negative aspect of spirituality (e.g., suppressive religious rules). Comments and body language reveal a lack of hope with depressive symptomatology. Deficiencies in the social network are identified and appear to affect the client's well-being and attitude toward recovery. Note: Not describing connections to a religious group does *not* indicate abnormal findings.
Observe nonverbal and verbal communication patterns in presence of others.	Eye contact is maintained (appropriate to cultural group) with nonverbal cues correlating with conversation.	Client displays poor eye contact. The presence of others strongly influences information client shares.
Begin to focus questions. Use spiritual assessment tools (Assessment Tools 11-2 and 11-3), if needed. Begin conversation with a general dialogue about global concepts such as hope, meaning, comfort, strength, peace, love, and connection: We have been discussing your support systems. What are your sources of hope, strength, comfort, and peace? What do you hold onto during difficult times? What sustains you and keeps you going? For some people, their religious or spiritual beliefs act as a source of comfort and strength in dealing with life's ups and downs; is this true for you? Use FICA assessment tool, Assessment Tool 11-1.	Reports spirituality giving a sense of peace that transcends illness or disease. Reports that meditation and exercise facilitate a sense of peace. Family frequently mentioned as source of strength and motivation. Client places a strong emphasis on spirituality as a guiding force in life.	Describes no connection to others such as God, nature, family, or peers. Shares pessimistic and fatalistic attitude toward recovery. Identifies limited coping resources with little desire to adapt new ones.
Continue to assess other dimensions of spirituality within groups. Ask about organizational (or formal) religious involvement. Reflect on previous conversations to direct questioning. Remember that not all persons who state they are religious and/or spiritual are involved with organized religious groups or ascribe to	Client may report regular attendance at a local mosque, church, or other religious meeting place and highlight importance of attendance as a recovery period in a very fast-paced life. States that involvement with others holding a similar worldview helps to give meaning and purpose to life.	Abnormal findings may include reporting involvement with "new religious group" in the area but being unable to provide details regarding affiliation or purpose of religious group. Client makes reference to extensive fasts and other activities that may be harmful to general health.

continued

Assessment Procedure	Normal Findings	Abnormal Findings
all the religious practices of that group. Note: If there is no connection to a religious group or faith tradition, skip or modify this section and the next. Ask the questions: Do you consider yourself part of an organized religion? How important is this to you? What aspects of your religion are helpful and not so helpful to you? Are you part of a religious or spiritual community? Does it help you? How?		
Ask transition question from organizational to personal beliefs. Ask client to specify differences or similarities in own beliefs and the beliefs of the faith or denomination with which affiliated. Ask questions: Do you have personal spiritual beliefs independent of organized religion? What are they? Do you believe in God? What kind of relationship do you have with God? What aspects of spirituality or spiritual practices do you find most helpful to you personally (e.g., prayer, meditation, reading scripture, attending religious services, listening to music, hiking, communing with nature)?	Describes personal beliefs that coincide with denominational beliefs. Denominational beliefs do not conflict with required medical care. Reports relationship with God healthy and positive. Desires to have time in the hospital to meditate and read scripture to gain focus and relieve stress.	Abnormal findings may include reporting very limited similarities between denomination and personal beliefs, past utilization of prayer and listening to religious music, but currently has no avenue for the fostering of spirituality.
Directly address beliefs that may conflict or affect one's health care. Assist clients with expression of spiritual practices if appropriate. Attend to end-of-life issues if the condition dictates. Ask the questions: Has being sick (or your current situation) affected your ability to do the things that usually help you spiritually? (Or affected your relationship with God?) As a [nurse], is there anything I can do to help you access the resources that usually help you? Are you worried about any conflicts between your beliefs and your medical situation/care/decisions? Would it be helpful for you to speak to a clinical chaplain/community spiritual leader? Are there any specific practices or restrictions I should know about in providing your medical care? (e.g., dietary restrictions, use of blood products) *If the client is dying:* How do your beliefs affect the kind of [nursing] care you would like me to provide over the next few days/weeks/months?	Client views present diagnosis of cancer as "part of God's will for her life" or/and desires to continue nature walks and other spiritual practices to develop a closer relationship with God. Client makes no reference to perceived abandonment or rejection that may lead to depression. Desires to have clergy from her local church for visitation time. Client asks the nurse to contact local clergy and provides telephone number.	Client appears traumatized with cancer diagnosis and views the illness as a fault of her past lifestyle or a punishment. Refuses visits from local clergy and hospital chaplains. Declines conversation and just wants to be sent home to die.

ASSESSMENT TOOL 11-2   Daily Spiritual Experiences Scale

The list that follows includes items you may or may not experience. Please consider if and how often you have these experiences; try to disregard whether you feel you should or should not have them. In addition, a number of items use the word "God." If this word is not a comfortable one, please substitute another idea that calls to mind the divine or holy for you.

Scoring:

1=Many times a day	4=Some Days
2=Every Day	5=Once in a While
3=Most Days	6=Never or Almost Never

	1	2	3	4	5	6
1. I feel God's presence.	1	2	3	4	5	6
2. I experience a connection to all of life.	1	2	3	4	5	6
3. During worship or at other times when connecting with God, I feel joy which lifts me out of my daily concerns.	1	2	3	4	5	6
4. I find strength in my religion or spirituality.	1	2	3	4	5	6
5. I find comfort in my religion or spirituality.	1	2	3	4	5	6
6. I feel deep inner peace and harmony.	1	2	3	4	5	6
7. I ask for God's help in the midst of daily activities.	1	2	3	4	5	6
8. I feel guided by God in the midst of daily activities.	1	2	3	4	5	6
9. I feel God's love for me directly.	1	2	3	4	5	6
10. I feel God's love for me through others.	1	2	3	4	5	6
11. I am spiritually touched by the beauty of creation.	1	2	3	4	5	6
12. I feel thankful for my blessings.	1	2	3	4	5	6
13. I feel a selfless caring for others.	1	2	3	4	5	6
14. I accept others even when they do things I think are wrong.	1	2	3	4	5	6
15. I desire to be closer to or in union with Him.*	1	2	3	4	5	6
16. In general, how close do you feel to God?*	1	2	3	4	5	6

*For questions 15 and 16, Scoring: 4=not close at all, 3=somewhat close, 2=very close, 1=as close as possible. Lower scores represent more daily spiritual experiences.

Adapted from Fetzer Institute. (1999). *Multidimensional measurement of religiousness/spirituality for use in health research*. Kalamazoo: John E. Fetzer Institute.

ASSESSMENT TOOL 11-3   Brief Religious Coping Questionnaire (RCOPE)

Instructions for administration: Think about how you try to understand and deal with major problems in your life. To what extent is each involved in the way you cope?

Positive Religious/Spiritual Coping Subscale

1. I think about how my life is part of a larger spiritual force.
   1. A great deal   3. Somewhat
   2. Quite a bit   4. Not at all
2. I work together with God as partners to get through hard times.
   1. A great deal   3. Somewhat
   2. Quite a bit   4. Not at all
3. I look to God for strength, support, and guidance in crisis.
   1. A great deal   3. Somewhat
   2. Quite a bit   4. Not at all

Negative Religious/Spiritual Coping Subscale

1. I feel that stressful situations are God's way of punishing me for my sins or lack of spirituality.
   1. A great deal   3. Somewhat
   2. Quite a bit   4. Not at all
2. I wonder if God has abandoned me.
   1. A great deal   3. Somewhat
   2. Quite a bit   4. Not at all
3. I try to make sense of the situation and decide what to do without relying on God.
   1. A great deal   3. Somewhat
   2. Quite a bit   4. Not at all

A more extensive form of the RCOPE exists and could be utilized for detailed analysis. Scale could be summed as a general screening tool or individual items could be identified (e.g. abandonment) and incorporated into the clinical setting.

Adapted from Fetzer Institute. (1999). *Multidimensional measurement of religiousness/spirituality for use in health research*. Kalamazoo: John E. Fetzer Institute.

VALIDATING AND DOCUMENTING FINDINGS

A client's spirituality often affects her health. There are numerous capacities in which this occurs and frequently will go unnoticed without assessment. Subjective and objective data will be collected during assessment. Noticeably the subjective data will be the primary source of information during a spiritual assessment, but the objective data can validate or call into question information presented to the nurse.

Sample Documentation of Subjective Data

75-year-old male recently admitted to the medical-surgical unit for diabetic foot ulcer. Family members present during initial assessment. The FICA spiritual assessment included in the initial exam. Client reports a strong sense of hope and comfort from God; attends church weekly. He states, "God just helps keep me going." Uses prayer as a coping mechanism to surmount the pain of diabetic neuropathy. No conflicts between the client's beliefs and his healthcare treatment, but he gladly accepts a visit from the hospital chaplain.

Sample Documentation of Objective Data

Client has an affect that correlates with his positive attitude. Makes direct eye contact while describing spiritual beliefs. Family members present nod in agreement with the client's responses.

Analysis of Data

DIAGNOSTIC REASONING: POSSIBLE CONCLUSIONS

After collecting subjective and objective data pertaining to spiritual assessment, identify abnormal findings and client's strengths. Then cluster the data to reveal any significant patterns or abnormalities. These data may be used to make clinical judgments about the status of the client's spirituality.

Selected Nursing Diagnoses

Following is a listing of selected nursing diagnoses (wellness, risk, actual) that you may identify when analyzing the cue clusters.

Wellness Diagnoses

- Readiness for enhanced Spiritual Well-Being

Risk Diagnoses

- Risk for Spiritual Distress

Actual Diagnoses

- Spiritual Distress

Selected Collaborative Problems

After grouping the data, certain collaborative problems may become apparent. Remember that collaborative problems differ from nursing diagnoses in that they cannot be prevented by nursing intervention. However, these physiologic or other complications of medical or other conditions can be detected and monitored by the nurse. In addition, the nurse can use physician- and nurse-prescribed interventions to minimize the complications of these problems. The nurse may also have to refer the client in such situations for further treatment of the problem. Following is an example of a collaborative problem that may be identified when assessing the spirituality. The collaborative problem is worded as Risk for Complications (or RC) followed by the problem.

- RC: Depression
- RC: Hypertension
- RC: Hypoglycemia
- RC: Opportunistic Infections

The RC related to spirituality is due to the psychologic or physiologic responses of the body under stress. Stress induced by states such as spiritual distress will create a cascade of events within the body that produce physiological responses and are influenced by the size and duration of the stressor as well as the client's ability to respond to that stressor.

Medical Problems

After grouping the data, it may become apparent that the client has signs and symptoms that require medical diagnosis and treatment. Referral to a primary care provider is necessary.

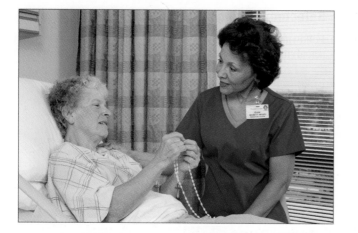

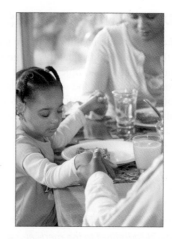

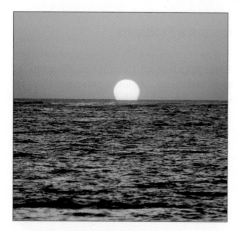

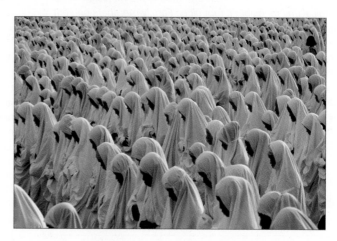

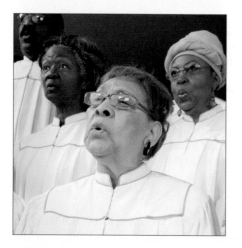

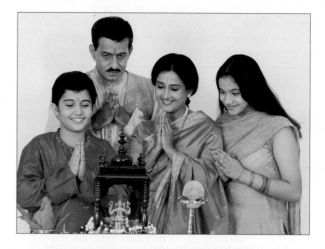

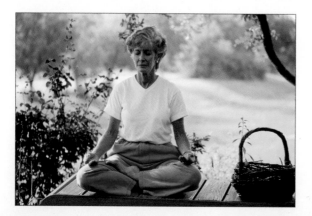

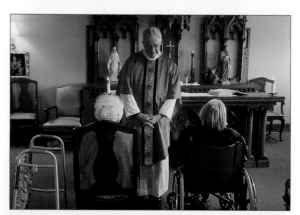

CASE STUDY

The case study demonstrates how to analyze spiritual assessment data for a specific client. The critical thinking exercises included in the study guide/lab manual that complement this text also offer opportunities to analyze assessment data.

Lindsay Baird is a 40-year-old woman who lives with her two children and husband outside of a rural community. Mrs. Baird presents at the clinic today for a routine check of her hypertension. Upon reviewing the past medical/family history, it is noted that Mrs. Baird is a Catholic and believes her spirituality to be a very important part of her medical care. Entering the room, Mrs. Baird greets you gracefully and continues to respond to general health questions with ease. After proceeding through relevant medical history since the last visit, a 5-pound weight gain is noted with a correlating blood pressure notably higher than the last visit. Questioning the recent changes in her medical condition, Mrs. Baird responds, "I just haven't felt like doing any exercise lately." Continuing to draw information out, you begin to ask particular questions related to stress levels, time restraints, and motivation. Eventually Mrs. Baird begins to tell the story of her family falling away from attending the church on a regular basis and the corresponding loss of support and motivation. She states, "I used to gain such strength going to our church meetings. It was such an encouragement. We used to walk with one another and talk about what God is doing in our lives . . . now I just feel overwhelmed and busy all of the time . . . and I can't talk with anyone."

The following concept map illustrates the diagnostic reasoning process.

Applying COLDSPA

Applying **COLDSPA** for client symptoms: "I just haven't felt like doing any exercise lately."

Mnemonic	Question	Data Provided	Missing Data
Character	Describe the sign or symptom (feeling, appearance, sound, smell, or taste if applicable).	Loss of motivation and social support network	
Onset	When did it begin?		"When were you first separated from your church (or support group)?"
Location	Where is it? Does it radiate? Does it occur anywhere else?	The patient reports negative physical and emotional consequences.	
Duration	How long does it last? Does it recur?		"Have you been separated from your church (or support group) before? If so, how long and what was the outcome?"
Severity	How bad is it? How much does it bother you?	Limited desire for exercise has resulted in weight gain.	
Pattern	What makes it better or worse?		"Has anything made it better or worse?"
Associated factors/How it **A**ffects the client	What other symptoms occur with it? How does it affect you?	The patient reports feeling overwhelmed and isolated.	

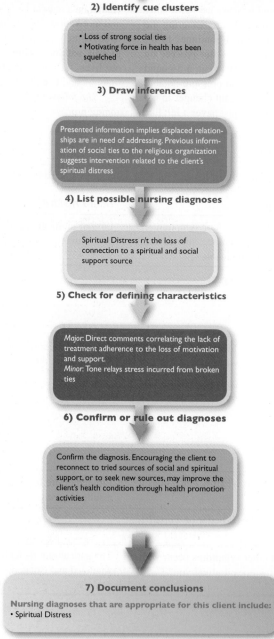

1) Identify abnormal findings and client strengths

Subjective Data

- Lack of adherence to the treatment regimen
- The information is not easily divulged
- Loss of previous strong ties to the religious group
- Client describes lack of motivation to participate in health promoting activities
- Heightened sense of stress due to the lost connections

Objective Data

- Blood pressure elevation between visits
- Weight increased 5 pounds from the previous visit
- Facial expressions changed to ones of concern as the conversation moved toward the client's struggles

2) Identify cue clusters

- Loss of strong social ties
- Motivating force in health has been squelched

3) Draw inferences

Presented information implies displaced relationships are in need of addressing. Previous information of social ties to the religious organization suggests intervention related to the client's spiritual distress

4) List possible nursing diagnoses

Spiritual Distress r/t the loss of connection to a spiritual and social support source

5) Check for defining characteristics

Major: Direct comments correlating the lack of treatment adherence to the loss of motivation and support.
Minor: Tone relays stress incurred from broken ties

6) Confirm or rule out diagnoses

Confirm the diagnosis. Encouraging the client to reconnect to tried sources of social and spiritual support, or to seek new sources, may improve the client's health condition through health promotion activities

7) Document conclusions

Nursing diagnoses that are appropriate for this client include:
- Spiritual Distress

References and Selected Readings

Anandarajah, G., & Hight, E. (2001). Spirituality and medical practice: Using the HOPE questions as a practical tool for spiritual assessment. *American Family Physician, 63*(1), 81–89.

Barnes, P., Powell-Griner, E., McFann, K., & Nahin, R. (2004). Complementary and alternative medicine use among adults: United States, 2002. *CDC Advance Data Report No. 343.*

Barnum, B. (2003). *Spirituality in nursing: From traditional to new age* (5th ed.). New York: Springer.

Barrett, D., Kurlan, G., & Johnson, T. (2001). *World Christian encyclopedia: A comparative survey of churches and religions in the modern world* (2nd ed.). New York: Oxford.

Beckman, S., Boxley-Harges, S., Bruick-Sorge, C., & Salmon B. (2007). Five strategies that heighten nurses' awareness of spirituality to impact client care. *Holistic Nursing Practice, 21*(3), 135–139.

Benson, H., & Klipper, M. (1975/2000). *The relaxation response.* New York: Hapertorch.

Buck, H. (2006). Spirituality: Concept analysis and model development. *Holistic Nursing Practice, 20*(6), 288–292.

Byrne, M. (2007). Spirituality in palliative care: What language do we need? Learning from pastoral care. *International Journal of Palliative Nursing, 13*(3), 118–124.

Dickinson, E. (2006). End-of-life issues in US nursing school curricula: 1984–2006. *Progress in Palliative Care, 14*(4), 165–167.

Esch, T., Fricchione, G., & Stefano, G. (2003). The therapeutic use of the relaxation response in stress-related diseases. *Medical Science Monitor, 9*(2), RA23–RA34.

Fetzer Institute. (1999). *Multidimensional measurement of religiousness/spirituality for use in health research.* Kalamazoo: John E. Fetzer Institute.

Gallup, G. (2006). *The spiritual state of the union: The role of spiritual commitment in the United States.* Princeton, NJ: The Gallup Organization.

Hoffert, D., Henshaw, C., & Mvududu, N. (2007). Enhancing the ability of nursing students to perform a spiritual assessment. *Nurse Educator, 32*(2), 66–72.

Kastenbaum, R. (2006). *Death, society, and the human experience* (9th ed.). Boston: Allyn & Bacon.

Koenig, H., & Cohen, H. (2002). *The link between religion and health: Psychoneuroimmunology and the faith factor.* New York: Oxford University Press.

Koenig, H., McCullough, M., & Larson, D. (2001). *Handbook of religion and health.* New York: Oxford University Press.

Koenig, H., Parkerson, G., & Meadon, K. (1997). Religion index for psychiatric research. *American Journal of Psychiatry, 154*(6), 885–886.

Kubler-Ross, E. (1996). *On death and dying: What the dying have to teach doctors, nurses, clergy and their own families.* New York: Macmillan.

Kubler-Ross, E. (1997). *The wheel of life: A memoir of living and dying.* New York: Touchstone.

Lantz, C. (2000). Teaching spiritual care in a public institution: Legal implications, standards of practice, and ethical obligations. *Journal of Nursing Education, 46*(1), 33–38.

Loustalot, F., Wyatt, S., May, W., Sims, M., & Ellison, C. (2006). Positive influence of religion and spirituality on blood pressure in the Jackson Heart Study. *Journal of Clinical Hypertension, Supplement A, 8*(5), 148.

Lovanio, K., & Wallace, M. (2007). Promoting spiritual knowledge and attitudes: A student nurse education project. *Holistic Nursing Practice, 21*(1), 42–47.

McCaffrey, A., Eisenberg, D., Legedza, A., Davis, R., & Phillips, R. (2004). Prayer for health concerns: Results from a national survey on prevalence and patterns of use. *Archives of Internal Medicine, 164,* 858–862.

McCord, G., Gilchrist, V., Grossman, S., King, B., McCormick, K., et al. (2004). Discussing spirituality with patients: A rational and ethical approach. *Annals of Family Medicine, 2*(4), 356–361.

McEwen, M. (2005). Spiritual nursing care: State of the art. *Holistic Nursing Practice, 19,* 161–168.

McSherry, W., & Ross, L. (2002). Dilemmas of spiritual assessment: Considerations for nursing practice. *Journal of Advanced Nursing, 38,* 479–488.

McSherry, W., & Smith, J. (2007). How do children express their spiritual needs? *Pediatric Nursing, 19*(3), 17–20.

Miller, W. (1999). *Integrating spirituality into treatment.* Washington, DC: American Psychological Association.

Miller, W., & Thoresen, C. (1999). Spirituality and health. In W. Miller (Ed.), *Integrating spirituality into treatment* (pp. 3–18). Washington, DC: American Psychological Association.

Mitchell. D., Bennett, M., & Manfrin-Ledet, L. (2006). Spiritual development of nursing students: Developing competence to provide spiritual care to patients at the end of life. *Journal of Nursing Education, 45*(9), 365–370.

Napier-Tibere, B. (2002). *Diversity, healing and health care.* Retrieved September 1, 2004, from http://www.gasi-ves.org/pdf/1-total-cohort.pdf

Nerburn, K. (2005). *The wisdom of the Native Americans.* Novato, CA: New World Library.

Neuman, B. (1995). *The Neuman systems model* (3rd ed.). Norwalk, CT: Appleton & Lange.

Nightingale, F. (1860/1996). *Notes on nursing.* New York, Dover.

O'Brien, M. (2007). *Spirituality in nursing: Standing on holy ground* (3rd ed.). Boston: Jones and Bartlett.

Pargament, K. (1997). *The psychology of religion and coping: Theory, research and practice.* New York: Guilford.

Puchalski, C. (2001). Taking a spiritual history allows clinicians to understand patients more fully. In M. Solomon, A. Romer, K. Heller, & D. Weissman (Eds.), *Innovations in end-of-life care: Practical strategies & international perspectives* (Vol. 2). Larchmont, NY: Mary Ann Liebert.

Rankin, E., & Delashmutt, M. (2006). Finding spirituality and nursing presence: The student's challenge. *Journal of Holistic Nursing, 24*(4), 282–288.

Stranahan, S. (2001). Spiritual perception, attitudes about spiritual care, and spiritual care practices among nurse practitioners. *Western Journal of Nursing Research, 23*(1), 90–104.

Tinley, S., & Kinney, A. (2007). Three philosophical approaches to the study of spirituality. *Advances in Nursing Science, 30*(1), 71–80.

Underwood, L., & Teresi, J. (2002). The Daily Spiritual Experience Scale: Development, theoretical description, reliability, exploratory factor analysis, and preliminary construct validity using health related data. *Annals of Behavioral Medicine, 24*(1), 22–33.

Websites

Benson-Henry Institute for Mind Body Medicine. Available at http://www.mbmi.org/

Center for Spirituality, Theology and Health, Duke University. Available at http://www.dukespiritualityandhealth.org/

Interfaith Health Program, Emory University. Available at http://ihpnet.org/

John Templeton Foundation. Available at http://www.templeton.org/

Larry Dossey. Available at http://www.dosseydossey.com/

The George Washington Institute for Spirituality and Health. Available at http://www.gwish.org/

University of Pennsylvania School of Medicine, Pastoral Care Faith Traditions and Health Care. Available at http://www.uphs.upenn.edu/pastoral/pubs/traditions.html

Yale University Guide to Native American Studies. Available at http://www.library.yale.edu/rsc/native/

Structure and Function

Information gathered during the nutritional assessment provides insight into the client's overall physical health. With obesity becoming a widespread health problem, nutritional assessment is vital. Obesity is a risk factor for numerous diseases/conditions such as heart disease, hypertension, and diabetes. Nutritional assessment helps to identify risk factors for obesity and to promote health. Conversely nutritional assessment can help to identify nutritional deficits, which also greatly impact the client's health.

Hydration is another important indicator of the client's general health status though it may be overlooked or confused with the signs and symptoms of nutritional changes. Hydration status must also be assessed.

NUTRITIONAL ASSESSMENT

The nutritional assessment is composed of an interview and anthropometric measurements, which are used to evaluate the client's physical growth, development, and nutritional status. The nurse works closely with the registered dietician (RD) through consultation and collaboration to evaluate the nutritional status and identify clients in need of instruction and/or nutritional support. **MyPyramid Tracker** is an online dietary and physical activity assessment tool that provides the client with an interactive approach to personalized food and daily calorie needs (Dietary Guidelines for Americans, 2005; U.S. Department of Agriculture and Center for Nutrition Policy and Promotion).

General Nutritional Status Interview

The nutritional assessment should begin with questions regarding the client's dietary habits. Questions should solicit information about average daily intake of food and fluids, types and quantities consumed, where and when food is eaten, and any conditions or diseases that affect intake or absorption. Collection of this information can add to the evaluation of the client's risk factors as well as point to health education needs. A **24-hour food recall** is an efficient and easy method of identifying a client's intake but must be used with an individual who is able to remember all types and quantities of foods and beverages taken in 24 hours. A variety of tools for assessing food habits and nutrition are available, including

- Sample form for a **nutrition history** (Assessment Tool 12-1)
- Checklist to use for nutritional screening (Assessment Tool 12-2)
- Estimated calorie requirements (Appendix G)
- Eating plan based on calorie level (Appendix H)
- USDA Food Guide and Canada's Food Guide (Appendices I and J)
- USDA food pyramid (Fig. 12-1) and traditional Asian, Latin American, Mediterranean, and Vegetarian diet pyramids (Fig. 12-2)

Anthropometric Measurements

As mentioned above, anthropometric measurements help to evaluate the client's physical growth, development, and nutritional status. First, height and weight are obtained. By comparing these findings to a standard table, the nurse can determine the client's **body mass index** (BMI) (Table 12-1). (Note: Adult calorie requirements and BMI can be quickly calculated by using the following website: http://www.bcm.edu/cnrc/caloriesneed.htm.) BMI is calculated based on height and weight regardless of gender. It is a practical measure for estimating total body fat and is calculated as weight in kilograms and divided by the square height in meters. Though a number of methods are available to evaluate weight status, the most commonly used screening method is the body mass index (Weight-control Information Network, March, 2006). Even though simple, quick, and inexpensive, use of BMI alone is not diagnostic of a client's health status. Because BMI does not differentiate between fat or muscle tissue, inaccurately high or low findings can result for individuals who are particularly muscular or the elderly who tend to lose muscle mass. The results will be erroneous if the individual is retaining fluid as with edema or ascites or if the client is pregnant. Additionally BMI may not accurately reflect body fat in adults, who are shorter than five feet (Weight-control Information Network, June, 2004). Therefore, further assessments using measurements

Nutrition History

1. How many meals and snacks do you eat each day?

   Meals _____   Snacks _____

2. How many times a week do you eat the following meals away from home?

   Breakfast _____   Lunch _____

   Dinner _____

   What types of eating places do you frequently visit? (Check all that apply)

   Fast-food _____   Restaurant _____

   Diner/cafeteria _____   Other _____

3. On average, how many pieces of fruit or glasses of juice do you eat or drink each day?

   Fresh fruit _____   Juice (8 oz. cup) _____

4. On average, how many servings of vegetables do you eat each day? _____

5. On average, how many times a week do you eat a high-fiber breakfast cereal? _____

6. How many times a week do you eat red meat (beef, lamb, veal) or pork? _____

7. How many times a week do you eat chicken or turkey? _____

8. How many times a week do you eat fish or shellfish? _____

9. How many hours of television do you watch every day? _____

Do you usually snack while watching television?

Yes _____ No _____

10. How many times a week do you eat desserts and sweets? _____

11. What types of beverages do you usually drink? How many servings of each do you drink a day?

    Water _____

    Juice _____

    Soda _____

    Diet soda _____

    Sports drinks _____

    Iced tea _____

    Iced tea with sugar _____

    Milk:

    Whole milk _____

    2% milk _____

    1% milk _____

    Skim milk _____

    Alcohol:

    Beer _____

    Wine _____

    Hard liquor _____

Used with permission from Hark, L. & Darwin, D. Jr. (1999). Taking a nutrition history: A practical approach for family physicians. *The American Family Physician,* 59 (6), 1521–36.

Speedy Checklist for Nutritional Health

Some warning signs of poor nutritional health are noted in this checklist. Use it to find out if your client is at nutritional risk. Read the statements below. Circle the number in the yes column for those that apply to the client. For each yes answer, score the number in the box. Total the nutrition score.

	YES
Illness or condition that made client change the kind and/or amount of food eaten	2
Eats fewer than two meals per day	3
Eats few fruits or vegetables, or milk products	2
Has three or more drinks of beer, liquor or wine almost every day	2
Tooth or mouth problems that make it hard to eat	2
Does not always have enough money to buy the food needed	4
Eats alone most of the time	1
Takes three or more different prescribed or over-the-counter drugs a day	1
Without wanting to, has lost or gained 10 lb in the last 6 months	2
Not physically able to shop, cook, and/or feed self	2
TOTAL	

Total the nutritional score.

0–2	Good. Recheck the score in 6 months.
3–5	Moderate nutritional risk. See what can be done to improve eating habits and lifestyle. Recheck score in 3 months.
6 or more	High nutritional risk. Consult with physician, dietitian, or other qualified health or social service professional.

Note: Remember that warning signs suggest risk but do not represent diagnosis of any condition.

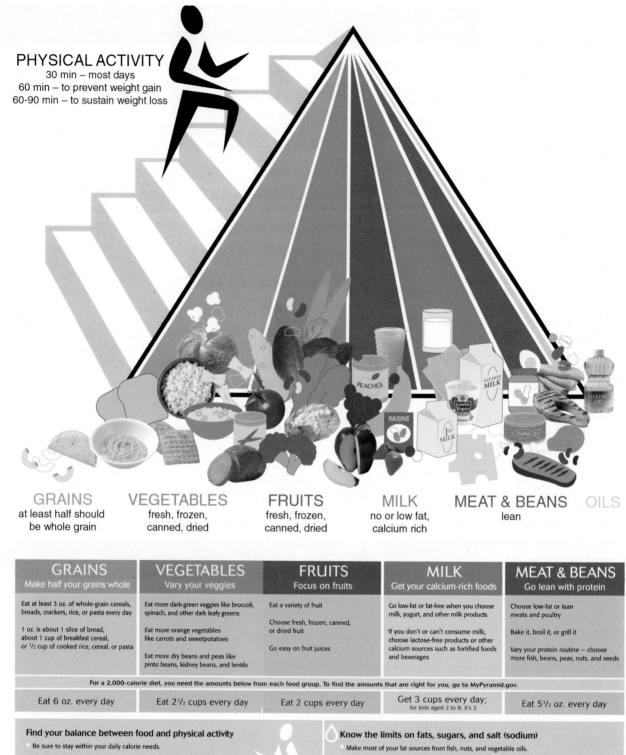

PHYSICAL ACTIVITY
30 min – most days
60 min – to prevent weight gain
60-90 min – to sustain weight loss

GRAINS	VEGETABLES	FRUITS	MILK	MEAT & BEANS	OILS
at least half should be whole grain	fresh, frozen, canned, dried	fresh, frozen, canned, dried	no or low fat, calcium rich	lean	

GRAINS Make half your grains whole	**VEGETABLES** Vary your veggies	**FRUITS** Focus on fruits	**MILK** Get your calcium-rich foods	**MEAT & BEANS** Go lean with protein
Eat at least 3 oz. of whole-grain cereals, breads, crackers, rice, or pasta every day 1 oz. is about 1 slice of bread, about 1 cup of breakfast cereal, or ½ cup of cooked rice, cereal, or pasta	Eat more dark-green veggies like broccoli, spinach, and other dark leafy greens Eat more orange vegetables like carrots and sweetpotatoes Eat more dry beans and peas like pinto beans, kidney beans, and lentils	Eat a variety of fruit Choose fresh, frozen, canned, or dried fruit Go easy on fruit juices	Go low-fat or fat-free when you choose milk, yogurt, and other milk products If you don't or can't consume milk, choose lactose-free products or other calcium sources such as fortified foods and beverages	Choose low-fat or lean meats and poultry Bake it, broil it, or grill it Vary your protein routine – choose more fish, beans, peas, nuts, and seeds

For a 2,000-calorie diet, you need the amounts below from each food group. To find the amounts that are right for you, go to MyPyramid.gov.

Eat 6 oz. every day	Eat 2½ cups every day	Eat 2 cups every day	Get 3 cups every day; for kids aged 2 to 8, it's 2	Eat 5½ oz. every day

Find your balance between food and physical activity
- Be sure to stay within your daily calorie needs.
- Be physically active for at least 30 minutes most days of the week.
- About 60 minutes a day of physical activity may be needed to prevent weight gain.
- For sustaining weight loss, at least 60 to 90 minutes a day of physical activity may be required.
- Children and teenagers should be physically active for 60 minutes every day, or most days.

Know the limits on fats, sugars, and salt (sodium)
- Make most of your fat sources from fish, nuts, and vegetable oils.
- Limit solid fats like butter, margarine, shortening, and lard, as well as foods that contain these.
- Check the Nutrition Facts label to keep saturated fats, *trans* fats, and sodium low.
- Choose food and beverages low in added sugars. Added sugars contribute calories with few, if any, nutrients.

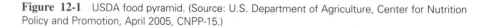

Figure 12-1   USDA food pyramid. (Source: U.S. Department of Agriculture, Center for Nutrition Policy and Promotion, April 2005, CNPP-15.)

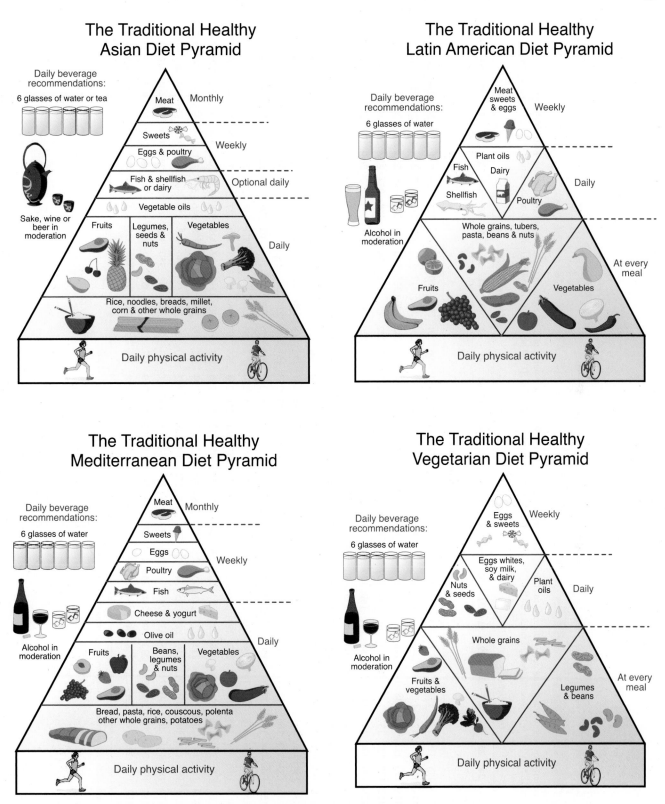

Figure 12-2 **(A)** The traditional healthy Asian diet pyramid, **(B)** the traditional healthy Latin-American diet pyramid, **(C)** the traditional healthy Mediterranean diet pyramid, and **(D)** the traditional healthy vegetarian diet pyramid.

Table 12-1   Adult Body Mass Index (BMI) Chart

Locate the height of interest in the left-most column and read across the row for that height to the weight of interest. Follow the column of the weight up to the top row that lists the BMI. BMI of below 18.5 is classified as underweight, BMI of 18.5 to 24.9 is the healthy weight range, BMI of 25–29.9 is the overweight range, and BMI of 30 and above is in the obese range. 40 or above is considered extreme obesity.

BMI	Normal						Overweight					Obese										Extreme Obesity														
	19	20	21	22	23	24	25	26	27	28	29	30	31	32	33	34	35	36	37	38	39	40	41	42	43	44	45	46	47	48	49	50	51	52	53	54
Height (inches)	Body Weight (pounds)																																			
58	91	96	100	105	110	115	119	124	129	134	138	143	148	153	158	162	167	172	177	181	186	191	196	201	205	210	215	220	224	229	234	239	244	248	253	258
59	94	99	104	109	114	119	124	128	133	138	143	148	153	158	163	168	173	178	183	188	193	198	203	208	212	217	222	227	232	237	242	247	252	257	262	267
60	97	102	107	112	118	123	128	133	138	143	148	153	158	163	168	174	179	184	189	194	199	204	209	215	220	225	230	235	240	245	250	255	261	266	271	276
61	100	106	111	116	122	127	132	137	143	148	153	158	164	169	174	180	185	190	195	201	206	211	217	222	227	232	238	243	248	254	259	264	269	275	280	285
62	104	109	115	120	126	131	136	142	147	153	158	164	169	175	180	186	191	196	202	207	213	218	224	229	235	240	246	251	256	262	267	273	278	284	289	295
63	107	113	118	124	130	135	141	146	152	158	163	169	175	180	186	191	197	203	208	214	220	225	231	237	242	248	254	259	265	270	278	282	287	293	299	304
64	110	116	122	128	134	140	145	151	157	163	169	174	180	186	192	197	204	209	215	221	227	232	238	244	250	256	262	267	273	279	285	291	296	302	308	314
65	114	120	126	132	138	144	150	156	162	168	174	180	186	192	198	204	210	216	222	228	234	240	246	252	258	264	270	276	282	288	294	300	306	312	318	324
66	118	124	130	136	142	148	155	161	167	173	179	186	192	198	204	210	216	223	229	235	241	247	253	260	266	272	278	284	291	297	303	309	315	322	328	334
67	121	127	134	140	146	153	159	166	172	178	185	191	198	204	211	217	223	230	236	242	249	255	261	268	274	280	287	293	299	306	312	319	325	331	338	344
68	125	131	138	144	151	158	164	171	177	184	190	197	203	210	216	223	230	236	243	249	256	262	269	276	282	289	295	302	308	315	322	328	335	341	348	354
69	128	135	142	149	155	162	169	176	182	189	196	203	209	216	223	230	236	243	250	257	263	270	277	284	291	297	304	311	318	324	331	338	345	351	358	365
70	132	139	146	153	160	167	174	181	188	195	202	209	216	222	229	236	243	250	257	264	271	278	285	292	299	306	313	320	327	334	341	348	355	362	369	376
71	136	143	150	157	165	172	179	186	193	200	208	215	222	229	236	243	250	257	265	272	279	286	293	301	308	315	322	329	338	343	351	358	365	372	379	386
72	140	147	154	162	169	177	184	191	199	206	213	221	228	235	242	250	258	265	272	279	287	294	302	309	316	324	331	338	346	353	361	368	375	383	390	397
73	144	151	159	166	174	182	189	197	204	212	219	227	235	242	250	257	265	272	280	288	295	302	310	318	325	333	340	348	355	363	371	378	386	393	401	408
74	148	155	163	171	179	186	194	202	210	218	225	233	241	249	256	264	272	280	287	295	303	311	319	326	334	342	350	358	365	373	381	389	396	404	412	420
75	152	160	168	176	184	192	200	208	216	224	232	240	248	256	264	272	279	287	295	303	311	319	327	335	343	351	359	367	375	383	391	399	407	415	423	431
76	156	164	172	180	189	197	205	213	221	230	238	246	254	263	271	279	287	295	304	312	320	328	336	344	353	361	369	377	385	394	402	410	418	426	435	443

Source: Adapted from *Clinical Guidelines on the Identification, Evaluation, and Treatment of Overweight and Obesity in Adults: The Evidence Report.* (1998)

that determine body fat composition should be performed to determine health status and associated risk factors.

Body composition measurements are useful in determining location of body fat. Waist circumference is the most common measurement used to determine the extent of abdominal visceral fat in relation to body fat. According to a recent study, adding waist circumference to body mass index (BMI) increases the predictive ability for health risk more so than using BMI alone (Meisinger, et al, 2006). Excess fat deep within the abdominal cavity known as visceral fat (Fig. 12-3) is associated with higher health risks than subcutaneous fat and may be an independent predictor of health risks even when BMI falls within the normal range (Weight-control Information Network, 2004). Women with 35 inches or greater waist circumference or men with 40 inches or greater waist circumference are at an increased risk for such disorders as diabetes, hypertension, hyperlipidemia, and cardiovascular disease. The three "vital signs" of obesity are waist circumference, weight, and body mass index (McDonald, 2007). As with BMI, waist circumference guidelines may not be accurate with adult clients who are shorter than five feet in height (Defining Overweight and Obesity, 2004).

Though used less often, the following measurements may also be obtained. Body composition measurements include mid-arm circumference, triceps skin-fold measurements, and mid-arm muscle circumference calculations. Mid-arm circumference helps to assess skeletal muscle mass. The triceps skin-fold helps to evaluate subcutaneous fat stores. The mid-arm circumference and triceps skin fold are used in a formula to calculate the mid-arm muscle circumference to evaluate muscle

reserve stores. These measurements are also used to evaluate the client's nutritional status.

Nutritional Problems

Malnutrition and Biochemical Indicators

Certain diseases, disorders, or lifestyle behaviors can place clients at risk for **under nutrition** or **malnutrition** and can exacerbate or facilitate disease processes. The following is a selected list of risk factors:

- Lower socioeconomic status whereby nutritious foods are unaffordable
- Lifestyle of long work hours and obtaining one or more meals from a fast-food chain or vending machine
- Poor food choices by children, teens, and adults include lots of fatty or fried meats, sugary foods, but few fruits and vegetables
- Chronic dieting, particularly with fad diets, to meet perceived societal norms for weight and appearance
- Chronic diseases (e.g., Crohn's disease, cirrhosis, or cancer) that may interfere with absorption or use of nutrients
- Dental and other factors such as difficulty chewing, loss of taste sensation, depression
- Limited access to sufficient food regardless of socioeconomic status such as being physically unable to shop, cook, or feed self
- Disorders whereby food is self limited or refused (e.g., anorexia nervosa, bulimia, depression, dementia, or other psychiatric disorders)
- Illness or trauma that increases client's nutritional needs dramatically but that interferes with his or her ability to ingest adequate nourishment (e.g., extensive burns)

The clinical signs and symptoms of malnutrition are often confused with those of other diseases or conditions. In addition, the signs and symptoms may not manifest until the malnutrition is profound. The nurse needs to collect as much data as possible, especially in clients who are at risk for malnutrition or show some early clinical signs. All of the information should then be evaluated in context to avoid making judgments based on one or two isolated signs or symptoms. Table 12-2 provides data collected during the complete health history and during physical assessment that help identify nutritional disorders; Assessment Tool 12-3 compares indicators of good nutritional status with indicators of poor nutritional status.

Reviewing certain laboratory tests can yield valuable information about the client's nutritional status. These tests can identify under-nutrition or malnutrition, especially subtle changes before they are clinically evident. For example, a person can be obese yet undernourished because of poor food choices. In this situation, laboratory tests such as hemoglobin or protein levels may indicate anemia or other nutritional disorders. Laboratory studies such as high cholesterol and triglyceride values can indicate risk factors in undernourished, normal, overweight, and obese people because these factors can be related to inherited tendencies, lack of exercise, and unhealthful dietary habits.

When people are malnourished, the body's protein stores are affected. The proteins usually sacrificed early are those that the body considers to be less essential to survival: albumen

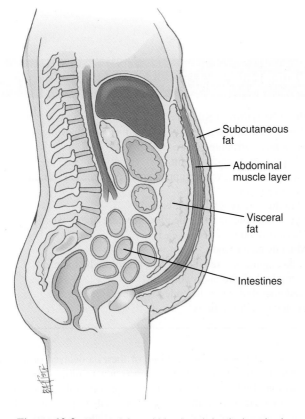

Figure 12-3 Visceral fat within the abdominal cavity increases health risks.

Subcutaneous fat

Abdominal muscle layer

Visceral fat

Intestines

Table 12-2   Evaluating Nutritional Disorders

This table can help you interpret your nutritional assessment findings. Body systems are listed below with signs or symptoms and the implications for each.

Body System or Region	Sign or Symptom	Implications
General	• Weakness and fatigue • Weight loss	• Anemia or electrolyte imbalance • Decreased calorie intake, increased calorie use, or inadequate nutrient intake or absorption
Skin, hair, and nails	• Dry, flaky skin • Dry skin with poor turgor • Rough, scaly skin with bumps • Petechiae or ecchymoses • Sore that won't heal • Thinning, dry hair • Spoon-shaped, brittle, or ridged nails	• Vitamin A, vitamin B-complex, or linoleic acid deficiency • Dehydration • Vitamin A deficiency • Vitamin C or K deficiency • Protein, vitamin C, or zinc deficiency • Protein deficiency • Iron deficiency
Eyes	• Night blindness; corneal swelling, softening, or dryness; Bitot's spots (gray triangular patches on the conjunctiva) • Red conjunctiva	• Vitamin A deficiency • Riboflavin deficiency
Throat and mouth	• Cracks at the corner of mouth • Magenta tongue • Beefy, red tongue • Soft, spongy, bleeding gums • Swollen neck (goiter)	• Riboflavin or niacin deficiency • Riboflavin deficiency • Vitamin B_{12} deficiency • Vitamin C deficiency • Iodine deficiency
Cardiovascular	• Edema • Tachycardia, hypotension	• Protein deficiency • Fluid volume deficit
GI	• Ascites	• Protein deficiency
Musculoskeletal	• Bone pain and bow leg • Muscle wasting	• Vitamin D or calcium deficiency • Protein, carbohydrate, and fat deficiency
Neurological	• Altered mental status • Paresthesia	• Dehydration and thiamine or vitamin B_{12} deficiency • Vitamin B_{12}, pyridoxine, or thiamine deficiency

Nutrition made incredibly easy. (2007) 2nd ed. Philadelphia: Lippincott Williams & Wilkins.

ASSESSMENT TOOL 12-3   General Indicators of Nutritional Status

Good Nutritional Status
Alert, energetic, good endurance, good posture
Good attention span, psychological stability
Weight within range for height, age, body size
Firm, well-developed muscles, healthy reflexes
Skin glowing, elastic, good turgor, smooth
Eyes bright, clear without fatigue circles
Hair shiny, lustrous, minimal loss
Mucous membranes:
    pink-red, gums pink and firm, tongue pink and
    moderately smooth, no swelling
Abdomen flat, firm
No skeletal changes

Poor Nutritional Status
Withdrawn, apathetic easily fatigued, stooped posture
Inattentive, irritable
Overweight or underweight
Flaccid muscles, wasted appearance, paresthesias, diminished reflexes
Skin dull, pasty, scaly, dry, bruised
Eyes dull, conjunctiva pale, discoloration under eyes
Hair brittle, dull, falls out easily
Mucous membranes:
    pale, gums are red, boggy and bleed easily, tongue
    bright dark red and swollen
Abdomen flaccid or distended (ascites)
Skeletal malformations

and globulins, transport proteins, skeletal muscle proteins, blood proteins, and immunoglobulins. These can be easily evaluated by blood tests. Additional tests to evaluate general immunity (immunocompetence) consist of small-dose intradermal injections of recall antigens such as those used to test for tuberculosis, mumps, and *Candida* (yeast). Because everyone has been exposed to at least one of these, a delayed or absent reaction can indicate immunosuppression resulting from malnutrition. Table 12-3 summarizes laboratory values and other tests that can alert health care professionals to possible malnutrition. Please note that there may be slight variations in lab value ranges depending on the reference you use.

Table 12-3	Laboratory Values That Reflect Malnutrition

Laboratory Value	Normal Range	Abnormal Range	
Fasting blood sugar (FBS) or blood glucose level	Adult: 65–99 mg/dL	Pre-diabetes 100–125 mg/dL **Critical:** <40 mg/dL or >400 mg/dL	
Hemoglobin A$_{1c}$	Nondiabetic: 4%–6%	Optimal diabetic control: <7%	
Hemoglobin and Hematocrit Hemoglobin (identifies iron-carrying capacity of the blood; test helps identify anemia, malnutrition, and hydration status)	Males: 13–18 g/dL Females: 12–16 g/dL	Males: ≤12 g/dL Females: ≤11 g/dL	Increased with dehydration or polycythemia
Hematocrit (identifies volume of red blood cells/liter of blood)	Males: 40%–52% Females: 36%–48% (Normal is usually about three times the hemoglobin level [ie., the Hct–Hgb ratio is 1:3])	Males: ≤39% Females: ≤35%	Decreased with overhydration and blood loss, poor dietary intake of iron, protein, certain vitamins
Visceral Proteins Serum albumin level (half-life of 14–20 days)	3.5–5.5 g/dL	Mild depletion: 2.8–3.5 Moderate depletion: 2.1–2.7 Severe depletion <2.1	Increased with dehydration Decreased with overhydration, malnutrition, liver disease
Total protein level (includes globulins)	6–8 g/dL	<5.0 g/dL	
Prealbumin: Transport protein for thyroxin (T4); short half-life makes it more sensitive to changes in protein stores (half life of 3–5 days)	15–30 mg/dL	Mild depletion: 10–15 Moderate depletion: 5–10 Severe depletion: <5	Decreased with undernutrition malnutrition
Transferrin: Transport protein for iron; may be more sensitive indicator of visceral protein stores than albumin because of its shorter half-life	200–400 mg/dL	Mild depletion: 150–199 Moderate depletion: 100–149 Severe depletion: <100	Increased with pregnancy or iron deficiency Decreased with chronic infection or cirrhosis
Creatinine Height Index (CHI) Retinol binding protein, responds rapidly to nutritional depletion due to short half-life	3–6 mg/L	Decreased with overhydration and liver disease	
Immune Function Tests Total lymphocyte count (TLC): % of lymphocytes in the white blood cell count with differential multiplied by 100	>2000 mm^3	Mild immuno-incompetence: 1200–2000 Moderate immuno-incompetence: 800–1199 Severe immuno-incompetence: <800	
Delayed cutaneous hypersensitivity reactions (to common antigens injected intradermally and observed after 24 to 48 hours)	>5–10 mm	<5 mm induration indicates immuno-incompetence	

Overnutrition

Increased caloric consumption, especially food high in fat and sugar, with decreased energy expenditure has led to near-epidemic obesity. Approximately two-thirds of the adult population in the United States is **overweight** and nearly a third of this group is **obese,** according to data from the 2001–2004 National Health and Nutrition Examination Survey (NHANES). Obesity is defined as excessive body fat in relation to lean body mass. The amount of body fat or adipose tissue includes concern for both the fat distribution throughout the body as well as the size of the fat deposits. The health risks of obesity include diabetes, heart disease, stroke, and hypertension, some forms of cancers, osteoarthritis, and sleep apnea.

Generally a person who is 10% over ideal body weight (IBW) is considered overweight, whereas one who is 20% over IBW is considered obese (see Table 12-4 for a determination of obesity based on body mass index). However, weight alone is not a completely reliable criterion. Muscle, bone, fat, and body fluid can account for excess body weight. For example because muscle is heavier than fat, an athlete who has increased muscle mass may be inaccurately categorized as overweight when referring to a standard weight chart. Therefore, although evaluating nutritional status by a client's weight can inform you about obvious alterations at either end of the weight—nutrition continuum, the client with subtle deviations from a healthy-appearing body may benefit from more extensive and varied examination.

| Table 12-4 | Classification of Overweight and Obesity by BMI, Waist Circumference, and Associated Disease Risk* |

	BMI (kg/m²)	Obesity Class	Disease Risk* (Relative to Normal Weight and Waist Circumference)	
			Men < 40 in (≤ 102 cm) Women ≤ 35 in (≤ 88 cm)	> 40 in (> 102 cm) > 35 in (> 88 cm)
Underweight	<18.5			
Normal†	18.5–24.9			
Overweight	25.0–29.9		Increased	High
Obesity	30.0–34.9	I	High	Very High
	35.0–39.9	II	Very High	Very High
Extreme Obesity	≥40	III	Extremely High	Extremely High

* Disease risk for type 2 diabetes, hypertension, and CVD.

† Increased waist circumference can also be a marker for increased risk even in persons of normal weight.

Adapted from "Preventing and Managing the Global Epidemic of Obesity. Report of the World Health Organization Consultation of Obesity." WHO, Geneva, June 1997.

Reprinted from *The practical guide: Identification, evaluation, and treatment of overweight and obesity in adults,* NIH Publication Number 00-4084, October 2000. http://www.nhlbi.nih.gov/guidelines/obesity/prctgd_c.pdf

HYDRATION ASSESSMENT

Hydration is another important indicator of the client's general health status but may be overlooked or confused with the signs and symptoms of nutritional changes. The signs of hydration changes may also be confused with certain disease states if only one or two indicators are evaluated. For this reason, the nurse needs to look for clusters of signs and symptoms that may indicate changes in hydration status. Adequate hydration can be affected by various situations in all age groups. Some examples in adults include

- Exposure to excessively high environmental temperatures
- Inability to access adequate fluids, especially water (e.g., clients who are unconscious, confused, or physically or mentally disabled)
- Excessive intake of alcohol or other diuretic fluids (coffee, sugar-rich and/or caffeine-rich soft drinks)
- People with impaired thirst mechanisms
- People taking diuretic medications
- Diabetic clients with severe hyperglycemia
- People with high fevers

Dehydration can have a seriously damaging effect on body cells and the execution of body functions. Because the thirst mechanism is poorly developed in humans, dehydration can develop unnoticed in normal persons under adverse conditions. Often a person may experience a sense of thirst only after dangerous excess or deficit of various serum electrolyte levels has occurred. A chronically and seriously ill client who is not receiving adequate fluids either orally or parenterally is at high risk for dehydration unless monitored carefully.

Overhydration in a healthy person is usually not a problem because the body is effective in maintaining a correct fluid balance. It does this by shifting fluids in and out of physiologic third spaces, such as extracellular tissues, the pleural and pericardial spaces, the tongue and the eyeball, and by excreting fluid in the urine, stool, and through respiration and perspiration. Clients at risk for overhydration or fluid retention are those with

kidney, liver, and cardiac diseases in which the fluid dynamic mechanisms are impaired.

In addition, seriously ill clients who are on humidified ventilation or who are receiving large volumes of parenteral fluids without close monitoring of their hydration status are also at risk. The health history interview provides an ideal time to teach home care clients and their caregivers how to monitor hydration by keeping records of fluid intake and output.

Health Assessment

COLLECTING SUBJECTIVE DATA: THE NURSING HEALTH HISTORY

The client interview provides invaluable information about the client's nutritional status.

COLLECTING OBJECTIVE DATA: PHYSICAL EXAMINATION

Physical examination includes observing body build, measuring weight and height, taking anthropometric measurements, and assessing hydration.

Preparing the Client

After the interview, ask the client to put on an examination gown. The client should be in a comfortable sitting position on the examination table (or on a bed in the home setting). Unless the client is bed-bound in the hospital, nursing home, or home care setting, explain that he will need to stand and sit during the assessment—particularly during anthropometric assessments. Keep in mind that some clients may be embarrassed to be measured like this, especially if they are overweight or underweight.

(text continues on page 160)

HISTORY OF PRESENT HEALTH CONCERN

Question	Rationale
Height and Weight What are your height and usual weight?	Answer provides a baseline for comparing client's perception with actual and current measurements. Answer also indicates client's knowledge of own health status.
Have you lost or gained a considerable amount of weight recently? How much? Over what period of time?	Weight changes may point to changes in nutrition or hydration status or to an illness causing weight changes.
Diet Are you now or have you been on a diet recently? How did you decide which diet to follow?	Whether or not the client is following his or her own diet or a medically prescribed diet, the answer to the question helps to identify chronic dieters and clients with eating disorders.
How much fluid do you drink each day? How much of it is water? How many sugary, caffeinated, or alcoholic beverages do you have each day?	Answers to these questions identify clients in terms of adequate, moderate, or excessive consumption of various kinds of fluids; they also identify those at risk for dehydration.
Can you recall what you ate in the last 24 hours? In the last 72 hours?	The client's typical daily diet indicates his or her level of nourishment, likes and dislikes, and dietary habits. As such, it provides a basis for planning healthful menu choices.
Any recent changes in appetite, taste, or smell? Any recent difficulties chewing or swallowing?	Changes to taste and smell and difficulty chewing or swallowing may reduce the client's intake of food.
Have you had any recent occurrences of vomiting, diarrhea, or constipation?	Each of these affects nutritional status.

continued on page 160

COLDSPA Example for Weight Gain

Use the **COLDSPA** mnemonic as a guideline to collect needed information for each symptom the client shares. In addition, the following questions help elicit important information.

Mnemonic	Question	Client Response Example
Character	Describe the sign or symptom (feeling, appearance, sound, smell, or taste if applicable).	Weight of 175 lb, height of 5'3″ with a BMI of 31
Onset	When did it begin?	"My weight has steadily increased over the past 5 years."
Location	Where is it? Does it radiate? Does it occur anywhere else?	"Mostly in my abdomen and thighs."
Duration	How long does it last? Does it recur?	N/A
Severity	How bad is it? How much does it bother you?	"I'm so tired of struggling with my weight. I look in the mirror and I can't believe it's me."
Pattern	What makes it better or worse?	"I have tried almost every diet. Some work for a while and then I gain weight again."
Associated factors/How it **A**ffects the client	What other symptoms occur with it? How does it affect you?	"I'm too tired to exercise. I don't even like to shop anymore because I hate trying on clothes. I look so fat."

PAST HEALTH HISTORY

Question	Rationale
Do you have any chronic illnesses?	Chronic illnesses, such as diabetes, may impact the client's nutritional status.
Have you experienced any recent trauma, surgery, or serious illness?	Each of these may increase the client's nutritional needs but decrease the client's ability to meet these needs.

FAMILY HISTORY

Question	Rationale
Are any members of your family obese?	Obesity often runs in families. In addition, families may have unhealthy eating patterns that contribute to obesity.
Do any members have heart disease or diabetes?	Heart disease and diabetes run in families.

LIFESTYLE AND HEALTH PRACTICES

Question	Rationale
Does your religion or culture have diet restrictions or requirements?	Some cultures and religions dictate diet.
What current medications/vitamins/supplements are you taking?	Some medications may decrease the client's absorption of nutrients.
Do you prepare your own meals? What do you eat on a typical day? What fluids and how much do you drink?	A daily account of dietary and fluid intake provides insight into the client's nutrition and hydration.
Do you have sufficient income for food?	Low income may compromise the client's ability to purchase food or make healthy food choices (i.e., foods high in fat and low in nutrients are often inexpensive.)
Do you follow an exercise regimen?	Physical exercise is important to maintaining health.

To reassure the client, explain that the examination is necessary for evaluating overall health status. Proceed with the examination in a straightforward, nonjudgmental manner.

Equipment

- Balance beam scale with height attachment
- Metric measuring tape
- Marking pencil
- Skin fold calipers

Physical Assessment

During examination of the client, remember these key points:

- Identify the equipment needed to take anthropometric measurements and the equipment's proper use.
- Explain the importance of anthropometric measurements to general health status.
- Educate the client regarding nutritional concerns and health-related risks.

(text continues on page 168)

PHYSICAL ASSESSMENT

Assessment Procedure	Normal Findings	Abnormal Findings

Body Build

Observe body build as well as muscle mass and fat distribution. Note body type (Fig. 12-4).

A wide variety of body types fall within a normal range—from small amounts of both fat and muscle to large amounts of muscle and/or fat. In general, the normal body is proportional. Bilateral muscles are firm and well developed. There is equal distribution of fat with some subcutaneous fat. Body parts are intact and appear equal without obvious deformities.

A lack of subcutaneous fat with prominent bones is seen in the undernourished. Abdominal ascites is seen in starvation and liver disease. Abundant fatty tissue is noted in obesity.

Muscle tone and mass decrease with aging. There is a loss of subcutaneous fat, making bones and muscles more prominent. Fat is also redistributed with aging. Fat is lost from the face and neck and redistributed to the arms, abdomen, and hips.

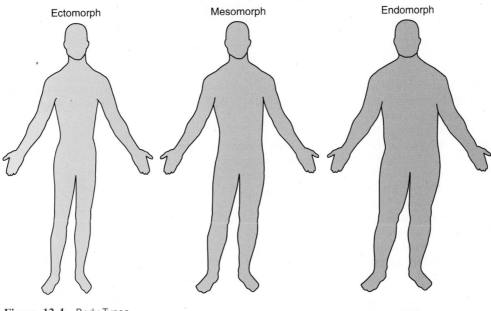

Ectomorph   Mesomorph   Endomorph

Figure 12-4 Body Types.

Measurements

Measure height. Measure the client's height by using the L-shaped measuring attachment on the balance scale. Instruct the client to stand shoeless on the balance scale platform with heels together and back straight and to look straight ahead. Raise the attachment above the client's head. Then lower it to the top of the client's head (Fig. 12-5). Record the client's height.

Height is within range for age, ethnic and genetic heritage. Children are usually within the range of parents' height.

Height begins to wane in the fifth decade of life because the intervertebral discs become thinner and spinal kyphosis increases.

Extreme shortness is seen in achondroplastic dwarfism and Turner's syndrome. Extreme tallness is seen in gigantism (excessive secretion of growth hormone) and in Marfan's syndrome.

continued

PHYSICAL ASSESSMENT *Continued*

Assessment Procedure	Normal Findings	Abnormal Findings

➤ **Clinical Tip** • *Without a scale, have the client stand shoeless with the back and heels against the wall. Balance a straight, level object (ruler) atop the client's head—parallel to the floor—and mark the object's position on the wall. Measure the distance between the mark and the floor. If the client cannot stand, measure the arm span to estimate height. Have the client stretch one arm straight out sideways. Measure from the tip of one middle finger to the tip of the nose. Multiply by 2 and record the arm span height.*

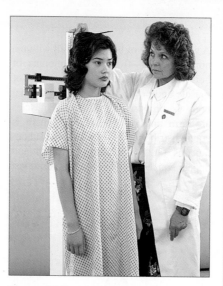

Figure 12-5 Measuring height. (© B. Proud.)

Measure weight. Level the balance beam scale at zero before weighing the client. Do this by moving the weights on the scale to zero and adjusting the knob by turning it until the balance beam is level. Ask the client to remove shoes and heavy outer clothing and to stand on the scale. Adjust the weights to the right and left until the balance beam is level again (Fig. 12-6). Record weight (2.2 lb = 1 kg). If you are weighing a client at home, you may have to use a scale with an automatically adjusting true zero.

Desirable weights for men and women are listed in the BMI table (see Table 12-4).

 Body weight may decrease with aging because of a loss of muscle or lean body tissue.

Weight does not fall within range of desirable weights for women and men.

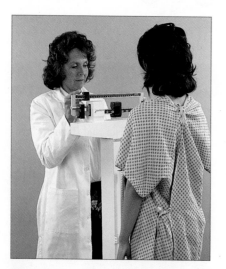

Figure 12-6 Measuring weight. (© B. Proud.)

continued

Assessment Procedure	Normal Findings	Abnormal Findings
Determine Ideal Body Weight (IBW) and percentage of IBW. Use this formula to calculate the client's IBW: *Female:* 100 lb for 5 ft + 5 lb for each inch over 5 ft ± 10% for small or large frame *Male:* 106 lb for 5 ft + 6 lb for each inch over 5 ft ± 10% for small or large frame. Calculate the client's percentage of IBW by the following formula: $$\frac{\text{actual weight}}{\text{IBW}} \times 100 = \%\text{IBW}$$	Body weight is within 10% of ideal range.	A current weight that is 80% to 90% of IBW indicates a lean client and possibly mild malnutrition. Weight that is 70% to 80% indicates moderate malnutrition; less than 70% may indicate severe malnutrition possibly from systemic disease, eating disorders, cancer therapies, and other problems. Weight exceeding 10% of the IBW range is considered overweight; weight exceeding 20% of IBW is considered obesity.
Measure Body Mass Index (BMI). Quickly determine BMI by accessing the National Institutes of Health's web site: http://nhlbisupport.com/bmi/bmicalc.htm or determine BMI using one of these formulas: $$\frac{\text{Weight in kilograms}}{\text{Height in meters}^2} = \text{BMI}$$ or $$\frac{\text{Weight in pounds}}{\text{Height in inches}^2} \times 703 = \text{BMI}$$	BMI is between 18.5 and 24.9 (see Table 12-1).	BMI <18.5 is considered underweight. BMI between 25.0 and 29.9 is considered overweight and increases risk for health problems. A BMI of 30 or greater is considered obese and places the client at a much higher risk for type 2 diabetes, cardiovascular disease, osteoarthritis, and sleep apnea.
Determine waist circumference. Have client stand straight with feet together and arms at sides. Place the measuring tape snuggly around the waist at the umbilicus, yet not compressing the skin (Fig. 12-7). Instruct the client to relax the abdomen and take a normal breath. When the client exhales, record the waist circumference. See Table 12-4 for an interpretation of waist circumference, BMI, and associated risks.	*Females:* Equal to or less than 35 inches (88 cm) *Males:* Equal to or less than 40 inches (102 cm) These findings are associated with reduced disease risk.	*Females:* Greater than 35 inches (88 cm) *Males:* Greater than 40 inches (102 cm) Adults with large visceral fat stores located mainly around the waist (android obesity) are more likely to develop health related problems than if the fat is located in the hips or thighs (gynoid obesity). These problems include an increased risk of type 2 diabetes, abnormal cholesterol and triglyceride levels, hypertension, and cardiovascular disease such as heart attack or stroke.
Measure mid-arm circumference (MAC). This evaluates skeletal muscle mass and fat stores. Have the client fully extend and dangle the nondominant arm freely next to the body. Locate the arm's midpoint (halfway between the top of the acromion process	Compare the client's current MAC to prior measurements and compare to the standard mid-arm circumference measurements for the client's age and sex listed in Table 12-5. Standard reference is 29.3 cm for men and 28.5 for women.	Measurements less than 90% of the standard reference are in the category of moderately malnourished. Less than 60% of the standard reference indicates sever malnourishment.

continued

PHYSICAL ASSESSMENT *Continued*

Assessment Procedure	Normal Findings	Abnormal Findings
and the olecranon process). Mark the midpoint and measure the MAC, holding the tape measure firmly around, but not pinching, the arm (Fig. 12-8). Record the measurement in centimeters. Refer to Table 12-5 to compare with the standard reference. For example: Record both the MAC and the standard reference number. "MAC = 25 cm; 88% of standard. Standard = 28.5" (25/28.5 = 88%)		
Measure triceps skinfold thickness (TSF). Take the TSF measurement to evaluate the degree of fat stores. Instruct the client to stand and hang the nondominant arm freely. Grasp the skinfold and subcutaneous fat between the thumb and forefinger midway between the	Compare the client's current measurement to past measurements and to the standard TSF measurements for the client's sex listed in Table 12-6. Standard reference is 12.5 mm for men and 16.5 mm for women.	Measurements less than 90% of the standard reference indicate a loss of fat stores and place the client in the moderately malnourished category. Less than 60% of the standard reference indicates severe malnourishment. Measurements greater than 120% of the standard indicate obesity.

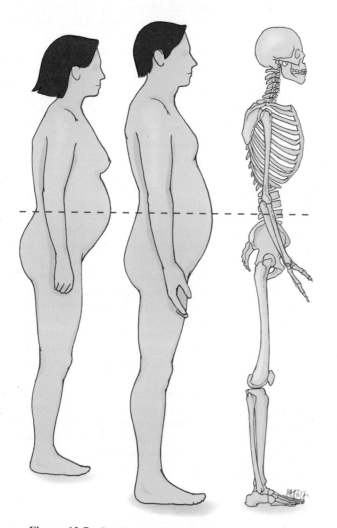

Figure 12-7 Positioning of measuring tape for waist circumference.

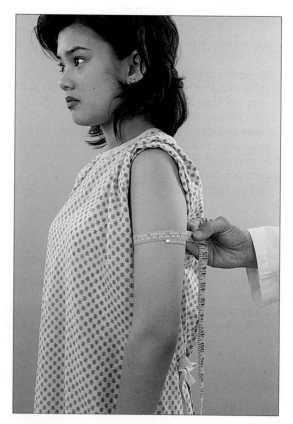

Figure 12-8 Measuring mid-arm circumference. (© B. Proud.)

continued

Assessment Procedure	Normal Findings	Abnormal Findings

acromion process and the tip of the elbow. Pull the skin away from the muscle (ask client to flex arm: If you feel a contraction with this maneuver, you still have the muscle) and apply the calipers (Fig. 12-9). Repeat three times and average the three measurements. Record the measurements in millimeters. Refer to Table 12-6 to compare with the standard reference. For example: Record both the TSF and the standard reference number: "TSF = 15mm; 91% of standard. Standard = 16.5" (15/16.5 = 91%).

➤ *Clinical Tip • A more accurate measurement can be obtained from the suprailiac region of the abdomen or the subscapular area.*

Calculate mid-arm muscle circumference (MAMC). To determine skeletal muscle reserves or the amount of lean body mass and evaluate malnourishment in clients, calculate the midarm muscle circumference (MAMC). MAMC is derived from MAC and TSF by the following formula:

$$MAMC = MAC(cm) - [0.314 \times TSF(mm)]$$

For example: Record the MAC and TSF and the standard reference number: "MAMC = 25 − [0.314 × 15] = 20.29; 87% of standard." Standard = 23.2. (20.29/23.2 = 87%).

➤ *Clinical Tip • When evaluating anthropometric data, base conclusions on a data cluster, not on individual findings. Factor in any special considerations and general health status. Although general standards are useful for making estimates, the client's overall health and well-being may be equal or more useful indicators of nutritional status.*

Compare the client's current MAMC to past measurements and to the data for MAMCs for the client's age and sex listed in Table 12-7. Standard reference is 25.3 cm for men and 23.2 cm for women.

The MAMC decreases to the lower percentiles with malnutrition and in obesity if TSF is high. If the MAMC is in a lower percentile and the TSF is in a higher percentile, the client may benefit from muscle-building exercises that increase muscle mass and decrease fat.

Malnutrition:

Mild—MAMC of 90% to 99%

Moderate—MAMC 60% to 90%

Severe—MAMC <60% as seen in protein-calorie malnutrition.

Table 12-5 Mid-arm Circumference (MAC) Standard Reference

Adult MAC (cm)	Standard Reference	90% of Standard Reference—Moderately Malnourished	60% of Standard Reference—Severely Malnourished
Men	29.3	26.3	17.6
Women	28.5	25.7	17.1

continued on page 167

PHYSICAL ASSESSMENT *Continued*

7Assessment Procedure	Normal Findings	Abnormal Findings

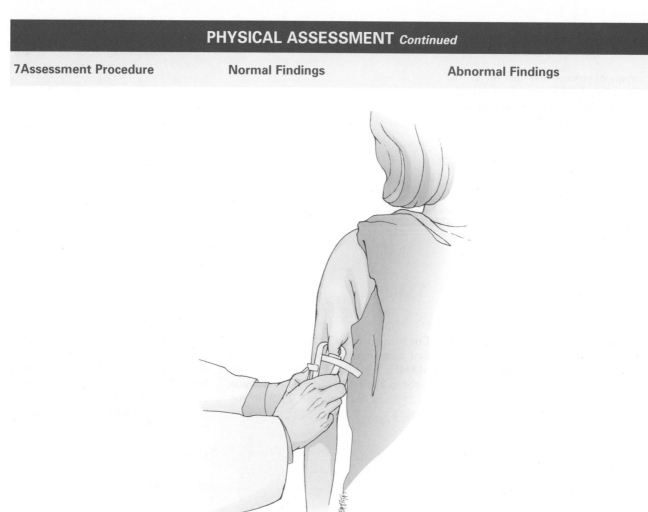

Figure 12-9 Measuring triceps skinfold thickness.

Table 12-6	Triceps Skinfold Thickness (TSF) Standard Reference		
Adult TSF (mm)	**Standard Reference**	**90% of Standard Reference— Moderately Malnourished**	**60% of Standard Reference— Severely Malnourished**
Men	12.5	11.3	7.5
Women	16.5	14.9	9.9

Table 12-7	Mid-arm Muscle Circumference (MAMC) Standard Reference		
Adult MAMC (cm)	**Standard Reference**	**90% of Standard Reference— Moderately Malnourished**	**60% of Standard Reference— Severely Malnourished**
Men	25.3	22.8	15.2
Women	23.2	20.9	13.9

continued

Assessment Procedure	Normal Findings	Abnormal Findings

Hydration

Inpatient Setting: Intake and Output **Measure intake and output (I & O) in inpatient settings.** Measure all fluids taken in by oral and parenteral routes, through irrigation tubes, as medications in solution, and through tube feedings. Also measure all fluid output (urine, stool, drainage from tubes, perspiration). Calculate insensible loss at 800 to 1000 mL daily, and add to total output.	Intake and output are closely balanced over 72 hours when insensible loss is included. ➤ *Clinical Tip • Fluid is normally retained during acute stress, illness, trauma, and surgery. Expect diuresis to occur in most clients in 48 to 72 hours.*	Imbalances in either direction suggest impaired organ function and fluid overload or inability to compensate for losses resulting in dehydration.
All Settings: Fluid-Related Changes **Weigh clients at risk for hydration changes daily.**	Weight is stable or changes less than 2 to 3 lb over 1 to 5 days.	Weight gains or losses of 6 to 10 lb in 1 week or less indicate a major fluid shift. A change of 2.2 lb (1 kg) is equal to a loss or gain of 1 L of fluid.
Check skin turgor. Pinch a small fold of skin, observing elasticity, and watch how quickly the skin returns to its original position.	There is no tenting and skin returns to original position.	Tenting can indicate fluid loss but is also present in malnutrition and loss of collagen in aged individuals. This finding must be correlated with other hydration findings.
Check for pitting edema.	No edema is present.	Pitting edema is a sign of fluid retention especially in cardiac and renal diseases.
Observe skin for moisture.	Skin is not excessively dry.	Abnormally dry and flaky skin. Corroborate such a finding with other findings because heredity and cholesterol and hormone levels determine skin moistness.
Assess venous filling. Lower the client's arm or leg and observe how long it takes to fill. Then raise the arm or leg and watch how long it takes to empty.	Veins fill in 3 to 5 seconds. Veins empty in 3 to 5 seconds.	Filling or emptying that takes more than 6 to 10 seconds suggests fluid volume deficit.
Observe neck veins with client in the supine position then with the head elevated above 45 degrees.	Neck veins are softly visible in supine position. With head elevated above 45 degrees, the neck veins flatten or are slightly visible but soft.	Flat veins in supine client may indicate dehydration. Visible firm neck veins indicate distention possibly resulting from fluid retention and heart disease.
Inspect the tongue's condition and furrows.	Tongue is moist, plump with central sulcus and no additional furrows.	Tongue is dry with visible papillae and several longitudinal furrows, suggesting loss of normal third-space fluid and dehydration.

continued

PHYSICAL ASSESSMENT Continued

Assessment Procedure	Normal Findings	Abnormal Findings
Gently palpate eyeball.	Eyeball is moderately firm to touch but not hard.	Eyeball is boggy and lacks normal tension, suggesting loss of normal third-space fluid and dehydration. ➤ **Clinical Tip** • *A hard eyeball is more indicative of eye disease than of hydration abnormalities.*
Observe eye position and surrounding coloration.	Eyes are not sunken and no dark circles appear under them.	Sunken eyes, especially with deep dark circles, point to dehydration.
Auscultate lung sounds.	No crackles, friction rubs, or harsh lung sounds are auscultated.	Loud or harsh breath sounds indicate decreased pleural fluid. Friction rubs may also be heard. Crackling indicates increased fluid, as in interstitial fluid sequestration, (i.e., pulmonary edema).
Take blood pressure with client in standing, sitting, and lying positions. Also palpate radial pulse.	There are no orthostatic changes; blood pressure and pulse rate remain within normal range for client's activity level and status.	Blood pressure registers lower than usual and/or drops more than 20 mmHg from lying to standing position, thereby indicating fluid volume deficit, especially if the pulse rate is also elevated. Radial pulse rate +1 and thready denotes dehydration. Elevated pulse rate and blood pressure indicate overhydration.

VALIDATING AND DOCUMENTING FINDINGS

Validate the nutritional assessment data you have collected. This is necessary to verify that the data are reliable and accurate. Following the health care facility or agency policy, document the assessment data.

Sample of Subjective Data

Sarah Bostic is a Caucasian female, stated age 42 years. Reports she had a fever for 2 days a week ago. Treated with Tylenol. No recurrences of fever. Lost 5 pounds over last 3 months with daily walking and low-fat diet. Drinks 4 to 6 glasses of water daily. Avoids concentrated sugars, alcohol, and caffeinated drinks. Has a bowl of cereal with skim milk and banana for breakfast; a sandwich of low-fat meat, cheese, lettuce and low-fat chips for lunch. Eats moderate amount of meat, rice, and vegetables for dinner. Reports one to two daily snacks of fruit, vegetables, pretzels, or popcorn. Allergic to seafood.

Sample of Objective Data

Well-developed body build for age with even distribution of fat and firm muscle. Height: 5 feet, 5 inches (165 cm); body frame: medium; weight: 128 lb (58 kg); BMI: 21.3; ideal body weight: 125; waist circumference 30 inches; MAC: 28 cm; TSF: 16.8 mm; MAMC: 22.7 cm.

Analysis of Data

DIAGNOSTIC REASONING: POSSIBLE CONCLUSIONS

After collecting subjective and objective data pertaining to the nutritional assessment, identify abnormal findings and client strengths. Then cluster the data to reveal any significant patterns or abnormalities. These data may then be used to make clinical judgments about the status of the client's nutritional health.

Selected Nursing Diagnoses

Following is a listing of selected nursing diagnoses (wellness, risk, or actual) that you may observe when analyzing the cue clusters.

Wellness Diagnoses

- Health-Seeking Behaviors related to desire and request to learn more about attaining ideal body weight
- Readiness for Enhanced Fluid Balance related to a desire for information pertaining to a need for increased fluids while shoveling snow

Risk Diagnoses

- Risk for Deficient Fluid Volume related to impending dehydration secondary to nausea and vomiting
- Risk for Imbalanced Fluid Volume related to lack of adequate home cooling system and high environmental temperatures forecasted
- Risk for Imbalanced Nutrition: More Than Body Requirements related to increasing sedentary lifestyle and decreasing metabolic demands

Actual Diagnoses

- Disturbed Body Image related to recent increase in weight
- Hopelessness related to inability to lose weight and remain on prescribed diet
- Impaired Swallowing related to muscle weakness and chewing difficulties secondary to a recent stroke
- Deficient Fluid Volume related to nausea and vomiting secondary to chemotherapy

- Excess Fluid Volume related to edema in ankles secondary to congestive heart failure
- Imbalanced Nutrition: More Than Body Requirements related to excessive caloric intake and sedentary lifestyle
- Imbalanced Nutrition: Less Than Body Requirements related to inadequate caloric/nutrient intake secondary to lack of access and ability to prepare or obtain nutritious foods to meet caloric and nutritive requirements

Selected Collaborative Problems

After grouping the data, certain collaborative problems may become apparent. Remember that collaborative problems differ from nursing diagnoses in that they cannot be prevented by nursing interventions. However, these physiologic complications of medical conditions can be detected and monitored by the nurse. In addition, the nurse can use physician- and nurse-prescribed interventions to minimize the complications of these problems. In such situations, the nurse may also have to refer the client for further treatment of the problem. Following is a list of collaborative problems that may be identified when obtaining a nutritional assessment. These problems are worded as Risk for Complications (or RC) followed by the problem.

- RC: Type 2 diabetes mellitus
- RC: Hypertension
- RC: Hyperlipidemia
- RC: Stroke

Medical Problems

After you group the data, it may become apparent that the client has signs and symptoms that require medical diagnosis and treatment. Refer to a primary care provider as necessary.

CASE STUDY

The case study demonstrates how to analyze nutritional assessment data for a specific client. The critical thinking exercises included in the study guide/lab manual and interactive product that complement this text also offer opportunities to analyze assessment data.

Mrs. Helen Jones, 78 years old, has a history of insulin-dependent diabetes mellitus (IDDM), also known as type 1 diabetes. When you weigh her during your weekly home visit, you find that she weighs 98 lb, which is 12 lb less than she weighed at your last visit. You try to weigh her at the same time of day each week—9:30 AM. She usually has breakfast at 6:30 AM and takes her morning NPH, 40 units at 7:30 AM. Today she tells you that she has been urinating "a lot" and that she feels like she has the flu for about 3 days with nausea and "just a little vomiting." She says she has not been eating well but adds, "I'm keeping my blood sugar up by drinking orange juice."

On assessment, you find that she has soft, sunken eyeballs and her tongue is dry and furrowed. Her blood pressure is 104/86 (usual is 150/88); her pulse is 92, and respirations are 22. Her temperature is 99.4°F. Her blood glucose level, tested by fingerstick, is 468 mg/dL (usual is 250 to 300 mg/dL). Mrs. Jones refuses to check her blood glucose level herself. When asked why she did not call the nurse or doctor when she became ill, she stated, "I didn't think it was that serious. I didn't have a high temperature."

The following concept map illustrates the diagnostic reasoning process.

continued on page 170

Applying COLDSPA

Applying **COLDSPA** for client symptoms: "urinating a lot and feels like she has a flu."

Mnemonic	Question	Data Provided	Missing Data
Character	Describe the sign or symptom (feeling, appearance, sound, smell, or taste if applicable).	12-lb weight loss; frequent urination; flu-like symptoms; nausea with some vomiting; soft, sunken eyeballs; dry, furrowed tongue; lower blood pressure than usual; increased respirations; low-grade fever; elevated blood glucose level, but not monitoring her glucose level (not eating much so reasons that she needs to keep "blood sugar up by drinking orange juice")	
Onset	When did it begin?	Began sometime after last week's visit. Reports 3 days of flu-like symptoms including nausea and vomiting.	
Location	Where is it? Does it radiate? Does it occur anywhere else?		Can you describe your flu-like symptoms? Are you thirsty? Are you having problems seeing?
Duration	How long does it last? Does it recur?		How often are you nauseated? How often do you urinate?
Severity	How bad is it? How much does it bother you?		How much do you urinate at a time? How much do you vomit at a time?
Pattern	What makes it better or worse?		What are you eating and when? How do you feel before you drink orange juice? How much juice do you have and how often? How much insulin are you taking and when do you take it?
Associated factors/How it **A**ffects the client	What other symptoms occur with it? How does it affect you?	Without a high fever, she didn't think her symptoms were very serious.	

1) Identify abnormal findings and client strengths

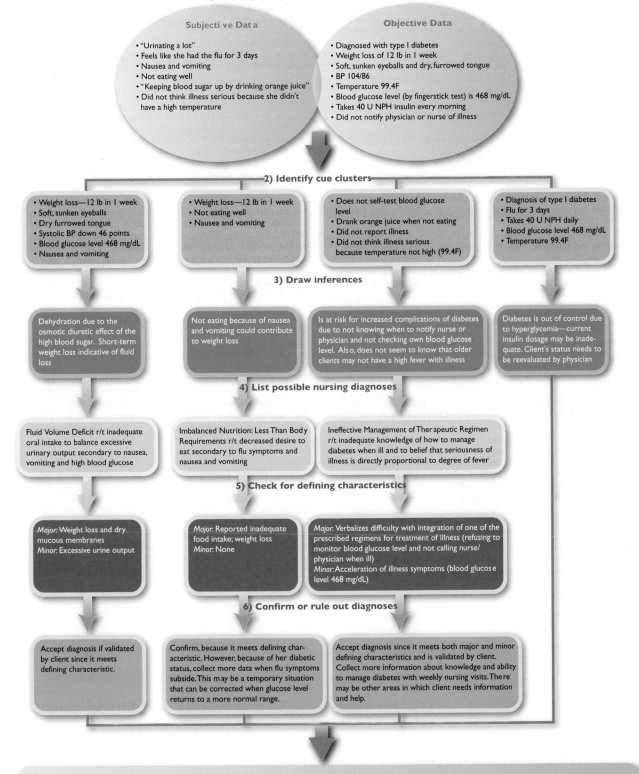

Subjective Data

- "Urinating a lot"
- Feels like she had the flu for 3 days
- Nausea and vomiting
- Not eating well
- "Keeping blood sugar up by drinking orange juice"
- Did not think illness serious because she didn't have a high temperature

Objective Data

- Diagnosed with type I diabetes
- Weight loss of 12 lb in 1 week
- Soft, sunken eyeballs and dry, furrowed tongue
- BP 104/86
- Temperature 99.4F
- Blood glucose level (by fingerstick test) is 468 mg/dL
- Takes 40 U NPH insulin every morning
- Did not notify physician or nurse of illness

2) Identify cue clusters

- Weight loss—12 lb in 1 week
- Soft, sunken eyeballs
- Dry furrowed tongue
- Systolic BP down 46 points
- Blood glucose level 468 mg/dL
- Nausea and vomiting

- Weight loss—12 lb in 1 week
- Not eating well
- Nausea and vomiting

- Does not self-test blood glucose level
- Drank orange juice when not eating
- Did not report illness
- Did not think illness serious because temperature not high (99.4F)

- Diagnosis of type I diabetes
- Flu for 3 days
- Takes 40 U NPH daily
- Blood glucose level 468 mg/dL
- Temperature 99.4F

3) Draw inferences

Dehydration due to the osmotic diuretic effect of the high blood sugar. Short-term weight loss indicative of fluid loss

Not eating because of nausea and vomiting could contribute to weight loss

Is at risk for increased complications of diabetes due to not knowing when to notify nurse or physician and not checking own blood glucose level. Also, does not seem to know that older clients may not have a high fever with illness

Diabetes is out of control due to hyperglycemia—current insulin dosage may be inadequate. Client's status needs to be reevaluated by physician

4) List possible nursing diagnoses

Fluid Volume Deficit r/t inadequate oral intake to balance excessive urinary output secondary to nausea, vomiting and high blood glucose

Imbalanced Nutrition: Less Than Body Requirements r/t decreased desire to eat secondary to flu symptoms and nausea and vomiting

Ineffective Management of Therapeutic Regimen r/t inadequate knowledge of how to manage diabetes when ill and to belief that seriousness of illness is directly proportional to degree of fever

5) Check for defining characteristics

Major: Weight loss and dry mucous membranes
Minor: Excessive urine output

Major: Reported inadequate food intake; weight loss
Minor: None

Major: Verbalizes difficulty with integration of one of the prescribed regimens for treatment of illness (refusing to monitor blood glucose level and not calling nurse/physician when ill)
Minor: Acceleration of illness symptoms (blood glucose level 468 mg/dL)

6) Confirm or rule out diagnoses

Accept diagnosis if validated by client since it meets defining characteristic.

Confirm, because it meets defining characteristic. However, because of her diabetic status, collect more data when flu symptoms subside. This may be a temporary situation that can be corrected when glucose level returns to a more normal range.

Accept diagnosis since it meets both major and minor defining characteristics and is validated by client. Collect more information about knowledge and ability to manage diabetes with weekly nursing visits. There may be other areas in which client needs information and help.

7) Document conclusions

Nursing diagnoses that are appropriate for this client include:

- Fluid Volume Deficit r/t oral intake inadequate to balance excessive urinary output secondary to nausea and vomiting and high blood glucose
- Imbalanced Nutrition: Less Than Body Requirements r/t decreased desire to eat secondary to flu symptoms and nausea and vomiting
- Ineffective Management of Therapeutic Regimen r/t inadequate knowledge of how to manage diabetes when ill and that seriousness of illness is directly proportional to degree of fever

Potential collaborative problems include the following:

Collaborative problems to be alert for include ketoacidosis, hyperglycemic hyperosmolar nonketotic (HHNK) syndrome, infection, vascular disease, diabetic retinopathy, diabetic neuropathy, and nephropathy. Mrs. Jones needs an immediate referral to her physician to manage the acute episode of hyperglycemia, to treat her "flu," and to evaluate her diabetic treatment regimen.

References and Selected Readings

American Cancer Society. Cancer prevention and early detection: Facts and figures. (2007). Atlanta, GA: Author. Available at http://www.cancer.org/docroot/stt/stt_0.asp

Department of Health and Human Services, Centers for Disease Control and Prevention (BMI Information and Calculations for Adults, Teens, and Children). Body mass index. Available at http://www.cdc.gov/nccdphp/dnpa/bmi/adult_BMI/about_adult_BMI.htm

Dewey, A., & Dean, T. (2007). Assessment and monitoring of nutritional status in patients with advanced cancer: Part 1. *International Journal of Palliative Nursing, 13*(6), 258–265.

Dudek, S. G. (2006). *Nutrition essentials for nursing practice* (5th ed.). Philadelphia: Lippincott Williams & Wilkins.

Health Canada, Food and Nutrition. Eating well with Canada's Food Guide. Available at http://www.hc-sc.gc.ca/fn-an/food-guide-aliment/index_e.html

Johnstone, C., Farley, A., & Hendry, C. (2006). Nurses' role in nutritional assessment and screening: Part one of a two-part series. *Nursing Times, 102*(49), 28–29.

Johnstone, C., Farley, A., & Hendry, C. (2007). Nurses' role in nutritional assessment and screening: Second of a two-part series. *Nursing Times, 102*(50), 28–29.

Kubrak, C., & Jensen, L. (2007). Malnutrition in acute care patients: A narrative review. *International Journal of Nursing Studies, 44*(6), 1036–1054.

McDonald, S. D. (2007). Management and prevention of obesity in adults and children. *Canadian Medical Association Journal, 176*(8), 1103–1106.

Meisinger, C., Thorand, B., Heier, M., & Lowel, H. (2006). Body fat distribution and risk of type 2 diabetes in the general population: Are there differences between men and women? The MONICA/KORA Augsburg cohort study. *American Journal of Clinical Nutrition, 84*(3), 483–489.

National Institutes of Health; National Heart, Lung, and Blood Institute. Calculate your body mass index. Available at http://nhlbisupport.com/bmi/bmicalc.htm

National Institutes of Health, National Heart, Lung, and Blood Institute, NHLBI Obesity Education Initiative, and the North American Association for the Study of Obesity (2000). The practice guide: Identification, evaluation, and treatment of overweight and obesity in adults. (NHI Publication No. 00-4084.) Washington, DC Available at http://www.nhlbi.nih.gov/guidelines/obesity

Nayer, B. H., Tubker, L., & Williams, S. (Eds.). (2007). *Nutrition made incredibly easy!* (2nd ed.). Philadelphia: Lippincott Williams & Wilkins.

Odencrants, S., Ehnfors, M., & Gorbe, S. J. (2007). Living with chronic obstructive pulmonary disease (COPD): Part II. RN's experience of nursing care for patients with COPD and impaired nutritional status. *Scandinavian Journal of Caring Sciences, 21*(1), 56–63.

Office of Disease Prevention and Health Promotion, U.S. Department of Health and Human Services. Healthy people 2010: Understanding and improving health. Washington, D.C. Available at http://www.healthypeople.gov/Document/

Poulsen, I., Peterson, H. V., Hallberg, I. R., & Schroll, M. (2007). Lack of nutritional and functional effects of nutritional supervision by nurses: A quasi-experimental study in geriatric patients. *Scandinavian Journal of Food & Nutrition, 51*(1), 6–12.

U.S. Centers for Disease Control, National Center for Chronic Disease Prevention and Health Promotion. (2007). Defining overweight and obesity. Available at http://www.cdc.gov.nccdphp/dnpa/obesity/

U.S. Department of Agriculture (USDA). Adult energy needs and BMI calculator. Baylor College of Medicine, Houston, TX. Available at http://www.bcm.edu/cnrc/caloriesneed.htm

U.S. Department of Agriculture (USDA) and Department of Health and Human Services. (2005). Dietary guidelines for Americans. Available at http://www.health.gov/dietaryguidelines

U.S. Department of Agriculture (USDA) and Department of Health and Human Services. (2005). Finding your way to a healthier you: Based on the dietary guidelines for Americans, 2005. (Publication No. 001-000-04718-3.) Available at http://www.healthierus.gov/dietaryguidelines

U.S. Department of Agriculture. MyPyramid food intake patterns. Available at http://www.mypyramid.gov/global_nav/pdf_food_intake.html

U.S. Department of Agriculture and Center for Nutrition Policy and Promotion. MyPyramid Tracker. Available at http://www.mypyramidtracker.gov/

Watts, S. A., & Anselmo, J. (2006). Nutrition for diabetes—all in a day's work. *Nursing 2006, 36*(6), 46–48.

Weight-control Information Network (WIN). An information service of the National Institutes of Diabetes and Digestive and Kidney Diseases (NIDDK). (2004). Statistics related to overweight and obesity, National Health and Nutrition Examination Survey (NHANES) 2001–2004. Available at http://win.niddk.nih.gov/publications/tools.htm#circumf

Weight-control Information Network (WIN), an information service of the National Institutes of Diabetes and Digestive and Kidney Diseases (NIDDK). Weight and waist measurement: Tools for adults. Available at http://win.niddk.nih.gov

Websites

American Diabetic Association, 216 W. Jackson Boulevard, Suite 800, Chicago, IL 60606; Consumer Nutrition Hotline: 800-366-1655. Available at http://www.eatright.org

American Heart Association, 7320 Greenville Ave., Dallas, TX 75231; National Center: 214-373-6300, Nutrition Information: 214-706-1179. Available at http://americanheart.org

National Cancer Institute, Cancer Information Service, 9000 Rockville Pike, Building 31, Room 10A-24, Bethesda, MD 20892; 1-800-4-CANCER. Available at http://www.cancer.gov/

Nursing Assessment of Physical Systems

13

Skin, Hair, and Nails

Structure and Function

The skin, hair, and nails are external structures that serve a variety of specialized functions. The sebaceous and sweat glands originating within the skin also have many vital functions. Each structure's function is described separately.

SKIN

The skin is composed of three layers: the epidermis, dermis, and subcutaneous tissue (Fig. 13-1a). The skin is thicker on the palms of the hands and soles of the feet and is continuous with the mucous membranes at the orifices of the body. Subcutaneous tissue, which contains varying amounts of fat, connects the skin to underlying structures.

The skin is a physical barrier that protects the underlying tissues and structures from microorganisms, physical trauma, ultraviolet radiation, and dehydration. It plays a vital role in temperature maintenance, fluid and electrolyte balance, absorption, excretion, sensation, immunity, and vitamin D synthesis. The skin also provides an individual identity to a person's appearance.

Epidermis

The **epidermis** (Fig. 13-1b), the outer layer of skin, is composed of four distinct layers: the **stratum corneum, stratum lucidum, stratum granulosum,** and **stratum germinativum.** The outermost layer consists of dead, keratinized cells that render the skin waterproof. (Keratin is a scleroprotein that is insoluble in water. The epidermis, hair, nails, dental enamel, and horny tissues are composed of keratin.) The epidermal layer is almost completely replaced every 3 to 4 weeks. The innermost layer of the epidermis (stratum germinativum) is the only layer that undergoes cell division and contains melanin (brown pigment) and keratin-forming cells. Skin color depends on the amount of melanin and carotene (yellow pigment) contained in the skin and the volume of blood containing hemoglobin, the oxygen-binding pigment that circulates in the dermis.

Dermis

The inner layer of skin is the **dermis** (see Fig. 13-1). It is connected to the epidermis by means of papillae. These papillae form the base for the visible swirls or friction ridges that provide the unique pattern of fingerprints with which we are familiar. Ridges also appear on the palms of the hands, the toes, and the soles of the feet. The dermis is a well-vascularized connective tissue layer containing collagen and elastic fibers, nerve endings, and lymph vessels. It is also the origin of hair follicles, sebaceous glands, and sweat glands.

Sebaceous Glands

The **sebaceous glands** (see Fig. 13-1a) develop from hair follicles and, therefore, are present over most of the body, excluding the soles and palms. They secrete an oily substance called **sebum** that lubricates hair and skin and reduces water loss through the skin. Sebum also has some fungicidal and bactericidal effects.

Sweat Glands

Sweat glands (see Fig. 13-1a) are of two types: eccrine and apocrine. The **eccrine glands** are located over the entire skin surface and secrete an odorless, colorless fluid, the evaporation of which is vital to the regulation of body temperature. The **apocrine glands** are concentrated in the axillae, perineum, and areolae of the breast and are usually open through a hair follicle. They secrete a milky sweat. The interaction of sweat with skin bacteria produces a characteristic body odor. Apocrine glands are dormant until puberty, at which time they become active. In women, apocrine secretions are linked with the menstrual cycle.

Subcutaneous Tissue

Merging with the dermis is the **subcutaneous tissue,** which is a loose connective tissue containing fat cells, blood vessels, nerves, and the remaining portions of sweat glands and hair follicles (see Fig. 13-1a). The subcutaneous tissue assists with heat regulation and contains the vascular pathways for

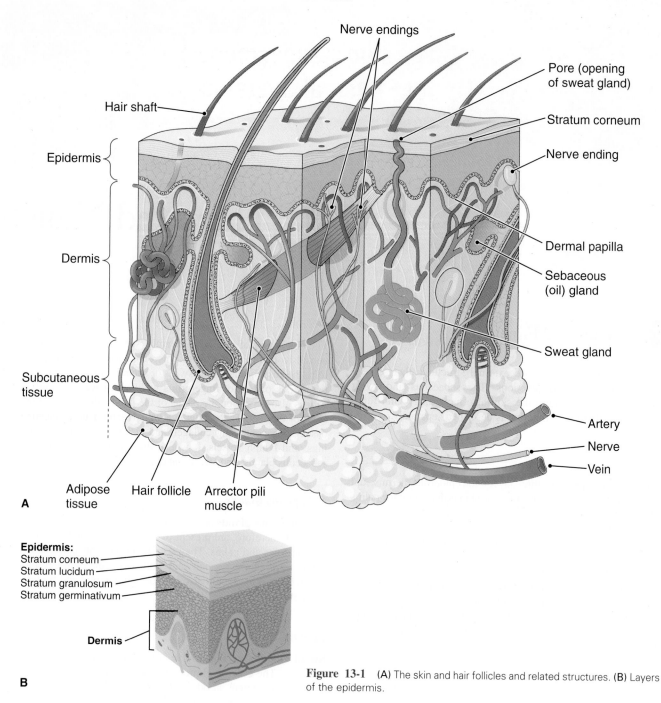

Nerve endings

Hair shaft

Epidermis

Dermis

Subcutaneous tissue

A

Adipose tissue

Hair follicle

Arrector pili muscle

Pore (opening of sweat gland)

Stratum corneum

Nerve ending

Dermal papilla

Sebaceous (oil) gland

Sweat gland

Artery

Nerve

Vein

Epidermis:
Stratum corneum
Stratum lucidum
Stratum granulosum
Stratum germinativum

Dermis

B

Figure 13-1 **(A)** The skin and hair follicles and related structures. **(B)** Layers of the epidermis.

the supply of nutrients and removal of waste products from the skin.

HAIR

Hair consists of layers of keratinized cells and is found over much of the body except for the lips, nipples, soles of the feet, palms of the hands, labia minora, and penis. Hair develops within a sheath of epidermal cells called the **hair follicle.** Hair growth occurs at the base of the follicle, where cells in the hair bulb are nourished by dermal blood vessels. The hair shaft is visible above the skin; the hair root is surrounded by the hair follicle (see Fig. 13-1). Attached to the follicle are the erector pili muscles, which contract in response to cold or

fright, decreasing skin surface area and causing the hair to stand erect.

There are two general types of hair: vellus and terminal. **Vellus hair** is short, pale, and fine and is present over much of the body. The **terminal hair** (particularly scalp and eyebrows) is longer, generally darker, and coarser than the vellus hair. Puberty initiates the growth of additional terminal hair in both sexes on the axillae, perineum, and legs. Hair color varies and is determined by the type and amount of pigment production. The absence of pigment or the inclusion of air spaces within the layers of the hair shaft results in gray or white hair.

Hair serves useful functions. Scalp hair is a protective covering. Nasal hair and ear hair, as well as eyelashes and eyebrows, filter dust and other airborne debris.

NAILS

The nails, located on the distal phalanges of fingers and toes, are hard, transparent plates of keratinized epidermal cells that grow from a root underneath the skin fold called the **cuticle** (Fig. 13-2). The **nail body** extends over the entire nailbed and has a pink tinge as a result of the rich blood supply underneath. At the base of the nail is the **lunula,** a paler, crescent-shaped area. The nails protect the distal ends of the fingers and toes.

Health Assessment

COLLECTING SUBJECTIVE DATA: THE NURSING HEALTH HISTORY

Diseases and disorders of the skin, hair, and nails can be local or they may be caused by an underlying systemic problem. To perform a complete and accurate assessment, the nurse needs to collect data about current symptoms, the client's past and family history, and lifestyle and health practices. The information obtained provides clues to the client's overall level of functioning in relation to the skin, hair, and nails.

When interviewing a client for information regarding skin, hair, and nails, ask questions in a straightforward manner. Keep in mind that a nonjudgmental and sensitive approach is needed if the client has abnormalities that may be associated with poor

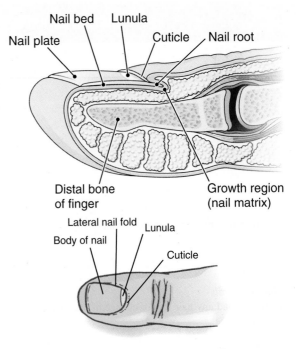

Figure 13-2   The nail and related structures.

hygiene or unhealthful behaviors. Also, some skin disorders might be highly visible and potentially damaging to the person's body image and self-concept.

(text continues on page 180)

HISTORY OF PRESENT HEALTH CONCERN

Question	Rationale
Skin Are you experiencing any current skin problems such as rashes, lesions, dryness, oiliness, drainage, bruising, swelling, or increased pigmentation? What aggravates the problem? What relieves it?	Any of these symptoms may be related to a pathologic skin condition. Bruises, welts, or burns may indicate accidents or trauma or abuse. If these injuries cannot be explained or the client's explanation seems unbelievable or vague, physical abuse should be suspected. Dry, itchy skin is a common concern in obese clients (Brown et al., 2004).
Describe any birthmarks or moles you now have. Have any of them changed color, size, or shape?	You need to know what is normal for the client so that future variations can be detected. A change in the appearance or bleeding of any skin mark, especially a mole, may indicate cancer. Asymmetry, irregular borders, color variations, diameter greater than 0.5 cm, and elevation are characteristics of cancerous lesions.
Have you noticed any change in your ability to feel pain, pressure, light touch, or temperature changes? Are you experiencing any pain, itching, tingling, or numbness?	Changes in sensation may indicate vascular or neurologic problems such as peripheral neuropathy related to diabetes mellitus or arterial occlusive disease. Sensation problems may put the client at risk for developing pressure ulcers (see Promote Health—Pressure Ulcers).
Do you have trouble controlling body odor? How much do you perspire?	Uncontrolled body odor or excessive or insufficient perspiration may indicate an abnormality with the sweat glands or an endocrine problem such as hypothyroidism or hyperthyroidism. Poor hygiene practices may account for body odor, and health education may be indicated.

continued on page 176

HISTORY OF PRESENT HEALTH CONCERN *Continued*

Question	Rationale
	Perspiration decreases with aging because sweat gland activity decreases.
	Because of decreased sweat production, most Asians and Native Americans have mild to no body odor, whereas Caucasians and African Americans tend to have a strong body odor (Andrews & Boyle, 1999) unless they use antiperspirant or deodorant products. Any strong body odor may indicate an abnormality.
Do you have any body piercings or tattoos?	Piercing needles place clients at risk for infection. Tattooing pigments can cause allergic reactions, keloids, and scars. Clients should be informed regarding these risks. Piercings and tatoos are gaining popularity.
Hair and Nails Have you had any hair loss or change in the condition of your hair? Describe.	Patchy hair loss may accompany infections, stress, hairstyles that put stress on hair roots, and some types of chemotherapy. Generalized hair loss may be seen in various systemic illnesses such as hypothyroidism and in clients receiving certain types of chemotherapy or radiation therapy.
	A receding hairline or male pattern baldness may occur with aging.
Have you had any change in the condition or appearance of your nails? Describe.	Nail changes may be seen in systemic disorders such as malnutrition or with local irritation (e.g., nail biting). (See Promote Health—Nail Infections.)
	Bacterial infections cause green, black, or brown nail discoloration. Yellow, thick, crumbling nails are seen in fungal infections. Yeast infections cause a white color and separation of the nail plate from the nail bed.

continued on page 178

COLDSPA Example

Use the **COLDSPA** mnemonic as a guideline to collect needed information for each symptom the client shares. In addition, the following questions help elicit important information.

Mnemonic	Question	Client Response Example
Character	Describe the sign or symptom (feeling, appearance, sound, smell, or taste if applicable).	Small, ¼ inch diameter raised brown spot
Onset	When did it begin?	3 months ago
Location	Where is it? Does it radiate? Does it occur anywhere else?	"On my right cheek next to my nose. I have had one like it on my lower back for a year."
Duration	How long does it last? Does it recur?	"It never goes away."
Severity	How bad is it? How much does it bother you?	"It scares me that it may be cancer."
Pattern	What makes it better or worse?	"I cover the one on my face with a cosmetic. It bleeds if I scrub it."
Associated factors/How it **A**ffects the client	What other symptoms occur with it? How does it affect you?	"It is ugly and embarrassing. It itches sometimes."

PROMOTE HEALTH

Pressure Ulcers

Overview

Pressure ulcers are one of the most preventable skin problems. When a patient develops a pressure ulcer while in a medical facility, it is usually due to nurses not assessing skin adequately and not teaching or following preventive procedures. Prevalence of pressure ulcers ranges from 10% to 17% in acute care, from 0% to 17% in home care, and from 2.2% to 23.9% in long-term care facilities (Ayello, 2004). Since pressure ulcers are extremely expensive to treat, both for the patient and for the medical facility, it is essential that

nurses learn how to assess for and prevent them. Ulcers can lead to sepsis and even to death.

For an initial assessment of the potential to develop a pressure ulcer, use the Braden Scale (see Assessment Tool 13-1).

Conditions that lead to pressure ulcers:

- Pressure
- Shear
- Friction

Assess Risk Factors

- Perception: inability to perceive pressure
- Mobility: inability to move self, decreased activity level, unable to reposition
- Moisture: diaphoresis, incontinences, sweating from climate
- Nutrition: deficient (especially protein deficit) or excessive (obesity)
- Friction or shear against surfaces
- Tissue tolerance decreased: age, vascular incompetence, blood sugar levels of diabetes mellitus, body weight/malnutrition

Teach Risk Reduction Tips

- Inspect the skin at least daily and more often if at greater risk using risk assessment tool (such as Braden Scale or PUSH tool) and keep a flow chart to document
- Bathe with mild soap or other agent; limit friction; use warm not hot water; set a bath schedule that is individualized
- For dry skin: use moisturizers; avoid low humidity and cold air
- Avoid vigorous massage

- Use careful positioning, turning, and transferring techniques to avoid shear and friction or prolonged pressure on any point
- Refer nutritional supplementation needs to primary care provider or dietitian, especially if protein deficient
- Refer incontinence condition to primary care provider
- Use incontinence skin cleansing methods as needed: frequency and methods of cleaning, avoiding dryness with protective barrier products

For bed- or chair-bound patients:

- Reposition or teach to self-reposition every 15 minutes (chair) or 2 hours (bed)
- Use repositioning schedule
- Use pressure mattress or chair cushion
- Use lifting devices if available to reduce shear
- Use positioning with pillows or wedges to avoid bony prominence contact with surfaces and to maintain body alignment
- For bed bound, avoid elevated head of bed except for brief periods

Provide structured teaching for patient, family, and caregivers as necessary.

PROMOTE HEALTH

Nail Infections

Overview

Nails, both toe and fingernails, are susceptible to infections with bacteria and fungi. Infections occur along the nail skin fold (paronychia), between the nail plate and the nail bed, or in the nail bed. Many other abnormal conditions cause nail changes; however, nail infections are often preventable. There are differences in how common conditions affect the nail. For instance, bacterial infections such as pseudomonas

cause a green, brown, or black discoloration with thickening and crumbling of the nail plate, and often separation of the plate from the bed. Yeast infections cause a white color in the nail plate and may involve separation but without the debris or crumbling seen in the other conditions. When a nail is injured and a hematoma forms, blood accumulates under the plate and can allow infections to enter (see Abnormal Findings 13-7).

Assess Risk Factors

- Nails in moist environment, especially walking in damp public locales (swimming pools, showers) or continuously wearing closed shoes; excessive perspiration

- Nail injury, trauma, or irritation (tight footwear, exercise trauma, artificial nails, excessive hand washing, nail biting)
- Repeated irritation (especially water, detergents)

PROMOTE HEALTH

Nail Infections *Continued*

- Immune system disorders such as diabetes mellitus and AIDS, or being on immunosuppressive medications
- Skin conditions such as psoriasis or lichen
- Some trades or professions (damp environments or shoe type required)
- Contagion from one digit to another or one person to another
- Possibly family predisposition

Teach Risk Reduction Tips
- Wear leather shoes except for sports
- Avoid wearing closed shoes all the time
- Wear socks that wick away moisture
- Avoid going barefoot in damp public areas
- Avoid too much perspiration or water (wear gloves on hands)
- Avoid trauma to nails
- Avoid unsanitary or unsafe nail care practices
- If treatment has been started, do not stop until recovery is complete

PAST HEALTH HISTORY

Question	Rationale
Describe any previous problems with skin, hair, or nails, including any treatment or surgery and its effectiveness.	Current problems may be a recurrence of previous ones. Visible scars may be explained by previous problems.
Have you ever had any allergic skin reactions to food, medications, plants, or other environmental substances?	Various types of allergens can precipitate a variety of skin eruptions.
Have you had a fever, nausea, vomiting, gastrointestinal (GI), or respiratory problems?	Some skin rashes or lesions may be related to viruses or bacteria.
For female clients: Are you pregnant? Are your menstrual periods regular?	Some skin and hair conditions can result from hormonal imbalance.
For male clients: Do you have a history of smoking and/or drinking alcohol?	A significant association between cigarette smoking, alcohol consumption, and psoriatic males has been found (Al-Rubaiy & Al-Rubiah, 2006).
Do you have a history of anxiety, depression, or any psychiatric problems?	Over one-third of dermatologic disorders have significant psychiatric comorbidity (Gupta, Gupta, Ellis, & Koblenzer, 2005). Depression often occurs in association with dermatologic disease (Fried, Gupta, & Gupta, 2005).

FAMILY HISTORY

Question	Rationale
Has anyone in your family had a recent illness, rash, or other skin problem or allergy? Describe.	Acne and atopic dermatitis tend to be familial. Viruses (e.g., chickenpox, measles) can be highly contagious. Some allergies may be identified from family history.
Has anyone in your family had skin cancer?	A genetic component is associated with skin cancer, especially malignant melanoma (see Promote Health—Skin Cancer).
Do you have a family history of keloids?	Ear piercing, if desired, should be performed before age 11 if there is a history to avoid keloid formation (Lane, Waller, & Davis, 2005).

continued

LIFESTYLE AND HEALTH PRACTICES

Question	Rationale
Do you sunbathe? How much sun or tanning-booth exposure do you get? What type of protection do you use?	Sun exposure can cause premature aging of skin and increase the risk of cancer. Hair can also be damaged by too much sun.
In your daily activities, are you regularly exposed to chemicals that may harm the skin (e.g., paint, bleach, cleaning products, weed killers, insect repellents, petroleum)?	Any of these substances have the potential to irritate or damage the skin, hair, or nails.
Do you spend long periods of time sitting or lying in one position?	Older, disabled, or immobile clients who spend long periods of time in one position are at risk for pressure ulcers.
Have you had any exposure to extreme temperatures?	Temperature extremes affect the blood supply to the skin and can damage the skin layers. Examples include frostbite and burns.
What is your daily routine for skin, hair, and nail care? What products do you use (e.g., soaps, lotions, oils, cosmetics, self-tanning products, razor type, hair spray, shampoo, coloring, nail enamel)? How do you cut your nails?	Regular habits provide information on hygiene and lifestyle. The products used may also be a cause of an abnormality. Improper nail-cutting technique can lead to ingrown nails or infection. Decreased flexibility and mobility may impair the ability of some elderly clients to maintain proper hygiene practices, such as nail cutting, bathing, and hair care.
What kinds of foods do you consume in a typical day? How much fluid do you drink each day?	A balanced diet is necessary for healthy skin, hair, and nails. Adequate fluid intake is required to maintain skin elasticity.
Do skin problems limit any of your normal activities?	Certain activities such as hiking, camping, and gardening may expose the client to allergens such as poison ivy. Moreover, exposure to the sun can aggravate conditions such as scleroderma. In addition, general home maintenance (e.g., cleaning, car washing) may expose the client to certain cleaning products to which he is sensitive or allergic.
Describe any skin disorder that prevents you from enjoying your relationships.	Skin, hair, or nail problems, especially if visible, may impair the client's ability to interact comfortably with others because of embarrassment or rejection by others. Social stigma toward some dermatologic disorders is widespread in Indian society (Chaturvedi, Singh, & Gupta, 2005).
How much stress do you have in your life? Describe.	Stress can cause or exacerbate skin abnormalities.
Do you perform a skin self-examination once a month?	If clients do not know how to inspect the skin, teach them how to recognize suspicious lesions early. (Self Assessment 13-1).

PROMOTE HEALTH

Skin Cancer

Overview

Skin cancer is the most common of cancers. It occurs in three types: melanoma, basal cell carcinoma (BCC), and squamous cell carcinoma (SCC). BCC and SCC are nonmelanomas. BCC is the most common skin cancer in whites and SCC in darker skin. Blacks and Hispanics, as well as whites, are susceptible to melanoma (Hu et al., 2004). Asians are less susceptible to skin cancers (Lee & Lim, 2003).

Nonmelanocyte skin cancers are the most common worldwide and are also increasing in populations heavily exposed to sunlight, especially in areas of ozone depletion. Malignant melanoma is the most serious skin cancer. It is the most rapidly increasing form of cancer in the United States with approximately 55,100 cases diagnosed in 2004 (CDC, 2007).

Intermittent exposure to the sun or ultraviolet radiation is associated with greatest risk for melanoma and for BCC, but overall amount of exposure is thought to be associated with SCC. SCC is most common on body sites with very heavy sun exposure, whereas BCC is most common on sites with moderate exposure (e.g., upper trunk or women's lower legs).

Precursor lesions occur for some melanomas (benign or dysplastic nevi) and for invasive SCC (actinic keratoses or SCC in situ) but there are no precursor lesions for BCC.

continued on page 180

PROMOTE HEALTH
Skin Cancer *Continued*

Assess Risk Factors

- Sun exposure, especially intermittent pattern with sunburn; risk increases if excessive sun exposure and sunburns began in childhood
- Nonsolar sources of ultraviolet radiation (tanning booth, sunlamps, high-UV geographical areas)
- Medical therapies such as PUBA and ionizing radiation
- Family or personal history and genetic susceptibility (especially for malignant melanoma)
- Moles, especially atypical lesions
- Pigmentation irregularities (albinism, burn scars)
- Fair skin that burns and freckles easily; light hair; light eyes
- Age; risk increases with increasing age
- Actinic keratoses
- Male gender (for nonmelanoma cancers)
- Chemical exposure (arsenic, tar, coal, paraffin, some oils for nonmelanoma cancers)
- Human papillomavirus (nonmelanoma cancers)
- Xeroderma pigmentosum (rare, inherited condition)
- Long-term skin inflammation or injury (nonmelanoma)
- Alcohol intake (BCC); smoking (SCC)
- Inadequate niacin (vitamin B_3) in diet
- Bowen's disease (scaly or thickened patch) (SCC)
- Depressed immune system

Teach Risk Reduction Tips
(For All Clients Including Asians and African Americans)

- Reduce sun exposure; seek shade
- Always use sunscreen (SPF 15 or higher) when sun exposure is anticipated.
- Wear long-sleeved shirts and wide-brimmed hats.
- Wear sunglasses that wrap around.
- Avoid sunburns.
- Understand the link between sun exposure and skin cancer and the accumulating effects of sun exposure on developing cancers.
- Examine the skin for suspected lesions. If there is anything unusual, seek professional advice as soon as possible. Use the ABCDE mnemonic to assess suspicious lesions.

    Asymmetry
    Border
    Color
    Diameter
    Elevation

(See Abnormal Findings 13-5)

- Have annual skin cancer screenings by a professional.
- Ensure diet is adequate in vitamin B_3.
- Talk with primary care provider about taking a vitamin D supplement (Lappe et al., 2007).

COLLECTING OBJECTIVE DATA: PHYSICAL EXAMINATION

Physical assessment of the skin, hair, and nails provides the nurse with data that may reveal local or systemic problems or alterations in a client's self-care activities. Local irritation, trauma, or disease can alter the condition of the skin, hair, or nails. Systemic problems related to impaired circulation, endocrine imbalances, allergic reactions, or respiratory disorders may also be revealed with alterations in the skin, hair, or nails. The appearance of the skin, hair, and nails also provides the nurse with data related to health maintenance and self-care activities such as hygiene, exercise, and nutrition.

A separate, comprehensive skin, hair, and nail examination, preferably at the beginning of a comprehensive physical examination, ensures that you do not inadvertently omit part of the examination. As you inspect and palpate the skin, hair, and nails, pay special attention to lesions and growths.

Preparing the Client

To prepare for the skin, hair, and nail examination, ask the client to remove all clothing and jewelry and put on an examination gown. In addition, ask the client to remove nail enamel, artificial nails, wigs, toupees, or hairpieces as appropriate.

Have the client sit comfortably on the examination table or bed for the beginning of the examination. The client may remain in a sitting position for most of the examination. However, to assess the skin on the buttocks and dorsal surfaces of the legs properly, the client may lie on her side or abdomen.

During the skin examination, ensure privacy by exposing only the body part being examined. Make sure that the room is a comfortable temperature. If available, sunlight is best for inspecting the skin. However, a bright light that can be focused on the client works just as well. Keep the room door closed or the

(text continues on page 182)

SELF-ASSESSMENT 13-1 How to Examine Your Own Skin

Coupled with a yearly skin exam by a doctor, self-examination of your skin once a month is the best way to detect early warning signs of the three main types of skin cancer: basal cell carcinoma, squamous cell carcinoma, and melanoma. *Look for a new growth or any skin change.*

What you'll need: a bright light, a full-length mirror, a hand mirror, 2 chairs or stools, a blow dryer, body maps and a pencil.

Examine your face, especially the nose, lips, mouth, and ears – front and back. Use one or both mirrors to get a clear view.

Thoroughly inspect your scalp, using a blow dryer and mirror to expose each section to view. Get a friend or family member to help, if you can.

Check your hands carefully: palms and backs, between the fingers and under the fingernails. Continue up the wrists to examine both front and back of your forearms.

Standing in front of the full-length mirror, begin at the elbows and scan all sides of your upper arms. Don't forget the underarms

Next focus on the neck, chest, and torso. Women should lift breasts to view the underside.

With your back to the full-length mirror, use the hand mirror to inspect the back of your neck, shoulders, upper back, and any part of the back of your upper arms you could not view in step 4.

Still using both mirrors, scan your lower back, buttocks, and backs of both legs.

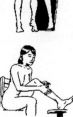

Sit down; prop each leg in turn on the other stool or chair. Use the hand mirror to examine the genitals. Check front and sides of both legs, thigh to shin, ankles, tops of feet, between toes and under toenails. Examine soles of feet and heels.

(Used with permission from The Skin Cancer Foundation. http://www.skincancer.org/step-by-step-self-examination.html)

bed curtain drawn to provide privacy as necessary. Explain what you are going to do, and answer any questions the client may have. Wear gloves when palpating any lesions because you may be exposed to drainage.

Clients from conservative religious groups (e.g., Orthodox Jews or Muslims) may require that the nurse be the same sex as the client. Also, to respect the client's modesty or desire for privacy, provide a long examination gown or robe.

Equipment

- Examination light
- Penlight
- Mirror for client's self-examination of skin
- Magnifying glass
- Centimeter ruler
- Gloves

- Wood's light
- Examination gown or drape
- Braden Scale for Predicting Pressure Sore Risk
- Pressure Ulcer Scale for Healing (PUSH) tool to measure pressure ulcer healing

Physical Assessment

When preparing to examine the skin, hair, and nails, remember these key points:

- Inspect skin color, temperature, moisture, texture.
- Check skin integrity.
- Be alert for skin lesions.
- Evaluate hair condition; loss or unusual growth.
- Note nail bed condition and capillary refill.

(text continues on page 203)

PHYSICAL ASSESSMENT

Assessment Procedure	Normal Findings	Abnormal Findings

Skin

Inspection

Inspect general skin coloration (Fig. 13-3). Keep in mind that the amount of pigment in the skin accounts for the intensity of color as well as hue.

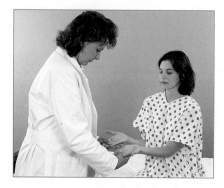

Figure 13-3 Inspecting the palms is an opportunity to assess overall coloration. (© B. Proud.)

Inspection reveals evenly colored skin tones without unusual or prominent discolorations.

Small amounts of melanin are common in whiter skins, while large amounts of melanin are common in olive and darker skins. Carotene accounts for a yellow cast.

👓 The older client's skin becomes pale due to decreased melanin production and decreased dermal vascularity.

Pallor (loss of color) is seen in arterial insufficiency, decreased blood supply, and anemia. Pallid tones vary from pale to ashen without underlying pink.

Cyanosis (Fig. 13-4A) may cause white skin to appear blue-tinged, especially in the perioral, nailbed, and conjunctival areas. Dark skin may appear blue, dull and lifeless in the same areas.

Central cyanosis results from a cardiopulmonary problem whereas peripheral cyanosis may be a local problem resulting from vasoconstriction.

To differentiate between central and peripheral cyanosis, look for central cyanosis in the oral mucosa.

Jaundice (Fig. 13-4B) in light- and dark-skinned people is characterized by yellow skin tones, from pale to pumpkin, particularly in the sclera, oral mucosa, palms, and soles.

Acanthosis nigricans (Fig. 13-4C) is roughening and darkening of skin in localized areas, especially the posterior neck (Stuart et al., 1999).

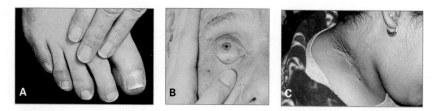

Figure 13-4 Abnormal findings for skin coloration: **(A)** Bluish cyanotic skin associated with oxygen deficiency. **(B)** Jaundice associated with hepatic dysfunction. **(C)** Acanthosis nigricans (AN), a linear streak-like pattern in dark-skinned people, suggests diabetes mellitus. (Source: Goodheart, H. P. [1999]. *A photoguide of common skin disorders: Diagnosis and management.* Baltimore: Williams & Wilkins.)

continued

Assessment Procedure	Normal Findings	Abnormal Findings
While inspecting skin coloration, note any odors emanating from the skin.	Client has slight or no odor of perspiration, depending on activity.	A strong odor of perspiration or foul odor may indicate disorder of sweat glands. Poor hygiene practices may indicate a need for client teaching or assistance with activities of daily living.
Inspect for color variations. Inspect localized parts of the body, noting any color variation.	Keep in mind that some clients have suntanned areas, freckles, or white patches known as vitiligo (Common Variations 13-1). The variations are due to different amounts of melanin in certain areas. A generalized loss of pigmentation is seen in albinism. Dark-skinned clients have lighter-colored palms, soles, nailbeds, and lips. Frecklelike or dark streaks of pigmentation are also common in the sclera and nailbeds of dark-skinned clients.	Abnormal findings include rashes, such as the reddish (in light-skinned people) or darkened (in dark-skinned people) butterfly rash across the bridge of the nose and cheeks (Fig. 13-5), characteristic of discoid lupus erythematosus (DLE). **Albinism** is a generalized loss of pigmentation. **Erythema** (skin redness and warmth) is seen in inflammation, allergic reactions, or trauma.
	White-skinned clients have darker pigment around nipples, lips, and genitalia.	Erythema in the dark-skinned client may be difficult to see. However, the affected skin feels swollen and warmer than the surrounding skin.
Check skin integrity, especially carefully in pressure point areas (see Fig. 13-6). Use the Braden Scale (see Assessment Tool 13-1) to predict pressure sore risk. If any skin breakdown is noted, use the PUSH tool (see Assessment Tool 13-2) to document the degree of skin breakdown. ➤ *Clinical Tip* • *In the obese client, carefully inspect skin on the limbs, under breasts, and in the groin area where problems are frequent.*	Skin is intact, and there are no reddened areas.	Skin breakdown is initially noted as a reddened area on the skin that may progress to serious and painful pressure ulcers (see Abnormal Findings 13-1 for stages of pressure ulcer development). Depending on the color of the client's skin, reddened areas may not be prominent, although the skin may feel warmer in the area of breakdown than elsewhere.
Inspect for lesions. Observe the skin surface to detect abnormalities. Note color, shape, and size of lesion. For very small lesions, use a magnifying glass to note these characteristics.	Smooth, without lesions. Stretch marks (striae), healed scars, freckles, moles, or birthmarks are common findings (see Common Variations 13-1).	Lesions may indicate local or systemic problems. Primary lesions (Abnormal Findings 13-2) arise from normal skin due to irritation or disease. Secondary lesions (Abnormal Findings 13-3) arise

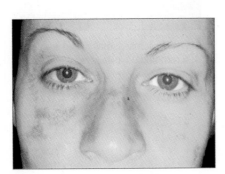

Figure 13-5 Characteristic butterfly rash of lupus erythematosus.

continued on page 189

Common Variations 13-1   Common Skin Variations

Many skin assessment findings are considered normal variations in that they are not health- or life-threatening. For example, freckles are common variations in fair-skinned clients, whereas unspotted skin is considered the ideal. Scars and vitiligo, on the other hand, are not exactly normal findings because scars suggest a healed injury or surgical intervention and vitiligo may be related to a dysfunction of the immune system. However, they are common and usually insignificant. Other common findings appear below.

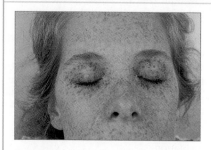
Freckles—flat, small macules of pigment that appear following sun exposure. (© B. Proud.)

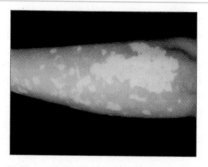
Vitiligo of forearm in an African American client. (Courtesy Neutrogena Care Institute.)

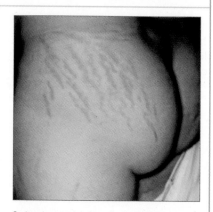
Striae (sometimes called stretch marks). (Courtesy E. R. Squibb.)

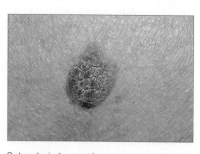
Seborrheic keratosis, a warty or crusty pigmented lesion. (With permission from Goodheart, H. P. [1999]. *A photo guide of common skin disorders: Diagnosis and management*. Baltimore: Williams & Wilkins.)

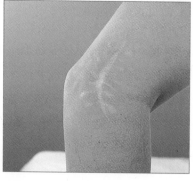
Scar.

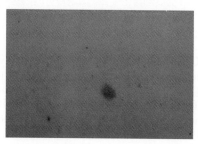
Mole (also called nevus), a flat or raised tan/brownish marking up to 6 mm wide.

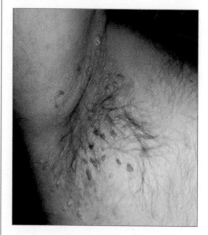
Cutaneous tags, raised yellow papules with a depressed center. (Courtesy of Steifel Laboratories, Inc.)

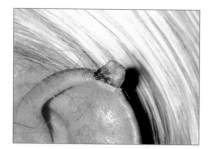
Cutaneous horn.

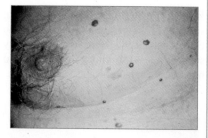
Cherry angiomas, small raised spots (1–5 mm wide) typically seen with aging.

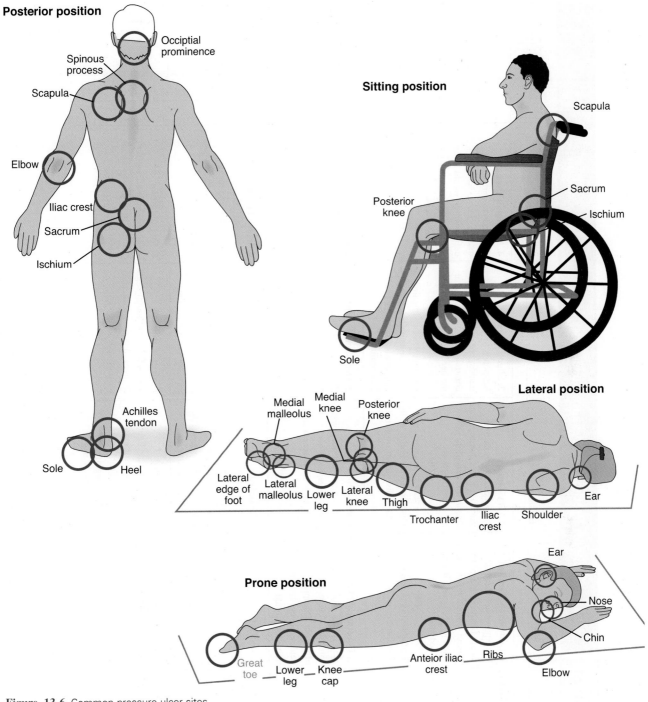

Posterior position

Occipital prominence
Spinous process
Scapula
Elbow
Iliac crest
Sacrum
Ischium
Achilles tendon
Sole
Heel

Sitting position

Scapula
Sacrum
Ischium
Posterior knee
Sole

Lateral position

Medial malleolus
Medial knee
Posterior knee
Lateral edge of foot
Lateral malleolus
Lower leg
Lateral knee
Thigh
Trochanter
Iliac crest
Shoulder
Ear

Prone position

Ear
Nose
Chin
Elbow
Great toe
Lower leg
Knee cap
Anteior iliac crest
Ribs

Figure 13-6 Common pressure ulcer sites.

ASSESSMENT TOOL 13-1   Braden Scale for Predicting Pressure Sore Risk

Patient's Name _____   Evaluator's Name _____   Date of Assessment

	1	2	3	4				
SENSORY PERCEPTION Ability to respond meaningfully to pressure-related discomfort	**1. Completely Limited** Unresponsive (does not moan, flinch, or grasp) to painful stimuli, due to diminished level of consciousness or sedation OR limited ability to feel pain over most of body.	**2. Very Limited** Responds only to painful stimuli. Cannot communicate discomfort except by moaning or restlessness OR has a sensory impairment which limits the ability to feel pain or discomfort over half of body.	**3. Slightly Limited** Responds to verbal commands, but cannot always communicate discomfort of the need to be turned. OR has some sensory impairment which limits ability to feel pain or discomfort in 1 or 2 extremities.	**4. No Impairment** Responds to verbal commands. Has no sensory deficit which would limit ability to feel or voice pain or discomfort.				
MOISTURE Degree to which skin is exposed to moisture	**1. Constantly Moist** Skin is kept moist almost constantly by perspiration, urine, etc. Dampness is detected every time patient is moved or turned.	**2. Very Moist** Skin is often, but not always moist. Linen must be changed at least once a shift.	**3. Occasionally Moist** Skin is occasionally moist, requiring an extra linen change approximately once a day.	**4. Rarely Moist** Skin is usually dry. Linen only requires changing at routine intervals.				
ACTIVITY Degree of physical activity	**1. Bedfast** Confined to bed.	**2. Chairfast** Ability to walk severely limited or non-existent. Cannot bear own weight and/or must be assisted into chair or wheelchair.	**3. Walks Occasionally** Walks occasionally during day, but for very short distances, with or without assistance. Spends majority of each shift in bed or chair.	**4. Walks Frequently** Walks outside room at least twice a day and inside room at least once every two hours during waking hours.				
MOBILITY Ability to change and control body position	**1. Completely Immobile** Does not make even slight changes in body or extremity position without assistance.	**2. Very Limited** Makes occasional slight changes in body or extremity position but unable to make frequent or significant changes independently.	**3. Slightly Limited** Makes frequent though slight changes in body or extremity position independently.	**4. No Limitation** Makes major and frequent changes in position without assistance.				

NUTRITION Usual food intake pattern	**1. Very Poor** Never eats a complete meal. Rarely eats more than half of any food offered. Eats 2 servings or less of protein (meat or dairy products) per day. Takes fluids poorly. Does not take a liquid dietary supplement OR Is NPO and/or maintained on clear liquids or IVs for more than 5 days.	**2. Probably Inadequate** Rarely eats a complete meal and generally eats only about half of any food offered. Protein intake includes only 3 servings of meat or dairy products per day. Occasionally will take a dietary supplement. OR Receives less than optimum amount of liquid diet or tube feeding.	**3. Adequate** Eats over half of most meals. Eats a total of 4 servings of protein (meat, dairy products) per day. Occasionally will refuse a meal, but will usually take a supplement when offered OR Is on a tube feeding or TPN regimen which probably meets most nutritional needs.	**4. Excellent** Eats most of every meal. Never refuses a meal. Usually eats a total of 4 or more servings of meat and dairy products. Occasionally eats between meals. Does not require supplementation.
FRICTION AND SHEAR	**1. Problem** Requires moderate to maximum assistance in moving. Complete lifting without sliding against sheets is impossible. Frequently slides down in bed or chair, requiring frequent repositioning with maximum assistance. Spasticity, contractures, or agitation leads to almost constant friction.	**2. Potential Problem** Moves feebly or requires minimum assistance. During a move skin probably slides to some extent against sheets, chair, restraints, or other devices. Maintains relatively good position in chair or bed most of the time but occasionally slides down.	**3. No Apparent Problem** Moves in bed and in chair independently and has sufficient muscle strength to lift up completely during move. Maintains good position in bed or chair.	
				Total Score

(Copyright: Barbara Braden and Nancy Bergstrom, 1988. Reprinted with permission.)

ASSESSMENT TOOL 13-2 | **PUSH Tool to Measure Pressure Ulcer Healing**

PUSH Tool 3.0

Patient Name _____ Patient ID# _____

Ulcer Location _____ Date _____

Directions:

Observe and measure the pressure ulcer. Categorize the ulcer with respect to surface area, exudate, and type of wound tissue. Record a sub-score for each of these ulcer characteristics.

Add the sub-scores to obtain the total score. A comparison of total scores measured over time provides an indication of the improvement or deterioration in pressure ulcer healing.

LENGTH × WIDTH (in cm²)	0	1	2	3	4	5	Sub-score
	0	<0.3	0.3−0.6	0.7−1.0	1.1−2.0	2.1−3.0	
		6	7	8	9	10	
		3.1−4.0	4.1−8.0	8.1−12.0	12.1−24.0	>24.0	
EXUDATE AMOUNT	0	1	2	3			Sub-score
	None	Light	Moderate	Heavy			
TISSUE TYPE	0	1	2	3	4		Sub-score
	Closed	Epithelial Tissue	Granulation Tissue	Slough	Necrotic Tissue		
							TOTAL SCORE

Length × Width: Measure the greatest length (head to toe) and the greatest width (side to side) using a centimeter ruler. Multiply these two measurements (length × width) to obtain an estimate of surface area in square centimeters (cm²). Caveat: Do not guess! Always use a centimeter ruler and always use the same method each time the ulcer is measured.

Exudate Amount: Estimate the amount of exudate (drainage) present after removal of the dressing and before applying any topical agent to the ulcer. Estimate the exudate (drainage) as none, light, moderate, or heavy.

Tissue Type: This refers to the types of tissue that are present in the wound (ulcer) bed. Score as a "4" if there is any necrotic tissue present. Score as a "3" if there is any amount of slough present and necrotic tissue is absent. Score as a "2" if the wound is clean and contains granulation tissue. A superficial

wound that is reepithelializing is scored as a "1". When the wound is closed, score as a "0".

4 – Necrotic Tissue (Eschar): black, brown, or tan tissue that adheres firmly to the wound bed or ulcer edges and may be either firmer or softer than surrounding skin.

3 – Slough: yellow or white tissue that adheres to the ulcer bed in strings or thick clumps, or is mucinous.

2 – Granulation Tissue: pink or beefy red tissue with a shiny, moist, granular appearance.

1 – Epithelial Tissue: for superficial ulcers, new pink or shiny tissue (skin) that grows in from the edges or as islands on the ulcer surface.

0 – Closed/Resurfaced: the wound is completely covered with epithelium (new skin).

Source: National Pressure Ulcer Advisory Panel. www.npuap.org/PDF/**push**3.pdf.

Assessment Procedure	Normal Findings	Abnormal Findings
➤ **Clinical Tip** • *When examining female or obese clients, lift the breasts (or ask the client to lift them) and skin folds to inspect all areas for lesions. Perspiration and friction often cause skin problems in these areas in obese clients (Brown et al., 2004).*	Older clients may have skin lesions because of aging. Some examples are seborrheic or senile keratoses, senile lentigines, cherry angiomas, purpura, and cutaneous tags and horns.	from changes in primary lesions. Vascular lesions (Abnormal Findings 13-4), reddish-bluish lesions, are seen with bleeding, venous pressure, aging, liver disease, or pregnancy. Skin cancer lesions can be either primary or secondary lesions and are classified as squamous cell carcinoma, basal cell carcinoma, or malignant melanoma (Abnormal Findings 13-5).
If you suspect a fungus, shine a Wood's light (an ultraviolet light filtered through a special glass) on the lesion.	Lesion does not fluoresce.	Blue-green fluorescence indicates fungal infection.
If you observe a lesion, note its location, distribution, and configuration. Measure the lesion with a centimeter ruler.	Normal lesions may be moles, freckles, birthmarks, and the like. They may be scattered over the skin in no particular pattern.	In abnormal findings, distribution may be diffuse (scattered all over), localized to one area, or in sun-exposed areas. Configuration (see Abnormal Findings 13-6) may be discrete (separate and distinct), grouped (clustered), confluent (merged), linear (in a line), annular and arciform (circular or arcing), or zosteriform (linear along a nerve route).
Palpation **Palpate skin to assess texture.** Use the palmar surface of your three middle fingers to palpate skin texture.	Skin is smooth and even.	Rough, flaky, dry skin is seen in hypothyroidism. Obese clients often report dry, itchy skin.
Palpate to assess thickness. If lesions are noted when assessing skin thickness, put gloves on and palpate the lesion between the thumb and finger. Observe for drainage or other characteristics.	Skin is normally thin but calluses (rough, thick sections of epidermis) are common on areas of the body that are exposed to constant pressure.	Very thin skin may be seen in clients with arterial insufficiency or in those on steroid therapy.
Palpate to assess moisture. Check under skin folds and in unexposed areas.	Skin surfaces vary from moist to dry depending on the area assessed. Recent activity or a warm environment may cause increased moisture.	Increased moisture or diaphoresis (profuse sweating) may occur in conditions such as fever or hyperthyroidism. Decreased moisture occurs with dehydration or hypothyroidism.
➤ **Clinical Tip** • *Some nurses believe that using the dorsal surfaces of the hands to assess moisture leads to a more accurate result.*	The older client's skin may feel dryer than a younger client's skin because sebum production decreases with age.	Clammy skin is typical in shock or hypotension.
Palpate to assess temperature. Use the dorsal surfaces of your hands to palpate the skin (Fig. 13-7).	Skin is normally a warm temperature.	Cold skin may accompany shock or hypotension. Cool skin may accompany arterial disease. Very warm skin may indicate a febrile state or hyperthyroidism.
➤ **Clinical Tip** • *You may also want to palpate with the palmar surfaces of your hands because current research indicates that these surfaces of the hands and fingers may be more sensitive to temperature (Cantwell-Gab, 1996).*		

continued

PHYSICAL ASSESSMENT *Continued*

Assessment Procedure	Normal Findings	Abnormal Findings

Palpate to assess mobility and turgor.
Ask the client to lie down. Using two fingers, gently pinch the skin on the sternum or under the clavicle (Fig. 13-8). *Mobility* refers to how easily the skin can be pinched. *Turgor* refers to the skin's elasticity and how quickly the skin returns to its original shape after being pinched.

Skin pinches easily and immediately returns to its original position.

⊙⊙ The older client's skin loses its turgor because of a decrease in elasticity and collagen fibers. Sagging or wrinkled skin appears in the facial, breast, and scrotal areas.

Decreased mobility is seen with edema. Decreased turgor (a slow return of the skin to its normal state taking longer than 30 seconds) is seen in dehydration.

Palpate to detect edema. Use your thumbs to press down on the skin of the feet or ankles to check for edema (swelling related to accumulation of fluid in the tissue).

Skin rebounds and does not remain indented when pressure is released.

Indentations on the skin may vary from slight to great and may be in one area or all over the body. See Chapter 21, Peripheral Vascular System, for a full discussion of edema.

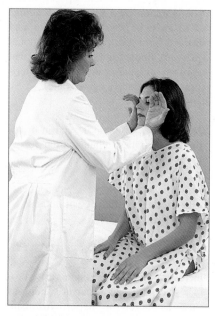

Figure 13-7 Assessing temperature and moisture. (© B. Proud.)

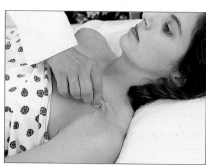

Figure 13-8 Palpating to assess skin turgor and mobility. (© B. Proud.)

Scalp and Hair

Inspection and Palpation
Have the client remove any hair clips, hair pins, or wigs. **Then inspect the scalp and hair for general color and condition.**

Natural hair color, as opposed to chemically colored hair, varies among clients from pale blond to black to gray or white. The color is determined by the amount of melanin present.

⊙⊙ Nutritional deficiencies may cause patchy gray hair in some clients. Severe malnutrition in African-American children may cause a copper-red hair color (Andrews & Boyle, 1999).

continued

Assessment Procedure	Normal Findings	Abnormal Findings
At 1-inch intervals, separate the hair from the scalp and inspect and palpate the hair and scalp for cleanliness, dryness or oiliness, parasites, and lesions (Fig. 13-9). Wear gloves if lesions are suspected or if hygiene is poor.	Scalp is clean and dry. Sparse dandruff may be visible. Hair is smooth and firm, somewhat elastic. However, as people age, hair feels coarser and drier. Individuals of black African descent often have very dry scalps and dry, fragile hair, which the client may condition with oil or a petroleum jelly-like product. (This kind of hair is of genetic origin and not related to thyroid disorders or nutrition. Such hair needs to be handled very gently.)	Excessive scaliness may indicate dermatitis. Raised lesions may indicate infections or tumor growth. Dull, dry hair may be seen with hypothyroidism and malnutrition. Poor hygiene may indicate a need for client teaching or assistance with activities of daily living. Pustules with hair loss in patches are seen in tinea capitis, a contagious fungal disease (ringworm, Fig. 13-10). Infections of the hair follicle (folliculitis) appear as pustules surrounded by erythema (Fig. 13-11).

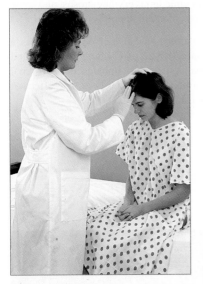

Figure 13-9 Inspecting the scalp and hair. (© B. Proud.)

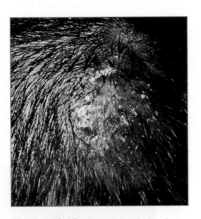

Figure 13-10 Tinea capitis (scalp ringworm).

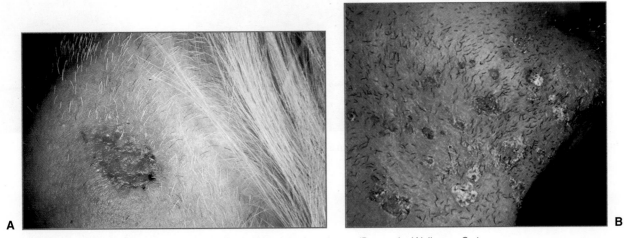

Figure 13-11 **(A)** Folliculitis of the scalp. **(B)** Folliculitis of the beard area. (Burroughs Wellcome Co.)

continued

PHYSICAL ASSESSMENT *Continued*

Assessment Procedure	Normal Findings	Abnormal Findings
Inspect amount and distribution of scalp, body, axillae, and pubic hair. Look for unusual growth elsewhere on the body.	Varying amounts of terminal hair cover the scalp, axillary, body, and pubic areas according to normal gender distribution. Fine vellus hair covers the entire body except for the soles, palms, lips, and nipples. Normal male pattern balding is symmetric (Fig. 13-12). Older clients have thinner hair because of a decrease in hair follicles. Pubic, axillary, and body hair also decrease with aging. Alopecia is seen, especially in men. Hair loss occurs from the periphery of the scalp and moves to the center. Elderly women may have terminal hair growth on the chin owing to hormonal changes.	Excessive generalized hair loss may occur with infection, nutritional deficiencies, hormonal disorders, thyroid or liver disease, drug toxicity, hepatic or renal failure (Sabbagh, 1999). It may also result from chemotherapy or radiation therapy. Patchy hair loss (Fig. 13-13) may result from infections of the scalp, discoid or systemic lupus erythematosus, and some types of chemotherapy. Hirsutism (facial hair on females) is a characteristic of Cushing's disease and results from an imbalance of adrenal hormones or it may be a side effect of steroids.

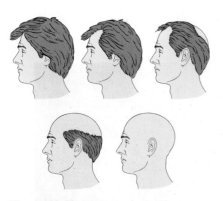

Figure 13-12   Male pattern balding.

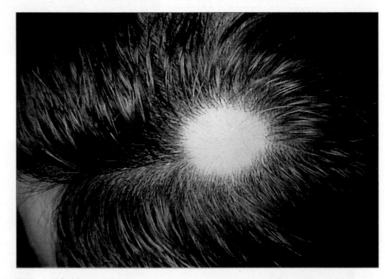

Figure 13-13   Patchy hair loss. (Courtesy Neutrogena Skin Care Institute.)

Nails

Inspection		
Inspect nail grooming and cleanliness.	Nails are clean and manicured.	Dirty, broken, or jagged fingernails may be seen with poor hygiene. They may also result from the client's hobby or occupation.

continued

Assessment Procedure	Normal Findings	Abnormal Findings
Inspect nail color and markings.	Pink tones should be seen. Some longitudinal ridging is normal. Dark-skinned clients may have freckles or pigmented streaks in their nails.	Pale or cyanotic nails may indicate hypoxia or anemia. Splinter hemorrhages may be caused by trauma. Beau's lines occur after acute illness and eventually grow out. Yellow discoloration may be seen in fungal infections or psoriasis. Nail pitting is also common in psoriasis (Abnormal Findings 13-7).
Inspect shape of nails.	There is normally a 160-degree angle between the nail base and the skin.	Early clubbing (180-degree angle with spongy sensation) and late clubbing (greater than 180-degree angle) can occur from hypoxia. Spoon nails (concave) may be present with iron deficiency anemia (Abnormal Findings 13-7).
Palpation **Palpate nail to assess texture.**	Nails are hard and basically immobile. Dark-skinned clients may have thicker nails. Older clients' nails may appear thickened, yellow, and brittle because of decreased circulation in the extremities.	Thickened nails (especially toenails) may be caused by decreased circulation.
Palpate to assess texture and consistency, noting whether nailplate is attached to nailbed.	Nails are smooth and firm; nailplate should be firmly attached to nailbed.	Paronychia (inflammation) indicates local infection. Detachment of nailplate from nailbed (onycholysis) is seen in infections or trauma.
Test capillary refill in nailbeds by pressing the nail tip briefly and watching for color change (Fig. 13-14).	Pink tone returns immediately to blanched nailbeds when pressure is released.	There is slow (greater than 2 seconds) capillary nailbed refill (return of pink tone) with respiratory or cardiovascular diseases that cause hypoxia.

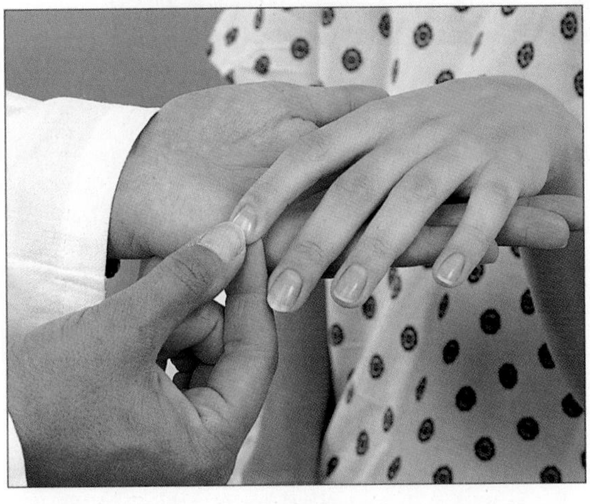

Figure 13-14   Testing capillary refill. (© B. Proud.)

Abnormal Findings 13-1   Identification of Pressure Ulcer Stage

During any skin assessment, the nurse remains watchful for signs of skin breakdown, especially in cases of limited mobility or fragile skin (e.g., in elderly or bedridden clients). Pressure ulcers, which lead to complications such as infection, are easier to prevent than to treat. Some risk factors for skin breakdown leading to pressure ulcers include poor circulation, poor hygiene, infrequent position changes, dermatitis, infection, or traumatic wounds. The stages of pressure ulcers appear below.

Stage I

Intact skin with nonblanchable redness of a localized area usually over a bony prominence. Darkly pigmented skin may not have visible blanching; its color may differ from the surrounding area. The area may be painful, firm, soft, warmer, or cooler as compared to adjacent tissue. Stage I may be difficult to detect in individuals with dark skin tones.

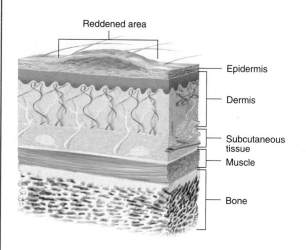

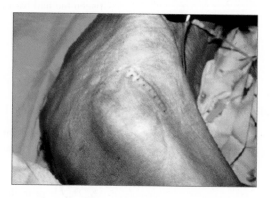

Stage II

Partial thickness loss of dermis presenting as a shallow open ulcer with a red-pink wound bed, without slough. May also present as an intact or open/ruptured serum-filled blister. Presents as a shiny or dry shallow ulcer without slough or bruising; bruising indicates suspected deep tissue injury. This stage should not be used to describe skin tears, tape burns, perineal dermatitis, maceration, or excoriation.

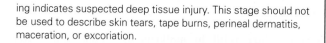

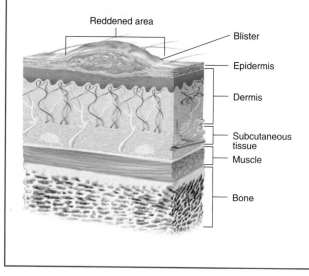

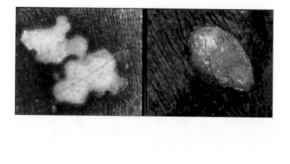

continued

Stage III

Full-thickness tissue loss. Subcutaneous fat may be visible but bone, tendon, or muscle is not exposed. Slough may be present but does not obscure the depth of tissue loss. May include undermining and tunneling. The depth of a stage III pressure ulcer varies by anatomical location. The bridge of the nose, ear, occiput, and malleolus do not have subcutaneous tissue, and stage III ulcers can be shallow. In contrast, areas of significant adiposity can develop extremely deep stage III pressure ulcers. Bone/tendon is not visible or directly palpable.

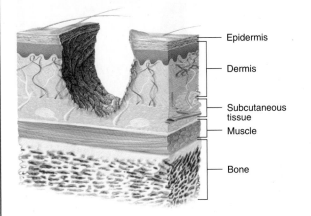

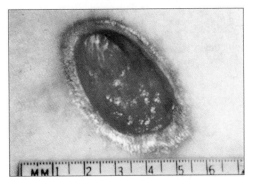

Epidermis

Dermis

Subcutaneous tissue

Muscle

Bone

Stage IV

Full-thickness tissue loss with exposed bone, tendon, or muscle. Slough or eschar may be present on some parts of the wound bed. Often includes undermining and tunneling. The depth of a stage IV pressure ulcer varies by anatomical location (see stage III). Stage IV ulcers can extend into muscle and/or supporting structures (e.g., fascia, tendon, or joint capsule) making osteomyelitis possible. Exposed bone/tendon is visible or directly palpable.

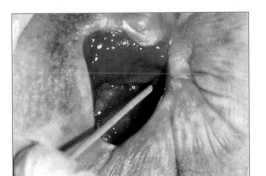

Epidermis

Dermis

Subcutaneous tissue

Muscle

Bone

Unstageable

Full-thickness tissue loss in which the base of the ulcer is covered by slough (yellow, tan, gray, green, or brown) and/or eschar (tan, brown, or black) in the wound bed. Until enough slough and/or eschar is removed to expose the base of the wound, the true depth, and therefore stage, cannot be determined. Stable (dry, adherent, intact without erythema or fluctuance) eschar on the heels serves as "the body's natural (biological) cover" and should not be removed.

(Text Source: National Pressure Ulcer Advisory Panel [2007]. Available at www.npuap.org/pr2.htm)

Abnormal Findings 13-2   Primary Skin Lesions

Primary skin lesions are original lesions arising from previously normal skin. Secondary lesions can originate from primary lesions.

Type and Description	Examples	Illustration	Photograph of Example
Macule, Patch • Flat, non-palpable skin color change (skin color may be brown, white, tan, purple, red) • Macule: < 1 cm, circumscribed border • Patch: > 1 cm, may have irregular border	• Freckles • Flat moles • Petechiae • Rubella • Vitiligo • Port wine stains • Ecchymosis	Macule Patch	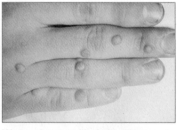 Ecchymoses (from prolonged topical corticosteroid use).
Papule. Plaque • Elevated, palpable, solid mass; circumscribed border • Papule: < 0.5 cm • Plaque: > 0.5 cm (may be coalesced papules with flat top)	Papules: • Elevated nevi • Warts • Lichen planus Plaques: • Psoriasis • Actinic keratosis	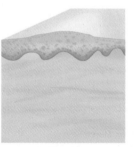Papule 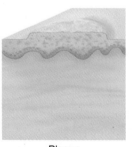Plaque	Warts, circumscribed elevations caused by a virus. (Courtesy of Reed and Carnick Pharmaceuticals.) 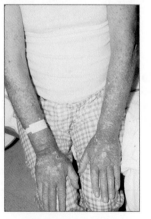Actinic Keratoses

continued

Abnormal Findings 13-2 | **Primary Skin Lesions** *Continued*

Type and Description	Examples	Illustration	Photograph of Example

Nodule, Tumor

- Elevated, solid, palpable mass
- Extends deeper into dermis than a papule
- Nodule: 0.5–2 cm; circumscribed
- Tumor: > 1–2 cm; does not always have sharp borders

Nodules:
- Lipoma
- Squamous cell carcinoma
- Poorly absorbed injection
- Dermatofibroma

Tumors:
- Larger lipoma
- Carcinoma

Nodule

Tumor

Lipomas. Multiple rubbery flesh-colored nodules are palpable on this patient.
(Source: Goodheart, H.G. [2005]. *Goodheart's Photo guide of common skin disorders.* Philadelphia: Lippincott Williams & Wilkins.)

Vesicle, Bulla

- Circumscribed elevated, palpable mass containing serous fluid
- Vesicle: < 0.5 cm
- Bulla: > 0.5 cm

Vesicles:
- Herpes simplex/zoster
- Varicella (chickenpox)
- Poison ivy
- Second-degree burn

Bulla:
- Pemphigus, contact dermatitis, large burn blisters, poison ivy, bullous impetigo

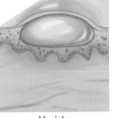

Vesicle

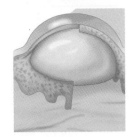

Bulla

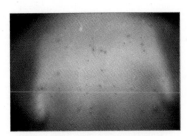

Varicella. Vesicles and crusts.
(Source: Goodheart, H.G. [2005]. *Goodheart's Photo guide of common skin disorders.* Philadelphia: Lippincott Williams & Wilkins.)

continued on page 198

Abnormal Findings 13-2 **Primary Skin Lesions** *Continued*

Type and Description	Examples	Illustration	Photograph of Example
Wheal • Elevated mass with transient borders • Often irregular • Size and color vary • Caused by movement of serous fluid into the dermis • Does not contain free fluid in a cavity (e.g., vesicle)	• Urticaria (hives) • Insect bites	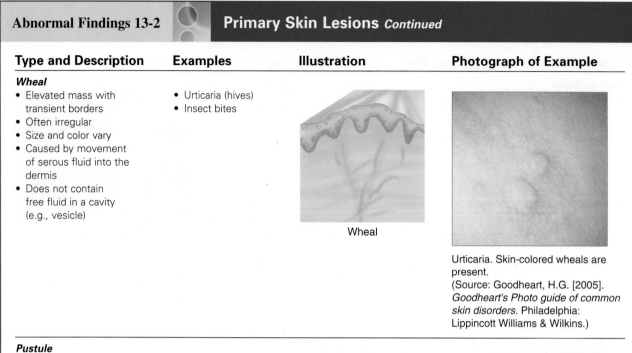 Wheal	Urticaria. Skin-colored wheals are present. (Source: Goodheart, H.G. [2005]. *Goodheart's Photo guide of common skin disorders*. Philadelphia: Lippincott Williams & Wilkins.)
Pustule • Pus-filled vesicle or bulla	• Acne • Impetigo • Furuncles • Carbuncles	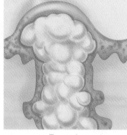 Pustule	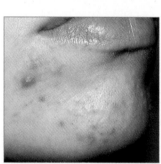 Inflammatory acne lesions. Papules, pustules, and closed comedones are all present on this patient. (Source: Goodheart, H.G. [2005] *Goodheart's Photo guide of common skin disorders*. Philadelphia: Lippincott Williams & Wilkins.)
Cyst • Encapsulated fluid-filled or semisolid mass • Located in the subcutaneous tissue or dermis	• Sebaceous cyst • Epidermoid cyst	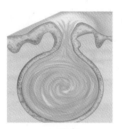 Cyst	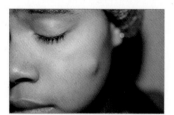 Epidermoid cysts are nodular.

Abnormal Findings 13-3   Secondary Skin Lesions

Secondary skin lesions result from changes in primary lesions.

Type and Description	Examples	Illustration	Photograph of Example
Erosion • Loss of superficial epidermis • Does not extend to the dermis • Depressed, moist area	• Rupture vesicles • Scratch marks • Aphthous ulcer	Erosion	Aphthous ulcer. (Source: Goodheart, H.P. [1999]. *A Photo guide of common skin disorders: Diagnosis and management.* Baltimore: Williams & Wilkins.)
Ulcer • Skin loss extending past epidermis • Necrotic tissue loss • Bleeding and scarring possible	• Stasis ulcer of venous insufficiency • Pressure ulcer	Ulcer	Ulcer from venous stasis.
Scar (Cicatrix) • Skin mark left after healing of wound or lesion • Represents replacement by connective tissue of the injured tissue • Young scars: red or purple • Mature scars: white or glistening	• Healed wound • Healed surgical incision	Scar	Mature healed wound.
Fissure • Linear crack in the skin • May extend to the dermis	• Chapped lips or hands • Athlete's foot	Fissure	Athlete's foot.

Abnormal Findings 13-4 | Vascular Skin Lesions

Vascular skin lesions are associated with bleeding, aging, circulatory conditions, diabetes, pregnancy and hepatic disease among other problems.

Type and Description	Illustration	Photograph
Petechia (Pl. Petechiae) • Round red or purple macule • Small: 1–2 mm • Secondary to blood extravasation • Associated with bleeding tendencies or emboli to skin	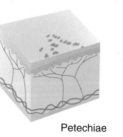 Petechiae	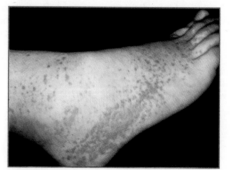 Petechiae. (Dermik Laboratories.)
Ecchymosis (Pl. Ecchymoses) • Round or irregular macular lesion • Larger than petechia • Color varies and changes: black, yellow, and green hues • Secondary to blood extravasation • Associated with trauma, bleeding tendencies	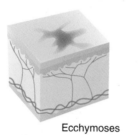 Ecchymoses	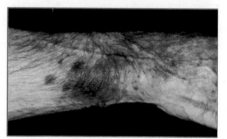 Purpura (hemorrhagic disease that produces ecchymoses and petechiae). (Syntex Laboratories, Inc.)
Hematoma • A localized collection of blood creating an elevated ecchymosis • Associated with trauma	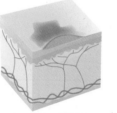 Hematoma	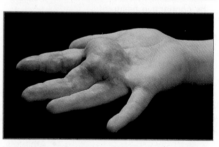 Hematoma. (© 1991 Patricia Barbara, RBP.)
Cherry Angioma • Papular and round • Red or purple • Noted on trunk, extremities • May blanch with pressure • Normal age-related skin alteration • Usually not clinically significant	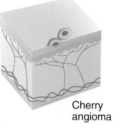 Cherry angioma	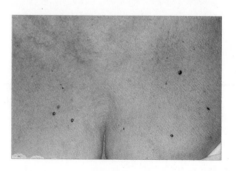

continued

Abnormal Findings 13-4 — Vascular Skin Lesions *Continued*

Type and Description	Illustration	Photograph
Spider Angioma • Red, arteriole lesion • Central body with radiating branches • Noted on face, neck, arms, trunk • Rare below waist • May blanch with pressure • Associated with liver disease, pregnancy, and vitamin B deficiency	Spider angioma	Spider angioma. (Dr. H. C. Robinson/Science Photo Library.)
Telangiectasis (Venous Star) • Shape varies: spiderlike or linear • Color bluish or red • Does not blanch when pressure is applied • Noted on legs, anterior chest • Secondary to superficial dilation of venous vessels and capillaries • Associated with increased venous pressure states (varicosities)	Telangiectasis	Spider telangiectasias. (Source: Goodheart, H. G. [2003]. *Goodheart's photo guide of common skin disorders.* Philadelphia: Lippincott Williams & Wilkins.)

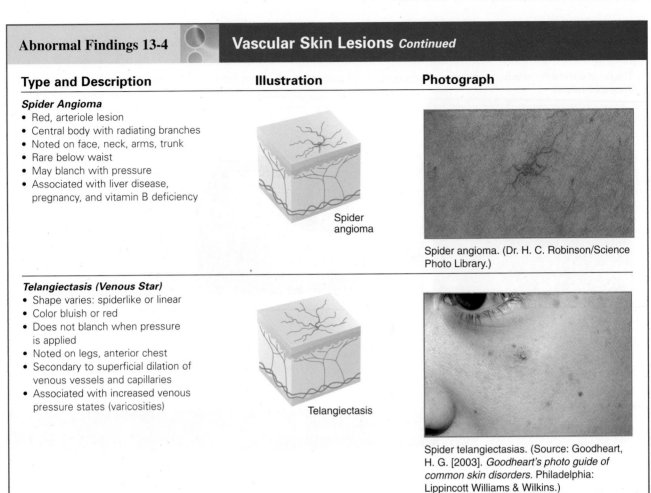

Abnormal Findings 13-5 — Skin Cancer

With the exception of malignant melanoma, most skin cancers are easily seen and easily cured, or at least controlled. Malignant melanoma can be deadly if not discovered and treated early, which is one reason why professional health assessment and skin self-assessment can be life-saving procedures.

Malignant melanoma is usually evaluated according to the mnemonic ABCDE: A for asymmetrical; B for borders that are irregular (uneven or notched); C for color variations; D for diameter exceeding ⅛ to ¼ of an inch; and E for elevated, not flat (See Figure A). Danger signs of malignant melanoma include any of the above factors. However, smaller areas may indicate early stage melanomas. Other warning signs include itching, tenderness, or pain, and a change in size or bleeding of a mole. New pigmentations are also warning signs. (American Cancer Society; American Academy of Dermatology.)

Asymmetry	Borders	Color	Diameter, Elevated

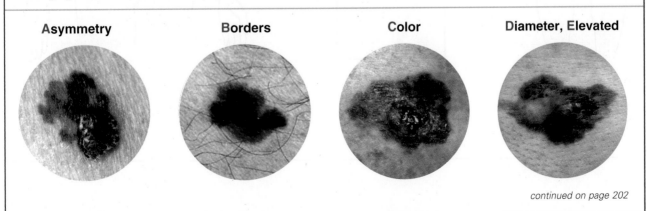

continued on page 202

Abnormal Findings 13-5   **Skin Cancer** *Continued*

The most commonly detected skin cancers include basal cell carcinoma, squamous cell carcinoma, and Kaposi's sarcoma (all illustrated below).

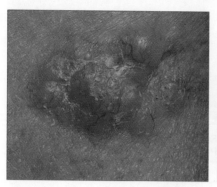
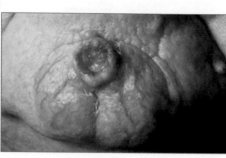
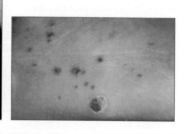

Abnormal Findings 13-6   **Configurations of Skin Lesions**

Describing lesions by shape, distribution, or configuration is one way to communicate specific characteristics that can help to identify causes and treatments. Some common configurations include the following:

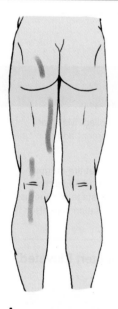
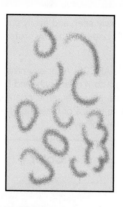
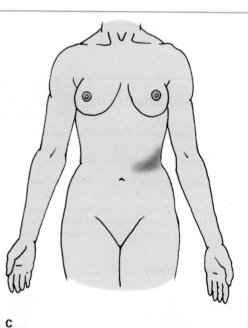

A
Linear configuration: straight line as in a scratch or streak.

B
Annular configuration: circular lesions.

C
Zosteriform configuration: linear lesions clustered along a nerve route.

continued

Abnormal Findings 13-6 | Configurations of Skin Lesions *Continued*

D
Discrete configuration: individual and distinct lesions.

E
Polycyclic configuration: circular lesions that tend to run together.

F
Confluent configuration: lesions run together.

Abnormal Findings 13-7 | Common Nail Disorders

Many clients have nails with lines, ridges, spots, and uncommon shapes that suggest an underlying disorder. Some examples follow:

A. Beau's lines (acute illness)

B. Spoon nails (from deficiency anemia)

180°
C. Early clubbing (oxygen deficiency)

>180°
D. Late clubbing (oxygen deficiency)

E. Pitting (psoriasis)

F. Paronychia (local infection)

VALIDATING AND DOCUMENTING FINDINGS

Validate your normal and abnormal findings with the client, other health care workers, or your instructors. Next, document the skin, hair, and nail assessment data that you have collected on the appropriate form your school or agency uses.

The following is a summary of areas of coverage and findings that are considered normal in a skin, hair, and nail assessment. Of course, abnormal findings would be carefully documented too. Normal findings can act as a baseline for findings that may change later.

Sample of Subjective Data

Thirty-five-year-old woman with no history of skin lesions, excessive hair loss, or nail disorders. Reports one episode of fine, raised, reddened rash on trunk after taking ampicillin for ear infection. Rash cleared within 3 days after discontinuation of ampicillin and administration of antihistamine. Showers in AM and bathes in PM with deodorant soap. Shampoos with baby shampoo each AM Applies moisturizer to skin after each cleansing; conditions hair after shampoo. Uses antiperspirant twice daily. Shaves legs and axillae with electric razor twice weekly. Weekly, trims toenails and fingernails and applies nail enamel to fingernails. Denies exposure to chemicals, abrasives, or excessive sunlight.

Sample of Objective Data

Skin pink, warm, dry, and elastic. No lesions or excoriations noted. Old appendectomy scar right lower abdomen, 4 inches long, thin, and white. Sprinkling of freckles noted across nose and cheeks. Hair brown, shoulder-length, clean, shiny. Normal distribution of hair on scalp and perineum. Hair has been removed from legs, axillae. Nails form 160-degree angle at base; are hard, smooth, and immobile. Nailbeds pink without clubbing. Cuticles smooth; no detachment of nail plate. Fingernails well manicured with clear enamel. Toenails clean and well trimmed.

After you have collected your assessment data, analyze the data, using diagnostic reasoning skills.

Analysis of Data

DIAGNOSTIC REASONING: POSSIBLE CONCLUSIONS

After collecting subjective and objective data pertaining to the skin, hair, and nails, identify abnormal findings and client strengths. Then cluster the data to reveal any significant patterns or abnormalities. Listed below are some possible conclusions that the nurse may make after assessing a client's skin, hair, and nails.

Selected Nursing Diagnoses

The following is a list of selected nursing diagnoses that may be identified when analyzing data from a skin, hair, and nail assessment.

Wellness Diagnoses

- Readiness for enhanced skin, hair, and nail integrity related to healthy hygiene and skin care practices, avoidance of overexposure to sun

- Health-Seeking Behavior: Requests information on skin reactions and effects of using a sun-tanning booth

Risk Diagnoses

- Risk for Impaired Skin Integrity related to excessive exposure to cleaning solutions and chemicals
- Risk for Impaired Skin Integrity related to prolonged sun exposure
- Risk for Imbalanced Body Temperature related to immobility, decreased production of natural oils, and thinning skin
- Risk for Impaired Tissue Integrity of toes related to thickened, dried toenails
- Risk for Imbalanced Body Temperature related to severe diaphoresis
- Risk for Infection related to scratching of rash
- Risk for Impaired Nail Integrity related to prolonged use of artificial nails
- Risk for Altered Nutrition: Less Than Body Requirements related to increased vitamin and protein requirements necessary for healing of a wound
- Risk for Infection related to multiple body piercings
- Risk for Infection related to periodic skin tattooing

Actual Diagnoses

- Ineffective Health Maintenance related to lack of hygienic care of the skin, hair, and nails
- Impaired Skin Integrity related to immobility and decreased circulation
- Impaired Skin Integrity related to poor nutritional intake and bowel/bladder incontinence
- Disturbed Body Image related to scarring, rash, or other skin condition that alters skin appearance
- Disturbed Sleep Pattern related to persistent itching of the skin
- Deficient Fluid Volume related to excessive diaphoresis secondary to excessive exercise and high environmental temperatures

Selected Collaborative Problems

After grouping the data, certain collaborative problems may become apparent. Remember that collaborative problems differ from nursing diagnoses in that they cannot be prevented or managed with independent nursing interventions. However, these physiologic complications of medical conditions can be detected and monitored by the nurse. In addition, the nurse can use physician- and nurse-prescribed interventions to minimize the complications of these problems. The nurse may also have to refer the client in such situations for further treatment of the problem. The following is a list of collaborative problems that may be identified when assessing the skin, hair, and nails. These problems are worded as Risk for Complications (or RC), followed by the problem.

- RC: Allergic reaction
- RC: Skin rash
- RC: Insect/animal bite
- RC: Septicemia
- RC: Hypovolemic shock
- RC: Skin infection

- RC: Skin lesion
- RC: Ischemic skin ulcers
- RC: Graft rejection
- RC: Hemorrhage
- RC: Burns

Medical Problems

After grouping the data, it may become apparent that the client has signs and symptoms that require medical diagnosis and treatment. Referral to a primary care provider is necessary.

CASE STUDY

The case study demonstrates how to analyze skin, hair, and nail data for a specific client. The critical thinking exercises included in the study guide/lab manual and interactive product that complement this text also offer opportunities to assess the data.

Mary Michaelson, a 29-year-old divorced woman, works as an office manager for a large, prestigious law firm. She reports she recently went to see a doctor because "my hair was falling out in chunks, and I have a red rash on my face and chest. It looks like a bad case of acne." After doing some blood work, her physician diagnosed her condition as discoid lupus erythematosus (DLE). She says she has come to see you, the occupational health nurse, because she feels "so ugly," and she is concerned that she may lose her job because of how she looks.

During the interview, she tells you that she is a surfer and is out in the sun all day nearly every weekend. She shares that she uses sunscreen but forgets to put it on at regular intervals during the day.

Your physical examination reveals an attractive, tanned, thin, anxious-appearing young woman. You note confluent and nonconfluent maculopapular lesions on her neck, chest above the nipple line, and over the shoulders and upper back to about the level of the T5 vertebra. Many of the lesions appear as red, scaling plaques with depressed, pale centers. A few of the lesions on her forehead and cheeks appear blistered. Patchy alopecia is also present. Her vital signs are within normal limits, and no other abnormalities are apparent at this time.

The following concept map illustrates the diagnostic reasoning process.

Applying COLDSPA

Applying **COLDSPA** for client symptoms: "I have a red rash on my face."

Mnemonic	Question	Data Provided	Missing Data
Character	Describe the sign or symptom (feeling, appearance, sound, smell, or taste if applicable).	Red, scaly, plaques with depressed pale center	
Onset	When did it begin?		When did this rash first appear?
Location	Where is it? Does it radiate? Does it occur anywhere else?	Confluent and nonconfluent on face, neck, chest, above nipple line, shoulders, and upper back	
Duration	How long does it last? Does it recur?		Has client ever had this type of rash or other rashes before?
Severity	How bad is it? How much does it bother you?	Blistered on face and forehead. May lose job due to appearance.	
Pattern	What makes it better or worse?		Has anything made it better or worse?
Associated factors/How it **A**ffects the client	What other symptoms occur with it? How does it affect you?	Client "feels ugly." Patchy alopecia	

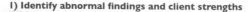

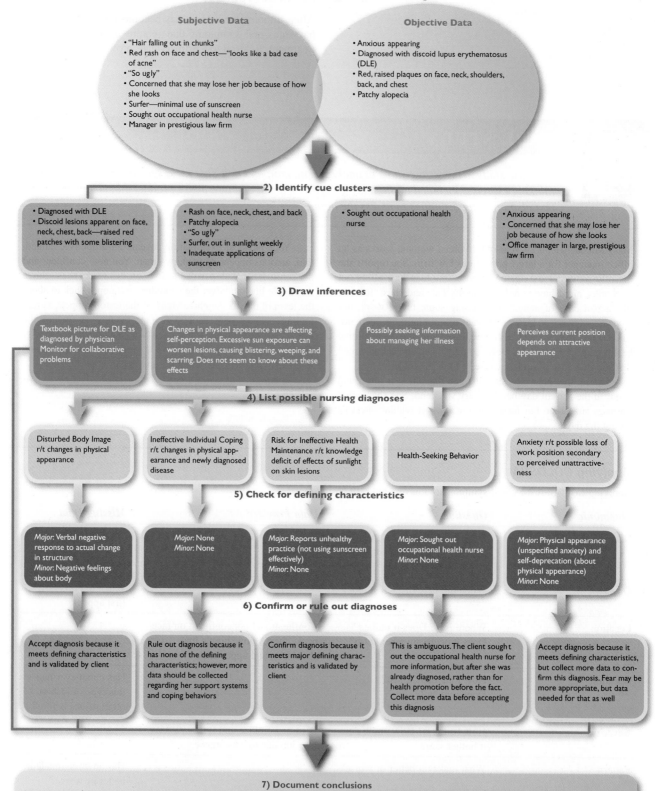

1) Identify abnormal findings and client strengths

Subjective Data

- "Hair falling out in chunks"
- Red rash on face and chest—"looks like a bad case of acne"
- "So ugly"
- Concerned that she may lose her job because of how she looks
- Surfer—minimal use of sunscreen
- Sought out occupational health nurse
- Manager in prestigious law firm

Objective Data

- Anxious appearing
- Diagnosed with discoid lupus erythematosus (DLE)
- Red, raised plaques on face, neck, shoulders, back, and chest
- Patchy alopecia

2) Identify cue clusters

- Diagnosed with DLE
- Discoid lesions apparent on face, neck, chest, back—raised red patches with some blistering

- Rash on face, neck, chest, and back
- Patchy alopecia
- "So ugly"
- Surfer, out in sunlight weekly
- Inadequate applications of sunscreen

- Sought out occupational health nurse

- Anxious appearing
- Concerned that she may lose her job because of how she looks
- Office manager in large, prestigious law firm

3) Draw inferences

Textbook picture for DLE as diagnosed by physician Monitor for collaborative problems

Changes in physical appearance are affecting self-perception. Excessive sun exposure can worsen lesions, causing blistering, weeping, and scarring. Does not seem to know about these effects

Possibly seeking information about managing her illness

Perceives current position depends on attractive appearance

4) List possible nursing diagnoses

Disturbed Body Image r/t changes in physical appearance

Ineffective Individual Coping r/t changes in physical appearance and newly diagnosed disease

Risk for Ineffective Health Maintenance r/t knowledge deficit of effects of sunlight on skin lesions

Health-Seeking Behavior

Anxiety r/t possible loss of work position secondary to perceived unattractiveness

5) Check for defining characteristics

Major: Verbal negative response to actual change in structure
Minor: Negative feelings about body

Major: None
Minor: None

Major: Reports unhealthy practice (not using sunscreen effectively)
Minor: None

Major: Sought out occupational health nurse
Minor: None

Major: Physical appearance (unspecified anxiety) and self-deprecation (about physical appearance)
Minor: None

6) Confirm or rule out diagnoses

Accept diagnosis because it meets defining characteristics and is validated by client

Rule out diagnosis because it has none of the defining characteristics; however, more data should be collected regarding her support systems and coping behaviors

Confirm diagnosis because it meets major defining characteristics and is validated by client

This is ambiguous. The client sought out the occupational health nurse for more information, but after she was already diagnosed, rather than for health promotion before the fact. Collect more data before accepting this diagnosis

Accept diagnosis because it meets defining characteristics, but collect more data to confirm this diagnosis. Fear may be more appropriate, but data needed for that as well

7) Document conclusions

The following nursing diagnoses appropriate for this client include:
- Body Image Disturbance r/t changes in physical appearance
- Risk for Altered Health Maintenance r/t knowledge deficit of effects of sunlight on skin lesions
- Anxiety r/t possible loss of work position secondary to perceived unattractiveness

Potential collaborative problems include the following:
- RC: Skin Infection/Scarring
- RC: Ischemic Ulcers
- RC: Systemic Lupus Erythematosus (SLE) and all related complications

References and Selected Readings

Abimelec, P. (2003). Fungal nail infections. Available at http://abimelec.com/dermatologist/fungal_nail_infection

Al-Rubaiy, L. K. Q., & Al-Rubiah, K. K. (2006). Alcohol consumption and smoking: A risk factor for psoriasis. *Internet Journal of Dermatology, 4*(2), 7.

Andrews, M., & Boyle, J. (2003). *Transcultural concepts in nursing care* (3rd ed.). Philadelphia: Lippincott Williams & Wilkins.

Bono, M. J., & Lyons, L. (2005). Cyanosis. *Emergency Medicine, 37*(9), 45–48.

Braden, B., & Bergstrom, B. (1988). Braden scale for predicting pressure sore risk. Available at www.bradenscale.com

Brannon, H. (2007). Fungal nail infections. Available at http://dermatology.about.com/cs/fungalinfections/a/Onychomycosis.htm

Brown, J., Wimpenney, P., & Maughan, H. (2004). Skin problems in people with obesity. *Nursing Standards, 18*(35), 38–42.

Butler, C. T. (2006). Pediatric skin care: Guidelines for assessment, prevention, and treatment. *Pediatric Nursing, 32*(5), 443–450, 452–454.

Caliendo, C., Armstrong, M. L., & Roberts, A. E. (2005). Self-reported characteristics of women and men with intimate body piercings. *Journal of Advanced Nursing, 49*(5), 474–484.

Centers for Disease Control and Prevention: Morbidity and Mortality Weekly Report. (2006). Methicillin-resistant *Staphylococcus aureus* skin infections among tattoo recipients—Ohio, Kentucky, and Vermont, 2004–2005. *Journal of the American Medical Association, 296*(4), 285–386.

Chaturvedi, S. K., Singh, G., & Gupta, N. (2005). Stigma experience in skin disorders: An Indian perspective. *Dermatologic Clinics, 23*(4), 635–642.

Choka, K. P., & Meyers, J. L. (2005). Teaching strategies. The skin challenge: A practical approach for teaching skin assessment and documentation. *Nurse Educator, 30*(5), 195–196.

Deci, D. M. (2005). The medical implications of body art. *Patient Care, 39*(4), 26–33.

Fried, R. G., Gupta, M. A., & Gupta, A. K. (2005). Depression and skin disease. *Dermatologic Clinics, 23*(4), 657–664.

Furlow, B. (2005). Systemic lupus erythematosus. *Radiologic Technology, 76*(4), 289–299.

Gottschalk, G. M. (2006). Pediatric HIV/AIDS and the skin: An update. *Dermatologic Clinics, 24*(4), 472–475.

Grey, J. E., Harding, K. G., & Enoch, S. (2006). Pressure ulcers. *British Medical Journal, 332*(7539), 472–475.

Gupta, M. A., Gupta, A. K., Ellis, C. N., & Koblenzer, C. S. (2005). Psychiatric evaluation of the dermatology patient. *Dermatologic Clinics, 23*(4), 591–599.

Guttman, C. (2000). Nail exam should be routine in elderly patients. *Dermatology Times, 21*(4), 40.

Holloway, S., & Jones, V. (2005). Skin care. The importance of skin care assessment. *British Journal of Nursing, 14*(22), 1172–1176.

Hooked on Nails. (2002). Nail diseases & disorders. Available at http://hooked-on-nails.com/naildisorders.html

Jalali, R., & Rezaie, M. (2005). Predicting pressure ulcer risk: Comparing the predictive validity of 4 scales. *Advances in Skin and Wound Care, 18*(2), 92–97.

Johannsen, L. L. (2005). Dermatology nursing essentials: Core knowledge. Skin assessment. *Dermatology Nursing, 17*(2), 165–166.

Kadawo, J. (2007). Vulval skin conditions. *Nursing Standards, 21*(7), 59.

Koblenzer, C. S. (2005). The emotional impact of chronic and disabling skin disease: A psychoanalytic perspective. *Dermatologic Clinics, 23*(4), 616–627.

Kwong, E., Pang, S., Wong, T., Ho, J., Shao-ling, X., & Li-jun, T. (2005). Predicting pressure ulcer risk with the modified Braden, Braden, and Norton scales in acute care hospital in Mainland China. *Applied Nursing Research, 18*(2), 122–128.

Lane, J. E., Waller, J. L., & Davis, L. S. (2005). Relationship between ear piercing and keloid formation. *Pediatrics, 115*(5), 1312–1314.

Laughlin, K., Tan, A. K. W., & Ellis, D. A. F. (2001). Evaluation system for facial skin assessment. *Journal of Otolaryngology, 28*(4), 238–241.

Lawton, S., & Littlewood, S. (2006). Vulval skin disease: Clinical features, assessment, and management. *Nursing Standards, 20*(42), 57–64, 68.

Leman, S. K., & Plattner, M. (2007). When beautification of the body turns ugly. *Clinical Advisor for Nurse Practitioners, 10*(2), 27–28, 31–33.

Mark, B. J., & Slavin, R. G. (2006). Allergic contact dermatitis. *Medical Clinics of North America, 90*(1), 169–185.

Massey, D. (2006). The value and role of skin and nail assessment in the critically ill. *Nursing in Critical Care, 11*(2), 80–85.

McCreath, H. E., Kono, A., Apleles, N. C. R., Howell, L., & Alessi, C. (2006). Subepidermal moisture measures and visual skin assessment of erythema and pressure ulcers. *Ostomy Wound Management, 52*(4), 101–102.

McMichael, A. J. (1999). A review of cutaneous disease in African-American patients. *Dermatology Nursing, 11*(1), 35–36, 41–47.

Muirhead, G. (1999). Common dermatologic problems in people of color. *Patient Care, 33*(20), 97.

National Institute of Health. (1992). The NIH Consensus Development Panel on Melanoma: Diagnosis and treatment of early melanoma. *Journal of the American Medical Association, 268*, 1314–1319.

National Pressure Ulcer Advisory Panel. (2007). Available at www.npuap.org/pr2.htm

Parhizgar, B. (2000). Skin signs of systemic disease. *Cortlandt Forum, 13*(1), 169.

Penzer, R., & Finch, M. (2002). Promoting healthy skin in older people. *Nursing Older People, 14*(5), 37.

Peterson, J. D., & Chan, L. S. (2006). A comprehensive management guide for atopic dermatitis. *Dermatology Nursing, 18*(6), 531–543.

Pierce, M., Rice, M., Fellows, J., & Salvadalena, G. (2006). Wet colostomy and peristomal skin breakdown . . . including commentary by Ginger Salvadalena. *Journal of Wound, Ostomy & Continence Nursing, 33*(5), 541–548.

Pullen, R. J. (2007). Assessing skin legions. Learn to identify different types and document their characteristics. *Nursing2007, 37*(8), 44–45.

Rogers, C. (2003). Skin assessment: Improving communication and recording. *Pediatric Nursing, 14*(5), 20–23.

Rose, P., Cohen, R., & Amsel, R. (2006). Development of a scale to measure the risk of skin breakdown in critically ill patients. *American Journal of Critical Care, 15*(3), 337.

Simpson, E. L., & Hanifin, J. M. (2006). Atopic dermatitis. *Medical Clinics of North America, 90*(1), 149–167.

Sinclair, R. (1998). Male pattern androgenetic alopecia. *British Medical Journal, 317*(7162), 865.

Stefanski, J. L., & Smith, K. J. (2006). The role of nutrition intervention in wound healing. *Home Health Care Management & Practice, 18*(4), 293–299.

Suddaby, E. C., Barnett, S. D., & Facteau, L. (2005). Skin breakdown in acute care pediatrics. *Pediatric Nursing, 31*(12), 132–138, 148.

Wall, S., Hunter, K., & Coleman-Miller, G. (2005). Development of an evidence-based specialty support surface decision tool. *Ostomy Wound Management, 51*(2), 80–86.

Wisser, D. Rennekamph, H. O., & Schaller, H. E. (2003). Skin assessment of burn wounds with a collagen based dermal substitute in a 2-year follow-up. *Burns, 30*(4), 399–401.

Wright, L. G. (2006). Maculopapular skin rashes associated with high-dose chemotherapy: Prevalence and risk factors. *Oncology Nursing Forum, 33*(6), 1095–1103.

Zulkowski, K., & Ayello, E. A. (2005). Urban and rural nurses' knowledge of pressure ulcers in the USA. *World Council of Enterostomal Therapists Journal, 25*(3), 24–26, 28–30.

Promote Health—Pressure Ulcers

Ayello, E. A. (2004). Predicting pressure ulcer risk. *The Hartford Institute for Geriatric Nursing, 1*(5). Available at http://www.hartfordign.org

Baranoski, S., & Ayello, E. A. (2004). *Wound care essentials: Practice principles.* Springhouse, PA: Lippincott.

National Pressure Ulcer Advisory Panel. (2001). PU Prevention-RN competency-based curriculum. Available at http://www.npuap.org

National Pressure Ulcer Advisory Panel. Cuddigan, J. Ayello, E. Sussman, C. (Eds.). (2001). *Pressure ulcers in America: Prevalence, incidence, and implications for the future.* Reston, VA: NPUAP.

Promote Health—Skin Cancer

American Academy of Family Physicians. (2000). Early detection and treatment of skin cancer. Available at http://www.aafp.org/afp/20000715/357.html

American Cancer Society (ACS). (2007). Cancer resource center. Available at www.cancer.org

Center for Disease Control and Prevention. (2007). Skin cancer. Available at http://www.cdc.gov/cancer/skin

Center for Disease Control and Prevention Division of Cancer Prevention and Control. (2006–2007). Skin cancer prevention and education initiative. Available at http://www.cdc.gov/cancer/skin/pdf/0607_skin_fs.pdf

Freedman, D. M., Sigurason, A., Doody, M., Mabuchi, K., & Linet, M. (2003). Risk of basal cell carcinoma in relation to alcohol intake and smoking. *Cancer Epidemiology Biomarkers Prevention, 12*(12), 1540–1543.

Goodheart, H. P. (1999). *A photoguide of common skin disorders: Diagnosis and management.* Baltimore: Williams & Wilkins.

Grant, W. B. (2004). Smoking overlooked as an important risk factor for squamous cell carcinomas. *Archives of Dermatology, 140*(3), 362–363.

Halder, R. M., & Ara, C. J. (2003). Skin cancer and photoaging in ethnic skin. *Dermatologic Clinics, 21*(4), 725–732.

Hu, S., Ma, F., Collado-Mesa, F., & Kirsner, R. (2004). UV radiation, latitude, and melanoma in U.S. Hispanics and blacks. *2004 Archives of Dermatology, 140*(7), 819–824.

Kirkland, J. B. (2003). Niacin and carcinogenesis. *Nutrition and Cancer, 46*(2), 110–118.

Lappe, J. M., Travers-Gustafson, D., Davies, K., Recker, R., Heaney, R., et al. (2007). Vitamin D and calcium supplementation reduces cancer risk: Results of a randomized trial. *American Journal of Clinical Nutrition, 85*, 1586–1591.

Lee, C. S., & Lim, H. (2003). Cutaneous diseases in Asians. *Dermatologic Clinics, 21*(4), 669–677.

Lens, M., & Dawes, M. (2004). Global perspectives of contemporary epidemiological trends of cutaneous malignant melanoma. *British Journal of Dermatology, 150*(2), 179–185.

McCarthy, W. H. (2004). The Australian experience in sun protection and screening for melanoma. *Journal of Surgical Oncology, 86*(4), 236–245.

Zak-Prelich, M., Narbutt, J., & Sepa-Jedrzefowska, A. (2004). Environmental risk factors predisposing to the development of basal cell carcinoma. *Dermatology Surgery, 30*(2, Pt. 2), 248–252.

Websites

American Academy of Family Physicians. Available at http://www.aafp.org

American Journal of Clinical Nutrition. Available at http://www.ajcn.org.

Centers for Disease Control and Prevention. Available at http://www.cdc.gov.

Mayo Clinic. Available at http://www.mayoclinic.com.

National Alopecia Areata Foundation (NAAF), P.O. Box 150760, San Rafael, CA 94915-0760; 415-472-3780. Available at http://www.alopeciaareta.com.

National Cancer Institute. Available at http://www.cancer.gov.

National Eczema Association for Science and Education, 1220 S.W. Morrison, Suite 433, Portland, OR 97205; 451-499-3474. Available at http://www.nationaleczema.org.

National Institute of Health. Available at http://www.nih.nlm.gov/medlineplus.

National Organization for Albinism and Hypopigmentation, P.O. Box 959, East Hampstead, NH 03826-0959; 1-800-473-2310. Available at http://www.albinism.org.

National Pressure Ulcer Advisory Panel. Available at www.npuap.org/PDF/**push**3.pdf.

National Psoriasis Foundation (USA), 6600 S.W. 92nd Ave., Suite 300, Portland, OR 97223-7195; 503-244-7404. Available at http://www.psoriasis.org.

National Vitiligo Foundation, 611 South Flieshel Ave., Tyler, TX 75701; 908-531-0074. Available at http://www.nvf.org.

Structure and Function

Head and neck assessment focuses on the cranium, face, thyroid gland, and lymph node structures contained within the head and neck.

THE HEAD

The framework of the head is the skull, which can be divided into two subsections: the cranium and the face (Fig. 14-1).

Cranium

The cranium houses and protects the brain and major sensory organs. It consists of eight bones:

- Frontal (1)
- Parietal (2)
- Temporal (2)
- Occipital (1)
- Ethmoid (1)
- Sphenoid (1)

In the adult client, the cranial bones are joined together by immovable sutures: the sagittal, coronal, squamosal, and lambdoid sutures.

Face

Facial bones give shape to the face. The face consists of 14 bones:

- Maxilla (2)
- Zygomatic (cheek) (2)
- Inferior conchae (2)
- Nasal (2)
- Lacrimal (2)
- Palatine (2)
- Vomer (1)
- Mandible (jaw) (1)

All of the facial bones are immovable except for the mandible, which has free movement (up, down, and sideways) at the temporomandibular joint. The face also consists of many muscles that produce facial movement and expressions. The **temporal artery,** a major artery, is located between the eye and the top of the ear. Two other important structures located in the facial region are the parotid and submandibular salivary glands. The **parotid glands** are located on each side of the face, anterior and inferior to the ears and behind the mandible. The **submandibular glands** are located inferior to the mandible, underneath the base of the tongue.

THE NECK

The structure of the neck is composed of muscles, ligaments, and the cervical vertebrae (Fig. 14-2). Contained within the neck are the hyoid bone, several major blood vessels, the larynx, trachea, and the thyroid gland, which is in the anterior triangle of the neck.

Muscles and Cervical Vertebrae

The sternomastoid (sternocleidomastoid) and trapezius muscles are two of the paired muscles that allow movement and provide support to the head and neck (Fig. 14-3). The **sternomastoid muscle** rotates and flexes the head, whereas the **trapezius muscle** extends the head and moves the shoulders. The **eleventh cranial nerve** is responsible for muscle movement that permits shrugging of the shoulders by the trapezius muscles and turning the head against resistance by the sternomastoid muscles. These two major muscles also form two triangles that provide important landmarks for assessment. The anterior triangle is located under the mandible, anterior to the sternomastoid muscle. The posterior triangle is located between the trapezius and sternomastoid muscles (see Fig. 14-3). The cervical vertebrae (C1 through C7) are located in the

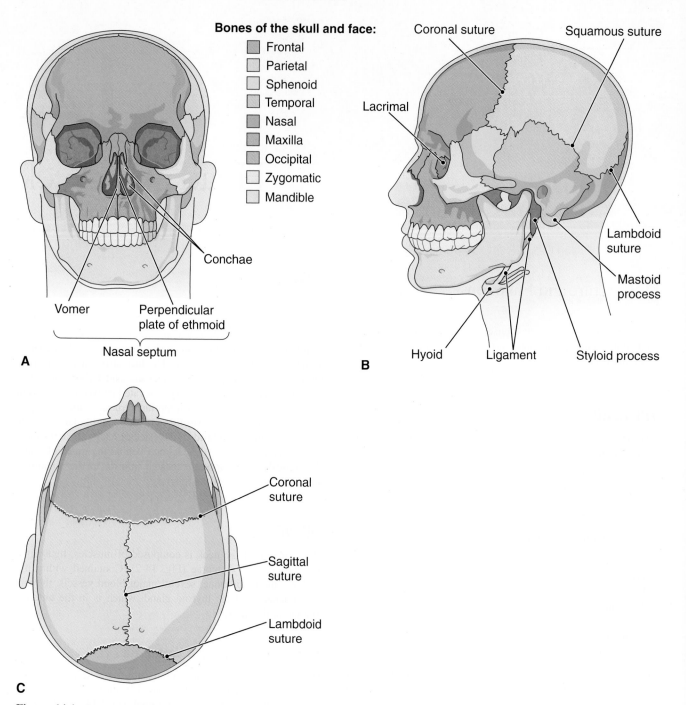

Figure 14-1   The skull. **(A)** Anterior view. **(B)** Left lateral view. **(C)** Superior view.

posterior neck and support the cranium (Fig. 14-4). The vertebra prominens is C7, which can easily be palpated when the neck is flexed. Using C7 as a landmark will help you to locate other vertebrae.

Blood Vessels

The **internal jugular veins** and **carotid arteries** are located bilaterally, parallel and anterior to the sternomastoid muscles. The external jugular vein lies diagonally over the surface of these muscles. The purpose and assessment of these major blood vessels are discussed in Chapter 21. However, you need to know the location of the carotid arteries when assessing the neck to avoid bilateral compression of the vessels, which can reduce the blood supply to the brain.

Thyroid Gland

The thyroid gland is the largest endocrine gland in the body. It produces thyroid hormones that increase the metabolic rate of most body cells. The thyroid gland is surrounded by several

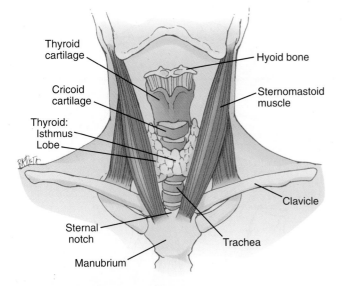

Figure 14-2 Structures of the neck.

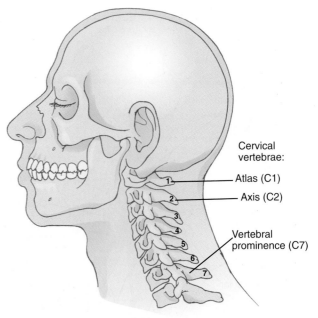

Figure 14-4 Cervical vertebrae.

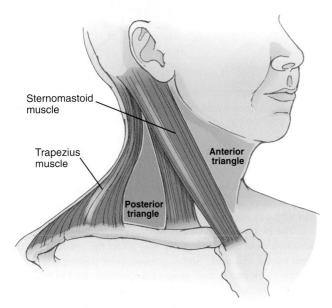

Figure 14-3 Neck muscles and landmarks.

LYMPH NODES OF THE HEAD AND NECK

Several lymph nodes are located in the head and neck (Fig. 14-5). **Lymph nodes** filter lymph, a clear substance composed mostly of excess tissue fluid, after the lymphatic vessels collect it but before it returns to the vascular system. This filtering action removes bacteria and tumor cells from lymph. In addition, lymphocytes and antibodies are produced in the lymph nodes as a defense against invasion by foreign substances. The size and shape of lymph nodes vary but most are less than 1 cm long and are buried deep in the connective tissue, which makes them nonpalpable in normal situations. They usually appear in clusters that vary in size from 2 to 100 individual nodes.

If the nodes become overwhelmed by microorganisms, as happens with an infection such as mononucleosis, they swell and become painful, but if cancer metastasizes to the lymph nodes, they may enlarge but not be painful. Normally lymph nodes are either not palpable or they may feel like very small beads. Sources vary in their reference to the names of lymph nodes. The most common head and neck lymph nodes are referred to as follows:

- Preauricular
- Postauricular
- Tonsillar
- Occipital
- Submandibular
- Submental
- Superficial cervical
- Posterior cervical
- Deep cervical
- Supraclavicular

When an enlarged lymph node is detected during assessment, the nurse needs to know from which part of the head or neck the lymph node receives drainage to assess if an abnormality (e.g., infection, disease) is in that area.

structures that are important to palpate for accurate location of the thyroid gland. The trachea, through which air enters the lungs, is composed of C-shaped hyaline cartilage rings. The first upper tracheal ring, called the cricoid cartilage, has a small notch in it. The thyroid cartilage (Adam's apple) is larger and located just above the cricoid cartilage. The hyoid bone, which is attached to the tongue, lies above the thyroid cartilage and under the mandible (see Fig. 14-2).

The thyroid gland consists of two lateral lobes that curve posteriorly on both sides of the trachea and esophagus and are mostly covered by the sternomastoid muscles. These two thyroid lobes are connected by an isthmus that overlies the second and third tracheal rings below the cricoid cartilage. In about one-third of the population, there is a third lobe that extends upward from the isthmus or from one of the two lobes.

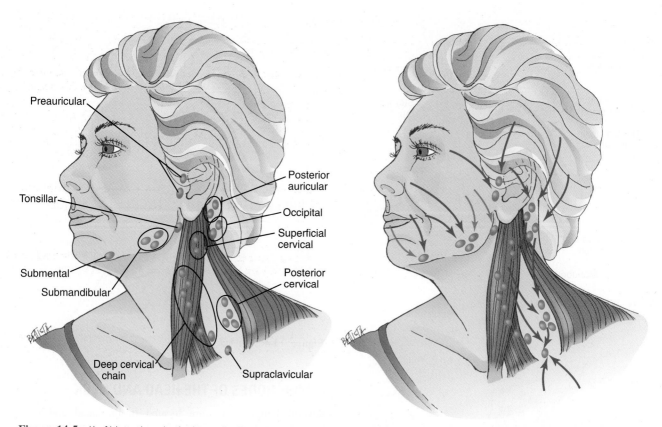

Figure 14-5 (*Left*) Lymph nodes in the neck. (*Right*) Direction of lymph flow. *Note*: Lymph nodes (represented by *green dots*) that are covered by hair may be palpated in the scalp under the hair.

Health Assessment

COLLECTING SUBJECTIVE DATA: THE NURSING HEALTH HISTORY

Abnormalities that cannot be directly observed in the physical appearance of the head and neck are often detected in the client's history. For example, a client may have no visible signs of any problems but may complain of frequent headaches. A detailed description of the type of headache pain and its location, intensity, and duration provides the nurse with valuable clues as to what the underlying problem might be.

In addition because of the overlap of several body systems in this area, a thorough nursing history is needed to detect the cause of possible underlying systemic problems. For example, the client experiencing dizziness, spinning, lightheadedness, or loss of consciousness may perceive the problems as related to

her head. However, these symptoms may indicate problems with the heart and neck vessels, peripheral vascular system, or neurologic system.

The history also provides an opportunity for you to evaluate activities of daily living that may affect the condition of the client's head and neck. Stress, tension, poor posture while performing work and lack of proper exercise may lead to head and neck discomfort. To prevent head and neck injuries, the nurse may inform the client of protective measures, such as wearing helmets, seat belts, and hard hats, during the history portion of the assessment.

Finally when discussing the client's head, neck, and facial structures, recognize that the appearance of these structures often has a great influence on the client's self-image.

The following is a selection of questions you may ask and areas you may cover with an average client.

(text continues on page 216)

HISTORY OF PRESENT HEALTH CONCERN

Question	Rationale
Pain	
Do you experience neck pain?	Neck pain may accompany muscular problems or cervical spinal cord problems. Stress and tension may increase neck pain. Sudden head and neck pain seen with elevated temperature and neck stiffness may be a sign of meningeal inflammation.
	Older clients who have arthritis or osteoporosis may experience neck pain and a decreased range of motion.
Do you experience headaches? Describe.	A precise description of the symptoms can help to determine possible causes of the discomfort. Temporomandibular joint syndrome is a major cause of chronic headaches. See Table 14-1 for a discussion of typical findings for migraine, tension, cluster, and tumor-related headaches.
Do you have any facial pain? Describe.	Trigeminal neuralgia (tic douloureux) is manifested by sharp, shooting, piercing facial pains that last from seconds to minutes. Pain occurs over the divisions of the fifth trigeminal cranial nerve (the ophthalmic, maxillary, and mandibular areas).
Do you have any difficulty moving your head or neck?	Diseases and disorders involving head and neck muscles may limit mobility and affect daily functioning.
Other Symptoms	
Have you noticed any lumps or lesions on your head or neck that do not heal or disappear? Describe their appearance and location.	Lumps and lesions that do not heal or disappear may indicate cancer.
Have you experienced any dizziness, lightheadedness, spinning sensation, or loss of consciousness? Describe.	Problems with the neck vessels (such as carotid artery occlusion), neurologic system, such as inner ear disease, cardiovascular system (heart block) may cause these symptoms. These symptoms imply a risk for injury.
Have you noticed a change in the texture of your skin, hair, or nails?	Alterations in thyroid function are manifested in several ways. An increase in thyroid hormone production (hyperthyroidism) can result in insomnia, thinning hair, palpitations, and weight loss. A decrease in thyroid hormone production (hypothyroidism) can result in insomnia and will have the opposite effects of thickening skin and nails, decreased energy levels, and constipation.
Have you noticed changes in your energy level, sleep habits, or emotional stability?	
Have you experienced any palpitations, blurred vision or changes in bowel habits?	

continued on page 215

COLDSPA Example

Use the **COLDSPA** mnemonic as a guideline to collect needed information for each symptom the client shares. In addition, the following questions help elicit important information.

Mnemonic	*Question*	*Client Response Example*
Character	Describe the sign or symptom (feeling, appearance, sound, smell, or taste if applicable).	"I have trouble turning my head to the right."
Onset	When did it begin?	"Two days ago when I woke up in the morning, and it is getting worse."
Location	Where is it? Does it radiate? Does it occur anywhere else?	"In the back of my neck and it radiates to my right shoulder with movement."
Duration	How long does it last? Does it recur?	"It is OK if I just sit still, but it hurts more if I turn."
Severity	How bad is it? How much does it bother you?	"It is difficult to drive because I can't see over my shoulder to change lanes."
Pattern	What makes it better or worse?	"Ibuprofen and a heating pad or warm shower helps a little."
Associated factors/How it **A**ffects the client	What other symptoms occur with it? How does it affect you?	"I can't do my work on the computer without being irritated with it."

Table 14-1 — Kinds and Characteristics of Headaches

Migraine	Cluster	Tension	Tumor Related
Character Accompanied by nausea, vomiting, and sensitivity to noise or light	May be accompanied by tearing, eyelid drooping, reddened eye, or runny nose	Symptoms of anxiety, tension, and depression may be present	Neurologic and mental symptoms and nausea and vomiting may develop
Onset and Precipitating Factors • May have prodromal stage (visual disturbances, vertigo, tinnitus, numbness or tingling of fingers or toes) • Precipitated by emotional disturbances, anxiety, or ingestion of alcohol, cheese, chocolate, or other foods and substances to which client is sensitive	• Sudden onset • May be precipitated by ingesting alcohol	• No prodromal stage • May occur with stress, anxiety, or depression	• No prodromal stage • May be aggravated by coughing, sneezing, or sudden movements of the head
Location Located around eyes, temples, cheeks, or forehead	Localized in the eye and orbit and radiating to the facial and temporal regions	Usually located in the frontal, temporal, or occipital region	Varies with location of tumor
Duration Lasts up to 3 days	Typically occurs in the late evening or night	Lasts days, months, or years	Commonly occurs in the morning and lasts for several hours
Severity Throbbing, severe, recurring	Intense and stabbing	Dull, aching, tight, diffuse	Aching, steady, variable in intensity
Pattern Rest may bring relief	Movement or walking back and forth may relieve the discomfort	Symptomatic relief may be obtained by local heat, massage, analgesics, anti-depressants, and muscle relaxants	Headache usually subsides later in the day.
Associated Factors Migraines occur more often in women	Cluster headaches occur more in young males	Tension headaches affect women more often than men	

PAST HEALTH HISTORY

Question	Rationale
Describe any previous head or neck problems (trauma, injury, falls) you have had. How were they treated (surgery, medication, physical therapy)? What were the results?	Previous head and neck trauma may cause chronic pain and limitation of movement. This may affect functioning.
Have you ever undergone radiation therapy for a problem in your neck region?	Radiation therapy has been linked to the development of thyroid cancer. Radiation to the neck area may also cause esophageal strictures leading to difficulty with swallowing.

FAMILY HISTORY

Question	Rationale
Is there a history of head or neck cancer in your family?	Genetic predisposition is a risk factor for head and neck cancers.
Is there a history of migraine headaches in your family?	Migraine headaches commonly have a familial association.

LIFESTYLE AND HEALTH PRACTICES

Question	Rationale
Do you smoke or chew tobacco? If yes, how much?	Tobacco use increases the risk of head and neck cancer.
Do you wear a helmet when riding a horse, bicycle, motorcycle, or other open sports vehicle (e.g., four-wheeler, go-cart)? Do you wear a hard hat for hazardous occupations?	Failure to use safety precautions increases the risk for head and neck injury (see Promote Health—Traumatic Brain Injury for more information).
What is your typical posture when relaxing, during sleep, and when working?	Poor posture or body alignment can lead to or exacerbate head and neck discomfort.
In what kinds of recreational activity do you participate? Describe the activity.	Contact or aggressive sports may increase the risk for a head or neck injury.
Have any problems with your head or neck interfered with your relationships with others or the role you occupy at home or at work?	Head and neck pain may interfere with relationships or prevent clients from completing their usual activities of daily living.

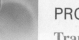

PROMOTE HEALTH
Traumatic Brain Injury

Overview

In 2007, the Centers for Disease Control and Prevention (CDC) estimated that the yearly impact of traumatic brain injury (TBI) in the United States is 1.1 million people treated and released from emergency rooms, 235,000 hospitalized and surviving, and 50,000 dead (NCIPC, 2007). Males have 1.5 times as much risk as females. The leading causes of TBI are falls (28%), motor vehicle accidents (20%), strikes by or against objects (19%), and assaults (11%). Outcomes of these injuries vary depending on cause: 91% of firearm-related TBIs result in death and 11% of fall-related TBIs are fatal (NCIPC, 2000). Each year, however, more than 80,000 Americans survive TBI to be discharged from the hospital with disabilities. Approximately 5.3 million Americans were alive in 1997 with TBI-related disabilities, which include impaired cognition (concentration, memory, judgment, and mood), movement (strength, coordination, and balance), seizure activity, or persistent unconsciousness (1% of TBI survivors) (NCIPC, 2000).

Risk Factors
- Transportation accidents
- Violence (often firearm related)
- Falls (especially in the elderly and children)
- Male gender
- Failure to use protective equipment (helmets, seat belts)
- Participation in contact or other sports, such as soccer, football, boxing, ice hockey, baseball, skiing, skate or snowboarding, horseback riding, or motorcycle riding

Teach Risk Reduction Tips
- Use safe driving techniques
- Never drive while under the influence of alcohol, drugs, or medications that cause drowsiness
- Wear protective gear such as helmets and seat belts
- Avoid violent or potentially violent environments when possible
- Work with community agencies to modify violent environments; develop anger management programs, drug-free programs, and firearm safety programs
- Modify one's residence to prevent falls, especially for the elderly and children
- Acquire and learn safe use of adaptive equipment for safe mobility inside and outside the home
- Avoid dangerous contact sports likely to cause brain injury; wear protective equipment when engaging in such activity
- Make sure children's playgrounds are shock absorbent (hardwood mulch or sand)

COLLECTING OBJECTIVE DATA: PHYSICAL EXAMINATION

Examining the head allows the nurse to evaluate the overlying protective structures (cranium and facial bones) before evaluating the underlying special senses (vision, hearing, smell, and taste) and the functioning of the neurologic system. This examination can detect head and facial shape abnormalities, asymmetry, structural changes, or tenderness. Assessment of both the head and neck assists the nurse to detect enlarged or tender lymph nodes. Thyroid enlargement, nodules, masses, or tenderness may be detected by palpating the thyroid gland. Palpation may also detect abnormalities of the neck and facial muscles.

Preparing the Client

Prepare the client for the head and neck examination by instructing him or her to remove any wig, hat, hair ornaments, pins, rubber bands, jewelry, and head or neck scarves.

 Take care to consider cultural norms for touch when assessing the head. Some cultures (e.g., Southeast Asian) prohibit touching the head or touching the feet before touching the head (Purnell & Paulanka, 2003).

Ask the client to sit in an upright position with the back and shoulders held back and straight. Explain the importance of remaining still during most of the inspection and palpation of the head and neck. However, explain she will be requested to move and bend the neck for examination of muscles and for palpation of the thyroid gland. Be aware that some clients may be anxious as you palpate the neck for lymph nodes, especially if they have a history of cancer that caused lymph node enlargement. Tell the client what you are doing and share your assessment findings.

 Another important thing to keep in mind as you examine the head and neck is that normal facial structures and features tend to vary widely among individuals and cultures.

Equipment

- Gloves
- Small cup of water
- Stethoscope

(text continues on page 223)

PHYSICAL ASSESSMENT

Assessment Procedure	Normal Findings	Abnormal Findings

Head and Face

Inspection and Palpation

Inspect the head. Inspect for size, shape, and configuration.

Head size and shape vary, especially in accord with ethnicity. Usually the head is symmetric, round, erect, and in midline. No lesions are visible.

The skull and facial bones are larger and thicker in acromegaly, which occurs when there is an increased production of growth hormone (Abnormal Findings 14-1).

Acorn-shaped, enlarged skull bones are seen in Paget's disease of the bone.

Inspect for involuntary movement.

Head should be held still and upright.

Tremors associated with neurologic disorders may cause a horizontal jerking movement. An involuntary nodding movement may be seen in patients with aortic insufficiency. Head tilted to one side may indicate unilateral vision or hearing deficiency or shortening of the sternomastoid muscle.

Palpate the head. Palpate for consistency.

> **Clinical Tip** • *Wear gloves to protect yourself from possible drainage.*

The head is normally hard and smooth without lesions.

Lesions or lumps on the head may indicate recent trauma or cancer.

Inspect the face. Inspect for symmetry, features, movement, expression, and skin condition.

> **Clinical Tip** • *The nasolabial folds and palpebral fissures are ideal places to check facial features for symmetry.*

The face is symmetric with a round, oval, elongated, or square appearance. No abnormal movements noted.

 In older clients, facial wrinkles are prominent because subcutaneous fat decreases with age. In addition, the lower face may shrink and the mouth may be drawn inward as a result of resorption of mandibular bone, also an age-related process.

Asymmetry in front of the earlobes occurs with parotid gland enlargement from an abscess or tumor. Unusual or asymmetric orofacial movements may be from an organic disease or neurologic problem, which should be referred for medical follow-up.

Drooping of one side of the face may result from a stroke—or cerebrovascular accident (CVA)—or a neurologic condition known as Bell's palsy (Fig. 14-6).

A "masklike" face marks Parkinson's disease; a "sunken" face with depressed eyes and hollow cheeks is typical of cachexia (emaciation or wasting); and a pale, swollen face may result from nephrotic syndrome.

See Abnormal Findings 14-1 for additional abnormalities of the face.

Palpate the temporal artery, which is located between the top of the ear and the eye (Fig. 14-7).

The temporal artery is elastic and not tender.

The strength of the pulsation of the temporal artery may be decreased in the older client.

The temporal artery is hard, thick, and tender with inflammation as seen with temporal arteritis (inflammation of the temporal arteries that may lead to blindness).

continued

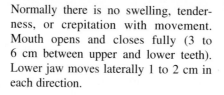

PHYSICAL ASSESSMENT *Continued*

Assessment Procedure	Normal Findings	Abnormal Findings
Palpate the temporomandibular joint. To assess the temporomandibular joint (TMJ), place your index finger over the front of each ear as you ask the client to open her mouth (Fig. 14-8). ➤ *Clinical Tip • When assessing TMJ syndrome, be sure to explore the client's history of headaches, if any.*	Normally there is no swelling, tenderness, or crepitation with movement. Mouth opens and closes fully (3 to 6 cm between upper and lower teeth). Lower jaw moves laterally 1 to 2 cm in each direction.	Limited range of motion, swelling, tenderness, or crepitation may indicate TMJ syndrome.

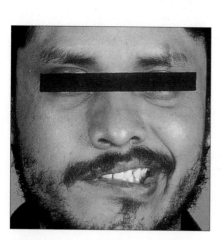

Figure 14-6 One-sided facial paralysis characterizes Bell's palsy. (© Chet Childs/CMSP.)

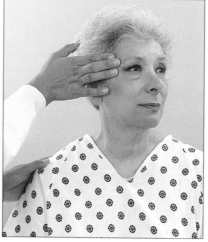

Figure 14-7 Palpating the temporal artery. (© B. Proud.)

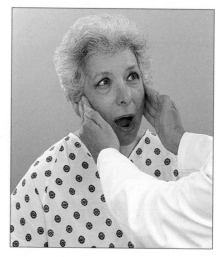

Figure 14-8 Palpating the TMJ. (© B. Proud.)

The Neck

Inspection

Inspect the neck. Observe the client's slightly extended neck for position, symmetry, and lumps or masses. Shine a light from the side of the neck across to highlight any swelling.	Neck is symmetric with head centered and without bulging masses.	Swelling, enlarged masses, or nodules may indicate an enlarged thyroid gland (Fig. 14-9), inflammation of lymph nodes, or a tumor.
Inspect movement of the neck structures. Ask the client to swallow a small sip of water. Observe the movement of the thyroid cartilage, thyroid gland (Fig. 14-10).	The thyroid cartilage, cricoid cartilage, and thyroid gland move upward symmetrically as the client swallows.	Asymmetric movement or generalized enlargement of the thyroid gland is considered abnormal.
Inspect the cervical vertebrae. Ask the client to flex the neck (chin to chest, ear to shoulder, twist left to right and right to left, and backward and forward). 👓 In older clients, cervical curvature may increase because of kyphosis of the spine. Moreover, fat may accumulate around the cervical vertebrae (especially in women). This is sometimes called a "dowager's hump."	C7 (vertebrae prominens) is usually visible and palpable.	Prominence or swellings other than the C7 vertebrae may be abnormal.

continued

Assessment Procedure	Normal Findings	Abnormal Findings
Inspect range of motion. Ask the client to turn the head to the right and to the left (chin to shoulder), touch each ear to the shoulder, touch chin to chest, and lift the chin to the ceiling.	Normally neck movement should be smooth and controlled with 45-degree flexion, 55-degree extension, 40-degree lateral abduction, and 70-degree rotation. 👓 Older clients usually have somewhat decreased flexion, extension, lateral bending, and rotation of the neck. This is usually due to arthritis.	Muscle spasms, inflammation, or cervical arthritis may cause stiffness, rigidity, and limited mobility of the neck, which may affect daily functioning.
Palpation **Palpate the trachea.** Place your finger in the sternal notch. Feel each side of the notch and palpate the tracheal rings (Fig. 14-11). The first upper ring above the smooth tracheal rings is the cricoid cartilage.	Trachea is midline.	The trachea may be pulled to one side in cases of a tumor, thyroid gland enlargement, aortic aneurysm, pneumothorax, atelectasis, or fibrosis.
Palpate the thyroid gland. Locate key landmarks with your index finger and thumb: *Hyoid bone* (arch-shaped bone that does not articulate directly with any other bone; located high in anterior neck). *Thyroid cartilage* (under the hyoid bone; the area that widens at the top of the trachea), also known as the "Adam's apple." *Cricoid cartilage* (smaller upper tracheal ring under the thyroid cartilage).	Landmarks are positioned midline.	Landmarks deviate from midline or are obscured because of masses or abnormal growths.

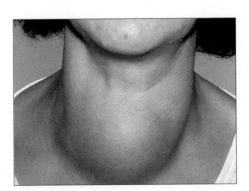

Figure 14-9 Diffuse enlargement of the thyroid gland.

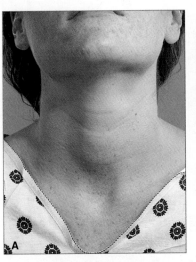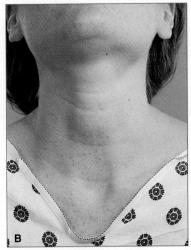

Figure 14-10 Inspecting the neck. **(A)** Slightly extended neck discloses internal structure. **(B)** Neck structures move (rise and fall). (© B. Proud.)

continued

PHYSICAL ASSESSMENT Continued

Assessment Procedure	Normal Findings	Abnormal Findings
To palpate the thyroid, use a posterior approach. Stand behind the client and ask her or him to lower the chin to the chest and turn the neck slightly to the right. This will relax the client's neck muscles. Then place your thumbs on the nape of the client's neck with your other fingers on either side of the trachea below the cricoid cartilage. Use your left fingers to push the trachea to the right. Then use your right fingers to feel deeply in front of the sternomastoid muscle (Fig. 14-12).	Unless the client is extremely thin with a long neck, the thyroid gland is usually not palpable. However, the isthmus may be palpated in midline. If the thyroid can be palpated, the lobes are smooth, firm, and nontender. The right lobe is often 25% larger than the left lobe. 👓 *If palpable,* the older client's thyroid may feel more nodular or irregular because of fibrotic changes that occur with aging; the thyroid may also be felt lower in the neck because of age-related structural changes.	In cases of diffuse enlargement; such as hyperthyroidism, Graves' disease, or an endemic goiter, the thyroid gland may be palpated. An enlarged, tender gland may result from thyroiditis. Multiple nodules of the thyroid may be seen in metabolic processes. However, rapid enlargement of a single nodule suggests a malignancy and must be evaluated further.
Ask the client to swallow as you palpate the right side of the gland. Reverse the technique to palpate the left lobe of the thyroid.	Glandular thyroid tissue may be felt rising underneath your fingers. Lobes should feel smooth, rubbery, and free of nodules.	Coarse tissue or irregular consistency may indicate an inflammatory process. Nodules should be described in terms of location, size, and consistency (see Spotlight Technique 14-1).
Auscultation **Auscultate the thyroid only if you find an enlarged thyroid gland during inspection or palpation.** Place the bell of the stethoscope over the lateral lobes of the thyroid gland (Fig. 14-13). Ask the client to hold his breath (to obscure any tracheal breath sounds while you auscultate).	No bruits are auscultated.	A soft, blowing, swishing sound auscultated over the thyroid lobes is often heard in hyperthyroidism because of an increase in blood flow through the thyroid arteries.

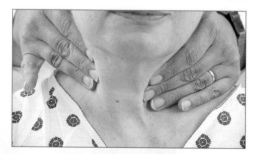

Figure 14-12   Palpating the thyroid. (© B. Proud.)

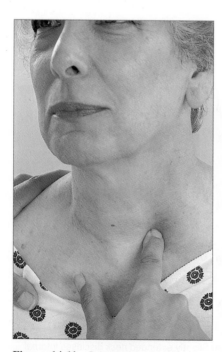

Figure 14-11   Palpating the trachea. (© B. Proud.)

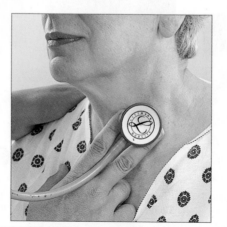

Figure 14-13   Auscultating for bruits over the thyroid gland. (© B. Proud.)

continued

SPOTLIGHT TECHNIQUE 14-1   Palpating Lymph Nodes

General Guidelines for Palpation

Have the client remain seated upright. Then palpate the lymph nodes with your fingerpads in a slow walking, gentle, circular motion. Ask the client to bend the head slightly toward the side being palpated to relax the muscles in that area. Compare lymph nodes that occur bilaterally. As you palpate each group of nodes, assess their size and shape, delimitation (whether they are discrete or confluent), mobility, consistency, and tenderness. Choose a particular palpation sequence. This chapter presents a sequence that proceeds in a superior to inferior order (from 1 to 10).

➤ *Clinical Tip • Which sequence you choose is not important. What is important is that you establish a specific sequence that does not vary from assessment to assessment. This helps to guard against skipping a group of nodes.*

Characteristics of the Lymph Nodes

While palpating the lymph nodes, note the following:

- Size and shape
- Delimitation
- Mobility
- Consistency
- Tenderness and location

Size and Shape

Normally lymph nodes, which are round and smaller than 1 cm, are not palpable. In older clients especially, the lymph nodes become fibrotic, fatty, and smaller because of a loss of lymphoid elements related to aging. (This may decrease the older person's resistance to infection.)

When lymph node enlargement exceeds 1 cm, the client is said to have lymphadenopathy, which may be caused by acute or chronic infection, an autoimmune disorder, or metastatic disease. If one or two lymphatic groups enlarge, the client is said to have *regional lymphadenopathy*. Enlargement of three or more groups is *generalized lymphadenopathy*. Generalized lymphadenopathy that persists for more than 3 months may be a sign of human immunodeficiency virus (HIV) infection.

Delimitation

Normally lymph node delimitation (the lymph node's position or boundary) is discrete. In chronic infection, however, the lymph nodes become confluent (they merge). In acute infection, they remain discrete.

Mobility

Typical lymph nodes are mobile both from side to side and up and down. In metastatic disease, the lymph nodes enlarge and become fixed in place.

Consistency

Somewhat more fibrotic and fatty in older clients, the normal lymph node is soft, whereas the abnormal node is hard and firm. Hard, firm, unilateral nodes are seen with metastatic cancers.

Tenderness and Location

Tender, enlarged nodes suggest acute infections; normally lymph nodes are not sore or tender. Of course, you need to document the location of the lymph node being assessed.

Lymph Nodes of the Head and Neck

Assessment Procedure	Normal Findings	Abnormal Findings
Spotlight Technique 14.1 describes general technique for palpating the lymph nodes.		
Palpate the **preauricular nodes** (in front of the ear), **postauricular nodes** (behind the ears), **occipital nodes** (at the posterior base of the skull).	There is no swelling or enlargement and no tenderness.	Enlarged nodes are abnormal.
Palpate the **tonsillar nodes** at the angle of the mandible on the anterior edge of the sternomastoid muscle (Fig. 14-14).	No swelling, no tenderness, no hardness is present.	Swelling, tenderness, hardness, immobility are abnormal.
Palpate the **submandibular nodes** located on the medial border of the mandible (Fig. 14-15).	No enlargement or tenderness is present.	Enlargement and tenderness are abnormal.

continued

PHYSICAL ASSESSMENT *Continued*

Assessment Procedure	Normal Findings	Abnormal Findings
➤ *Clinical Tip* • *Do not confuse the submandibular nodes with the lobulated submandibular gland.*		
Palpate the **submental nodes,** which are a few centimeters behind the tip of the mandible	No enlargement or tenderness is present.	Enlargement and tenderness are abnormal.
➤ *Clinical Tip* • *It is easier to palpate these nodes using one hand.*		
Palpate the **superficial cervical nodes** in the area superficial to the sternomastoid muscle.	No enlargement or tenderness is present.	Enlargement and tenderness are abnormal.
Palpate the **posterior cervical nodes** in the area posterior to the sternomastoid and anterior to the trapezius in the posterior triangle.	No enlargement or tenderness is present.	Enlargement and tenderness are abnormal.
Palpate the **deep cervical chain nodes** deeply within and around the sternomastoid muscle.	No enlargement or tenderness is present.	Enlargement and tenderness are abnormal.
Palpate the **supraclavicular nodes** by hooking your fingers over the clavicles and feeling deeply between the clavicles and the sternomastoid muscles (Fig. 14-16).	No enlargement or tenderness is present.	An enlarged, hard, nontender node, particularly on the left side, may indicate a metastasis from a malignancy in the abdomen or thorax.

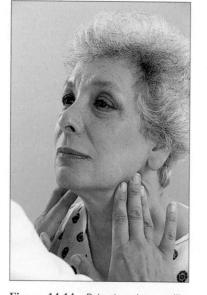

Figure 14-14 Palpating the tonsillar nodes. (© B. Proud.)

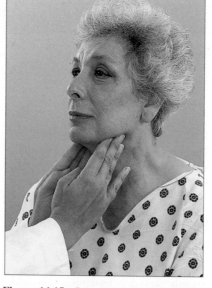

Figure 14-15 Palpating the submandibular nodes. (© B. Proud.)

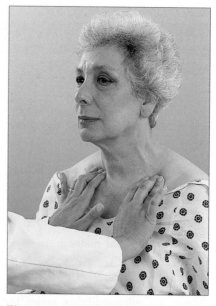

Figure 14-16 Palpating the supraclavicular nodes. (© B. Proud.)

Abnormal Findings 14-1 | Head and Neck Abnormalities

During any physical examination of the head, the nurse may encounter many variations from normal as well as many abnormalities. Some of the most common abnormalities are pictured here.

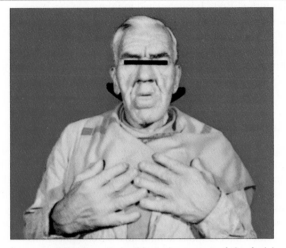

Acromegaly is characterized by enlargement of the facial features (nose, ears) and the hands and feet.

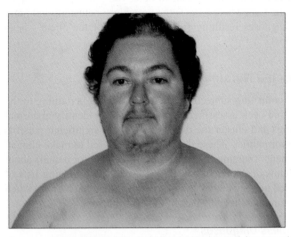

A moon-shaped face with reddened cheeks and increased facial hair may indicate Cushing's syndrome.

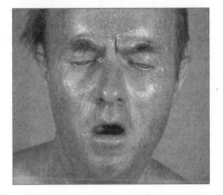

A tightened-hard face with thinning facial skin is seen in scleroderma. (With permission from Clements, P.J., & Furst, D.E. [1996]. Systemic sclerosis. Baltimore: Williams & Wilkins.)

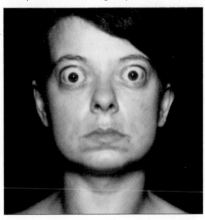

Exophthalmos is seen in hyperthyroidism.

VALIDATING AND DOCUMENTING FINDINGS

Validate the head and neck assessment data that you have collected. This is necessary to verify that the data are reliable and accurate. Document the assessment data following the health care facility or agency policy.

Sample of Subjective Data

No history of head or neck problems, trauma, or surgery. No head or facial pain. Has not experienced episodes of lightheadedness or dizziness. Does not chew or smoke tobacco. Works as secretary. Has good work setting and equipment to promote correct posture. Rides bikes 10 miles four times a week to relieve stress. Wears a bike helmet. Has no complaints about current condition of head and neck.

Sample of Objective Data

Head symmetrically round, hard, and smooth without lesions or bumps. Face oval, smooth, and symmetric. Temporal artery elastic and nontender. Temporomandibular joint palpated with full range of motion without tenderness. Neck symmetric with centered head position and no bulging masses. C7 is visible and palpable with neck flexed. Has smooth, controlled, full range of motion of neck. Thyroid gland nonvisible but palpable when swallowing. Trachea in midline. Lymph nodes nonpalpable except for a few deep cervical less than 1 cm bilaterally.

Analysis of Data

DIAGNOSTIC REASONING: POSSIBLE CONCLUSIONS

After collecting the assessment data, you will need to analyze the data. Listed below are some possible conclusions and nursing diagnoses resulting from assessment of the client's head and neck.

Selected Nursing Diagnoses

After collecting subjective and objective data pertaining to the head and neck assessment, you will need to identify abnormal findings and cluster the data to reveal any significant patterns or abnormalities. These data will then be used to make clinical judgments (nursing diagnoses: wellness, risk, or actual) about the status of the client's head and neck. The following lists of selected nursing diagnoses may be some that you identify when analyzing data for this part of the assessment.

Wellness Diagnoses

- Health-Seeking Behavior: Requests assistance information on how to quit smoking

Risk Diagnoses

- Risk for Injury to head and neck related to poor posture
- Risk for Injury to head and neck related to not wearing protective devices (e.g., head gear during contact sports, seat belts, eye goggles)

Actual Diagnoses

- Ineffective Health Maintenance related to lack of knowledge of the importance of wearing protective gear during contact sports and wearing seat belt while driving or riding as a passenger
- Ineffective Health Maintenance related to lack of knowledge of the effects and dangers associated with smoking and using smokeless tobacco
- Ineffective Tissue Perfusion: Cerebral related to impaired circulation to brain
- Imbalanced Nutrition: Less Than Body Requirements related to increased metabolism secondary to hyperthyroidism
- Imbalanced Nutrition: More Than Body Requirements related to decreased metabolism secondary to hypothyroidism
- Imbalanced Nutrition: Less Than Body Requirements related to irritated oral cavity that prevents consumption of food
- Activity Intolerance related to fatigue and weakness secondary to slowed metabolic rate secondary to hypothyroidism or to surgery of head, neck, or face
- Constipation related to hyperthyroidism or hypothyroidism
- Disturbed Body Image related to injury
- Impaired Swallowing related to mechanical obstruction of the head and neck secondary to tissue swelling, tracheostomy, or abnormal growth
- Impaired Swallowing related to lack of gag reflex, paralysis of facial muscles, or decreased cognition

Selected Collaborative Problems

After grouping the data, certain collaborative problems may become apparent. Remember that collaborative problems differ from nursing diagnoses in that they cannot be prevented by nursing interventions. However, these physiologic complications of medical conditions can be detected and monitored by the nurse. In addition, the nurse can use physician- and nurse-prescribed interventions to minimize the complications of these problems. The nurse may also have to refer the client in such situations for further treatment of the problem. Following is a list of collaborative problems that may be identified when assessing the head and neck of a patient. These problems are worded as Risk for Complications (or RC), followed by the problem.

- RC: Hypocalcemia
- RC: Hypercalcemia
- RC: Corneal abrasion (related to inability to close eyelids secondary to exophthalmos)
- RC: Thyroid crisis
- RC: Thyroid dysfunction
- RC: Cerebral vascular accident
- RC: Seizures
- RC: Cranial nerve impairment (fifth trigeminal, seventh facial, eleventh spinal accessory)
- RC: Increased intracranial pressure

Medical Problems

After the data are grouped, it may become apparent that the client has signs and symptoms that may require medical diagnosis and treatment. Referral to a primary care provider is necessary.

CASE STUDY

The case study presents assessment data for a specific client. It is followed by an analysis of the data to arrive at specific conclusions. The critical thinking exercises included in the study guide/lab manual and interactive product that complement this text also offer opportunities to analyze assessment data.

You are volunteering to do health screening assessments at a neighborhood clinic. You observe Margy Kase, who is 19 years old, and notice a diffuse swelling of her anterior neck. Margy is thin and fidgety. She has beads of perspiration on her forehead and upper lip, even though the room is cool. She denies any throat pain or difficulty swallowing, but she says that she is hungry all of the time lately and thinks she has lost some weight. She says she has come to the clinic today for a physical examination because she wants to stay healthy, even though she doesn't have health insurance and cannot afford a doctor. She tells you that somehow she manages to obtain a yearly checkup.

Margy's height is 5 ft. 9 in., and her weight is 110 lb. She states, "This is about 7 pounds lower than my normal weight." As you consult the standard weight charts, you discover that she is in about the fifth percentile for her age, with a medium frame. Her vital signs: BP 132/78, pulse 96, respirations 18. She does not know what her usual blood pressure is. Her thyroid gland appears slightly enlarged when palpated, and a bruit is detected upon auscultation. The rest of the physical examination findings appear to be within normal limits.

The following concept map illustrates the diagnostic reasoning process.

Applying COLDSPA

Applying **COLDSPA** for client symptoms: "hungry all the time, diffuse swelling in neck."

Mnemonic	Question	Data Provided	Missing Data
Character	Describe the sign or symptom (feeling, appearance, sound, smell, or taste if applicable).	"I am hungry all the time." Client appears thin, fidgety, and is perspiring on her forehead and upper lip in a cool exam room.	
Onset	When did it begin?		"When did you first start feeling hungry all the time? When did you first start losing weight?"
Location	Where is it? Does it radiate? Does it occur anywhere else?		"Have you noticed the swelling in your neck? When did this begin?"
Duration	How long does it last? Does it recur?		"What times of the day are you more or less hungry?"
Severity	How bad is it? How much does it bother you?	"I have lost weight."	"How much weight have you lost?"
Pattern	What makes it better or worse?		"Is there anything that relieves your hunger?"
Associated factors/How it **A**ffects the client	What other symptoms occur with it? How does it affect you?	"I want to stay healthy, but I do not have any health insurance and cannot afford a doctor."	"What other symptoms have you noticed with the weight loss?" Any excessive thirst or urinating?"

1) Identify abnormal findings and client strengths

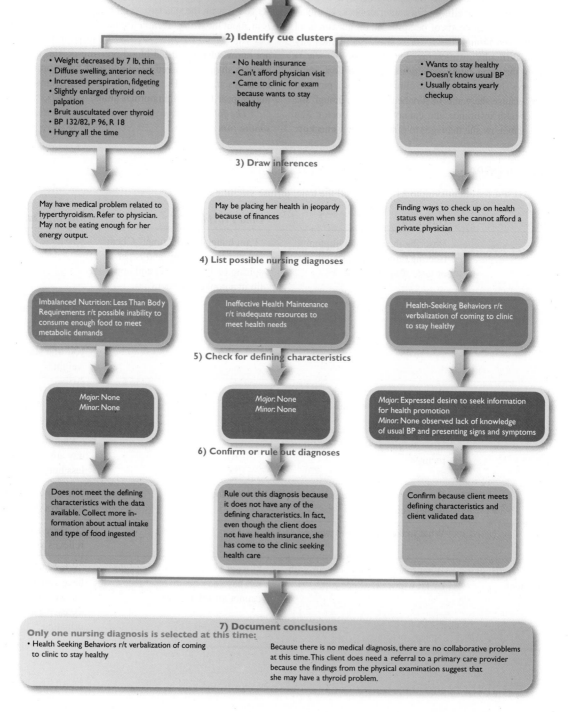

Subjective Data

- 7-lb weight loss
- Does not know her usual blood pressure
- Hungry all the time
- Came to clinic for physical examination because she wants to stay healthy
- No health insurance and cannot afford a doctor
- Usually obtains a yearly checkup
- Denies throat pain and difficulty swallowing

Objective Data

- Thin, 19-year-old woman
- Weight at 110 lb is in fifth percentile for height
- Excessive perspiration and fidgeting
- Diffuse swelling of anterior neck
- Slightly enlarged thyroid on palpation
- BP 132/82, P 96, R 18

2) Identify cue clusters

- Weight decreased by 7 lb, thin
- Diffuse swelling, anterior neck
- Increased perspiration, fidgeting
- Slightly enlarged thyroid on palpation
- Bruit auscultated over thyroid
- BP 132/82, P 96, R 18
- Hungry all the time

- No health insurance
- Can't afford physician visit
- Came to clinic for exam because wants to stay healthy

- Wants to stay healthy
- Doesn't know usual BP
- Usually obtains yearly checkup

3) Draw inferences

May have medical problem related to hyperthyroidism. Refer to physician. May not be eating enough for her energy output.

May be placing her health in jeopardy because of finances

Finding ways to check up on health status even when she cannot afford a private physician

4) List possible nursing diagnoses

Imbalanced Nutrition: Less Than Body Requirements r/t possible inability to consume enough food to meet metabolic demands

Ineffective Health Maintenance r/t inadequate resources to meet health needs

Health-Seeking Behaviors r/t verbalization of coming to clinic to stay healthy

5) Check for defining characteristics

Major: None
Minor: None

Major: None
Minor: None

Major: Expressed desire to seek information for health promotion
Minor: None observed lack of knowledge of usual BP and presenting signs and symptoms

6) Confirm or rule out diagnoses

Does not meet the defining characteristics with the data available. Collect more information about actual intake and type of food ingested

Rule out this diagnosis because it does not have any of the defining characteristics. In fact, even though the client does not have health insurance, she has come to the clinic seeking health care

Confirm because client meets defining characteristics and client validated data

7) Document conclusions

Only one nursing diagnosis is selected at this time:
- Health Seeking Behaviors r/t verbalization of coming to clinic to stay healthy

Because there is no medical diagnosis, there are no collaborative problems at this time. This client does need a referral to a primary care provider because the findings from the physical examination suggest that she may have a thyroid problem.

References and Selected Readings

Al-Absi, A. I., Wall, B. M., & Cooke, C. R. (2004). Medial arterial calcification mimicking temporal arteritis. *American Journal of Kidney Diseases, 44*(4), e73–78.

Argueta, R. (2000). When a thyroid abnormality is palpable. Symposium. First of four articles on thyroid diseases. *Postgraduate Medicine, 107*(1), 100–104, 109–110, 155–156.

Atassi, K. A., & Harris, M. L. (2000). Action stat: Subarachnoid hemorrhage. *Nursing, 30*(1), 33.

Bell, S. (2002). Headaches: Assessment and management. *Ohio Nurses Review, 77*(10), 4–7, 12–13, quiz 13–14.

Brach, J. (1999). Not all facial paralysis is Bell's palsy: A case report. *Archives of Physical Medicine and Rehabilitation, 80*(7), 857–859.

Bruce, S. D. (2004). Radiation induced xerostomia: How dry is your patient? *Clinical Journal of Oncology Nursing, 8*(1), 61–67.

Byard, E. (2000). Exertional headaches: Misdiagnosis can have long-lasting effects. *Advance for Nurse Practitioners, 8*(11), 87–88.

Charters, A. (2004). Can nurses, working in the emergency department, independently clear cervical spines? A review of the literature. *Accident and Emergency Nursing.* 12(1), 19–23.

Deschler, D. G., Walsh, K., & Hayden, R. E. (2004). Follow-up quality of life assessment in patients after head and neck surgery as evaluated by lay caregivers. *ORL Head and Neck Nursing, 22*(1), 26–32.

Duckett, K. (2004). The right assessments = the right PPS payment. *Home Health Nurse, 22*(5), 312–316.

Facial paralysis. (2007). Available at http://www.nlm.nih.gov/medlineplus/.

Goiter. (2007). Available at http://mayoclinic.com/health/goiter/DS00217

Holm, G. B. (2004). Office management of back and neck pain. Principles of diagnosis and treatment. *Advance for Nurse Practitioners, 12*(7), 38–43.

Kappes, J. N., & McNair, R. S. (2003). Headache and visual changes at triage: Do not allow the patient assumptions to cloud your critical thinking. *Journal of Emergency Nursing, 29*(6), 584–586.

Kunkel, R. (2000). Managing primary headache symptoms. *Patient Care, 34*(2), 100–117.

Moloney, M. (2000). Caring for the women with migraine headaches. *Nurse Practitioner: American Journal of Primary Health Care, 25*(2), 17–18, 21–22, 24.

National Institute of Neurological Disorders and Stroke (NINDS). (2008). NINDS headache information page. Available at http://ninds.nih.gov/disorders/headache.

[No authors listed] (2003). What you need to know about . . . hyperthyroidism. *Nursing Times, 99*(24), 32.

Sakai, O., Curtain, H. D., Romo, L. V., & Som, P. M. (2000). Lymph node pathology. Benign proliferative, lymphoma, & metastatic disease. *Radiology Clinics of North America, 38*(5), 979–998.

Schori-Ahmed, D. (2003). Defenses gone awry. Thyroid disease. *RN, 66*(6), 38–43; quiz 44.

Voog, U., Alstergren, P., Leibur, E., Kallikorm, R., & Kopp, S. (2003). Impact of temporomandibular joint pain on activities of daily living in patients with rheumatoid arthritis. *Acta Odontologica Scandinavica, 61*(5), 278–282.

Zimmerman, P. G. (2002). Triage and differential diagnosis of patients with headaches, dizziness, low back pain, and rashes: a basic primer. *Journal of Emergency Nursing, 28*(3), 209–215.

Promote Health—Traumatic Brain Injury

Centers for Disease Control and Prevention (CDC). National Center for Injury Prevention and Control. (2000). *Epidemiology of traumatic brain injury in the United States.* Available: www.cdc.gov/ncipc.

National Center for Injury Prevention and Control (NCIPC). (2007). TBI—Traumatic brain injury. Available at http://www.cdc.gov/ncipc/tbi/TBI.htm.

National Institute of Neurological Disorders and Stroke (NINDS). (2007). Traumatic brain injury information page. Available at http://www.ninds.nih.gov/disorders/tbi/tbi.htm.

Structure and Function

The eye transmits visual stimuli to the brain for interpretation and, in doing so, functions as the organ of vision. The eyeball is located in the eye orbit, a round, bony hollow formed by several different bones of the skull. In the orbit, the eye is surrounded by a cushion of fat. The bony orbit and fat cushion protect the eyeball.

To perform a thorough assessment of the eye, you need a good understanding of the external structures of the eye, the internal structures of the eye, the visual fields and pathways, and the visual reflexes.

EXTERNAL STRUCTURES OF THE EYE

The **eyelids** (upper and lower) are two movable structures composed of skin and two types of muscle: striated and smooth. Their purpose is to protect the eye from foreign bodies and limit the amount of light entering the eye. In addition, they serve to distribute tears that lubricate the surface of the eye (Fig. 15-1). The upper eyelid is larger, more mobile, and contains *tarsal plates* made up of connective tissue. These plates contain the *meibomian glands,* which secrete an oily substance that lubricates the eyelid.

The eyelids join at two points: the **lateral (outer) canthus** and **medial (inner) canthus.** The medial canthus contains the puncta, two small openings that allow drainage of tears into the lacrimal system, and the **caruncle,** a small, fleshy mass that contains sebaceous glands. The white space between open eyelids is called the **palpebral fissure.** When closed, the eyelids should touch. When open, the upper lid position should be between the upper margin of the iris and the upper margin of the pupil. The lower lid should rest on the lower border of the iris. No sclera should be seen above or below the limbus (the point where the sclera meets the cornea).

Eyelashes are projections of stiff hair curving outward along the margins of the eyelids that filter dust and dirt from air entering the eye.

The **conjunctiva** is a thin, transparent, continuous membrane that is divided into two portions: a *palpebral* and a *bulbar* portion. The palpebral conjunctiva lines the inside of the eyelids, and the bulbar conjunctiva covers most of the anterior eye, merging with the cornea at the limbus. The point at which the palpebral and bulbar conjunctivae meet creates a folded recess that allows movement of the eyeball. This transparent membrane allows for inspection of underlying tissue and serves to protect the eye from foreign bodies.

The **lacrimal apparatus** consists of glands and ducts that serve to lubricate the eye (Fig. 15-2). The *lacrimal gland,* located in the upper outer corner of the orbital cavity just above the eye, produces tears. As the lid blinks, tears wash across the eye then drain into the *puncta,* which are visible on the upper and lower lids at the inner canthus. Tears empty into the *lacrimal canals* and are then channeled into the *nasolacrimal sac* through the *nasolacrimal duct.* They drain into the nasal meatus.

The **extraocular muscles** are the six muscles attached to the outer surface of each eyeball (Fig. 15-3). These muscles control six different directions of eye movement. Four rectus muscles are responsible for straight movement, and two oblique muscles are responsible for diagonal movement. Each muscle coordinates with a muscle in the opposite eye. This allows for parallel movement of the eyes and thus the binocular vision characteristic of humans. Innervation for these muscles is supplied by three cranial nerves: the oculomotor (III) trochlear (IV), and abducens (VI).

INTERNAL STRUCTURES OF THE EYE

The eyeball is composed of three separate coats or **layers** (Fig. 15-4). The external layer consists of the *sclera* and *cornea.* The **sclera** is a dense, protective, white covering that physically supports the internal structures of the eye. It is continuous anteriorly with the transparent cornea (the "window of the eye"). The **cornea** permits the entrance of light, which passes through the lens to the retina. It is well supplied with nerve endings, making it responsive to pain and touch.

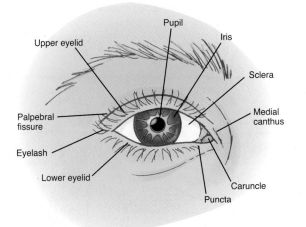

Figure 15-1 External structures of the eye.

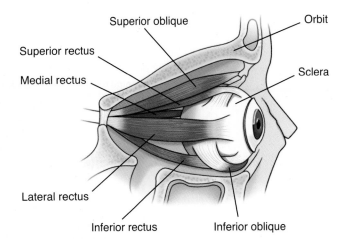

Figure 15-3 Extraocular muscles control the direction of eye movement.

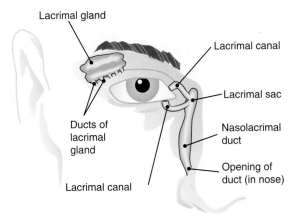

Figure 15-2 The lacrimal apparatus consists of tear (lacrimal) glands and ducts.

➤ **Clinical Tip** • *Because of this sensory property, contact with a wisp of cotton stimulates a blink in both eyes known as the* corneal reflex. *This reflex is supported by the trigeminal nerve, which carries the afferent sensation into the brain, and the facial nerve, which carries the efferent message that stimulates the blink.*

The middle layer contains both an anterior portion, which includes the *iris* and the *ciliary body,* and a posterior layer, which includes the *choroid.* The *ciliary body* consists of muscle tissue that controls the thickness of the lens, which must be adapted to focus on objects near and far away.

The **iris** is a circular disc of muscle containing pigments that determine eye color. The central aperture of the iris is called the **pupil.** Muscles in the iris adjust to control the pupil's size, which controls the amount of light entering the eye. The muscle fibers of the iris also decrease the size of the pupil to accommodate for near vision and dilate the pupil when far vision is needed.

The **lens** is a biconvex, transparent, avascular, encapsulated structure located immediately posterior to the iris. Suspensory ligaments attached to the ciliary body support the position of the lens. The lens functions to refract (bend) light rays onto the retina. Adjustments must be made in refraction depending on the distance of the object being viewed. Refractive ability of the lens can be changed by a change in shape of the lens (which is controlled by the ciliary body). The lens bulges to focus on close objects and flattens to focus on far objects.

The **chorioid layer** contains the vascularity necessary to provide nourishment to the inner aspect of the eye and prevents light from reflecting internally. Anteriorly, it is continuous with the ciliary body and the iris.

The innermost layer, the **retina,** extends only to the ciliary body anteriorly. It receives visual stimuli and sends it to the brain. The retina consists of numerous layers of nerve cells, including the cells commonly called rods and cones. These specialized nerve cells are often referred to as "photoreceptors" because they are responsive to light. The rods are highly sensitive to light, regulate black and white vision, and function in dim light. The cones function in bright light and are sensitive to color.

The **optic disc** is a cream-colored, circular area located on the retina toward the medial or nasal side of the eye. It is where the optic nerve enters the eyeball. The optic disc can be seen with the use of an ophthalmoscope and is normally round or oval in shape, with distinct margins. A smaller circular area that appears slightly depressed is referred to as the **physiologic cup.** This area is approximately one-third the size of the entire optic disc and appears somewhat lighter/whiter than the disc borders.

The **retinal vessels** can be readily viewed with the aid of an ophthalmoscope. Four sets of *arterioles* and *venules* travel through the optic disc, bifurcate, and extend to the periphery of the fundus. Vessels are dark red and grow progressively narrower as they extend out to the peripheral areas. Arterioles carry oxygenated blood and appear brighter red and narrower than the veins. The general background, or fundus (Fig. 15-5),

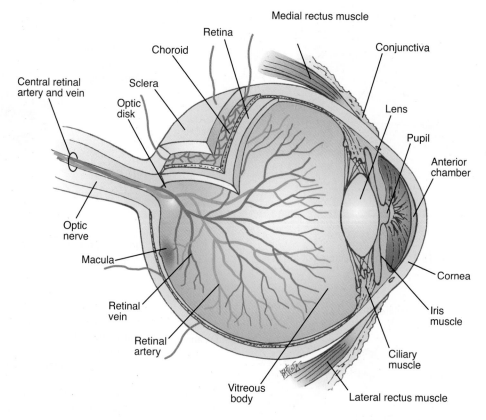

Figure 15-4 Anatomy of the eye.

varies in color, depending on skin color. A retinal depression known as the fovea centralis is located adjacent to the optic disc in the temporal section of the fundus. This area is surrounded by the macula, which appears darker than the rest of the fundus. The fovea centralis and macular area are highly concentrated with cones and form the area of highest visual resolution and color vision.

The eyeball contains several chambers that serve to maintain structure, protect against injury, and transmit light rays. The **anterior chamber** is located between the cornea and iris, and the **posterior chamber** is the area between the iris and the lens. These chambers are filled with aqueous humor, a clear liquid substance produced by the ciliary body. **Aqueous humor** helps to cleanse and nourish the cornea and lens as well as maintain intraocular pressure. The aqueous humor filters out of the eye from the posterior to the anterior chamber then into the *canal of Schlemm* through a filtering site called the *trabecular meshwork.* Another chamber, the **vitreous chamber,** is located in the area behind the lens to the retina. It is the largest of the chambers and is filled with a vitreous humor that's clear and gelatinous.

VISION

Visual Fields and Visual Pathways

A **visual field** refers to what a person sees with one eye. The visual field of each eye can be divided into four quadrants: upper temporal, lower temporal, upper nasal, and lower nasal (Fig. 15-6). The temporal quadrants of each visual field extend farther than the nasal quadrants. Thus, each eye sees a slightly different view but their visual fields overlap quite a bit. As a result of this, humans have binocular vision ("two-eyed" vision) in which the visual cortex fuses the two slightly different images and provides depth perception or three-dimensional vision.

Visual perception occurs as light rays strike the retina, where they are transformed into nerve impulses, conducted to the brain through the optic nerve, and interpreted. In the eye, light must pass through transparent media (cornea, aqueous humor, lens, and vitreous body) before reaching the retina.

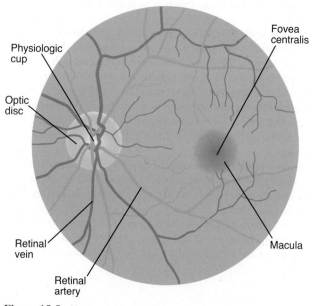

Figure 15-5 Normal ocular fundus.

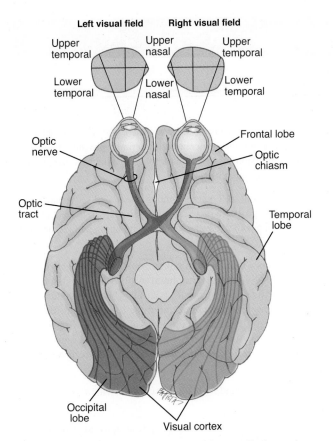

Figure 15-6 Visual fields and visual pathways. Each eye has a slightly different view of the same field. However, the views overlap significantly, which accounts for binocular vision.

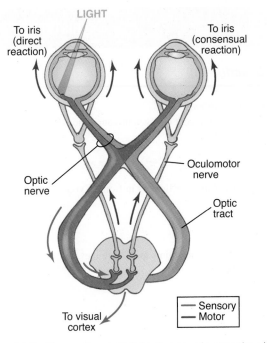

Figure 15-7 The pupils admit light that travels over the visual pathways. If a light focuses on only one eye, the pupil responds to ensure that the light needed for vision can enter but not so much that eye damage would result. The other pupil responds in the same manner. This phenomenon of direct pupillary response and consensual pupillary response is a reflex governed by the oculomotor nerve.

The cornea and lens are the main eye components that refract (bend) light rays on the retina. The image projected on the retina is upside down and reversed right to left from the actual image. For example, an image from the lower temporal visual field strikes the upper temporal quadrant of the retina. At the point where the optic nerves from each eyeball cross—the **optic chiasma**—the nerve fibers from the nasal quadrant of each retina (from both temporal visual fields) cross over to the opposite side. At this point, the right optic tract contains only nerve fibers from the right side of the retina and the left optic tract contains only nerve fibers from the left side of the retina. Therefore, the left side of the brain views the right side of the world.

Visual Reflexes

The **pupillary light reflex** causes pupils immediately to constrict when exposed to bright light. This can be seen as a *direct reflex,* in which constriction occurs in the eye exposed to the light, or as an *indirect or consensual reflex,* in which exposure to light in one eye results in constriction of the pupil in the opposite eye (Fig. 15-7). These protective reflexes, mediated by the oculomotor nerve, prevent damage to the delicate photoreceptors by excessive light.

Accommodation is a functional reflex allowing the eyes to focus on near objects. This is accomplished through movement of the ciliary muscles causing an increase in the curvature of the lens. This change in shape of the lens is not visible.

However, convergence of the eyes and constriction of the pupils occur simultaneously and can be seen.

Health Assessment

COLLECTING SUBJECTIVE DATA: THE NURSING HEALTH HISTORY

Beginning when the nurse first meets the client, assessment of vision provides important information about the client's ability to interact with the environment. Changes in vision are often gradual and go unrecognized by clients until a severe problem develops. Therefore, asking the client specific questions about his vision may help with early detection of disorders. With recent advances in medicine and surgery, early detection and intervention are increasingly important.

First gather data from the client about his or her current level of eye health. Also discuss any past and family history problems that are related to the eye. Collecting data concerning environmental influences on vision as well as how any problems are influencing or affecting the client's usual activities of daily living is also important. Answers to these types of questions help to evaluate a client's risk for vision loss and, in turn, present ways that the client may modify or reduce the risk of eye problems.

(text continues on page 235)

HISTORY OF PRESENT HEALTH CONCERN

Question	*Rationale*
Visual Problems	
Describe any recent changes in your vision. Were they sudden or gradual?	Sudden changes in vision are associated with acute problems such as head trauma or increased intracranial pressure. Gradual changes in vision may be related to aging, diabetes, hypertension, or neurologic disorders.
Do you see spots or floaters in front of your eyes?	Spots or floaters are common among clients with myopia or in clients over age 40. In most cases, they are due to normal physiologic changes in the eye associated with aging and require no intervention.
Do you experience blind spots? Are they constant or intermittent?	A scotoma is a blind spot that is surrounded by either normal or slightly diminished peripheral vision. It may be from glaucoma. Intermittent blind spots may be associated with vascular spasms (ophthalmic migraines) or pressure on the optic nerve by a tumor or intracranial pressure. Consistent blind spots may indicate retinal detachment. Any report of a blind spot requires immediate attention and referral to a physician.
Do you see halos or rings around lights?	Seeing halos around lights is associated with narrow-angle glaucoma.
Do you have trouble seeing at night?	Night blindness is associated with optic atrophy, glaucoma, and vitamin A deficiency.
Do you experience double vision?	Double vision (diplopia) may indicate increased intracranial pressure due to injury or a tumor.
Other Symptoms	
Do you have any eye pain or itching? Describe.	Burning or itching pain is usually associated with allergies or superficial irritation. Throbbing, stabbing, or deep, aching pain suggests a foreign body in the eye or changes within the eye.
	Most common eye disorders are not associated with actual pain; therefore, any reported eye pain should be referred immediately.
Do you have any redness or swelling in your eyes?	Redness or swelling of the eye is usually related to an inflammatory response caused by allergy, foreign body, or bacterial or viral infection.
Do you experience excessive watering or tearing of the eye? One eye or both eyes?	Excessive tearing (epiphora) is caused by exposure to irritants or obstruction of the lacrimal apparatus. Unilateral epiphora is often associated with foreign body or obstruction. Bilateral epiphora is often associated with exposure to irritants, such as makeup or facial cleansers, or it may be a systemic response.
Have you had any eye discharge? Describe.	Discharge other than tears from one or both eyes suggests a bacterial or viral infection.

continued

COLDSPA Example for Eye Pain

Use the **COLDSPA** mnemonic as a guideline to collect needed information for each symptom the client shares. In addition, the following questions help elicit important information.

Mnemonic	Question	Client Response Example
Character	Describe the sign or symptom (feeling, appearance, sound, smell, or taste if applicable).	"My right eye really hurts."
Onset	When did it begin?	"A couple of hours ago, when I accidentally poked my key in my eye."
Location	Where is it? Does it radiate? Does it occur anywhere else?	"Only my right eye."
Duration	How long does it last? Does it recur?	"It hurts constantly."
Severity	How bad is it? or How much does it bother you?	"It makes it difficult to drive and is quite painful."
Pattern	What makes it better or worse?	"It hurts when I blink and feels better if I keep my eye shut."
Associated factors/How it **A**ffects the client	What other symptoms occur with it? How does it affect you?	"My right eye is watery and my vision is blurry."

PAST HEALTH HISTORY

Question	Rationale
Have you ever had problems with your eyes or vision?	A history of eye problems or changes in vision provides clues to the current health of the eye.
Have you ever had eye surgery?	Surgery may alter the appearance of the eye and the results of future examinations.
Describe any past treatments you have received for eye problems (medication, surgery, laser treatments, corrective lenses). Were these successful? Were you satisfied?	Client may not be satisfied with past treatments for vision problems.

FAMILY HISTORY

Question	Rationale
Is there a history of eye problems or vision loss in your family?	Many eye disorders have familial tendencies. Examples include glaucoma, refraction errors, and allergies.

LIFESTYLE AND HEALTH PRACTICES

Question	Rationale
Are you exposed to conditions or substances in the workplace or home that may harm your eyes or vision (e.g., chemicals, fumes, smoke, dust, or flying sparks)? Do you wear safety glasses during exposure to harmful substances?	Injuries or diseases may be related to exposure in the workplace or home. These problems can be minimized or avoided altogether with hazard identification and implementation of safety measures.

continued on page 234

LIFESTYLE AND HEALTH PRACTICES *Continued*

Question	Rationale
Do you wear sunglasses during exposure to the sun?	Exposure to ultraviolet radiation puts the client at risk for the development of cataracts (opacities of the lenses of the eyes; see Promote Health—Cataracts, Glaucoma, and Macular Degeneration). Consistent use of sunglasses during exposure minimizes the client's risk.
What types of medications do you take?	Some medications have ocular side effects such as corticosteroids, lovastatin, pyridostigmine, quinidine, risperidone, and rifampin.
Has your vision loss affected your ability to care for yourself? To work?	Vision problems may interfere with the client's ability to perform usual activities of daily living. The client may be unable to read medication labels or fill insulin syringes. If the vision problem is severe, the client's ability to perform hygiene practices or prepare food may be affected. Vision problems may affect a client's ability to work if the job is one that depends on sight, such as pilot or bus driver.
When was your last eye examination?	A thorough eye examination is recommended for healthy clients every 2 years. Clients with eye disorders or vision problems should be examined more frequently according to their physician's recommendations.
Do you have a prescription for corrective lenses (glasses or contacts)? Do you wear them regularly? If you wear contacts, how long do you wear them? How do you clean them?	The amount of time the client wears the corrective lenses provides information on the severity of the visual problem. Clients who do not wear the prescribed corrective lenses are susceptible to eye strain. Improper cleaning or prolonged wearing of contact lenses can lead to infection and corneal damage.

PROMOTE HEALTH

Cataracts, Glaucoma, and Macular Degeneration

Overview

Cataracts are the leading cause of blindness worldwide, followed by glaucoma. Part of the VISION 2020 Global Initiative of the WHO is devoted to reducing cataract, glaucoma, and macular degeneration which cause approximately 161 million people worldwide to be visually impaired (WHO, 2007).

Cataract is the name given to opacity or clouding of the eye's lens. The opacity can develop in various parts of the lens. Glaucoma is a group of diseases that may begin with no symptoms but lead to vision loss through optic nerve damage. Glaucoma involves loss of retinal ganglion cells causing optic neuropathy. Increased intraocular pressure is often but not always associated with glaucoma. Macular degeneration is a group of diseases characterized by breakdown of the center portion of the retina known as the macula.

Risk Factors—Cataracts

- Increasing age, especially over age 50
- Prolonged exposure to ultraviolet B (UV-B) light, especially in latitudes closer to the equator
- Diabetes mellitus
- Cigarette smoking
- Alcohol use
- Diet low in antioxidants, especially vitamins E and B
- High blood pressure
- Eye injury/surgery
- Steroid use
- Female gender

Risk Factors—Glaucoma

- Increased intraocular pressure (IOP)
- Age, usually over age 40

continued

PROMOTE HEALTH

Cataracts, Glaucoma, and Macular Degeneration *Continued*

- Family history (genetics or similar environment)
- Race or ethnicity: African ancestry (increased IOP; develops at earlier age)
- Race or ethnicity: Caucasian of northern Europe ancestry (pseudoexfoliative type)
- Race or ethnicity: Asian (angle closure type)
- Arteriosclerosis
- Near or far sightedness (each predisposes to different type)

Risk Factors—Macular Degeneration
- Age (25% of those 65–74 and 33% of those over 74 years)
- Cigarette smoking
- Female gender and early menopause
- High blood pressure or cardiovascular disease
- Diet high in mono- or polyunsaturated fats, or linoleic vegetable fats, especially those found in snack foods
- Prolonged sun exposure

Teach Risk Reduction Tips
As many of the same causes result in these three eye diseases, preventive strategies overlap.
- Wear sunglasses and hats in the sun (even on cloudy days. Squinting does not eliminate ultraviolet light entering the eye).

- Quit smoking.
- Limit alcohol intake.
- Eat a diet high in antioxidant vitamins.
- Take a vitamin supplement of vitamin C (400 IU), vitamin E (15 IU), vitamin A (25,000 IU), zinc (80 mg), and copper (2 mg) if supported by your physician.
- Avoid high fat intake, even monounsaturated fats.
- Avoid eye injuries.
- Eat fish (for macular degeneration in particular)
- Have eyes examined regularly (every 4 years for 40–65 year olds; every 1–2 years for those over 65 years of age); new therapies have been developed to slow glaucoma if detected early.
- Seek medical care for the following symptoms:
  - Painless blurring of vision
  - Light sensitivity
  - Poor night vision
  - Double vision in one eye
  - Need for brighter light to read
  - Fading or yellowing of colors

(American Academy of Ophthalmology, 2003)

COLLECTING OBJECTIVE DATA: PHYSICAL EXAMINATION

The purpose of the eye and vision examination is to identify any changes in vision or signs of eye disorders in an effort to initiate early treatment or corrective procedures. Collected objective data should include assessment of eye function through specific vision tests, inspection of the external eye, and inspection of the internal eye using an ophthalmoscope.

For the most part, inspection and palpation of the external eye are straightforward and simple to perform. The vision tests and use of the ophthalmoscope require a great deal of skill, and thus practice, for the examiner to be capable and confident during the examination. It is a good idea for the beginning examiner to practice on friends, family, or classmates to gain experience and to become comfortable performing the examinations.

Preparing the Client

Explain each vision test thoroughly to guarantee accurate results. For the eye examination, position the client so she is seated comfortably. During examination of the internal eye with the ophthalmoscope, you will move very close to the client's face to view the retina and internal structures. Explain to the client that this may be slightly uncomfortable. To ease

any client anxiety, explain in detail what you will be doing and answer any questions the client may have.

Equipment

- Snellen or E chart
- Hand-held Snellen card or near vision screener
- Penlight
- Opaque cards
- Ophthalmoscope
- Disposable gloves (wear as needed to prevent spreading infection or coming in contact with exudate)

Physical Assessment

Before performing eye examination, review and recognize structures and functions of the eyes. While performing the examination, remember these key points:

- Administer vision tests competently and record the results.
- Use the ophthalmoscope correctly and confidently.
- Recognize and distinguish normal variations from abnormal findings.

(text continues on page 259)

PHYSICAL ASSESSMENT

Assessment Procedure	Normal Findings	Abnormal Findings

Evaluating Vision

Test distant visual acuity. Position the client 20 feet from the Snellen or E chart (see Equipment Spotlight 15-1) and ask her to read each line until she cannot decipher the letters or their direction (Fig. 15-8). Document the results.

> ➤ **Clinical Tip** • *If the client wears glasses, they should be left on unless they are reading glasses (reading glasses blur distance vision).*

During this vision test, note any client behaviors (i.e., leaning forward, head tilting or squinting) that could be unconscious attempts to see better.

Normal distant visual acuity is 20/20 with or without corrective lenses. This means the client can distinguish what the person with normal vision can distinguish from 20 feet away.

Myopia (impaired far vision) is present when the second number in the test result is larger than the first (20/40). The higher the second number, the poorer the vision. A client is considered legally blind when vision in the better eye with corrective lenses is 20/200 or less. Any client with vision worse than 20/30 should be referred for further evaluation.

 Visual acuity varies by race in U.S. populations. Japanese and Chinese Americans have the poorest corrected visual acuity (especially myopia) followed by African Americans and Hispanics. Native

---

EQUIPMENT SPOTLIGHT 15-1   Vision Charts

Snellen Chart
Used to test distant visual acuity, the Snellen chart consists of lines of different letters stacked one on top of the other. The letters are large at the top and decrease in size from top to bottom. The chart is placed on a wall or door at eye level in a well-lighted area. The client stands 20 feet from the chart and covers one eye with an opaque card (which prevents the client from peeking through the fingers). Then the client reads each line of letters until he or she can no longer distinguish them.

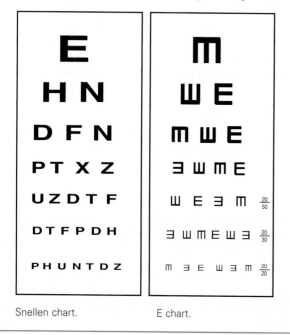

Snellen chart.   E chart.

E Chart
If the client cannot read or has a handicap that prevents verbal communication, the E chart is used. The E chart is configured just like the Snellen chart but the characters on it are only Es, which face in all directions. The client is asked to indicate by pointing which way the open side of the E faces. If the client wears glasses, they should be left on, unless they are reading glasses (reading glasses blur distance vision).

Test Results
Acuity results are recorded somewhat like blood pressure readings—in a manner that resembles a fraction (but in no way is interpreted as a fraction). A common example of an acuity test score is 20/20. The top, or first, number is always 20, indicating the distance from the client to the chart. The bottom, or second, number refers to the last full line the client could read. Usually the last line on the chart is the 20/20 line. The examiner needs to document whether the client wore glasses during the test. If any letters on a line are missed, encourage the client to continue reading until he or she cannot distinguish any letters, but record the number of letters missed by using a minus sign. If the client missed two letters on the 20/30 line, the recorded score would be 20/30 -2.

continued

Assessment Procedure	Normal Findings	Abnormal Findings

Americans and Caucasians have the best corrected acuity. Eskimos are undergoing an epidemic of myopia (Overfield, 1995; The Eye Digest, 2006; The Eye Disease Prevalence Group, 2004).

Test near visual acuity. Use this test for middle-aged clients and others who complain of difficulty reading.

Give the client a hand-held vision chart (e.g., Jaeger reading card, Snellen card, or comparable chart) to hold 14 inches from the eyes. Have the client cover one eye with an opaque card before reading from top (largest print) to bottom (smallest print). Repeat test for other eye.

> **Clinical Tip** • The client who wears glasses should keep them on for this test.

Normal near visual acuity is 14/14 (with or without corrective lenses). This means the client can read what the normal eye can read from a distance of 14 inches.

Presbyopia (impaired near vision) is indicated when the client moves the chart away from the eyes to focus on the print. It is caused by decreased accommodation.

 Presbyopia is a common condition in clients over age 45.

Test visual fields for gross peripheral vision. To perform the confrontation test, position yourself approximately 2 feet away from the client at eye level. Have the client cover his left eye while you cover your right eye (Fig. 15-9). Look directly at each other with your uncovered eyes. Next fully extend your left arm at midline and slowly move one finger (or a pencil) upward from below until the client sees your finger (or pencil). Test the remaining three visual fields of the client's right eye (i.e., superior, temporal, and nasal). Repeat the test for the opposite eye.

With normal peripheral vision, the client should see the examiner's finger at the same time the examiner sees it. Normal visual field degrees are approximately as follows:

Inferior: 70 degrees

Superior: 50 degrees

Temporal: 90 degrees

Nasal: 60 degrees

A delayed or absent perception of the examiner's finger indicates reduced peripheral vision (Abnormal Findings 15-1). The client should be referred for further evaluation.

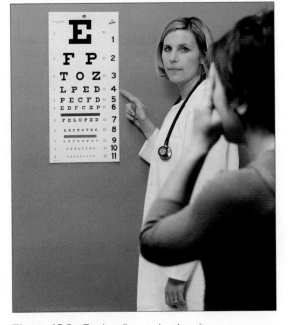

Figure 15-8 Testing distant visual acuity.

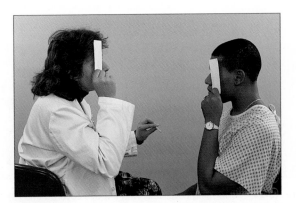

Figure 15-9 Performing confrontation test to assess visual fields (©B. Proud).

continued

PHYSICAL ASSESSMENT Continued

Assessment Procedure	Normal Findings	Abnormal Findings

Testing Extraocular Muscle Function

Perform corneal light reflex test. This test assesses parallel alignment of the eyes. Hold a penlight approximately 12 inches from the client's face. Shine the light toward the bridge of the nose while the client stares straight ahead. Note the light reflected on the corneas.

The reflection of light on the corneas should be in the exact same spot on each eye, which indicates parallel alignment.

Asymmetric position of the light reflex indicates deviated alignment of the eyes. This may be due to muscle weakness or paralysis (Abnormal Findings 15-2).

Perform cover test. The cover test detects deviation in alignment or strength and slight deviations in eye movement by interrupting the fusion reflex that normally keeps the eyes parallel.

The uncovered eye should remain fixed straight ahead. The covered eye should remain fixed straight ahead after being uncovered.

The uncovered eye will move to establish focus when the opposite eye is covered. When the covered eye is uncovered, movement to reestablish focus occurs. Either of these findings indicates a deviation in alignment of the eyes and muscle weakness (Abnormal Findings 15-2).

Ask the client to stare straight ahead and focus on a distant object. Cover one of the client's eyes with an opaque card (Fig. 15-10). As you cover the eye, observe the uncovered eye for movement. Now remove the opaque card and observe the previously covered eye for any movement. Repeat test on the opposite eye.

Phoria is a term used to describe misalignment that occurs only when fusion reflex is blocked.

Strabismus is constant malalignment of the eyes.

Tropia is a specific type of misalignment: *esotropia* is an inward turn of the eye, and *exotropia* is an outward turn of the eye.

Perform the positions test assesses eye muscle strength and cranial nerve function.

Eye movement should be smooth and symmetric throughout all six directions.

Failure of eyes to follow movement symmetrically in any or all directions indicates a weakness in one or more extraocular muscles or dysfunction of the cranial nerve that innervates the particular muscle (see Abnormal Findings 15-2).

Instruct the client to focus on an object you are holding (approximately 12 inches from the client's face). Move the object through the six cardinal positions of gaze in a clockwise direction, and observe the client's eye movements (Fig. 15-11).

Nystagmus, an oscillating (shaking) movement of the eye may be associated with an inner ear disorder, multiple sclerosis, brain lesions, or narcotics use.

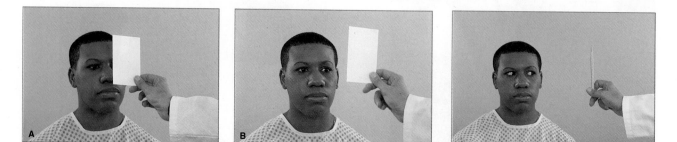

Figure 15-10 Performing cover test with **(A)** eye covered and **(B)** eye uncovered (© B. Proud).

Figure 15-11 Performing positions test (© B. Proud).

continued

Assessment Procedure	Normal Findings	Abnormal Findings

External Eye Structures

Inspection and Palpation
Inspect the eyelids and eyelashes.

Assessment Procedure	Normal Findings	Abnormal Findings
Note width and position of palpebral fissures.	The upper lid margin should be between the upper margin of the iris and the upper margin of the pupil. The lower lid margin rests on the lower border of the iris. No white sclera is seen above or below the iris. Palpebral fissures may be horizontal.	Drooping of the upper lid, called *ptosis*, may be attributed to oculomotor nerve damage, myasthenia gravis, weakened muscle or tissue, or a congenital disorder (see Abnormal Findings 15-3). Retracted lid margins, which allow for viewing of the sclera when the eyes are open, suggest hyperthyroidism.
Assess ability of eyelids to close.	The upper and lower lids close easily and meet completely when closed.	Failure of lids to close completely puts client at risk for corneal damage.
Note the position of the eyelids in comparison with the eyeballs. Also note any unusual • Turnings • Color • Swelling • Lesions • Discharge	The lower eyelid is upright with no inward or outward turning. Eyelashes are evenly distributed and curve outward along the lid margins. Xanthelasma, raised yellow plaques located most often near the inner canthus, are a normal variation associated with increasing age and high lipid levels.	An inverted lower lid is a condition called an *entropion,* which may cause pain and injure the cornea as the eyelash brushes against the conjunctiva and cornea. *Ectropion,* an everted lower eyelid, results in exposure and drying of the conjunctiva. Both conditions (see Abnormal Findings 15-3) interfere with normal tear drainage. 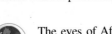 Though usually abnormal, entropion and ectropion are common in older clients.
Observe for redness, swelling, discharge, or lesions.	Skin on both eyelids is without redness, swelling, or lesions.	Redness and crusting along the lid margins suggest seborrhea or blepharitis, an infection caused by *Staphylococcus aureus.* Hordeolum (stye), a hair follicle infection, causes local redness, swelling, and pain. A chalazion, an infection of the meibomian gland (located in the eyelid), may produce extreme swelling of the lid, moderate redness, but minimal pain (see Abnormal Findings 15-3).
Observe the position and alignment of the eyeball in the eye socket.	Eyeballs are symmetrically aligned in sockets without protruding or sinking. The eyes of African Americans protrude slightly more than those of Caucasians, and African Americans of both sexes may have eyes protruding beyond 21 mm. A difference of more than 2 mm between the two eyes is abnormal (Mercandetti, 2007).	Protrusion of the eyeballs accompanied by retracted eyelid margins is termed *exophthalmos* (see Abnormal Findings 15-3) and is characteristic of Graves' disease (a type of hyperthyroidism). A sunken appearance of the eyes may be seen with severe dehydration or chronic wasting illnesses.

continued

PHYSICAL ASSESSMENT *Continued*

Assessment Procedure	Normal Findings	Abnormal Findings

Inspect the bulbar conjunctiva and sclera. Have the client keep her head straight while looking from side to side then up toward the ceiling (Fig. 15-12). Observe clarity, color, and texture.	Bulbar conjunctiva is clear, moist, and smooth. Underlying structures are clearly visible. Sclera is white.
	
	  Yellowish nodules on the bulbar conjunctiva are called *pinguecula*. These harmless nodules are common in older clients and appear first on the medial side of the iris and then on the lateral side.
	
	  Darker-skinned clients may have sclera with yellow or pigmented freckles.
		Generalized redness of the conjunctiva suggests *conjunctivitis* (pink eye).
		
		 Areas of dryness are associated with allergies or trauma.
		
		 Episcleritis is a local, noninfectious inflammation of the sclera. The condition is usually characterized by either a nodular appearance or by redness with dilated vessels (see Abnormal Findings 15-3).

Inspect the palpebral conjunctiva. ➤ *Clinical Tip* • *This procedure is stressful and uncomfortable for the client, It is usually only done if the client complains of pain or "something in the eye."*		
Put on gloves for this assessment procedure. First inspect the palpebral conjunctiva of the lower eyelid by placing your thumbs bilaterally at the level of the lower bony orbital rim and gently pulling down to expose the palpebral conjunctiva (Fig. 15-13). Avoid pressuring the eye. Ask the client to look up as you observe the exposed areas.	The lower and upper palpebral conjunctivae are clear and free of swelling or lesions.	Cyanosis of the lower lid suggests a heart or lung disorder.
Evert the upper eyelid. Ask the client to look down with his or her eyes slightly open. Gently grasp the client's upper eyelashes and pull the lid downward (Fig. 15-14A). Place a cotton-tipped applicator approximately 1 cm above the eyelid margin and push down with the applicator while still holding the eyelashes (Fig. 15-14B). Hold the eyelashes against the upper ridge of the bony orbit just below the eyebrow, to maintain the everted position of the eyelid. Examine the palpebral conjunctiva for swelling, foreign bodies, or trauma. Return the eyelid to normal by moving the lashes forward and asking the client to look up and blink. The eyelid should return to normal.	Palpebral conjunctiva is free of swelling, foreign bodies, or trauma.	A foreign body or lesion may cause irritation, burning, pain and/or swelling of the upper eyelid.

continued

Assessment Procedure	Normal Findings	Abnormal Findings
Inspect the lacrimal apparatus. Assess the areas over the lacrimal glands (lateral aspect of upper eyelid) and the puncta (medial aspect of lower eyelid).	No swelling or redness should appear over areas of the lacrimal gland. The puncta is visible without swelling or redness and is turned slightly toward the eye.	Swelling of the lacrimal gland may be visible in the lateral aspect of the upper eyelid. This may be caused by blockage, infection, or an inflammatory condition. Redness or swelling around the puncta may indicate an infectious or inflammatory condition. Excessive tearing may indicate a nasolacrimal sac obstruction.
Palpate the lacrimal apparatus. Put on disposable gloves to palpate the nasolacrimal duct to assess for blockage. Use one finger and palpate just inside the lower orbital rim (Fig. 15-15).	No drainage should be noted from the puncta when palpating the nasolacrimal duct.	Expressed drainage from the puncta on palpation occurs with duct blockage.

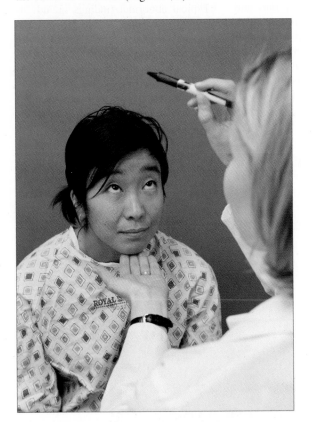

Figure 15-12 Inspecting the bulbar conjunctiva.

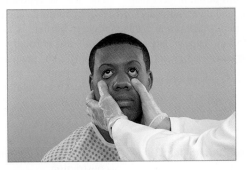

Figure 15-13 Inspecting palpebral conjunctiva: lower eyelid (© B. Proud).

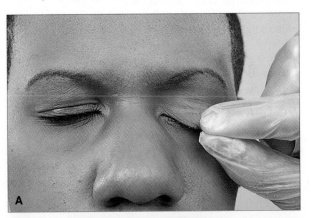

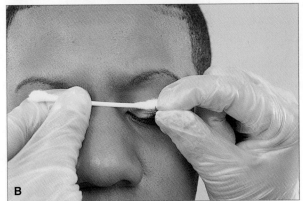

Figure 15-14 Everting the upper eyelid.

continued

PHYSICAL ASSESSMENT Continued

Assessment Procedure	Normal Findings	Abnormal Findings
Inspect the cornea and lens. Shine a light from the side of the eye for an oblique view. Look through the pupil to inspect the lens.	The cornea is transparent with no opacities. The oblique view shows a smooth and overall moist surface; the lens is free of opacities. 👓 *Arcus senilis*, a normal condition in older clients, appears as a white arc around the limbus (Fig. 15-16). The condition has no effect on vision.	Areas of roughness or dryness on the cornea are often associated with injury or allergic responses. Opacities of the lens are seen with cataracts (Abnormal Findings 15-4).
Inspect the iris and pupil. Inspect shape and color of iris and size and shape of pupil. Measure pupils against a gauge (Fig. 15-17) if they appear larger or smaller than normal or if they appear to be two different sizes.	The iris is typically round, flat, and evenly colored. The pupil, round with a regular border, is centered in the iris. Pupils are normally equal in size (3 to 5 mm). An inequality in pupil size of less than 0.5 mm occurs in 20% of clients. This condition, called *anisocoria*, is normal.	Typical abnormal findings include irregularly shaped irises, miosis, mydriasis, and anisocoria. (For a description of these abnormalities and their implications, see Abnormal Findings 15-5). If the difference in pupil size changes throughout pupillary response tests, the inequality of size is abnormal.
Test pupillary reaction to light. Test for direct response by darkening the room and asking the client to focus on a distant object. To test direct pupil reaction, shine a light obliquely into one eye and observe the pupillary reaction. Shining the light obliquely into the pupil and asking the client to focus on an object in the distance ensures that	The normal direct pupillary response is constriction.	Monocular blindness can be detected when light directed to the blind eye results in no response in either pupil. When light is directed into the unaffected eye, both pupils constrict.

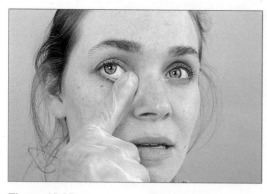

Figure 15-15 Palpating the lacrimal apparatus (© B. Proud).

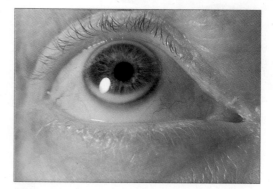

Figure 15-16 Arcus senilis.

Pupil Gauge (mm)

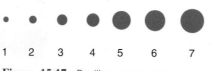

1 2 3 4 5 6 7

Figure 15-17 Pupillary gauge measures pupils (dilation or constriction) in millimeters (mm).

continued

Assessment Procedure	Normal Findings	Abnormal Findings
pupillary constriction is a reaction to light and not a near reaction. ➤ **Clinical Tip** • *Use a pupillary gauge to measure the constricted pupil. Then, document the finding in a format similar to (but not) a fraction. The top (or first) number indicates the pupil's eye at rest, and the bottom (or second) number indicates the constricted size; for example, O.S. (left eye, oculus sinister) 3/2; O.D. (right eye, oculus dexter) 3/1.*		
Assess consensual response at the same time as direct response by shining a light obliquely into one eye and observing the pupillary reaction in the opposite eye. ➤ **Clinical Tip** • *When testing for consensual response, place your hand or another barrier to light (e.g., index card) between the client's eyes to avoid an inaccurate finding.*	The normal consensual pupillary response is constriction.	Pupils do not react at all to direct and consensual pupillary testing.
Test accommodation of pupils. Accommodation occurs when the client moves his focus of vision from a distant point to a near object, causing the pupils to constrict. Hold your finger or a pencil about 12 to 15 inches from the client. Ask the client to focus on your finger or pencil and to remain focused on it as you move it closer in toward the eyes (Fig. 15-18).	The normal pupillary response is constriction of the pupils and convergence of the eyes when focusing on a near object (accommodation and convergence).	Pupils do not constrict; eyes do not converge.

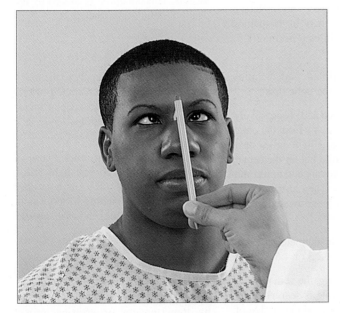

Figure 15-18 Testing accommodation of pupils (© B. Proud).

continued

PHYSICAL ASSESSMENT Continued

Assessment Procedure	Normal Findings	Abnormal Findings

Internal Eye Structures

Using an ophthalmoscope (see Equipment Spotlight 15-2), inspect the internal eye. To observe the red reflex, set the diopter at zero and stand 10 to 15 inches from the client's right side at a 15-degree angle. Place your free hand on the client's head, which helps limit head movement (Fig. 15-19). Shine the light beam toward the client's pupil.

The red reflex should be easily visible through the ophthalmoscope. The red area should appear round with regular borders.

Abnormalities of the red reflex most often result from cataracts. These usually appear as black spots against the background of the red light reflex. Two types of age-related cataracts are nuclear cataracts and peripheral cataracts (Abnormal Findings 15-4).

Inspect the optic disc. Keep the light beam focused on the pupil and move closer to the client from a 15-degree angle. You should be very close to the client's eye (about 3 to 5 cm), almost touching the eyelashes. Rotate the diopter setting to bring the retinal structures into sharp focus. The diopter should be zero if neither the examiner nor the client has refractive errors. Note shape, color, size, and physiologic cup.

> ➤ **Clinical Tip** • *The diameter of the optic disc (DD) is used as the standard of measure for the location and size of other structures and any abnormalities or lesions within the ocular fundus. When documenting a structure within the ocular fundus, also note the position of the structure as it relates to numbers on the clock. For example, lesion is at 2:00, 1 DD in size, 2 DD from disc.*

The optic disc should be round to oval with sharp, well-defined borders (Fig. 15-20).

The nasal edge of the optic disc may be blurred. The disc is normally creamy, yellow-orange to pink, and approximately 1.5 mm wide.

The physiologic cup, the point at which the optic nerve enters the eyeball, appears on the optic disc as slightly depressed and a lighter color than the disc. The cup occupies less than half of the disc's diameter. The disc's border may be surrounded by rings and crescents, consisting of white sclera or black retinal pigment. These normal variations are not considered in the optic disc's diameter.

 Optic nerve discs are larger in blacks, Asians, and Native Americans than in Hispanics and non-Hispanic whites (Girkin, 2005; Overfield, 1995).

Papilledema, or swelling of the optic disc, appears as a swollen disc with blurred margins, a hyperemic (blood-filled) appearance, more visible and more numerous disc vessels, and lack of visible physiologic cup. The condition may result from hypertension or increased intracranial pressure (Abnormal Findings 15-6).

The intraocular pressure associated with *glaucoma* interferes with the blood supply to optic structures and results in the following characteristics: an enlarged physiologic cup that occupies more than half of the disc's diameter, pale base of enlarged physiologic cup, and obscured or displaced retinal vessels.

Optic atrophy is evidenced by the disc being white in color and a lack of disc vessels. This condition is caused by the death of optic nerve fibers.

Inspect the retinal vessels. Remain in the same position as described previously. Inspect the sets of retinal vessels by following them out to the periphery of each section of the eye. Note the number of sets of arterioles and venules.

Also note color and diameter of the arterioles.

Four sets of arterioles and venules should pass through the optic disc.

Arterioles are bright red and progressively narrow as they move away from the optic disc. Arterioles have a light reflex that appears as a thin, white line in the center of the arteriole. Venules are darker red and larger than arterioles. They also progressively narrow as they move away from the optic disc.

Changes in the blood supply to the retina may be observed in constricted arterioles, dilated veins, or absence of major vessels (Abnormal Findings 15-7).

Initially hypertension may cause a widening of the arterioles' light reflex and the arterioles take on a copper color. With long-standing hypertension, arteriole walls thicken and appear opaque or silver.

Observe the arteriovenous (AV) ratio.

The ratio of arteriole diameter to vein diameter (AV ratio) is 2:3 or 4:5.

Look at AV crossings.

In a normal AV crossing, the vein passing underneath the arteriole is seen right up to the column of blood on either side of the arteriole (the arteriole wall itself is normally transparent).

Arterial nicking, tapering, and banking are abnormal AV crossings caused by hypertension or arteriosclerosis (Abnormal Findings 15-7).

continued on page 246

EQUIPMENT SPOTLIGHT 15-2   Ophthalmoscope

The ophthalmoscope is a hand-held instrument that allows the examiner to view the fundus of the eye by the projection of light through a prism that bends the light 90 degrees. There are several lenses arranged on a wheel that affect the focus on objects in the eye. The examiner can rotate the lenses with his or her index finger. Each lens is labeled with a negative or positive number, a unit of strength called a diopter. Red numbers indicate a negative diopter and are used for myopic (nearsighted) clients. Black numbers indicate a positive diopter and are used for hyperopic (farsighted) clients. The zero lens is used if neither the examiner nor the client has refractive errors.

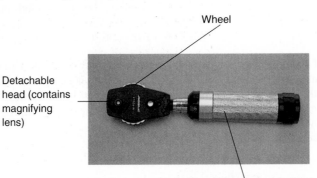

Wheel

Detachable head (contains magnifying lens)

Body (contains light source)

Basics of Operation

1. Turn the ophthalmoscope "on" and select the aperture with the large round beam of white light. The small round beam of white light may be used if the client has smaller pupils. There are other apertures but they are not typically used for basic ophthalmologic screening.
2. Ask the client to remove eyeglasses but keep contact lenses in place. You should also remove your glasses. Any refractive errors can be accommodated for by rotating the lenses (if errors are severe, glasses should be left on). Removing glasses enables you to get closer to the client's eye, allowing for a more accurate inspection. Keep your contact lenses in place.
3. Ask the client to fix his or her gaze on an object that is straight ahead and slightly upward.
4. Darken the room to allow pupils to dilate (for a more thorough examination, eyedrops are used to dilate pupils).
5. Hold the ophthalmoscope in your right hand with your index finger on the lens wheel and place it to your right eye (braced between the eyebrow and the nose) if you are examining the client's right eye. Use your left hand and left eye if you are examining the client's left eye. This allows you to get as close to the client's eye as possible without bumping noses with the client.

Some Do's and Don'ts

Do

- Begin about 10 to 15 inches from the client at a 15-degree angle to the client's side.
- Pretend that the ophthalmoscope is an extension of your eye. Keep focused on the red reflex as you move in closer, then rotate the diopter setting to see the optic disk.

Don't

- Do not use your right eye to examine the client's left eye or your left eye to examine the client's right eye (your noses will bump).
- Do not move the ophthalmoscope around; ask the client to look into light to view the fovea and macula.
- Do not get frustrated—the ophthalmologic examination requires practice.

PHYSICAL ASSESSMENT Continued

Assessment Procedure	Normal Findings	Abnormal Findings
Inspect retinal background. Remain in the same position described previously and search the retinal background from the disc to the macula, noting the color and the presence of any lesions.	General background appears consistent in texture. The red-orange color of the background is lighter near the optic disc.	Cotton-wool patches (soft exudates) and hard exudates from diabetes and hypertension appear as light-colored spots on the retinal background. Hemorrhages and microaneurysms appear as red spots and streaks on the retinal background (Abnormal Findings 15-7).
Inspect fovea (sharpest area of vision) and macula. Remain in the same position described previously. Shine the light beam toward the side of the eye or ask the client to look directly into the light. Observe the fovea and the macula that surrounds it.	The macula is the darker area, one disc diameter in size, located to the temporal side of the optic disc. Within this area is a starlike light reflex called the fovea.	Excessive clumped pigment appears with detached retinas or retinal injuries. Macular degeneration may be due to hemorrhages, exudates, or cysts.
Inspect anterior chamber. Remain in the same position and rotate the lens wheel slowly to +10, +12, or higher to inspect the anterior chamber of the eye.	The anterior chamber is transparent.	*Hyphemia* occurs when injury causes red blood cells to collect in the lower half of the anterior chamber (Fig. 15-21).
		Hypopyon usually results from an inflammatory response in which white blood cells accumulate in the anterior chamber and produce cloudiness in front of the iris (Fig. 15-22).

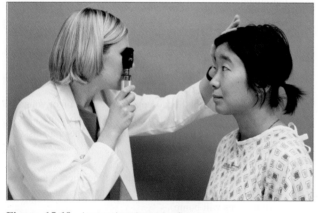

Figure 15-19 Inspecting the red reflex.

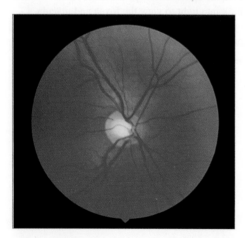

Figure 15-20 Normal ocular fundus (also called the optic disc).

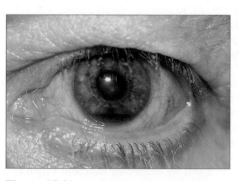

Figure 15-21 Hyphemia (© 1995 Science Photo Library/CMSP).

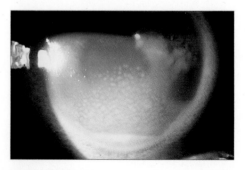

Figure 15-22 Hypopyon.

Abnormal Findings 15-1

Visual Field Defects

When a client reports losing full or partial vision in one or both eyes, the nurse can usually anticipate a lesion as the cause. Some abnormal findings associated with visual field defects are illustrated here. The darker areas signify vision loss.

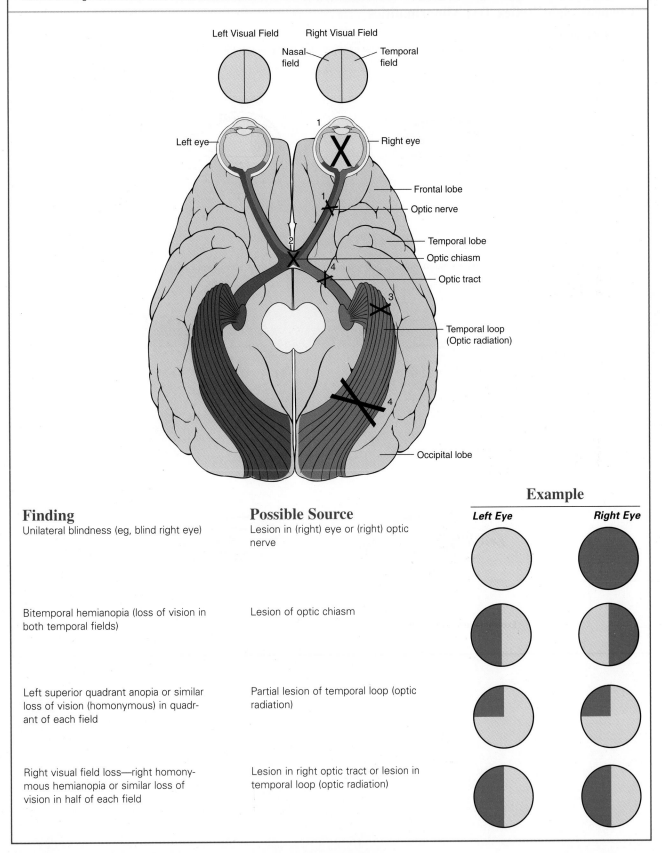

Finding	Possible Source	Example
		Left Eye / Right Eye
Unilateral blindness (eg, blind right eye)	Lesion in (right) eye or (right) optic nerve	
Bitemporal hemianopia (loss of vision in both temporal fields)	Lesion of optic chiasm	
Left superior quadrant anopia or similar loss of vision (homonymous) in quadrant of each field	Partial lesion of temporal loop (optic radiation)	
Right visual field loss—right homonymous hemianopia or similar loss of vision in half of each field	Lesion in right optic tract or lesion in temporal loop (optic radiation)	

Abnormal Findings 15-2   **Extraocular Muscle Dysfunction**

Abnormalities found during an assessment of extraocular muscle function are described below:

Corneal Light Reflex Test Abnormalities

Pseudostrabismus

Normal in young children, the pupils will appear at the inner canthus (due to the epicanthic fold).

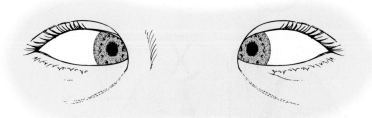

Strabismus (or Tropia)

A constant malalignment of the eye axis, strabismus is defined according to the direction toward which the eye drifts and may cause amblyopia.

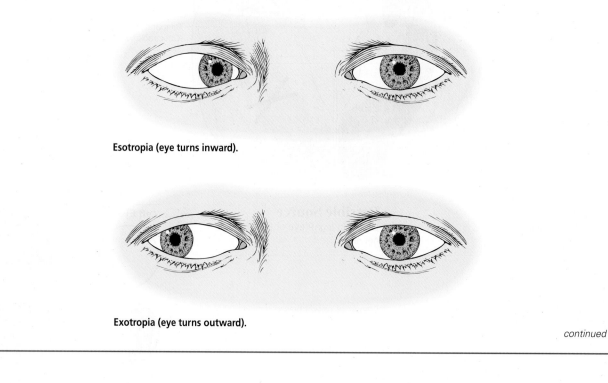

Esotropia (eye turns inward).

Exotropia (eye turns outward).

continued

Abnormal Findings 15-2 | **Extraocular Muscle Dysfunction** *Continued*

Cover Test Abnormalities

Phoria (Mild Weakness)

Noticeable only with the cover test, phoria is less likely to cause amblyopia than strabismus. Esophoria is an inward drift and exophoria an outward drift of the eye.

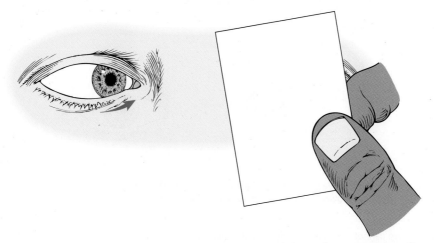

The uncovered eye is weaker; when the stronger eye is covered, the weaker eye moves to refocus.

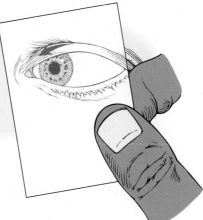

When the weaker eye is covered, it will drift to a relaxed position.

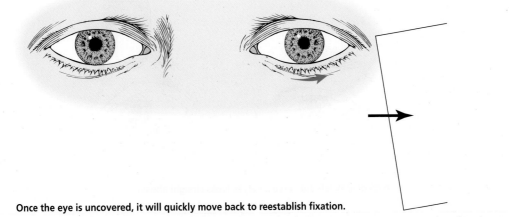

Once the eye is uncovered, it will quickly move back to reestablish fixation.

continued on page 250

Abnormal Findings 15-2   **Extraocular Muscle Dysfunction** *Continued*

Positions Test Abnormalities

Paralytic Strabismus

Noticeable with the positions test, paralytic strabismus is usually the result of weakness or paralysis of one or more extraocular muscles. The nerve affected will be on the same side as the eye affected (for instance, a right eye paralysis is related to a right-side cranial nerve). The position in which the maximum deviation appears indicates the nerve involved.

6th nerve paralysis: The eye cannot look to the outer side.

In left 6th nerve paralysis, the client tries to look to the left. The right eye moves left, but the left eye cannot move left.

4th nerve paralysis: The eye cannot look down when turned inward.

A client with left 4th nerve paralysis looks down and to the right.

3rd nerve paralysis: Upward, downward, and inward movements are lost. Ptosis and pupillary dilation may also occur.

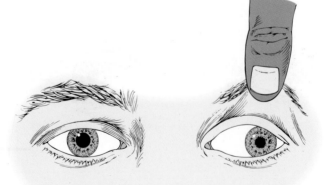

A client with left 3rd nerve paralysis looks straight ahead.

Abnormal Findings 15-3 Abnormalities of the External Eye

Some easily recognized abnormalities that affect the external eye are illustrated below.

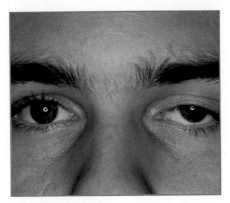

Ptosis (drooping eye).

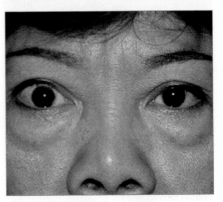

Exophthalmos (protruding eyeballs and retracted eyelids).

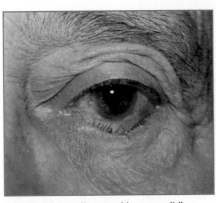

Entropion (inwardly turned lower eyelid).

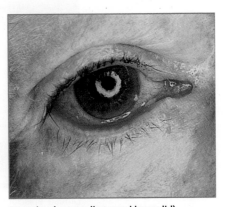

Ectropion (outwardly turned lower lid).

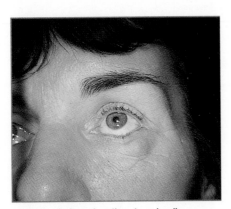

Chalazion (infected meibomian gland).

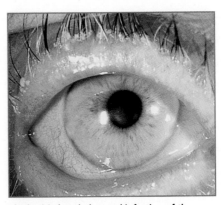

Blepharitis (staphylococcal infection of the eyelid).

continued on page 252

Abnormal Findings 15-3   **Abnormalities of the External Eye** *Continued*

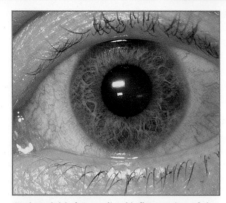

Conjunctivitis (generalized inflammation of the conjunctiva). (© 1995 Dr. P. Marazzi/Science photo Library/CMSP.)

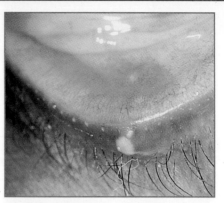

Hordeolum (stye).

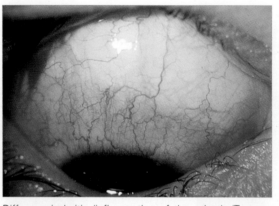

Diffuse episcleritis (inflammation of the sclera). (Tasman, W., & Jaeger, E. [Eds.], [2001]. *The Wills Eye Hospital atlas of clinical ophthalmology* [2nd ed.]. Philadelphia: Lippincott Williams & Wilkins.)

Abnormal Findings 15-4   **Abnormalities of the Cornea and Lens**

Representative abnormalities of the cornea are illustrated below as a corneal scar and a pterygium. Lens abnormalities are represented by a nuclear cataract and a peripheral cataract. Usually, cataracts are most easily seen by the naked eye.

Corneal Abnormalities

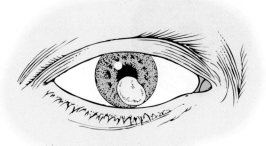

A corneal scar, which appears grayish white, usually is due to an old injury or inflammation.

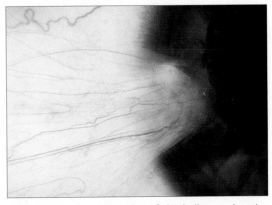

Early pterygium, a thickening of the bulbar conjunctiva that extends across the nasal side. (Tasman, W., & Jaeger, E. [Eds.], [2001]. *The Wills Eye Hospital atlas of clinical ophthalmology* [2nd ed.]. Philadelphia: Lippincott Williams & Wilkins.)

Lens Abnormalities

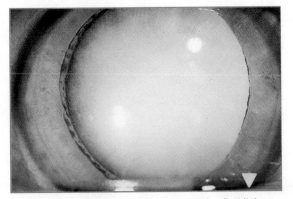

Nuclear cataracts appear gray when seen with a flashlight; they appear as a black spot against the red reflex when seen through an ophthalmoscope.

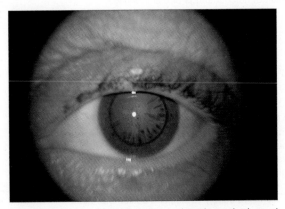

Peripheral cataracts look like gray spokes that point inward when seen with a flashlight; they look like black spokes that point inward against the red reflex when seen through an ophthalmoscope. (Tasman, W., & Jaeger, E. [Eds.], [2001]. *The Wills Eye Hospital atlas of clinical ophthalmology* [2nd ed.]. Philadelphia: Lippincott Williams & Wilkins.)

Abnormal Findings 15-5 **Abnormalities of the Iris and Pupils**

Irregularly Shaped Iris

An irregularly shaped iris causes a shallow anterior chamber, which may increase the risk for narrow-angle (closed-angle) glaucoma.

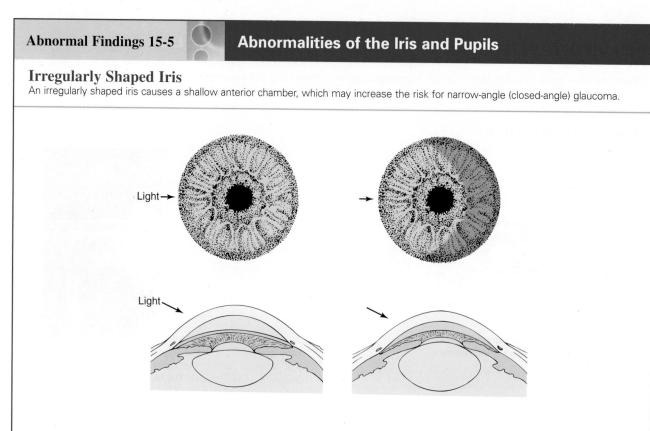

Miosis

Also known as pinpoint pupils, miosis is characterized by constricted and fixed pupils—possibly a result of narcotic drugs or brain damage.

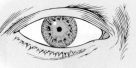
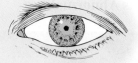

Anisocoria

Anisocoria is pupils of unequal size. In some cases, the condition is normal; in other cases, it is abnormal. For example, if anisocoria is greater in bright light compared with dim light, the cause may be trauma, tonic pupil (caused by impaired parasympathetic nerve supply to iris), and oculomotor nerve paralysis. If anisocoria is greater in dim light compared with bright light, the cause may be Horner's syndrome (caused by paralysis of the cervical sympathetic nerves and characterized by ptosis, sunken eyeball, flushing of the affected side of the face, and narrowing of the palpebral fissure).

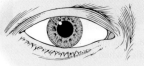
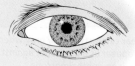

Mydriasis

Dilated and fixed pupils, typically resulting from central nervous system injury, circulatory collapse, or deep anesthesia.

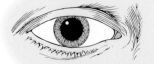
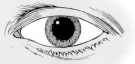

Abnormal Findings 15-6 | Abnormalities of the Optic Disc

Characteristic abnormal findings during an ophthalmoscopic examination include signs and symptoms of papilledema, glaucoma, and optic atrophy as described below.

Papilledema
- Swollen optic disc
- Blurred margins
- Hyperemic appearance from accumulation of excess blood
- Visible and numerous disc vessels
- Lack of visible physiologic cup

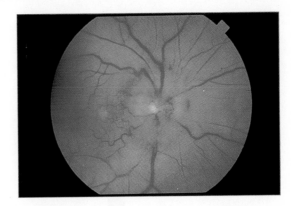

Glaucoma
- Enlarged physiologic cup occupying more than half of the disc's diameter
- Pale base of enlarged physiologic cup
- Obscured and/or displaced retinal vessels

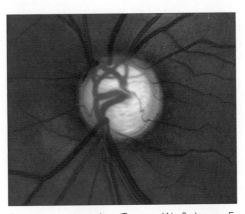

Glaucomatous cupping. (Tasman, W., & Jaeger, E. [Eds.], [2001]. *The Wills Eye Hospital atlas of clinical ophthalmology* [2nd ed.]. Philadelphia: Lippincott Williams & Wilkins.)

Optic Atrophy
- White optic disc
- Lack of disc vessels

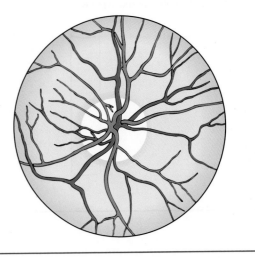

Abnormal Findings 15-7

Abnormalities of the Retinal Vessels and Background

Characteristic abnormal findings during an ophthalmoscopic examination of the retinal vessels include constricted arterioles, copper wire arterioles, silver wire arteriole, arteriovenous (AV) nicking, AV tapering, and AV banking. Signs and symptoms are described below.

Constricted Arteriole
- Narrowing of the arteriole
- Occurs with hypertension

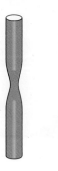

Copper Wire Arteriole
- Widening of the light reflex and a coppery color
- Occurs with hypertension

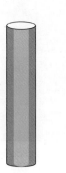

Silver Wire Arteriole
- Opaque or silver appearance caused by thickening of arteriole wall
- Occurs with long-standing hypertension

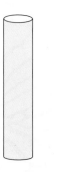

Arteriovenous Nicking
- Arteriovenous crossing abnormality characterized by vein appearing to stop short on either side of arteriole
- Caused by loss of arteriole wall transparency from hypertension

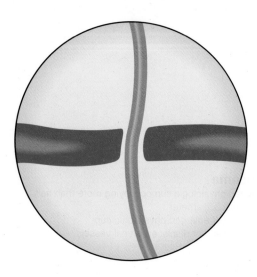

Arteriovenous Tapering
- Arteriovenous crossing abnormality characterized by vein appearing to taper to a point on either side of the arteriole
- Caused by loss of arteriole wall transparency from hypertension

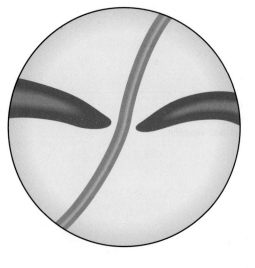

continued

Abnormal Findings 15-7

Abnormalities of the Retinal Vessels and Background *Continued*

Arteriovenous Banking

- Arteriovenous crossing abnormality characterized by twisting of the vein on the arteriole's distal side and formation of a dark, knuckle-like structure
- Caused by loss of arteriole wall transparency from hypertension

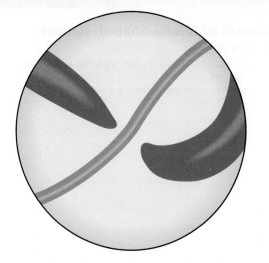

Cotton Wool Patches

- Also known as *soft exudates,* cotton wool patches have a fluffy cotton ball appearance with irregular edges
- Appear as white or gray moderately sized spots on retinal background
- Caused by arteriole microinfarction
- Associated with diabetes mellitus and hypertension

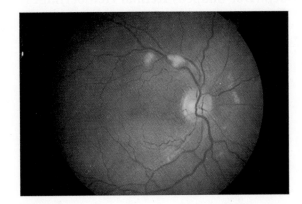

Hard Exudate

- Solid, smooth surface and well-defined edges
- Creamy yellow-white, small, round spots typically clustered in circular, linear, or star pattern
- Associated with diabetes mellitus and hypertension

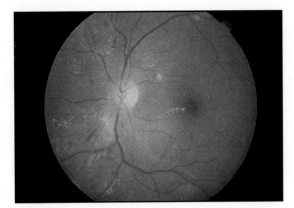

(Tasman, W., & Jaeger, E. [Eds.], [2001]. *The Wills Eye Hospital atlas of clinical ophthalmology* [2nd ed.]. Philadelphia: Lippincott Williams & Wilkins.)

continued on page 258

Abnormal Findings 15-7   **Abnormalities of the Retinal Vessels and Background** *Continued*

Superficial (Flame-Shaped) Retinal Hemorrhages
- Appear as small, flame-shaped, linear red streaks on retinal background
- Hypertension and papilledema are common causes

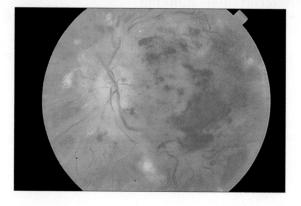

Deep (Dot-Shaped) Retinal Hemorrhages
- Appear as small, irregular red spots with blurred edges on retinal background
- Lie deeper in retina than superficial retinal hemorrhages
- Associated with diabetes mellitus

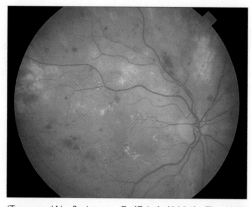

(Tasman, W., & Jaeger, E. [Eds.], [2001]. *The Wills Eye Hospital atlas of clinical ophthalmology* [2nd ed.]. Philadelphia: Lippincott Williams & Wilkins.)

Microaneurysms
- Round, tiny red dots with smooth edges on retinal background
- Localized dilations of small vessels in retina, but vessels are too small to see
- Associated with diabetic retinopathy

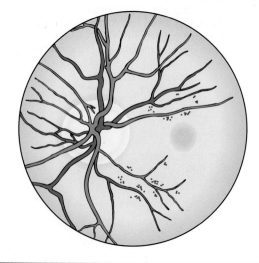

VALIDATING AND DOCUMENTING FINDINGS

Validate the eye assessment data that you have collected. This is necessary to verify that the data are reliable and accurate. Document the assessment data following the health care facility or agency policy.

Sample of Subjective Data

Client denies recent changes in vision. Denies excessive tearing, redness, swelling, or pain of eyes. Denies spots, floaters, or blind spots. States no problem with seeing at night. No previous eye surgeries. No family history of eye problems. Denies exposure to conditions or substances that harm the eyes. Wears sunglasses regularly. Does not wear corrective lenses. Last eye examination was 1 year ago.

Sample of Objective Data

Acuity tested by Snellen chart: O.D. (right eye) 20/20, O.S. (left eye) 20/20. Visual fields full by confrontation. Corneal light reflex shows equal position of reflection. Eyes remain fixed throughout cover test. Extraocular movements smooth and symmetric with no nystagmus. Eyelids in normal position with no abnormal widening or ptosis. No redness, discharge, or crusting noted on lid margins. Conjunctiva and sclera appear moist and smooth. Sclera white with no lesions or redness. No swelling or redness over lacrimal gland; puncta is visible without swelling or redness; no drainage noted when nasolacrimal duct is palpated. Cornea is transparent, smooth, and moist with no opacities; lens is free of opacities. Irises are round, flat, and evenly colored. Pupils are equal in size and reactive to light and accommodation. Pupils converge evenly. Red reflex present bilaterally. Both optic discs visualized easily, creamy white in color, with distinct margins and vessels noted with no crossing defects. Retinal background free of lesions and orange-red in color. Macula visualized within normal limits. Anterior chamber is transparent.

Analysis of Data

DIAGNOSTIC REASONING: POSSIBLE CONCLUSIONS

After collecting subjective and objective data pertaining to the eyes, identify abnormal findings and client strengths. Then cluster the data to reveal any significant patterns or abnormalities.

Listed below are some possible conclusions that the nurse may make after assessing a client's eyes.

Selected Nursing Diagnoses

The following is a list of selected nursing diagnoses that may be identified when analyzing data from eye assessment.

Wellness Diagnoses

- Readiness for enhanced visual integrity

Risk Diagnoses

- Risk for Eye Injury related to hazardous work area or participation in high-level contact sports
- Risk for Injury related to impaired vision secondary to the aging process
- Risk for Eye Injury related to decreased tear production secondary to the aging process
- Risk for Self-Care Deficit (specify) related to vision loss

Actual Diagnoses

- Ineffective Health Maintenance related to lack of knowledge of necessity for eye examinations
- Self-Care Deficit (specify) related to poor vision
- Acute Pain related to injury from eye trauma, abrasion, or exposure to chemical irritant
- Social Isolation related to inability to interact effectively with others secondary to vision loss

Selected Collaborative Problems

After grouping the data, it may become apparent that certain collaborative problems emerge. Remember that collaborative problems differ from nursing diagnoses in that they cannot be prevented by nursing interventions. However, these physiologic complications of medical conditions can be detected and monitored by the nurse. In addition, the nurse can use physician- and nurse-prescribed interventions to minimize the complications of these problems. The nurse may also have to refer the client in such situations for further treatment of the problem. Following is a list of collaborative problems that may be identified when assessing the eye. These problems are worded as Risk for Complications (or RC), followed by the problem.

- RC: Increased intraocular pressure
- RC: Corneal ulceration or abrasion

Medical Problems

After grouping the data, it may become apparent that the client has signs and symptoms that require medical diagnosis and treatment. Referral to a primary care provider is necessary.

CASE STUDY

The case study demonstrates how to analyze eye data for a specific client. The critical thinking exercises included in the study guide/lab manual and interactive products that complement this text also offer opportunities to assess the data.

You are preparing to discharge Mr. Luther Johnson (LJ), a 68-year-old African American man, after a 2-day hospital stay for management of an acute asthma attack. His history indicates that he has been taking oral and inhaled corticosteroids intermittently for the last 17 years for asthma. You ask him if he has any other concerns he wants to discuss before he leaves. "Yes," he says, "I have noticed some strange things that are happening with my vision. I'm concerned, although my doctor says it's nothing to worry about—but I am worried." When you ask for an example of what is unusual about his vision, he tells you that he doesn't always see stairs in front of him ("I trip a lot lately.") and when he is reading, words on the page seem to be missing sometimes. "At first I thought I was just distracted, but then I almost hit another car when I made a left turn—I didn't see it at all. I got more concerned after that. My wife says that she has noticed more problems with my driving but didn't want to upset me by

saying something." He indicates he does a lot of driving for his work as a computer hardware trouble-shooter. "I have to work to pay the rent and support my wife."

When you examine his eyes, you note the following: conjugate gaze without ptosis; slight protrusion of eyeballs and firm to touch; pupils are small, equal, round and constrict with both direct and consensual illumination 2/1 OU (each eye). Corneas appear smooth with normal corneal light reflex and spontaneous blink reflex; sclera slightly yellow (appropriate for ethnicity), iris dark brown without defect; EOMs—parallel tracking through six cardinal positions of gaze; with confrontation, defects noted in left, right, and inferior peripheral visual fields; central and superior visual fields appear intact; visual acuity 20/30 OU (using a vision screener). Negative for pain, redness, discharge, swelling.

The following concept map illustrates the diagnostic reasoning process.

Applying COLDSPA

Applying **COLDSPA** for client symptoms: "vision changes."

Mnemonic	Question	Data Provided	Missing Data
Character	Describe the sign or symptom (feeling, appearance, sound, smell, or taste if applicable).	"I have strange things with my vision. I do not always see stairs in front of me and words seem to be missing on a page when I am reading."	
Onset	When did it begin?		"When did this first begin?"
Location	Where is it? Does it radiate? Does it occur anywhere else?		"Is your vision worse in your right or left eye or the same in both eyes?"
Duration	How long does it last? Does it recur?	"I notice the problem more when I am reading, walking, or driving."	
Severity	How bad is it? or How much does it bother you?	"I almost hit another car when I made a left turn and got distracted. I did not see it at all."	
Pattern	What makes it better or worse?	n/a	
Associated factors/How it **A**ffects the client	What other symptoms occur with it? How does it affect you?	"I work as a troubleshooter for computers and have to drive and read a lot on the computer. I have to work to support my wife and pay bills."	

1) Identify abnormal findings and client strengths

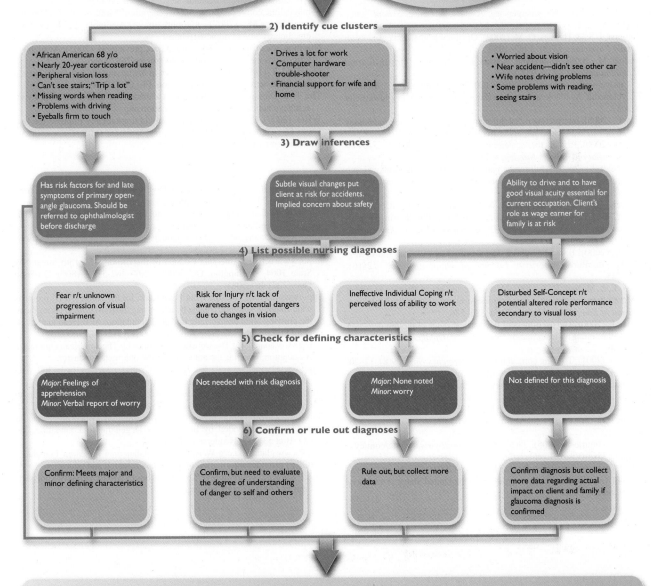

Subjective Data

- "Strange things are happening with my vision"
- Can't always see stairs in front of him
- "I trip a lot lately"
- Words missing on page when reading
- Almost hit a car making a left turn—didn't see car
- Wife noticed problems with his driving
- Worried about vision; has mentioned to doctor
- Work involves much driving—trouble-shooting computer hardware
- Financial support for wife and home

Objective Data

- African American man, 68 years old
- Recent hospitalization with acute asthma attack
- On oral and inhaled corticosteroids for almost 20 years
- Visual acuity 20/30 OU with gross screening
- PERRL 2/1 OU
- Conjugate gaze, parallel tracking
- Intact corneal light and blink reflexes
- Sclera slightly yellow, iris dark brown
- Visual field defects in right, left, and inferior peripheral fields
- Intact central and superior visual fields
- Slight protrusion of eyeballs, firm to touch

2) Identify cue clusters

- African American 68 y/o
- Nearly 20-year corticosteroid use
- Peripheral vision loss
- Can't see stairs; "Trip a lot"
- Missing words when reading
- Problems with driving
- Eyeballs firm to touch

- Drives a lot for work
- Computer hardware trouble-shooter
- Financial support for wife and home

- Worried about vision
- Near accident—didn't see other car
- Wife notes driving problems
- Some problems with reading, seeing stairs

3) Draw inferences

Has risk factors for and late symptoms of primary open-angle glaucoma. Should be referred to ophthalmologist before discharge

Subtle visual changes put client at risk for accidents. Implied concern about safety

Ability to drive and to have good visual acuity essential for current occupation. Client's role as wage earner for family is at risk

4) List possible nursing diagnoses

Fear r/t unknown progression of visual impairment

Risk for Injury r/t lack of awareness of potential dangers due to changes in vision

Ineffective Individual Coping r/t perceived loss of ability to work

Disturbed Self-Concept r/t potential altered role performance secondary to visual loss

5) Check for defining characteristics

Major: Feelings of apprehension
Minor: Verbal report of worry

Not needed with risk diagnosis

Major: None noted
Minor: worry

Not defined for this diagnosis

6) Confirm or rule out diagnoses

Confirm: Meets major and minor defining characteristics

Confirm, but need to evaluate the degree of understanding of danger to self and others

Rule out, but collect more data

Confirm diagnosis but collect more data regarding actual impact on client and family if glaucoma diagnosis is confirmed

7) Document conclusions

Nursing diagnoses that are appropriate for this client include:
- Fear r/t unknown progression of visual impairment
- Risk for Injury r/t lack of awareness of potential dangers due to changes in vision
- Disturbed Self-Concept r/t potential altered role performance secondary to visual loss

Potential collaborative problems include the following:
- RC: Blindness
- RC: Increased intraocular pressure
Medical diagnosis is yet to be made. Client should be referred to an ophthalmologist for further examination.

References and Selected Readings

Bass, S. J., & Sherman, J. (2004). Optic disk evaluation and utility of high-tech devices in the assessment of glaucoma. *Optometry, 75*(5), 277–296.

Bickerton, R. (2000). Identifying and treating ocular emergencies. *Journal of Ophthalmic Nursing and Technology, 19*(5), 225–229.

Bremner, F. D. (2004). Pupil assessment in optic nerve disorders. *Eye, 18*(11), 1175–1181.

Buchan, J. C., Saihan, Z., & Reynolds, A. G. (2003). Nurse triage, diagnosis and treatment of eye casualty patients: A study of quality and utility. *Accident and Emergency Nursing, 22*(4), 226–228.

Center for Disease Control. (2004). Prevalence of visual impairment and selected eye diseases among persons aged ≥ 50 years with and without diabetes – United States, 2002, *MMWR Weekly, 53*(45), 1069–1071, available at http://www.cdc.gov/mmwr/preview/mmwrhtml/mm5345a3.html

Davis, R. (2002). Ocular emergencies: A quick reference. *School Nurse News, 19*(2), 34–37.

Distelhorst, J. S., & Hughes, G. M. (2003). Open-angle glaucoma. *American Family Physicians, 67*(9), 1937–1950.

El Mallah, M. (2000). Amblyopia: Is visual loss permanent? *British Journal of Ophthalmology, 84*(9), 952–956.

Eye movements—uncontrollable. (2007). MedlinePlus Medical Encyclopedia. Available at http://www.nlm.nih.goiv/medilineplus/article/003037

Girkin, C. (2005). Interpreting racial differences in glaucoma. *Ophthalmology Management,* available at http://www.ophmanagement.com.

Glenn, G. (2000). Risk factors screening and treatment of diabetic eye disease. *Journal of Diabetes Nursing, 4*(1), 28–31.

Goldschmidt, L. (2000). Multimedia patient education in the office: Going where few patients have gone before. *Ophthalmology Clinics of North America, 13*(2), 239–247.

Goldzweig, C. L., Rowe, S., Wenger, N. S., MacLean, C. H., & Shekelle, P. G. (2004). Preventing and managing visual disability in primary care: Clinical application. *Journal of the American Medical Association, 291*(12), 1497–1502.

Harris, E. (2000). Bacterial subretinal abscess: A case report and review of the literature. *American Journal of Ophthalmology, 129*(6), 778–785.

Kappes, J., & McNair, R. S. (2003). Headache and visual changes at triage: Do not allow the patient's assumptions to cloud your critical thinking. *Journal of Emergency Nursing, 29*(6), 584–586.

Kushner, F. (2000). The usefulness of the cervical range of motion device in the ocular motility examination. *Archives of Ophthalmology, 118*(7), 946–950.

Marsden, J. (2001). Treating corneal trauma. *Emergency Nurse, 9*(8), 17–20.

McCarty, C., & Taylor, H. (2000). Age-specific causes of bilateral visual impairment. *Archives of Ophthalmology, 118*(2), 264–269.

Moss, S. (2000). Prevalence of the risk factors for dry eye syndrome. *Archives of Ophthalmology, 118*(9), 1264–1268.

Rapaport, M. (2000). Eyelid dermatitis. *Dermatology Nursing, 12*(5), 352–354.

Sports eye injuries. (2005). Available at http://www.uic.edu/com/eye/LearningAboutVision/EyeFacts/SportsEyeInjuries

The Eye Diseases Prevalence Research Group. (2004). Causes and prevalence of visual impairment among adults in the United States. *Archives of Ophthalmology, 122,* 477–485.

The Eye Digest: Myopia inherited? (2006). In *The Myopia Manual.* Available at http://www.agingeye.net/myopia

Promote Health—Cataracts, Glaucoma, and Macular Degeneration

American Academy of Ophthalmology. (2003). Cataract. Available at http://www.medem.com/medlb/article_detaillb.cfm/article

Foundation Fighting Blindness. (2007). Macular degeneration—What environmental and behavioral factors increase the risk? Available at http://www.blindness.org/disease/riskfactors.asp/type=2

International Glaucoma Association (IGA). (2007). Glaucoma – risk factors. Available at http://www.glaucoma-association.com/nqcontent.cfm/a_ id=728&=fromcfc&tt=article&lang=en&site_id=483

Mayo Clinic. (2007). Glaucoma. Available at http://www.mayoclinic.com/health/glaucoma/DS00283/DSECTION=8

Mayo Clinic. (2007). Macular degeneration. Available at http://www.mayoclinic.com/health/macular-degeneration/DS00284/DSECTION=8

Mercandetti, M. (2007). Exophthalmos. Available at http://www.emedicine.com/oph/topics616.htm

Nutrition scientists take a look at cataract prevention. (2005). Available at http://www.medicalnewstoday.com/articles/28920.php

Overfield, T. (1995). *Biologic variation in health and illness: Race, age and sex differences* (2nd ed.). Boca Raton, FL: CRC Press.

The Eye Digest. (2003). What is a cataract? Available at http://www.agingeye.net/cataract/cataractinformation.php

WHO. (2007). Sight tests and glasses could dramatically improve the lives of 150 million people with poor vision. Available at http://www.who.int/mediacentre/news/releases/2006/pr55

Websites

http://www.aafp.org/afp.xml Produced by the American Academy of Family Physicians, this site strives to preserve and promote the science and art of family medicine and to ensure high-quality, cost-effective health care for patients of all ages. Online journal is available.

http://www.aao.org/news/eynet American Academy of Ophthalmology website source for clinical insights.

http://www.acb.org American Council of the Blind, 1155 15th Street NW, Suite 1004, Washington, DC 20005, (202) 467-5081, (800) 424-8666, Fax: (202) 467-5085.

http://www.afb.org The American Foundation for the Blind (AFB) promotes wide-ranging, systemic change by addressing the most critical issues facing the growing blind and visually impaired population. AFB Headquarters, 11 Penn Plaza, Suite 300, New York, NY 10001, (212) 502-7600.

http://www.aoanet.org The website is produced by The American Optometric Association, which is the authority for the optometric industry.

http://www.biomedcentral.com BioMed Central provides over 100 open access journals covering all areas of biology and medicine.

http://www.blindness.org Informational website produced by The Foundation Fighting Blindness, 11435 Cronhill Drive, Owings Mills, MD 21117-2220.

http://www.eyesight.org Resource for information concerning macular degeneration provided by the Macular Degeneration Foundation, Inc. P.O. Box 531313, Henderson, NV 89053.

http://www.glaucoma.org Website of The Glaucoma Research Foundation (GRF) provides information on glaucoma research and education.

http://www.uic.edu/com/eye/LearningAboutVision/EyeFacts/SportsEye Injuries (2005). Sports eye injuries.

16
Ears

Structure and Function

The ear is the sense organ of hearing and equilibrium. It consists of three distinct parts: the **external ear,** the **middle ear,** and the **inner ear.** The tympanic membrane separates the external ear from the middle ear. Both the external ear and the tympanic membrane can be assessed by direct inspection and by using an otoscope. However, the middle and inner ear cannot be directly inspected. Instead, these parts of the ear are assessed by testing hearing acuity and the conduction of sound. Before learning assessment techniques, it is important to understand the anatomy and physiology of the ear.

STRUCTURES OF THE EAR

External Ear

The external ear is composed of the auricle or **pinna** and the **external auditory canal** (Fig. 16-1). The external auditory canal is S-shaped in the adult. The outer part of the canal curves up and back and the inner part of the canal curves down and forward. Modified sweat glands in the external ear canal secrete **cerumen,** a wax-like substance that keeps the tympanic membrane soft. Cerumen has bacteriostatic properties, and its sticky consistency serves as a defense against foreign bodies. The **tympanic membrane,** or eardrum, has a translucent, pearly gray appearance and serves as a partition stretched across the inner end of the auditory canal, separating it from the middle ear. The membrane itself is concave and located at the end of the auditory canal in a tilted position such that the top of the membrane is closer to the auditory meatus than the bottom. The distinct landmarks (Fig. 16-2) of the tympanic membrane include

- Handle and short process of the malleus—the nearest auditory ossicle that can be seen through the translucent membrane
- Umbo—the base of the malleus but also serves as a center point landmark
- Cone of light—the reflection of the otoscope light seen as a cone due to the concave nature of the membrane
- Pars flaccida—the top portion of the membrane that appears to be less taut than the bottom portion
- Pars tensa—the bottom of the membrane that appears to be taut

Middle Ear

The middle ear, or **tympanic cavity,** is a small, air-filled chamber in the temporal bone. It is separated from the external ear by the eardrum and from the inner ear by a bony partition containing two openings, the round and oval windows. The middle ear contains three auditory ossicles: the **malleus,** the **incus,** and the **stapes** (see Fig. 16-1). These tiny bones are responsible for transmitting sound waves from the eardrum to the inner ear through the oval window. Air pressure is equalized on both sides of the tympanic membrane by means of the **eustachian tube,** which connects the middle ear to the nasopharynx (see Fig. 16-1).

Inner Ear

The inner ear, or **labyrinth,** is fluid filled and is made up of the bony labyrinth and an inner membranous labyrinth. The bony labyrinth has three parts: the **cochlea,** the **vestibule,** and the **semicircular canals** (see Fig. 16-1). The inner cochlear duct contains the spiral organ of Corti, which is the sensory organ for hearing. **Sensory receptors,** located in the vestibule and in the membranous semicircular canals, sense position and head movements to help maintain both static and dynamic equilibrium. Nerve fibers from these areas form the **vestibular nerve,** which connects with the cochlear nerve to form the eighth cranial nerve (acoustic or vestibulocochlear nerve).

HEARING

Sound vibrations traveling through air are collected by and funneled through the external ear and cause the eardrum to vibrate. Sound waves are then transmitted through auditory ossicles as the vibration of the eardrum causes the malleus, the incus, and then the stapes to vibrate. As the stapes vibrates at the oval window, the sound waves are passed to the fluid in the inner ear. The movement of this fluid stimulates the hair cells of the spiral organ of Corti and initiates the nerve impulses that travel to the brain by way of the acoustic nerve.

The transmission of sound waves through the external and middle ear is referred to as "**conductive hearing,**" and the transmission of sound waves in the inner ear is referred to as "perceptive" or "**sensorineural hearing**." Therefore, a conductive hearing loss would be related to a dysfunction of the external or middle ear (e.g., impacted ear wax, otitis media, foreign object, perforated eardrum, drainage in the middle ear, or otosclerosis). A "sensorineural loss" would be related to

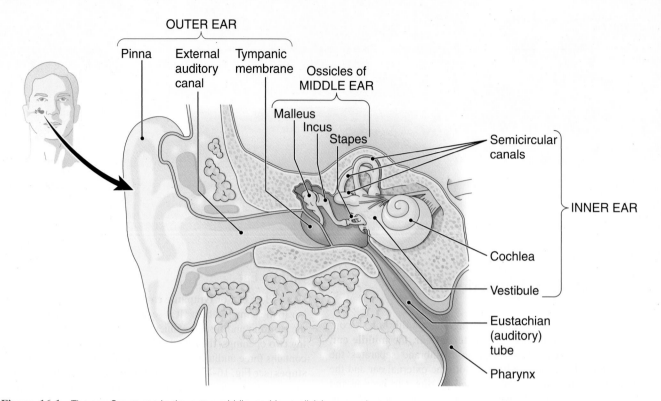

OUTER EAR

Pinna External auditory canal Tympanic membrane

Ossicles of MIDDLE EAR

Malleus
Incus
Stapes

Semicircular canals

INNER EAR

Cochlea

Vestibule

Eustachian (auditory) tube

Pharynx

Figure 16-1 The ear. Structures in the outer, middle, and inner divisions are shown.

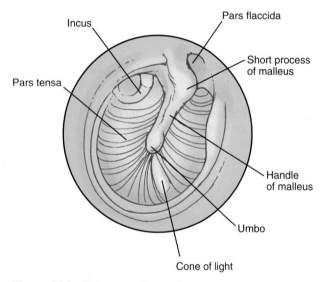

Incus Pars flaccida

Short process of malleus

Pars tensa

Handle of malleus

Umbo

Cone of light

Figure 16-2 Right tympanic membrane.

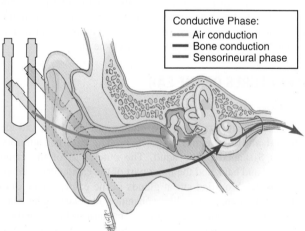

Conductive Phase:
—— Air conduction
—— Bone conduction
—— Sensorineural phase

Figure 16-3 Pathways of hearing.

dysfunction of the inner ear (i.e., organ of Corti, cranial nerve VIII, or temporal lobe of brain).

In addition to the usual pathway for sound vibrations detailed previously, the bones of the skull also conduct sound waves. This bone conduction, though less efficient, serves to augment the usual pathway of sound waves through air, bone, and finally fluid (Fig. 16-3).

Health Assessment

Beginning when the nurse first meets the client, assessment of hearing provides important information about the client's ability to interact with the environment. Changes in hearing are often gradual and go unrecognized by clients until a severe problem develops. Therefore, asking the client specific questions about hearing may help in detecting disorders at an early stage.

COLLECTING SUBJECTIVE DATA: THE NURSING HEALTH HISTORY

First it is important to gather data from the client about the current level of hearing and ear health as well as past and family health history problems related to the ear. During data collection, the examiner should be alert to signs of hearing loss such as inappropriate answers, frequent requests for repetition, etc. Collecting data concerning environmental influences on hearing and how these problems affect the client's usual activities of daily living is also important. Answers to these types of questions help you to evaluate a client's risk for hearing loss and, in turn, present ways that the client may modify or lower the risk of ear and hearing problems.

(text continues on page 268)

HISTORY OF PRESENT HEALTH CONCERN

Question	Rationale
Changes in Hearing Describe any recent changes in your hearing.	A sudden decrease in ability to hear in one ear may be associated with otitis media. A client reporting any sudden hearing loss should be referred to a physician for evaluation. Presbycusis, a gradual hearing loss, is common after the age of 50 years.
Are all sounds affected with this change or just some sounds?	Presbycusis often begins with a loss of the ability to hear high-frequency sounds.
Other Symptoms Do you have any ear drainage? Describe the amount and any odor.	Drainage (otorrhea) usually indicates infection. Purulent, bloody drainage suggests an infection of the external ear (external otitis). Purulent drainage associated with pain and a popping sensation is characteristic of otitis media with perforation of the tympanic membrane.
Do you have any ear pain? If so, do you have an accompanying sore throat, sinus infection, or problem with your teeth or gums?	Earache (otalgia) can occur with ear infections, cerumen blockage, sinus infections, or teeth and gum problems.
Do you experience any ringing or crackling in your ears?	Ringing in the ears (tinnitus) may be associated with excessive ear wax buildup, high blood pressure, or certain ototoxic medications (such as streptomycin, gentamicin, kanamycin, neomycin, ethacrynic acid, furosemide, indomethacin, or aspirin).
Do you ever feel like you are spinning or that the room is spinning? Do you ever feel dizzy or unbalanced?	Vertigo (true spinning motion) may be associated with an inner ear problem. It is termed *subjective vertigo* when the client feels that he is spinning around and *objective vertigo* when the client feels that the room is spinning around him. It is important to distinguish vertigo from dizziness.

continued on page 266

COLDSPA Example

Use the **COLDSPA** mnemonic as a guideline to collect needed information for each symptom the client shares. In addition, the following questions help elicit important information.

Mnemonic	Question	Client Response Example
Character	Describe the sign or symptom (feeling, appearance, sound, smell, or taste if applicable).	"Throbbing ear pain"
Onset	When did it begin?	"Last night around 7 PM"
Location	Where is it? Does it radiate? Does it occur anywhere else?	"Inside my right ear"
Duration	How long does it last? Does it recur?	"The pressure is constant but the pain varies depending on when I last took Ibuprofen"
Severity	How bad is it? or How much does it bother you?	"It kept me awake last night"
Pattern	What makes it better or worse?	"I took an Ibuprofen last night at around 8 PM and I woke up with the pain again at around 11 PM. It hurts a lot when I cough."
Associated factors/ How it **A**ffects the client	What other symptoms occur with it? How does it affect you?	"Everything sounds muffled— I can hardly hear. I had a cold about a week ago and it went away, but now I have this earache."

PAST HEALTH HISTORY

Question	Rationale
Have you ever had any problems with your ears such as infections, trauma, or earaches?	A history of repeated infections can affect the tympanic membrane and hearing (see Promote Health—Otitis Media).
Describe any past treatments you have received for ear problems (medication, surgery, hearing aids). Were these successful? Were you satisfied?	Client may be dissatisfied with past treatments for ear or hearing problems. The older client may have had a bad experience with certain hearing aids and may refuse to wear one. The client may also associate a negative self-image with a hearing aid.

FAMILY HISTORY

Question	Rationale
Is there a history of hearing loss in your family?	In many cases, hearing loss is hereditary.

LIFESTYLE AND HEALTH PRACTICES

Question	Rationale
Do you work or live in an area with frequent or continuous loud noise? How do you protect your ears from the noise?	Continuous loud noises (e.g., machinery, music, explosives) can cause a hearing loss unless the ears are protected with ear guards (see Promote Health—Hearing Loss).
Do you spend a lot of time swimming or in water? How do you protect your ears?	Swimmer's ear (infection of the ear canal) may be seen when contaminated water is left in the ear. Earplugs may help to keep water out and over-the-counter ear drops may be used to dry out the water in the ears.
Has your hearing loss affected your ability to care for yourself? To work?	Hearing loss or ear pain may interfere with the client's ability to perform usual activities of daily living. Clients may not be able to drive, talk on the telephone, or operate machinery safely because of poor hearing ability. The ability to perform in occupations that rely heavily on hearing, such as a receptionist or telephone operator, may be affected.
Has your hearing loss affected your socializing with others?	Clients who have decreased hearing may withdraw, isolate themselves, or become depressed because of the stress of verbal communication.
When was your last hearing examination?	Yearly hearing tests are recommended for clients who are exposed to loud noises for long periods. Knowing the date of the examination helps to determine recent changes.
How do you care for your ears?	Use of cotton-tipped applicators inside the ear can cause ear wax to become impacted and cause ear damage.

PROMOTE HEALTH
Otitis Media

Overview

Otitis media is an inflammation or infection of the middle ear, which often causes fluid to build up behind the ear drum. Otitis media often begins when a throat or respiratory viral infection spreads to the middle ear. Ear infections are often associated with dysfunction or swelling of the eustachian tube. By age three, 75% of children will have had at least one episode of otitis media and many children will have many recurrent ear infections. The fact that children are more susceptible than adults to otitis media is due mostly to the shorter, straighter, narrower eustachian tubes of children. This tube structure also applies to Native Americans, Eskimos, New Zealand Maoris, and some other aborigines (Casselbrandt et al., 1995). Blacks have lower rates of both otitis media and noise-induced or other forms of hearing loss (News24, 2006).

Risk Factors

- Age (highest rate between 6 and 18 months old, but occur from 4 months to 4 years; rarely in adults)
- Group child care
- Poor air quality (tobacco smoke and air pollution)
- Family history
- Race/ethnic group (American Indian or Eskimo)

Teach Risk Reduction Tips

- Keep child away from sick children (limit time in group care)
- Protect child from secondhand smoke
- Breast feed baby for at least 6 months
- If bottle fed, hold baby in upright position
- Ask child's primary caregiver about preventive pneumococcal vaccine.

PROMOTE HEALTH
Hearing Loss

Overview

Hearing loss is a common problem today due to the effects of noise, disease, aging, heredity, and exposure to traumatic injury. There are three types of hearing loss: conductive, sensorineural, and mixed. Conductive hearing loss results in sound not being conducted through the canal to the drum and ossicles in the middle ear. This affects the hearing of faint sounds. Sensorineural hearing loss occurs when there is damage to the cochlea of the inner ear and to the nerve pathways to the brain. This loss affects faint sounds and the ability to hear clearly and understand speech. Mixed hearing loss occurs when both middle ear and nerves are damaged. There are many descriptors of hearing loss, including degree and configuration. Genetic hearing loss occurs in about 1/1,000 births. Also of genetic origin is late onset hearing loss, which occurs with age (presbycusis) and which affects 25% of persons between 65 and 75 and 75% of those over 75 years of age. Blacks are less affected by hearing loss than Caucasians. Causes of hearing loss include the gradual loss from noise over time, ear wax buildup, ear drum rupture, infections, tumors, and damage to bones or nerves in ear.

Risk Factors

- Age (greater than 65 years)
- Loud noises (decibel levels above 85: occupations; recreation: firearms, motorcycles, loud music, snowmobiles
- Heredity
- Otitis media (especially if chronic or untreated)
- Some medications (gentamicin, some chemotherapy drugs; tinnitus or loss with high dose aspirin or NSAIDS, antimalarials, and loop diuretics)
- Some illnesses (with high temperatures, e.g., meningitis; viral infections, e.g., mumps, measles, chicken pox; brain diseases, e.g., multiple sclerosis, tumor, stroke)
- Child of mother who contracted rubella while pregnant

Teach Risk Reduction Tips

- Use ear protection when working or spending time in noise levels above 85 decibels. Follow federal guidelines for time spent in high noise environments (see Mayo Clinic, 2007).
- Have regular ear examinations, especially if spending time in noisy environments.
- Avoid medications associated with ototoxicity, if possible.
- Obtain treatment for otitis media; seek treatment for recurrent sinusitis, which can lead to otitis media.
- Have a sudden hearing loss, dizziness, and tinnitus evaluated as soon as possible.

COLLECTING OBJECTIVE DATA: PHYSICAL EXAMINATION

The purpose of the ear and hearing examination is to evaluate the condition of the external ear, the condition and patency of the ear canal, the status of the tympanic membrane, bone and air conduction of sound vibrations, hearing acuity, and equilibrium. The external ear structures and ear canal are relatively easy to assess through inspection. Using the tuning fork to evaluate bone and air conduction is also a fairly simple procedure. However, more practice and expertise are needed to use the otoscope correctly to examine the condition of the structures of the tympanic membrane.

Preparing the Client

Make sure the client is seated comfortably during the ear examination. This helps to promote the client's participation, which is very important in this examination. In addition, the test should be explained thoroughly to guarantee accurate results. To ease any client anxiety, explain in detail what you will be doing. Also answer any questions the client may have. As you prepare the client for the ear examination, carefully note how she responds to your explanations. Does the client appear to hear you well or does it seem she is straining to catch everything you say? Does the client respond to you verbally or nonverbally or do you have to repeat what you say to get a response? This initial observation provides you with clues as to the status of the client's hearing.

Equipment

- Watch with a second-hand for Romberg test
- Tuning fork (512 or 1,024 Hz)
- Otoscope

Physical Assessment

Before performing examination make sure to

- Recognize the role of hearing in communication and adaptation to the environment particularly in regard to aging.
- Know how to use the otoscope effectively when performing the ear examination (Equipment Spotlight—Otoscope).
- Understand the usefulness and significance of basic hearing tests.

(text continues on page 275)

EQUIPMENT SPOTLIGHT 16-1   Otoscope

The otoscope is a flashlight-type viewer used to visualize the eardrum and external ear canal. Some guidelines for using it effectively follow.

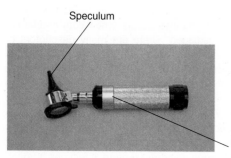

Speculum

Body (contains light source)

1. Ask the client to sit comfortably with the back straight and the head tilted slightly away from you toward his or her opposite shoulder.
2. Choose the largest speculum that fits comfortably into the client's ear canal (usually 5 mm in the adult) and attach it to the otoscope. Holding the instrument in your dominant hand, turn the light on the otoscope to "on."
3. Use the thumb and fingers of your opposite hand to grasp the client's auricle firmly but gently. Pull out, up, and back to straighten the external auditory canal. Do not alter this positioning at any time during the otoscope examination.
4. Grasp the handle of the otoscope between your thumb and fingers and hold the instrument up or down. Handle up is preferred because it is easier then to brace your hand against the client's face.
5. Position the hand holding the otoscope against the client's head or face. This position prevents forceful insertion of the instrument and helps to steady your hand throughout the examination, which is especially helpful if the client makes any unexpected movements.
6. Insert the speculum gently down and forward into the ear canal (approximately 0.5 inch). As you insert the otoscope, be careful not to touch either side of the inner portion of the canal wall. This area is bony and covered by a thin, sensitive layer of epithelium. Any pressure will cause the client pain.
7. Move your head in close to the otoscope and position your eye to look through the lens.

PHYSICAL ASSESSMENT

Assessment Procedure	Normal Findings	Abnormal Findings

External Ear Structures

Inspection and Palpation
Inspect the auricle, tragus, and lobule. Note size, shape and position (Fig. 16-4).

Ears are equal in size bilaterally (normally 4 to 10 cm). The auricle aligns with the corner of each eye and within a 10-degree angle of the vertical position. Earlobes may be free, attached, or soldered (tightly attached to adjacent skin with no apparent lobe).

 Most African Americans and Caucasians have free lobes, whereas most Asians have attached or soldered lobes although any type is possible in all cultural groups (Overfield, 1995).

 The older client often has elongated earlobes with linear wrinkles.

Ears are smaller than 4 cm or larger than 10 cm.

Malaligned or low-set ears may be seen with genitourinary disorders or chromosomal defects.

Continue inspecting the auricle, tragus, and lobule. Observe for lesions, discolorations, and discharge.

The skin is smooth with no lesions, lumps, or nodules. Color is consistent with facial color. Darwin's tubercle, which is a clinically insignificant projection, may be seen on the auricle (Fig. 16-5). No discharge should be present.

Some abnormal findings suggest various disorders, including

Enlarged preauricular and postauricular lymph nodes—infection

Tophi (nontender, hard, cream-colored nodules on the helix or antihelix, containing uric acid crystals)—gout

Blocked sebaceous glands—postauricular cysts

Ulcerated, crusted nodules that bleed—skin cancer (most often seen on the helix due to skin exposure)

Redness, swelling, scaling, or itching—otitis externa

Pale blue ear color—frostbite (see Abnormal Findings 16-1)

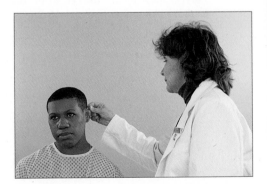

Figure 16-4 Inspecting the external ear (© B. Proud).

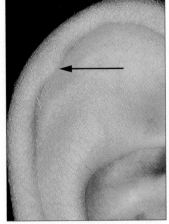

Figure 16-5 Darwin's tubercle.

continued

PHYSICAL ASSESSMENT *Continued*

Assessment Procedure	Normal Findings	Abnormal Findings
Palpate the auricle and mastoid process.	Normally the auricle, tragus, and mastoid process are not tender.	A painful auricle or tragus is associated with otitis externa or a postauricular cyst.
		Tenderness over the mastoid process suggests mastoiditis.
		Tenderness behind the ear may occur with otitis media.

Internal Ear: Otoscopic Examination

Inspection

Inspect the external auditory canal. Use the otoscope (see Equipment Spotlight—Otoscope and Fig. 16-6).

Note any discharge along with the color and consistency of cerumen (ear wax).

A small amount of odorless cerumen (ear wax) is the only discharge normally present. Cerumen may be yellow, orange, red, brown, gray, or black and soft, moist, dry, flaky, or even hard.

 Most Europeans and Africans, 97% or more, have wet earwax; Asians and Native Americans have dry, with transition in southern Asia. The gene accounting for this has been isolated and is associated with lower sweat production of the apocrine glands, possibly an adaptation to cold (Wade, 2006).

 In some older clients, harder, drier cerumen tends to build as cilia in the ear canal become more rigid. Coarse, thick, wirelike hair may grow at the ear canal entrance as well. This is an abnormal finding only if it impairs hearing.

Abnormal findings associated with specific disorders include

Foul-smelling, sticky, yellow discharge—otitis externa or impacted foreign body

Bloody, purulent discharge—otitis media with ruptured tympanic membrane

Blood or watery drainage (cerebrospinal fluid)—skull trauma (refer client to physician immediately)

Impacted cerumen blocking the view of the external ear canal—conductive hearing loss

Observe the color and consistency of the ear canal walls and inspect the character of any nodules.

The canal walls should be pink and smooth and without nodules.

Abnormal findings in the ear canal may include

Reddened, swollen canals—otitis externa

Exostoses (nonmalignant nodular swellings)

Polyps may block the view of the eardrum (Abnormal Findings 16-2).

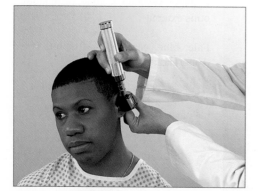

Figure 16-6 Inspecting the external canal and tympanic membrane (© B. Proud).

continued

Assessment Procedure	Normal Findings	Abnormal Findings
Inspect the tympanic membrane (eardrum). Note color, shape, consistency, and landmarks.	The tympanic membrane should be pearly, gray, shiny, and translucent with no bulging or retraction. It is slightly concave, smooth and intact. A cone-shaped reflection of the otoscope light is normally seen at 5 o'clock in the right ear and at 7 o'clock in the left ear. The short process and handle of the malleus and the umbo are clearly visible (see Fig. 16-2). The older client's eardrum may appear cloudy. The landmarks may be more prominent because of atrophy of the tympanic membrane associated with the normal process of aging.	Abnormal findings in the tympanic membrane may include Red, bulging eardrum and distorted, diminished or absent light reflex—acute otitis media Yellowish, bulging membrane with bubbles behind—serous otitis media Bluish or dark red color—blood behind the eardrum from skull trauma White spots—scarring from infections Perforations—trauma from infection Prominent landmarks—eardrum retraction from negative ear pressure resulting from an obstructed eustachian tube Obscured or absent landmarks—eardrum thickening from chronic otitis media (see Abnormal Findings 16-2)

Hearing and Equilibrium Tests

Display 16-1 describes hearing loss and testing.	In general, African Americans have slightly better hearing at low and high frequencies (250 and 6000 Hz); Caucasians have better hearing at middle frequencies (2000 and 4000 Hz). African Americans are less susceptible to noise-induced hearing loss (Overfield, 1995).	
Perform Weber's Test if the client reports diminished or lost hearing in one ear. The test helps to evaluate the conduction of sound waves through bone to help distinguish between conductive hearing (sound waves transmitted by the external and middle ear) and sensorineural hearing (sound waves transmitted by the inner ear). Strike a tuning fork softly with the back of your hand and place it in the center of the client's head or forehead (Fig. 16-7). Centering is the important part. Ask whether the client hears the sound better in one ear or the same in both ears.	Vibrations are heard equally well in both ears. No lateralization of sound to either ear.	With *conductive hearing loss*, the client reports lateralization of sound to the poor ear—that is, the client "hears" the sounds in the poor ear. The good ear is distracted by background noise, conducted air, which the poor ear has trouble hearing. Thus the poor ear receives most of the sound conducted by bone vibration. With *sensorineural hearing loss*, the client reports lateralization of sound to the good ear. This is because of limited perception of the sound due to nerve damage in the bad ear, making sound seem louder in the unaffected ear.

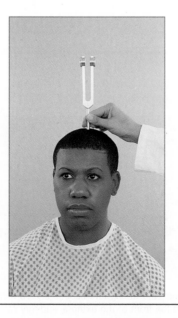

Figure 16-7 The Weber test assesses sound conducted via bone (© B. Proud).

continued

DISPLAY 16-1   Hearing Loss and Testing

Sensoneural Hearing and Hearing Loss

Actual hearing takes place when sound waves are channeled through the auditory canal, causing the tympanic membrane to vibrate. These vibrations are transmitted through the middle ear by the auditory ossicles to the inner ear, where they are converted into nerve impulses that travel to the brain for interpretation.

A sensoneural hearing loss results when damage is located in the inner ear. Conduction of sound waves is occurring through normal pathways, but the impaired inner ear cannot make the conversion into nerve impulses. Possible causes of sensoneural hearing loss are prolonged exposure to loud noises or using ototoxic medications.

Presbycusis, a gradual sensoneural hearing loss due to degeneration of the cochlea or vestibulocochlear nerve, is common in older (over age 50) clients. The client with presbycusis has difficulty hearing consonants and whispered words; this difficulty increases over time.

Conductive Hearing and Loss

Bone conduction occurs when the temporal bone vibrates with sound waves and the vibrations are picked up by the tympanic membrane and/or auditory ossicles. This type of conduction results in the perception of sound but is virtually ineffective for interpretation of sounds.

A conductive hearing loss occurs when something blocks or impairs the passage of vibrations from getting to the inner ear. While a number of causes exist, cerumen buildup and fluid in the middle ear are the most common barriers to "vibration" transmission.

Conductive hearing impairment is not uncommon in the older client due to greater incidence of cerumen buildup and/or atrophy or sclerosis of the tympanic membrane. A condition called otosclerosis often occurs with aging as the auditory ossicles develop a spongy consistency that results in conductive hearing loss.

Hearing Tests

The tests discussed in this chapter are performed to give the examiner a basic idea of whether the client has hearing loss, what type (conduction or sensorineural) of hearing loss it might be, and whether there is a problem with equilibrium. These tests present an opportunity to educate clients about risk factors for hearing loss. These tests are not completely accurate and do not provide the examiner with any exact percentage of hearing loss. Therefore, the client should be referred to a hearing specialist for more accurate testing if a problem is suspected.

Auditory testing performed with a tuning fork is meant for screening only and should not be used for diagnostic purposes. Variations from expected findings in any tests using a tuning fork are simply an indication of the need for more elaborate testing and referral.

PHYSICAL ASSESSMENT Continued

Assessment Procedure	Normal Findings	Abnormal Findings
Perform the Rinne test. The Rinne test compares air and bone conduction sounds. Strike a tuning fork and place the base of the fork on the client's mastoid process (Fig. 16-8). Ask the client to tell you when the sound is no longer heard. Move the prongs of the tuning fork to the front of the external auditory canal. Ask the client to tell you if they hear the sound and when they are no longer able to hear the sound, then note the length of time.	Air conduction sound is normally heard longer than bone conduction sound (AC > BC).	With *conductive hearing loss,* bone conduction sound is heard longer than or equally as long as air conduction sound (BC ≥ AC). With *sensorineural hearing loss,* air conduction sound is heard longer than bone conduction sound (AC > BC) if anything is heard at all.

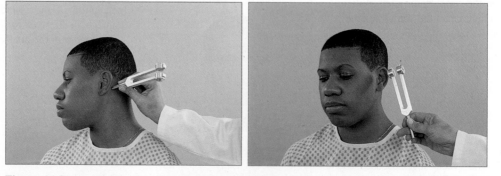

Figure 16-8 For the Rinne test, the tuning fork base is placed first on the mastoid process (left), after which the prongs are moved to the front of the external auditory canal (right) (© B. Proud).

continued

Assessment Procedure	Normal Findings	Abnormal Findings
Perform the Romberg Test. This tests the client's equilibrium. Ask the client to stand with feet together and arms at sides and eyes open and then with the eyes closed. ➤ *Clinical Tip • Put your arms around the client without touching him or her to prevent falls.*	Client maintains position for 20 seconds without swaying or with minimal swaying.	Client moves feet apart to prevent falls or starts to fall from loss of balance. This may indicate a vestibular disorder.

Abnormal Findings 16-1   Abnormalities of the External Ear and Ear Canal

Many abnormalities may affect the external ear and ear canal; among them are infections and abnormal growths. Some are pictured below.

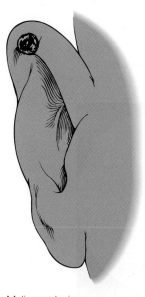

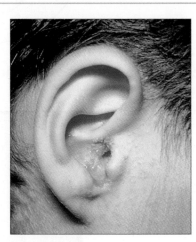

Otitis externa. (© 1992 Science Photo Library/CMSP.)

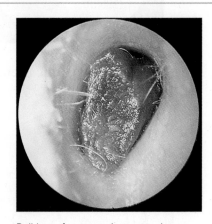

Build-up of cerumen in ear canal.

Malignant lesion.

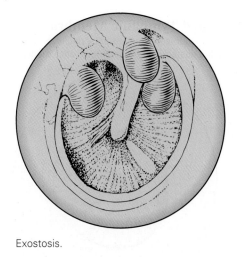

Exostosis.

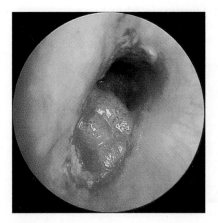

Polyp.

Abnormal Findings 16-2

Abnormalities of the Tympanic Membrane

The thin, drumlike structure of the tympanic membrane is essential for hearing. It is also essential for promoting equilibrium and barring infection. Damage to the membrane may have grave and serious consequences.

Acute Otitis Media

Note the red, bulging membrane; decreased or absent light reflex.

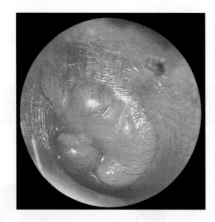

Serous Otitis Media

Note the yellowish, bulging membrane with bubbles behind it.

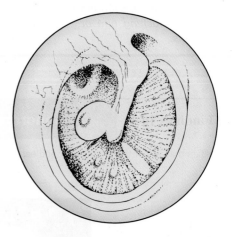

Blue/Dark Red Tympanic Membrane

Indicates blood behind eardrum due to trauma.

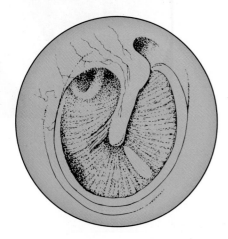

Scarred Tympanic Membrane

White spots and streaks indicate scarring from infections.

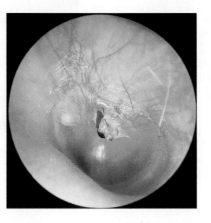

Perforated Tympanic Membrane

Perforation results from rupture caused by increased pressure usually from untreated infection or trauma.

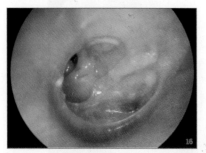

(© 1992 Science Photo Library/CMSP.)

Retracted Tympanic Membrane

Prominent landmarks are caused by negative ear pressure due to obstructed eustachian tube or chronic otitis media.

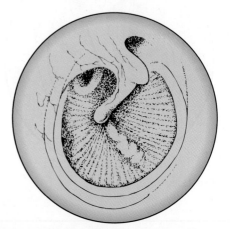

VALIDATING AND DOCUMENTING FINDINGS

Validate the ear assessment data that you have collected. This is necessary to verify that the data are reliable and accurate. Document the assessment data following the health care facility or agency policy.

Sample Subjective Data

Client denies recent changes in hearing. No drainage, pain, or ringing. Has not experienced any spinning sensations. States history of one ear infection several years ago. Has had no surgery, does not use a hearing aid device. Denies frequent exposure to loud noises. Last hearing examination was 3 years ago.

Sample Objective Data

Equal in size bilaterally, auricles aligned with the corner of each eye within a 10-degree angle of vertical position. Skin smooth, no lumps, lesions, nodules. No discharge. Nontender on palpation. Small amount of moist yellow cerumen in external canal, no nodules present. Tympanic membrane pearly gray, shiny, transparent, no bulging or retraction, smooth, intact. Cone-shaped reflection at 5 o'clock position in right ear, 7 o'clock position in left ear. Short process, handle of malleus and umbo clearly visible. Whisper test: Client repeats two-syllable word. Weber's test: Hears vibration equally well in both ears. Rinne test: AC > BC. Romberg test: Maintains position for 20 seconds without swaying.

After you have collected your assessment data, you will need to analyze the data using diagnostic reasoning skills. Refer to the discussion of diagnostic reasoning skills in Chapter 6.

Analysis of Data

DIAGNOSTIC REASONING: POSSIBLE CONCLUSIONS

After collecting subjective and objective data pertaining to the ears, identify abnormal findings and client strengths. Then cluster the data to reveal any significant patterns or abnormalities. These data will then be used to make clinical judgments (nursing diagnoses: wellness, risk, or actual) about the status of the client's ears. Listed below are some possible conclusions that the nurse may make after assessing a client's ears.

Selected Nursing Diagnoses

The following is a list of selected nursing diagnoses that may be identified when analyzing data from ear assessment.

Wellness Diagnoses

- Readiness for enhanced communication related to use of hearing aid

Risk Diagnoses

- Risk for Injury related to hearing impairment
- Risk for Loneliness related to hearing loss

Actual Diagnoses

- Disturbed Sensory Perception: Auditory related to conductive or sensorineural hearing loss
- Acute Pain related to infection of external or middle ear
- Impaired Social Interaction related to inability to interact effectively with others secondary to hearing loss
- Disturbed Body Image related to concern over appearance and with hearing aid

Selected Collaborative Problems

After grouping the data, it may become apparent that certain collaborative problems emerge. Remember that collaborative problems differ from nursing diagnoses in that they cannot be prevented by nursing interventions. However, these physiologic complications of medical conditions can be detected and monitored by the nurse. In addition, the nurse can use physician- and nurse-prescribed interventions to minimize the complications of these problems. The nurse may also have to refer the client in such situations for further treatment of the problem. The following is a list of collaborative problems that may be identified when assessing the ear. These problems are worded Risk for Complications (or RC), followed by the problem.

- RC: Otitis media (acute, chronic, or serous)
- RC: Otitis externa
- RC: Perforated tympanic membrane

Medical Problems

If after grouping the data it becomes apparent that the client has signs and symptoms that may require medical diagnosis and treatment, referral to a primary care provider is necessary.

CASE STUDY

The case study demonstrates how to analyze ear data for a specific client. The critical thinking exercises included in the study guide/lab manual and interactive product that complement this text also offer opportunities to assess the data.

Josephine Carmino is a 57-year-old woman who lives alone in a small urban apartment. She lives on a fixed income from her deceased husband's Social Security pension. She has come to the clinic for her routine checkup. During the initial interview, you notice that she does not always answer your questions appropriately and she talks very softly when she offers information spontaneously. When you check her hearing with the whisper test, she asks you to repeat the word several times, and finally tells you with annoyance in her voice, "You just have to speak up if you expect people to hear you!" When you do the Rinne test, the results show BC > AC. When you question her about problems, she denies having any hearing loss. She says she has never had audiometric studies and she can't afford them now. She also tells you that she doesn't talk to friends on the telephone anymore because they don't talk loudly enough.

The following concept map illustrates the diagnostic reasoning process.

Applying COLDSPA

Applying **COLDSPA** for client symptoms: "Client answers questions inappropriately and speaks very softly."

Mnemonic	Question	Data Provided	Missing Data
Character	Describe the sign or symptom (feeling, appearance, sound, smell, or taste if applicable).	During routine checkup, client answers questions inappropriately and speaks very softly	
Onset	When did it begin?	Denies hearing loss and has never had any audiometric studies.	"When did you first notice your friends were not speaking loud enough on the phone?"
Location	Where is it? Does it radiate? Does it occur anywhere else?		Test for conductive and sensory hearing loss in both ears.
Duration	How long does it last? Does it recur?	Asks examiner to repeat the whispered word several times	"When do you find talking with others the most comfortable or beneficial to you?"
Severity	How bad is it? or How much does it bother you?	Seems annoyed when unable to hear your questions	"Do you find it easier to visit in a group or with just one other person?"
Pattern	What makes it better or worse?	"You just have to speak up if you expect people to hear you!"	"What is your preferred way of communicating with others?"
Associated factors/How it **A**ffects the client	What other symptoms occur with it? How does it affect you?	"I never talk on the phone because my friends do not speak loudly enough."	

1) Identify abnormal data and client strengths

Subjective Data

- Denies any hearing loss
- Never has had audiometry and cannot afford it
- Doesn't talk to friends on telephone anymore
- Friends do not talk loud enough on the telephone

Objective Data

- Does not answer questions appropriately
- Speaks very softly
- Fails whisper test
- Rinne test: BC>AC

2) Identify cue clusters

- Does not answer questions appropriately
- Fails whisper test
- Speaks very softly
- Friends do not talk loud enough on telephone
- Rinne test: BC>AC

- Denies hearing loss
- Has never had audiometric studies and cannot afford them

- Does not talk to friends on telephone anymore
- Friends do not talk loud enough on the telephone

3) Draw inferences

Data suggest a conduction hearing loss. Soft speaking voice indicates that she hears her own voice loudly, which also points to conductive loss in the middle ear

At risk for progression of hearing loss because she denies evident hearing problem, although it could just be lack of understanding if her voice sounds loud to her

Limiting social contacts because she cannot hear well on the telephone

4) List possible nursing diagnoses

Impaired Verbal Communication r/t lack of understanding of hearing deficit

Ineffective Health Maintenance r/t denial of hearing problem and inadequate resources to get additional testing

Impaired Social Interaction r/t decreased ability to maintain contact with friends secondary to probable hearing deficit

5) Check for defining characteristics

Major: Inappropriate response, does not answer nurse's questions appropriately
Minor: Does not talk to friends on telephone because she cannot hear them (not understanding)

Major: No specific characteristics, but implied because of denial of health problem and lack of financial resources for additional diagnostic measures
Minor: None

Major: Reports insecurity in social situations (implied because refuses to talk with friends on phone because cannot hear them well enough)
Minor: None specific

6) Confirm or rule out diagnoses

Confirm because it meets the major and minor defining characteristics

Rule out at this time because not enough data to validate major defining characteristics. However, important to collect more information about this diagnosis because client may be at risk for deterioration of hearing without follow-up care

Accept diagnosis because it meets major defining characteristic

7) Document conclusions

Two diagnoses are appropriate at this time:
- Impaired Communication r/t lack of understanding of hearing deficit
- Impaired Social Interaction r/t decreased ability to maintain contact with friends secondary to probable hearing deficit

No collaborative problems could be identified because there is no medical diagnosis at this time. Mrs. Carmino should be referred to a physician whose services she can afford and who can evaluate and recommend treatment for hearing loss. (In addition, it would be useful also to refer her to a social worker for evaluation of her financial status and to help her to locate resources to assist with medical care.)

References and Selected Readings

Austen, S., & Lynch, C. (2004). Non-organic hearing loss redefined: Understanding categorizing and managing non-organic behavior. *International Journal of Audiology, 43*(8), 449–457.

Battista, R. (2004). Audiometric findings of patients with migraine-associated dizziness. *Otology and Neurotology, 25*(6), 987–992.

Ferrite, S., & Santana, V. (2005). Joint effects of smoking, noise exposure and age on hearing loss. *Occupational Medicine, 55*(1), 48–53.

Fischer, T., Singer, S., Gulla, J., Garra, G., & Rosenfeld, R. (2005). Reaction toward a new treatment paradigm for acute otitis media. *Pediatric Emergency Care, 21*(3), 170–172.

Folmer, R., & Shi, B. (2004). Chronic tinnitus resulting from cerumen removal procedures. *International Tinnitus Journal, 10*(1), 42–46.

Guest, J., Greener, M., Robinson, A., & Smith, A. (2004). Impacted cerumen: composition, production, epidemiology and management. *QIM: An International Journal of Medicine, 97*(8), 477–488.

Jacobson, J., & Jacobson, C. (2004). Evaluation of hearing loss in infants and young children. *Pediatric Annals, 33*(12), 811–821.

Kadhim, A., Colweavy, M., O'Donovan, C., & Blayney, A. (2004). Bone anchored hearing aids: Reality, failure and current status. *Irish Medical Journal, 97*(10), 312–314.

Rotteveel, L., Proops, D., Ramsdenm, R., Saeed, S., vanOlphen, A., & Mylanus, E. (2004). Cochlear implantation in 53 patients with otosclerosis: Demographics, computed tomographic scanning, surgery, and complications. *Otology and Neurotology, 25*(6), 943–952.

Schilder, A., Feuth, T., Rijkers, G., & Zielhuis, G. (2005). Eustachian tube function before recurrence of otitis media with effusion. *Archives of Otolaryngology-Head Neck Surgery, 131*(2), 118–123.

Spilman, L. (2002). Examination of the external ear. *Advances in Neonatal Care, 2*(2), 72–80.

Straetemans, M., vanHeerbeek, N., Wilson, C., Roberts, A., & Stephens, D. (2005). Aetiological investigation of sensorineural hearing loss in children. *Archives of Disease in Childhood, 90*(3), 307–309.

Sweat, T. (2004). Alternatives to ear syringing for removal of earwax. *American Family Physician, 69*(8), 1860, 1862; author reply 1862–1863.

Promote Health—Otitis Media and Hearing Loss

American Speech and Hearing Association (ASHA). (2004). The prevalence and incidence of hearing loss in adults. Available at http://www.asha.org

American Speech-Language Hearing Association. (2007). Type, degree, and configuration of hearing loss. Available at http://www.asha.org/public/hearing/disorders/types.htm

BUPA Foundation. (2003). Hearing loss. Health fact sheet from BUPA. Available at http://hcd2.bupa.co.uk/fact_sheets

Casselbrandt, M., Mandel, E., Kurs-Lasky, M., Rockette, H., & Bluestone, C. (1995). Otitis media in a population of black American and white American infants, 0-2 years of age. *International Journal of Pediatric Otorhinolaryngology, 33*(1), 1–16.

Causes of acquired deafness: Prevalence of acquired or "late" deafness. (May 2004). Available at http://deafened.org

Mayo Clinic. (2006). Ear infection (Middle ear). Available at http://www.mayoclinic.com/health/ear-infections/DS00303/DSECTION=3

Mayo Clinic. (2006). Hearing loss. Available at http://www.mayoclinic.com/health/hearing-loss/DS00172/DSECTION=8

National Institute of Deafness and Other Communication Disorders (NIDCD). (2004). Statistics about hearing disorders, ear infections, and deafness. Available at http://www.nidcde.nih.gov/health/statistics/hearing

National Institute on Deafness and Other Communication Disorders (NIDCD). (2002). Otitis media (Ear infection). Available at http://www.nidcd.nih.gov/health/hearing/otitism.htm#children

News24. (2006). Blacks hear better than whites. Available at http://www.health24.com/news/Hearing_managment/1-1239,36212.asp

Overfield, T. (1995). *Biological variation in health and illness* (2nd ed.). Boca Raton, FL: CRC Press.

Wade, N. (2006, January 29). Japanese scientists identify ear wax gene. *New York Times.* Available at http://www.nytimes.com/2006/01/29/science/29cnd-ear.html

Websites

Acoustic Neuroma Association, P.O. Box 12402, Atlanta, GA 30355. Available at http://ANAusa.org

Alexander Graham Bell Association for the Deaf, Inc., 3417 Volta Place, NW, Washington, DC 20007-2778. Available at http://www.agbel.org

American Academy of Audiology, 8201 Greensboro Dr., Suite 300, McLean, VA 22102. Available at http://www.audiology.com

American Academy of Otolaryngology – Head and Neck Surgery, One Prince Street, Alexandria, VA 22314-3357. Available at http://www.entnet.org

American Tinnitus Association, P.O. Box 5, Portland, OR 97207-0005. Available at http://www.ata.org

National Institute on Deafness and Other Communication Disorders, National Institutes of Health, Building 31, Room 3c35 9000, Rockville Pike, Bethesda, MD 20892. Available at http://www.nidcd.nih.gov

17

Mouth, Throat, Nose, and Sinuses

Structure and Function

The mouth and throat make up the first part of the digestive system and are responsible for receiving food (ingestion), taste, preparing food for digestion, and aiding in speech. Cranial nerves V (trigeminal), VII (facial), IX (glossopharyngeal), and XII (hypoglossal) assist with some of these functions (the cranial nerves are discussed in Chapter 25). The nose and **paranasal sinuses** constitute the first part of the respiratory system and are responsible for receiving, filtering, warming, and moistening air to be transported to the lungs. Receptors of cranial nerve I (olfactory) are also located in the nose. These receptors are related to the sense of smell.

MOUTH

The mouth or **oral cavity** is formed by the lips, cheeks, hard and soft palates, uvula, and the tongue and its muscles (Fig. 17-1). The mouth is the beginning of the digestive tract and serves as an airway for the respiratory tract. The upper and lower lips form the entrance to the mouth and serve as a protective gateway to the digestive and respiratory tracts. The roof of the oral cavity is formed by the anterior hard **palate** and the posterior soft palate. An extension of the soft palate is the **uvula**, which hangs in the posterior midline of the oropharynx. The cheeks form the lateral walls of the mouth, whereas the tongue and its muscles form the floor of the mouth. The **mandible** (jaw bone) provides the structural support for the floor of the mouth.

Contained within the mouth are the tongue, teeth, gums, and the openings of the salivary glands (parotid, submandibular, and sublingual). The tongue is a mass of muscle and is attached to the hyoid bone and styloid process of the temporal bone and is connected to the floor of the mouth by a fold of tissue called the frenulum. The tongue assists with moving food, swallowing, and speaking. The gums (**gingiva**) are covered by mucous membrane and normally hold 32 permanent teeth in the adult (Fig. 17-2). The top, visible, white enameled part of each tooth is the crown. The portion of the tooth that is embedded in the gums is the root. The crown and root are connected by the region of the tooth referred to as the neck. Small bumps called

papillae cover the dorsal surface of the tongue. Taste buds, scattered over the tongue's surface, carry sensory impulses to the brain. The three pairs of **salivary glands** secrete saliva (watery, serous fluid containing salts, mucus, and salivary amylase) into the mouth (Fig. 17-3). **Saliva** helps break down and lubricates food. **Amylase** digests carbohydrates. The parotid glands, located below and in front of the ears, empty through Stensen's ducts, which are located inside the cheek across from the second upper molar. The **submandibular glands,** located in the lower jaw, open under the tongue on either side of the frenulum through openings called Wharton's ducts. The **sublingual glands,** located under the tongue, open through several ducts located on the floor of the mouth.

THROAT

The throat (**pharynx**), located behind the mouth and nose, serves as a muscular passage for food and air. The upper part of the throat is the nasopharynx. Below the **nasopharynx** lies the **oropharynx,** and below the oropharynx lies the **laryngopharynx.** The soft palate, anterior and posterior pillars, and uvula connect behind the tongue to form arches. Masses of lymphoid tissue referred to as the **palatine tonsils** are located on both sides of the oropharynx at the end of the soft palate between the anterior and posterior pillars. The **lingual tonsils** lie at the base of the tongue. **Pharyngeal tonsils** or adenoids are found high in the nasopharynx. Because tonsils are masses of lymphoid tissue, they help protect against infection (Fig. 17-4).

NOSE

The nose consists of an external portion covered with skin and an internal nasal cavity. It is composed of bone and cartilage and is lined with mucous membrane. The **external nose** consists of a bridge (upper portion), tip, and two oval openings called **nares.** The **nasal cavity** is located between the roof of the mouth and the cranium. It extends from the anterior nares (nostrils) to the posterior nares, which open into the nasopharynx. The nasal septum separates the cavity into two halves. The front of the nasal **septum** contains a rich supply of blood vessels and is known as Kiesselbach's area. This is a common site for nasal bleeding.

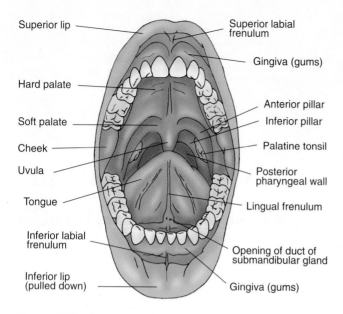

Figure 17-1   Structures of the mouth.

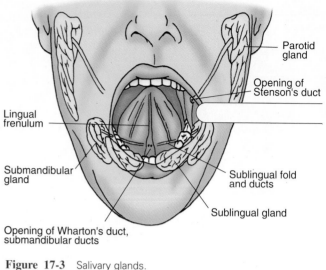

Figure 17-3   Salivary glands.

The superior, middle, and inferior **turbinates** are bony lobes, sometimes called conchae, that project from the lateral walls of the nasal cavity. These three turbinates serve to increase the surface area that is exposed to incoming air (see Fig. 17-4). As the person inspires air, nasal hairs (vibrissae) filter large particles from the air. Ciliated mucosal cells then capture and propel debris toward the throat, where it is swallowed. The rich blood supply of the nose warms the inspired air as it is moistened by the mucous membrane. A meatus underlies each turbinate and receives drainage from the **paranasal sinuses** and the **nasolacrimal duct.** Receptors for the first cranial nerve (olfactory) are located in the upper part of the nasal cavity and septum.

SINUSES

Four pairs of **paranasal sinuses** (frontal, maxillary, ethmoidal, and sphenoidal) are located in the skull (Fig. 17-5). These air-filled cavities decrease the weight of the skull and act as resonance chambers during speech. The paranasal sinuses are also lined with ciliated mucous membrane that traps debris and propels it toward the outside. The sinuses are often a primary site of infection because they can easily become blocked. The **frontal sinuses** (above the eyes) and the **maxillary sinuses** (in the upper jaw) are accessible to examination by the nurse. The **ethmoidal and sphenoidal sinuses** are smaller, located deeper in the skull, and are not accessible for examination.

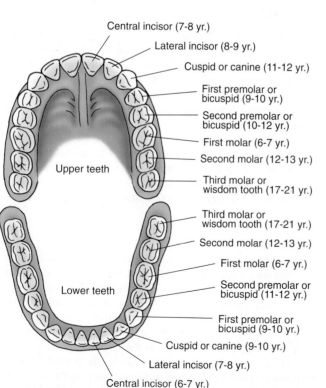

Figure 17-2   Teeth.

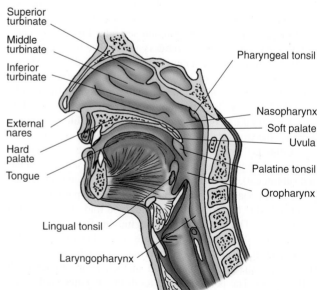

Figure 17-4   Nasal cavity and throat structures.

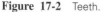

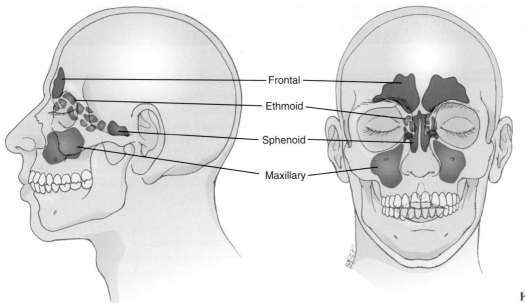

Figure 17-5 Paranasal sinuses.

Nursing Assessment

COLLECTING SUBJECTIVE DATA: THE NURSING HEALTH HISTORY

Subjective data related to the mouth, throat, nose, and sinus can aid in detecting diseases and abnormalities that may affect the client's activities of daily living. Screening for cancer of the mouth, throat, nose, and sinuses is an important area of this assessment. These cancers are highly preventable (see Promote Health—Cancer of the Oral Cavity). Use of tobacco and heavy alcohol consumption increases one's risk for cancer. Data collected regarding the client's risk factors may form the basis for preventive teaching.

Other problems may cause discomfort and loss of function and can lead to serious systemic disorders. For example, malnutrition may develop in a client who cannot eat certain foods because of poorly fitting dentures. A client with frequent sinus infections and headaches may have impaired concentration, which affects job or school performance.

This examination also allows the nurse to evaluate the client's health practices. For example, improper use of nasal decongestants may explain recurrent sinus congestion, and infection and improper oral hygiene practices may cause tooth decay or gum disease. The nurse should provide teaching for a client with these health practices.

(text continues on page 285)

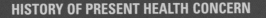

HISTORY OF PRESENT HEALTH CONCERN

Question	*Rationale*
Tongue and Mouth Do you experience tongue or mouth sores or lesions? Are they painful? How long have you had them? Do they recur? Is it single or do you have many?	Painful, recurrent ulcers in the mouth are seen with aphthous stomatitis (canker sores) and herpes simplex (cold sores). Mouth or tongue sores that do not heal; red or white patches that persist; a lump or thickening; or rough, crusty, or eroded areas are warning signs of cancer and need to be referred for further evaluation (see Promote Health—Cancer of the Oral Cavity).
Do you experience redness, swelling, bleeding, or pain of the gums or mouth? How long has this been happening? Do you have any toothache? Have you lost any permanent teeth?	Red, swollen gums that bleed easily occur in early gum disease (gingivitis), whereas destruction of the gums with tooth loss occurs in more advanced gum disease (periodontitis). Pain can accompany inflammation and is a later sign of oral cancer.

continued on page 282

HISTORY OF PRESENT HEALTH CONCERN *Continued*

Question	Rational
	The gums recede, become ischemic, and undergo fibrotic changes as a person ages. Tooth surfaces may be worn from prolonged use. These changes make the older client more susceptible to periodontal disease and tooth loss.
Nose and Sinuses Do you have pain over your sinuses?	Sinusitis may cause pressure and pain over the sinuses (see Promote Health—Sinusitis).
Do you experience nosebleeds? How much bleeding? What color is the blood?	Nosebleeds may be seen with overuse of nasal sprays, excessively dry nasal mucosa, hypertension, leukemia, thrombocytopenia, and other blood disorders. A client who experiences frequent nosebleeds should be referred for further evaluation.
Do you experience frequent clear or mucous drainage from your nose?	Thin, watery, clear nasal drainage (rhinorrhea) can indicate a chronic allergy or, in a person with a past head injury, a cerebrospinal fluid leak. Mucous drainage, especially yellow, is typical of a cold, rhinitis, or a sinus infection.
Can you breathe through both of your nostrils? Do you have a stuffy nose at times during the day or night?	Inability to breathe through both nostrils may indicate sinus congestion, obstruction, or a deviated septum. Nasal congestion can interfere with daily activities or a restful sleep.
Do you have seasonal allergies, i.e., hay fever? Describe the timing of the allergies (e.g., spring, summer) and symptoms (e.g., sinus problems, runny nose, or watery eyes).	Pollens cause seasonal rhinitis, whereas dust may cause rhinitis year round.
Have you experienced a change in your ability to smell or taste?	A decrease in the ability to smell may occur with upper respiratory infections, smoking, cocaine use, or a neurologic lesion or tumor in the frontal lobe of the brain or in the olfactory bulb or tract. A decreased ability to taste may be reported by clients with upper respiratory infections or lesions of the facial nerve (VII). Changes in perception of smell also occur from a zinc deficiency and from menopause in some women.
	The ability to smell and taste decreases with age. Medications can also decrease sense of smell and taste in older people.
Throat Do you have difficulty chewing or swallowing food? How long have you had this? Do you have any pain?	Dysphagia (difficulty swallowing) may be seen in esophageal disorders, anxiety, poorly fitting dentures, or a neurologic disorder. Dysphagia increases the risk for aspiration, and clients with dysphagia may require consultation with a speech therapist. Difficulty chewing, swallowing, or moving the tongue or jaws may be a late sign of oral cancer. Malocclusion may also cause difficulty chewing or swallowing.
Do you have a sore throat? How long have you had it? Describe. How often do you get sore throats?	Throat irritation and soreness are common with sinus drainage and may also occur with a viral or bacterial infection. A sore throat that persists without healing may signal throat cancer.
Do you experience hoarseness? How long?	Hoarseness is associated with upper respiratory infections, allergies, hypothyroidism, overuse of the voice, smoking or inhaling other irritants, and cancer of the larynx. If hoarseness lasts 2 weeks or longer, refer the client for further evaluation.

continued

COLDSPA Example

Use the **COLDSPA** mnemonic as a guideline to collect needed information for each symptom the client shares. In addition, the following questions help elicit important information.

Mnemonic	Question	Client Response Example
Character	Describe the sign or symptom (feeling, appearance, sound, smell, or taste if applicable).	"My throat is sore and it hurts to swallow."
Onset	When did it begin?	"Last night."
Location	Where is it? Does it radiate? Does it occur anywhere else?	"Just in my throat."
Duration	How long does it last? Does it recur?	"The pain is constant, and getting worse."
Severity	How bad is it? or How much does it bother you?	"I'm miserable."
Pattern	What makes it better or worse?	"Ibuprofen helps some but it never goes away completely."
Associated factors/How it **A**ffects the client	What other symptoms occur with it? How does it affect you?	"Headache, 101 fever, and my boyfriend says I have bad breath."

PAST HEALTH HISTORY

Question	Rationale
Have you ever had any oral, nasal, or sinus surgery?	Present symptoms may be related to past problems.
Do you have a history of sinus infections? Describe your symptoms. Do you use nasal sprays? (What type? How much? How often?)	Some clients are more susceptible to sinus infections, which tend to recur. Overuse of nasal sprays may cause nasal irritation, nosebleeds, and rebound swelling.

FAMILY HISTORY

Question	Rationale
Is there a history of mouth, throat, nose, or sinus cancer in your family?	There is a genetic risk factor for mouth, throat, nose, and sinus cancers.

LIFESTYLE AND HEALTH PRACTICES

Question	Rationale
Do you smoke or use smokeless tobacco? If so, how much? Are you interested in quitting this habit?	Cigarette, pipe, or cigar smoking and use of smokeless tobacco increase a person's risk for oral cancer. Tobacco use and heavy alcohol consumption are responsible for 75% of the oral cancers (Weinberg & Estefan, 2002). Cancer of the cheek is linked to chewing tobacco. Smoking a pipe is a risk factor for lip cancer. Clients who want to quit using tobacco may benefit from a referral to a smoking cessation program (see Promote Health—Cancer of the Oral Cavity).
Do you drink alcohol? How much and how often?	Excessive use of alcohol increases a person's risk for oral cancer.
Do you grind your teeth?	Grinding the teeth (bruxism) may be a sign of stress or of slight malocclusion. The practice may also precipitate temporomandibular joint (TMJ) problems and pain.

continued on page 284

LIFESTYLE AND HEALTH PRACTICES *Continued*

Question	*Rationale*
Describe how you care for your teeth or dentures. How often do you brush and use dental floss? When was your last dental examination?	Proper brushing, flossing, and oral hygiene can prevent dental caries and gum disease. Regular dental checkups and screening can help to detect the early signs of gum disease and oral cancer, which promotes early treatment.
If the client wears braces: How do you care for your braces? Do you avoid any specific types of foods? Describe your usual dietary intake for a day.	Clients with braces should avoid crunchy, sticky, and chewy foods when wearing braces. These foods can damage the braces and the teeth. Poor nutrition also increases one's risk for oral cancers.
If the client wears dentures: How do your dentures fit? **Elderly and some disabled clients may have difficulty caring properly for teeth or dentures because of poor vision or impaired dexterity.**	Poorly fitting dentures may lead to poor eating habits, a reluctance to speak freely, and mouth sores or leukoplakia (thick white patches of cells). Leukoplakia is a precancerous condition.
Do you brush your tongue?	Cleaning the tongue is a way to prevent bad breath resulting from bacteria that accumulates on the posterior tongue.
How often are you in the sun? Do you use lip sunscreen products?	Exposure to the sun is the primary risk factor associated with lip cancer.

PROMOTE HEALTH

Cancer of the Oral Cavity

Overview
More than 90% of oral cavity and oropharyngeal cancers are squamous cell cancers. Cancers develop in the lining, in the salivary glands, tonsils, or base of the tongue, but only squamous cell cancers of the oral and oropharyngeal cavity are discussed here. As of the year 2007, experts estimated that 34,360 new cases would be diagnosed in the United States with 7,550 deaths resulting. The incidence of oral cancer has slowly decreased in the United States since the early 1980s. Most cases (90%) occur in people who are heavy users of tobacco (smoking and smokeless) and alcohol and whose ages range in the fifties and sixties.

However, cases of oral cavity and tongue cancers are beginning to appear more frequently in people in their thirties and forties. Incidence is higher in men but is increasing in women. People with oral and oropharyngeal cancer often have another cancer or develop one at a later time. Follow-up examinations and avoidance of risk factors are extremely important for these clients (American Cancer Society [ACS], 2007).

Risk Factors (ACS, 2007)
- Tobacco use, smoking and smokeless
- Alcohol consumption
- Combined tobacco and alcohol use
- Alcohol dependence accompanied with nutritional deficiencies
- Age over 40
- Male gender (twice as likely to affect males as females, but incidence is rising in females)
- Genetic predisposition, family history
- Occupation related to nickel refining, woodworking, or textile fibers
- Diet low in fruits and vegetables; Vitamin A deficiency
- Ultraviolet light exposure (especially the lips)
- Long term irritation (i.e., poorly fitted dentures)

Possible Risk Factors
- Human papillomavirus (HPV) infection
- Immune system suppression
- Marijuana use
- Mouthwash

Teach Risk Reduction Tips (ACS, 2007)
- Stop smoking
- Limit alcohol consumption
- Eat a healthy, balanced diet
- Take precautions when working in an environment where substances or particles could be inhaled
- Avoid excessive exposure to ultraviolet light
- Avoid sources of oral irritation

Assessment Procedure	Normal Findings	Abnormal Findings
Inspect the buccal mucosa. Use a penlight and tongue depressor to retract the lips and cheeks to check color and consistency (Fig. 17-8). Also note Stenson's ducts (parotid ducts) located on the buccal mucosa across from the second upper molars.	It should appear pink in light-skinned clients; tissue pigmentation typically increases in dark-skinned clients. In both, tissue is smooth and moist without lesions. Stenson's ducts are visible with flow of saliva and with no redness, swelling, pain, or moistness in area. Fordyce spots or granules, yellowish-whitish raised spots, are normal ectopic sebaceous glands. 👓 Oral mucosa is often drier and more fragile in the older client because the epithelial lining of the salivary glands degenerates.	Leukoplakia may be seen in chronic irritation and smoking. ➤ *Clinical Tip • Smokers may also have a yellow-brown coating on the tongue, which is not leukoplakia.* Leukoplakia is a precancerous lesion, and the client should be referred for evaluation. Whitish, curdlike patches that scrape off over reddened mucosa and bleed easily indicate "thrush" (*Candida albicans*) infection. Koplik's spots (tiny whitish spots that lie over reddened mucosa) are an early sign of the measles. Canker sores may be seen as may brown patches inside the cheeks of clients with adrenocortical insufficiency. See Abnormal Findings 17-1.
Inspect and palpate the tongue. Ask client to stick out the tongue. Inspect for color, moisture, size, and texture. Observe for fasciculations (fine tremors), and check for midline protrusion. Palpate any lesions present for induration (hardness).	Tongue should be pink, moist, a moderate size with papillae (little protuberances) present. A common variation is a fissured, topographic-map–like tongue, which is not unusual in older clients (Fig. 17-9). No lesions are present.	Among possible abnormalities are deep longitudinal *fissures* seen in dehydration; a *black tongue* indicative of bismuth (PeptoBismol) toxicity: *black, hairy tongue;* a smooth, reddish, shiny tongue without papillae indicative of niacin or vitamin B^{12} deficiencies, certain anemias, and antineoplastic therapy (see Abnormal Findings 17-1). An enlarged tongue suggests hypothyroidism, acromegaly, or Down's syndrome, and angioneurotic edema of anaphylaxis. A very small tongue suggests malnutrition. An atrophied tongue or fasciculations point to cranial nerve (hypoglossal, CN 12) damage.

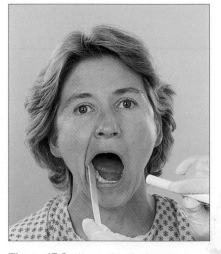

Figure 17-8   Inspecting the buccal mucosa.

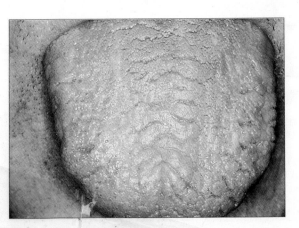

Figure 17-9   Fissured tongue (courtesy of Dr. Michael Bennett).

continued

PHYSICAL ASSESSMENT *Continued*

Assessment Procedure	Normal Findings	Abnormal Findings
Assess the ventral surface of the tongue. Ask the client to touch the tongue to the roof of mouth, and use a penlight to inspect ventral surface of tongue, frenulum, and the area under the tongue. Palpate the area (Fig. 17-10) if you see lesions, if the client is over age 50, or if the client uses tobacco or alcohol. Note any induration. Check also for a short frenulum that limits tongue motion (the origin of "tongue-tied").	The tongue's ventral surface is smooth, shiny, pink or slightly pale with visible veins and no lesions. The older client may have varicose veins on the ventral surface of the tongue (Fig. 17-11).	Leukoplakia, persistent lesions, ulcers, or nodules may indicate cancer and should be referred. Induration increases the likelihood of cancer. ➤ *Clinical Tip* • *The area underneath the tongue is the most common site of oral cancer.*
Inspect for Wharton's ducts—openings from the submandibular salivary glands—located on either side of the frenulum on the floor of the mouth.	The frenulum is midline; Wharton's ducts are visible with salivary flow or moistness in the area. The client has no swelling, redness, or pain.	Abnormal findings include lesions, ulcers, nodules, or hypertrophied duct openings on either side of frenulum.
Observe the sides of the tongue; use a square gauze pad to hold the client's tongue to each side (Fig. 17-12). Palpate any lesions, ulcers, or nodules for induration.	No lesions, ulcers, or nodules are apparent.	Canker sores may be seen on the sides of the tongue in clients receiving certain kinds of chemotherapy. Leukoplakia, persistent lesions, ulcers, or nodules may indicate cancer and should be further evaluated medically. Induration increases the likelihood of cancer (see Abnormal Findings 17-1). ➤ *Clinical Tip* • *The side of the tongue is the most common site of tongue cancer.*

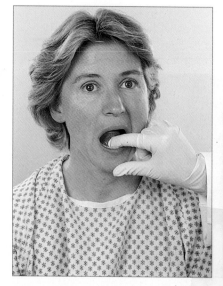

Figure 17-10 Palpating area under tongue.

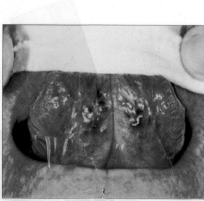

Figure 17-11 Varicose veins on ventral surface of tongue.

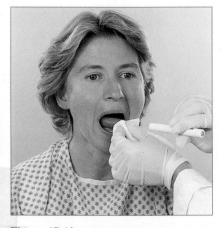

Figure 17-12 Inspecting side of tongue.

continued

Assessment Procedure	Normal Findings	Abnormal Findings
Check the strength of the tongue. Place your fingers on the external surface of the client's cheek. Ask the client to press the tongue's tip against the inside of the cheek to resist pressure from your fingers. Repeat on the opposite cheek.	The tongue offers strong resistance.	Decreased tongue strength may occur with a defect of the twelfth cranial nerve—hypoglossal—or with a shortened frenulum that limits motion.
Check the anterior tongue's ability to taste by placing drops of sugar and salty water on the tip and sides of tongue with a tongue depressor.	The client can distinguish between sweet and salty.	Loss of taste discrimination occurs with zinc deficiency, a seventh cranial nerve (facial) defect, and certain medication use.
Inspect the hard (anterior) and soft (posterior) palates and uvula. Ask the client to open the mouth wide while you use a penlight to look at the roof. Observe color and integrity.	The hard palate is pale or whitish with firm, transverse rugae (wrinklelike folds). 🌐 A bony protuberance in the midline of the hard palate, called a torus palatinus, is a normal variation seen more often in females, Eskimos, Native Americans, and Asians (Fig. 17-13). Palatine tissues are intact; the soft palate should be pinkish, movable, spongy, and smooth.	A candidal infection may appear as thick white plaques on the hard palate. Deep purple, raised, or flat lesions may indicate a Kaposi's sarcoma (seen in clients with AIDS; see Abnormal Findings 17-1). A yellow tint to the hard palate may indicate jaundice because bilirubin adheres to elastic tissue (collagen). An opening in the hard palate is known as a cleft palate.
Note odor. While the mouth is wide open, note any unusual or foul odor.	No unusual or foul odor is noted.	Fruity or acetone breath is associated with diabetic ketoacidosis. An ammonia odor is often associated with kidney disease. Foul odors may indicate an oral or respiratory infection, or tooth decay. Alcohol or tobacco use may be identified by breath odor. Fecal breath odor occurs in bowel obstruction; sulfur odor (fetor hepaticus) occurs in end-stage liver disease.
Assess the uvula. Apply a tongue depressor to the tongue (halfway between the tip and back of the tongue) and shine a penlight into the client's wide-open mouth (Fig. 17-14). Note the characteristics and positioning of the uvula. Ask the client to say "aaah" and watch for the uvula and soft palate to move.	The uvula is a fleshy, solid structure that hangs freely in the midline. No redness of or exudate from uvula or soft palate. Midline elevation of uvula and symmetric elevation of the soft palate.	A bifid uvula looks like it is split in two or partially severed. Clients with a bifid uvula may have a submucous cleft palate.

> **Clinical Tip** • *Depress the tongue slightly off center to avoid eliciting the gag response.*

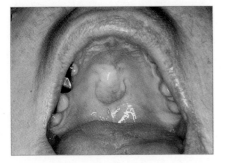

Figure 17-13 Torus palatinus (courtesy of Dr. Michael Benett).

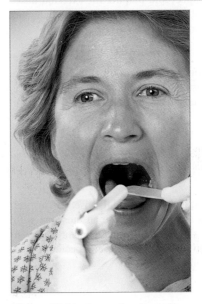

Figure 17-14 Inspecting the uvula.

continued

PHYSICAL ASSESSMENT *Continued*

Assessment Procedure	Normal Findings	Abnormal Findings
		A bifid uvula is common in Native Americans (Bifid uvula, 2005) (see Abnormal Findings 17-1). Asymmetric movement or loss of movement may occur after a cerebrovascular accident (stroke). Palate fails to rise and uvula deviates to normal side with cranial nerve X (vagus) paralysis.
Inspect the tonsils. Using the tongue depressor to keep the mouth open wide, inspect the tonsils for color, size, and presence of exudate or lesions. Tonsils should be graded.	Tonsils may be present or absent. They are normally pink and symmetric and may be enlarged to 1+ in healthy clients. No exudate, swelling, or lesions should be present.	Tonsils are red, enlarged (to 2+, 3+, or 4+), and covered with exudate in tonsillitis. Abnormal Findings 17-2 depicts grading of tonsils. They also may be indurated with patches of white or yellow exudate.
Inspect the posterior pharyngeal wall. Keeping the tongue depressor in place, shine the penlight on the back of the throat. Observe the color of the throat, and note any exudate or lesions. Before inspecting the nose, discard gloves and perform hand hygiene.	Throat is normally pink without exudate or lesions. Atrophy of tonsils in adults is normal.	A bright red throat with white or yellow exudate indicates pharyngitis. Yellowish mucus on throat may be seen with postnasal sinus drainage.

Nose

Inspection and palpation

Inspect and palpate the external nose. Note nasal color, shape, consistency, and tenderness.	Color is the same as the rest of the face; the nasal structure is smooth and symmetric; the client reports no tenderness.	Nasal tenderness on palpation accompanies a local infection.
Check patency of air flow through the nostrils by occluding one nostril at a time and asking client to sniff.	Client is able to sniff through each nostril while other is occluded.	Client cannot sniff through a nostril that is not occluded, nor can he or she sniff or blow air through the nostrils. This may be a sign of swelling, rhinitis, or a foreign object obstructing the nostrils. A line across the tip of the nose just above the fleshy tip is common in clients with chronic allergies.
Inspect the internal nose. To inspect the internal nose, use an otoscope with a short wide-tip attachment (or you can also use a nasal speculum and penlight).	The nasal mucosa is dark pink, moist, and free of exudate. The nasal septum is intact and free of ulcers or perforations. Turbinates are dark pink (redder than oral mucosa), moist, and free of lesions	Nasal mucosa is swollen and pale pink or bluish gray in clients with allergies. Nasal mucosa is red and swollen with upper respiratory infection. Exudate is common with infection and may

continued

Assessment Procedure	Normal Findings	Abnormal Findings
Use your nondominant hand to stabilize and gently tilt the client's head back. Insert the short wide tip of the otoscope into the client's nostril without touching the sensitive nasal septum (Fig. 17-15). Slowly direct the otoscope back and up to view the nasal mucosa, nasal septum, the inferior and middle turbinates, and the nasal passage (the narrow space between the septum and the turbinates). ➤ *Clinical Tip • Position the otoscope's handle to the side to improve your view of the structures. If an otoscope is unavailable, use a penlight and hold the tip of the nose slightly up. A nasal speculum with a penlight also facilitates good visualization.*	(Fig. 17-16). The superior turbinate will not be visible from this point of view. A deviated septum may appear to be an overgrowth of tissue (Fig. 17-17). This is a normal finding as long as breathing is not obstructed.	range from large amounts of watery discharge to thick yellow-green purulent discharge. Purulent nasal discharge is seen with acute bacterial rhinosinusitis. Bleeding (epistaxis) or crusting may be noted on lower anterior part of nasal septum with local irritation. Ulcers of the nasal mucosa or a perforated septum may be seen with use of cocaine, trauma, chronic infection, or chronic nose picking. Small, pale, round, firm overgrowths or masses on mucosa (polyps) are seen in clients with chronic allergies (see Abnormal Findings 17-3).

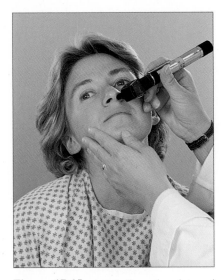

Figure 17-15 Inspecting the internal nose using an otoscope and wide-tipped attachment.

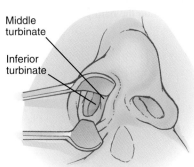

Figure 17-16 Normal internal nose.

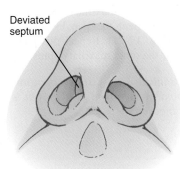

Figure 17-17 Deviated septum.

Sinuses

Palpation **Palpate the sinuses.** When an infection is suspected, the nurse can examine the sinuses through palpation, percussion, and transillumination. Palpate the frontal sinuses by using your thumbs to press up on the brow on each side of nose (Fig. 17-18).	Frontal and maxillary sinuses are nontender to palpation, and no crepitus is evident.	Frontal or maxillary sinuses are tender to palpation in clients with allergies or acute bacterial rhinosinusitis. If the client has a large amount of exudate, you may feel crepitus upon palpation over the maxillary sinuses.

continued

PHYSICAL ASSESSMENT *Continued*

Assessment Procedure	Normal Findings	Abnormal Findings
Palpate the maxillary sinuses by pressing with thumbs up on the maxillary sinuses (Fig. 17-19).		

Percussion

Assessment Procedure	Normal Findings	Abnormal Findings
Percuss the sinuses. Lightly tap (percuss) over the frontal sinuses and over the maxillary sinuses for tenderness.	The sinuses are not tender on percussion.	The frontal and maxillary sinuses are tender upon percussion in clients with allergies or sinus infection.

Transillumination

Assessment Procedure	Normal Findings	Abnormal Findings
Transilluminate the sinuses. If sinus tenderness was detected during palpation and percussion, transillumination will let you see if the sinuses are filled with fluid or pus. Transilluminate the frontal sinuses by holding a strong, narrow light source snugly under the eyebrows (the room should be dark). Use your other hand to shield the light. Repeat this technique for the other frontal sinus. Figure 17-20 illustrates the technique.	A red glow transilluminates the frontal sinuses. This indicates a normal, air-filled sinus.	Absence of a red glow usually indicates a sinus filled with fluid or pus.
Transilluminate the maxillary sinuses by holding a strong, narrow light source over the maxillary sinus and asking the client to open his or her mouth (Fig. 17-21). Repeat this technique for the other maxillary sinus.	A red glow transilluminates the maxillary sinuses (Fig. 17-22). The red glow will be seen on the hard palate.	Absence of a red glow usually indicates a sinus filled with fluid, pus, or thick mucus (from chronic sinusitis; see Promote Health—Sinusitis).

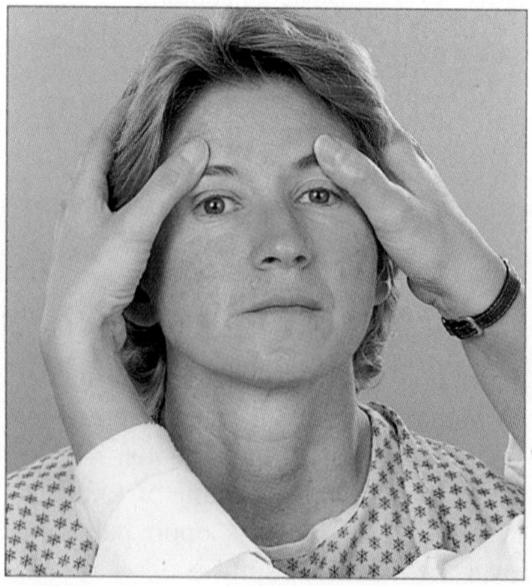

> ➤ **Clinical Tip** • Upper dentures should be removed so the light is not blocked.

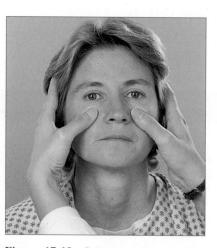

Figure 17-18 Palpating the frontal sinuses.

Figure 17-19 Palpating the maxillary sinuses.

continued

Assessment Procedure	Normal Findings	Abnormal Findings

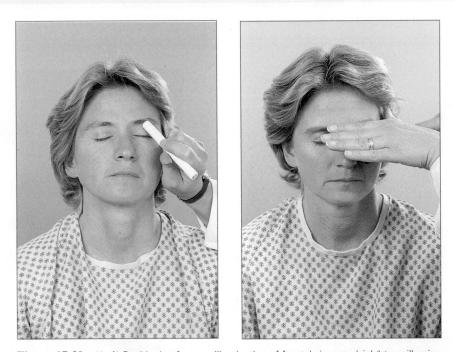

Figure 17-20 (*Left*) Positioning for transillumination of frontal sinuses; (*right*) transillumination of frontal sinuses; note the red glow. (This photograph shows a lighted room because of a special photographic technique. In practice, the room must be dark to show the red glow. © B. Proud.)

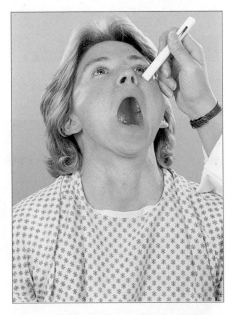

Figure 17-21 Positioning for transillumination of maxillary sinuses.

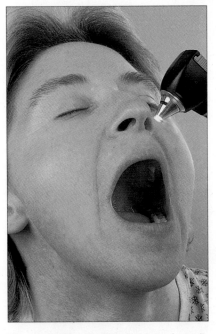

Figure 17-22 Transillumination of maxillary sinuses; note the red glow. (This photograph shows a lighted room because of a special photographic technique. In practice, the room must be dark to show the red glow. © B. Proud.)

Abnormalities of the Mouth and Throat

This display depicts common abnormalities of the mouth and throat.

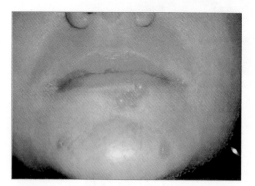

Herpes simplex type I.

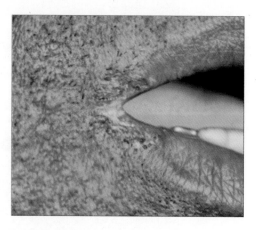

Cheilosis of lips.

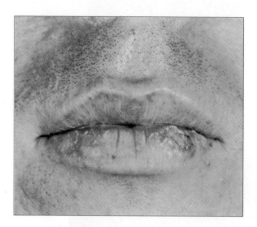

Carcinoma of lip.

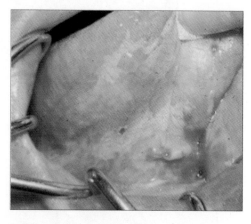

Leukoplakia (ventral surface.)

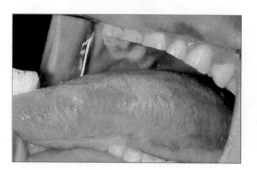

Hairy leukoplakia (lateral surface.)

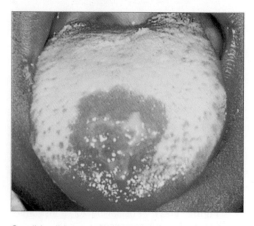

Candida albicans infection (thrush).

continued

Abnormal Findings 17-1

Abnormalities of the Mouth and Throat *Continued*

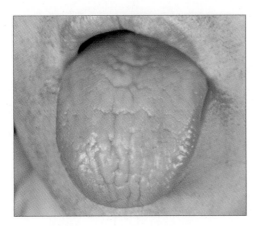

Smooth, reddish, shiny tongue without papillae due to vitamin B12 deficiency.

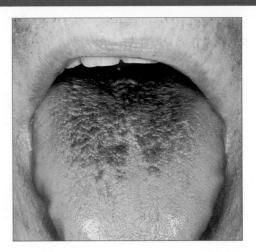

Black hairy tongue. (Dr. Michael Bennett.)

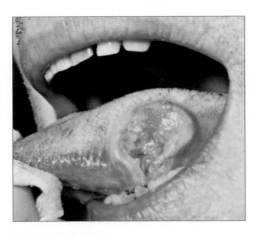

Carcinoma of tongue.

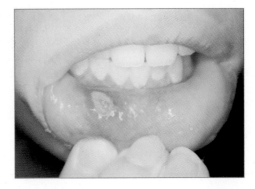

Canker sore.

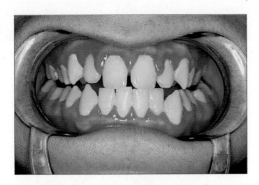

Gingivitis. (Dr. Michael Bennett.)

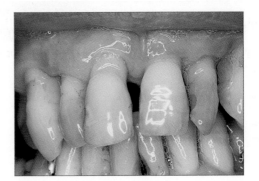

Receding gums (periodontitis). (Dr. Michael Bennett.)

continued on page 296

Abnormal Findings 17-1 — Abnormalities of the Mouth and Throat *Continued*

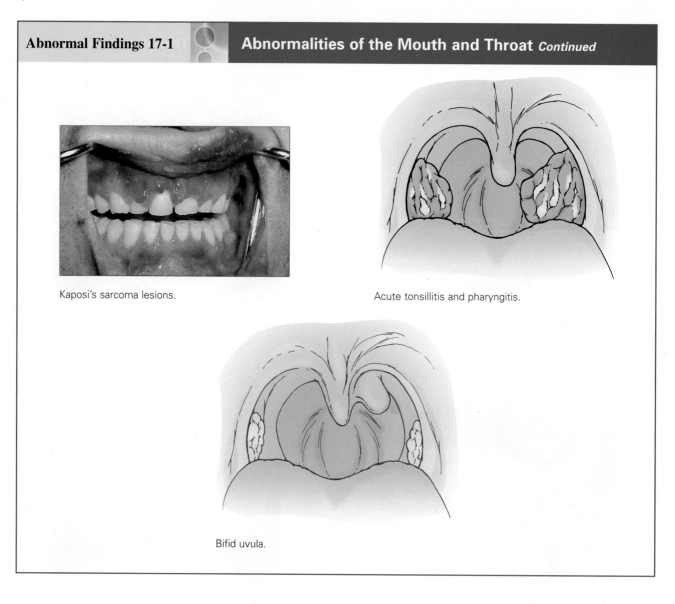

Kaposi's sarcoma lesions.

Acute tonsillitis and pharyngitis.

Bifid uvula.

Abnormal Findings 17-2 — Tonsillitis (Detecting and Grading)

In a client who has both tonsils and a sore throat, tonsillitis can be identified and ranked with a grading scale from 1 to 4 as follows:

1+   Tonsils are visible.
2+   Tonsils are midway between tonsillar pillars and uvula.
3+   Tonsils touch the uvula.
4+   Tonsils touch each other.

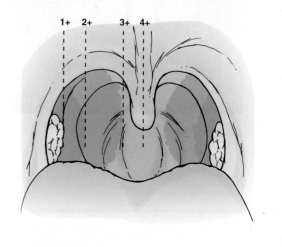

Abnormal Findings 17-3   Abnormalities of the Nose

The following are common abnormalities of the nose.

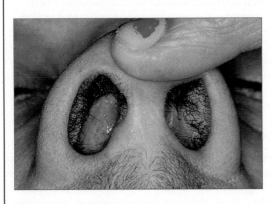

Nasal polyp. (© 1992 J. Barrabe.)

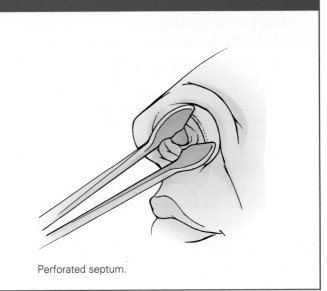

Perforated septum.

VALIDATING AND DOCUMENTING FINDINGS

Validate the mouth, throat, nose, and sinus assessment data that you have collected. This is necessary to verify that the data are reliable and accurate. Document the assessment data following the health care facility or agency policy.

Sample Documentation of Subjective Data

Client describes the condition of mouth, throat, and nose as "adequate." No history of past oral or nasal surgery. Has 32 permanent teeth. Had four teeth filled for cavities several years ago as a child. Brushes teeth twice a day and uses dental floss each evening. Occasional mild bleeding with flossing. Never needed braces. Receives regular dental checkups twice a year. Has occasional sinus headaches (one to two per year) and minor sore throats due to sinus drainage. Relieved with over-the-counter oral decongestants and acetaminophen (Tylenol). Nasal discharge clear to purulent occasionally. No oral or nasal lesions noted by client. Does not smoke or chew tobacco. No difficulty breathing through either nostril. Able to chew and swallow without difficulty. No oral or nasal pain or tenderness.

Sample Documentation of Objective Data

Lips pink, smooth, and moist without lesions. Buccal mucosa pink, moist, and without exudate. Parotid ducts visible with no redness or swelling. Moist bubbles are seen near ducts. Thirty-two white to yellowish teeth present. Gums pink without redness or swelling. Protrudes geographic tongue in midline with no tremors. Equal bilateral strength in tongue. Ventral surface of tongue smooth and shiny pink with small visible veins present. Frenulum in midline with visible submandibular ducts on each side. Torus palatinus visible on whitish hard palate. Soft palate smooth and pink. Midline and symmetric elevation of uvula and soft palate with phonation. Tonsillar pillars pink and symmetric. Tonsils absent.

Nose somewhat large but smooth and symmetric. Able to sniff and blow through each nostril. Nasal septum slightly deviated to left but does not obstruct air flow. Inferior and middle turbinates dark pink, moist, and free of lesions. No purulent drainage noted. Frontal and maxillary sinuses transilluminate and are nontender to palpation and percussion.

Analysis of Data

DIAGNOSTIC REASONING: POSSIBLE CONCLUSIONS

After collecting subjective and objective data pertaining to the mouth, throat, nose, and sinuses, identify abnormal findings and client strengths. Then cluster the data to reveal any significant patterns or abnormalities. These data may be used to make clinical judgments about the status of the client's mouth, throat, nose, and sinuses.

Selected Nursing Diagnoses

Following is a listing of selected nursing diagnoses (wellness, risk, or actual) that you may identify when analyzing the cue clusters.

Wellness Diagnoses

- Readiness for Enhanced Effective Management of the teeth and gums
- Health-Seeking Behaviors: Requests information on how to quit smoking

Risk Diagnoses

- Risk for Aspiration related to decreased or absent gag reflex
- Risk for Imbalanced Nutrition: Less Than Body Requirements related to poorly fitting dentures or gum disease
- Risk for Infection of gums related to poor oral hygiene
- Risk for Injury to teeth and gums related to participation in active sports and lack of knowledge of protective mouth gear

Actual Diagnoses

- Ineffective Health Maintenance related to poor oral hygiene
- Bathing/Hygiene Self-Care Deficit: Oral mouth care related to paralysis or decreased cognitive functions
- Disturbed Sensory Perception: Olfactory related to local irritation of nasal mucosa, impairment of cranial nerve I, decrease in olfactory bulb function secondary to nasal obstruction
- Impaired Oral Mucous Membranes related to poor oral hygiene or dehydration
- Impaired Swallowing related to impaired neurologic or neuromuscular function (i.e., CVA; damage to cranial nerves V, VII, IX, or X; cerebral palsy; myasthenia gravis; muscular dystrophy; cerebral palsy)
- Pain related to chronic sinusitis or inflammation of oral mucous membranes (gingivitis, periodontitis, canker sores)
- Disturbed Sensory Perception: Gustatory related to impairment of cranial nerve VII or IX, reduction of number of taste buds secondary to the aging process
- Imbalanced Nutrition: Less Than Body Requirements related to decreased appetite secondary to decreased sense of taste and smell and social isolation

Selected Collaborative Problems

After grouping the data, certain collaborative problems may become apparent. Remember that collaborative problems differ from nursing diagnoses in that they cannot be prevented by nursing intervention. However, these physiologic complications of medical conditions can be detected and monitored by the nurse. In addition, the nurse can use physician- and nurse-prescribed interventions to minimize the complications of these problems. The nurse may also have to refer the client in such situations for further treatment of the problem. Following is a list of collaborative problems that may be identified when obtaining a general impression. These problems are worded as Risk for Complications (or RC) followed by the problem.

- RC: Nosebleed
- RC: Sinus infection
- RC: Stomatitis
- RC: Gum infection (gingivitis, periodontitis)
- RC: Oral lesions
- RC: Laryngeal edema

Medical Problems

After grouping the data, the client's signs and symptoms may clearly require medical diagnosis and treatment. Referral to a primary care provider is necessary.

CASE STUDY

The case study demonstrates how to analyze mouth, throat, nose, and sinus assessment data for a specific client. The critical thinking exercises included in the study guide/lab manual and interactive product that complement this text also offer opportunities to analyze assessment data.

Jonathan Miller (JM), a 22-year-old college student, visits the student health service in mid-December complaining of severe throat pain ("like swallowing razor blades"), swollen lymph nodes, chills, fever, general fatigue, and anorexia. He admitted that he had been studying "day and night" for final exams and had "only one more to go." "This is the third time I've had this problem this year," he related. "I didn't even bother coming in the first or second time. I just stayed in bed between classes and treated myself."

Upon examination, you note that his face and neck are flushed, with dark circles underlying his eyes. His blood pressure is 126/72 rt. arm; pulse is 104; respirations are 24; and oral temperature reads 103.2°F/39.6°C. When inspecting his throat, you find erythema and edema of the pharynx and uvula with white, patchy exudate on the tonsillar areas. Tonsils are 3+ and injected. Cervical and retropharyngeal lymph nodes are grossly palpable and very tender.

The following concept map illustrates the diagnostic reasoning process.

continued

Applying COLDSPA

Applying **COLDSPA** for client symptoms: "severe throat pain."

Mnemonic	Question	Data Provided	Missing Data
Character	Describe the sign or symptom (feeling, appearance, sound, smell, or taste if applicable).	Severe throat pain	
Onset	When did it begin?		"When did this pain first begin?"
Location	Where is it? Does it radiate? Does it occur anywhere else?		"Do you have any pain in your sinuses or neck?"
Duration	How long does it last? Does it recur?	"Third time I have had this during the past year, but I have always just stayed in bed and treated it myself."	
Severity	How bad is it? or How much does it bother you?	"Feels like I am swallowing razor blades."	
Pattern	What makes it better or worse?		"Are you taking anything that makes the pain go away?"
Associated factors/How it **A**ffects the client	What other symptoms occur with it? How does it affect you?	"Swollen lymph nodes, chills, fever, fatigue, and loss of appetite."	

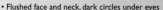

1) Identify abnormal findings and client strengths

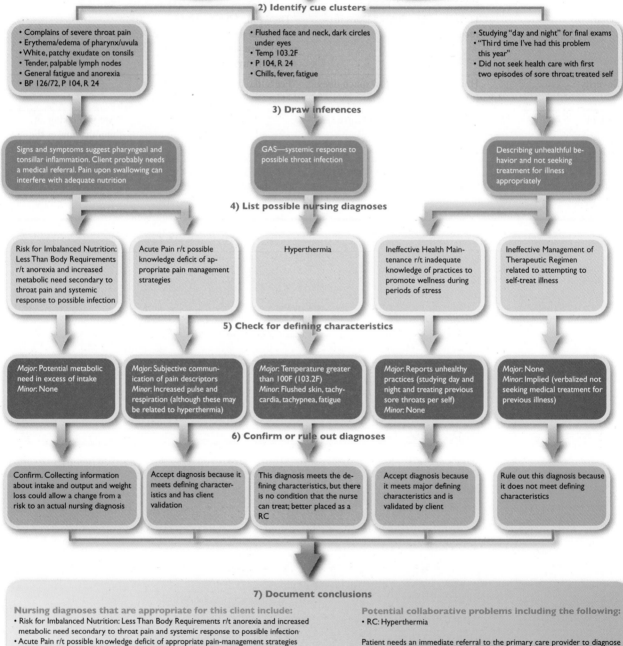

Subjective Data

- Complains of severe throat pain ("like swallowing razor blades")
- Complains of swollen, tender lymph nodes; chills; fever; general fatigue; and anorexia
- Studying "day and night" for final exams
- "Third time I've had this problem this year"
- Did not seek health care with first two episodes of sore throat; treated self

Objective Data

- Flushed face and neck, dark circles under eyes
- BP 126/72, P 104, R 24
- Temp. 103.2F
- Erythema and edema of the pharynx and uvula
- Tonsils are 3+ and infected
- White, patchy exudate on the tonsilar areas
- Cervical and retropharyngeal lymph nodes grossly palpable

2) Identify cue clusters

- Complains of severe throat pain
- Erythema/edema of pharynx/uvula
- White, patchy exudate on tonsils
- Tender, palpable lymph nodes
- General fatigue and anorexia
- BP 126/72, P 104, R 24

- Flushed face and neck, dark circles under eyes
- Temp 103.2F
- P 104, R 24
- Chills, fever, fatigue

- Studying "day and night" for final exams
- "Third time I've had this problem this year"
- Did not seek health care with first two episodes of sore throat; treated self

3) Draw inferences

Signs and symptoms suggest pharyngeal and tonsillar inflammation. Client probably needs a medical referral. Pain upon swallowing can interfere with adequate nutrition

GAS—systemic response to possible throat infection

Describing unhealthful behavior and not seeking treatment for illness appropriately

4) List possible nursing diagnoses

Risk for Imbalanced Nutrition: Less Than Body Requirements r/t anorexia and increased metabolic need secondary to throat pain and systemic response to possible infection

Acute Pain r/t possible knowledge deficit of appropriate pain management strategies

Hyperthermia

Ineffective Health Maintenance r/t inadequate knowledge of practices to promote wellness during periods of stress

Ineffective Management of Therapeutic Regimen related to attempting to self-treat illness

5) Check for defining characteristics

Major: Potential metabolic need in excess of intake
Minor: None

Major: Subjective communication of pain descriptors
Minor: Increased pulse and respiration (although these may be related to hyperthermia)

Major: Temperature greater than 100F (103.2F)
Minor: Flushed skin, tachycardia, tachypnea, fatigue

Major: Reports unhealthy practices (studying day and night and treating previous sore throats per self)
Minor: None

Major: None
Minor: Implied (verbalized not seeking medical treatment for previous illness)

6) Confirm or rule out diagnoses

Confirm. Collecting information about intake and output and weight loss could allow a change from a risk to an actual nursing diagnosis

Accept diagnosis because it meets defining characteristics and has client validation

This diagnosis meets the defining characteristics, but there is no condition that the nurse can treat; better placed as a RC

Accept diagnosis because it meets major defining characteristics and is validated by client

Rule out this diagnosis because it does not meet defining characteristics

7) Document conclusions

Nursing diagnoses that are appropriate for this client include:
- Risk for Imbalanced Nutrition: Less Than Body Requirements r/t anorexia and increased metabolic need secondary to throat pain and systemic response to possible infection
- Acute Pain r/t possible knowledge deficit of appropriate pain-management strategies
- Ineffective Health Maintenance r/t inadequate knowledge of practices to promote wellness during periods of stress

Potential collaborative problems including the following:
- RC: Hyperthermia

Patient needs an immediate referral to the primary care provider to diagnose and treat his throat condition

References and Selected Readings

Arkell, S. (2003). Update on oral candidosis. *Nursing Times, 99*(48), 52–3.

Bifid uvula. (2005). Available at http://www.biology-online.org/dictionary/Bifid_uvula

Daniel, B. T., Damato, K. L., & Johnson, J. (2004). Education issues in oral care. *Seminars in Oncology Nursing, 20*(1), 48–52.

Eilers, J., & Epstein, J. B. (2004). Assessment and measurement of oral mucositis. *Seminars in Oncology Nursing, 20*(1), 22–29.

Freer, S. K. (2000). Use of an oral assessment tool to improve practice. *Professional Nurse, 15*(10), 635–637.

Gilmurry, B. (2000). Wheezing, breathlessness, and cough – Is it really asthma? A look at vocal cord dysfunction. *Canadian Journal of Respiratory Therapy, 35*(4), 28–31.

Hamdy, S. (2004). The diagnosis and management of adult neurogenic dysphagia. *Nursing Times, 100*(18), 52–54.

Keefe, D. M., Gibson, R. J., & Hauer-Jensen, M. (2004). Gastrointestinal mucositis. *Seminars in Oncology Nursing, 20*(1), 38–47.

Krejci, C. B., & Bissada, N. F. (2000). Periodontitis—The risks for its development. *General Dentistry, 48*(4), 430–436.

Landry, S. T. (2000). Alternatives: Healthy teeth from the inside out. *Health (San Francisco), 14*(2), 82, 86, 89.

Olson, K., Hanson, J., Hamilton, J., Stacey, D., Eades, M., Gue, D., et al. (2004). Assessing the reliability and validity of the revised WCCNR stomatitis staging system for cancer therapy-induced stomatis. *Canadian Oncology Nursing Journal, 14*(3), 168–174, 176–182.

Overfield, T. (1995). *Biological variation in health and illness: Race, age, and sex differences* (2nd ed.). Boca Raton, FL: CRC Press.

Reynolds, T. (2004). Ear, nose, and throat problems in accident and emergency. *Nursing Standards, 18*(26), 47–53, quiz, 54–55.

Scheid, D. C., & Hamm, R. H. (2004). Acute bacterial rhinosinusitis in adults: Part I. Evaluation. *American Family Physician, 70,* 1685–1692.

Sjogren, R., & Nordstrom, G. (2000). Oral health status of psychiatric patients. *Journal of Clinical Nursing, 9*(4), 632–638.

Weinberg, M. A., & Estefan, D. J. (2002). Assessing oral malignancies. *American Family Physician, 65*(7), 1379–1384.

Promote Health—Sinusitis and Cancer of the Oral Cavity

American Cancer Society. (2007). What are the risk factors for oral cavity and oropharyngeal cancer? Available at http://www.cancer.org/docroot/CRI

Hicks, R. (2006). Sinusitis. Available at http://www.bbc.co.uk/health

Mayo Clinic. (2006). Chronic sinusitis. Available at http://www.mayoclinic.com/health/chronic-sinusitis/DS00232/DSECTION=3

Sinusitis. (2005). Available at http://www.familydoctor.org/online/famdocen/home/common/infections/cold-flu/686.html

Websites

American Dental Association, 211 E Chicago Ave., Chicago, IL. 60611; 312-440-2806; http://www.ada.org

Centers for Disease Control and Prevention, 1600 Clifton Road, Atlanta, GA. 30333; 404-639-7000; http://www.cdc.gov/health

National Oral Health Information Clearinghouse, 1 NOHIC Way, Bethesda, MD. 20892-3500; 1-301-401-7364; http://www.pho.com/node/9826

18

Thorax and Lungs

Structure and Function

The term **thorax** identifies the portion of the body extending from the base of the neck superiorly to the level of the diaphragm inferiorly. The lungs, distal portion of the trachea, and the bronchi, are located in the thorax and constitute the **lower respiratory system.** The outer structure of the thorax is referred to as the *thoracic cage;* the *thoracic cavity* contains the respiratory components. A thorough assessment of the lower respiratory system focuses on the external chest as well as the respiratory components in the thoracic cavity.

THORACIC CAGE

The **thoracic cage** is constructed of the sternum, 12 pairs of ribs, 12 thoracic vertebrae, muscles, and cartilage. It provides support and protection for many important organs including those of the lower respiratory system. Structures and landmarks of the anterior thoracic cage (Fig. 18-1) and the posterior thoracic cage (Fig. 18-2) are discussed below.

Sternum and Clavicles

The **sternum,** or breastbone, lies in the center of the chest anteriorly and is divided into three parts: the manubrium, the body, and the xiphoid process. The manubrium connects laterally with the clavicles (collar bones) and the first two pairs of ribs. The clavicles extend from the manubrium to the acromion of the scapula.

A U-shaped indentation located on the superior border of the manubrium is an important landmark known as the **suprasternal notch.** A few centimeters below the suprasternal notch, a bony ridge can be palpated at the point where the manubrium articulates with the body of the sternum. This landmark, often referred to as the *sternal angle* (or angle of Louis), is also the location of the second pair of ribs and becomes a reference point for counting ribs and intercostal spaces.

Ribs and Thoracic Vertebrae

The 12 pairs of ribs constitute the main structure of the thoracic cage. They are numbered superiorly to inferiorly, the uppermost pair being number one. Each pair of ribs has a corresponding pair of intercostal spaces located immediately inferior to it. Anteriorly the first seven pairs articulate with the sternum by way of costal cartilages. The first pair of ribs curves up immediately under the clavicles so only a small portion of these ribs and the first interspaces are palpable. The second ribs and intercostal spaces are easily located adjacent to the sternal angle. Ribs two through six are easy to count anteriorly because of their articulation with the sternal body.

The next four pairs of ribs (seven through ten) connect to the cartilages of the pair lying superior to them rather than to the sternum (see Fig. 18-1). This configuration forms an angle between the right and left costal margins meeting at the level of the xiphoid process. This angle, commonly referred to as the *costal angle,* is an important landmark for assessment. It is normally less than 90 degrees but may be increased in instances of long-standing hyperinflation of the lungs as in emphysema. The 11th and 12th pairs of ribs are called **"floating" ribs** because they do not connect to either the sternum or another pair of ribs anteriorly. Instead they are attached posteriorly to the vertebra and their anterior tips are free and palpable (see Fig. 18-2).

The ribs are more difficult to palpate posteriorly. Each pair of ribs articulates with its respective **thoracic vertebra.** The spinous process of the seventh cervical vertebra (C7), also called the **vertebra prominens,** can be easily felt with the client's neck flexed. The process immediately inferior to the vertebra prominens is the first thoracic vertebra, which is adjacent to the posterior aspect of the first rib.

➤ **Clinical Tip •** *When counting the spinous processes, it is helpful to know that they align with their corresponding ribs only to the fourth thoracic vertebra (T4). After this, the spinous processes angle downward from their own vertebral body and can be palpated over the vertebral body and rib below.*

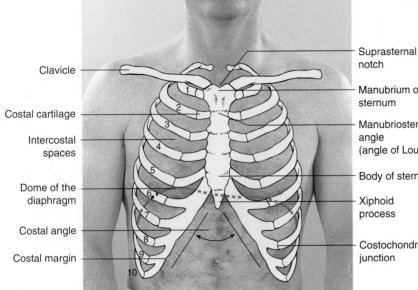

Clavicle

Costal cartilage

Intercostal spaces

Dome of the diaphragm

Costal angle

Costal margin

Suprasternal notch

Manubrium of sternum

Manubriosternal angle (angle of Louis)

Body of sternum

Xiphoid process

Costochondral junction

Figure 18-1   Anterior thoracic cage.

The lower tip of each scapula is at the level of the seventh or eighth rib when the client's arms are at his or her side (see Fig. 18-2).

Vertical Reference Lines

By counting the ribs, an examiner can describe the location of a finding vertically. However, to describe a location around the circumference of the chest wall, the examiner uses imaginary lines running vertically on the chest wall. On the anterior chest, these lines are known as the **midsternal line** and the **right and left midclavicular lines** (Fig. 18-3).

The posterior thorax includes the **vertebral (or spinal) line** and the **right and left scapular lines,** which extend through the inferior angle of the scapulae when the arms are at the client's side (Fig. 18-4).

The lateral aspect of the thorax is divided into three parallel lines. The **midaxillary line** runs from the apex of the axillae to the level of the 12th rib. The **anterior axillary line** extends from the anterior axillary fold along the anterolateral aspect of the thorax, whereas the **posterior axillary line** runs from the posterior axillary fold down the posterolateral aspect of the chest wall (Fig. 18-5).

THORACIC CAVITY

The thoracic cavity consists of the **mediastinum** and the lungs. The mediastinum refers to a central area in the thoracic cavity that contains the trachea, esophagus, heart, and great vessels. These structures are discussed in separate chapters (Chapters 17 and 20). The lungs lie on each side of the mediastinum.

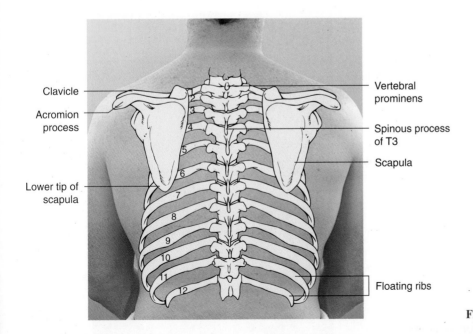

Clavicle

Acromion process

Lower tip of scapula

Vertebral prominens

Spinous process of T3

Scapula

Floating ribs

Figure 18-2   Posterior thoracic cage.

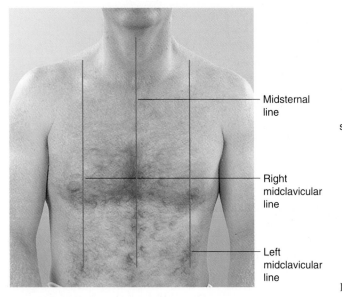

Figure 18-3   Anterior vertical lines (imaginary landmarks).

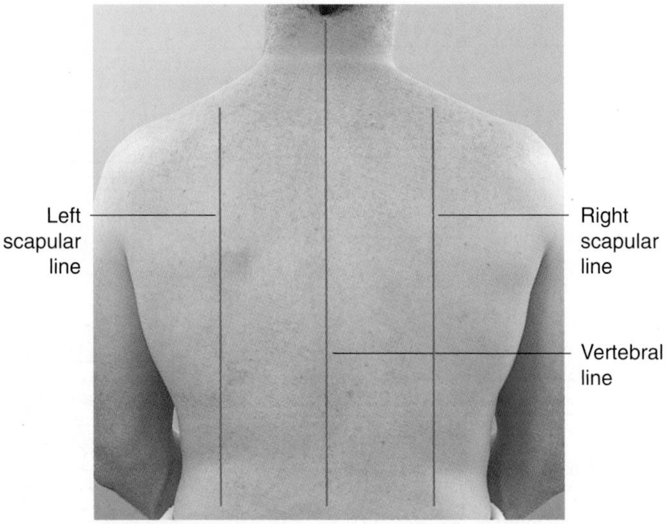

Figure 18-4   Posterior vertical lines (imaginary landmarks).

Lungs

The **lungs** are two cone-shaped, elastic structures suspended within the thoracic cavity. The **apex** of each lung extends slightly above the clavicle; the **base** is at the level of the **diaphragm.** At the point of the midclavicular line on the anterior surface of the thorax, the lung extends to approximately the sixth rib. Laterally lung tissue reaches the level of the eighth rib, and posteriorly the lung base lies at about the tenth rib (Fig. 18-6).

Although the lungs are paired, they are not completely symmetric. Both are divided into lobes by fissures. The right lung is made up of three lobes, whereas the left lung contains only two lobes. Fissures separating the lobes run obliquely through the chest, making the lobes appear as diagonal sloping segments. Anteriorly the horizontal fissure separating the right upper lobe from the middle lobe extends from the fifth rib in the right mid-axillary line to the third intercostal space or fourth rib

at the right sternal border. Posteriorly oblique fissures extend on both the right and left lungs from the level of T3 to the sixth rib at the midclavicular line.

In the healthy adult, during deep inspiration the lungs extend down to about the eighth intercostal space anteriorly and the twelfth intercostal space posteriorly. During expiration, the lungs rise to the fifth or sixth intercostal space anteriorly and tenth posteriorly.

➤ **Clinical Tip •** *Remember that most lung tissue in the upper lobes of both lungs is located on the anterior surface of the chest. Similarly the lower lobes of both lungs are primarily located toward the posterior surface of the chest wall. In addition, the right middle lobe of the lung does not extend to the posterior side of the thoracic wall and, thus, must be assessed from the anterior surface alone.*

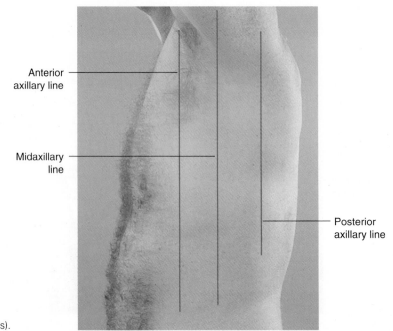

Figure 18-5   Lateral vertical lines (imaginary landmarks).

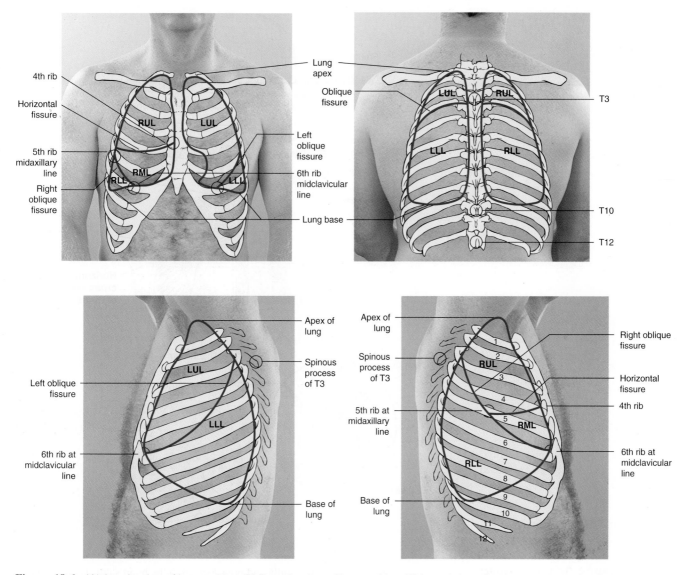

Figure 18-6 (**A**) Anterior view of lung position. (**B**) Posterior view of lung position. (**C**) Lateral view of left lung position. (**D**) Lateral view of right lung position.

Pleural Membranes

The thoracic cavity is lined by a thin, double-layered serous membrane collectively referred to as the pleura (Fig. 18-7). The **parietal pleura** line the chest cavity, and the **visceral pleura** covers the external surfaces of the lungs. The **pleural space** lies between the two pleural layers. In the healthy adult, the lubricating serous fluid between the layers allows movement of the visceral layer over the parietal layer during ventilation without friction. Because the pleural space is one of the physiologic third spaces for body fluid storage, severe dehydration will reduce the volume of pleural fluid, resulting in the increased transmission of lung sounds and a possible friction rub.

Trachea and Bronchi

The **trachea** is a flexible structure that lies anterior to the esophagus, begins at the level of the cricoid cartilage in the neck, and is approximately 10 to 12 cm long in an adult (see Fig. 18-7). C-shaped rings of **hyaline cartilage** compose the trachea; they help to maintain its shape and prevent its collapse during respiration.

At the level of the sternal angle, the trachea bifurcates into the right and left main **bronchi.** Both bronchi are at an oblique position in the mediastinum and enter the lungs at the hilum. The **right main bronchus** is shorter and more vertical than the **left main bronchus,** making aspirated objects more likely to enter the right lung than the left.

The bronchi and trachea represent "dead space" in the respiratory system, where air is transported but no gas exchange takes place. They function primarily as a passageway for both inspired and expired air. In addition, the trachea and bronchi are lined with mucous membranes containing **cilia.** These hairlike projections help sweep dust, foreign bodies, and bacteria that have been trapped by the mucus toward the mouth for removal.

Inspired air travels through the trachea into the main bronchi and continues through the system. The bronchi repeatedly bifurcate into smaller passageways known as **bronchioles.** Eventually the bronchioles terminate at the alveolar ducts, and air is channeled into the alveolar sacs, which contain the **alveoli** (see Fig. 18-7). Alveolar sacs contain a number of alveoli in a cluster formation (resembling grapes), creating millions of interalveolar walls that serve to increase the surface area available for gas exchange.

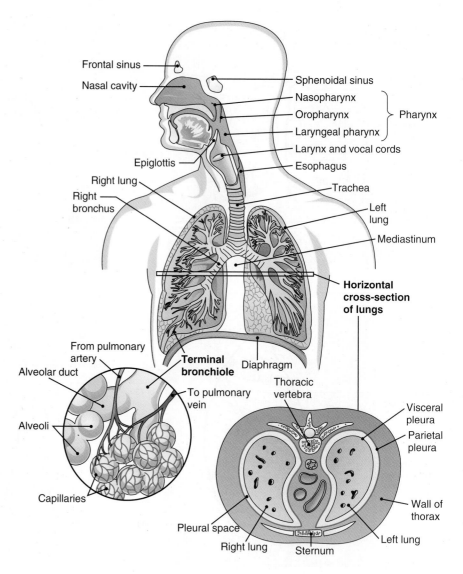

Figure 18-7 Major structures of the respiratory system.

MECHANICS OF BREATHING

The purpose of respiration is to maintain an adequate oxygen level in the blood to support cellular life. By providing oxygen and eliminating carbon dioxide, respiration assists in the rapid compensation for metabolic acid–base defects; however, changes in the respiratory pattern can cause acid–base imbalances.

External respiration, or ventilation, is the mechanical act of breathing and is accomplished by expansion of the chest, both vertically and horizontally. Vertical expansion is accomplished through contraction of the diaphragm. Horizontal expansion occurs as intercostal muscles lift the sternum and elevate the ribs, resulting in an increase in anteroposterior diameter.

As a result of this enlargement of the chest cavity, a slight negative pressure is created in the lungs in relation to the atmospheric pressure, resulting in an inflow of air into the lungs. This process, called **inspiration,** is shown in Figure 18-8. **Expiration** is mostly passive in nature and occurs with relaxation of the intercostal muscles and the diaphragm. As the diaphragm relaxes, it assumes a domed shape. The resultant decrease in the size of the chest cavity creates a positive pressure, forcing air out of the lungs.

Breathing patterns change according to cellular demands—often without awareness on the part of the individual. Such involuntary control of respiration is the work of the medulla and pons located in the brain stem. The hypothalamus and the sympathetic nervous system also play a role in involuntary control of respiration in response to emotional changes such as fear or excitement.

Hormonal regulation, changes in oxygen or carbon dioxide levels in the blood, or changes in the hydrogen ion (pH) level cause changes in breathing patterns. Under normal circumstances, the strongest stimulus to breathe is an increase of carbon dioxide in the blood (hypercapnia). A decrease in oxygen (hypoxemia) also increases respiration but is less effective than a rise in carbon dioxide levels.

Health Assessment

COLLECTING SUBJECTIVE DATA: THE NURSING HEALTH HISTORY

Subjective data related to the thoracic and lung assessment provide many clues about underlying respiratory problems and associated nursing diagnoses as well as clues about risk for the development of lung disorders. Information about the client's level of functioning is also important because certain respiratory problems greatly impact a person's ability to perform activities of daily living. When collecting subjective data, remember to

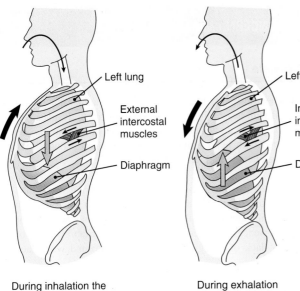

During inhalation the diaphragm presses the abdominal organs downward and forward.

During exhalation the diaphragm rises and recoils to the resting position.

Action of rib cage in inhalation

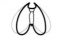

Action of rib cage in exhalation

Figure 18-8 Mechanics of normal—not deep, not shallow—inspiration (*left*) and expiration (*right*).

follow up on the client's related signs and symptoms to determine specific respiratory problems and associated nursing diagnoses.

Be careful to avoid judgmental approaches to poor health practices. Smoking, for example, has become a stigmatized addiction in our society. Avoid conveying feelings of intolerance when caring for a smoker with respiratory complaints. Based on the client's readiness for teaching, the nurse may offer information about smoking cessation methods.

(text continues on page 311)

HISTORY OF PRESENT HEALTH CONCERN

Question	Rationale
Difficulty Breathing Do you ever experience difficulty breathing? Describe the difficulty.	Dyspnea (difficulty breathing) can indicate a number of health problems, most of which are related to the respiratory system. Gradual onset of dyspnea is usually indicative of lung changes such as emphysema, whereas sudden onset is associated with viral or bacterial infections.
Do you experience any other symptoms when you have difficulty breathing?	Associated symptoms provide clues to the underlying problem. Certain associated symptoms suggest problems in other body systems. For example, edema or angina that occurs with dyspnea may indicate a cardiovascular problem.
Do you have difficulty breathing when you are resting or do any specific activities cause the difficulty?	Older adults may experience dyspnea with certain activities related to aging changes of the lungs (loss of elasticity, fewer functional capillaries, and loss of lung resiliency).

continued on page 308

HISTORY OF PRESENT HEALTH CONCERN *Continued*

Question	Rationale
Do you have difficulty breathing when you sleep? Do you use more than one pillow or elevate the head of the bed when you sleep?	Orthopnea (difficulty breathing when lying supine) may be associated with heart failure. Paroxysmal nocturnal dyspnea (severe dyspnea that awakens the person from sleep) also may be associated with heart failure. Changes in sleep patterns may cause the client to feel fatigued during the day.
Do you snore when you sleep? Have you been told that you stop breathing at night when you snore?	Sleep apnea (periods of breathing cessation during sleep) may be the source of snoring and gasping sounds. In general, sleep apnea diminishes the quality of sleep, which may account for fatigue or excessive tiredness, depression, irritability, loss of memory, lack of energy, and a risk for auto and workplace accidents.
Chest pain Do you have chest pain? Is the pain associated with a cold, fever, or deep breathing?	Pain-sensitive nerve endings are located in the parietal pleura, thoracic muscles, and tracheobronchial tree but not in the lungs. Thus chest pain associated with a pulmonary origin may be a late sign of pulmonary disease. Chest pain related to pleuritis may be absent in older clients because of age-related alterations in pain perception.
Cough Do you have a cough? When and how often does it occur?	Continuous coughs are usually associated with acute infections, whereas those occurring only early in the morning are often associated with chronic bronchial inflammation or smoking. Coughs late in the evening may be the result of exposure to irritants during the day. Coughs occurring at night are often related to postnasal drip or sinusitis. The ability to cough effectively may be decreased in the older client because of weaker muscles and increased rigidity of the thoracic wall.
Do you produce any sputum when you cough? If so, what color is the sputum? How much sputum do you cough up? Has this amount increased or decreased recently? Does the sputum have an odor?	Nonproductive coughs are often associated with upper respiratory irritations and early congestive heart failure. White or mucoid sputum is often seen with common colds, viral infections, or bronchitis. Yellow or green sputum is often associated with bacterial infections. Blood in the sputum (hemoptysis) is seen with more serious respiratory conditions. Rust-colored sputum is associated with tuberculosis or pneumococcal pneumonia. Pink, frothy sputum may be indicative of pulmonary edema. An increase in the amount of sputum is often seen in an increase in exposure to irritants, chronic bronchitis, and pulmonary abscess. Clients with excessive, tenacious secretions may need instruction on controlled coughing and measures to reduce viscosity of secretions.
Do you wheeze when you cough or when you are active?	Wheezing indicates narrowing of the airways due to spasm or obstruction. Wheezing is associated with congestive heart failure (CHF), asthma (reactive airway disease), or excessive secretions.
Gastrointestinal symptoms Do you have any gastrointestinal symptoms such as heartburn, frequent hiccups, or chronic cough?	Studies have shown that patients with asthma often have GERD (gastroesophageal reflux disease) or are more susceptible to GERD.

continued

COLDSPA Example for Chest Pain

Use the **COLDSPA** mnemonic as a guideline to collect needed information for each symptom the client shares. In addition, the following questions help elicit important information.

Mnemonic	Question	Client Response Example
Character	Describe the sign or symptom (feeling, appearance, sound, smell, or taste if applicable).	"I have pain in my chest when I cough or take a deep breath."
Onset	When did it begin?	"About six days ago."
Location	Where is it? Does it radiate? Does it occur anywhere else?	"It is on my right side." *Client points to right lower back side of chest.*
Duration	How long does it last? Does it recur?	"It hurts when I cough or take a deep breath."
Severity	How bad is it? How much does it bother you?	"I can't sleep at night and have trouble going up stairs because I am short-winded."
Pattern	What makes it better or worse?	"Mucinex helps me to cough up phlegm but I still have the pain."
Associated factors/How it **A**ffects the client	What other symptoms occur with it? How does it affect you?	"A 102 fever for the last 2 days. I am coughing up thick tan sputum. I smoke 1 pack a day but have quit for the last 2 days."

PAST HEALTH HISTORY

Question	Rationale
Have you had prior respiratory problems?	A history of respiratory disease increases the risk for a recurrence. In addition, some respiratory diseases may imitate other disorders. For example, asthma symptoms may mimic symptoms commonly associated with emphysema or heart failure.
Have you ever had any thoracic surgery, biopsy, or trauma?	Previous surgeries may alter the appearance of the thorax and cause changes in respiratory sounds. Trauma to the thorax can result in lung tissue changes.
Have you been tested for or diagnosed with allergies?	Many allergic responses are manifested with respiratory symptoms such as dyspnea, cough, or hoarseness. Clients may need education on controlling the amount of allergens in their environment.
Have you ever had a chest x-ray, tuberculosis (TB) skin test, or influenza immunization? Have you had any other pulmonary studies in the past?	Information on previous chest x-rays, TB skin tests, influenza immunizations, and so forth is useful for comparison with current findings and gives information on self-care practices and possible teaching needs.
Have you recently traveled outside of the United States? Have you been in close contact with anyone known or suspected to have SARS?	Travel to high-risk areas such as mainland China; Hong Kong; Hanoi, Vietnam; Singapore; or Toronto, Canada, may have exposed the client to SARS (severe acute respiratory syndrome).

continued on page 310

FAMILY HISTORY

Question	Rationale
Is there a history of lung disease in your family?	The development of lung cancer is thought to be partially based on genetics. A history of certain respiratory diseases (asthma, emphysema) in a family may increase the risk for development of the disease. Exposure to viral or bacterial respiratory infections in the home increases the risk for development of these conditions.
Did any family members in your home smoke when you were growing up?	Second-hand smoke puts individuals at risk for emphysema or lung cancer later in life.
Is there a history of other pulmonary illnesses/disorders in the family, e.g., asthma?	Some pulmonary disorders, such as asthma, tend to run in families.

LIFESTYLE AND HEALTH PRACTICES

Question	Rationale
Have you ever smoked cigarettes or other tobacco products? Do you currently smoke? At what age did you start? How much do you smoke and how much have you smoked in the past? What activities do you usually associate with smoking? Have you ever tried to quit?	Smoking is linked to a number of respiratory conditions, including lung cancer (see Promote Health—Lung Cancer). The number of years a person has smoked and the number of cigarettes per day influence the risk for development of smoking-related respiratory problems. Information on smoking behavior and previous efforts to quit may be helpful later in identifying measures to assist with smoking cessation.
Are you exposed to any environmental conditions that affect your breathing? Where do you work? Are you around smokers?	Exposure to certain environmental inhalants can result in an increased incidence of certain respiratory conditions. Environmental irritants commonly associated with occupations include coal dust, insecticides, paint, pollution, asbestos fibers, and the like. For example, inhaling dust contaminated with *Histoplasma capsulatum* may cause histoplasmosis, a systemic fungal disease. This disease is common in the rural midwestern United States. Second-hand smoke is another irritant that can seriously affect a person's respiratory health.
Do you have difficulty performing your usual daily activities? Describe any difficulties.	Respiratory problems can negatively affect a person's ability to perform the usual activities of daily living.
What kind of stress are you experiencing at this time? How does it affect your breathing?	Shortness of breath can be a manifestation of stress. Client may need education about relaxation techniques.
Are you currently taking medications for breathing problems or other medications (prescription or OTC) that affect your breathing? Do you use any other treatments at home for your respiratory problems?	Consider all medications when determining if respiratory problems could be attributed to adverse reactions. Certain medications, for example, beta-adrenergic antagonists (beta blockers) such as atenolol (Tenormin) or metoprolol (Lopressor) and angiotensin-converting enzyme (ACE) inhibitors such as enalapril (Vasotec) or lisinopril (Zestril), are associated with the side effect of persistent cough. These medications are contraindicated with some respiratory problems such as asthma. If the client is using oxygen or other respiratory therapy at home, it is important to evaluate knowledge of proper use and precautions as well as the client's ability to afford the therapy.
Have you used any herbal medicines or alternative therapies to manage colds or other respiratory problems?	Many people use herbal therapies, such as Echinacea, or alternative therapies, such as zinc lozenges, to decrease cold symptoms. Knowing what clients are using enables you to check for side effects or adverse interactions with prescribed medications.

PROMOTE HEALTH
Lung Cancer

Overview

Lung cancer is the leading cause of death in the United States and Europe. Both incidence and mortality rates for lung cancer continue to increase despite decreasing mortality rates for most other cancers. However, the rates for men and women have changed. The incidence of lung cancer among women in the United States and Europe is soaring to epidemic proportions (CancerConsultants.com, 1998–2004).

In 2005, there are expected to be 172,500 new lung cancer cases and 163,510 deaths in the United States with 73,020 of the deaths being women (nearly twice as many as those caused by breast cancer). The average age of diagnosis is 60; a lung cancer diagnosis is unusual under age 40. For people whose cancer is found early and treated with surgery, the 5-year survival rate is about 42% but only 15% of cases are diagnosed in the early stages.

Risk Factors

- Cigarette smoking
- Genetic predisposition possibly associated with interaction of genetics and smoking
- Beta carotene supplements esp. in presence of heavy smoking, moderate alcohol intake
- Asbestos exposure
- Radon exposure
- Exposure to workplace pollutants: radioactive ores, mining chemicals (e.g., arsenic, vinyl chloride, nickel, coal, mustard gas, chloromethyl esters, and fuels such as gasoline)
- Other environmental exposure: air pollution, passive tobacco smoke, marijuana smoking
- History of previous lung cancer, silicosis, berylliosis
- Recurring inflammation that leaves scars (e.g., tuberculosis, some types of pneumonia)
- African American heritage, especially men
- Gender; women's lung cells may have a predisposition to lung cancer when exposed to tobacco smoke
- History of Hodgkin's disease treated with chemotherapy, radiation or both
- Smokers who have been treated with chemotherapy or radiation
- Eating a poor diet with few fruits and vegetables

Teach Risk Reduction Tips

- Do not start smoking, and stop smoking if you do smoke.
- Join a smoking cessation program.
- Eat a healthy, low-cholesterol diet with adequate amounts of fruits and vegetables.
- If you smoke, avoid beta carotene supplements or diet high in beta carotene.
- Limit exposure to air pollution and harmful substances.
- Wear a mask when exposed to air pollution or dangerous airborne substances.

Collecting Objective Data: Physical Examination

Examination of the thorax and lungs begins when the nurse first meets the client and observes any obvious breathing difficulties. However, complete examination of the thorax and lungs consists of inspection, palpation, percussion, and auscultation of the posterior and anterior thorax to evaluate functioning of the lungs. Inspection and palpation are fairly simple skills to acquire; however practice and experience are the best ways to become proficient with percussion and auscultation.

Preparing the Client

Have the client remove all clothing from the waist up and put on an examination gown or drape. The gown should open down the back and is used to limit exposure. Examination of a female client's chest may create anxiety because of embarrassment related to breast exposure. Explain that exposure of the entire chest is necessary during some parts of the examination; to further ease client anxiety, explain the procedures before initiating the examination.

For the beginning of the examination, ask the client to sit in an upright position with arms relaxed at the sides. Provide explanations during the examination as you perform the various assessment techniques. The client should be encouraged to ask questions and to inform the examiner of any discomfort or fatigue he experiences during the examination. Try to make sure that the room temperature is comfortable for the client.

Equipment

- Examination gown and drape
- Gloves
- Stethoscope
- Light source
- Mask
- Skin marker
- Metric ruler

Physical Assessment

During examination of the client, remember these key points:

- Provide privacy for the client.
- Keep your hands warm to promote the client's comfort during examination.
- Remain nonjudgmental regarding client's habits and lifestyle, particularly smoking. At the same time, educate and inform about risks, such as lung cancer and chronic obstructive pulmonary disease (COPD), related to habits.

(text continues on page 325)

PHYSICAL ASSESSMENT

Assessment Procedure	Normal Findings	Abnormal Findings

General

Inspection

Inspect for nasal flaring and pursed lip breathing.

Nasal flaring is not observed. Normally the diaphragm and the external intercostal muscles do most of the work of breathing. This is evidenced by outward expansion of the abdomen and lower ribs on inspiration and return to resting position on expiration.

Nasal flaring is seen with labored respirations (especially in small children) and is indicative of hypoxia.

Pursed lip breathing may be seen in asthma, emphysema, or CHF as a physiologic response to help slow down expiration and keep alveoli open longer.

Observe color of face, lips, and chest.

The client has evenly colored skin tone without unusual or prominent discoloration.

Ruddy to purple complexion may be seen in clients with COPD or CHF as a result of polycythemia. Cyanosis may be seen if client is cold or hypoxic.

Cyanosis makes white skin appear blue-tinged, especially in the perioral, nailbed, and conjunctival areas. Dark skin appears blue, dull, and lifeless in the same areas.

Inspect color and shape of nails.

Pink tones should be seen in the nailbeds. There is normally a 160-degree angle between the nail base and the skin.

Pale or cyanotic nails may indicate hypoxia. Early clubbing (180-degree angle) and late clubbing (greater than a 180-degree angle) can occur from hypoxia.

Posterior Thorax

Inspection

Inspect configuration. While the client sits with her arms at her sides, stand behind her and observe the position of scapulae and the shape and configuration of the chest wall (Fig. 18-9).

➤ *Clinical Tip • Some clinicians prefer to inspect the entire thorax first, followed by palpation of the anterior and posterior thorax, then percussion and auscultation of the anterior and posterior thorax.*

Scapulae are symmetric and nonprotruding. Shoulders and scapulae are at equal horizontal positions. The ratio of anteroposterior to transverse diameter is 1:2.

Spinous processes appear straight, and thorax appears symmetric with ribs sloping downward at approximately a 45-degree angle in relation to the spine.

 Kyphosis (an increased curve of the thoracic spine) is common in older clients (see Abnormal Findings 18-1). It results from a loss of lung resiliency and a loss of skeletal muscle; it may be a normal finding.

 The size of the thorax, which affects pulmonary function, differs by race. Compared with African Americans, Asians and Native Americans, adult Caucasians have a larger thorax and greater lung capacity (Overfield, 1995).

Spinous processes that deviate laterally in the thoracic area may indicate scoliosis.

Spinal configurations may have respiratory implications. Ribs appearing horizontal at an angle greater than 45 degrees with the spinal column are frequently the result of an increased ratio between the anteroposterior–transverse diameter (barrel chest). This condition is commonly the result of emphysema due to hyperinflation of the lungs.

Abnormal Findings 18-1 depicts various thoracic configurations.

continued

Assessment Procedure	Normal Findings	Abnormal Findings
Observe use of accessory muscles. Watch as the client breathes and note use.	The client does not use accessory (trapezius/shoulder) muscles to assist breathing. The diaphragm is the major muscle at work. This is evidenced by expansion of the lower chest during inspiration.	Trapezius, or shoulder, muscles are used to facilitate inspiration in cases of acute and chronic airway obstruction or atelectasis.
Inspect the client's positioning. Note the client's posture and his ability to support weight while breathing comfortably.	Client should be sitting up and relaxed, breathing easily with arms at sides or in lap.	Client leans forward and uses arms to support weight and lift chest to increase breathing capacity, referred to as the *tripod position* (Fig. 18-10). This is often seen in chronic obstructive pulmonary disease (COPD). See Promote Health—COPD.
Palpation **Palpate for tenderness and sensation.** Palpation may be performed with one or both hands; however, the sequence of palpation is established (Fig. 18-11). Use your fingers to palpate for tenderness, warmth, pain, or other sensations. Start toward the midline at the level of the left scapula (over the apex of the left lung) and move your hand left to right, comparing findings bilaterally. Move systematically downward and out to cover the lateral portions of the lungs at the bases.	Client reports no tenderness, pain, or unusual sensations. Temperature should be equal bilaterally.	Tender or painful areas may indicate inflamed fibrous connective tissue. Pain over the intercostal spaces may be from inflamed pleurae. Pain over the ribs, especially at the costal chondral junctions, is a symptom of fractured ribs. Muscle soreness from exercise or the excessive work of breathing (as in COPD) may be palpated as tenderness. Increased warmth may be related to local infection.

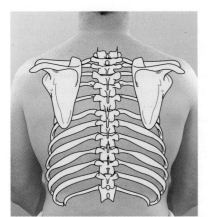

Figure 18-9 Observing the posterior thorax.

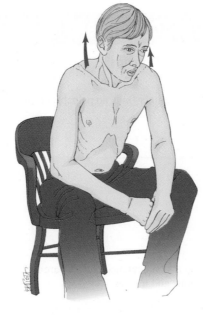

Figure 18-10 Tripod position.

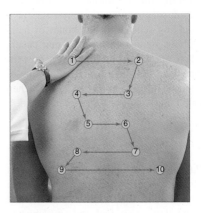

Figure 18-11 Sequence for palpating the posterior thorax.

continued

PROMOTE HEALTH
COPD

Overview
Chronic obstructive pulmonary disease (COPD) is used to describe several conditions that obstruct airflow to and from the alveoli. The two most common conditions are emphysema and chronic bronchitis. Active and passive smoking and fumes from biomass fuels are thought to cause most cases of COPD. In China, where about 50% of men smoke, respiratory diseases are the fourth leading cause of death in urban areas, but the biomass fuel fumes increase the rural rate to the leading cause of death (COPD statistical, 2002–2004). These statistics estimate that COPD is the fourth leading cause of death in the Unites States, but will rise to the third for both men and women by 2020.

Risk Factors
- Smoking, both active and passive
- Exposure to biomass fumes
- Male (current rate is markedly higher in males but female rate is increasing)
- Age (increases in those over 50 years)
- Chronic respiratory irritation
- Recurrent respiratory illnesses
- Cold, dry air; hot, humid air; or high altitudes

Teach Risk Reduction Tips
- If smoking, STOP.
- Avoid passive smoke.
- Avoid air pollution and smog.
- Avoid chronic respiratory irritation (fumes, illnesses, allergens).
- Avoid respiratory illnesses (seek primary care advice regarding influenza vaccine).
- Avoid cold, dry air; hot, humid air; or high altitudes when possible (especially prolonged exposure to these).
- Seek early diagnosis if symptoms develop so that treatment and further preventive strategies can be initiated.

PHYSICAL ASSESSMENT Continued

Assessment Procedure	Normal Findings	Abnormal Findings
Palpate for crepitus. Crepitus, also called subcutaneous emphysema, is a crackling sensation (like bones or hairs rubbing against each other) that occurs when air passes through fluid or exudate. Use your fingers and follow the sequence in Fig 18-11 (p. 313) when palpating.	The examiner finds no palpable crepitus.	Crepitus can be palpated if air escapes from the lung or other airways into the subcutaneous tissue as occurs after an open thoracic injury, around a chest tube, or tracheostomy. It also may be palpated in areas of extreme congestion or consolidation. In such situations, mark margins and monitor to note any decrease or increase in the crepitant area.
Palpate surface characteristics. Put on gloves and use your fingers to palpate any lesions that you noticed during inspection. Also feel for any unusual masses.	Skin and subcutaneous tissue are free of lesions and masses.	Any unusual palpable mass should be evaluated further by a physician or other appropriate professional.

continued

Assessment Procedure	Normal Findings	Abnormal Findings
Palpate for fremitus. Following the above sequence, use the ball or ulnar edge of one hand to assess for fremitus (vibrations of air in the bronchial tubes transmitted to the chest wall). As you move your hand to each area, ask the client to say "ninety-nine." Assess all areas for symmetry and intensity of vibration. ➤ **Clinical Tip** • *The ball of the hand is best for assessing tactile fremitus because the area is especially sensitive to vibratory sensation.*	Fremitus is symmetric and easily identified in the upper regions of the lungs. If fremitus is not palpable on either side, the client may need to speak louder. A decrease in the intensity of fremitus is normal as the examiner moves toward the base of the lungs. However, fremitus should remain symmetric for bilateral positions.	Unequal fremitus is usually the result of consolidation (which increases fremitus) or bronchial obstruction, air trapping in emphysema, pleural effusion, or pneumothorax (which all decrease fremitus). Diminished fremitus even with a loud spoken voice may indicate an obstruction of the tracheobronchial tree.
Assess chest expansion. Place your hands on the posterior chest wall with your thumbs at the level of T9 or T10 and pressing together a small skin fold. As the client takes a deep breath, observe the movement of your thumbs (Fig. 18-12).	When the client takes a deep breath, the examiner's thumbs should move 5 to 10 cm apart symmetrically. 👓 Because of calcification of the costal cartilages and loss of the accessory musculature, the older client's thoracic expansion may be decreased although it should still be symmetric.	Unequal chest expansion can occur with severe atelectasis (collapse or incomplete expansion), pneumonia, chest trauma, or pneumothorax (air in the pleural space). Decreased chest excursion at the base of the lungs is characteristic of chronic obstructive pulmonary disease (COPD). This is due to decreased diaphragmatic function.
Percussion **Percuss for tone.** Start at the apices of the scapulae and percuss across the tops of both shoulders. Then percuss the intercostal spaces across and down, comparing sides. Percuss to the lateral aspects at the bases of the lungs, comparing sides. Figure 18-13 depicts the sequence for percussion.	*Resonance* is the percussion tone elicited over normal lung tissue (Fig. 18-14). Percussion elicits flat tones over the scapula.	Hyperresonance is elicited in cases of trapped air such as in emphysema or pneumothorax. Dullness is present when fluid or solid tissue replaces air in the lung or occupies the pleural space such as in lobar pneumonia, pleural effusion, or tumor.

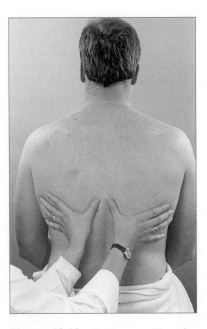

Figure 18-12 Starting position for assessing symmetry of chest expansion.

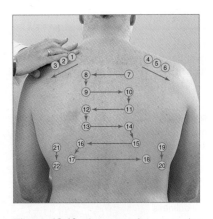

Figure 18-13 Sequence for percussing the posterior thorax.

continued

PHYSICAL ASSESSMENT Continued

Assessment Procedure	Normal Findings	Abnormal Findings

Percuss for diaphragmatic excursion. Ask the client to *exhale* forcefully and hold the breath. Beginning at the scapular line (T7), percuss the intercostal spaces of the right posterior chest wall. Percuss downward until the tone changes from resonance to dullness. Mark this level and allow the client to breathe. Next ask the client to *inhale* deeply and hold it. Percuss the intercostal spaces from the mark downward until resonance changes to dullness. Mark the level and allow the client to breathe. Measure the distance between the two marks (Fig. 18-15). Perform on both sides of the posterior thorax.

Excursion should be equal bilaterally and measure 3 to 5 cm in adults.

The level of the diaphragm may be higher on the right because of the position of the liver.

In well-conditioned clients, excursion can measure up to 7 or 8 cm.

Diaphragmatic descent may be limited by atelectasis of the lower lobes or by emphysema in which diaphragmatic movement and air trapping are minimal. The diaphragm remains in a low position on inspiration and expiration.

Other possible causes for limited descent can be pain or abdominal changes such as extreme ascites, tumors, or pregnancy.

Uneven excursion may be seen with inflammation from unilateral pneumonia, damage to the phrenic nerve, or splenomegaly.

Auscultation

Auscultate for breath sounds. To best assess lung sounds, you will need to hear the sounds as directly as possible. Do not attempt to listen through clothing or a drape, which may produce additional sound or muffle lung sounds that exist. To begin, place the diaphragm of the stethoscope firmly and directly on the posterior chest wall at the apex of the lung at C7. Ask the client to breathe deeply through his or her mouth for each area of auscultation (each placement of the stethoscope) in the auscultation sequence so you can best hear inspiratory and expiratory sounds. Be alert to the client's comfort and offer times for rest and normal breathing if fatigue is becoming a problem.

Three types of normal breath sounds may be auscultated—bronchial, bronchovesicular, and vesicular (Table 18-1).

➤ *Clinical Tip • Breath sounds are considered normal only in the area specified. Heard elsewhere, they are considered abnormal sounds. For example, bronchial breath sounds are abnormal if heard over the peripheral lung fields.*

Figure 18-16 depicts locations of normal breath sounds.

Sometimes breath sounds may be hard to hear with obese or heavily muscled clients due to increased distance to underlying lung tissue.

Diminished or absent breath sounds often indicate that little or no air is moving in or out of the lung area being auscultated. This may indicate obstruction within the lungs as a result of secretions, mucus plug, or a foreign object. It may also indicate abnormalities of the pleural space such as pleural thickening, pleural effusion, or pneumothorax. In cases of emphysema, the hyperinflated nature of the lungs, together with a loss of elasticity of lung tissue, may result in diminished inspiratory breath sounds. Increased (louder) breath sounds often occur when consolidation or compression results in a denser lung area that enhances the transmission of sound.

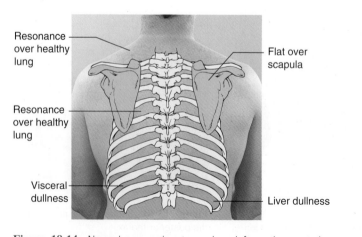

Figure 18-14 Normal percussion tones heard from the posterior thorax.

Resonance over healthy lung

Resonance over healthy lung

Visceral dullness

Flat over scapula

Liver dullness

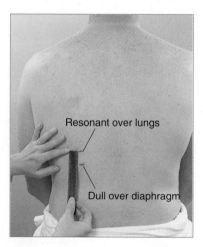

Figure 18-15 Measuring diaphragmatic excursion.

Resonant over lungs

Dull over diaphragm

continued

Assessment Procedure	Normal Findings	Abnormal Findings

Deep breathing may be especially difficult for the older client, who may fatigue easily. Thus offer rest as needed.

Auscultate from the apices of the lungs at C7 to the bases of the lungs at T10 and laterally from the axilla down to the seventh or eighth rib. Listen at each site for at least one complete respiratory cycle. Follow the auscultating sequence shown in Figure 18-17.

Table 18-1 Normal Breath Sounds

Type	Pitch	Quality	Amplitude	Duration	Location	Illustration
Bronchial	High	Harsh or hollow	Loud	Short during inspiration, long in expiration	Trachea and thorax	
Bronchovesicular	Moderate	Mixed	Moderate	Same during inspiration and expiration	Over the major bronchi—*posterior:* between the scapulae; *anterior:* around the upper sternum in the first and second intercostal spaces	
Vesicular	Low	Breezy	Soft	Long in inspiration, short inexpiration	Peripheral lung fields	

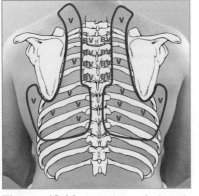

Figure 18-16 Location of breath sounds for the posterior thorax. V, vesicular sounds; BV, bronchovesicular sounds.

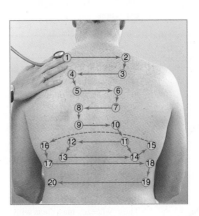

Figure 18-17 Sequence for auscultating the posterior thorax.

continued

PHYSICAL ASSESSMENT *Continued*

Assessment Procedure	Normal Findings	Abnormal Findings
Auscultate for adventitious sounds. Adventitious sounds are sounds added or superimposed over normal breath sounds and heard during auscultation. Be careful to note the location on the chest wall where adventitious sounds are heard as well as the location of such sounds within the respiratory cycle.	No adventitious sounds, such as crackles (discrete and discontinuous sounds) or wheezes (musical and continuous), are auscultated.	Adventitious lung sounds, such as crackles (formerly called rales) and wheezes (formerly called rhonchi) are evident. See Table 18-2 for a complete description of each type of adventitious breath sound.

Table 18-2 Adventitious Breath Sounds

Abnormal Sound	Characteristics	Source	Associated Conditions
Discontinuous Sounds Crackles (fine)	High-pitched, short, popping sounds heard during inspiration and not cleared with coughing; sounds are discontinuous and can be simulated by rolling a strand of hair between your fingers near your ear.	Inhaled air suddenly opens the small deflated air passages that are coated and sticky with exudate.	Crackles occurring late in inspiration are associated with restrictive diseases such as pneumonia and congestive heart failure. Crackles occurring early in inspiration are associated with obstructive disorders such as bronchitis, asthma, or emphysema.
Crackles (coarse)	Low-pitched, bubbling, moist sounds that may persist from early inspiration to early expiration; also described as softly separating Velcro.	Inhaled air comes into contact with secretions in the large bronchi and trachea.	May indicate pneumonia, pulmonary edema, and pulmonary fibrosis. "Velcro rales" of pulmonary fibrosis are heard louder and closer to stethoscope, usually do not change location, and are more common in clients with long-term COPD.
Continuous Sounds Pleural friction rub	Low-pitched, dry, grating sound; sound is much like crackles, only more superficial and occurring during both inspiration and expiration.	Sound is the result of rubbing of two inflamed pleural surfaces.	Pleuritis
Wheeze (sibilant)	High-pitched, musical sounds heard primarily during expiration but may also be heard on inspiration.	Air passes through constricted passages (caused by swelling, secretions, or tumor).	Sibilant wheezes are often heard in cases of acute asthma or chronic emphysema.
Wheeze (sonorous)	Low-pitched snoring or moaning sounds heard primarily during expiration but may be heard throughout the respiratory cycle. These wheezes may clear with coughing.	Same as sibilant wheeze. The pitch of the wheeze cannot be correlated to the size of the passageway that generates it.	Sonorous wheezes are often heard in cases of bronchitis or single obstructions and snoring before an episode of sleep apnea. *Stridor* is a harsh honking wheeze with severe broncholaryngospasm, such as occurs with croup.

continued

Assessment Procedure	Normal Findings	Abnormal Findings
➤ **Clinical Tip** • *If you hear an abnormal sound during auscultation, always have the client cough, then listen again and note any change. Coughing may clear the lungs.*		
Auscultate voice sounds. *Bronchophony:* Ask the client to repeat the phrase "ninety-nine" while you auscultate the chest wall.	Voice transmission is soft, muffled, and indistinct. The sound of the voice may be heard but the actual phrase cannot be distinguished.	The words are easily understood and louder over areas of increased density. This may indicate consolidation from pneumonia, atelectasis, or tumor.
Egophony: Ask the client to repeat the letter "E" while you listen over the chest wall.	Voice transmission will be soft and muffled but the letter "E" should be distinguishable.	Over areas of consolidation or compression, the sound is louder and sounds like "A."
Whispered Pectoriloquy: Ask the client to whisper the phrase "one–two–three" while you auscultate the chest wall.	Transmission of sound is very faint and muffled. It may be inaudible.	Over areas of consolidation or compression, the sound is transmitted clearly and distinctly. In such areas, it sounds as if the client is whispering directly into the stethoscope.

Anterior Thorax

Inspection

Inspect for shape and configuration. Have the client sit with her arms at her sides. Stand in front of the client and assess shape and configuration.	The anteroposterior diameter is less than the transverse diameter. The ratio of anteroposterior diameter to the transverse diameter is 1:2.	Anteroposterior equals transverse diameter, resulting in a barrel chest (see Abnormal Findings 18-1). This is often seen in emphysema because of hyperinflation of the lungs.
Inspect position of the sternum. Observe the sternum from an anterior and lateral viewpoint.	Sternum is positioned at midline and straight. The sternum and ribs may be more prominent in the older client because of loss of subcutaneous fat.	*Pectus excavatum* is a markedly sunken sternum and adjacent cartilages (often referred to as funnel chest). It is a congenital malformation that seldom causes symptoms other than self-consciousness. *Pectus carinatum* is a forward protrusion of the sternum causing the adjacent ribs to slope backward (often referred to as pigeon chest). (See Abnormal Findings 18-1 for illustrations of both conditions.) Both conditions may restrict expansion of the lungs and decrease the lung capacity.
Watch for sternal retractions.	Retractions not observed.	Sternal retractions are noted with severely labored breathing.
Inspect slope of the ribs. Assess the ribs from an anterior and lateral viewpoint.	Ribs slope downward with symmetric intercostal spaces. Costal angle is within 90 degrees.	Barrel-chest configuration results in a more horizontal position of the ribs and costal angle of more than 90 degrees. This often results from long-standing emphysema.

continued

PHYSICAL ASSESSMENT Continued

Assessment Procedure	Normal Findings	Abnormal Findings
Observe quality and pattern of respiration. Note breathing characteristics as well as rate, rhythm, and depth. Table 18-3 describes respiration patterns. ➤ *Clinical Tip • When assessing respiratory patterns, it is more objective to describe the breathing pattern, rather than just labeling the pattern.*	Respirations are relaxed, effortless, and quiet. They are of a regular rhythm and normal depth at a rate of 10 to 20 per minute in adults. Tachypnea and bradypnea may be normal in some clients.	Labored and noisy breathing is often seen with severe asthma or chronic bronchitis. Abnormal breathing patterns include tachypnea, bradypnea, hyperventilation, hypoventilation, Cheyne-Stokes respiration, and Biot's respiration.

Table 18-3 Respiration Patterns

Type	Description	Pattern	Clinical Indication
Normal	12 to 20/min and regular		Normal breathing pattern
Tachypnea	>24/min and shallow		May be a normal response to fever, anxiety, or exercise Can occur with respiratory insufficiency, alkalosis, pneumonia, or pleurisy
Bradypnea	<10/min and regular		May be normal in well-conditioned athletes Can occur with medication-induced depression of the respiratory center, diabetic coma, neurologic damage
Hyperventilation	Increased rate and increased depth		Usually occurs with extreme exercise, fear, or anxiety Kussmaul's respirations are a type of hyperventilation associated with diabetic ketoacidosis. Other causes of hyperventilation include disorders of the central nervous system, an overdose of the drug salicylate, or severe anxiety.
Hypoventilation	Decreased rate, decreased depth, irregular pattern		Usually associated with overdose of narcotics or anesthetics
Cheyne-Stokes respiration	Regular pattern characterized by alternating periods of deep, rapid breathing followed by periods of apnea		May result from severe congestive heart failure, drug overdose, increased intracranial pressure, or renal failure May be noted in elderly persons during sleep, not related to any disease process
Biot's respiration	Irregular pattern characterized by varying depth and rate of respirations followed by periods of apnea		May be seen with meningitis or severe brain damage

continued

Assessment Procedure	Normal Findings	Abnormal Findings
Inspect intercostal spaces. Ask the client to breathe normally and observe the intercostal spaces.	No retractions or bulging of intercostal spaces are noted.	Retraction of the intercostal spaces indicates an increased inspiratory effort. This may be the result of an obstruction of the respiratory tract or atelectasis. Bulging of the intercostal spaces indicates trapped air such as in emphysema or asthma.
Observe for use of accessory muscles. Ask the client to breathe normally and observe for use of accessory muscles.	Use of accessory muscles (sternomastoid and rectus abdominis) is not seen with normal respiratory effort. After strenuous exercise or activity, individuals with normal respiratory status may use neck muscles for a short time to enhance breathing.	Neck muscles (sternomastoid, scalene, and trapezius) are used to facilitate inspiration in cases of acute or chronic airway obstruction or atelectasis. The abdominal muscles and the internal intercostal muscles are used to facilitate expiration in COPD.

Palpation

Assessment Procedure	Normal Findings	Abnormal Findings
Palpate for tenderness, sensation, and surface masses. Use your fingers to palpate for tenderness and sensation. Start with your hand positioned over the left clavicle (over the apex of the left lung) and move your hand left to right, comparing findings bilaterally. Move your hand systematically downward toward the midline at the level of the breasts and outward at the base to include the lateral aspect of the lung. The established sequence for palpating the anterior thorax (Fig. 18-18) serves as a guide for positioning your hands. ➤ *Clinical Tip* • *Anterior thoracic palpation is best for assessing the right lung's middle lobe.*	No tenderness or pain is palpated over the lung area with respirations.	Tenderness over thoracic muscles can result from exercising (e.g., push ups and the like) especially in a previously sedentary client.
Palpate for tenderness at costochondral junctions of ribs.	Palpation does not elicit tenderness.	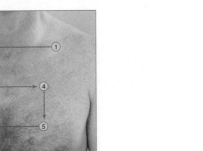 Tenderness or pain at the costochondral junction of the ribs is seen with fractures, especially in older clients with osteoporosis.

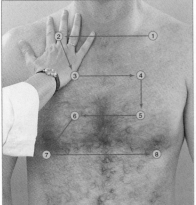

Figure 18-18 Sequence for palpating the anterior thorax.

continued

PHYSICAL ASSESSMENT *Continued*

Assessment Procedure	Normal Findings	Abnormal Findings
Assess for crepitus as you would on the posterior thorax (described previously).	No crepitus is palpated.	In areas of extreme congestion or consolidation, crepitus may be palpated particularly in clients with lung disease.
Also palpate any surface masses or lesions.	No unusual surface masses or lesions are palpated.	Surface masses or lesions may indicate cysts or tumors.
Palpate for fremitus. Using the sequence for the anterior chest above, palpate for fremitus using the same technique as for the posterior thorax. ➤ *Clinical Tip • When you assess for fremitus on the female client, avoid palpating the breast. Breast tissue dampens the vibrations.*	Fremitus is symmetric and easily identified in the upper regions of the lungs. A decreased intensity of fremitus is expected toward the base of the lungs; however, fremitus should be symmetric bilaterally.	Diminished vibrations, even with a loud spoken voice, may indicate an obstruction of the tracheobronchial tree. Clients with emphysema may have considerably decreased fremitus as a result of air trapping.
Palpate anterior chest expansion. Place your hands on the client's anterolateral wall with your thumbs along the costal margins and pointing toward the xiphoid process (Fig. 18-19). As the client takes a deep breath, observe the movement of your thumbs.	Thumbs move outward in a symmetric fashion from the midline.	Unequal chest expansion can occur with severe atelectasis, pneumonia, chest trauma, pleural effusion, or pneumothorax. Decreased chest excursion at the bases of the lungs is seen with COPD.
Percussion **Percuss for tone.** Percuss the apices above the clavicles. Then percuss the intercostal spaces across and down, comparing sides (Fig. 18-20).	Resonance is the percussion tone elicited over normal lung tissue. Figure 18-21 depicts normal tones and their locations. Percussion elicits dullness over breast tissue, the heart, and the liver. Tympany is detected over the stomach, and flatness is detected over the muscles and bones.	Hyperresonance is elicited in cases of trapped air such as in emphysema or pneumothorax. Dullness may characterize areas of increased density such as consolidation, pleural effusion, or tumor.

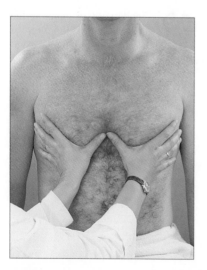

Figure 18-19 Palpating anterior chest expansion.

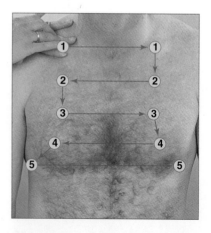

Figure 18-20 Sequence for percussing the anterior thorax.

continued

Assessment Procedure	Normal Findings	Abnormal Findings

Auscultation

Auscultate for anterior breath sounds, adventitious sounds, and voice sounds. Place the diaphragm of the stethoscope firmly and directly on the anterior chest wall. Auscultate from the apices of the lungs slightly above the clavicles to the bases of the lungs at the sixth rib. Ask the client to breathe deeply through his mouth in an effort to avoid transmission of sounds that may occur with nasal breathing. Be alert to the client's comfort and offer times for rest and normal breathing if fatigue is becoming a problem, particularly for the older client.

Listen at each site for at least one complete respiratory cycle. Follow the sequence for anterior auscultation shown in Figure 18-22.

> ➤ *Clinical Tip • Again, do not attempt to listen through clothing or other materials. However, if the client has a large amount of hair on the chest, listening through a thin T-shirt can decrease extraneous sounds that may be misinterpreted as crackles.*

Figure 18-23 depicts locations for normal breath sounds.

Refer to text in the posterior thorax section for normal voice sounds.

Refer to Table 18-2 for adventitious breath sounds. Refer to text in the posterior thorax section for normal voice sounds.

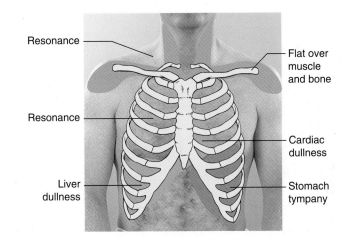

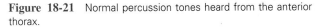

Figure 18-21 Normal percussion tones heard from the anterior thorax.

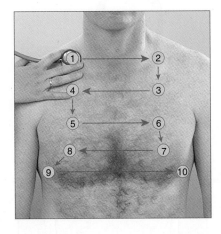

Figure 18-22 Sequence for auscultating the anterior thorax.

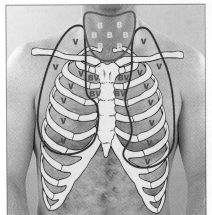

Figure 18-23 Location of breath sounds for the anterior thorax. B, bronchial sounds; V, vesicular sounds; BV, bronchovesicular sounds.

Abnormal Findings 18-1   **Thoracic Deformities and Configurations**

Normal chest configuration.

Cross section
of thorax

Barrel chest.

Cross section of
barrel-shaped thorax

Pectus excavatum (funnel chest).

Pectus carinatum (pigeon chest).

continued

Abnormal Findings 18-1 | Thoracic Deformities and Configurations *Continued*

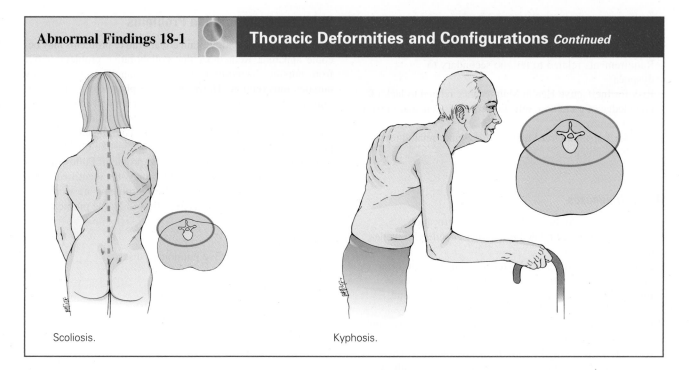

Scoliosis.

Kyphosis.

VALIDATING AND DOCUMENTING FINDINGS

If there are discrepancies between objective and subjective data or if abnormal findings are inconsistent with other data, validate your data. This is necessary to verify that the data are reliable and accurate. Document the assessment data following the health care facility or agency policy.

Sample Documentation of Subjective Data

No dyspnea, cough, or chest pain with breathing at rest or with activity. No past history or family history of respiratory diseases. Has never smoked and works in well-ventilated factory. Reports "one or two" colds per year. No known allergies. Last TB skin test performed 5 months ago with negative results. Last chest x-ray 4 years ago after "minor" car accident. X-ray report at that time was normal.

Sample Documentation of Objective Data

Respirations 18/minute, relaxed and even. Anteroposterior less than transverse diameter. Chest expansion symmetric. No retracting or bulging of intercostal spaces. No pain or tenderness noted on palpation. Tactile fremitus symmetric. Percussion tones resonant over all lung fields. Diaphragmatic excursion 4 cm and equal bilaterally. Vesicular breath sounds auscultated over lung fields. No adventitious sounds present.

After you have collected your assessment data, you will need to use diagnostic reasoning skills to analyze the data.

Analysis of Data

DIAGNOSTIC REASONING: POSSIBLE CONCLUSIONS

After collecting subjective and objective data pertaining to the thorax and lung assessment, identify abnormal findings and client strengths. Then cluster the data to reveal any significant patterns or abnormalities. These data may then be used to make clinical judgments about the status of the client's thorax and lungs.

Selected Nursing Diagnoses

Following is a listing of selected nursing diagnoses (wellness, risk, or actual) that you may identify when analyzing the clue clusters.

Wellness Diagnoses

- Readiness for Enhanced Breathing Patterns
- Health-Seeking Behaviors: Requests information on TB skin testing, how to quit smoking, or on exercises to improve respiratory status

Risk Diagnoses

- Risk for Respiratory Infection related to exposure to environmental pollutants and lack of knowledge of precautionary measures

- Risk for Activity Intolerance related to imbalance between oxygen supply and demand
- Risk for Imbalanced Nutrition: Less Than Body Requirements related to fatigue secondary to dyspnea
- Risk for Ineffective Health Maintenance related to lack of knowledge of condition, infection transmission, and prevention of recurrence
- Risk for Impaired Oral Mucous Membranes related to mouth breathing

Actual Diagnoses

- Anxiety related to dyspnea and fear of suffocation
- Activity Intolerance related to fatigue secondary to inadequate oxygenation
- Ineffective Airway Clearance related to inability to clear thick, mucous secretions secondary to pain and fatigue
- Impaired Gas Exchange related to chronic lung tissue damage secondary to chronic smoking
- Ineffective Airway Clearance related to bronchospasm and increased pulmonary secretions
- Ineffective Breathing Pattern: Hyperventilation related to hypoxia and lack of knowledge of controlled breathing techniques
- Disturbed Sleep Pattern related to excessive coughing
- Impaired Gas Exchange related to poor muscle tone and decreased ability to remove secretions secondary to the aging process

Selected Collaborative Problems

After grouping the data, certain collaborative problems may become apparent. Remember that collaborative problems differ from nursing diagnoses in that they cannot be prevented by nursing intervention. However, these physiologic complications of medical conditions can be detected and monitored by the nurse. In addition, the nurse can use physician- and nurse-prescribed interventions to minimize the complications of these problems. The nurse may also have to refer the client in such situations for further treatment of the problem. Following is a list of collaborative problems that may be identified when obtaining a general impression. These problems are worded as Risk for Complications (or RC), followed by the problem.

- RC: Atelectasis
- RC: Pneumonia
- RC: Chronic obstructive pulmonary disease
- RC: Asthma
- RC: Bronchitis
- RC: Pleural effusion
- RC: Pneumothorax
- RC: Pulmonary edema
- RC: Tuberculosis

Medical Problems

Development of RC and/or other signs and symptoms may clearly require medical treatment and referral to a primary care provider.

CASE STUDY

The case study demonstrates how to analyze thoracic and lung assessment data for a specific client. The critical thinking exercises included in the study guide/lab manual and interactive product that complement this text also offer opportunities to analyze assessment data.

This is your third weekly home visit with George Burney, a 60-year-old Caucasian man who was discharged after being hospitalized for 10 days with acute respiratory failure secondary to chronic obstructive pulmonary disease (COPD).

His eyes sparkling, he tells you he is feeling great and that he was able to walk outside on his patio for a few minutes today without his oxygen. He uses oxygen at 2 L/min when he exercises and prn for shortness of breath. He reports a "chronic cough, as usual" but denies sputum production. He says he still has difficulty "getting off a good cough" because "I just don't have the energy anymore."

Upon inspection, you note his facial color and lips are ruddy, but nail beds are pink. His breathing pattern is regular, unlabored, but tachypneic at 28 respirations per minute, which is his usual rate. Examining his thorax, you note he is barrel-chested with a transverse-to-lateral ratio of about 2.5 to 3. Although he is not using accessory muscles to breathe, you observe slight intercostal bulging and rigidly upright posture in the chair. While auscultating his lungs, you note diminished breath sounds bilaterally in most of lower lobes and a small, discrete area of coarse crackles in the upper portion of the left lower lobe. You also smell the odor of cigarettes on his breath, and, when you confront him with this information, he says, "I didn't think one would hurt when I was outside."

The following concept map illustrates the diagnostic reasoning process.

Applying COLDSPA

Applying **COLDSPA** for client symptoms: "chronic cough."

Mnemonic	Question	Data Provided	Missing Data
Character	Describe the sign or symptom (feeling, appearance, sound, smell, or taste if applicable).	"Chronic cough."	
Onset	When did it begin?		"When did you notice you could not bring up sputum when you cough?"
Location	Where is it? Does it radiate? Does it occur anywhere else?		"Do you have any chest pain?"
Duration	How long does it last? Does it recur?		"Are you short of breath when you walk or do other activities? How often do you use your oxygen?"
Severity	How bad is it? or How much does it bother you?	"I am feeling great and I went outside on the patio today for a few minutes without my oxygen."	
Pattern	What makes it better or worse?		"What makes your shortness of breath and cough worse? Or better?"
Associated factors/How it **A**ffects the client	What other symptoms occur with it? How does it affect you?	Lacks energy to cough up any real sputum; smokes an occasional cigarette outside.	

1) Identify abnormal data and client strengths

Subjective Data

- "Chronic cough, as usual" but denies sputum production
- Difficulty coughing effectively R/T decreased energy
- Didn't think having one cigarette while outside would hurt him
- Feels great today
- Walked on patio for a few minutes without oxygen

Objective Data

- Recent hospitalization for respiratory failure
- Ruddy facial and lip color, pink nail beds
- Tachypnea, but regular and unlabored
- Barrel chest, intercostal bulging, rigid posture
- Diminished breath sounds in lower lobes
- Discrete, coarse crackles in upper segment of LLL

2) Identify cue clusters

- Ruddy coloring
- Intercostal bulging
- Barrel chest

- Chronic cough
- No sputum
- Discrete crackles
- Diminished breath sounds
- Tachypnea
- Verbalizes decreased energy

- Odor of cigarettes on breath
- "Didn't think one (cigarette) would hurt when I was outside"
- Chronic cough

3) Draw inferences

Refer for: signs consistent with COPD diagnosis

Airway clearance impaired due to ineffective cough. May need instruction in energy-conserving cough techniques.

Denying hazardous effects of smoking on current health status

4) List possible nursing diagnoses

Ineffective Airway Clearance r/t knowledge of deficit of energy-conserving and possibly appropriate coughing techniques

Activity Intolerance r/t decreased energy secondary to compromised gas exchange from COPD

Ineffective Health Maintenance r/t denial of effects of cigarette smoking on current health status

Ineffective Management of Therapeutic Regimen r/t denial of effect of smoking on current health status

5) Check for defining characteristics

Major: Ineffective cough (no sputum produced) and inability to remove airway secretions
Minor: Abnormal breath sounds (crackles) and abnormal respiratory rate (tachypnea)

Major: None identified (dyspnea implied)
Minor: Weakness (verbalized decreased energy)

Major: Reports smoking cigarettes; denies significance
Minor: Chronic cough

Major: None
Minor: Verbalized did not take action (in this case, did forbidden action—smoking) to reduce risk factor

6) Confirm or rule out diagnoses

Accept diagnosis because it was validated by the client and because it meets all the defining characteristics

Rule out diagnosis because it does not meet the major defining characteristic. Needs further data for validation

Accept diagnosis because it meets major and minor defining characteristics

Rule out because it does not meet major defining characteristics

7) Document conclusions

Nursing diagnoses that are appropriate for this client include:
- Ineffective Airway Clearance r/t knowledge deficit of energy-conserving and possibly appropriate coughing techniques
- Ineffective Health Maintenance r/t denial of effects of cigarette smoking on current health status

Potential collaborative problems include the following:
- RC: Respiratory failure
- RC: Hypoxemia
- RC: Upper respiratory infection
- Refer to physician for signs of COPD

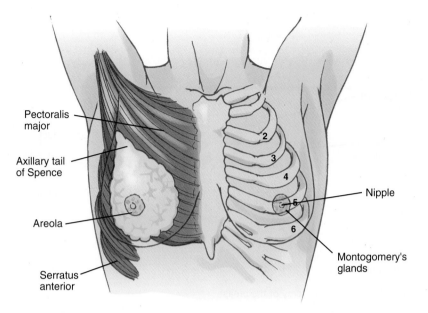

Figure 19-1   Anatomic breast landmarks and their position in the thorax.

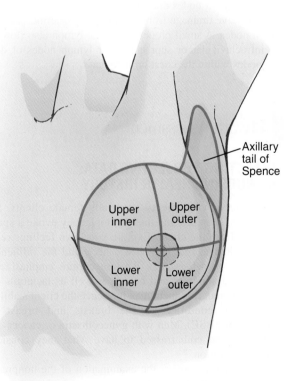

Figure 19-2   Breast quadrants. The upper outer quadrant is the area most targeted by breast cancer.

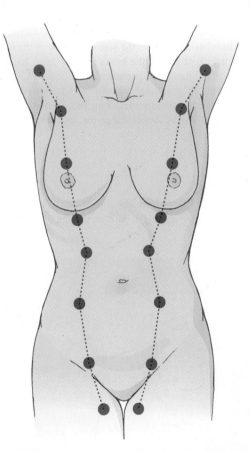

Figure 19-3   Supernumerary nipples along the "milk line," which extends bilaterally from the axilla to the groin.

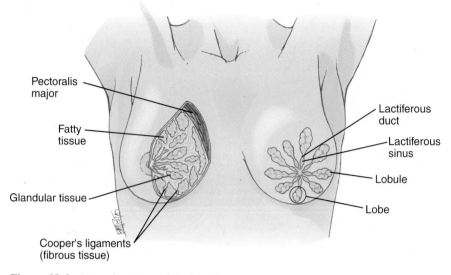

Figure 19-4   Internal anatomy of the breast.

Fatty tissue is the third component of the breast. The glandular tissue is embedded in the fatty tissue. This subcutaneous and retromammary fat provides most of the substance to the breast and thus determines the size and shape of the breasts. The functional capability of the breast is not related to size but rather to the glandular tissue present.

The amount of glandular, fibrous, and fatty tissue varies according to various factors including the client's age, body build, nutritional status, hormonal cycle, and whether she is pregnant or lactating.

LYMPH NODES

The major **axillary lymph nodes** consist of the anterior (pectoral), posterior (subscapular), lateral (brachial), and central

(midaxillary) nodes (Fig. 19-5). The anterior nodes drain the anterior chest wall and breasts. The posterior chest wall and part of the arms are drained by the posterior nodes.

The lateral nodes drain most of the arms, and the central nodes receive drainage from the anterior, posterior, and lateral lymph nodes. A small proportion of the lymph also flows into the infraclavicular or supraclavicular lymph nodes or deeper into nodes within the chest or abdomen.

Health Assessment

COLLECTING SUBJECTIVE DATA: THE NURSING HEALTH HISTORY

When interviewing clients, especially female clients, about the breasts, keep in mind that this topic may evoke a spate of emotions from the client. Explore your own feelings regarding body image, fear of breast cancer, and the influence of the breasts on self-esteem. Western culture emphasizes the breasts for femininity and beauty as well as lactation. Fear, anxiety, or embarrassment may influence the client's ability to discuss the condition of the breasts and breast self-examination (BSE). Men with gynecomastia or cancer of the breast may be embarrassed to have what they consider a "female condition."

This chapter covers the examination of the nonpregnant woman's breasts. Subjective data related to breast changes associated with pregnancy are covered in Chapter 29. Remember, if the client reports any symptom, you need to explore it further by performing a symptom analysis using the following guide.

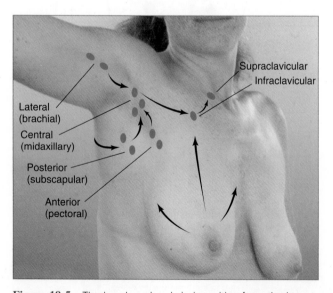

Figure 19-5   The lymph nodes drain impurities from the breasts (*arrows* show direction).

(text continues on page 337)

HISTORY OF PRESENT HEALTH CONCERNS

Question	Rationale
Have you noticed any lumps or swelling in your breasts? If so, where? When did you first notice it? Has the lump grown or swelling increased? Is the lump or swelling associated with other problems? Does the lump or swelling change during your menstrual cycle?	Lumps may be present with benign breast disease (fibrocystic breast disease), fibroadenomas, or malignant tumors (see Promote Health—Breast Cancer). Any lumps should be assessed further, and the client should be referred to a physician. Premenstrual breast lumpiness and soreness that subside after the end of the menstrual cycle may indicate benign breast disease (fibrocystic breast disease).
Have you noticed any lumps or swelling in the underarm area?	
Have you noticed any redness, warmth, or dimpling of your breasts? Any rash on the breast, nipple, or axillary area?	Redness and warmth indicate inflammation. A dimpling or retraction of the nipple or fibrous tissue may indicate breast cancer.
Have you noticed any change in the size or firmness of your breasts?	A recent increase in the size of one breast may indicate inflammation or abnormal growth. The older client may notice a decrease in the size and firmness of the breast as she ages because of a decrease in estrogen levels. Glandular tissue decreases whereas fatty tissue increases. A well-fitting supportive bra can reduce breast discomfort related to sagging breasts.
Do you experience any pain in your breasts? If so, where? Does it occur at any specific time during your menstrual cycle? Is there a certain activity that seems to initiate the pain?	Pain and tenderness of the breasts are common in benign breast disease and just before and during menstruation. This is especially true for clients taking oral contraceptives. Breast pain can also be a late sign of breast cancer.
Do you have any discharge from the nipples? If so, describe its color, consistency, and odor, if any. When did it start? Which nipple has the discharge?	If the client reports any blood or blood-tinged discharge, she should be referred to a physician for further evaluation. Sometimes, a clear benign discharge may be manually expressed from a breast that is frequently stimulated. Certain medications (oral contraceptives, phenothiazines, steroids, digitalis, and diuretics) are also associated with a clear discharge.

continued on page 334

COLDSPA Example for Lump in Breast

Use the **COLDSPA** mnemonic as a guideline to collect needed information for each symptom the client shares. In addition, the following questions help elicit important information.

Mnemonic	Question	Client Response Example
Character	Describe the sign or symptom (feeling, appearance, sound, smell, or taste if applicable).	"I found a lump in my left breast the size of a quarter."
Onset	When did it begin?	"I just noticed it yesterday when I took a shower."
Location	Where is it? Does it radiate? Does it occur anywhere else?	"It is in the left upper side of my left breast."
Duration	How long does it last? Does it recur?	"It does not hurt."
Severity	How bad is it? or How much does it bother you?	"I am worried about what it might be because my mother had breast cancer."
Pattern	What makes it better or worse?	"It seems to get bigger the more I feel it, but it does not go away."
Associated factors/How it **A**ffects the client	What other symptoms occur with it? How does it affect you?	"I try to work, but I just keep thinking about this lump in my breast."

PAST HEALTH HISTORY

Question	Rationale
Have you had any prior breast disease? Have you ever had breast surgery, a breast biopsy, breast implants, or breast trauma? If so, when did this occur? What was the result?	A personal history of breast cancer increases the risk for recurrence of cancer. Previous surgeries may alter the appearance of the breasts. Breast problems may occur with silicone breast implants. Trauma to the breasts from sports, accidents, or physical abuse can result in breast tissue changes.
How old were you when you began to menstruate? Have you experienced menopause?	Early menses (before age 13) or delayed menopause (after age 52) increases the risk for breast cancer.
Have you given birth to any children? At what age did you have your first child?	The risk of breast cancer is greater for women who have never given birth or for those who had their first child after age 30.
When was the first and last day of your menstrual cycle?	This information will inform you if this is the optimal time to examine the breasts. Hormone-related swelling, breast tenderness, and generalized lumpiness are reduced right after menstruation.

FAMILY HISTORY

Question	Rationale
Is there a history of breast cancer in your family? Who (sister, mother, maternal grandmother)?	A history of breast cancer in one's family increases one's risk for breast cancer.

LIFESTYLE AND HEALTH PRACTICES

Question	Rationale
Are you taking any hormones, contraceptives, or antipsychotic agents?	Hormones and some antipsychotic agents can cause breast engorgement in women. Hormones and oral contraceptives also increase the risk of breast cancer. Haloperidol (Haldol), an antipsychotic drug, can cause galactorrhea (persistent milk secretion whether or not the woman is breast-feeding or not) and lactation. This is also a side effect of medroxyprogesterone (Depo-Provera) injections.
Do you live or work in an area where you have excessive exposure to radiation, benzene, or asbestos?	Exposure to these environmental hazards can increase the risk of breast cancer.
What is your typical daily diet?	A high-fat diet may increase the risk for breast cancer.
How much alcohol do you drink each day?	Alcohol intake exceeding two drinks per day has been associated with a higher risk for breast cancer.
How much coffee, tea, cola (or other forms of caffeine) do you consume each day?	Caffeine can aggravate fibrocystic breast disease.
Do you engage in any type of regular exercise? If so, what type of bra do you wear when you exercise?	Breast tissue can lose its elasticity if vigorous exercise (i.e., running, aerobics) is performed without support for the breast. A well-fitting, supportive bra can also reduce discomfort in the breasts during exercise.

continued

LIFESTYLE AND HEALTH PRACTICES *Continued*

Question	*Rationale*
How important are your breasts to you in relation to a positive feeling about yourself and your physical appearance? Do you have any fears regarding breast disease?	The condition of the breasts may significantly influence how a woman feels about herself. Alterations in the breasts may threaten a woman's body image and feelings of self-worth, and men may be embarrassed to have enlarged breasts.
Do you examine your own breasts? Describe when you do this. Have you noted any changes in your breasts such as a lump, swelling, skin irritation, or dimpling, nipple pain or retraction (turning inward), redness or scaliness or nipple or breast skin, or discharge? If yes, have you reported this to your health care provider? ➤ *Clinical Tip* • *Older clients and others who no longer menstruate may find it helpful to pick a set day of the month for BSE, a date they will remember each month such as the day of the month they were born.*	Women should be told about the benefits and limitations of BSE beginning at age 20. Emphasize the importance of reporting any new breast symptoms to a health professional. It is acceptable for women to choose not to do BSE or to do BSE irregularly. If a woman chooses to do BSE, instruct on proper technique (Self-Assessment 19-1) allowing time for questions and review of their technique (American Cancer Society, 2003). The best time for BSE is right after menstruation or between the fourth and seventh day of the cycle if the cycle is regular. If the client is on cyclic estrogen therapy, she should examine her breasts on the last day that the medicine is not being taken. It is important for women to know their breasts and report any breast changes promptly to their health care providers. Remember that most of the time breast changes are not cancer but it is important to detect breast cancer early for effective treatment. Women who have had a breast lumpectomy, augmentation, or breast reconstruction may also perform BSE. Some women may choose not to do BSE even if knowledgeable of the benefits and limitations. This choice needs to be accepted by the examiner.
Have you ever had your breasts examined by a physician? When was your last examination?	The ACS recommends a clinical breast examination by a health care professional every 3 years for women ages 20 to 39 and every year for women age 40 and older (ACS, 2008).
Have you ever had a mammogram? If so, when was your last one?	The ACS recommends an annual mammogram for women age 40 and continuing for as long as a woman is in good health. Women at increased risk (e.g., family history, genetic tendency, past breast cancer) should talk to their doctors about the benefits and limitations of starting mammography screening earlier, having additional tests (i.e., breast ultrasound and MRI) and having more frequent exams (ACS, 2008).

PROMOTE HEALTH
Breast Cancer

Overview
Breast cancer is the most common cancer among women, and the incidence is rising. Breast cancer is the second leading cause of cancer death among white American women. Breast cancer deaths are highest among African-American women. However, early detection and treatment have resulted in increased survival rates. A 4% yearly increase during the 1980s has now leveled off at about 101 diagnosed cases per 100,000 women (American Cancer Society, 2007).

Risk Factors
- Gender (100 times more common in women)
- Age (Risk increases with increasing age, especially after age 50 years.)
- Genetics (In 10% of breast cancers, mutations of BRCA1 and BRCA2 genes are identified. In addition, a p53 tumor suppressor gene has been identified in some breast cancers.)

continued on page 336

PROMOTE HEALTH

Breast Cancer *Continued*

- Family history of breast cancer or ovarian cancer
- Personal history of breast cancer or certain precursor conditions
- Early menarche and late menopause
- No natural children
- First child born to a mother older than age 30
- Oral contraceptive use (slight risk)
- Regular alcohol intake, especially with two to five drinks daily
- Higher education or socioeconomic status
- Previous breast irradiation
- Hormone replacement therapy with progesterone
- Wet ear wax
- Chest exposed to radiation therapy as child
- Alcohol consumption
- Smoking

Possible Risk Factors for Breast Cancer
- Taller height
- High waist-to-hip ratio; obesity beginning as adult or after menopause
- High-fat diet (ambivalent findings; ACS, 2000)
- Low number of births
- No breast-feeding (ACS, 2000)
- Low level of physical activity
- Exposure to pesticides
- Long-term antibiotic use

Possible Risk Factors for Mortality
- No (or poor) breast self-examination
- Poor screening (physical examination or mammography)

Teach Risk Reduction Tips
- Do not delay pregnancy until after 30 years of age.
- Breast-feed.
- Perform monthly breast self-examination (BSE).
- Follow the American Cancer Society Guidelines for clinical evaluation and mammography.
- Avoid weight gain in adulthood, especially around menopause.
- Strenuous exercise, especially in youth, but also in adulthood; stay active.
- Nonsteroidal anti-inflammatory drug (NSAID) therapy (may have protective effect).
- Research: natural or synthetic vitamin A.
- Eat well-rounded diet low in fat and including flaxseed.
- Limit alcohol intake.
- Reduce antibiotic use except when absolutely necessary.
- Avoid use of birth control pills and hormone replacement unless necessary; discuss with your physician.
- Avoid exposure to pesticides.
- Maintain regular sleep schedule; 9 hours/night in a dark room.
- Avoid exposure to bright light at night. Avoid night shift if possible.

SELF ASSESSMENT 19-1   Breast Self-Examination

- Lie down and place your right arm behind your head. The exam is done while lying down, and not standing up, because when lying down the breast tissue spreads evenly over the chest wall as thinly as possible, making it much easier to feel all the breast tissue.

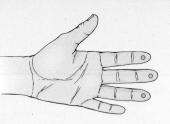

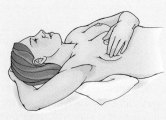

- Use the finger pads of the three middle fingers on your left hand to feel for lumps in the right breast. Use overlapping dime-sized circular motions of the finger pads to feel the breast tissue.

- Use three different levels of pressure to feel all the breast tissue. Light pressure is needed to feel the tissue closest to the skin; medium pressure to feel a little deeper; and firm pressure to feel the tissue closest to the chest and ribs. A firm ridge in the lower curve of each breast is normal. If you're not sure how hard to press, talk with your doctor or nurse. Use each pressure level to feel the breast tissue before moving on to the next spot.

Move around the breast in an up-and-down pattern starting at an imaginary line drawn straight down your side from the underarm

continued

and moving across the breast to the middle of the chest bone (sternum or breastbone). Be sure to check the entire breast area going down until you feel only ribs and up to the neck or collar bone (clavicle).

There is some evidence to suggest that the up-and-down pattern (sometimes called the vertical pattern) is the most effective pattern for covering the entire breast and not missing any breast tissue.

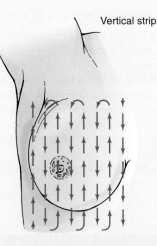

Vertical strip

Repeat the exam on your left breast, using the finger pads of the right hand. While standing in front of a mirror with your hands pressing firmly down on your hips, look at your breasts for any changes of size, shape, contour, or dimpling. (The pressing down on the hips position contracts the chest wall muscles and enhances any breast changes.)

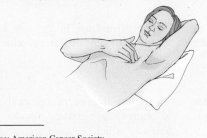

Source: American Cancer Society.

Examine each underarm while sitting up or standing and with your arm only slightly raised so you can easily feel in this area. Raising your arm straight up tightens the tissue in this area and makes it very difficult to examine.

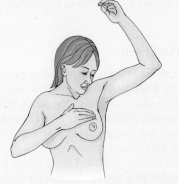

This procedure for doing breast self-exam represents changes in previous procedure recommendations. These changes represent an extensive review of the medical literature and input from an expert advisory group. There is evidence that the woman's position (lying down), area felt, pattern of coverage of the breast, and use of different amounts of pressure increase the sensitivity of BSE as measured with silicon models and for CBE using patient models with known small noncancerous lumps in their breasts (ACS, 2008).

Remember, if you find any changes, see your doctor right away.

COLLECTING OBJECTIVE DATA: PHYSICAL EXAMINATION

The purpose of breast assessment is to identify signs of breast disease and then to initiate early treatment. The incidence of breast cancer in women is rising, but early detection and treatment have resulted in increased survival rates.

It is often convenient to assess the breasts immediately after assessment of the thorax and lungs. Female breast examinations are also performed by the nurse before a mammogram or by the gynecologist or nurse practitioner before a routine pelvic examination. A breast examination should also be a routine part of the complete male assessment. However, the male breast examination is not as detailed as the female breast examination.

Keep in mind that breast palpation requires practice and skill because the consistency of the breasts varies widely from client to client. Some breasts are more difficult to palpate than others. For example, it is more difficult to palpate and inspect large, pendulous breasts to ensure adequate evaluation of all breast tissue. It may also be difficult to detect new lumps in women who have fibrocystic breast disease and who have granular, singular, or multiple mobile, tender lumps in their breasts.

The actual hands-on physical examination of the breast may create client anxiety. The client may be embarrassed about exposing his or her breasts and may be anxious about what the assessment will reveal. Explain in detail what is happening throughout the assessment and answer any questions the client might have. In addition, attempt to provide the client with as much privacy as possible during the examination.

This chapter covers the examination of the nonpregnant woman's breasts. Objective data related to breast changes associated with pregnancy are covered in Chapter 29.

Preparing the Client

Prepare for the breast examination by having the client sit in an upright position. Explain that it will be necessary to expose both breasts to compare for symmetry during inspection. One breast may be draped while the other breast is palpated. Be sensitive to the fact that many women may feel embarrassed to have their breasts examined.

The breasts are first inspected in the sitting position while the client is asked to hold arms in different positions. The breasts are then palpated while the client assumes a supine position.

The final part of the examination involves teaching clients how to perform BSE and asking them to demonstrate what they have learned. If the client states that she or he already knows how to perform BSE, then ask the client to demonstrate how this is done.

Equipment

- Centimeter ruler
- Small pillow
- Gloves
- Client handout for BSE
- Slide for specimen

Physical Assessment

Key points for physical assessment include the following:

- Explain to the client what the steps of the examination are and the rationale for them.
- Warm your hands.
- Observe and inspect breast skin, areolas, and nipples for size, shape, rashes, dimpling, swelling, discoloration, retraction, asymmetry and other unusual findings.
- Palpate breasts and axillary lymph nodes for swelling, lumps, masses, warmth or inflammation, tenderness, and other abnormalities.
- Perform the physical assessment just as carefully on male clients.

(text continues on page 346)

PHYSICAL ASSESSMENT

Assessment Procedure	Normal Findings	Abnormal Findings
Female Breasts		

Inspection

Assessment Procedure	Normal Findings	Abnormal Findings
Inspect size and symmetry. Have the client disrobe and sit with arms hanging freely (Fig. 19-6). Explain what you are observing to help ease client anxiety.	Breasts can be a variety of sizes and are somewhat round and pendulous. One breast may normally be larger than the other. The older client often has more pendulous, less firm, and saggy breasts.	A recent increase in the size of one breast may indicate inflammation or an abnormal growth. A pigskin-like or orange-peel (peau d'orange) appearance results from edema, which is seen in metastatic breast disease (Fig. 19-7). The edema is caused by blocked lymphatic drainage.

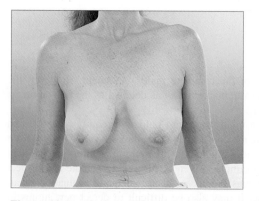

Figure 19-6 Client should sit with arms hanging freely at sides during assessment of breast size and symmetry.

continued

Assessment Procedure	**Normal Findings**	**Abnormal Findings**
Inspect color and texture. Be sure to note client's overall skin tone when inspecting the breast skin. Note any lesions.	Color varies depending on the client's skin tone. Texture is smooth with no edema. Linear stretch marks may be seen during and after pregnancy or with significant weight gain or loss.	Redness is associated with breast inflammation.
Inspect superficial venous pattern Observe visibility and pattern of breast veins.	Veins radiate either horizontally and toward the axilla (transverse) or vertically with a lateral flare (longitudinal). Veins are more prominent during pregnancy. These two patterns are seen in varying proportions among different cultural groups. However, both patterns are normal and the transverse pattern predominates.	A prominent venous pattern may occur as a result of increased circulation due to a malignancy. An asymmetric venous pattern may be due to malignancy.
Inspect the areolas. Note the color, size, shape, and texture of the areolas of both breasts.	Areolas vary from dark pink to dark brown, depending on the client's skin tones. They are round and may vary in size. Small Montgomery tubercles are present.	Peau d'orange skin, associated with carcinoma, may be first seen in the areola, whereas red, scaly, crusty areas are indicative of Paget's disease (Fig. 19-8).

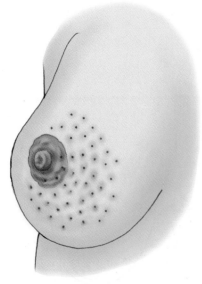

Figure 19-7 Resulting from edema, an orange peel (peau d'orange) appearance of the breast is associated with cancer.

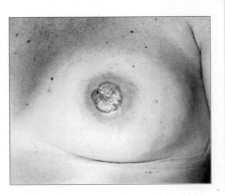

Figure 19-8 Paget's disease is typified by a crusty, red scaliness of the nipple.

continued

PHYSICAL ASSESSMENT *Continued*

Assessment Procedure	Normal Findings	Abnormal Findings

Female Breasts

Inspect the nipples. Note the size and direction of the nipples of both breasts. Also note any dryness, lesions, bleeding, or discharge.

Nipples are nearly equal bilaterally in size and are in the same location on each breast. Nipples are usually everted, but they may be inverted or flat. Supernumerary nipples (Fig. 19-9) may appear along the embryonic "milk line." No discharge should be present.

👓 The older client may have smaller, flatter nipples that are less erectile on stimulation.

A recently retracted nipple that was previously everted suggests malignancy (Fig. 19-10). Any type of spontaneous discharge should be referred for cytologic study and further evaluation.

Inspect for retraction and dimpling. To inspect the breasts accurately for retraction and dimpling, ask the client to remain seated while performing several different maneuvers. Ask the client to raise her arms overhead (Fig. 19-11A); then press her hands against her hips (Fig. 19-11B). Next ask her to press her hands together (Fig. 19-11C). These actions contract the pectoral muscles.

The client's breasts should rise symmetrically with no sign of dimpling or retraction.

Dimpling or retraction (Fig. 19-12) is usually caused by a malignant tumor that has fibrous strands attached to the breast tissue and the fascia of the muscles. As the muscle contracts, it draws the breast tissue and skin with it, causing dimpling or retraction.

Finally ask the client to lean forward from the waist (Fig. 19-13). The nurse should support the client by the hands or forearms. This is a good position to use in women who have large, pendulous breasts.

Breasts should hang freely and symmetrically.

Restricted movement of breast or retraction of the skin (Fig. 19-14) or nipple indicates fibrosis and fixation of the underlying tissues. This is usually due to an underlying malignant tumor.

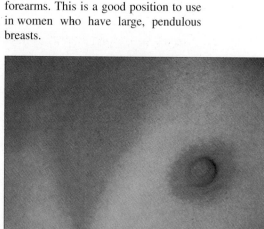

Figure 19-9 Supernumerary nipple (Logan-Young, W., & Hoffman, N.Y. [1994]. *Breast cancer: A practical guide to diagnosis*. Rochester, NY: Mt. Hope Publishing.).

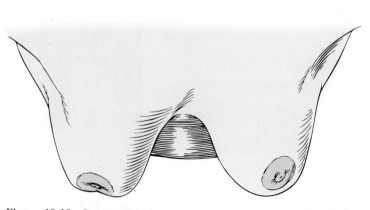

Figure 19-10 Retracted nipple.

continued

Assessment Procedure	Normal Findings	Abnormal Findings
Palpation **Palpate texture and elasticity.** See Assessment Tool 19-1.	Smooth, firm, elastic tissue. 👓 The older client's breasts may feel more granular, and the inframammary ridge may be more easily palpated as it thickens.	Thickening of the tissues may occur with an underlying malignant tumor.
Palpate tenderness and temperature. See Assessment Tool 19-1.	A generalized increase in nodularity and tenderness may be a normal finding associated with the menstrual cycle or hormonal medications. Breasts should be a normal body temperature.	Painful breasts may be indicative of benign breast disease but can also occur with a malignant tumor. The client should be referred for further evaluation. Heat in the breasts of women who have not just given birth or who are not lactating indicates inflammation.

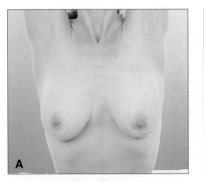

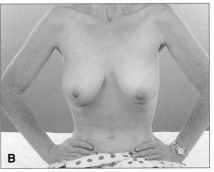

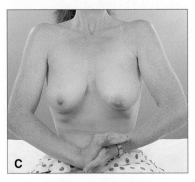

Figure 19-11 During assessment for retraction and dimpling, the client first (A) raises her arms over her head, (B) lowers them and presses them against the hips, and then (C) presses the hands together with the fingers of one hand pointing opposite to the fingers of the other hand.

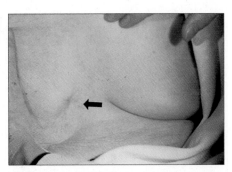

Figure 19-12 Dimpling of the breast nipple (Logan-Young, W., & Hoffman, N.Y. [1994]. *Breast cancer: A practical guide to diagnosis.* Rochester, NY: Mt. Hope Publishing.).

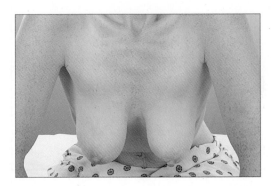

Figure 19-13 Forward-leaning position for breast inspection.

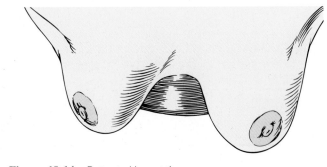

Figure 19-14 Retracted breast tissue.

continued on page 343

ASSESSMENT TOOL 19-1   Guidelines for Palpating the Breasts

1. Ask the client to lie down and to place overhead the arm on the same side as the breast being palpated. Place a small pillow or rolled towel under the breast being palpated.
2. Use the flat pads of three fingers to palpate the client's breasts (Figure A).
3. Palpate the breasts using one of three different patterns (Figures B, C, and D). Choose one that is most comfortable for you, but be consistent and thorough with the method chosen.
4. Be sure to palpate every square inch of the breast, from the nipple and areola to the periphery of the breast tissue and up into the tail of Spence. Vary the levels of pressure as you palpate.

   Light—superficial
   Medium—mid-level tissue
   Firm—to the ribs

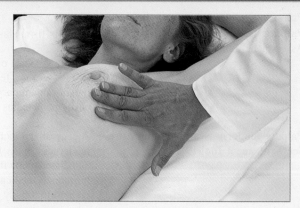

Figure A.

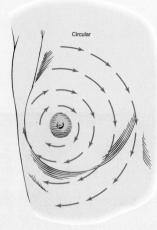

Figure B. Circular or clockwise.

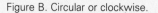

Figure C. Wedged.

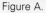

Figure D. Vertical strip.

5. Use the bimanual technique (Figure E) if the client has large breasts. Support the breast with your nondominant hand and use your dominant hand to palpate.

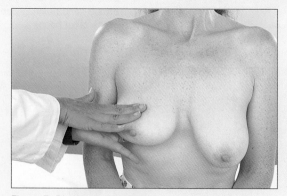

Figure E. Bimanual palpation.

Assessment Procedure	Normal Findings	Abnormal Findings
Palpate for masses. Note location, size in centimeters, shape, mobility, consistency, and tenderness (see Assessment Tool 19-1). Also note the condition of the skin over the mass. If you detect any lump, refer the client for further evaluation.	No masses should be palpated. However, a firm inframammary transverse ridge may normally be palpated at the lower base of the breasts.	Malignant tumors are most often found in the upper outer quadrant of the breast. They are usually unilateral with irregular, poorly delineated borders. They are hard and nontender and fixed to underlying tissues. Fibroadenomas are usually 1- to 5-cm, round or oval, mobile, firm, solid, elastic, nontender, single or multiple benign masses found in one or both breasts. Benign breast disease consists of bilateral, multiple, firm, regular, rubbery, mobile nodules with well-demarcated borders. Pain and fullness occurs just before menses (Abnormal Findings 19-1).
Palpate the nipples. Wear gloves to compress the nipple gently with your thumb and index finger (Fig. 19-15). Note any discharge. If spontaneous discharge occurs from the nipples, a specimen must be applied to a slide and the smear sent to the laboratory for cytologic evaluation.	The nipple may become erect and the areola may pucker in response to stimulation. A milky discharge is usually normal only during pregnancy and lactation. However, some women may normally have a clear discharge.	Discharge may be seen in endocrine disorders and with certain medications (i.e., antihypertensives, tricyclic antidepressants, and estrogen). Discharge from one breast may indicate benign intraductal papilloma, fibrocystic disease, or cancer of the breast.
Palpate mastectomy or lumpectomy site. If the client has had a mastectomy or lumpectomy, it is still important to perform a thorough examination. Palpate the scar and any remaining breast or axillary tissue for redness, lesions, lumps, swelling, or tenderness (Fig. 19-16).	Scar is whitish with no redness or swelling. No lesions, lumps, or tenderness noted.	Redness and inflammation of the scar area may indicate infection. Any lesions, lumps, or tenderness should be referred for further evaluation.

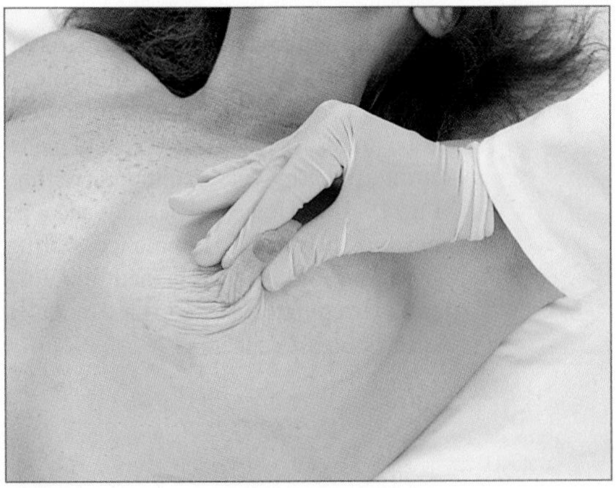

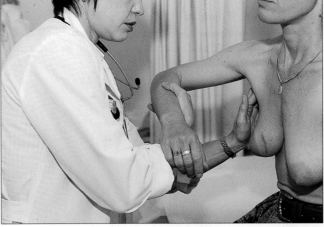

Figure 19-15 Palpating nipples for masses and discharge.

Figure 19-16 Palpating surgical site (© Dorothy Littell Greco 1993, Stock Boston).

continued

PHYSICAL ASSESSMENT Continued

Assessment Procedure	Normal Findings	Abnormal Findings

The Axillae

Inspection and Palpation

Inspect and palpate the axillae. Ask the client to sit up. Inspect the axillary skin for rashes or infection.

No rash or infection noted.

Redness and inflammation may be seen with infection of the sweat gland. Dark, velvety pigmentation of the axillae (acanthosis nigricans) may indicate an underlying malignancy.

Hold the client's elbow with one hand, and use the three fingerpads of your other hand to palpate firmly the axillary lymph nodes (Fig. 19-17).

No palpable nodes or one to two small (less than 1 cm), discrete, nontender, movable nodes in the central area.

Enlarged (greater than 1 cm) lymph nodes may indicate infection of the hand or arm. Large nodes that are hard and fixed to the skin may indicate an underlying malignancy.

First palpate high into the axillae, moving downward against the ribs to feel for the central nodes. Continue to move down the posterior axillae to feel for the posterior nodes. Use bimanual palpation to feel for the anterior axillary nodes. Finally palpate down the inner aspect of the upper arm.

Finally ask the client to demonstrate how she performs BSE if she chooses to receive feedback on her technique and method. This should be offered as an option and the client's choice accepted. This time offers the nurse an opportunity to teach BSE. Give clients printed instructions (see Self-Assessment 19-1).

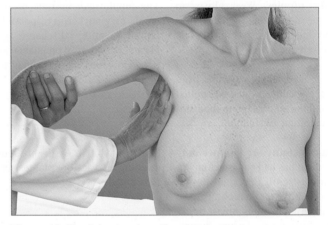

Figure 19-17   Palpating the axillary lymph nodes.

The Male Breasts

Inspection and Palpation

Inspect and palpate the breasts, areolas, nipples, and axillae. Note any swelling, nodules, or ulceration. Palpate the flat disc of undeveloped breast tissue under the nipple.

No swelling, nodules, or ulceration should be detected.

Soft, fatty enlargement of breast tissue is seen in obesity. Gynecomastia, a smooth, firm, movable disc of glandular tissue, may be seen in one breast in males during puberty for a temporary time (Fig. 19-18). However, it may also be seen in hormonal imbalances, drug abuse, cirrhosis, leukemia, and thyrotoxicosis. Irregularly shaped, hard nodules occur in breast cancer.

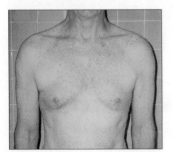

Figure 19-18   Gynecomastia.

Abnormal Findings 19-1 | **Abnormalities of the Breasts**

Whereas some abnormalities of the breast are readily apparent, such as peau d' orange and Paget's disease, some breast internal changes are detected only by palpation and mammography. The following illustrations represent breast abnormalities characteristic of tumors, fibroadenomas, and benign disease (fibrocystic breasts).

Cancerous Tumors

These are irregular, firm, hard, not defined masses that may be fixed or mobile. They are not usually tender and usually occur after age 50.

Fibroadenomas

These lesions are lobular, ovoid, or round. They are firm, well defined, seldom tender, and usually singular and mobile. They occur more commonly between puberty and menopause.

Benign Breast Disease

Also called fibrocystic breast disease, benign breast disease is marked by round, elastic, defined, tender, and mobile cysts. The condition is most common from age 30 to menopause, after which it decreases.

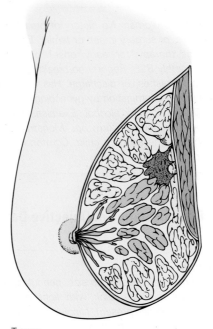
Tumor.

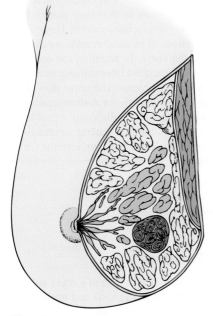
Fibroadenoma.

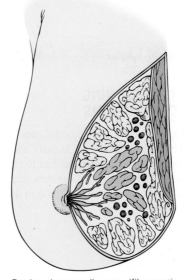
Benign breast disease (fibrocystic breast disease).

VALIDATING AND DOCUMENTING FINDINGS

Validate the breast and lymph node assessment data you have collected. This is necessary to verify that the data are reliable and accurate. Document the assessment data following the health care facility or agency policy.

Sample Documentation of Subjective Data

Forty-year-old woman. No history of breast disease, biopsies, or surgery in self or family. Takes hormone replacement therapy for early onset of menopause. Performs monthly BSE. Reports no breast lesions, lumps, swelling, pain, rashes, or discharge. Has yearly mammogram and breast examination by gynecologist. Eats a low-fat diet. Does not drink alcohol. Exercises four times a week wearing supportive, firm bra. Menstruation started at age 14. Has one adopted child. Comfortable with discussing condition of breasts.

Sample Documentation of Objective Data

Inspection
Bilateral breasts moderate in size, pendulant, and symmetric. Breast skin pale pink with light brown areola. Montgomery tubercles present. Nipples everted bilaterally. Free movement of breasts with position changes of arms and hands. No dimpling, retraction, lesions, or inflammation noted. Axillae free of rashes or inflammation.

Palpation
No masses or tenderness palpated. Bilateral mammary ridge present. No discharge from nipples. Axillary (central, anterior, or posterior) and lateral arm lymph nodes nonpalpable. Demonstrates appropriate technique for BSE.

Analysis of Data

DIAGNOSTIC REASONING: POSSIBLE CONCLUSIONS

After collecting subjective and objective data pertaining to the breast and lymphatic assessment, identify abnormal findings and client strengths. Then cluster the data to reveal any significant patterns or abnormalities. These data many then be used to make clinical judgments about the status of the client's breast and lymphatic health.

Selected Nursing Diagnoses

Following is a listing of selected nursing diagnoses (wellness, risk, or actual) that you may identify when analyzing the cue clusters.

Wellness Diagnoses

- Readiness for enhanced health management of breasts
- Health-Seeking Behavior: Requests information on BSE

Risk Diagnoses

- Risk for Ineffective Management of Therapeutic Regimen related to busy lifestyle and lack of knowledge of monthly BSE

Actual Diagnoses

- Fear of breast cancer related to increased risk factors
- Ineffective Individual Coping related to diagnoses of breast cancer
- Disturbed Body Image related to mastectomy
- Anticipatory Grieving related to anticipation of poor outcome of breast biopsy
- Ineffective Management of Therapeutic Regimen related to lack of knowledge of BSE

Selected Collaborative Problems

After grouping the data, certain collaborative problems may become apparent. Remember that collaborative problems differ from nursing diagnoses in that they cannot be prevented or treated by nursing interventions alone. However, these physiologic complications of medical conditions can be detected and monitored by the nurse. In addition, the nurse can use physician- and nurse-prescribed interventions to minimize the complications of these problems. The nurse may also have to refer the client in such situations for further treatment of the problem. Following is a list of collaborative problems that may be identified when obtaining a general impression. These problems are worded as Risk for Complications (or RC), followed by the problem.

- RC: Infection (abscess)
- RC: Hematoma
- RC: Benign breast disease

Medical Problems

After grouping the data, the client's signs and symptoms may clearly require medical diagnosis and treatment. Referral to a primary care provider is necessary.

CASE STUDY

The case study demonstrates how to analyze breast and lymphatic assessment data for a specific client. The critical thinking exercises included in the study guide/lab manual and interactive product that complement this text also offer opportunities to analyze assessment data.

During her routine physical examination ("I schedule one every year now because I want to live to a healthy old age"), Mrs. Nicole Barnes, a 42-year-old African American, tells you that she is concerned with the lumps and tenderness that occur in her breasts each month, just a few days before her menstrual period. In response to questioning, she relates that she is a "heavy coffee drinker" and is under a great deal of stress in her job. She reports that a maternal aunt died of breast cancer. She wants to know if the lumps could be cancerous or what can be done to eliminate this breast problem. On examination, you note that her breasts feel nodular but without discrete masses. Other findings include no evidence of inflammation, no axillary node enlargement, and no lesions or nipple drainage. You suspect that she has fibrocystic changes characteristic of benign breast disease.

The following concept map illustrates the diagnostic reasoning process.

Applying COLDSPA

Applying **COLDSPA** for client symptoms: "lumps and tenderness in breasts each month."

Mnemonic	Question	Data Provided	Missing Data
Character	Describe the sign or symptom (feeling, appearance, sound, smell, or taste if applicable).	"Lumps and tenderness in breasts."	
Onset	When did it begin?	"Each month before menstrual period."	
Location	Where is it? Does it radiate? Does it occur anywhere else?		"Where are the lumps and tenderness? In both or one breast? In one specific area or all over the breasts?
Duration	How long does it last? Does it recur?		How long do the tenderness and lumps last after they appear? Do they come and go or is it persistent?
Severity	How bad is it? or How much does it bother you?	"Can this be cancerous? What can I do to make this go away?"	
Pattern	What makes it better or worse?	Client drinks a lot of coffee and has a lot of work-related stress.	
Associated factors/How it **A**ffects the client	What other symptoms occur with it? How does it affect you?	Client's maternal aunt died of breast cancer.	

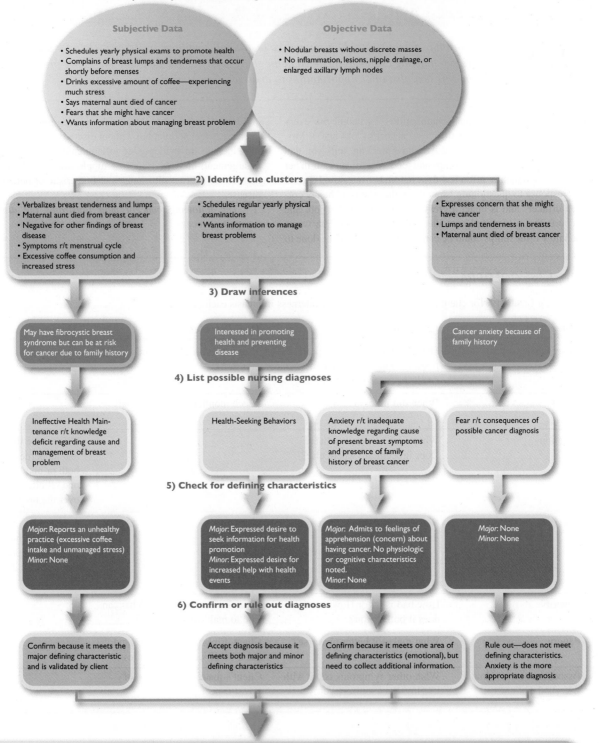

1) Identify abnormal findings and client strengths

Subjective Data
- Schedules yearly physical exams to promote health
- Complains of breast lumps and tenderness that occur shortly before menses
- Drinks excessive amount of coffee—experiencing much stress
- Says maternal aunt died of cancer
- Fears that she might have cancer
- Wants information about managing breast problem

Objective Data
- Nodular breasts without discrete masses
- No inflammation, lesions, nipple drainage, or enlarged axillary lymph nodes

2) Identify cue clusters

- Verbalizes breast tenderness and lumps
- Maternal aunt died from breast cancer
- Negative for other findings of breast disease
- Symptoms r/t menstrual cycle
- Excessive coffee consumption and increased stress

- Schedules regular yearly physical examinations
- Wants information to manage breast problems

- Expresses concern that she might have cancer
- Lumps and tenderness in breasts
- Maternal aunt died of breast cancer

3) Draw inferences

May have fibrocystic breast syndrome but can be at risk for cancer due to family history

Interested in promoting health and preventing disease

Cancer anxiety because of family history

4) List possible nursing diagnoses

Ineffective Health Maintenance r/t knowledge deficit regarding cause and management of breast problem

Health-Seeking Behaviors

Anxiety r/t inadequate knowledge regarding cause of present breast symptoms and presence of family history of breast cancer

Fear r/t consequences of possible cancer diagnosis

5) Check for defining characteristics

Major: Reports an unhealthy practice (excessive coffee intake and unmanaged stress)
Minor: None

Major: Expressed desire to seek information for health promotion
Minor: Expressed desire for increased help with health events

Major: Admits to feelings of apprehension (concern) about having cancer. No physiologic or cognitive characteristics noted.
Minor: None

Major: None
Minor: None

6) Confirm or rule out diagnoses

Confirm because it meets the major defining characteristic and is validated by client

Accept diagnosis because it meets both major and minor defining characteristics

Confirm because it meets one area of defining characteristics (emotional), but need to collect additional information.

Rule out—does not meet defining characteristics. Anxiety is the more appropriate diagnosis

7) Document conclusions

Nursing diagnoses that are appropriate for this client include:
- Ineffective Health Maintenance r/t knowledge deficit regarding cause and management of breast problem
- Health-Seeking Behaviors
- Anxiety r/t inadequate knowledge regarding cause of present breast symptoms and presence of family history of breast cancer

Potential collaborative problems include the following:
No collaborative problems could be identified because there is no medical diagnosis at this time.
Mrs. Barnes needs a referral to her physician for evaluation, diagnosis, and possible biopsy of her breast lumps.

References and Selected Readings

Allison, V. (2004). Breast cancer: Evaluation of a nurse-led family history clinic. *Journal of Clinical Nursing, 13*(6), 765.

American Cancer Society. (2003). *Cancer facts and figures—2003.* Atlanta: Author.

American Cancer Society. (2007). Can breast cancer be found early? Available at http://www.cancer.org

American Cancer Society. (2008). How to perform a breast self-exam. Available http://www.cancer.org

Bernard, L. L., & Guarnaccia, C. A. (2003). Two models of caregiver strain and bereavement adjustment in comparison of husband and daughter caregivers of breast cancer hospice patients. *Gerontologist, 43*(60), 808–816.

Brooks, J. (2006). A patient's journey: Living with breast cancer. *British Medical Journal, 333,* 31–33.

Budin, W. (2004). Sexual adjustment to breast cancer in unmarried women. *The Research Connection: The Psychosocial & Nursing Advisory Board to the New Jersey Commission on Cancer Research.* Available at http://www.state.nh.us

DeHaven, M. J., Hunter, I. B., Wilder, L., et al. (2004). Health programs in faith-based organizations: Are they effective? *American Journal of Public Health, 94,* 1030–1036.

Dest, V. M. (2004). Mammograms and how often? *RN, 67*(6), 26–31; quiz 31.

George, S. A. (2004). Barriers to breast cancer screening: An integrative review. *Health Care for Women International, 21*(1), 53–65.

Greifzu, S. P. (2004). Breast cancer. *RN, 67*(2), 36–42.

Lacovara, J., & Ray, J. (2007). Deciphering the diagnostics of breast cancer. *Medsurg Nursing 16*(6), 391–399.

Luszczynska, A. (2004). Change in breast self-examination behavior: Effects of intervention on enhancing self-efficacy. *Journal of International Behavioral Medicine, 11*(2), 95–103.

Pritt, B., Pang, Y., Kellogg, M., St. John, T., & Elhosseiny, A. (2004). Diagnostic value of nipple cytology: Study of 466 cases. *Cancer 102*(4), 233–238.

Secginli, S., & Nahcivan, N. (2004). Reliability and validity for the breast cancer screening belief scale among Turkish women. *Cancer Nursing: An International Journal for Cancer Care, 27*(4), 287–294.

Susan G. Komen for the cure. (2008). Available at http://www.komen.org/bse

Szwajcer, A., Hannan, R., Donoghue, J., & Mitten-Lewis, S. (2004). Evaluating key dimensions of the breast cancer nurse role in Australia. *Cancer Nursing, 27*(1), 79–84.

Taylor, R. (1999). Protocols in practice. Case management program for breast cancer education. *Nursing Case Management, 4*(3), 135–144.

Turner, J., Kelly, B., Swanson, C., Allison, R., & Wetzig, N. (2004). Psychosocial impact of newly diagnosed advanced breast cancer. Paper in *Psycho-Oncology (articles online in advance of print).* Published online: September 13, 2004.

U.S. Prevention Services Task Force. (2002). Screening for breast cancer. Available at http://www.ahrq.gov

WebMD. (2004). Breast cancer husband. Available at http://www.webmd.com/content/chat_transcripts

Wood, R. Y., & Duffy, M. E. (2004). Video breast health kits: Testing a cancer education innovation in older high-risk populations. *Journal of Cancer Education, 19*(2), 98–104.

Zuckerman, D. (2002). The breast cancer information gap. *RN, 65*(2), 39–41.

Promote Health—Breast Cancer

American Cancer Society. (2008). ACS breast screening resource center. Available at http://www.cancer.org

Breast cancer: Statistics. (2007). Available at http://www.imaginis.com/breasthealth/statistics.asp

Mayo Clinic. (2007). Breast cancer prevention: Lifestyle choices and more. Available at http://www.mayoclinic.com/health/breast-cancer-prevention/WO00091

Overfield, T. (1995). *Biologic variation in health and illness: Race, age, and sex differences* (2nd ed.). Boca Raton, FL: CRC Press.

WebMD. (2007). Breast cancer and weight changes. Available http://www.webmd.com/breast-cancer/news/20071022/weight-gain-ups-breast-cancer-risk

Websites

American Cancer Society. ACS Breast Cancer Resource Center. Available at http://www.cancer.org

National Cancer Institute. Available at http://www.cancer.gov

The National Cancer Institute (NCI) Breast Cancer Risk Assessment Tool. Available at http://bcra.nci.nih.gov/brc/start.htm

Washington University School of Medicine. Available at http://www.yourdiseaserisk.wustl.edu/

Structure and Function

The **cardiovascular system** is a highly complex system that includes the heart and a closed system of blood vessels. To collect accurate data and correctly interpret that data, the examiner must have an understanding of the structure and function of the heart, the great vessels, the electrical conduction system of the heart, the cardiac cycle, the production of heart sounds, cardiac output, and the neck vessels. This information helps the examiner to differentiate between normal and abnormal findings as they relate to the cardiovascular system.

HEART AND GREAT VESSELS

The heart is a hollow, muscular, four-chambered (left and right atria and left and right ventricles) organ located in the middle of the thoracic cavity between the lungs in the space called the *mediastinum.* It is about the size of a clenched fist and weighs approximately 255 g (9 oz) in women and 310 g (10.9 oz) in men. The heart extends vertically from the left second to the left fifth intercostal space (ICS) and horizontally from the right edge of the sternum to the left midclavicular line (MCL). The heart can be described as an inverted cone. The upper portion, near the left second ICS, is the base and the lower portion, near the left fifth ICS and the left MCL, is the apex. The anterior chest area that overlies the heart and great vessels is called the *precordium* (Fig. 20-1). The right side of the heart pumps blood to the lungs for gas exchange (pulmonary circulation); the left side of the heart pumps blood to all other parts of the body (systemic circulation).

The large veins and arteries leading directly to and away from the heart are referred to as the **great vessels. The superior and inferior vena cava** return blood to the right atrium from the upper and lower torso respectively. The **pulmonary artery** exits the right ventricle, bifurcates, and carries blood to the lungs. The **pulmonary veins** (two from each lung) return oxygenated blood to the left atrium. The *aorta* transports oxygenated blood from the left ventricle to the body (Fig. 20-2).

Heart Chambers and Valves

The heart consists of four chambers or cavities: two upper chambers, the **right and left atria,** and two lower chambers,

the **right and left ventricles.** The right and left sides of the heart are separated by a partition called the **septum.** The thin-walled atria receive blood returning to the heart and pump blood into the ventricles. The thicker-walled ventricles pump blood out of the heart. The left ventricle is thicker than the right ventricle because the left side of the heart has a greater workload.

The entrance and exit of each ventricle are protected by one-way valves that direct the flow of blood through the heart. The **atrioventricular (AV) valves** are located at the entrance into the ventricles. There are two AV valves: the **tricuspid valve** and the **bicuspid (mitral) valve.** The tricuspid valve is composed of three cusps or flaps and is located between the right atrium and the right ventricle; the bicuspid (mitral) valve is composed of two cusps or flaps and is located between the left atrium and the left ventricle. Collagen fibers, called **chordae tendineae,** anchor the AV valve flaps to papillary muscles within the ventricles.

Open AV valves allow blood to flow from the atria into the ventricles. However, as the ventricles begin to contract, the AV valves snap shut, preventing the regurgitation of blood into the atria. The valves are prevented from blowing open in the reverse direction (i.e., toward the atria) by their secure anchors to the papillary muscles of the ventricular wall. The **semilunar valves** are located at the exit of each ventricle at the beginning of the great vessels. Each valve has three cusps or flaps that look like half-moons, hence the name "semilunar." There are two semilunar valves: the **pulmonic valve** is located at the entrance of the pulmonary artery as it exits the right ventricle and the **aortic valve** is located at the beginning of the ascending aorta as it exits the left ventricle. These valves are open during ventricular contraction and close from the pressure of blood when the ventricles relax. Blood is thus prevented from flowing backward into the relaxed ventricles (see Fig. 20-2).

Heart Covering and Walls

The **pericardium** is a tough, inextensible, loose-fitting, fibroserous sac that attaches to the great vessels and, thereby, surrounds the heart. A serous membrane lining, the **parietal pericardium,** secretes a small amount of pericardial fluid that allows for smooth, friction-free movement of the heart. This same type of serous membrane covers the outer surface of the heart and is known as the **epicardium. The myocardium** is the thickest layer of the heart and is made up of contractile cardiac

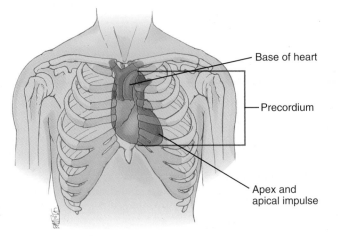

Figure 20-1 The heart and major blood vessels lie centrally in the chest behind the protective sternum.

Base of heart

Precordium

Apex and apical impulse

muscle cells. The **endocardium** is a thin layer of endothelial tissue that forms the innermost layer of the heart and is continuous with the endothelial lining of blood vessels (see Fig. 20-2).

ELECTRICAL CONDUCTION OF THE HEART

Cardiac muscle cells have a unique inherent ability. They can spontaneously generate an electrical impulse and conduct it through the heart. The generation and conduction of electrical impulses by specialized sections of the myocardium regulate the events associated with the filling and emptying of the cardiac chambers. The process is called the **cardiac cycle** (see description below).

Pathways

The **sinoatrial (SA) node** (or sinus node) is located on the posterior wall of the right atrium near the junction of the superior and inferior vena cava. The SA node, with inherent rhythmicity, generates impulses (at a rate of 60 to 100 per minute) that are conducted over both atria, causing them to contract simultaneously and send blood into the ventricles. The current, initiated by the SA node, is conducted across the atria to the **AV node** located in the lower interatrial septum (Fig. 20-3). The AV node slightly delays incoming electrical impulses from the atria then relays the impulse to the AV bundle (bundle of His) in the upper interventricular septum. The electrical impulse then travels down the right

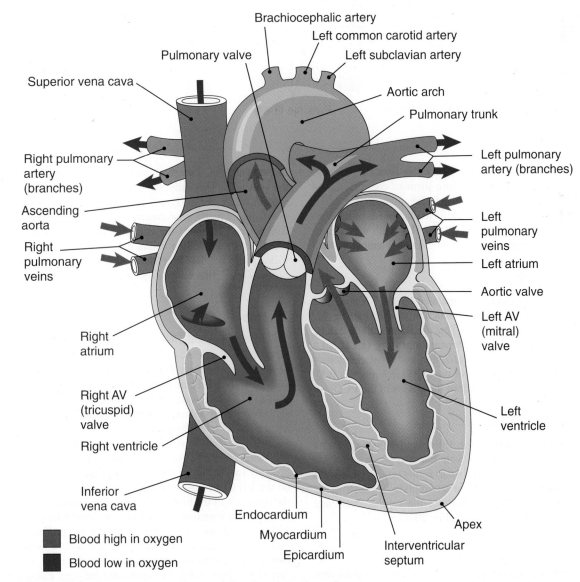

Figure 20-2 Heart chambers, valves, and direction of circulatory flow.

Brachiocephalic artery

Left common carotid artery

Left subclavian artery

Pulmonary valve

Aortic arch

Superior vena cava

Pulmonary trunk

Right pulmonary artery (branches)

Left pulmonary artery (branches)

Ascending aorta

Left pulmonary veins

Right pulmonary veins

Left atrium

Aortic valve

Left AV (mitral) valve

Right atrium

Right AV (tricuspid) valve

Left ventricle

Right ventricle

Inferior vena cava

Endocardium

Myocardium

Epicardium

Apex

Interventricular septum

■ Blood high in oxygen

■ Blood low in oxygen

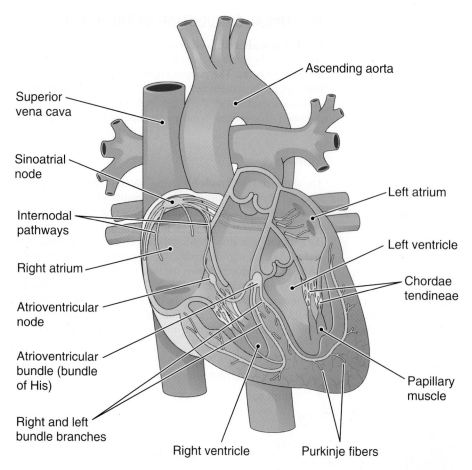

Superior vena cava

Sinoatrial node

Internodal pathways

Right atrium

Atrioventricular node

Atrioventricular bundle (bundle of His)

Right and left bundle branches

Right ventricle

Purkinje fibers

Ascending aorta

Left atrium

Left ventricle

Chordae tendineae

Papillary muscle

Figure 20-3 The electrical conduction system of the heart begins with impulse generated by the sinoatrial node (*green*) and circuited continuously over the heart.

and left bundle branches and the **Purkinje fibers** in the myocardium of both ventricles, causing them to contract almost simultaneously. Although the SA node functions as the "pacemaker of the heart," this activity shifts to other areas of the conduction system, such as the **Bundle of His** (with an inherent discharge of 40 to 60 per minute), if the SA node cannot function.

Electrical Activity

Electrical impulses, which are generated by the SA node and travel throughout the cardiac conduction circuit, can be detected on the surface of the skin. This electrical activity can be measured and recorded by **electrocardiography (ECG, aka EKG),** which records the depolarization and repolarization of the cardiac muscle. The phases of the ECG are known as P, Q, R, S, and T. Display 20-1 describes the phases of the ECG.

THE CARDIAC CYCLE

The **cardiac cycle** refers to the filling and emptying of the heart's chambers. The cardiac cycle has two phases: **diastole** (relaxation of the ventricles, known as filling) and **systole** (contraction of the ventricles, known as emptying). Diastole endures for approximately two-thirds of the cardiac cycle and systole is the remaining one-third (Fig. 20-4).

Diastole

During ventricular diastole, the AV valves are open and the ventricles are relaxed. This causes higher pressure in the atria than

in the ventricles. Therefore, blood rushes through the atria into the ventricles. This early, rapid, passive filling is called *early or protodiastolic filling.* This is followed by a period of slow passive filling. Finally, near the end of ventricular diastole, the atria contract and complete the emptying of blood out of the upper chambers by propelling it into the ventricles. This final active filling phase is called *presystole, atrial systole,* or sometimes the *"atrial kick."* This action raises left ventricular pressure.

Systole

The filling phases during diastole result in a large amount of blood in the ventricles, causing the pressure in the ventricles to be higher than in the atria. This causes the AV valves (mitral and tricuspid) to shut. Closure of the AV valves produces the first heart sound (S_1), which is the beginning of systole. This valve closure also prevents blood from flowing backward (a process known as *regurgitation*) into the atria during ventricular contraction.

At this point in systole, all four valves are closed and the ventricles contract (isometric contraction). There is now high pressure inside the ventricles, causing the aortic valve to open on the left side of the heart and the pulmonic valve to open on the right side of the heart. Blood is ejected rapidly through these valves. With ventricular emptying, the ventricular pressure falls and the semilunar valves close. This closure produces the second heart sound (S_2), which signals the end of systole. After closure of the semilunar valves, the ventricles relax. Atrial pressure is now higher than the ventricular pressure, causing the AV valves to open and diastolic filling to begin again.

DISPLAY 20-1 Phases of the Electrocardiogram

The phases of the electrocardiogram (ECG), which records depolarization and repolarization of the heart, are assigned letters: P, Q, R, S, and T.

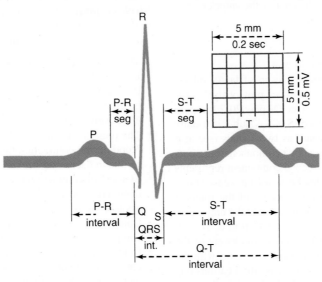

- **P wave:** Atrial depolarization; conduction of the impulse throughout the atria.
- **PR interval:** Time from the beginning of the atrial depolarization to the beginning of ventricular depolarization, that is, from the beginning of the P wave to the beginning of the QRS complex.
- **QRS complex:** Ventricular depolarization (also atrial repolarization); conduction of the impulse throughout the ventricles, which then triggers contraction of the ventricles; measured from the beginning of the Q wave to the end of the S wave.

- **ST segment:** Period between ventricular depolarization and the beginning of ventricular repolarization.
- **T wave:** Ventricular repolarization; the ventricles return to a resting state.
- **QT interval:** Total time for ventricular depolarization and repolarization, that is, from the beginning of the Q wave to the end of the T wave; the QT interval varies with heart rate.
- **U wave:** May or may not be present; if it is present, it follows the T wave and represents the final phase of ventricular repolarization.

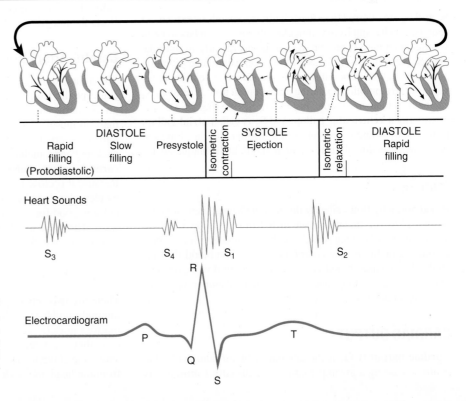

Figure 20-4 The cardiac cycle consists of filling and ejection. Heart sounds S_2, S_3, and S_4 are associated with diastole, while S_1 is associated with systole. The electrical activity of the heart is measured throughout diastole and systole by electrocardiography.

HEART SOUNDS

Heart sounds are produced by valve closure, as described above. The opening of valves is silent. Normal heart sounds, characterized as "lub dubb" (S_1 and S_2), and, occasionally, extra heart sounds and murmurs can be auscultated with a stethoscope over the precordium, the area of the anterior chest overlying the heart and great vessels.

Normal Heart Sounds

The **first heart sound (S_1)** is the result of closure of the AV valves: the mitral and tricuspid valves. As mentioned previously, S_1 correlates with the beginning of systole (see Display 20-2 for more information about S_1 and variations of S_1). S_1 ("lub") is usually heard as one sound but may be heard as two sounds (see also Fig. 20-4). If heard as two sounds, the first component represents mitral valve closure (M_1), and the second component represents tricuspid closure (T_1). M_1 occurs first because of increased pressure on the left side of the heart and because of the route of myocardial depolarization. S_1 may be heard over the entire precordium but is heard best at the apex (left MCL, fifth ICS).

The **second heart sound (S_2)** results from closure of the semilunar valves (aortic and pulmonic) and correlates with the beginning of diastole. S_2 ("dubb") is also usually heard as one sound but may be heard as two sounds. If S_2 is heard as two sounds, the first component represents aortic valve closure (A_2) and the second component represents pulmonic valve closure (P_2). A_2 occurs first because of increased pressure on the left side of the heart and because of the route of myocardial depolarization. If S_2 is heard as two distinct sounds, it is called a *split* S_2. A splitting of S_2 may be exaggerated during inspiration and disappear during expiration. S_2 is heard best at the base of the heart. See Display 20-3 for more information about variations of S_2.

Extra Heart Sounds

S_3 and S_4 are referred to as diastolic filling sounds or extra heart sounds, which result from ventricular vibration secondary to rapid ventricular filling. If present, S_3 can be heard early in diastole, after S_2 (see Fig. 20-4). S_4 also results from ventricular vibration but, contrary to S_3, the vibration is secondary to ventricular resistance (noncompliance) during atrial contraction. If present, S_4 can be heard late in diastole, just before S_1 (see Fig. 20-4). S_3 is often termed **ventricular gallop,** and S_4 is called **atrial gallop.** Extra heart sounds are described further in the Physical Assessment section of the text and in Spotlight Technique 20-1.

Murmurs

Blood normally flows silently through the heart. There are conditions, however, that can create turbulent blood flow in which a swooshing or blowing sound may be auscultated over the precordium. Conditions that contribute to turbulent blood flow include (1) increased blood velocity, (2) structural valve defects, (3) valve malfunction, and (4) abnormal chamber openings (e.g., septal defect).

CARDIAC OUTPUT

Cardiac output (CO) is the amount of blood pumped by the ventricles during a given period of time (usually 1 min) and is determined by the stroke volume (SV) multiplied by the heart rate (HR): $SV \times HR = CO$. The normal adult cardiac output is 5 to 6 L/min.

Stroke Volume

Stroke volume is the amount of blood pumped from the heart with each contraction (stroke volume from the left ventricle is usually 70 mL). Stroke volume is influenced by several factors:

- The degree of stretch of the heart muscle up to a critical length before contraction (preload); the greater the preload, the greater the stroke volume. This holds true unless the heart muscle is stretched so much that it cannot contract effectively.
- The pressure against which the heart muscle has to eject blood during contraction (afterload); increased afterload results in decreased stroke volume.
- Synergy of contraction (i.e., the uniform, synchronized contraction of the myocardium); conditions that cause an asynchronous contraction decrease stroke volume.
- Compliance or distensibility of the ventricles; decreased compliance decreases stroke volume.
- Contractility or the force of contractions of the myocardium under given loading conditions; increased contractility increases stroke volume.

Although cardiac muscle has an innate pattern of contractility, cardiac activity is also mediated by the autonomic nervous system to respond to changing needs. The sympathetic impulses increase heart rate and, therefore, cardiac output. The parasympathetic impulses, which travel to the heart by the vagus nerve, decrease the heart rate and, therefore, decrease cardiac output.

NECK VESSELS

Assessment of the cardiovascular system includes evaluation of the vessels of the neck: the **carotid artery** and the **jugular veins** (Fig. 20-5). Assessment of the pulses of these vessels reflects the integrity of the heart muscle.

Carotid Artery Pulse

The right and left common carotid arteries extend from the brachiocephalic trunk and the aortic arch and are located in the groove between the trachea and the right and left sternocleidomastoid muscles. Slightly below the mandible, each bifurcates into an internal and external carotid artery. They supply the neck and head, including the brain, with oxygenated blood. The **carotid artery pulse** is a centrally located arterial pulse. Because it is close to the heart, the pressure wave pulsation coincides closely with ventricular systole. The carotid arterial pulse is good for assessing amplitude and contour of the pulse wave. The pulse should normally have a smooth, rapid upstroke that occurs in early systole and a more gradual downstroke.

Jugular Venous Pulse and Pressure

There are two sets of jugular veins: internal and external. The internal jugular veins lie deep and medial to the sternocleidomastoid muscle. The external jugular veins are more superficial; they lie lateral to the sternocleidomastoid muscle and above the clavicle. The jugular veins return blood to the heart from the head and neck by way of the superior vena cava.

DISPLAY 20-2   Understanding Normal S₁ Sounds and Variations

S_1, which is the first heart sound, is produced by the atrioventricular (AV) closing. S_1 (the "lub" portion of "lub dubb") correlates with the beginning of systole.

The intensity of S_1 depends on the position of the mitral valve at the start of systole, the structure of the valve leaflets, and how quickly pressure rises in the ventricles. All of these factors influence the speed and amount of closure the valve experiences, which, in turn, determine the amount of sound produced.

➤ **Clinical Tip** • *Normal variations in S_1 are heard at the base and the apex of the heart. S_1 is softer at the base and louder at the apex of the heart. An S_1 may be split along the lower left sternal border, where the tricuspid component of the sound, usually too faint to be heard, can be auscultated. A split S_1 heard over the apex may be an S_4.*

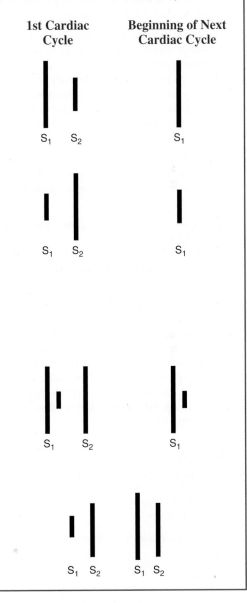

Accentuated S₁

An accentuated S_1 sound is louder than an S_2. This occurs when the mitral valve is wide open and closes quickly. Examples include

- Hyperkinetic states in which blood velocity increases such as fever, anemia, and hyperthyroidism
- Mitral stenosis in which the leaflets are still mobile but increased ventricular pressure is needed to close the valve

Diminished S₁

Sometimes the S_1 sound is softer than the S_2 sound. This occurs when the mitral valve is not fully open at the time of ventricular contraction and valve closing. Examples include

- Delayed conduction from the atria to the ventricles as in first-degree heart block, which allows the mitral valve to drift closed before ventricular contraction closes it
- Mitral insufficiency in which extreme calcification of the valve limits mobility
- Delayed or diminished ventricular contraction arising from forceful atrial contraction into a noncompliant ventricle as in severe pulmonary or systemic hypertension.

Split S₁

As named, a split S_1 occurs as a split sound. This occurs when the left and right ventricles contract at different times (asynchronous ventricular contraction). Examples include

- Conduction delaying the cardiac impulse to one of the ventricles as in bundle branch block
- Ventricular ectopy in which the impulse starts in one ventricle, contracting it first, and then spreading to the second ventricle

Varying S₁

This occurs when the mitral valve is in different positions when contraction occurs. Examples include

- Rhythms in which the atria and ventricles are beating independently of each other
- Totally irregular rhythm such as atrial fibrillation

Assessment of the **jugular venous pulse** is important for determining the hemodynamics of the right side of the heart. The level of the jugular venous pressure reflects right atrial (central venous) pressure and, usually, right ventricular diastolic filling pressure. Right-sided heart failure raises pressure and volume, thus raising jugular venous pressure.

Decreased **jugular venous pressure** occurs with reduced left ventricular output or reduced blood volume. The right internal jugular vein is most directly connected to the right atrium and provides the best assessment of pressure changes. Components of the jugular venous pulse follow:

a wave—reflects rise in atrial pressure that occurs with atrial contraction

x descent—reflects right atrial relaxation and descent of the atrial floor during ventricular systole

(text continues on page 359)

DISPLAY 20-3   Variations in S_2

The S_2 sound depends on the closure of the aortic and the pulmonic valves. Closure of the pulmonic valve is delayed by inspiration, resulting in a split S_2 sound. The components of the split sound are referred to as A_2 (aortic valve sound) and P_2 (pulmonic valve sound). If either sound is absent, no split sounds are heard. The A_2 sound is heard best over the second right intercostal space. P_2 is normally softer than A_2.

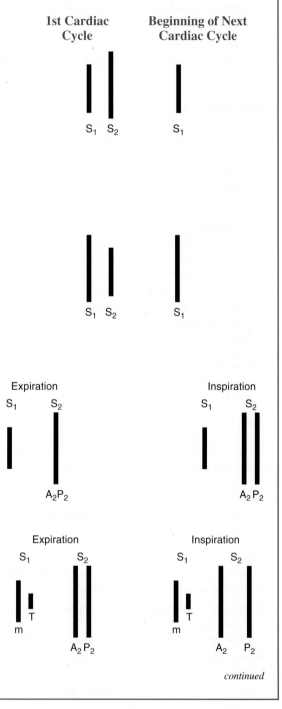

Accentuated S_2

An accentuated S_2 means that S_2 is louder than S_1. This occurs in conditions in which the aortic or pulmonic valve has a higher closing pressure. Examples include

- Increased pressure in the aorta from exercise, excitement, or systemic hypertension (a booming S_2 is heard with systemic hypertension)
- Increased pressure in the pulmonary vasculature, which may occur with mitral stenosis or congestive heart failure
- Calcification of the semilunar valve in which the valve is still mobile as in pulmonic or aortic stenosis

Diminished S_2

A diminished S_2 means that S_2 is softer than S_1. This occurs in conditions in which the aortic or pulmonic valves have decreased mobility. Examples include

- Decreased systemic blood pressure, which weakens the valves, as in shock
- Aortic or pulmonic stenosis in which the valves are thickened and calcified, with decreased mobility

Normal (Physiologic) Split S_2

A normal split S_2 can be heard over the second or third left intercostal space. It is usually heard best during inspiration and disappears during expiration. Over the aortic area and apex, the pulmonic component of S_2 is usually too faint to be heard and S_2 is a single sound resulting from aortic valve closure. In some patients, S_2 may not become single on expiration unless the patient sits up. Splitting that does not disappear during expiration is suggestive of heart disease.

Wide Split S_2

This is an increase in the usual splitting that persists throughout the entire respiratory cycle and widens on expiration. It occurs when there is delayed electrical activation of the right ventricle. Example includes

- Right bundle branch block, which delays pulmonic valve closing

continued

| DISPLAY 20-3 | Variations in S_2 *Continued* |

Fixed Split S_2

This is a wide splitting that does not vary with respiration. It occurs when there is delayed closure of one of the valves. Example includes

- Atrial septal defect and right ventricular failure, which delay pulmonic valve closing

1st Cardiac Cycle — Expiration: S_1 S_2 ($A_2 P_2$)

Beginning of Next Cardiac Cycle — Inspiration: S_1 S_2 ($A_2 P_2$)

Reversed Split S_2

This is a split S_2 that appears on expiration and disappears on inspiration—also known as paradoxical split. It occurs when closure of the aortic valve is abnormally delayed, causing A_2 to follow P_2 in expiration. Normal inspiratory delay of P_2 makes the split disappear during inspiration. Example includes

- Left bundle branch block

Expiration: S_1 S_2 ($A_2 P_2$)

Inspiration: S_1 S_2

Accentuated A_2

An accentuated A_2 is loud over the right, second intercostal space. This occurs with increased pressure as in systemic hypertension and aortic root dilation because of the closer position of the aortic valve to the chest wall.

Diminished A_2

A diminished A_2 is soft or absent over the right, second intercostal space. This occurs with immobility of the aortic valve in calcific aortic stenosis.

Accentuated P_2

An accentuated P_2 is louder than or equal to an A_2 sound. This occurs with pulmonary hypertension, dilated pulmonary artery, and atrial septal defect. A wide split S_2, heard even at the apex, indicates an accentuated P_2.

Diminished P_2

A soft or absent P_2 sound occurs with an increased anteroposterior diameter of the chest (barrel chest), which is associated with aging, pulmonic stenosis, or COPD (chronic obstructive pulmonary disease).

| SPOTLIGHT TECHNIQUE 20-1 | **Auscultating Heart Sounds** |

Most nurses need many hours of practice in auscultating heart sounds to assess a client's health status and interpret findings proficiently and confidently. Practitioners may be able to recognize an abnormal heart sound but may have difficulty determining what and where it is exactly. Continued exposure and experience increase one's ability to determine the exact nature and characteristics of abnormal heart sounds. An added difficulty involves palpation, particularly of the apical impulse in clients who are obese or barrel chested. These conditions increase the distance from the apex of the heart to the precordium.

Where to Auscultate

Heart sounds can be auscultated in the traditional five areas on the precordium, which is the anterior surface of the body overlying the heart and great vessels. The traditional areas include the aortic area, the pulmonic area, Erb's point, the tricuspid area, and the mitral or apical area. The four valve areas do not reflect the anatomic location of the valves. Rather, they reflect the way in which heart sounds radiate to the chest wall. Sounds always travel in the direction of blood flow. For example, sounds that originate in the tricuspid valve are usually best heard along the left lower sternal border at the fourth or fifth intercostal space.

continued on page 358

SPOTLIGHT TECHNIQUE 20-1   Auscultating Heart Sounds *Continued*

Traditional Areas of Auscultation

- Aortic area: Second intercostal space at the right sternal border—the base of the heart
- Pulmonic area: Second or third intercostal space at the left sternal border—the base of the heart
- Erb's point: Third to fifth intercostal space at the left sternal border
- Mitral (apical): Fifth intercostal space near the left midclavicular line—the apex of the heart
- Tricuspid area: Fourth or fifth intercostal space at the left lower sternal border

Alternative Areas

In reality, the areas described above overlap extensively and sounds produced by the valves can be heard all over the precordium. Therefore, it is important to listen to more than just five specific points on the precordium. Keep the fact of overlap in mind and use the names of the chambers instead of Erb's point, mitral, and tricuspid areas when auscultating over the pre-

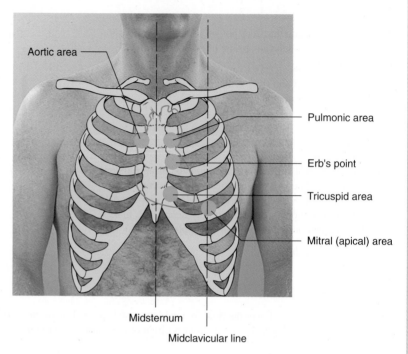

cordium. "Alternative" (versus the traditional) areas of auscultation overlap and are not as discrete as the traditional areas. The alternative areas are the aortic area, pulmonic area, left atrial area, right atrial area, left ventricular area, and right ventricular area.

Cover the entire precordium. As you auscultate in all areas, concentrate on systematically moving the stethoscope from left to right across the entire heart area from the base to the apex (top to bottom) or from the apex to the base (bottom to top).

Alternative Areas of Auscultation

- Aortic area: Right second intercostal space to apex of heart
- Pulmonic area: second and third left intercostal spaces close to sternum but may be higher or lower
- Left atrial area: Second to fourth intercostal space at the left sternal border
- Right atrial area: Third to fifth intercostal space at the right sternal border
- Left ventricular area: Second to fifth intercostal spaces, extending from the left sternal border to the left midclavicular line
- Right ventricular area: Second to fifth intercostal spaces, centered over the sternum

How to Auscultate

Position yourself on the client's right side. The client should be supine with the upper trunk elevated 30 degrees. Use the diaphragm of the stethoscope to auscultate all areas of the precordium for high-pitched sounds. Use the bell of the stethoscope to detect (differentiate) low-pitched sounds or gallops. The diaphragm should be applied firmly to the chest, whereas the bell should be applied lightly.

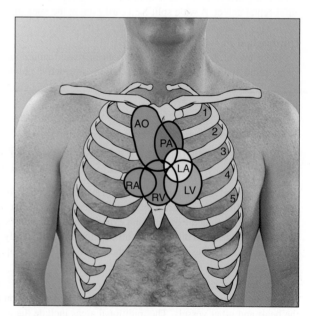

Focus on one sound at a time as you auscultate each area of the precordium. Start by listening to the heart's rate and rhythm. Then identify the first and second heart sounds, concentrate on each heart sound individually, listen for extra heart sounds, listen for murmurs, and finally listen with the client in different positions.

➤ **Clinical Tip** • *Closing your eyes reduces visual stimuli and distractions and may enhance your ability to concentrate on auditory stimuli.*

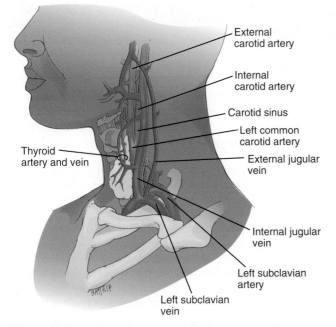

Figure 20-5 Major neck vessels, including the carotid arteries and jugular veins.

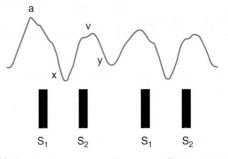

Figure 20-6 Jugular venous pulse wave reflects pressure levels in the heart.

v wave—reflects right atrial filling, increased volume, and increased atrial pressure

y descent—reflects right atrial emptying into the right ventricle and decreased atrial pressure

Figure 20-6 illustrates the jugular venous pulse.

Health Assessment

COLLECTING SUBJECTIVE DATA: THE NURSING HEALTH HISTORY

Subjective data collected about the heart and neck vessels helps the nurse to identify abnormal conditions that may affect the client's ability to perform activities of daily living and to fulfill his role and responsibilities. Data collection also provides information on the client's risk for cardiovascular disease and helps to identify area where health education is needed. The client may not be aware of the significant role that health promotion activities can play in preventing cardiovascular disease.

When compiling the nursing history of current complaints or symptoms, personal and family history, and lifestyle and health practices, remember to thoroughly explore signs and symptoms that the client brings to your attention either intentionally or inadvertently.

(text continues on page 363)

HISTORY OF PRESENT HEALTH CONCERN

Question	Rationale
Chest Pain and Palpitations Do you experience chest pain? When did it start? Describe the type of pain, location, radiation, duration, and how often you experience the pain. Rate the pain on a scale of 0 to 10, with 10 being the worst possible pain. Does activity make the pain worse? Did you have perspiration (diaphoresis) with the chest pain?	Chest pain can be cardiac, pulmonary, muscular, or gastrointestinal in origin. Angina (cardiac chest pain) is usually described as a sensation of squeezing around the heart; a steady, severe pain; and a sense of pressure. It may radiate to the left shoulder and down the left arm or to the jaw. Diaphoresis and pain worsened by activity are usually related to cardiac chest pain.
Do you experience palpitations?	Palpitations may occur with an abnormality of the heart's conduction system or during the heart's attempt to increase cardiac output by increasing the heart rate. Palpitations may cause the client to feel anxious.
Other Symptoms Do you tire easily? Do you experience fatigue? Describe when the fatigue started. Was it sudden or gradual? Do you notice it at any particular time of day?	Fatigue may result from compromised cardiac output. Fatigue related to decreased cardiac output is worse in the evening or as the day progresses.

continued on page 360

HISTORY OF PRESENT HEALTH CONCERN *Continued*

Question	Rationale
Do you have difficulty breathing or shortness of breath (dyspnea)?	Dyspnea may result from congestive heart failure, pulmonary disorders, coronary artery disease, myocardial ischemia, and myocardial infarction. Dyspnea may occur at rest, during sleep, or with mild, moderate, or extreme exertion.
Do you wake up at night with an urgent need to urinate (nocturia)? How many times a night?	Increased renal perfusion during periods of rest or recumbency may cause nocturia. Decreased frequency may be related to decreased cardiac output.
Do you experience dizziness?	Dizziness may indicate decreased blood flow to the brain due to myocardial damage; however, there are several other causes for dizziness such as inner ear syndromes, decreased cerebral circulation, and hypotension. Dizziness may put the client at risk for falls.
Do you experience swelling (edema) in your feet, ankles, or legs?	Edema of the lower extremities may occur as a result of heart failure.
Do you have frequent heart burn? When does it occur? What relieves it? How often do you experience it?	Cardiac pain may be overlooked or misinterpreted as gastrointestinal problems. Gastrointestinal pain may occur after meals and is relieved with antacids, whereas cardiac pain may occur anytime, is not relieved with antacids, and worsens with activity.

COLDSPA Example for Chest Pain

Use the **COLDSPA** mnemonic as a guideline to collect needed information for each symptom the client shares. In addition, the following questions help elicit important information.

Mnemonic	Question	Client Response Example
Character	Describe the sign or symptom (feeling, appearance, sound, smell, or taste if applicable).	"Pressure, chest pain."
Onset	When did it begin?	"Last night after dinner."
Location	Where is it? Does it radiate? Does it occur anywhere else?	"Center of chest and radiates down left arm."
Duration	How long does it last? Does it recur?	"The pressure is constant but the amount of pressure gets worse when I walk or move around."
Severity	How bad is it? or How much does it bother you?	"It bothers me a lot and sometimes it really hurts a lot."
Pattern	What makes it better or worse?	"It goes away a little when I sit down for a while."
Associated factors/ How it **A**ffects the client	What other symptoms occur with it? How does it affect you?	"Sometimes I feel lightheaded, sweaty, and cold. It scares me because I can't do anything."

PAST HEALTH HISTORY

Question	Rationale
Have you been diagnosed with a heart defect or a murmur?	Congenital or acquired defects affect the heart's ability to pump, decreasing the oxygen supply to the tissues.

continued

PAST HEALTH HISTORY *Continued*

Question	Rationale
Have you ever had rheumatic fever?	Approximately 40% of people with rheumatic fever develop rheumatic carditis. Rheumatic carditis develops after exposure to group A beta-hemolytic streptococci and results in inflammation of all layers of the heart, impairing contraction and valvular function.
Have you ever had heart surgery or cardiac balloon interventions?	Previous heart surgery may change the heart sounds heard during auscultation. Surgery and cardiac balloon interventions indicate prior cardiac compromise.
Have you ever had an electrocardiogram (ECG)? When was the last one performed? Do you know the results?	A prior ECG allows the health care team to evaluate for any changes in cardiac conduction or previous myocardial infarction.
Have you ever had a blood test called a lipid profile? Based on your last test, do you know what your cholesterol levels were?	Dyslipidemia presents the greatest risk for the developing coronary artery disease. Elevated cholesterol levels have been linked to the development of atherosclerosis (Lichtenstein et al., 2006).
Do you take medications or use other treatments for heart disease? How often do you take them? Why do you take them?	Clients may have medications prescribed for heart disease but may not take them regularly. Clients may skip taking their diuretics because of having to urinate frequently. Beta-blockers may be omitted because of the adverse effects on sexual energy. Education about medications may be needed.
Do you monitor your own heart rate or blood pressure?	Self-monitoring of heart rate or blood pressure is recommended if the client is taking cardiotonic or antihypertensive medications respectively. A demonstration is necessary to ensure appropriate technique.

FAMILY HISTORY

Question	Rationale
Is there a history of hypertension, myocardial infarction (MI), coronary heart disease (CHD), elevated cholesterol levels, or diabetes mellitus (DM) in your family?	A genetic predisposition to these risk factors increases a client's chance for developing heart disease.

LIFESTYLE AND HEALTH PRACTICES

Question	Rationale
Do you smoke? How many packs of cigarettes per day and for how many years?	Cigarette smoking greatly increases the risk of heart disease (see Promote Health—Coronary Heart Disease).
What type of stress do you have in your life? How do you cope with it?	Stress has been identified as a possible risk factor for heart disease.
Describe what you usually eat in a 24-hour period.	An elevated cholesterol level increases the chance of fatty plaque formation in the coronary vessels.
How much alcohol do you consume each day/week?	Excessive intake of alcohol has been linked to hypertension. More than two drinks per day for men, or one for women, is associated with high blood pressure and other diseases (AHA, 2007).

continued on page 362

LIFESTYLE AND HEALTH PRACTICES *Continued*

Question	*Rationale*
Do you exercise? What type of exercise and how often?	A sedentary lifestyle is a known modifiable risk factor contributing to heart disease. Aerobic exercise three times per week for 30 min is more beneficial than anaerobic exercise or sporadic exercise in preventing heart disease.
Describe your daily activities. How are they different from your routine 5 or 10 years ago? Does fatigue, chest pain, or shortness of breath limit your ability to perform daily activities? Describe. Are you able to care for yourself?	Heart disease may impede the ability to perform daily activities. Exertional dyspnea or fatigue may indicate heart failure. An inability to complete activities of daily living may necessitate a referral for home care.
Has your heart disease had any effect on your sexual activity?	Many clients with heart disease are afraid that sexual activity will precipitate chest pain. If the client can walk one block or climb two flights of stairs without experiencing symptoms, it is generally acceptable for the client to engage in sexual intercourse. Nitroglycerin can be taken before intercourse as a prophylactic for chest pain. In addition, the side-lying position for sexual intercourse may reduce the workload on the heart.
How many pillows do you use to sleep at night? Do you get up to urinate during the night? Do you feel rested in the morning?	If heart function is compromised, cardiac output to the kidneys is reduced during episodes of activity. At rest, cardiac output increases, as does glomerular filtration and urinary output. Orthopnea (the inability to breathe while supine) and nocturia may indicate heart failure. In addition, these two conditions may also impede the ability to get adequate rest.
How important is having a healthy heart to your ability to feel good about yourself and your appearance? What fears about heart disease do you have?	A person's feeling of self-worth may depend on his or her ability to perform usual daily activities and fulfill his or her usual roles.

PROMOTE HEALTH
Coronary Heart Disease

Overview

Coronary heart disease (CHD) is caused by atherosclerosis of the coronary arteries, which restricts blood flow to the coronary tissues. Too much pressure in the arteries makes the walls thick and stiff (arteriosclerosis, or hardening of the arteries). When the coronary arteries are affected, chest pain (angina) or heart attack (myocardial infarction) can occur. Signs and symptoms develop gradually and often do not appear until angina or an MI occurs due to the formation of a blood clot resulting in an inadequate blood supply to the heart tissues. Atherosclerosis may begin as early as childhood and causes are still not clear. It is thought that damage to the inner layer of an artery begins the process. Risk factors may cause the damage or make it worse. The damage causes fatty deposits (plaques) made of cholesterol and other cellular waste products to accumulate and then harden. Thus the space inside the artery is narrowed. Pieces of the fatty deposit may break off and enter the blood stream, and can cause a blood clot to form and further narrow the artery, leading to tissue damage such as a heart attack.

Women have been thought to be less susceptible to coronary heart disease until after menopause. New evidence shows that more women die from heart disease and stroke (480,000 per year) than the total number of cardiovascular-related deaths in men, or from the next five leading causes of death in women (AHA, 2006; Sherrod et al., 2007).

Age is a factor in cardiovascular disease. The World Health Organization (WHO, 2004) has reported that 85% of persons who die of a heart attack are 65 or older, but 80% of heart attack deaths among individuals under 65 years of age occur during the first attack. The lifetime risk of developing CHD after age 40 is 49% for men and 32% for women. About 25% of men and 38% of women are expected to die within 1 year of an initial recognized heart attack.

Ethnicity also plays a role in developing CHD. African Americans, Mexican Americans, American Indians, native Hawaiians, and some Asian Americans have a higher risk of heart disease (AHA, 2006). These rates are thought to be due to more severe hypertension, and higher rates of obesity and diabetes in these populations.

continued

PROMOTE HEALTH
Coronary Heart Disease *Continued*

Risk Factors

- Age: Male over 45; female over 55 (postmenopausal or ovaries removed, and not using estrogen replacement therapy)
- Family history, especially of aneurysm or early heart disease: father or brother diagnosed with CHD before age 55; mother or sister before age 65 (National Heart Lung and Blood Institute, 2007)
- African American, Mexican American, American Indian, native Hawaiian, Asian American (AHA, 2006)
- The metabolic syndrome:
  - Abdominal obesity
  - Blood fat disorders: high triglycerides; low HDL and high LDL cholesterol (total cholesterol above 200 mg/dL; HDL less than 40 mg/dL; LDL above 130 mg/dL)
  - High blood pressure
  - Insulin resistance or glucose intolerance (e.g., diabetes mellitus, especially NIDDM)
  - High fibrinogen or plasminogen activator inhibitor in blood
  - Low grade infection or inflammation (e.g., elevated C-reactive protein in blood) (AHA, 2007)
- Body weight: 20 or more pounds overweight; upper body adiposity (Azevedo et al., 1999).
- Smoking
- Sedentary lifestyle/limited physical activity
- Dietary intake low in antioxidants (especially fruit), high in saturated fat, and low in fiber
- Low birth weight (Lesson et al., 2001)
- Excessive alcohol consumption (more than two drinks per day for men and one for women; leads to obesity, high blood pressure, and other cardiac diseases) (AHA, 2007).
- Stress: Psychological/emotional or physical stress; family relationship stresses; burnout; and daily hassles, especially in women (AHA, 2006)

Teach Risk Reduction Tips
General Tips:

- Stop smoking.
- Lower high blood cholesterol.
- Control high blood pressure.
- Maintain tight control of diabetes.
- Follow a regular exercise plan.
- Achieve and maintain your ideal body weight.
- Control stress and anger.
- Eat a diet low in saturated fat and cholesterol.

More Detailed Tips:

- Stop smoking or seek help from smoking cessation groups to stop smoking.
- Get moving: Establish a regular exercise program with moderate activity such as brisk walking for at least 30 minutes a day.
- Eat a healthy diet: Include fruits, vegetables, and whole grains. Eat foods low in saturated fat, trans fatty acids, cholesterol, and sodium; minimize intake of foods with added sugars. If eating a low carbohydrate diet, make sure most of the fats and proteins are from plant sources rather than meat and dairy sources (Halton et al., 2007).
- Eat 3½ ounces equivalent of cocoa, such as dark chocolate, per day (if not contraindicated) to help lower blood pressure (Taubert, Rpoesen, & Schomig, 2007).
- If overweight, start a weight reduction program.
- Manage stress by reducing personal stress as much as possible. Try muscle relaxation and deep breathing. Seek help from your health care provider if necessary.
- Work with your health care provider to control high blood pressure, diabetes, or blood glucose levels, and other chronic diseases.
- Work with your health care provider to control elevated blood cholesterol.
- Know your family risk of atherosclerosis and CHD.
- If you drink alcohol, limit to one drink per day (women) or two drinks per day (men), especially of red wine. If you do not drink alcohol, do not start (AHA, 2007).
- Women: Consult your primary care provider or your gynecologist about the risk of taking postmenopausal hormone replacement.
- Learn about heart disease and the signs of heart attack:
  - Uncomfortable pressure, fullness, squeezing, or pain in center of chest that lasts for more than a few minutes that may come and go.
  - Pain spreading to shoulders, arms, neck, jaw, or back.
  - Chest discomfort with lightheadedness, fainting, sweating, nausea, or shortness of breath.
  - Women: Shortness of breath, with or without chest discomfort
  - Women: Extreme fatigue; sudden cold sweat

Risk Assessment Tool for Estimating 10-Year Risk of Developing CHD
Self-assessment can be found at the National Cholesterol Education Program website: http://hp2010.nhlbihin.net/atpiii/calculator.asp

COLLECTING OBJECTIVE DATA: PHYSICAL EXAMINATION

A major purpose of this examination is to identify any sign of heart disease and thereby initiate early referral and treatment. Since 1900, cardiovascular disease (CVD) has been the number one killer in the United States every year except 1918 and more than 2,600 Americans die of CVD every day, for an average of one death every 33 seconds (AHA, 2000). Some 60.8 million Americans have one or more types of CVD (AHA, 2001). The National Cholesterol Education Project (NCEP) recommends that all adults age 20 years or older have their total cholesterol and HDL cholesterol levels checked at least once every 5 years.

Assessment of the heart and neck vessels is an essential part of the total cardiovascular examination. It is important to remember that additional data gathered during assessment of the blood pressure, skin, nails, head, thorax and lungs, and peripheral pulses all play a part in the complete cardiovascular assessment. These additional assessment areas are covered in Chapters 7, 13, 14, 18, and 21.

The part of the cardiovascular assessment covered in this chapter involves inspection, palpation, and auscultation of the neck and anterior chest area (precordium). Inspection is a fairly easy skill to acquire. However, auscultation requires a lot of practice to develop expert proficiency. Novice practitioners may be able to recognize an abnormal heart sound but may have difficulty determining what and where it is exactly. Continued exposure and experience increase the practitioner's ability to determine the exact nature and characteristics of abnormal heart sounds. In addition, it may be difficult to palpate the apical impulse in clients who are obese or barrel chested because these conditions increase the distance from the apex of the heart to the precordium.

Heart and neck vessel assessment skills are useful to the nurse in all types of health care settings, including acute, clinical, and home health care.

> **Clinical Tip** • *When performing a total body system examination (see Chapter 26), it is often convenient to assess the heart and neck vessels immediately after assessment of the thorax and lungs.*

Preparing the Client

Prepare clients for the examination by explaining that they will need to expose the anterior chest. Female clients may keep their breasts covered and may simply hold the left breast out of the way when necessary. Explain to the client that she will need to assume several different positions for this examination. Auscultation and palpation of the neck vessels and inspection, palpation, and auscultation of the precordium are performed with the client in the supine position with the head elevated to about 30 degrees. The client will be asked to assume a left lateral position for palpation of the apical impulse if the examiner is having trouble locating the pulse with the client in the supine position. In addition, the client will be asked to assume a left lateral and a sitting-up and leaning-forward position so the examiner can auscultate for the presence of any abnormal heart sounds. These positions may bring out an abnormal sound not detected with the client in the supine position. Make sure you explain to the client that you will be listening to the heart in a number of places and that this does not necessarily mean that anything is wrong. Provide the client with as much modesty as possible during the examination, describe the steps of the examination, and answer any questions the client may have. These actions will help to ease any client anxiety.

Equipment

- Stethoscope with a bell and diaphragm
- Small pillow
- Penlight or movable examination light
- Watch with second hand
- Centimeter rulers (two)

Physical Assessment

Remember these key points during examination:

- Understand the anatomy and function of the heart and major coronary vessels to identify and interpret heart sounds and electrocardiograms accurately.
- Know normal variations of the cardiovascular system in the elderly client.

(text continues on page 378)

PHYSICAL ASSESSMENT

Assessment Procedure	Normal Findings	Abnormal Findings
Neck Vessels		
Inspection **Observe the jugular venous pulse.** Inspect the jugular venous pulse by standing on the right side of the client. The client should be in a supine position with the torso elevated 30 to 45 degrees. Make sure the head and torso are on the same plane. Ask the client to turn the head slightly to the left. Shine a tangential light source onto the neck to increase visualization of pulsations as well as shadows. Next inspect the suprasternal notch or the area around the clavicles for pulsations of the internal jugular veins. > *Clinical Tip* • *Be careful not to confuse pulsations of the carotid arteries with pulsations of the internal jugular veins.*	The jugular venous pulse is not normally visible with the client sitting upright. This position fully distends the vein, and pulsations may or may not be discernible.	Fully distended jugular veins with the client's torso elevated more than 45 degrees indicate increased central venous pressure that may be the result of right ventricular failure, pulmonary hypertension, pulmonary emboli, or cardiac tamponade.

continued

Assessment Procedure	Normal Findings	Abnormal Findings

Evaluate jugular venous pressure. Evaluate jugular venous pressure by watching for distention of the jugular vein. It is normal for the jugular veins to be visible when the client is supine; to evaluate jugular vein distention, position the client in a supine position with the head of the bed elevated 30, 45, 60, and 90 degrees. At each increase of the elevation, have the client's head turned slightly away from the side being evaluated. Using tangential lighting, observe for distention, protrusion, or bulging.

Note: In acute care settings, invasive cardiac monitors (pulmonary artery catheters) are used for precisely measuring pressures.

The jugular vein should not be distended, bulging, or protruding at 45 degrees or greater.

Distention, bulging, or protrusion at 45, 60, or 90 degrees may indicate right-sided heart failure. Document at which positions (45, 60, and/or 90 degrees) you observe distention.

Clients with obstructive pulmonary disease may have elevated venous pressure only during expiration.

An inspiratory increase in venous pressure, called Kussmaul's sign, may occur in clients with severe constrictive pericarditis.

Auscultation and Palpation

Auscultate the carotid arteries. Auscultate the carotid arteries if the client is middle-aged or older or if you suspect cardiovascular disease. Place the bell of the stethoscope over the carotid artery and ask the client to hold his or her breath for a moment so breath sounds do not conceal any vascular sounds (Fig. 20-7).

➤ *Clinical Tip • Always auscultate the carotid arteries before palpating because palpation may increase or slow the heart rate, therefore, changing the strength of the carotid impulse heard.*

Palpate the carotid arteries. Palpate each carotid artery alternately by placing the pads of the index and middle fingers medial to the sternocleidomastoid muscle on the neck (Fig. 20-8). Note amplitude and contour of the pulse, elasticity of the artery, and any thrills.

No blowing or swishing or other sounds are heard.

Pulses are equally strong; a 2+ or normal with no variation in strength from beat to beat. Contour is normally smooth and rapid on the upstroke and slower and less abrupt on the downstroke. Arteries are elastic and no thrills are noted.

The strength of the pulse is evaluated on a scale from 0 to 4 as follows:

Pulse Amplitude Scale
0 = Absent
1+ = Weak
2+ = Normal
3+ = Increased
4+ = Bounding

A bruit, a blowing or swishing sound caused by turbulent blood flow through a narrowed vessel, is indicative of occlusive arterial disease. However, if the artery is more than two-thirds occluded, a bruit may not be heard.

Pulse inequality may indicate arterial constriction or occlusion in one carotid.

Weak pulses may indicate hypovolemia, shock, or decreased cardiac output.

A bounding, firm pulse may indicate hypervolemia or increased cardiac output.

Variations in strength from beat to beat or with respiration are abnormal and may indicate a variety of problems (Abnormal Findings 20-1).

A delayed upstroke may indicate aortic stenosis.

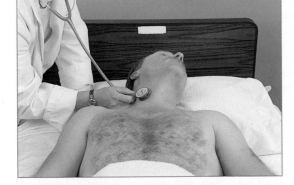

Figure 20-7 Auscultating the carotid artery (© B. Proud).

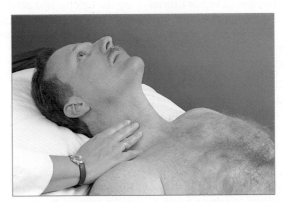

Figure 20-8 Palpating the carotid artery (© B. Proud).

continued

PHYSICAL ASSESSMENT Continued

Assessment Procedure	Normal Findings	Abnormal Findings
➤ **Clinical Tip** • *If you detect occlusion during auscultation, palpate very lightly to avoid blocking circulation or triggering vagal stimulation and bradycardia, hypotension, or even cardiac arrest.* Palpate the carotid arteries individually because bilateral palpation could result in reduced cerebral blood flow. Be cautious with older clients because atherosclerosis may have caused obstruction and compression may easily block circulation.		Loss of elasticity may indicate arteriosclerosis. Thrills may indicate a narrowing of the artery.

Heart (Precordium)

Inspection

Inspect pulsations. With the client in supine position with the head of the bed elevated between 30 and 45 degrees, stand on the client's right side and look for the apical impulse and any abnormal pulsations. ➤ **Clinical Tip** • *The apical impulse was originally called the point of maximal impulse (PMI). However, this term is not used any more because a maximal impulse may occur in other areas of the precordium as a result of abnormal conditions.*	The apical impulse may or may not be visible. If apparent, it would be in the mitral area (left midclavicular line, fourth or fifth intercostal space). The apical impulse is a result of the left ventricle moving outward during systole.	Pulsations, which may also be called heaves or lifts, other than the apical pulsation are considered abnormal and should be evaluated. A heave or lift may occur as the result of an enlarged ventricle from an overload of work. Abnormal Findings 20-2 describes abnormal ventricular impulses.

Palpation

Palpate the apical impulse. Remain on the client's right side and ask the client to remain supine. Use the palmar surfaces of your hand to palpate the apical impulse in the mitral area (fourth or fifth intercostal space at the midclavicular line) (Fig. 20-9A). After locating the pulse, use one finger pad for more accurate palpation (see Fig. 20-9B). ➤ **Clinical Tip** • *If this pulsation cannot be palpated, have the client assume a left lateral position. This displaces the heart toward the left chest wall and relocates the apical impulse farther to the left.*	The apical impulse is palpated in the mitral area and may be the size of a nickel (1 to 2 cm). Amplitude is usually small—like a gentle tap. The duration is brief, lasting through the first two-thirds of systole and often less. In obese clients or clients with large breasts, the apical impulse may not be palpable. In older clients the apical impulse may be difficult to palpate because of increased anteroposterior chest diameter.	The apical impulse may be impossible to palpate in clients with pulmonary emphysema. If the apical impulse is larger than 1 to 2 cm, displaced, more forceful, or of longer duration, suspect cardiac enlargement.
Palpate for abnormal pulsations. Use your palmar surfaces to palpate the apex, left sternal border, and base.	No pulsations or vibrations are palpated in the areas of the apex, left sternal border, or base.	A thrill, which feels similar to a purring cat, or a pulsation is usually associated with a grade IV or higher murmur.

continued

Assessment Procedure	Normal Findings	Abnormal Findings
Auscultation **Auscultate heart rate and rhythm.** Follow the guidelines given in Display 20-4. Place the diaphragm of the stethoscope at the apex and listen closely to the rate and rhythm of the apical impulse.	Rate should be 60 to 100 beats per minute with regular rhythm. A regularly irregular rhythm, such as sinus arrhythmia when the heart rate increases with inspiration and decreases with expiration, may be normal in young adults. Normally the pulse rate in females is 5 to 10 beats per minute faster than in males. Pulse rates do not differ by race or age in adults (Overfield, 1995).	Bradycardia (less than 60 beats/min) or tachycardia (more than 100 beats/min) may result in decreased cardiac output. Clients with irregular rhythms (i.e., premature atrial contraction or premature ventricular contractions) and irregular rhythms (i.e., atrial fibrillation and atrial flutter with varying block) should be referred for further evaluation. These types of irregular patterns may predispose the client to decreased cardiac output, heart failure, or emboli (see Abnormal Findings 20-3).
If you detect an irregular rhythm, auscultate for a pulse rate deficit. This is done by palpating the radial pulse while you auscultate the apical pulse. Count for a full minute.	The radial and apical pulse rates should be identical.	A pulse deficit (difference between the apical and peripheral/radial pulses) may indicate atrial fibrillation, atrial flutter, premature ventricular contractions, and varying degrees of heart block.
Auscultate to identify S_1 and S_2. Auscultate the first heart sound (S_1 or "lub") and the second heart sound (S_2 or "dubb"). Remember these two sounds make up the cardiac cycle of systole and diastole. S_1 starts systole, and S_2 starts diastole. The space, or systolic pause, between S_1 and S_2 is of short duration (thus S_1 and S_2 occur very close together), whereas the space, or diastolic pause, between S_2 and the start of another S_1 is of longer duration. ➤ *Clinical Tip • If you are experiencing difficulty differentiating S_1 from S_2, palpate the carotid pulse: the harsh sound that occurs with the carotid pulse is S_1 (Fig. 20-10).*	S_1 corresponds with each carotid pulsation and is loudest at the apex of the heart. S_2 immediately follows after S_1 and is loudest at the base of the heart.	See Displays 20-2 and 20-3.

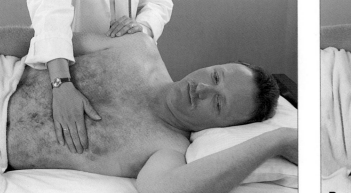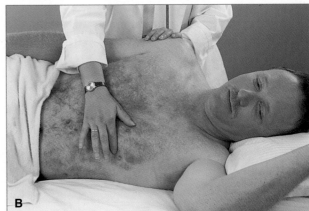

Figure 20-9 Locate the apical impulse with the palmar surface (**A**); then palpate the apical impulse with the finger pad (**B**) (© B. Proud).

continued

PHYSICAL ASSESSMENT *Continued*

Assessment Procedure	Normal Findings	Abnormal Findings
Listen to S_1. Use the diaphragm of the stethoscope to best hear S_1 (Fig. 20-11).	A distinct sound is heard in each area but loudest at the apex. May become softer with inspiration. A split S_1 may be heard normally in young adults at the left lateral sternal border.	Accentuated, diminished, varying, or split S_1 are all abnormal findings (see Display 20-2).
Listen to S_2. Use the diaphragm of the stethoscope. Ask the client to breath regularly. ➤ *Clinical Tip • Do not ask the client to hold his or her breath. Breath holding will cause any normal or abnormal split to subside.*	Distinct sound is heard in each area but is loudest at the base. A split S_2 (into two distinct sounds of its components—A_2 and P_2) is normal and termed *physiologic splitting*. It is usually heard late in inspiration at the second or third left interspaces (see Display 20-3).	Any split S_2 heard in expiration is abnormal. The abnormal split can be one of three types: wide, fixed, or reversed.
Auscultate for extra heart sounds. Use the diaphragm first then the bell to auscultate over the entire heart area. Note the characteristics (e.g., location, timing) of any extra sound heard. Auscultate during the systolic pause (space heard between S_1 and S_2).	Normally no sounds are heard.	Ejection sounds or clicks (e.g., a midsystolic click associated with mitral valve prolapse). A friction rub may also be heard during the systolic pause. Abnormal Findings 20-4 provides a full description of the extra heart sounds (normal and abnormal) of systole and diastole.
Auscultate during the diastolic pause (space heard between end of S_2 and the next S_1). ➤ *Clinical Tip • While auscultating, keep in mind that development of a pathologic S_3 may be the earliest sign of heart failure.*	Normally no sounds are heard. A physiologic S_3 heart sound is a benign finding commonly heard at the beginning of the diastolic pause in children, adolescents, and young adults. It is rare after age 40. The physiologic S_3 usually subsides upon standing or sitting up. A physiologic S_4 heart sound may be heard near the end of diastole in well-conditioned athletes and in adults older than age 40 or 50 with no evidence of heart disease, especially after exercise.	A pathologic S_3 (ventricular gallop) may be heard with ischemic heart disease, hyperkinetic states (e.g., anemia), or restrictive myocardial disease. A pathologic S_4 (atrial gallop) toward the left side of the precordium may be heard with coronary artery disease, hypertensive heart disease, cardiomyopathy, and aortic stenosis. A pathologic S_4 toward the right side of the precordium may be heard with pulmonary hypertension and pulmonic stenosis.

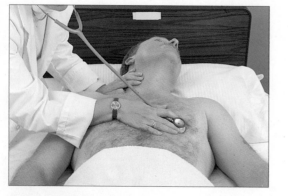

Figure 20-10   Palpating the carotid pulse while auscultating S_1 and S_2 (© B. Proud).

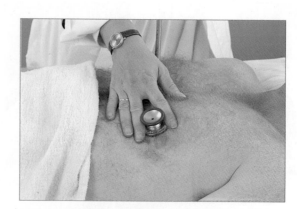

Figure 20-11   Auscultating S_1 (© B. Proud).

continued

Assessment Procedure	Normal Findings	Abnormal Findings
		S_3 and S_4 pathologic sounds together create a quadruple rhythm, which is called a *summation gallop*. Opening snaps occur early in diastole and indicate mitral valve stenosis. A friction rub may also be heard during the diastolic pause (see Abnormal Findings 20-4).
Auscultate for murmurs. A murmur is a swishing sound caused by turbulent blood flow through the heart valves or great vessels. Auscultate for murmurs across the entire heart area. Use the diaphragm and the bell of the stethoscope in all areas of auscultation because murmurs have a variety of pitches. Also auscultate with the client in different positions as described below because some murmurs occur or subside according to the client's position.	Normally no murmurs are heard. However, innocent and physiologic midsystolic murmurs may be present in a healthy heart.	Pathologic midsystolic, pansystolic, and diastolic murmurs. Abnormal Findings 20-5 describes pathologic murmurs.
Auscultate with the client assuming other positions. Ask the client to assume a left lateral position. Use the bell of the stethoscope and listen at the apex of the heart.	S_1 and S_2 heart sounds are normally present.	An S_3 or S_4 heart sound or a murmur of mitral stenosis that was not detected with the client in the supine position may be revealed when the client assumes the left lateral position.
Ask the client to sit up, lean forward, and exhale. Use the diaphragm of the stethoscope and listen over the apex and along the left sternal border (Fig. 20-12).	S_1 and S_2 heart sounds are normally present.	Murmur of aortic regurgitation may be detected when the client assumes this position.

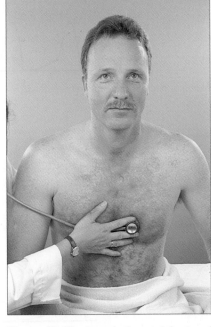

Figure 20-12 Auscultating at left sternal border with client sitting up, leaning forward, and exhaling (© B. Proud).

Abnormal Findings 20-1   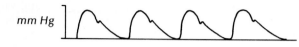   **Abnormal Arterial Pulse and Pressure Waves**

A normal pulse, represented below, has a smooth, rounded wave with a notch on the descending slope. The pulse should feel strong and regular. The notch is not palpable. The pulse pressure (the difference between the systolic and diastolic pressure) is 30 to 40 mmHg. Pulse pressure may be measured in waveforms, which are produced when a pulmonary artery catheter is used to evaluate arterial pressure.

mm Hg

The arterial pressure waveform consists of five parts: Anacrotic limb, systolic peak, dicrotic limb, dicrotic notch, and end diastole. The initial upstroke, or anacrotic limb, occurs as blood is rapidly ejected from the ventricle through the open aortic valve into the aorta. The anacrotic limb ends at the systolic peak, the waveform's highest point. Arterial pressure falls as the blood continues into the peripheral vessels and the waveform turns downward forming the dicrotic limb. When the pressure in the ventricle is less than the pressure in the aortic root, the aortic valve closes and a small notch (dicrotic notch) appears on the waveform. The closing of the aortic notch is the beginning of diastole. The pressure continues to fall in the aortic root until it reaches its lowest point, seen on the waveform as the diastolic peak.

Changes in circulation and heart rhythm affect the pulse and its waveform. Listed below are some of the variations you may find.

Small, Weak Pulse

Characteristics
- Diminished pulse pressure
- Weak and small on palpation
- Slow upstroke
- Prolonged systolic peak

Causes
- Conditions causing a decreased stroke volume
- Heart failure
- Hypovolemia
- Severe aortic stenosis
- Conditions causing increased peripheral resistance
- Hypothermia
- Severe congestive heart failure

Large, Bounding Pulse

Characteristics
- Increased pulse pressure
- Strong and bounding on palpation
- Rapid rise and fall with a brief systolic peak

Causes
- Conditions that cause an increased stroke volume or decreased peripheral resistance
- Fever
- Anemia
- Hyperthyroidism
- Aortic regurgitation
- Patent ductus arteriosus
- Conditions resulting in increased stroke volume due to decreased heart rate
- Bradycardia
- Complete heart block
- Conditions resulting in decreased compliance of the aortic walls
- Aging
- Atherosclerosis

Bisferiens Pulse

Characteristics
- Double systolic peak

Causes
- Pure aortic regurgitation
- Combined aortic stenosis and regurgitation
- Hypertrophic cardiomyopathy

continued

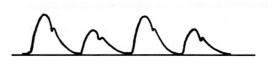

Abnormal Findings 20-1 | **Abnormal Arterial Pulse and Pressure Waves** *Continued*

Pulsus Alternans

Characteristics
- Regular rhythm
- Changes in amplitude (or strength) from beat to beat (you may need a sphygmomanometer to detect the difference)

Causes
- Left ventricular failure (usually accompanied by an S_3 sound on the left)

Bigeminal Pulse

Characteristics
- Regular, irregular rhythm (one normal beat followed by a premature contraction)
- Alternates in amplitude (one strong pulse followed by a quick, weaker one)

Causes
- Premature ventricular contractions

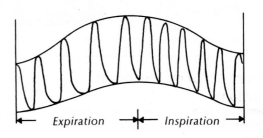

Premature contractions

Paradoxical Pulse

Characteristics
- Palpable decrease in pulse amplitude on quiet inspiration
- Pulse becomes stronger with expiration
- You may need a sphygmomanometer to detect the change (the systolic pressure will decrease by more than 10 mmHg during inspiration)

Causes
- Pericardial tamponade
- Constrictive pericarditis
- Obstructive lung disease

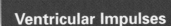

Expiration ◄——►◄ *Inspiration* ——►

Abnormal Findings 20-2 | **Ventricular Impulses**

Assessment of the chest may reveal abnormalities or variations of the ventricular impulse, signs of hypertension, hypertrophy, volume overload, and pressure overload. Some of the abnormalities or variations include the following:

Lift

A diffuse lifting left during systole at the left lower sternal border, a lift or heave is associated with right ventricular hypertrophy caused by pulmonic valve disease, pulmonic hypertension, and chronic lung disease. You may also see retraction at the apex, from the posterior rotation of the left ventricle caused by the oversized right ventricle.

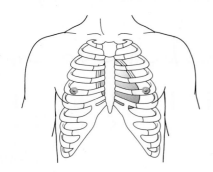

Thrill

A thrill is palpated over the second and third intercostal space; a thrill may indicate severe aortic stenosis and systemic hypertension. A thrill palpated over the second and third left intercostal spaces may indicate pulmonic stenosis and pulmonic hypertension.

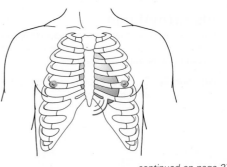

continued on page 372

Abnormal Findings 20-2 | Ventricular Impulses *Continued*

Accentuated Apical Impulse

A sign of pressure overload, the accentuated apical impulse has increased force and duration but is not usually displaced in left ventricular hypertrophy without dilatation associated with aortic stenosis or systemic hypertension.

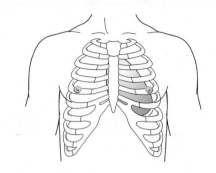

Laterally Displaced Apical Impulse

A sign of volume overload, an apical impulse displaced laterally and found over a wider area is the result of ventricular hypertrophy and dilatation associated with mitral regurgitation, aortic regurgitation, or left-to-right shunts.

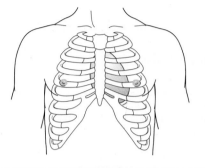

Abnormal Findings 20-3 | Abnormal Heart Rhythms

Changes in the heart rhythm alter the sounds heard on auscultation.

Premature Atrial or Junctional Contractions

These beats occur earlier than the next expected beat and are followed by a pause. The rhythm resumes with the next beat.

Auscultation Tip: The early beat has an S_1 of different intensity and a diminished S_2. S_1 and S_2 are otherwise similar to normal beats.

Premature Ventricular Contractions

These beats occur earlier than the next expected beat and are followed by a pulse. The rhythm resumes with the next beat.

Auscultation Tip: The early beat has an S_1 of different intensity and a diminished S_2. Both sounds are usually split.

Sinus Arrhythmia

With this dysrhythmia, the heart rate speeds up and slows down in a cycle, usually becoming faster with inhalation and slower with expiration.

Auscultation Tip: S_1 and S_2 sounds are usually normal. The S_1 may vary with the heart rate.

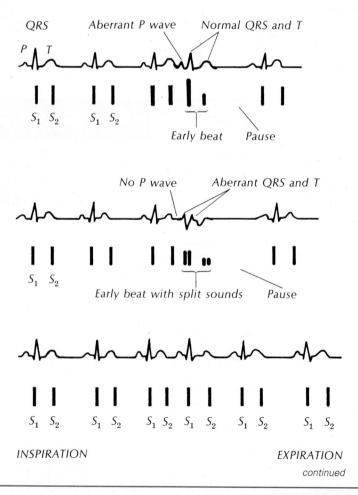

continued

Atrial Fibrillation and Atrial Flutter with Varying Ventricular Response

With this dysrhythmia, ventricular contraction occurs irregularly. At times, short runs of the irregular rhythm may appear regularly.

Auscultation Tip: S_1 varies in intensity.

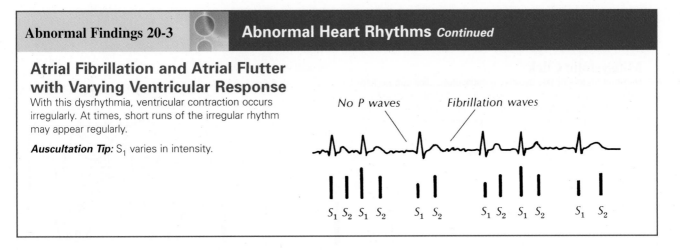

Abnormal Findings 20-4   **Extra Heart Sounds**

Additional heart sounds can be classified by their timing in the cardiac cycle. The presence of the sound during systole or diastole helps in its identification. Some sounds extend into both systole and diastole.

Extra Heart Sounds During Systole—Clicks

High-frequency sounds heard just after S_1 (ejection clicks) are produced by a functioning but diseased valve. Clicks can occur in early or mid-to-late systole and are best heard through the diaphragm of the stethoscope.

Aortic Ejection Click

Heard during early systole at the second right intercostal space and apex, the aortic ejection click occurs with the opening of the aortic valve and does not change with respiration.

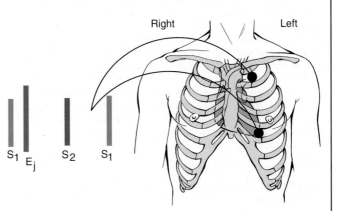

Pulmonic Ejection Click

Best heard at the second left intercostal space during early systole, the pulmonic ejection click often becomes softer with inspiration.

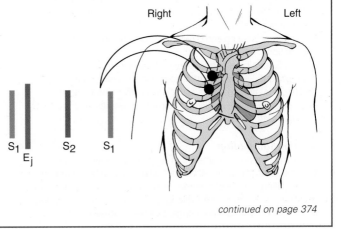

continued on page 374

Midsystolic Click

Heard in middle or late systole, a midsystolic click can be heard over the mitral or apical area and is the result of mitral valve leaflet prolapse during left ventricular emptying. A late systolic murmur typically follows, indicating mild mitral regurgitation.

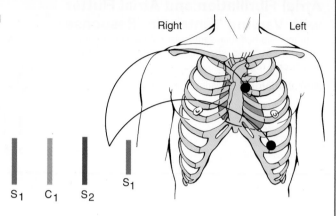

S_1 C_1 S_2 S_1

Right   Left

Extra Heart Sounds During Diastole

Opening Snap

Occurring in early diastole, an opening snap (OS) is heard with the opening of a stenotic or stiff mitral valve. Heard throughout the whole precordium, it does not vary with respirations. Often mistaken for a split S_2 or an S_3, the opening snap occurs earlier in diastole and has a higher pitch than an S_3.

S_3 *(Third Heart Sound)*

Also called a ventricular gallop, the S_3 has a low frequency and is heard best using the bell of the stethoscope at the apical area or lower right ventricular area of the chest with the patient in the left lateral position. The sound is often accentuated during inspiration and has the rhythm of the word "Ken-tuc-ky." S_3 is the result of vibrations caused by the blood hitting the ventricular wall during rapid ventricular filling.

The S_3 can be a normal finding in young children, people with a high cardiac output, and in the third trimester of pregnancy. It is rarely normal in people older than age 40 years and is usually associated with decreased myocardial contractility, myocardial failure, congestive heart failure, and volume overload of the ventricle from valvular disease.

S_4 *(Fourth Heart Sound)*

Also called an atrial gallop, S_4 is a low-frequency sound occurring at the end of diastole when the atria contract. It is caused by vibrations from blood flowing rapidly into the ventricles after atrial contraction. S_4 has the rhythm of the word "Ten-nes-see" and may increase during inspiration. It is best heard with the bell of the stethoscope over the apical area with the patient in a supine or left lateral position and is never heard in the absence of atrial contraction.

The S_4 can be a normal sound in trained athletes and some older patients, especially after exercise. However, it is usually an abnormal finding and is associated with coronary artery disease, hypertension, aortic and pulmonic stenosis, and acute myocardial infarction.

Summation Gallop

The simultaneous occurrence of S_3 and S_4 is called a summation gallop. It is brought about by rapid heart rates in which diastolic filling time is shortened, moving S_3 and S_4 closer together, resulting in one prolonged sound. Summation gallop is associated with severe congestive heart disease.

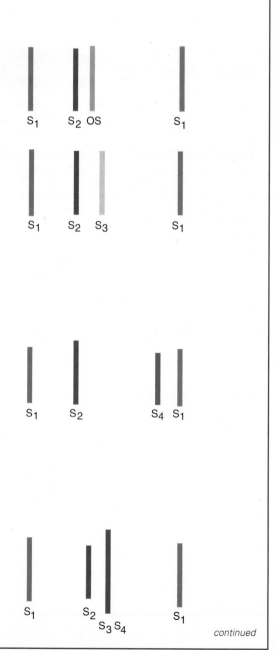

S_1 S_2 OS S_1

S_1 S_2 S_3 S_1

S_1 S_2 S_4 S_1

S_1 S_2 S_3 S_4 S_1

continued

Abnormal Findings 20-4 — Extra Heart Sounds *Continued*

Extra Heart Sounds in Both Systole and Diastole

Pericardial Friction Rub

Usually heard best in the third intercostal space to the left of the sternum, a pericardial friction rub is caused by inflammation of the pericardial sac. A high-pitched, scratchy, scraping sound, the rub may increase with exhalation and when the patient leans forward. For best results, use the diaphragm of the stethoscope and have the patient sit up, lean forward, exhale, and hold his or her breath.

The pericardial friction rub can have up to three components: atrial systole, ventricular systole, and ventricular diastole. These components are associated with cardiac movement. The first two components are usually present. If only one component is present, the rub may be confused with a murmur. Friction rubs are commonly heard during the first week after a myocardial infarction. If a significant pericardial effusion is present, S_1 and S_2 sounds will be distant.

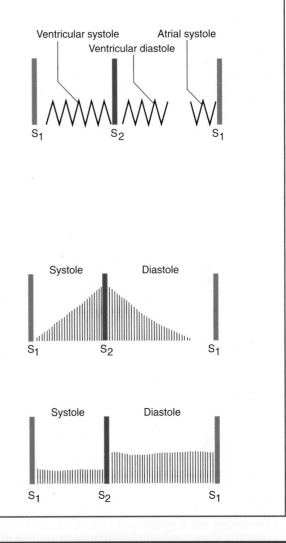

Patent Ductus Arteriosus

Patent ductus arteriosus (PDA) is a congenital anomaly that leaves an open channel between the aorta and pulmonary artery. Found over the second left intercostal space, the murmur of PDA may radiate to the left clavicle. It is classified as a continuous murmur because it extends through systole and into part of diastole. It has a medium pitch and a harsh, machinery-like sound. The murmur is loudest in late systole, obscures S_2, fades in diastole, and often has a silent interval in late diastole.

Venous Hum

Common in children, a venous hum is a benign sound caused by turbulence of blood in the jugular veins. It is heard above the medial third of the clavicles, especially on the right, and may radiate to the first and second intercostal spaces. A low-pitched sound, it is often described as a humming or roaring continuous murmur without a silent interval and is loudest in diastole. A venous hum can be obliterated by putting pressure on the jugular veins.

Abnormal Findings 20-5 — Heart Murmurs

Heart murmurs are typically characterized by turbulent blood flow, which creates a swooshing or blowing sound over the precordium. When listening to the heart, be alert for this turbulence and keep the characteristics of heart murmurs in mind.

Characteristics

Heart murmurs are assessed according to various characteristics, which include timing, intensity, pitch, quality, shape or pattern, location, transmission, and ventilation and position.

Timing

A murmur can occur during systole or diastole. In addition to determining when it occurs, it is important to determine where it occurs, because a systolic murmur can be present in a healthy heart whereas a diastolic murmur always indicates heart disease. Systolic murmurs can be divided into three categories: midsystolic, pansystolic, and late systolic. Diastolic murmurs can be divided into three categories: early diastolic, mid-diastolic, and late diastolic.

Intensity

Six grades describe the intensity of a murmur.

Grade 1: Very faint, heard only after the listener has "tuned in"; may not be heard in all positions
Grade 2: Quiet but heard immediately on placing the stethoscope on the chest
Grade 3: Moderately loud
Grade 4: Loud*
Grade 5: Very loud, may be heard with a stethoscope partly off the chest*
Grade 6: May be heard with the stethoscope entirely off the chest*

continued on page 376

Abnormal Findings 20-5 — Heart Murmurs *Continued*

Pitch
Murmurs can assume a high, medium, or low pitch.

Quality
The sound murmurs make has been described as blowing, rushing, roaring, rumbling, harsh, or musical.

Shape or Pattern
The shape of a murmur is determined by its intensity from beginning to end. There are four different categories of shape: crescendo (growing louder), decrescendo (growing softer), crescendo–decrescendo (growing louder and then growing softer), and plateau (staying the same throughout).

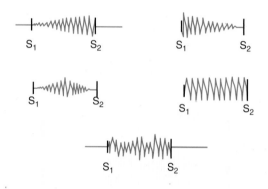

Location
Determine where you can best hear the murmur; this is the point where the murmur originates. Try to be as exact as possible in describing its location. Use the heart landmarks in your description (e.g., the second intercostal space at the left sternal border).

Transmission
The murmur may be felt in areas other than the point of origination. If you determine where the murmur transmits, you can determine the direction of blood flow and the intensity of the murmur.

Ventilation and Position
Determine if the murmur is affected by inspiration, expiration, or a change in body position.

Midsystolic Murmurs
The most common type of heart murmurs, midsystolic murmurs occur during ventricular ejection and can be innocent, physiologic, or pathologic. They have a crescendo-decrescendo shape and usually peak near midsystole and stop before S_2.

Innocent Murmur
Not associated with any physical abnormality, innocent murmurs occur when the ejection of blood into the aorta is turbulent. Very common in children and young adults, they may also be heard in older people with no evidence of cardiovascular disease. A patient may have an innocent murmur and another kind of murmur.

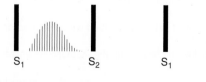

Location: Second to fourth left intercostal spaces between the left sternal border and the apex
Radiation: Little radiation
Intensity: Grade 1 to 2
Pitch: Medium
Quality: Variable
Position: Usually disappear when the patient sits

Physiologic Murmur
Caused by a temporary increase in blood flow, a physiologic murmur can occur with anemia, pregnancy, fever, and hyperthyroidism.

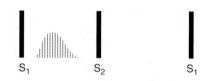

Location: Second to fourth left intercostal spaces between the left sternal border and the apex
Radiation: Little radiation
Intensity: Grade 1 to 2
Pitch: Medium
Quality: Harsh

Murmur of Pulmonic Stenosis
A pathologic murmur, the murmur of pulmonic stenosis occurs from impeded flow across the pulmonic valve and increased right ventricular afterload. Often occuring as a congenital anomaly, the murmur is commonly found in children. Pathologic changes in flow across the valve, as in atrial septal defect, may also mimic this condition.

With severe pulmonic stenosis, the S_2 is widely split and P_2 is diminished. An early pulmonic ejection sound is also common. A right-sided S_4 may also be present, and the right ventricular impulse is often stronger and may be prolonged.

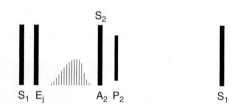

Location: Second and third intercostal spaces
Radiation: Toward the left shoulder and neck
Intensity: Soft to loud (may be associated with a thrill if loud)
Pitch: Medium
Quality: Harsh
Position: Loudest during inspiration

Murmur of Aortic Stenosis
The murmur of aortic stenosis occurs when stenosis of the aortic valve impedes blood flow across the valve and increases left ventricular afterload. Aortic stenosis may result from a congenital anomaly, rheumatic disease, or a degenerative process. Conditions that may mimic this murmur include aortic sclerosis, a bicuspid aortic valve, a dilated aorta, or any condition that mimics the flow across the valve, such as aortic regurgitation.

continued

Abnormal Findings 20-5 ● ● Heart Murmurs *Continued*

If valvular disease is severe, A_2 may be delayed, resulting in an unsplit S_2 or a paradoxical split S_2. An S_4 may occur as a result of decreased left ventricular compliance. An aortic ejection sound, if present, suggests a congenital cause.

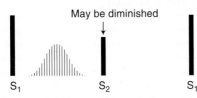

May be diminished

Location: Right second intercostal space
Radiation: May radiate to the neck and down the left sternal border to the apex
Intensity: Usually loud, with a thrill
Pitch: Medium
Quality: Harsh, may be musical at the apex
Position: Heard best with the patient sitting and leaning forward, loudest during expiration

Murmur of Hypertrophic Cardiomyopathy

Caused by unusually rapid ejection of blood from the left ventricle during systole, the murmur of cardiac hypertrophy results from massive hypertrophy of the ventricular muscle. There may be a coexisting obstruction to blood flow. If there is an accompanying distortion of the mitral valve, mitral regurgitation may result. The patient may also have an S_3 and an S_4. There may be a sustained apical impulse with two palpable components.

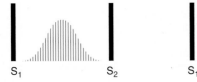

Location: Third and fourth left intercostal space, decreases with squatting, increases with straining down
Intensity: Variable
Pitch: Medium
Quality: Harsh

Pansystolic Murmurs

Occuring when blood flows from a chamber with high pressure to a chamber of low pressure through an orifice that should be closed, pansystolic murmurs are pathologic. Also called *holosystolic murmur,* these murmurs begin with S_1 and continue through systole to S_2.

Murmur of Mitral Regurgitation

Occuring when the mitral valve fails to close fully in systole, the murmur of mitral regurgitation is the result of blood flowing from the left ventricle back into the left atrium. Volume overload occurs in the left ventricle, causing dilatation and hypertrophy.

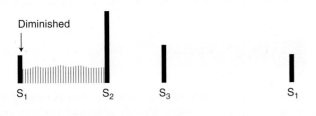

Diminished

The S_1 sound is often decreased, and the apical impulse is stronger and may be prolonged. Left ventricular volume overload should be suspected if an apical S_3 is heard.

Location: Apex
Radiation: To the left axilla, less often to the left sternal border
Intensity: Soft to loud, an apical thrill is associated with loud murmurs
Pitch: Medium to high
Quality: Blowing
Position: Heard best with patient in the left lateral decubitus position, does not become louder with inspiration

Murmur of Tricuspid Regurgitation

Blood flowing from the right ventricle back into the right atrium over a tricuspid valve that has not fully closed causes the murmur of tricuspid regurgitation. Right ventricular failure with dilatation is the most common cause and usually results from pulmonary hypertension or left ventricular failure.

With this murmur, the right ventricular impulse is stronger and may be prolonged. There may be an S_3 along the lower left sternal border and the jugular venous pressure is often elevated with visible *v* waves.

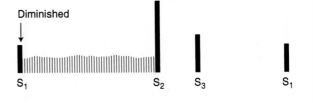

Diminished

Location: Lower left sternal border
Radiation: To the right of the sternum, to the xiphoid area, and sometimes to the midclavicular line; there is no radiation to the axilla
Intensity: Variable
Pitch: Medium to high
Quality: Blowing
Position: May increase slightly with inspiration

Ventricular Septal Defect

A congenital abnormality in which blood flows from the left ventricle into the right ventricle through a hole in the septum, a ventricular septal defect causes a loud murmur that obscures the A_2 sound. Other findings vary depending on the severity of the defect and any associated lesions.

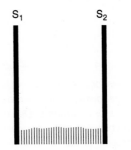

Location: Third, fourth, and fifth left intercostal space
Radiation: Often wide

continued on page 378

Abnormal Findings 20-5 | **Heart Murmurs** *Continued*

Intensity: Very loud, with a thrill
Pitch: High
Quality: Harsh
Position: Increase with exercise

Diastolic Murmurs

Usually indicative of heart disease, diastolic murmurs occur in two types. Early decrescendo diastolic murmurs indicate flow through an incompetent semilunar valve, commonly the aortic valve. Rumbling diastolic murmurs in mid- or late diastole indicate valve stenosis, usually of the mitral valve.

Aortic Regurgitation

Occuring when the leaflets of the aortic valve fail to close completely, the murmur of aortic regurgitation is the result of blood flowing from the aorta back into the left ventricle. This results in left ventricular volume overload. An ejection sound also may be present. Severe regurgitation should be suspected if an S_3 or S_4 is also present. The apical impulse becomes displaced downward and laterally with a widened diameter and increased duration. As the pulse pressure increases, the arterial pulses are often large and bounding.

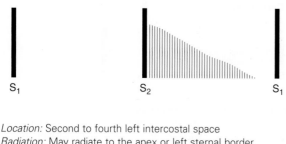

Location: Second to fourth left intercostal space
Radiation: May radiate to the apex or left sternal border
Intensity: Grade 1 to 3
Pitch: High

Quality: Blowing, sometime mistaken for breath sounds
Position: Heard best with the patient sitting, leaning forward. Have the patient exhale and then hold his or her breath.

Murmur of Mitral Stenosis

The murmur of mitral stenosis is the result of blood flow across a diseased mitral valve. Thickened, stiff, distorted leaflets are usually the result of rheumatic fever. The murmur is loud during mid-diastole as the ventricle fills rapidly, grows quiet, and becomes loud again immediately before systole, as the atria contract. In patients with atrial fibrillation, the second half of the murmur is absent because of the lack of atrial contraction.

The patient also has a loud S_1, which may be palpable at the apex. There is often an opening snap (OS) after S_2. P_2 becomes loud and the right ventricular impulse becomes palpable if pulmonary hypertension develops.

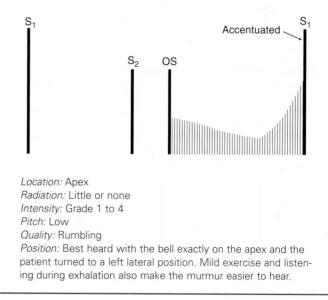

Location: Apex
Radiation: Little or none
Intensity: Grade 1 to 4
Pitch: Low
Quality: Rumbling
Position: Best heard with the bell exactly on the apex and the patient turned to a left lateral position. Mild exercise and listening during exhalation also make the murmur easier to hear.

VALIDATING AND DOCUMENTING FINDINGS

Validate the heart and neck vessel assessment data that you have collected. This is necessary to verify that the data are reliable and accurate. Document the assessment data following the health care facility or agency policy.

Sample of Subjective Data

No chest pain, dyspnea, dizziness, or palpitations. No previous history of cardiovascular disease. Denies rheumatic fever. No current medications or treatments. Denies family history of hypertension, myocardial infarction, coronary heart disease, high cholesterol levels, or diabetes mellitus. Client has never had an ECG. States he needs to exercise more and consume less fat. Client does not monitor own pulse or blood pressure. Denies the use of tobacco. Sleeps 6 to 8 h per night. Feels rested after sleep. States that job can be somewhat stressful.

Sample of Objective Data

Carotid pulse equal bilaterally, 2+, elastic. No bruits auscultated over carotids. Jugular venous pulsation disappears when upright. Jugular venous pressure × 2 cm. No visible pulsations, heaves, or lifts on precordium. Apical impulse palpated in the fifth ICS at the left MCL, approximately the size of a nickel, with no thrill. Apical heart rate auscultated, 70 beats/min, regular rhythm, S_1 heard best at apex, S_2 heard best at base. No S_3 or S_4 auscultated. No splitting of heart sounds, snaps, clicks, or murmurs noted.

Analysis of Data

After collecting subjective and objective data pertaining to the heart and neck vessels, identify abnormal findings and client strengths. Then cluster the data to reveal any significant patterns or abnormalities. These data may be used to make clinical judgments about the status of the client's heart and neck vessels.

DIAGNOSTIC REASONING: POSSIBLE CONCLUSIONS

Selected Nursing Diagnoses

The following is a listing of selected nursing diagnoses that you may identify when analyzing data for this part of the assessment.

Wellness Diagnoses

- Readiness for enhanced cardiac output
- Health-Seeking Behavior: Desired information on exercise and low-fat diet

Risk Diagnoses

- Risk for Sexual Dysfunction related to misinformation or lack of knowledge regarding sexual activity and heart disease
- Risk for Ineffective Denial related to smoking and obesity

Actual Diagnoses

- Fatigue related to decreased cardiac output
- Activity Intolerance related to compromised oxygen transport secondary to heart failure
- Acute Pain: Cardiac related to an inequality between oxygen supply and demand

- Anxiety
- Ineffective Tissue Perfusion: Cardiac related to impaired circulation

Selective Collaborative Problems

After grouping the data, you may see various collaborative problems emerge. Remember that collaborative problems differ from nursing diagnoses in that they cannot be prevented by nursing interventions. However, these physiologic complications of medical conditions can be detected and monitored by the nurse. In addition, the nurse can use physician- and nurse-prescribed interventions to minimize the complications of these problems. The nurse may also have to refer the client in such situations for further treatment of the problem. Following is a list of collaborative problems that may be identified when assessing the heart and neck vessels. These problems are worded as Risk for Complications (or RC) followed by the problem.

- RC: Decreased cardiac output
- RC: Dysrhythmias
- RC: Hypertension
- RC: Congestive heart failure
- RC: Angina
- RC: Cerebrovascular accident
- RC: Cerebral hemorrhage
- RC: Renal failure

Medical Problems

Once the data are grouped, certain signs and symptoms may become evident and may require medical diagnosis and treatment. Referral to a primary care provider is necessary.

CASE STUDY

The case study demonstrates how to analyze thoracic and lung assessment data for a specific client. The critical thinking exercises included in the study guide/lab manual and interactive product that complement this text also offer opportunities to analyze assessment data.

Malcolm Winchester is being admitted to the coronary care unit (CCU) with a diagnosis of hypertension, angina, R/O MI (myocardial infarction). He is a tall, slender black man who looks younger than his stated age of 45. He is in no acute distress. Mr. Winchester says, "I don't know why they brought me here— I guess my wife panicked and called 911. I have these pains all of the time, but my doc said they were from my high blood pressure. I don't hurt now."

His wife arrives, looking pale and anxious. "I don't know what to do with him. I work so hard to keep him healthy, but he goes out to that fast food place and eats burgers and fries. I'm so tired of dealing with him when he won't help himself." Mr. Winchester grins and says, "I just got to have my junk food! That low-fat, low-salt diet my doctor put me on is impossible."

Physical assessment reveals BP 210/110 right arm reclining and 200/108 left arm reclining, pulse 88 regular and strong, respirations 16 regular and moderately shallow, temperature 36.5°C (97.7°F). His apical beat is also 88 and strong; heart sounds: S_1 and S_2 with no murmurs and clicks, but an S_4 is noted. Evaluation of the thorax reveals no heaves or visible pulsation. Neck veins are flat at >45 degrees and no carotid bruits noted. Skin is warm and dry, dark brown with pink nail beds, palms, and oral mucous membranes. Pedal pulses strong; 1 + ankle edema present.

The following concept map illustrates the diagnostic reasoning process.

Applying COLDSPA

Applying **COLDSPA** for client symptoms: "high blood pressure/chest pain."

Mnemonic	Question	Data Provided	Missing Data
Character	Describe the sign or symptom (feeling, appearance, sound, smell, or taste if applicable).	"I have these pains all the time; I don't hurt now."	"Describe how the pains feel to you."
Onset	When did it begin?		"When did the chest pain first start this time?"
Location	Where is it? Does it radiate? Does it occur anywhere else?		"Point to where the pain was. Does it spread down your arm? To your back? Anywhere else?"
Duration	How long does it last? Does it recur?		"How long does the pain last when it occurs? How often does the pain recur?"
Severity	How bad is it? or How much does it bother you?		"Describe the intensity of the pain on a scale of 1 to 10 with 10 being the worst possible."
Pattern	What makes it better or worse?		"What makes the chest pains come and go?
Associated factors/How it **A**ffects the client	What other symptoms occur with it? How does it affect you?	"My doctor said these pains were from my high blood pressure."	"When you have the chest pain, does it affect what you are doing?"

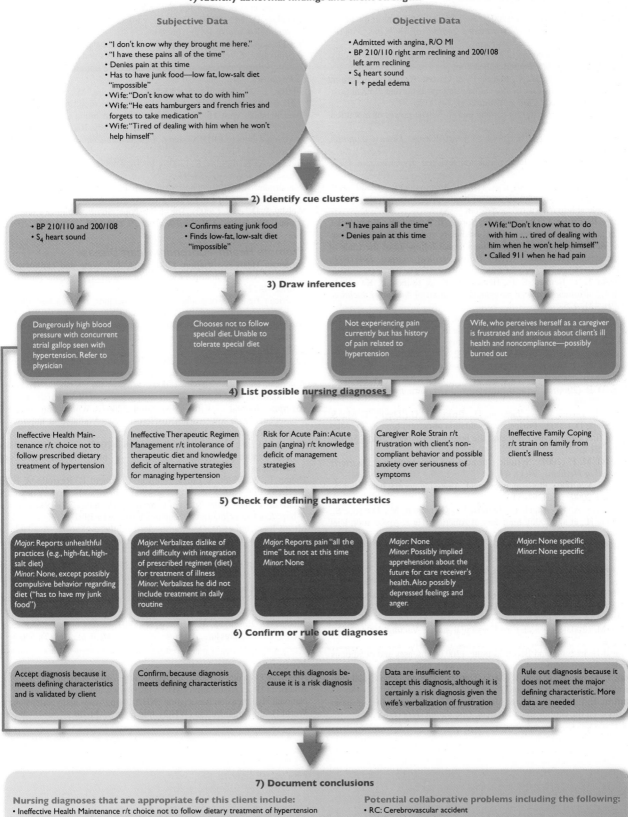

1) Identify abnormal findings and client strengths

Subjective Data
- "I don't know why they brought me here."
- "I have these pains all of the time"
- Denies pain at this time
- Has to have junk food—low fat, low-salt diet "impossible"
- Wife: "Don't know what to do with him"
- Wife: "He eats hamburgers and french fries and forgets to take medication"
- Wife: "Tired of dealing with him when he won't help himself"

Objective Data
- Admitted with angina, R/O MI
- BP 210/110 right arm reclining and 200/108 left arm reclining
- S_4 heart sound
- 1 + pedal edema

2) Identify cue clusters

- BP 210/110 and 200/108
- S_4 heart sound

- Confirms eating junk food
- Finds low-fat, low-salt diet "impossible"

- "I have pains all the time"
- Denies pain at this time

- Wife: "Don't know what to do with him … tired of dealing with him when he won't help himself"
- Called 911 when he had pain

3) Draw inferences

Dangerously high blood pressure with concurrent atrial gallop seen with hypertension. Refer to physician

Chooses not to follow special diet. Unable to tolerate special diet

Not experiencing pain currently but has history of pain related to hypertension

Wife, who perceives herself as a caregiver is frustrated and anxious about client's ill health and noncompliance—possibly burned out

4) List possible nursing diagnoses

Ineffective Health Maintenance r/t choice not to follow prescribed dietary treatment of hypertension

Ineffective Therapeutic Regimen Management r/t intolerance of therapeutic diet and knowledge deficit of alternative strategies for managing hypertension

Risk for Acute Pain: Acute pain (angina) r/t knowledge deficit of management strategies

Caregiver Role Strain r/t frustration with client's non-compliant behavior and possible anxiety over seriousness of symptoms

Ineffective Family Coping r/t strain on family from client's illness

5) Check for defining characteristics

Major: Reports unhealthful practices (e.g., high-fat, high-salt diet)
Minor: None, except possibly compulsive behavior regarding diet ("has to have my junk food")

Major: Verbalizes dislike of and difficulty with integration of prescribed regimen (diet) for treatment of illness
Minor: Verbalizes he did not include treatment in daily routine

Major: Reports pain "all the time" but not at this time
Minor: None

Major: None
Minor: Possibly implied apprehension about the future for care receiver's health. Also possibly depressed feelings and anger.

Major: None specific
Minor: None specific

6) Confirm or rule out diagnoses

Accept diagnosis because it meets defining characteristics and is validated by client

Confirm, because diagnosis meets defining characteristics

Accept this diagnosis because it is a risk diagnosis

Data are insufficient to accept this diagnosis, although it is certainly a risk diagnosis given the wife's verbalization of frustration

Rule out diagnosis because it does not meet the major defining characteristic. More data are needed

7) Document conclusions

Nursing diagnoses that are appropriate for this client include:
- Ineffective Health Maintenance r/t choice not to follow dietary treatment of hypertension
- Ineffective Therapeutic Regimen Management r/t intolerance of therapeutic diet and knowledge deficit of alternative strategies for managing hypertension
- Risk for Acute Pain: acute pain (angina) r/t knowledge deficit of management strategies

Potential collaborative problems including the following:
- RC: Cerebrovascular accident
- RC: Retinal hemorrhage
- RC: Myocardial infarction
- RC: Heart failure
- RC: Renal failure

References and Selected Readings

Adrogue, H. J., & Madias, N. (2007). Sodium and potassium in the pathogenesis of hypertension. *New England Journal of Medicine, 356*(19), 1966–1978.

American Heart Association. (2007). Alcohol, wine and cardiovascular disease. Available at http://americanheart.org

Archbold, R. A., Barakat, K., Magee, P., & Curzen, N. (2001). Screening for carotid artery disease before cardiac surgery: Is current clinical practice evidence based? *Clinical Cardiology, 24*(1), 26–32.

Barett et al. (2004). Mastering cardiac murmurs: The power of repetition. *Chest, 126,* 470–475.

Chizner, M. (2003). The diagnosis of heart disease. *Disease-a month, 48*(1), 7–98.

Chobanian, A. V. (2006). Prehypertension revisited. *Hypertension, 48*(5), 812–814.

Cinà, C., Clase, C., & Radan, A. (2006). Asymptomatic carotid bruit: Assessment of asymptomatic carotid bruit. From ACS Surgery Online. Available at http://www.medscape.com

Cook, N. R., Cutler, J., Obarzanek, E., Buring, J., Rexrode K., Kumanyika, S. et al. (2007). Long term effects of dietary sodium reduction on cardiovascular disease outcomes: Observational follow-up of the trials of hypertension prevention (TOHP). *British Medical Journal, 334*(7599), 885.

Davidson, L. J., Bennett, S. E., Hamera, E. K., & Raines, B. K. (2004). What constitutes advanced assessment? *Journal of Nursing Education, 43*(9), 421–425.

Daviglus, M. L., Stamler, J., Pirzada, A., Yan, L. L., Garside, D. B., Liu, K., et al. (2004). Favorable cardiac risk profile in young women and low risk of cardiovascular and all-cause mortality. *Journal of the American Medical Association, 292*(13), 1588–1592.

Dulak, S. B. (2004). Hands-on help: Assessing heart sounds. *RN, 67*(8), 241–244.

Fabius, D. B. (2000). Solving the mystery of heart murmurs. *Nursing 2000, 30*(7), 39–44.

Gillett, M., Davis, W. A., Jackson, D., Bruce, D. G., Davis, T. M., & Fremantle D. (2003). Prospective evaluation of carotid bruit as a predictor of first sign of type 2 diabetes: the Fremantle Diabetes Study. *Stroke, 34*(9), 2145–2151.

Jolobe, O. M. P. (2001). Systolic murmurs and aortic stenosis. *Quarterly Journal of Medicine, 94*(1), 49.

Kirton, C. A. (2000). Physical assessment. Assessing normal heart sounds. *Nursing 2000, 30*(2), 52–54.

Lichtenstein, A. H., Appel, L., Brands, M., Carnethon, M., Daniels, S., Franch, H., et al. (2006). Summary of American Heart Association Diet and Lifestyle Recommendations Revision 2006. *Arteriosclerosis, Thrombosis and Vascular Biology, 26*(7), 2186–2191.

Loveridge, M. (2003). Acquiring percussion and auscultation skills through experiential learning. *Emergency Nurse, 11*(6), 31–37.

McLean, D., Kingsbury, K., Costello, J., Cloutier, L., & Matheson, S. (2007). 2007 Hypertension Education Program (CHEP) recommendations: Management of hypertension by nurses. *Canadian Journal of Cardiovascular Nursing, 17*(2), 10–16.

Mehta, M. (2003). Assessing cardiovascular status. *Nursing 2003, 33*(1), 56–58.

National Heart Lung and Blood Institute. (2007). Diseases and conditions index: Atherosclerosis. Available at http://www.nhlbi.nih.gov

Nirav, J., Mehta, M., & Ijaz, A. (2003). Third heart sound: Genesis and clinical importance. *International Journal of Cardiology, 97*(2), 183–186.

Schiffrin, E. L., Lipman, M., & Mann, J. (2007). Chronic kidney disease: Effects on the cardiovascular system. *Circulation, 116*(1), 85–97.

Scott, C., & MacInnes, F. D. (2006). Cardiac patient assessment: Putting the patient first. *British Journal of Nursing, 15*(9), 502–508.

Shindler, D. M. (2007). Practical cardiac auscultation. *Critical Care Nursing Quarterly 30*(2), 166–80.

Soudarssanane, M. B., Karthigeyan, M., Mahalakshmy, T., Sahai, A., Srinivasan, S., et al. (2007). Rheumatic fever and rheumatic heart disease: Primary prevention is the cost effective option. *Indian Journal of Pediatrics, 74*(6), 567–570.

Steffen, L. M., Kroenke, C., Xinhua, Y., Pereira, M., Slattery, M., Van Hzorn, L., et al. (2005). Association of plant food, dairy product, and meat intake with 15-y incidence of elevated blood pressure in young black and white adults: The Coronary Artery Risk Development in Young Adults (CARDIA) study. *American Journal of Clinical Nutrition, 82*(6), 1169–1177.

Todd, B. A., & Higgins, K. (2005). Recognizing aortic & mitral valve disease. *Nursing, 35*(6), 58–93.

Wasserman, A. (2000). Chest pain. Is it life – threatening – or benign? *Consultant, 40*(7), 1204–1208.

Welsby, P. D., et al. (2003). The stethoscope: Some preliminary investigations. *Postgraduate Medical Journal 79,* 695–698.

Promote Health—Coronary Heart Disease

American Heart Association. (2007). Alcohol, wine and cardiovascular disease. Available at http://www.americanheart.org/presenter.jhtml?identifier=4422

American Heart Association. (2006). Association releases new diet and lifestyle recommendations. Available at http://americanheart.org

American Heart Association. (2006). Risk factors and coronary heart disease. Available at http://americanheart.org/presenter.jhtml?identifier=47265

American Heart Association. (2006). What are healthy levels of cholesterol? Available at http://americanheart.org/presenter.jhtml?identifier=183

American Heart Association. (2007). What is the metabolic syndrome? Available at http://americanheart.org/presenter.jhtml?identifier=4756

American Journal of Clinical Nutrition. (2007). Whole-grain intake is associated with lowered atherosclerosis risk. Available at http://www.ajcn.org/misc/release1.shtml

Cleveland Clinic Heart & Vascular Institute. (2007). Coronary artery disease treatment—Medical. Available at http://clevelandclinic.org/heartcenter

Halton T., W. Willet, S. Liu, J. Manson, C. Albert, K. Rexrode, & F. Hu (2006). Low-carbohydrate-diet score and the risk of coronary heart disease in women. *New England Journal of Medicine,* 355(19). Available http://content.nejm.org/cgi/content/short/355/19/1991

MayoClinic.com. (2007). Arteriosclerosis/atherosclerosis. Available at http://www.mayoclinic.com/health/arteriosclerosis-atherosclerosis/DS00525

National Heart Lung and Blood Institute. (2007). Who is at risk for atherosclerosis. Available at http://www.nhlbi.nih.gov/health/dci/Diseases/Atherosclerosis/atherosclerosis_risk

Sherrod, M., Albarez, Y., Brookshire, A., & Cheek, D. (2007). A woman's worst enemy. *American Nurse Today,* 2(2), 25–29.

Taubert, D., Rosen, R., & Schomig, E. (2007). Effect of cocoa and tea intake on blood pressure. *Archives of Internal Medicine,* 167(7), 626–634.

Websites

American Dietetics Association (ADA). http://www.eatright.org
American Heart Association (AHA). http://www.americanheart.org
National Hypertension Association (NHA). http://www.nathypertension.org
World Health Organization (WHO). http://www.who.int

Peripheral Vascular System

Structure and Function

To perform a thorough peripheral vascular assessment, the nurse needs to understand the structure and function of the arteries and veins of the arms and legs, the lymphatic system, and the capillaries. Equally important is an understanding of fluid exchange. The information provided on these pages can help you compile subjective and objective data related to the peripheral vascular system and differentiate normal vascular findings from normal variations and abnormalities.

ARTERIES

Arteries are the blood vessels that carry oxygenated, nutrient-rich blood from the heart to the capillaries. The arterial network is a high-pressure system. Blood is propelled under pressure from the left ventricle of the heart. Because of this high pressure, arterial walls must be thick and strong; the arterial walls also contain elastic fibers so they can stretch. Figure 21-1 illustrates the layers and the relative thickness of arterial walls. Each heartbeat forces blood through the arterial vessels under high pressure, creating a surge. This surge of blood is the **arterial pulse.** The pulse can be felt only by lightly compressing a superficial artery against an underlying bone. Many arteries are located in protected areas, far from the surface of the skin. Therefore, the arteries discussed in this chapter include only major arteries of the arms and legs—the **peripheral arteries**—that are accessible to examination. The other major arteries accessible to examination—temporal, carotid, and aorta—are discussed in Chapters 14, 20, and 22, respectively.

Major Arteries of the Arm

The **brachial artery** is the major artery that supplies the arm. The brachial pulse can be palpated medial to the biceps tendon in and above the bend of the elbow. The brachial artery divides near the elbow to become the **radial artery** (extending down the thumb side of the arm) and the **ulnar artery** (extending down the little finger side of the arm). Both of these arteries provide blood to the hand. The **radial pulse** can be palpated on the

lateral aspect of the wrist. The **ulnar pulse,** located on the medial aspect of the wrist, is a deeper pulse and may not be easily palpated. The radial and ulnar arteries join to form two arches just below their pulse sites. The superficial and deep **palmar arches** provide extra protection against arterial occlusion to the hands and fingers (Fig. 21-2).

Major Arteries of the Leg

The **femoral artery** is the major supplier of blood to the legs. Its pulse can be palpated just under the inguinal ligament. This artery travels down the front of the thigh then crosses to the back of the thigh, where it is termed the popliteal artery. The **popliteal pulse** can be palpated behind the knee. The **popliteal artery** divides below the knee into anterior and posterior branches. The anterior branch descends down the top of the foot, where it becomes the **dorsalis pedis artery.** Its pulse can be palpated on the great toe side of the top of the foot. The posterior branch is called the **posterior tibial artery.** The posterior tibial pulse can be palpated behind the medial malleolus of the ankle. The dorsalis pedis artery and posterior tibial artery form the **dorsal arch,** which, like the superficial and deep palmar arches of the hands, provides the feet and toes with extra protection from arterial occlusion (see Fig. 21-2). For a discussion of pulse measurement, see Assessment Tool 21-1.

VEINS

Veins are the blood vessels that carry deoxygenated, nutrient-depleted, waste-laden blood from the tissues back to the heart. The veins of the arms, upper trunk, head, and neck carry blood to the superior vena cava, where it passes into the right atrium. Blood from the lower trunk and legs drains upward into the inferior vena cava. The veins contain nearly 70% of the body's blood volume. Because blood in the veins is carried under much lower pressure than in the arteries, the vein walls are much thinner (see Fig. 21-1). In addition, veins are larger in diameter than arteries and can expand if blood volume increases. This helps to reduce the workload on the heart.

This chapter focuses on those veins that are most susceptible to dysfunction: the three types of veins in the legs. Two

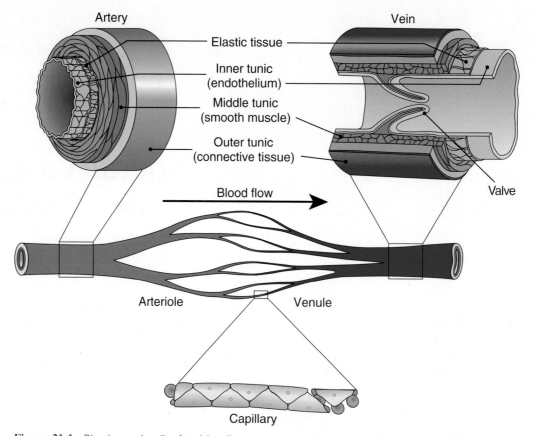

Figure 21-1 Blood vessel walls. Arterial walls are constructed to accommodate the high pulsing pressure of blood transported by the pumping heart, whereas venous walls are constructed with valves that promote the return of blood and prevent backflow.

other major veins that are important to assess—the internal and external jugular veins—are discussed in Chapter 20.

There are three types of veins: **deep veins, superficial veins,** and **perforator (or communicator) veins.** The two deep veins in the leg are the **femoral vein** in the upper thigh and the **popliteal vein** located behind the knee. These veins account for about 90% of venous return from the lower extremities. The superficial veins are the great and small **saphenous veins.** The great saphenous vein is the longest of all veins and extends from the medial dorsal aspect of the foot, crosses over the medial malleolus, and continues across the thigh to the medial aspect of the groin, where it joins the femoral vein. The small saphenous vein begins at the lateral dorsal aspect of the foot, travels up behind the lateral malleolus on the back of the leg, and joins the popliteal vein. The perforator veins connect the superficial veins with the deep veins (Fig. 21-3).

Veins differ from arteries in that there is no force that propels forward blood flow; the venous system is a low-pressure system. This fact is of special concern in the veins of the leg. Blood from the legs and lower trunk must flow upward with no help from the pumping action of the heart. Three mechanisms of venous function help to propel blood back to the heart. The first mechanism has to do with the structure of the veins. Deep, superficial, and perforator veins all contain one-way valves. These valves permit blood to pass through them on the way to the heart and they prevent blood from returning through them in the opposite direction. The second mechanism is muscular contraction. Skeletal muscles contract with movement and, in effect, squeeze blood toward the heart through the one-way valves. The third mechanism is the creation of a pressure

gradient through the act of breathing. Inspiration decreases intrathoracic pressure while increasing abdominal pressure, thus producing a pressure gradient.

If there is a problem with any of these mechanisms, venous return is impeded and **venous stasis** results. Risk factors for venous stasis include long periods of standing still, sitting, or lying down. Lack of muscular activity causes blood to pool in the legs, which, in turn, increases pressure in the veins. Other causes of venous stasis include varicose (tortuous and dilated) veins, which increase venous pressure. Damage to the vein wall can also contribute to venous stasis.

CAPILLARIES AND FLUID EXCHANGE

Capillaries are small blood vessels that form the connection between the arterioles and venules and allow the circulatory system to maintain the vital equilibrium between the vascular and interstitial spaces. Oxygen, water, and nutrients in the interstitial fluid are delivered by the arterial vessels to the microscopic capillaries (Fig. 21-4). Hydrostatic force (generated by the blood pressure) is the primary mechanism by which the interstitial fluid diffuses out of the capillaries and enters the tissue space. The interstitial fluid releases the oxygen, water, and nutrients and picks up waste products such as carbon dioxide and other by-products of cellular metabolism. The fluid then reenters the capillaries by osmotic pressure and is transported away from the tissues and interstitial spaces by venous circulation. As mentioned previously, the lymphatic capillaries function to remove any excess fluid left behind in

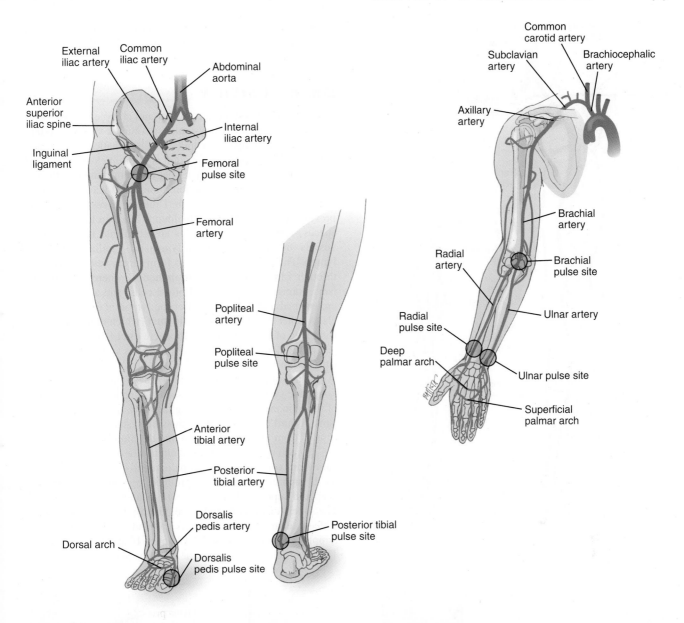

Figure 21-2 Major arteries of the arms and legs.

ASSESSMENT TOOL 21-1	Assessing Pulse Strength

Palpation of the pulses in the peripheral vascular examination is typically to assess amplitude or strength. Pulse amplitude is graded on a 0 to 4+ scale, with 4+ being the strongest. Elasticity of the artery wall may also be noted during the peripheral vascular examination, by palpating for a resilient (bouncy) quality rather than a more rigid arterial tone, whereas pulse rate and rhythm are best assessed during examination of the heart and neck vessels. (See Chapter 20.)

Pulse Amplitude

Pulse amplitude is typically graded as 0 to 4+:

0 (absent pulse)	Pulse cannot be felt, even with the application of extreme pressure.
1+ (thready pulse)	Pulse is very difficult to feel, and applying slight pressure causes pulse to disappear.
2+ (weak pulse)	Pulse is stronger than a thready pulse, but applying light pressure causes pulse to disappear.
3+ (normal pulse)	Pulse is easily felt and requires moderate pressure to make it disappear.
4+ (bounding pulse)	Pulse is strong and does not disappear with moderate pressure.

Lynn, P. (2008). *Taylor's clinical nursing skills: A nursing process approach* (2nd ed.). Wolters Kluwer/Lippincott Williams & Wilkins; p. 17.

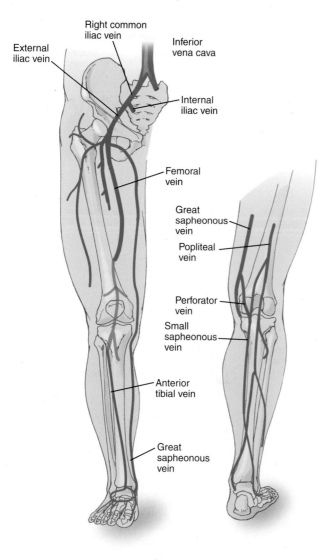

Figure 21-3 Major veins of the legs.

the interstitial spaces. Thus, the capillary bed is very important in maintaining the equilibrium of interstitial fluid and preventing edema.

LYMPHATIC SYSTEM

The **lymphatic system,** an integral and complementary component of the circulatory system, is a complex vascular system composed of lymphatic capillaries, lymphatic vessels, and lymph nodes. Its primary function is to drain excess fluid and plasma proteins from bodily tissues and return them to the venous system. During circulation, more fluid leaves the capillaries than the veins can absorb. Draining excess fluid action prevents edema, which is a buildup of fluid in the interstitial spaces. The fluids and proteins absorbed into the lymphatic vessels by the microscopic lymphatic capillaries become lymph. These capillaries join to form larger vessels that pass through filters known as **lymph nodes,** where microorganisms, foreign materials, dead blood cells, and abnormal cells are trapped and destroyed. After the lymph is filtered, it travels to either the **right lymphatic duct** (which drains the upper right side of the body) or the **thoracic duct** (which drains the rest of the body) then back into the venous system through the **subclavian veins** (Fig. 21-5).

This unique filtering feature of the lymph nodes allows the lymphatic system to perform a second function as a major part of the immune system defending the body against microorganisms. A third function of the lymphatic system is to absorb fats (lipids) from the small intestine into the bloodstream.

Lymph nodes are somewhat circular or oval. Normally they vary from very small and nonpalpable to 1 to 2 cm in diameter. Lymph nodes tend to be grouped together. They are both deep and superficial, and many are located near major joints. The superficial lymph nodes are the only lymph nodes accessible to examination. The cervical and axillary superficial lymph nodes are discussed in Chapters 14 and 19, respectively. The superficial lymph nodes of the arms and legs assessed in

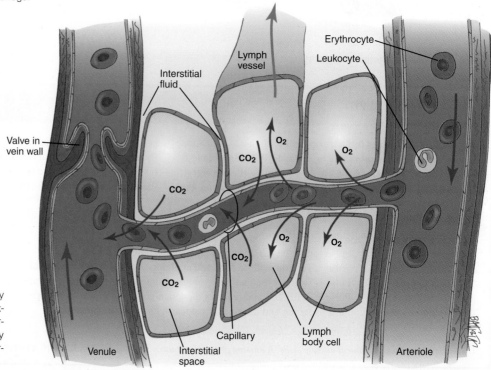

Figure 21-4 Normal capillary circulation ensures removal of excess fluid (edema) from the interstitial spaces as well as delivery of oxygen (O_2) and removal of carbon dioxide (CO_2).

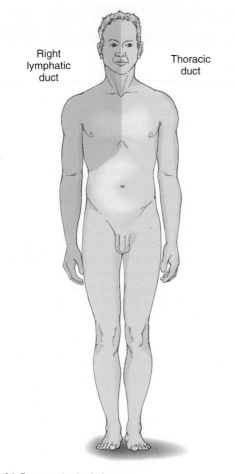

Figure 21-5 Lymphatic drainage.

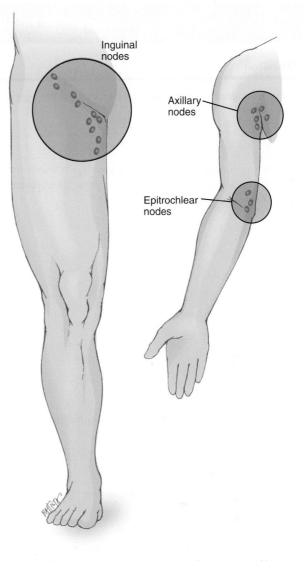

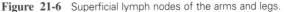

Figure 21-6 Superficial lymph nodes of the arms and legs.

this chapter include the epitrochlear nodes and the superficial inguinal nodes.

The **epitrochlear nodes** are located approximately 3 cm above the elbow on the inner (medial) aspect of the arm. These lymph nodes drain the lower arm and hand. Lymph from the remainder of the arm and hand drains to the axillary lymph nodes. The **superficial inguinal nodes** consist of two groups: a horizontal and a vertical chain of nodes. The horizontal chain is located on the anterior thigh just under the inguinal ligament, and the vertical chain is located close to the great saphenous vein. These nodes drain the legs, external genitalia, and lower abdomen and buttocks (Fig. 21-6).

Health Assessment

COLLECTING SUBJECTIVE DATA: THE NURSING HEALTH HISTORY

Disorders of the peripheral vascular system may develop gradually. Severe symptoms may not occur until there is extensive damage. Therefore, it is important for the nurse to ask questions about symptoms that the client may consider inconsequential. It is also important for the nurse to ask about personal and family history of vascular disease. This information provides insight into the client's risk for a recurrence or development of problems with the peripheral vascular system. It is especially important to evaluate aspects of the client's lifestyle and health factors that may impair peripheral vascular health. These questions provide the nurse with an avenue for discussing healthy lifestyles that can prevent or minimize peripheral vascular disease. Some of the history questions may overlap those asked when assessing the heart and the skin because of the close relationship between systems.

(text continues on page 391)

HISTORY OF PRESENT HEALTH CONCERN

Question	Rationale
Have you noticed any color, temperature, or texture changes in your skin?	Cold, pale, clammy skin on the extremities and thin, shiny skin with loss of hair, especially over the lower legs, are associated with arterial insufficiency. Warm skin and brown pigmentation around the ankles are associated with venous insufficiency.
Do you experience pain or cramping in your legs? Describe the pain (aching, stabbing). How often does it occur? Does it occur with activity? Does it wake you from sleep?	Intermittent claudication characterized by cramping pain in the calves, thighs, or buttocks and weakness that occurs with activity and is relieved with rest may indicate arterial disease (Scherer & Regensteiner, 2004). Heaviness and an aching sensation aggravated by standing or sitting for long periods of time and is relieved by rest are associated with venous disease. Leg pain that awakens a client from sleep is often associated with advanced chronic arterial occlusive disease. However, the lack of pain may signal neuropathy in a diabetic client. Reduced sensation or an absence of pain can result in a failure to recognize a problem or fully understand the problem's significance.
	Older clients with arterial disease may not have the classic symptoms of intermittent claudication, but may experience coldness, color change, numbness, and abnormal sensations.
Do you have any leg veins that are ropelike, bulging, or contorted?	Varicose veins are hereditary but may also develop from increased venous pressure and venous pooling (e.g., as happens during pregnancy). Standing in one place for long times also increases the risk for varicosities.
Do you have any sores or open wounds on your legs? Where are they located? Are they painful?	Ulcers associated with arterial disease are usually painful and are often located on the toes, foot, or lateral ankle. Venous ulcers are usually painless and occur on the lower leg or medial ankle.
Do you have any swelling (edema) in your legs or feet? At what time of day is swelling worst? Any pain with swelling?	Peripheral edema (swelling) results from an obstruction of the lymphatic flow or from venous insufficiency from such conditions as incompetent valves or decreased osmotic pressure in the capillaries. It may also occur with deep vein thrombosis. With leg or foot ulcers, edema can reduce tissue perfusion and wound oxygenation (see Promote Health—Deep Vein Thrombosis).
Do you have any swollen glands or lymph nodes? If so, do they feel tender, soft, or hard?	Enlarged lymph nodes may indicate a local or systemic infection.
	With aging, lymphatic tissue is lost, resulting in smaller and fewer lymph nodes.
For male clients: Have you experienced a change in your usual sexual activity? Describe.	Impotence may occur in clients with decreased blood flow or an occlusion of the blood vessels such as aortoiliac occlusion (Leriche's syndrome). Men may be reluctant to report or discuss difficulties they have achieving or maintaining an erection.

continued on page 390

COLDSPA Example for Swelling in Legs

Use the **COLDSPA** mnemonic as a guideline to collect needed information for each symptom the client shares. In addition, the following questions help elicit important information.

Mnemonic	Question	Client Response Example
Character	Describe the sign or symptom (feeling, appearance, sound, smell, or taste if applicable).	"I've gained 14 pounds even though I've been eating about the same foods. I have swelling in my legs."
Onset	When did it begin?	"About a week ago."
Location	Where is it? Does it radiate? Does it occur anywhere else?	"It's mostly in my legs, ankles, and feet. They seem heavy and puffy."
Duration	How long does it last? Does it recur?	"Most of the time, though it does seem worse at the end of the day."
Severity	How bad is it? or How much does it bother you?	"The swelling is getting worse and now I'm getting more and more short of breath."
Pattern	What makes it better or worse?	"It helps to lie down in the recliner and keep my feet up. The swelling is worse when I sit with my feet on the floor."
Associated factors/How it **A**ffects the client	What other symptoms occur with it? How does it affect you?	"My skin on my legs and feet feels so tight and now I can't wear anything but my old house shoes. I have to sit up at night in the recliner in order to breathe easier."

PROMOTE HEALTH
Deep Vein Thrombosis (DVT)

Overview

Deep vein thrombosis (DVT) is a blood clot in a deep leg vein. These clots can develop in the lower leg or the thigh, but the thigh is the more serious area for clots because these are more likely to travel to the lung. About 1 in 1,000 Americans develop DVT each year. The cause of DVT is not known but some risk factors and preventive strategies have been identified. For a more detailed form to assess risk, see the Caprini DVT Risk Stratification Tool (*Improving DVT prevention*, 2006).

Risk Factors

- Any condition that increases blood clotting, including inherited conditions
- Low blood flow to deep vein(s) from surgery, immobilization, injury, constriction
- Some cancers and cancer treatments
- Other vascular conditions such as varicose veins
- Sitting for long periods, especially in a car or airplane
- Pregnancy, especially the first 6 weeks after giving birth
- 60 years of age or older (although DVT can occur at younger ages)
- Overweight
- Birth control pills, hormone therapy, postmenopausal hormone replacement
- Having a central venous catheter in a vein
- Having more than one DVT risk factor above

Teach Risk Reduction Tips

- If sitting for long periods, stand up as often as possible or at least every hour. Exercise feet and lower leg muscles frequently.
- Get out of bed and walk as soon as possible after surgery or illness.
- Follow physician's orders for taking clot preventing medicines if required for some surgeries and follow up with physician as necessary. Report tenderness or pain, swelling, or warmth or redness in calf or thigh.
- When traveling long distances, especially by plane:
  - Exercise leg muscles frequently in airport as well as on plane; curl and press toes down to improve circulation.
  - Wear compression stockings (AHA recommendation).
  - Avoid socks with tight elastic bands around tops.
  - Drink plenty of fluids to avoid dehydration.
  - Take aspirin if advised by physician or not contraindicated by other medical conditions.
  - On long car trips, stop every two hours to get out and walk around.

PAST HEALTH HISTORY

Question	*Rationale*
Describe any problems you had in the past with the circulation in your arms and legs (e.g., blood clots, ulcers, coldness, hair loss, numbness, swelling, or poor healing).	A history of prior peripheral vascular disease increases a person's risk for a recurrence. Following deep vein thrombosis (DVT), post-thrombotic syndrome leading to tissue damage may develop and persist indefinitely (Date, 2007).
Have you had any heart or blood vessel surgeries or treatments such as coronary artery bypass grafting, repair of an aneurysm, or vein stripping?	Previous surgeries may alter the appearance of the skin and underlying tissues surrounding the blood vessels. Grafts for bypass surgeries are often taken from veins in the legs.

FAMILY HISTORY

Question	*Rationale*
Do you, or does your family, have a history of diabetes, hypertension, coronary heart disease, intermittent claudication, or elevated cholesterol or triglyceride levels?	These disorders or abnormalities tend to be hereditary and cause damage to blood vessels. An essential aspect of treating peripheral vascular disease is to identify and then modify risk factors (Muthu et al., 2007).

LIFESTYLE AND HEALTH PRACTICES

Question	*Rationale*
Do you (or did you in the past) smoke cigarettes or use any other form of tobacco? How much and for how long? If you have used tobacco, are you willing to quit?	Smoking cigarettes (and using other forms of tobacco) significantly increases a person's risk for chronic arterial insufficiency. The risk increases according to the length of time a person smokes and the amount of tobacco smoked. If willing to quit smoking, provide resources to assist in quitting. If unwilling to quit, provide information and help identify barriers to quitting (www.ahrq.gov/hlpsmksqt.pdf). Smoking cessation in middle age has the following benefits: reduced workload on the heart, improved respiratory function, and reduced risk for lung cancer (Maville & Huerta, 2008).
Do you exercise regularly?	Regular exercise improves peripheral vascular circulation and decreases stress, pulse rate, and blood pressure, thereby decreasing the risk for developing peripheral vascular disease.
For female clients: Do you take oral or transdermal (patch) contraceptives?	These contraceptives increase the risk for thrombophlebitis, Raynaud's disease, hypertension, and edema.
Are you experiencing any stress in your life at this time?	Stress increases the heart rate and blood pressure and can contribute to vascular disease.
How have problems with your circulation (i.e., peripheral vascular system) affected your ability to function?	Discomfort or pain associated with chronic arterial disease and the aching heaviness associated with venous disease may limit a client's ability to stand or walk for long periods. This, in turn, may affect job performance and the ability to care for a home and family or participate in social events.

continued

Question	Rationale
Do leg ulcers or varicose veins affect how you feel about yourself?	If clients perceive the appearance of their legs as disfiguring, their body image or feelings of self-worth may be negatively influenced.
Do you regularly take medications prescribed by your physician to improve your circulation?	Drugs that inhibit platelet aggregation, such as cilostazol (Pletal) or clopidogrel (Plavix), may be prescribed to increase blood flow. Aspirin also prevents blood clotting and is used to reduce the risks associated with peripheral vascular disease. Pentoxifylline (Trental) may be prescribed to reduce blood viscosity, improve blood flow to the tissues thus reducing tissue hypoxia. Topical medications such as xenaderm (Trypsin) can also improve wound oxygenation by increasing blood flow thus promoting wound healing. Clients who fail to take their medications regularly are at risk for developing peripheral vascular problems. These clients require teaching about their medication and the importance of taking it regularly.
Do you wear support hose to treat varicose veins?	Support stockings help to reduce venous pooling and increase blood return to the heart.

COLLECTING OBJECTIVE DATA: PHYSICAL EXAMINATION

The purpose of the peripheral vascular assessment is to identify any signs or symptoms of peripheral vascular disease including arterial insufficiency, venous insufficiency, or lymphatic involvement. This is accomplished by performing an assessment first of the arms then the legs, concentrating on skin color and temperature, major pulse sites, and major groups of lymph nodes.

Examination of the peripheral vascular system is very useful in acute care, extended care, and home health care settings. Early detection of peripheral vascular disease can prevent long-term complications. A complete peripheral vascular examination involves inspection, palpation, and auscultation. In addition, there are several special assessment techniques that are necessary to perform on clients with suspected peripheral vascular problems.

The arms and legs should be closely compared bilaterally. Better objective data can be gained by assessing a particular feature on one extremity and then the other. For example, evaluate the strength of the dorsalis pedis pulse on the right foot and compare your findings with those of the left foot.

Preparing the Client

Have the client wear an examination gown and sit upright on an examination table. Make sure the room is a comfortable temperature (about 72°F) without drafts. This helps to prevent vasodilation or vasoconstriction. Before you begin the assessment, inform the client that it will be necessary to inspect and palpate all four extremities and that the groin will also need to be exposed for palpation of the inguinal lymph nodes and palpation and auscultation of the femoral arteries. Explain that the client can sit for examination of the arms but will need to lie down for examination of the legs and groin and will need to follow your directions for several special assessment techniques toward the end of the examination. As you perform the examination, explain in detail what you are doing and answer any questions the client may have. This helps to ease any client anxiety.

Equipment

- Centimeter tape
- Stethoscope
- Doppler ultrasound device
- Conductivity gel
- Tourniquet
- Gauze or tissue
- Waterproof pen
- Blood pressure cuff

Physical Assessment

- Discuss risk factors for peripheral vascular disease with client.
- Accurately inspect arms and legs for edema and venous patterning.
- Observe carefully for signs of arterial and venous insufficiency (skin color, venous pattern, hair distribution, lesions or ulcers) and inadequate lymphatic drainage.
- Recognize characteristic clubbing.
- Palpate pulse points correctly.
- Use the Doppler ultrasound instrument correctly (Spotlight Equipment 21-1).

(text continues on page 408)

EQUIPMENT SPOTLIGHT 21.1   **How to Use the Doppler Ultrasound Device**

The Doppler ultrasound device transmits and receives ultrasound waves to evaluate blood flow. It works by transmitting ultra high frequency sound waves that strike red blood cells (RBCs) in an artery or vein. The rebounding ultrasound waves produce a whooshing sound when echoing from an artery and a nonpulsating rush when echoing from a vein. The strength of the sound is determined by the velocity of the RBCs. In partially occluded vessels, RBCs pass more slowly through the vessel, thus decreasing the sound. Fully occluded vessels produce no sound. The battery-operated hand-held Doppler device is used to

- Assess unpalpable pulses in the extremities
- Determine the patency of arterial bypass grafts
- Assess tissue perfusion in an extremity

Operating the Device

When assessing peripheral circulation with a Doppler ultrasound device, first inform the patient that the assessment is painless and noninvasive. Then the test can proceed as follows:

- Apply a fingertip-sized mound of lukewarm gel over the blood vessel to be assessed.
- At a 60- to 90-degree angle, lightly place the vascular probe at the top of the mound of gel.
- Listen for a whooshing (artery) or nonpulsating rushing (vein) sound.
- Clean the skin with a tissue.
- Clean the probe as recommended by the manufacturer.
- Mark the site with a permanent pen for easy re-assessment.
- Record findings.

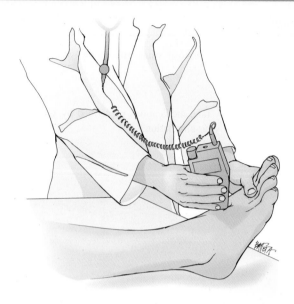

Improving Results

- A warm extremity will increase signal strength.
- Place the tube or packet of gel in warm water before use because cold gel will promote vasoconstriction and make it more difficult to detect a signal.
- Avoid pressing the probe too snugly against the skin because this may obliterate the signal.

PHYSICAL ASSESSMENT

Assessment Procedure	Normal Findings	Abnormal Findings
Arms		
Inspection **Observe arm size and venous pattern; also look for edema.** If there is an observable difference, measure bilaterally the circumference of the arms at the same locations with each re-measurement and record findings in centimeters. ➤ *Clinical Tip* • *Mark locations on arms with a permanent marker to ensure the exact same locations are used with each reassessment.*	Arms are bilaterally symmetric with minimal variation in size and shape. No edema or prominent venous patterning.	Lymphedema results from blocked lymphatic circulation, which may be caused by breast surgery. It usually affects one extremity, causing induration and non-pitting edema. Prominent venous patterning with edema may indicate venous obstruction. See Assessment Tool 21.2.

continued

ASSESSMENT TOOL 21-2   Stages of Lymphedema

Grade	Description	Measurement
Stage 0	No obvious signs or symptoms. Impaired lymph drainage is sub-clinical. Lymphedema (LE) may be present for months to years before progressing to later stages.	Edema is not evident. Clinical detection does not occur until the normal interstitial volume increases by 30% or more.
Stage I	Swelling is present. An affected area pits with pressure. Elevation relieves swelling. Skin texture is smooth. LE is spontaneously reversible.	<3 cm difference between extremities
Stage II	Skin tissue is firmer. Skin may look tight and shiny. Pitting may or may not occur. Elevation does not completely alleviate the swelling. Hair loss or nail changes may be experienced in an affected extremity. LE is spontaneously irreversible. Assistance will be needed to reduce edema.	3–5 cm difference between extremities
Stage III	LE has progressed to the elephantiasis stage. An affected area is nonpitting with a permanent eczema. Skin is firm and thick. Hyperkeratosis, fat deposits, and acanthosis are present. Skin folds develop. May be at risk for cellulitis, infections, or ulcerations. An affected area may ooze fluid. LE is irreversible. Elevation will not alleviate symptoms.	≥5 cm difference between extremities

Based on information from Dell & Doll, 2006; Holcomb, 2006; Quan & Petrek, 2004; Story, 2005. Compiled by Marr (2007). *Clinical journal of oncology nursing, 11*(1); 21.

Assessment Procedure	Normal Findings	Abnormal Findings
Observe coloration of the hands and arms (Fig. 21-7).	Color varies depending on the client's skin tone, although color should be the same bilaterally (see Chapter 13 for more information).	Raynaud's disease, a vascular disorder caused by vasoconstriction or vasospasm of the fingers or toes, is characterized by rapid changes of color (pallor, cyanosis, and redness), swelling, pain, numbness, tingling, burning, throbbing, and coldness. The disorder commonly occurs bilaterally; symptoms last minutes to hours (Fig. 21-8).
Palpation **Palpate the client's fingers, hands, and arms, and note the temperature.**	Skin is warm to the touch bilaterally from fingertips to upper arms.	A cool extremity may be a sign of arterial insufficiency. Cold fingers and hands, for example, are common findings with Raynaud's disease.
Palpate to assess capillary refill time. Compress the nailbed until it blanches. Release the pressure and calculate the time it takes for color to return. This test indicates peripheral perfusion and reflects cardiac output.	Capillary beds refill (and, therefore, color returns) in 2 seconds or less.	Capillary refill time exceeding 2 seconds may indicate vasoconstriction, decreased cardiac output, shock, arterial occlusion, or hypothermia.

continued

PHYSICAL ASSESSMENT *Continued*

Assessment Procedure	Normal Findings	Abnormal Findings

➤ *Clinical Tip • Inaccurate findings may result if the room is cool, if the client has edema, anemia, or if the client recently smoked a cigarette.*

Palpate the radial pulse. Gently press the radial artery against the radius (Fig. 21-9). Note elasticity and strength.

➤ *Clinical Tip • For difficult-to-palpate pulses, use a Doppler ultrasound device. (Spotlight Equipment 21.1).*

Radial pulses are bilaterally strong (3+). Artery walls have a resilient quality (bounce).

Increased radial pulse volume indicates a hyperkinetic state (4+ or bounding pulse). Diminished (1+ or 2+) or absent (0) pulse suggests partial or complete arterial occlusion (which is more common in the legs than the arms). The pulse could also be decreased from Buerger's disease or scleroderma. See Assessment Tool 21-1.

Obliteration of the pulse may result from compression by external sources, as in compartment syndrome.

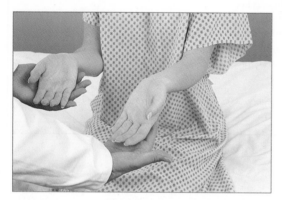

Figure 21-7   Inspecting color related to circulation (© B. Proud).

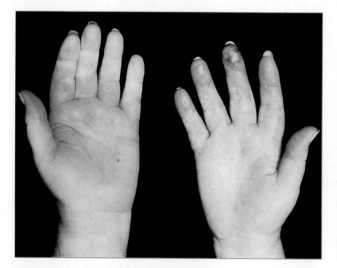

Figure 21-8   Hallmarks of Raynaud's disease are color changes (with permission from Effeney, D.J., & Stoney, R.J. [1993]. *Wylie's atlas of vascular surgery: Disorders of the extremities.* Philadelphia: Lippincott Williams & Wilkins.)

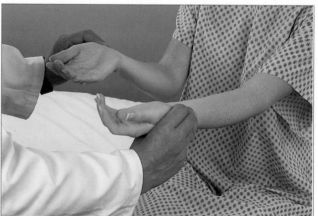

Figure 21-9   Palpating the radial pulse (© B. Proud).

continued

Assessment Procedure	Normal Findings	Abnormal Findings
Palpate the ulnar pulses. Apply pressure with your first three fingertips to the medial aspects of the inner wrists. The ulnar pulses are not routinely assessed because they are located deeper than the radial pulses and are difficult to detect. Palpate the ulnar arteries if you suspect arterial insufficiency (Fig. 21-10).	The ulnar pulses may not be detectable.	Lack of resilience or inelasticity of the artery wall may indicate arteriosclerosis.
You can also palpate the brachial pulses if you suspect arterial insufficiency. Do this by placing the first three fingertips of each hand at the client's right and left medial antecubital creases. Alternatively, palpate the brachial pulse in the groove between the biceps and triceps (Fig. 21-11).	Brachial pulses have equal strength bilaterally.	Brachial pulses are increased, diminished, or absent.
Palpate the epitrochlear lymph nodes. Take the client's left hand in your right hand as if you were shaking hands. Flex the client's elbow about 90 degrees. Use your left hand to palpate behind the elbow in the groove between the biceps and triceps muscles (Fig. 21-12). If nodes are detected, evaluate for size, tenderness, and consistency. Repeat palpation on the opposite arm.	Normally epitrochlear lymph nodes are not palpable.	Enlarged epitrochlear lymph nodes may indicate an infection in the hand or forearm or they may occur with generalized lymphadenopathy. Enlarged lymph nodes may also occur because of a lesion in the area.

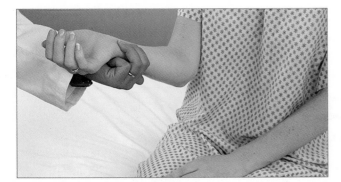

Figure 21-10 Palpating the ulnar pulse (© B. Proud).

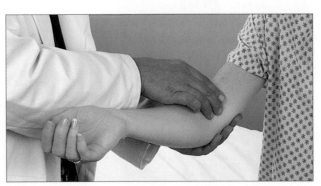

Figure 21-11 Palpating the brachial pulse (© B. Proud).

continued

PHYSICAL ASSESSMENT *Continued*

Assessment Procedure	Normal Findings	Abnormal Findings
Perform the Allen test. The Allen test evaluates patency of the radial or ulnar arteries. It is implemented when patency is questionable or before such procedures as a radial artery puncture. The test begins by assessing ulnar patency. Have the client rest the hand palm side up on the examination table and make a fist. Then use your thumbs to occlude the radial and ulnar arteries (Fig. 21-13A). Continue pressure to keep both arteries occluded and have the client release the fist (Fig. 21-13B). Note that the palm remains pale. Release the pressure on the ulnar artery and watch for color to return to the hand. To assess radial patency, repeat the procedure as before, but at the last step, release pressure on the radial artery (Fig. 21-13C).	Pink coloration returns to the palms within 3 to 5 seconds if the ulnar artery is patent. Pink coloration returns within 3 to 5 seconds if the radial artery is patent.	With arterial insufficiency or occlusion of the ulnar artery, pallor persists. With arterial insufficiency or occlusion of the radial artery, pallor persists.

> ➤ *Clinical Tip* • *Opening the hand into exaggerated extension may cause persistent pallor (false-positive Allen's test).*

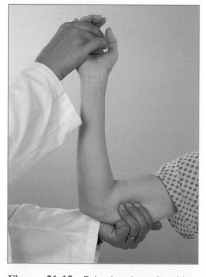

Figure 21-12 Palpating the epitrochlear lymph nodes located in the upper inside of the arm (© B. Proud).

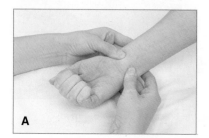

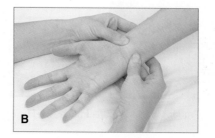

Figure 21-13 Performing the Allen test (© B. Proud).

continued

Assessment Procedure	Normal Findings	Abnormal Findings

Legs

Inspection, Palpation, and Auscultation Ask the client to lie supine. Then drape the groin area and place a pillow under the client's head for comfort. **Observe skin color while inspecting both legs from the toes to the groin.**	Pink color for lighter-skinned clients and pink or red tones visible under darker-pigmented skin. There should be no changes in pigmentation.	Pallor, especially when elevated, and rubor, when dependent, suggests arterial insufficiency. Cyanosis when dependent suggests venous insufficiency. A rusty or brownish pigmentation around the ankles indicates venous insufficiency.
Inspect distribution of hair.	Hair covers the skin on the legs and appears on the dorsal surface of the toes. 👓 Hair loss on the lower extremities occurs with aging and is, therefore, not an absolute sign of arterial insufficiency in the older client.	Loss of hair on the legs suggests arterial insufficiency. Often thin, shiny skin is noted as well.
Inspect for lesions or ulcers.	Legs are free of lesions or ulcerations.	Ulcers with smooth, even margins that occur at pressure areas, such as the toes and lateral ankle, result from arterial insufficiency. Ulcers with irregular edges, bleeding, and possible bacterial infection that occur on the medial ankle, result from venous insufficiency (Abnormal Findings 21-1).
Inspect for edema. Inspect the legs for unilateral or bilateral edema. Note veins, tendons, and bony prominences. If the legs appear asymmetric, use a centimeter tape to measure in four different areas: circumference at midthigh, largest circumference at the calf, smallest circumference above the ankle, and across the forefoot. Compare both extremities at the same locations (Fig. 21-14). ➤ **Clinical Tip** • Taking a measurement in centimeters from the patella to the location to be measured can aid in getting the exact location on both legs. If additional readings are necessary, use a felt-tipped pen to ensure exact placement of the measuring tape.	Identical size and shape bilaterally; no swelling or atrophy.	Bilateral edema may be detected by the absence of visible veins, tendons, or bony prominences. Bilateral edema usually indicates a systemic problem, such as congestive heart failure, or a local problem, such as lymphedema (abnormal or blocked lymph vessels) or prolonged standing or sitting (orthostatic edema). Unilateral edema is characterized by a 1-cm difference in measurement at the ankles, or a 2-cm difference at the calf, and a swollen extremity. It is usually caused by venous stasis due to insufficiency or an obstruction. It may also be caused by lymphedema (Abnormal Findings 21-2). A difference in measurement between legs may also be due to muscular atrophy. Muscular atrophy usually results from disuse due to stroke or from being in a cast for a prolonged time.

continued

PHYSICAL ASSESSMENT Continued

Assessment Procedure	Normal Findings	Abnormal Findings
Palpate edema. If edema is noted during inspection, palpate the area to determine if it is pitting or nonpitting (Abnormal Findings 21-2). Press the edematous area with the tips of your fingers, hold for a few seconds, then release. If the depression does not rapidly refill and the skin remains indented on release, pitting edema is present.	No edema (pitting or nonpitting) present in the legs.	Pitting edema is associated with systemic problems, such as congestive heart failure or hepatic cirrhosis, and local causes such as venous stasis due to insufficiency or obstruction or prolonged standing or sitting (orthostatic edema). A 1+ to 4+ scale is used to grade the severity of pitting edema with 4+ being most severe (Fig. 21-15).
Palpate bilaterally for temperature of the feet and legs. Use the backs of your fingers. Compare your findings in the same areas bilaterally (Fig. 21-16). Note location of any changes in temperature.	Toes, feet, and legs are equally warm bilaterally.	Generalized coolness in one leg or change in temperature from warm to cool as you move down the leg suggests arterial insufficiency. Increased warmth in the leg may be caused by superficial thrombophlebitis resulting from a secondary inflammation in the tissue around the vein. ➤ *Clinical Tip • Bilateral coolness of the feet and legs suggests one of the following: The room is too cool, the client may have recently smoked a cigarette, be anemic, or the client is anxious. All of these factors cause vasoconstriction, resulting in cool skin.*

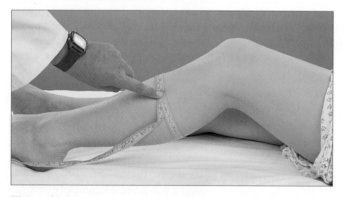

Figure 21-14 Measuring the calf circumference (© B. Proud).

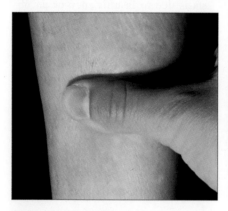

Figure 21-15 Pitting edema.

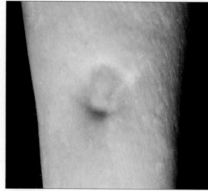

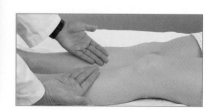

Figure 21-16 Palpating skin temperature (© B. Proud).

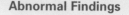

continued

Assessment Procedure	Normal Findings	Abnormal Findings
Palpate the superficial inguinal lymph nodes. First, expose the client's inguinal area, keeping the genitals draped. Feel over the upper medial thigh for the vertical and horizontal groups of superficial inguinal lymph nodes. If detected, determine size, mobility, or tenderness. Repeat palpation on the opposite thigh.	Nontender, movable lymph nodes up to 1 or even 2 cm are commonly palpated.	Lymph nodes larger than 2 cm with or without tenderness (lymphadenopathy) may be from a local infection or generalized lymphadenopathy. Fixed nodes may indicate malignancy.
Palpate the femoral pulses. Ask the client to bend the knee and move it out to the side. Press deeply and slowly below and medial to the inguinal ligament. Use two hands if necessary. Release pressure until you feel the pulse. Repeat palpation on the opposite leg. Compare amplitude bilaterally (Fig. 21-17).	Femoral pulses strong and equal bilaterally.	Weak or absent femoral pulses indicate partial or complete arterial occlusion.
Auscultate the femoral pulses. If arterial occlusion is suspected in the femoral pulse, position the stethoscope over the femoral artery and listen for bruits. Repeat for other artery (Fig. 21-18).	No sounds auscultated over the femoral arteries.	Bruits over one or both femoral arteries suggest partial obstruction of the vessel and diminished blood flow to the lower extremities.
Palpate the popliteal pulses. Ask the client to raise (flex) the knee partially. Place your thumbs on the knee while positioning your fingers deep in the bend of the knee. Apply pressure to locate the pulse. It is usually detected lateral to the medial tendon (Fig. 21-19). ➤ *Clinical Tip • If you cannot detect a pulse, try palpating with the client in a prone position. Partially raise the leg, and place your fingers deep in the bend of the knee. Repeat palpation in opposite leg, and note amplitude bilaterally.*	It is not unusual for the popliteal pulse to be difficult or impossible to detect, and yet for circulation to be normal.	Although normal popliteal arteries may be nonpalpable, an absent pulse may also be the result of an occluded artery. Further circulatory assessment such as temperature changes, skin-color differences, edema, hair distribution variations, and dependent rubor (dusky redness) distal to the popliteal artery assists in determining the significance of an absent pulse (Aliabadi, 2004).

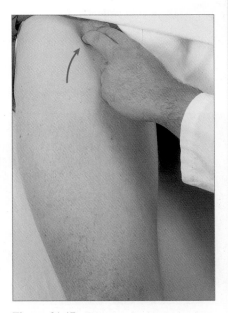

Figure 21-17 Palpating the femoral pulses.

continued

PHYSICAL ASSESSMENT Continued

Assessment Procedure	Normal Findings	Abnormal Findings
Palpate the dorsalis pedis pulses. Dorsiflex the client's foot and apply light pressure lateral to and along the side of the extensor tendon of the big toe. The pulses of both feet may be assessed at the same time to aid in making comparisons. Assess amplitude bilaterally (Fig. 21-20). ➤ *Clinical Tip • It may be difficult or impossible to palpate a pulse in an edematous foot. A Doppler ultrasound device may be useful in this situation.*	Dorsalis pedis pulses are bilaterally strong. This pulse is congenitally absent in 5% to 10% of the population.	A weak or absent pulse may indicate impaired arterial circulation. Further circulatory assessments (temperature and color) are warranted to determine the significance of an absent pulse.
Palpate the posterior tibial pulses. Palpate behind and just below the medial malleolus (in the groove between the ankle and the Achilles tendon) (Fig. 21-21). Palpating both posterior tibial pulses at the same time aids in making comparisons. Assess amplitude bilaterally.	The posterior tibial pulses should be strong bilaterally. However, in about 15% of healthy clients, the posterior tibial pulses are absent.	A weak or absent pulse indicates partial or complete arterial occlusion.

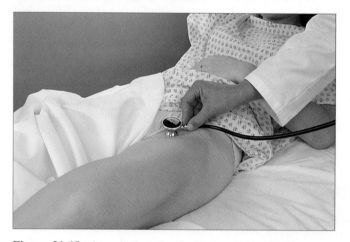

Figure 21-18 Auscultating the femoral pulse to detect bruits (© B. Proud).

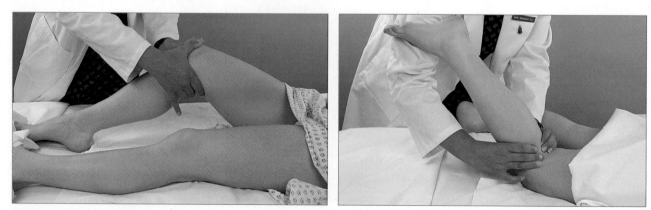

Figure 21-19 Palpating the popliteal pulse with the client (*left*) supine and (*right*) prone (© B. Proud).

continued

Assessment Procedure	Normal Findings	Abnormal Findings

> *Clinical Tip* • *Edema in the ankles may make it difficult or impossible to palpate a posterior tibial pulse. In this case, Doppler ultrasound may be used to assess the pulse.*

Inspect for varicosities and thrombophlebitis. Ask the client to stand because varicose veins may not be visible when the client is supine and not as pronounced when the client is sitting. As the client is standing, inspect for superficial vein thrombophlebitis. To fully assess for a suspected phlebitis, palpate for tenderness. If superficial vein thrombophlebitis is present, note redness or discoloration on the skin surface over the vein.

Veins are flat and barely seen under the surface of the skin.

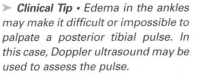 Varicosities are common in the older client.

Varicose veins may appear as distended, nodular, bulging, and tortuous, depending on severity. Varicosities are common in the anterior lateral thigh and lower leg, the posterior lateral calf, or anus (known as hemorrhoids). Varicose veins result from incompetent valves in the veins, weak vein walls, or an obstruction above the varicosity. Despite venous dilation, blood flow is decreased and venous pressure is increased. Superficial vein thrombophlebitis is marked by redness, thickening, and tenderness along the vein. Aching or cramping may occur with walking or dorsiflexion of the foot (positive Homans' sign). Swelling and inflammation are often noted (Fig. 21-22).

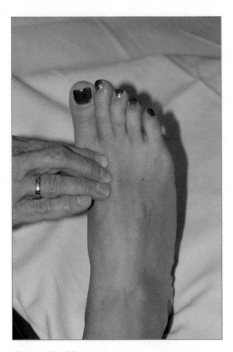

Figure 21-20 Palpating the dorsalis pedis pulse.

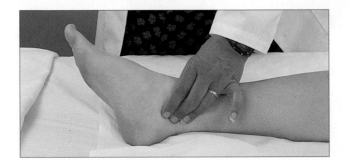

Figure 21-21 Palpating the posterior tibial pulse (© B. Proud).

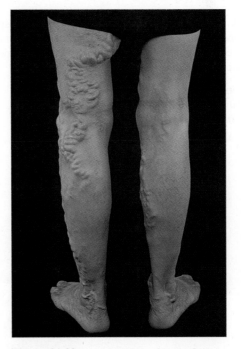

Figure 21-22 Varicose veins (© 1995 Science Photo Library).

continued

PHYSICAL ASSESSMENT *Continued*

Assessment Procedure	Normal Findings	Abnormal Findings
Homans' Sign: This test has been traditionally used but is controversial now, especially if the client has a history of deep vein thrombosis because this test may dislodge the clot. ➤ *Clinical Tip • Flexing the knee helps to eliminate confusion between calf pain and Achilles tendon pain. A second method calls for putting your hand under the knee, slightly flexing it, and sharply dorsiflexing the foot. Ask the client to report pain or tenderness. Repeat this on the opposite leg.*	No pain or tenderness elicited indicates a negative Homans' sign.	Calf pain and tenderness elicited are a positive Homans' sign. A positive sign may indicate deep vein thrombosis (blood clot in deep vein) or superficial thrombophlebitis (inflammation of a superficial vein). However, further diagnostic testing such as ultrasound of the legs and referral are indicated for a definitive diagnosis.

Special Tests for Arterial or Venous Insufficiency

Perform position change test for arterial insufficiency. If pulses in the legs are weak, further assessment for arterial insufficiency is warranted. The client should be in a supine position. Place both of your hands under both of the client's ankles. Raise the legs about 12 inches above the level of the heart. As you support the client's legs, ask the client to pump the feet up and down for about a minute to drain the legs of venous blood, leaving only arterial blood to color the legs (Fig. 21-23).	Feet pink to slightly pale in color in the light-skinned client with elevation. Inspect the soles in the dark-skinned client, although it is more difficult to see subtle color changes in darker skin. When the client sits up and dangles the legs, a pinkish color returns to the tips of the toes in 10 seconds or less. The superficial veins on top of the feet fill in 15 seconds or less.	Marked pallor with legs elevated is an indication of arterial insufficiency. Return of pink color that takes longer than 10 seconds and superficial veins that take longer than 15 seconds to fill suggest arterial insufficiency. Persistent rubor (dusky redness) of toes and feet with legs dependent also suggests arterial insufficiency.
Then ask the client to sit up and dangle legs off the side of the examination table. Note the color of both feet and the time it takes for color to return. ➤ *Clinical Tip • This assessment maneuver will not be accurate if the client has peripheral vascular disease of the veins with incompetent valves.*	Normal responses with absent pulses suggest that an adequate collateral circulation has developed around an arterial occlusion.	

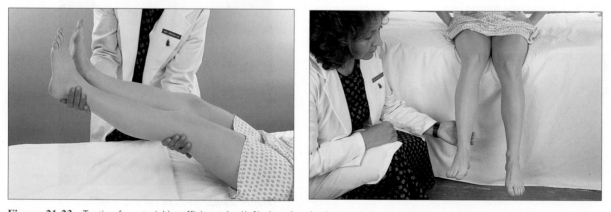

Figure 21-23   Testing for arterial insufficiency by (*left*) elevating the legs and then (*right*) having client dangle the legs (© B. Proud).

continued

Assessment Procedure	Normal Findings	Abnormal Findings

Determine ankle-brachial pressure index (ABPI), also known as Ankle-Brachial Index (ABI). If the client has symptoms of arterial occlusion, the ankle-brachial pressure index should be used to compare the upper and lower limbs systolic blood pressure. The ankle-brachial pressure index (ABPI) is the ratio of the ankle systolic blood pressure to the arm (brachial) systolic blood pressure. See Table 21.1. The ABPI is considered an accurate objective assessment for determining the degree of peripheral arterial disease. It detects decreased systolic pressure distal to the area of stenosis or arterial narrowing and allows the nurse to quantify this measurement. Use the following steps to measure ABPI:

- Have the client rest in a supine position for at least 5 minutes.
- Apply the blood pressure (BP) cuff to first one arm and then the other to determine the brachial pressure using the Doppler. First palpate the pulse and use the Doppler to hear the pulse. The "whooshing" sound indicates the brachial pulse. Pressures in both arms are assessed because asymptomatic stenosis in the subclavian artery can produce an abnormally low reading and should not be used in the calculations. Record the *higher reading*.
- Apply the BP cuff to the right ankle, then palpate the posterior tibial pulse at the medial aspect of the ankle and the dorsalis pedis pulse on the dorsal aspect of the foot. Using the same Doppler technique as in the arms, determine and record *both* systolic pressures. Repeat this procedure on the left ankle (Fig. 21-24). If you are unable to assess these pulses, use the peroneal—artery (Fig. 21-25).

Generally the ankle pressure in a healthy person is the same or slightly higher than the brachial pressure, resulting in an ABPI of approximately 1, or no arterial insufficiency (Holman, 2004). Comparable findings between an experienced nurse using a pocket Doppler and vascular lab results were noted in a recent study (Bonham et al., 2007).

In addition to the abnormal ABPI findings, reduced or absent pedal pulses, cool leg unilaterally, lack of hair, and shiny skin on leg suggests peripheral arterial occlusive disease (Holman, 2004). Early recognition of cardiovascular disease may be determined using ABPI measurements (Pearson, 2007).

Table 21.1	ABI (APBI) Guidelines	
1.0–1.2 ABI	Normal–No arterial insufficiency	
0.8–1.0 ABI	Mild insufficiency	
0.5–0.8 ABI	Moderate insufficiency	
<0.5 ABI	Severe insufficiency	
<0.3 ABI	Limb threatening	

(Smith, Duell, and Martin, 2008)

continued

PHYSICAL ASSESSMENT *Continued*

Assessment Procedure	Normal Findings	Abnormal Findings
• ABPI calculation: Divide the higher ankle pressure for each foot by the higher brachial pressure. For example, you may have measured the highest brachial pulse as 160, the highest pulse in the right ankle as 80, and the highest pulse in the left ankle as 94. Dividing each by 160 (80/160 and 94/160) will result in a right ABPI of 0.5 and a left ABPI of 0.59.		

➤ *Clinical Tip:*

• Make sure to use a correctly sized blood pressure cuff. The bladder of the cuff should be 20% wider than the diameter of the client's limb.
• Document blood pressure cuff sizes used on the nursing plan of care (e.g., "12-cm BP cuff used for brachial pressure: 10-cm BP cuff used for ankle pressure"). This minimizes the risk of shift-to-shift discrepancies in ABPIs.
• Inflate the blood pressure cuff enough to ensure complete closure of the artery. Inflation should be 20 to 30 mm Hg beyond the point at which the last arterial signal was detected.
• Avoid deflating the blood pressure cuff too rapidly. Instead, try to maintain a deflation rate of 2 to 4 mm Hg/s for clients without arrhythmias and 2 mm Hg/s or slower for clients with arrhythmias. Deflating the cuff more

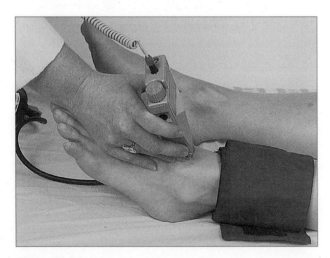

Figure 21-24 When measuring systolic pressure from the dorsalis pedis artery, apply the blood pressure cuff above the malleolus and the Doppler device at a 60- to 90-degree angle over the anterior tibial artery. Then move the device downward along the length of the vessel.

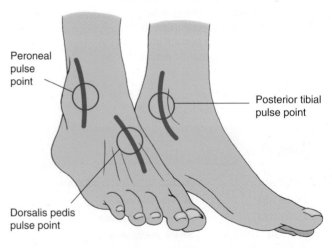

Figure 21-25 If you cannot measure pressure in the dorsalis pedis or posterior tibial artery, measure it in the peroneal artery. The blood pressure cuff can remain in place.

continued

Assessment Procedure	Normal Findings	Abnormal Findings

rapidly than that may cause you to miss the client's highest pressure and record an erroneous (low) blood pressure measurement.

- Be suspicious of arterial pressure recorded at less than 40 mm Hg. This may mean that the venous signal was mistaken for the arterial signal. If you measure arterial pressure, which is normally 120 mm Hg at below 40 mm Hg, ask a colleague to double-check your findings before you record the arterial pressure.
- Suspect medial calcific sclerosis any time you calculate an ABPI of 1.3 or greater or measure ankle pressure at more than 300 mm Hg. This condition is associated with diabetes mellitus, chronic renal failure, and hyperparathyroidism. Medial calcific sclerosis produces falsely elevated ankle pressure by making the vessels noncompressible.

Manual compression test. If the client has varicose veins, perform manual compression to assess the competence of the vein's valves. Ask the client to stand. Firmly compress the lower portion of the varicose vein with one hand. Place your other hand 6 to 8 inches above your first hand (Fig. 21-26). Feel for a pulsation to your fingers in the upper hand. Repeat this test in the other leg if varicosities are present.

No pulsation is palpated if the client has competent valves.

You will feel a pulsation with your upper fingers if the valves in the veins are incompetent.

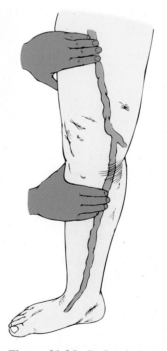

Figure 21-26 Performing manual compression to assess competence of venous valves in clients with varicose veins.

continued

PHYSICAL ASSESSMENT *Continued*

Assessment Procedure	Normal Findings	Abnormal Findings
Trendelenburg test. If the client has varicose veins, perform the Trendelenburg test to determine the competence of the saphenous vein valves and the retrograde (backward) filling of the superficial veins. The client should lie supine. Elevate the client's leg 90 degrees for about 15 seconds or until the veins empty. With the leg elevated, apply a tourniquet to the upper thigh. ➤ *Clinical Tip* • *Arterial blood flow is not occluded if there are arterial pulses distal to the tourniquet.* Assist the client to a standing position and observe for venous filling. Remove the tourniquet after 30 seconds, and watch for sudden filling of the varicose veins from above.	Saphenous vein fills from below in 30 seconds. If valves are competent, there will be no rapid filling of the varicose veins from above (retrograde filling) after removal of tourniquet.	Filling from above with the tourniquet in place and the client standing suggests incompetent valves in the saphenous vein. Rapid filling of the superficial varicose veins from above after the tourniquet has been removed also indicates retrograde filling past incompetent valves in the veins.

Abnormal Findings 21-1 — Characteristics of Arterial and Venous Insufficiency

Arterial Insufficiency
Pain: Intermittent claudication to sharp, unrelenting, constant
Pulses: Diminished or absent
Skin Characteristics: Dependent rubor

- Elevation pallor of foot
- Dry, shiny skin
- Cool-to-cold temperature
- Loss of hair over toes and dorsum of foot
- Nails thickened and ridged

Ulcer Characteristics:

- Location: Tips of toes, toe webs, heel or other pressure areas if confined to bed
- Pain: Very painful
- Depth of ulcer: Deep, often involving joint space
- Shape: Circular
- Ulcer base: Pale black to dry and gangrene
- Leg edema: Minimal unless extremity kept in dependent position constantly to relieve pain

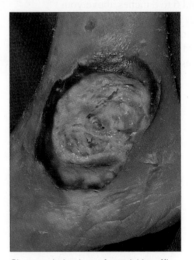

Characteristic ulcer of arterial insufficiency. (© 1994 Michael English, M.D.)

Venous Insufficiency
Pain: Aching, cramping
Pulses: Present but may be difficult to palpate through edema
Skin Characteristics:

- Pigmentation in gaitor area (area of medial and lateral malleolus)
- Skin thickened and tough
- May be reddish-blue in color
- Frequently associated with dermatitis

continued

Abnormal Findings 21-1

Characteristics of Arterial and Venous Insufficiency Continued

Ulcer Characteristics:
- Location: Medial malleolus or anterior tibial area
- Pain: If superficial, minimal pain; but may be very painful
- Depth of ulcer: Superficial
- Shape: Irregular border
- Ulcer base: Granulation tissue–beefy red to yellow fibrinous in chronic long-term ulcer
- Leg edema: Moderate to severe

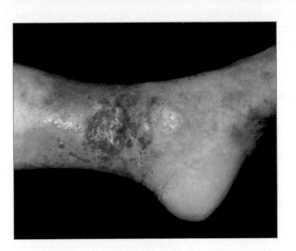

Characteristic ulcer of venous insufficiency. (Courtesy of Dermik Laboratories, Inc.)

(Used with permission from Smeltzer, S. C., Bare, B. G., Hinkle, J. H., & Cheever, K. H. [2008]. *Brunner and Suddarth's textbook of medical surgical nursing* [11th ed.]. Philadelphia: Lippincott Williams & Wilkins.)

Abnormal Findings 21-2

Types of Peripheral Edema

Edema Associated With Lymphedema
- Caused by abnormal or blocked lymph vessels
- Nonpitting
- Usually bilateral; may be unilateral
- No skin ulceration or pigmentation

Edema Associated With Chronic Venous Insufficiency
- Caused by obstruction or insufficiency of deep veins
- Pitting, documented as:

  1+ = slight pitting
  2+ = deeper than 1+
  3+ = noticeably deep pit; extremity looks larger
  4+ = very deep pit; gross edema in extremity

- Usually unilateral; may be bilateral
- Skin ulceration and pigmentation may be present

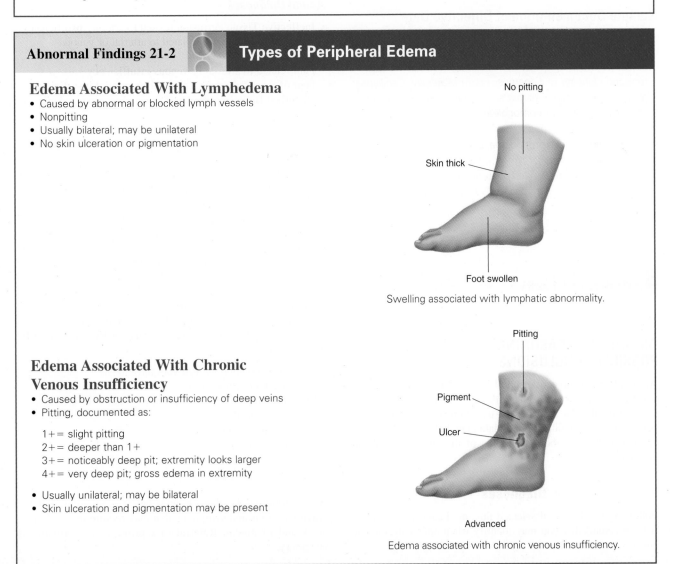

Swelling associated with lymphatic abnormality.

Edema associated with chronic venous insufficiency.

VALIDATING AND DOCUMENTING FINDINGS

Validate the peripheral vascular assessment data you have collected. This is necessary to verify that the data are reliable and accurate. Document the assessment data following the health care facility or agency policy.

Sample Documentation of Subjective Data

> A 43-year-old man reports no color or temperature changes in arms or legs, no pain in legs, no open sores on legs, no swelling of arms or legs. States no bulging veins, no swollen glands, no problems with sexual activity, no history of circulatory problems, no previous surgery on the veins or arteries. Explains that his mother has hypertension and his father's brother died from complications of diabetes. Client states he does not smoke, manages his stress well, and exercises regularly.

Sample Documentation of Objective Data

> Arms are equal in size, no swelling, pinkish skin tone, no clubbing of fingertips, warm bilaterally. Capillary refill time less than 2 seconds, radial and brachial pulses strong bilaterally, no epitrochlear lymph nodes palpated. Legs are pink from toes to groin bilaterally, normal distribution of hair, no ulcers or edema. Legs are warm bilaterally, 1-cm nontender inguinal lymph nodes palpated, femoral, popliteal, dorsalis pedis, and posterior tibial pulses strongly palpated bilaterally. No apparent varicosities or superficial thrombophlebitis.

Analysis of Data

DIAGNOSTIC REASONING: POSSIBLE CONCLUSIONS

After collecting subjective and objective data pertaining to the peripheral vascular assessment, identify abnormal findings and client strengths. Then cluster the data to reveal any significant patterns or abnormalities. These data may then be used to make clinical judgments about the status of the client's peripheral vascular system.

Selected Nursing Diagnoses

Following is a listing of selected nursing diagnoses (wellness, risk, or actual) that you may identify when analyzing the cue clusters.

Wellness Diagnoses

- Readiness for enhanced circulation to extremities
- Health-Seeking Behavior: Requests information on regular monitoring of pulse, blood pressure, cholesterol and triglyceride levels, regular exercise, and smoking cessation

Risk Diagnoses

- Risk for Ineffective Therapeutic Regimen Management (monitoring of pulse, blood pressure, cholesterol and triglyceride levels, regular exercise, and smoking cessation) related to a busy lifestyle, lack of knowledge and resources to follow healthy lifestyle
- Risk for Infection related to poor circulation to and impaired skin integrity of lower extremities
- Risk for Injury related to decreased sensation in lower extremities secondary to edema and/or neuropathies
- Risk for Impaired Skin Integrity related to poor circulation to extremities secondary to arterial or venous insufficiency
- Risk for Activity Intolerance related to leg pain on walking
- Risk for Peripheral Neurovascular Dysfunction related to venous or arterial occlusion secondary to trauma, surgery, or mechanical compression

Actual Diagnoses

- Ineffective Tissue Perfusion related to arterial insufficiency
- Impaired Skin Integrity related to arterial or venous insufficiency
- Pain related to arterial or venous insufficiency
- Fear of loss of extremities related to arterial insufficiency
- Disturbed Body Image related to leg ulcerations, edema, or varicosities

Selected Collaborative Problems

After grouping the data, certain collaborative problems may become apparent. Remember that collaborative problems differ from nursing diagnoses in that they cannot be prevented through nursing interventions. However, these physiologic complications of medical conditions can be detected and monitored by the nurse. In addition, the nurse can use physician- and nurse-prescribed interventions to minimize the complications of these problems. The nurse may also have to refer the client in such situations for further treatment of the problem. Following is a list of collaborative problems that may be identified when obtaining a general impression. These problems are worded as Risk for Complications (or RC), followed by the problem.

- RC: Thromboembolic/deep vein thrombosis
- RC: Arterial occlusion
- RC: Peripheral vascular (arterial or venous) insufficiency
- RC: Hypertension
- RC: Ischemic ulcers
- RC: Gangrene

Medical Problems

After grouping the data, it may become apparent that the client has signs and symptoms that may require medical diagnosis and treatment. Referral to a primary care provider is necessary.

CASE STUDY

The case study demonstrates how to analyze peripheral vascular assessment data for a specific client. The critical thinking exercises included in the study guide/lab manual and interactive product that complement this text also offer opportunities to analyze assessment data.

Mr. Lee is a 40-year-old, previously healthy but obese (250 lb at 5 feet, 9 inches tall) man who comes to see the nurse practitioner with the complaint, "I must have pulled something in my right leg. I was walking along and I heard a pop, and now, 3 days later, my right leg is very sore. It really hurts to walk." He states that he is self-employed, developing software programs for computers. He says that he usually sits at his computer for about 4 hours at a stretch, then he walks two blocks to his favorite coffee shop for lunch (a sandwich or a salad with cheese and fruit, and usually a piece of cake or pie). After lunch, he goes back to work for another 5 to 6 hours. At night, he eats dinner and watches television for a few hours. His medical history includes a coronary artery bypass graft (CABG) 5 years ago for angina, complicated postoperatively by a pulmonary embolus. However, he has not had any problems since then. The nurse's physical assessment reveals his right calf to be swollen, slightly flushed, red, warm, and tender to palpation. His right calf measures 42 cm at 20 cm above the ankle (medial malleolus); his left calf is 34.5 cm at the same location. Homans' sign is positive for pain in the right calf only. He denies numbness, tingling, or loss of mobility in either extremity.

The following concept map illustrates the diagnostic reasoning process.

Applying COLDSPA

Applying **COLDSPA** for client symptoms: "Leg is very sore and hurts after something popped in it 3 days ago."

Mnemonic	Question	Data Provided	Missing Data
Character	Describe the sign or symptom (feeling, appearance, sound, smell, or taste if applicable).	Client states he pulled something in his right leg and heard a popping sound. Now the leg is very sore and it hurts to walk.	"Describe the pain/soreness in your leg."
Onset	When did it begin?	3 days ago	
Location	Where is it? Does it radiate? Does it occur anywhere else?	Right calf is swollen, red, warm, and tender to touch. Right calf measures 42 cm while left calf is 34.5 cm. Positive Homans' sign in right calf only.	"Does your pain radiate? Any pain elsewhere?"
Duration	How long does it last? Does it recur?		"Is the pain constant or intermittent?"
Severity	How bad is it? or How much does it bother you?		"Rate your pain on a 10 point scale."
Pattern	What makes it better or worse?		"Have you taken any medication or other treatment for the pain? Anything else that seems to make it worse/better?"
Associated factors/How it **A**ffects the client	What other symptoms occur with it? How does it affect you?	Sits at desk for 4 to 6 hours at a time.	"Describe your activity/exercise currently and prior to 3 days ago. Are you having any shortness of breath?" (history of pulmonary embolism)

1) Identify abnormal findings and client strengths

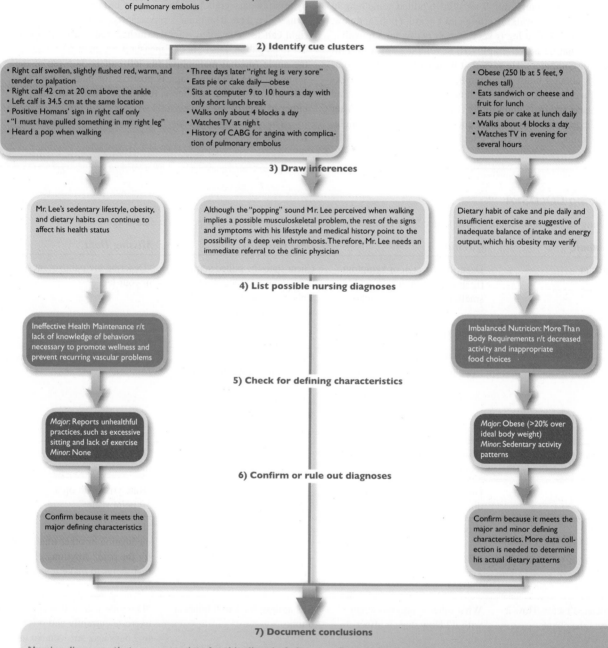

Subjective Data

- "I must have pulled something in my right leg."
- "I heard a pop when I was walking"
- 3 days later, "right leg is very sore."
- Pain in right calf with walking
- Sits at computer 9 to 10 hours a day with only short lunch break
- Walks about four blocks a day
- Watches television in evening for several hours
- Eats sandwich or salad with cheese and fruit for lunch
- Eats pie or cake at lunch daily
- History of CABG for angina with complication of pulmonary embolus

Objective Data

- Obese (250 lb at 5 feet, 9 inches tall)
- Right calf swollen, slightly flushed red, warm, and tender to palpation
- Right calf 42 cm at 20 cm above the ankle
- Left calf is 34.5 cm at the same location
- Positive Homans' sign in right calf only

2) Identify cue clusters

- Right calf swollen, slightly flushed red, warm, and tender to palpation
- Right calf 42 cm at 20 cm above the ankle
- Left calf is 34.5 cm at the same location
- Positive Homans' sign in right calf only
- "I must have pulled something in my right leg"
- Heard a pop when walking

- Three days later "right leg is very sore"
- Eats pie or cake daily—obese
- Sits at computer 9 to 10 hours a day with only short lunch break
- Walks only about 4 blocks a day
- Watches TV at night
- History of CABG for angina with complication of pulmonary embolus

- Obese (250 lb at 5 feet, 9 inches tall)
- Eats sandwich or cheese and fruit for lunch
- Eats pie or cake at lunch daily
- Walks about 4 blocks a day
- Watches TV in evening for several hours

3) Draw inferences

Mr. Lee's sedentary lifestyle, obesity, and dietary habits can continue to affect his health status

Although the "popping" sound Mr. Lee perceived when walking implies a possible musculoskeletal problem, the rest of the signs and symptoms with his lifestyle and medical history point to the possibility of a deep vein thrombosis. Therefore, Mr. Lee needs an immediate referral to the clinic physician

Dietary habit of cake and pie daily and insufficient exercise are suggestive of inadequate balance of intake and energy output, which his obesity may verify

4) List possible nursing diagnoses

Ineffective Health Maintenance r/t lack of knowledge of behaviors necessary to promote wellness and prevent recurring vascular problems

Imbalanced Nutrition: More Than Body Requirements r/t decreased activity and inappropriate food choices

5) Check for defining characteristics

Major: Reports unhealthful practices, such as excessive sitting and lack of exercise
Minor: None

Major: Obese (>20% over ideal body weight)
Minor: Sedentary activity patterns

6) Confirm or rule out diagnoses

Confirm because it meets the major defining characteristics

Confirm because it meets the major and minor defining characteristics. More data collection is needed to determine his actual dietary patterns

7) Document conclusions

Nursing diagnoses that are appropriate for this client include:
- Imbalanced Nutrition: More Than Body Requirements r/t decreased activity and possibly inappropriate food choices
- Ineffective Health Maintenance r/t lack of knowledge of behaviors necessary to promote wellness and prevent recurring vascular problems

Potential collaborative problems include the following:
- RC: Pulmonary embolism
- RC: Cellulitis

Mr. Lee should not be allowed to leave the clinic without seeing a physician for evaluation related to possible deep vein thrombosis.

References and Selected Readings

Bonham, P. A., Cappuccio, M., Hulsey, T., Michel, Y., Kelechi, T., Jenkins, C., & Robison, J. (2007). Are ankle and toe brachial indices (ABI-TBI) obtained by a pocket Doppler interchangeable with those obtained by standard laboratory equipment? *Journal of Wound, Ostomy and Continence Nursing, 34*(1), 35–44.

Date, M. (2007). Protect your patients from venous thromboembolism. *American Nurse Today, 2*(11), 25–27.

Dell, D. D., & Doll, C. (2006). Caring for a patient with lymphedema. *Nursing2006, 36*(6), 49–51.

Holman, J. R. (2004). Peripheral artery disease: Tips on diagnosis and management. *Consultant, 44*(1), 101–108.

Khawaja, F. J., Bailey, K., Turner, S., Kardia, S., Mosley, T. H., & Kullo, I. (2007). Association of novel risk factors with ankle brachial index in African American and non-Hispanic white populations. *Mayo clinic proceedings, 82*(6), 709–716.

Lynn, P. (2008). *Taylor's clinical nursing skills: A nursing process approach.* (2nd ed.). Philadelphia: Wolters Kluwer/Lippincott Williams & Wilkins.

Marrs, J. (2007). Lymphedema and implications for oncology nursing practice. *Clinical Journal of Oncology Nursing, 11*(1), 19–21.

Maville, J. A., & Huerta, C. G. (2008). *Health promotion in nursing.* (2nd ed.). Clifton Park, NY: Thomson; Delmar Learning.

Muthu, C., Chu, J. J., Le Heron, C., Roake, J. A., & Lewis, D. R. (2007). Patient awareness of risk factors for peripheral vascular disease. *Annuals of Vascular Surgery, 21*(4), 433–437.

Palmieri, R. L. (2006). Artery stenosis paves the way for stroke. *Nursing2006, 36*(6), 37–41.

Pearson, T. L. (2007). Correlation of ankle-brachial index values with carotid disease, coronary disease, and cardiovascular risk factors in women. *Journal of Cardiovascular Nursing, 22*(6), 436–439.

Sayre, E. K., Kelechi, T. J., & Neal, B. (2007). Sudden increase in temperature predicts venous ulcers: A case study. *Journal of Vascular Nursing, 25*(3), 46–58

Smeltzer, S., Bare, B., Hinkel, J. H., & Cheever, K. H. (2008). *Brunner & Suddarth's textbook of medical-surgical nursing.* (11th ed.). Philadelphia: Lippincott Williams & Wilkins.

Smith, S. F., Duell, D. J., & Martin, B. C. (2008). *Clinical nursing skills: Basic to advanced skills.* (7th ed.). Upper Saddle River, NJ: Pearson/Prentice Hall.

Promote Health—Deep Vein Thrombosis

Deep vein thrombosis. (2006–2007). Available at http://blood.emedtv.com/deep-vein-thrombosis/deep-vein-thrombosis.html

Improving DVT prevention. (2006). *Physician's Weekly, XXIII(48).* Available at http://www.physiciansweekly.com/article.asp?issueid=412&articleid=3861

Useful Website Resources

American Venous Forum, 13 Elm Street, Manchester, MA 01944; 978-526-8330; http://www.venous-info.com

Circle of Hope Lymphedema Foundation, Inc.: http://www.lymphedema-circleofhope.org

Helping Smokers Quit: A Guide for Nurses (March 2005). Agency for Healthcare Research and Quality. http://www.ahrq.gov/about/nursing

National Heart, Lung, and Blood Institute, Health Information Center, P.O. Box 30105, Bethesda, MD 20824-0105; 301-592-8573; http://www.nhlbi.nih.gov

National Lymphedema Network. www.lymphnet.org

Society of Vascular Nursing, 7794 Grow Drive, Pensacola, FL 32514; 888-536-4786; http://www.svnnet.org

Society of Vascular Surgery, 13 Elm Street, Manchester, MA 01944-1314; 078-526-8330; http://www.vascularweb.org

Vascular Disease Foundation, 3333 S. Wadsworth Boulevard, #B104-37, Lakewood, CO 80227; 1-866-723-4636; http://www.vdf.org

Structure and Function

The abdomen is bordered superiorly by the costal margins, inferiorly by the symphysis pubis and inguinal canals, and laterally by the flanks (Fig. 22-1). To perform an adequate assessment of the abdomen, the nurse needs to understand the anatomic divisions known as the abdominal quadrants, the abdominal wall muscles, and the internal anatomy of the abdominal cavity.

ABDOMINAL QUADRANTS

For the purposes of examination, the abdomen can be described as having four quadrants termed the right upper quadrant (**RUQ**), right lower quadrant (**RLQ**), left lower quadrant (**LLQ**), and left upper quadrant (**LUQ**). The quadrants are determined by an imaginary vertical line (midline) extending from the tip of the sternum (xiphoid) through the umbilicus to the symphysis pubis. This line is bisected perpendicularly by the lateral line, which runs through the umbilicus across the abdomen. Familiarization with the organs and structures in each quadrant is essential to accurate data collection, interpretation, and documentation of findings. Another, older method divides the abdomen into nine regions. Three of these regions are still commonly used to describe abdominal findings: epigastric, umbilical, and hypogastric or suprapubic. Assessment Tool 22-1 describes abdominal quadrants and regions.

ABDOMINAL WALL MUSCLES

The abdominal contents are enclosed externally by the abdominal wall musculature, which includes three layers of muscle extending from the back, around the flanks, to the front. The outermost layer is the external abdominal oblique; the middle layer is the internal abdominal oblique; and the innermost layer is the transverse abdominis (Fig. 22-2). Connective tissue from these muscles extends forward to encase a vertical muscle of the anterior abdominal wall called the rectus abdominis. The fibers and connective tissue extensions of these muscles (aponeuroses) diverge in a characteristic plywood-like pattern (several thin layers arranged at right angles to each other), which provides strength to the abdominal wall. The joining of these muscle fibers and aponeuroses at the midline of the abdomen forms a white line called the linea alba, which extends vertically from the xiphoid process of the sternum to the symphysis pubis. The abdominal wall muscles protect the internal organs and allow normal compression during functional activities such as coughing, sneezing, urination, defecation, and childbirth.

INTERNAL ANATOMY

A thin, shiny, serous membrane called the peritoneum lines the abdominal cavity (parietal peritoneum) and also provides a protective covering for most of the internal abdominal organs (visceral peritoneum). Within the abdominal cavity are structures of several different body systems: gastrointestinal, reproductive (female), lymphatic, and urinary. These structures are typically referred to as the abdominal viscera and can be divided into two types: solid viscera and hollow viscera (Fig. 22-3). Solid viscera are those organs that maintain their shape consistently: liver, pancreas, spleen, adrenal glands, kidneys, ovaries, and uterus. The hollow viscera consist of structures that change shape depending on their contents. These include the stomach, gallbladder, small intestine, colon, and bladder.

➤ **Clinical Tip** • *Whether or not abdominal viscera are palpable depends on location, structural consistency, and size.*

Solid Viscera

The liver is the largest solid organ in the body. It is located below the diaphragm in the **RUQ** of the abdomen. It is composed of four lobes that fill most of the **RUQ** and extend to the left midclavicular line.

➤ **Clinical Tip** • *In many people, the liver extends just below the right costal margin, where it may be palpated. If palpable, the liver has a soft consistency. The liver functions as an accessory digestive organ and has a variety of metabolic and regulatory functions as well, including glucose storage, formation of blood plasma proteins and clotting factors, urea synthesis, cholesterol production, bile formation, destruction of red blood cells, storage of iron and vitamins, and detoxification.*

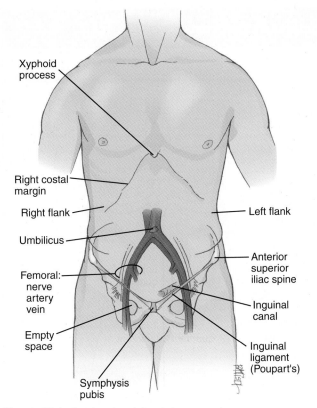

Xyphoid process

Right costal margin

Right flank

Umbilicus

Femoral:
nerve
artery
vein

Empty space

Symphysis pubis

Left flank

Anterior superior iliac spine

Inguinal canal

Inguinal ligament (Poupart's)

Figure 22-1 Landmarks of the abdomen.

The pancreas, located mostly behind the stomach deep in the upper abdomen, is normally not palpable. It is a long gland extending across the abdomen from the **RUQ** to the **LUQ**. The pancreas has two functions: it is an endocrine gland and an accessory organ of digestion. The spleen is approximately 7 cm wide and is located above the left kidney just below the diaphragm at the level of the ninth, tenth, and eleventh ribs. It is posterior to the left midaxillary line and posterior and lateral to the stomach. This soft, flat structure is normally not palpable. In some healthy clients, the lower tip can be felt below the left costal margin.

➤ **Clinical Tip** • *When the spleen enlarges, the lower tip extends down and toward the midline.*

The spleen functions primarily to filter the blood of cellular debris, to digest microorganisms, and to return the breakdown products to the liver.

The kidneys are located high and deep under the diaphragm. These glandular, bean-shaped organs measuring approximately $10 \times 5 \times 2.5$ cm are considered posterior organs and approximate with the level of the T12 to L3 vertebrae. The tops of both kidneys are protected by the posterior rib cage. Kidney tenderness is best assessed at the costovertebral angle (Fig. 22-4). The right kidney is positioned slightly lower because of the position of the liver. Therefore, in some thin clients, the bottom portion of the right kidney may be palpated anteriorly. The primary function of the kidneys is filtration and elimination of metabolic waste products. However, the kidneys also

play a role in blood pressure control and maintenance of water, salt, and electrolyte balances. In addition, they function as endocrine glands by secreting hormones.

The pregnant uterus may be palpated above the level of the symphysis pubis in the midline. The ovaries are located in the **RLQ** and **LLQ** and are normally palpated only during a bimanual examination of the internal genitalia (see Chapter 23).

Hollow Viscera

The abdominal cavity begins with the stomach. It is a distensible, flask-like organ located in the **LUQ** just below the diaphragm and between the liver and spleen. The stomach is not usually palpable. The stomach's main function is to store, churn, and digest food.

The gallbladder, a muscular sac approximately 10 cm long, functions primarily to concentrate and store the bile needed to digest fat. It is located near the posterior surface of the liver lateral to the midclavicular line. It is not normally palpated because it is difficult to distinguish between the gallbladder and the liver.

The small intestine is actually the longest portion of the digestive tract (approximately 7.0 m long) but is named for its small diameter (approximately 2.5 cm). Two major functions of the small intestine are digestion and absorption of nutrients through millions of mucosal projections lining its walls. The small intestine, which lies coiled in all four quadrants of the abdomen, is not normally palpated.

The colon, or large intestine, has a wider diameter than the small intestine (approximately 6.0 cm) and is approximately 1.4 m long. It originates in the **RLQ**, where it attaches to the small intestine at the ileocecal valve. The colon is composed of three major sections: ascending, transverse, and descending. The ascending colon extends up along the right side of the abdomen. At the junction of the liver in the **RUQ**, it flexes at a right angle and becomes the transverse colon. The transverse colon runs across the upper abdomen. In the **LUQ** near the spleen, the colon forms another right angle then extends downward along the left side of the abdomen as the descending colon. At this point, it curves in toward the midline to form the sigmoid colon in the **LLQ**. The sigmoid colon is often felt as a firm structure on palpation, whereas the cecum and ascending colon may feel softer. The transverse and descending colon may also be felt on palpation.

The colon functions primarily to secrete large amounts of alkaline mucus to lubricate the intestine and neutralize acids formed by the intestinal bacteria. Water is also absorbed through the large intestine, leaving waste products to be eliminated in stool.

The urinary bladder, a distensible muscular sac located behind the pubic bone in the midline of the abdomen, functions as a temporary receptacle for urine. A bladder filled with urine may be palpated in the abdomen above the symphysis pubis.

Vascular Structures

The abdominal organs are supplied with arterial blood by the abdominal aorta and its major branches (Fig. 22-5). Pulsations of the aorta are frequently visible and palpable midline in the upper abdomen. The aorta branches into the right and left iliac

ASSESSMENT TOOL 22-1   Locating Abdominal Structures by Quadrants

Abdominal assessment findings are commonly allocated to the quadrant in which they are discovered, or their location may be described according to the nine abdominal regions that some practitioners may still use as reference marks. Quadrants and contents are listed here.

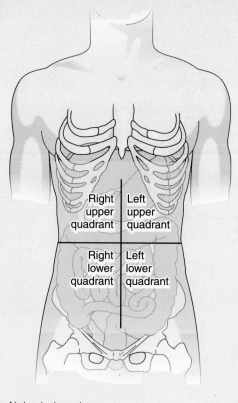

Right upper quadrant | Left upper quadrant
Right lower quadrant | Left lower quadrant

Abdominal quadrants.

Right Upper Quadrant (RUQ)
Ascending and transverse colon
Duodenum
Gallbladder
Hepatic flexure of colon
Liver
Pancreas (head)
Pylorus (the small bowel—or ileum—traverses
    all quadrants)
Right adrenal gland
Right kidney (upper pole)
Right ureter

Right Lower Quadrant (RLQ)
Appendix
Ascending colon
Cecum
Right kidney (lower pole)
Right ovary and tube
Right ureter
Right spermatic cord

Left Upper Quadrant (LUQ)
Left adrenal gland
Left kidney (upper pole)
Left ureter
Pancreas (body and tail)
Spleen
Splenic flexure of colon
Stomach
Transverse descending colon

Left Lower Quadrant (LLQ)
Left kidney (lower pole)
Left ovary and tube
Left ureter
Left spermatic cord
Descending and sigmoid colon

Midline
Bladder
Uterus
Prostate gland

continued

The older method of describing abdominal locations uses (9) nine regions, pictured below.

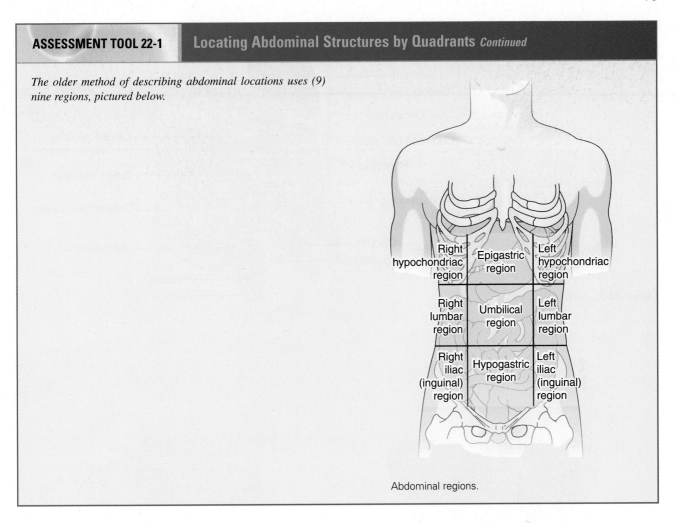

Abdominal regions.

---

arteries just below the umbilicus. Pulsations of the right and left iliac arteries may be felt in the **RLQ** and **LLQ**.

Health Assessment

COLLECTING SUBJECTIVE DATA: THE NURSING HEALTH HISTORY

The nurse may collect subjective data concerning the abdomen as part of a client's overall health history interview or as a focused history for a current abdominal complaint. The data focus on symptoms of particular abdominal organs and the function of the digestive system along with aspects of nutrition, usual bowel habits, and lifestyle.

Keep in mind that the client may be uncomfortable discussing certain issues such as elimination. Asking questions in a matter-of-fact way helps to put the client at ease. In addition, a client experiencing abdominal symptoms may have difficulty describing the nature of the problem. Therefore, the nurse may need to facilitate client responses and quantitative answers by encouraging descriptive terms and examples (i.e., pain as sharp or knifelike, headache as throbbing, or back pain as searing), rating scales, and accounts of effects on activities of daily living.

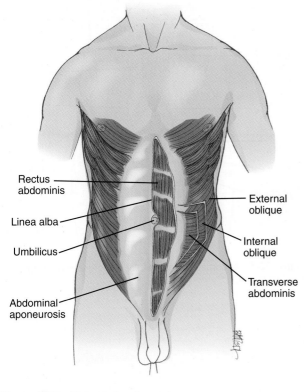

Figure 22-2 Abdominal wall muscles.

Rectus abdominis
Linea alba
Umbilicus
Abdominal aponeurosis
External oblique
Internal oblique
Transverse abdominis

(text continues on page 423)

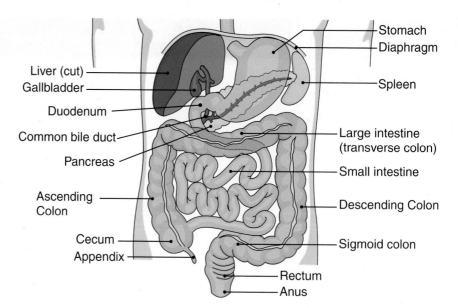

Stomach
Diaphragm
Liver (cut)
Gallbladder
Spleen
Duodenum
Common bile duct
Large intestine (transverse colon)
Pancreas
Small intestine
Ascending Colon
Descending Colon
Cecum
Sigmoid colon
Appendix
Rectum
Anus

Figure 22-3   Abdominal viscera.

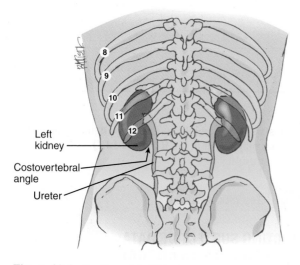

Left kidney
Costovertebral angle
Ureter

Figure 22-4   Position of the kidneys.

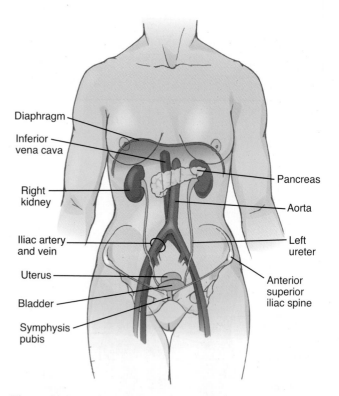

Diaphragm
Inferior vena cava
Pancreas
Right kidney
Aorta
Iliac artery and vein
Left ureter
Uterus
Anterior superior iliac spine
Bladder
Symphysis pubis

Figure 22-5   Abdominal and vascular structures (aorta and iliac artery and vein).

HISTORY OF PRESENT HEALTH CONCERN

Question	Rationale
Abdominal Pain Are you experiencing abdominal pain?	Abdominal pain occurs when specific digestive organs or structures are affected by chemical or mechanical factors such as inflammation, infection, distention, stretching, pressure, obstruction, or trauma.
How would you describe the pain? How bad is the pain (severity) on a scale of 1 to 10, with 10 being the worst?	The quality or character of the pain may suggest its origin (Display 22-1). The client's perception of pain provides data on his or her response and tolerance with pain. Sensitivity to pain varies greatly among individuals. Sensitivity to pain may diminish with aging. Therefore, elderly patients must be carefully assessed for acute abdominal conditions.
How did (does) the pain begin?	The onset of pain is a diagnostic clue to its origin. For example, acute pancreatitis produces sudden onset of pain, whereas the pain of pancreatic cancer may be gradual or recurrent.
Where is the pain located? Does it move or has it changed from the original location?	Location helps to determine the pain source and whether it is primary or referred (see Display 22-1).
When does the pain occur (timing and relation to particular events such as eating, exercise, bedtime)?	Timing and the relationship of particular events may be a clue to origin of pain (e.g., the pain of a duodenal ulcer may awaken the client at night).
What seems to bring on the pain (precipitating factors), make it worse (exacerbating factors), or make it better (alleviating factors)?	Various factors can precipitate or exacerbate abdominal pain such as alcohol ingestion with pancreatitis or supine position with gastroesophageal reflux disease. Lifestyle and stress factors may be implicated in certain digestive disorders such as peptic ulcer disease. Alleviating factors, such as using antacids or histamine blockers, may be a clue to origin.
Is the pain associated with any other symptoms such as nausea, vomiting, diarrhea, constipation, gas, fever, weight loss, fatigue, or yellowing of the eyes or skin?	Associated signs and symptoms may provide diagnostic evidence to support or rule out a particular origin of pain. For example, epigastric pain accompanied by tarry stools suggests a gastric or duodenal ulcer.
Indigestion Do you experience indigestion? Describe.	Indigestion (pyrosis), often described as heartburn, may be an indication of acute or chronic gastric disorders including hyperacidity, gastroesophageal reflux disease (GERD), peptic ulcer disease, and stomach cancer. Take time to determine the client's exact symptoms because many clients call gaseousness, belching, bloating, and nausea indigestion (see Promote Health—Peptic Ulcer Disease).
Does anything in particular seem to cause or aggravate this condition?	Certain factors (e.g., food, drinks, alcohol, medications, stress) are known to increase gastric secretion and acidity and cause or aggravate indigestion.

continued on page 419

DISPLAY 22-1   **Mechanisms and Sources of Abdominal Pain**

Types of Pain

Abdominal pain may be formally described as visceral, parietal, or referred.

- *Visceral pain* occurs when hollow abdominal organs, such as the intestines, become distended or contract forcefully or when the capsules of solid organs such as the liver and spleen are stretched. Poorly defined or localized and intermittently timed, this type of pain is often characterized as dull, aching, burning, cramping, or colicky.

- *Parietal pain* occurs when the parietal peritoneum becomes inflamed, as in appendicitis or peritonitis. This type of pain tends to localize more to the source and is characterized as a more severe and steady pain.

- *Referred pain* occurs at distant sites that are innervated at approximately the same levels as the disrupted abdominal organ. This type of pain travels, or refers, from the primary site and becomes highly localized at the distant site. The accompanying illustrations show common clinical patterns and referents of pain.

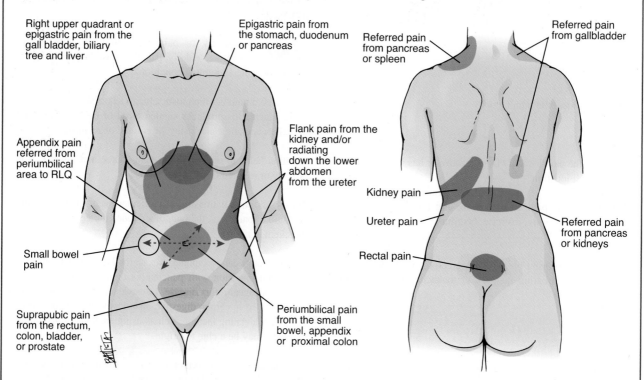

Patterns and referents of abdominal pain.

Character of Abdominal Pain and Implications

Dull, Aching

Appendicitis
Acute hepatitis
Biliary colic
Cholecystitis
Cystitis
Dyspepsia
Glomerulonephritis
Incarcerated or strangulated hernia
Irritable bowel syndrome
Hepatocellular cancer
Pancreatitis
Pancreatic cancer
Perforated gastric or duodenal ulcer
Peritonitis
Peptic ulcer disease
Prostatitis

Burning, Gnawing

Dyspepsia
Peptic ulcer disease
Cramping ("crampy")
Acute mechanical obstruction
Appendicitis
Colitis
Diverticulitis
Gastroesophageal reflux disease (GERD)

Pressure

Benign prostatic hypertrophy
Prostate cancer
Prostatitis
Urinary retention

Colicky

Colon cancer

Sharp, Knifelike

Splenic abscess
Splenic rupture
Renal colic
Renal tumor
Ureteral colic
Vascular liver tumor

Variable

Stomach cancer

HISTORY OF PRESENT HEALTH CONCERNS *Continued*

Question	Rationale
Nausea and Vomiting Do you experience nausea? Describe. Is it triggered by any particular activities, events, or other factors?	Nausea may reflect gastric dysfunction and is also associated with many digestive disorders and diseases of the accessory organs, such as the liver and pancreas, as well as with renal failure and drug intolerance. Nausea may also be precipitated by dietary intolerance, psychological triggers, or menstruation. Nausea may also occur at particular times such as early in the day with some pregnant clients ("morning sickness"), after meals with gastric disorders, or between meals with changes in blood glucose levels.
Have you been vomiting? Describe the vomitus. Is it associated with any particular trigger factors?	Vomiting is associated with impaired gastric motility or reflex mechanisms. Description of vomitus (emesis) is a clue to the source. For example, bright hematemesis is seen with bleeding esophageal varices and ulcers of the stomach or duodenum. Elderly or neuromuscular- or consciousness-impaired clients are at risk for lung aspiration with vomiting.
Appetite Have you noticed a change in your appetite? Has this change affected how much you eat or your normal weight?	Loss of appetite (anorexia) is a general complaint often associated with digestive disorders, chronic syndromes, cancers, and psychological disorders. Appetite changes should be carefully correlated with dietary history and weight monitoring. Significant appetite changes and food intake may adversely affect the client's weight and put the client at additional risk. Older clients may experience a decline in appetite from various factors such as altered metabolism, decreased taste sensation, decreased mobility, and possibly depression. If appetite declines, the client's risk for nutritional imbalance increases.
Bowel Elimination Have you experienced a change in bowel elimination patterns? Describe.	Changes in bowel patterns must be compared to usual patterns for the client. Normal frequency varies from two to three times per day to three times per week.
Do you have constipation? Describe. Do you have any accompanying symptoms?	Constipation is usually defined as a decrease in the frequency of bowel movements or the passage of hard and possibly painful stools. Signs and symptoms that accompany constipation may be a clue as to the cause of constipation such as bleeding with malignancies or pencil-shaped stools with intestinal obstruction.
Have you experienced diarrhea? Describe. Do you have any accompanying symptoms?	Diarrhea is defined as frequency of bowel movements producing unformed or liquid stools. It is important to compare these stools to the client's usual bowel patterns. Bloody and mucoid stools are associated with inflammatory bowel

continued on page 420

HISTORY OF PRESENT HEALTH CONCERN *Continued*

Question	*Rationale*
	diseases (e.g., ulcerative colitis, Crohn's disease); clay-colored, fatty stools may be from malabsorption syndromes. Associated symptoms or signs may suggest the disorder's origin. For example, fever and chills may result from an infection or weight loss and fatigue may result from a chronic intestinal disorder or a cancer.
	Older clients are especially at risk for potential complications with diarrhea, such as fluid volume deficit, dehydration, electrolyte, and acid–base imbalances, because they have a higher fat-to-lean muscle ratio.
Have you experienced any yellowing of your skin or whites of your eyes, itchy skin, dark urine (yellow-brown or tea colored), or clay-colored stools?	These symptoms should be evaluated to rule out possible liver disease.

continued

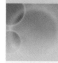

PROMOTE HEALTH
Peptic Ulcer Disease

Overview
Peptic ulcers are eroded areas of the mucosa in the stomach or first part of the intestine. The location determines the name of the ulcer: gastric or duodenal. The ulcerated area results from wear and irritation and causes pain and/or bleeding. The mucous coating that normally protects the mucosa can be disrupted by bacteria such as *H. pylori* or by eroding medications such as nonsteroidal anti-inflammatory medicines, allowing the digestive juices to erode the mucosa. Peptic ulcers can lead to perforation, obstruction, or gastric cancer. The actual causes of ulcers remain elusive. Why some people who have *H. pylori* develop ulcers and others do not is unclear. Risk factors include those that actually cause ulcers and those that irritate the mucosal lining, allowing more likely infection with *H. pylori*.

Risk Factors
- *H. pylori* infection
- Live in crowded, unsanitary conditions
- Take nonsteroidal anti-inflammatory or COX-2 inhibitor medications (or corticosteroids, but there is less research support for these)
- Prior ulcer disease
- Recent major surgery
- Zollinger-Ellison syndrome
- Recent severe injury or burn
- Head trauma
- Radiation therapy
- Congenital malformations of stomach or duodenum
- Some malignant diseases
- Age: duodenal for men (30–50 years of age); gastric for women (over 60 years of age)
- African American or Hispanic

- Type O blood
- Stress not a cause but can exacerbate symptoms and prolong healing
- Possible risk factors: cigarette smoking, alcohol, and acidic beverages (fruit juices, caffeine) increase irritation of stomach lining

Teach Risk Reduction Tips
- Avoid contracting *H. pylori* if possible; wash hands, use gloves when in contact with another's body fluids.
- Stop smoking.
- Reduce or stop using alcohol.
- Reduce intake of acidic foods and drinks, and caffeine.
- Ask primary health care provider about protective medications if taking irritating medications such as nonsteroidal anti-inflammatories.
- Consider stress management strategies.

COLDSPA Example for Abdominal Pain

Use the **COLDSPA** mnemonic as a guideline to collect needed information for each symptom the client shares. In addition, the following questions help elicit important information.

Mnemonic	Question	Client Response Example
Character	Describe the sign or symptom (feeling, appearance, sound, smell, or taste if applicable).	"It started hurting all over and then got worse in my right side."
Onset	When did it begin?	"Late last night"
Location	Where is it? Does it radiate? Does it occur anywhere else?	"On my right, lower part of my belly"
Duration	How long does it last? Does it recur?	"It is continual. The pain will not let up."
Severity	How bad is it? or How much does it bother you?	"It hurts so bad that I cannot focus on doing anything."
Pattern	What makes it better or worse?	"It is getting worse. I tried some Mylanta but it did not help."
Associated factors/How it **A**ffects the client	What other symptoms occur with it? How does it affect you?	"I'm nauseated, I can't move without it hurting, and I could not go to work this morning."

PAST HEALTH HISTORY

Question	Rationale
Have you ever had any of the following gastrointestinal disorders: ulcers, gastroesophageal reflux, inflammatory or obstructive bowel disease, pancreatitis, gallbladder or liver disease, diverticulosis, or appendicitis?	Presenting the client with a list of the more common disorders may help the client to identify any that he has or has had.
Have you had any urinary tract disease such as infections, kidney disease or nephritis, or kidney stones?	Urinary tract infections may become recurrent and chronic. Moreover, resistance to drugs used to treat infection must be evaluated. Chronic kidney infection may lead to permanent kidney damage. Older clients are prone to urinary tract infections because the activity of protective bacteria in the urinary tract declines with age.
Have you ever had viral hepatitis (type A, B, or C)? Have you ever been exposed to viral hepatitis?	Various populations (e.g., school and health care personnel) are at increased risk for exposure to hepatitis viruses. Any type of viral hepatitis may cause liver damage.
Have you ever had abdominal surgery or trauma to the abdomen?	Prior abdominal surgery or trauma may cause abdominal adhesions, thereby predisposing the client to future complications or disorders.
What prescription or over-the-counter medications do you take?	Medications may produce side effects that adversely affect the gastrointestinal tract. For example, aspirin, ibuprofen, and steroids may cause gastric bleeding. Chronic use of antacids or histamine-2 blockers may mask the symptoms of more serious stomach disorders. Overuse of laxatives may decrease intestinal tone and promote dependency. High iron intake may lead to chronic constipation.

continued on page 422

FAMILY HISTORY

Question	Rationale
Is there a history of any of the following diseases or disorders in your family: colon, stomach, pancreatic, liver, kidney, or bladder cancer; liver disease; gallbladder disease; kidney disease?	Family history of certain disorders increases the client's risk for those disorders. Genetic testing can now identify the risk for certain cancers (colon, pancreatic, and prostate) and other diseases. Client awareness of family history can serve as a motivation for health screening and positive health promotion behaviors.

LIFESTYLE AND HEALTH PRACTICES

Question	Rationale
Do you drink alcohol? How much? How often?	Alcohol ingestion can affect the gastrointestinal tract through immediate and long-term effects on such organs as the stomach, pancreas, and liver. Alcohol-related disorders include gastritis, esophageal varices, pancreatitis, and liver cirrhosis.
What types of foods and how much food do you typically consume each day? How much noncaffeinated fluid do you consume each day? How much caffeine do you think you consume each day (e.g., in tea, coffee, chocolate, and soft drinks)?	A baseline dietary and fluid survey helps to determine nutritional and fluid adequacy and risk factors for altered nutrition, constipation, diarrhea, and diseases such as cancer.
How much and how often do you exercise? Describe your activities during the day.	Regular exercise promotes peristalsis and thus regular bowel movements. In addition, exercise may help to reduce risk factors for various diseases such as cancer and hypertension (see Promote Health—Gallbladder Cancer).
What kind of stress do you have in your life? How does it affect your eating or elimination habits?	Lifestyle and associated stress and psychological factors can affect gastrointestinal function through effects on secretion, tone, and motility.
If you have a gastrointestinal disorder, how does it affect your lifestyle and how you feel about yourself?	Certain gastrointestinal disorders and their effects (e.g., weight loss) or treatment (e.g., drugs, surgery) may produce physiologic or anatomic effects that affect the client's perception of self, body image, social interaction and intimacy, and life goals and expectations.

PROMOTE HEALTH
Gallbladder Cancer

Overview
Of the several types of tumors that affect the gallbladder, about 80% are adenocarcinomas (ACS, 2006). The American Cancer Society reports that gallbladder cancer is the fifth most common gastrointestinal cancer and that between 5,000 and 7,000 new cases are diagnosed each year in the United States. Only 10% of patients survive 5 years due to late discovery after the cancer has advanced.

Women are affected two and one half times as often as men. Gallstones are the most common risk factor, especially when onset is at or before middle age or when there is one large stone. Many risk factors for gallbladder cancer are associated with gallstones, including high parity, obesity, and abnormalities of the biliary system promoting chronic inflammation.

continued

PROMOTE HEALTH
Gallbladder Cancer *Continued*

Risk Factors
- Age (over 70 years)
- Female gender (gallbladder)
  - Postmenopause
  - Increased parity
- Male gender (bile duct)
- Ethnicity
  - Native American (North, Central, and South America)
  - Hispanic
  - New Zealand Maori (Lowenfels et al., 1999)
- Gallstone, especially early onset of large gallstone
- Chronic inflammation of gallbladder
- Porcelain gallbladder (calcium deposits)
- Gallbladder polyps
- Common bile duct abnormalities
- Typhoid carrier
- Obesity
- Diet high in carbohydrates and fats and low in fiber
- Cigarette smoking

- Environmental exposure to industrial chemicals used in rubber and metal manufacturing
- Autoimmune disorder primary sclerosing cholangitis (PSC)
- Ulcerative colitis
- Certain parasitic flatworm cysts (Asian fish)

Teach Risk Reduction Tips
- Stop smoking.
- Prevent obesity. Follow ACS diet and exercise suggestions. Diet consists of five servings of fruits and vegetables; six servings of bread, grains, and legumes; and fewer fatty foods. Exercise consists of 30 minutes most days.
- Avoid industrial chemical exposure.
- Schedule periodic medical examinations to assess gallbladder and general status, especially if a history of risk factors is identified.

COLLECTING OBJECTIVE DATA: PHYSICAL EXAMINATION

The abdominal examination is performed for a variety of different reasons: as part of a comprehensive health examination; to explore gastrointestinal complaints; to assess abdominal pain, tenderness, or masses; or to monitor the client postoperatively. Assessing the abdomen can be challenging, considering the number of organs of the digestive system and the need to distinguish the source of clinical signs and symptoms.

The sequence for assessment of the abdomen differs from the typical order of assessment. Auscultate after you inspect so as not to alter the client's pattern of bowel sounds. Percussion then palpation follow auscultation. Adjust the bed level as necessary throughout the examination and approach the client from the right side. Use tangential lighting, if available, for optimal visualization of the abdomen.

The nurse needs to understand and anticipate various concerns of the client by listening and observing closely for verbal and nonverbal cues. Commonly clients feel anxious and modest during the examination, possibly from anticipated discomfort or fear that the examiner will find something seriously wrong. As a result, the client may tense the abdominal muscles, voluntarily guarding the area. Ease anxiety by explaining each aspect of the examination, answering the client's questions, and draping the client's genital area and breasts (in women) when these are not being examined.

Another potential factor to deal with is ticklishness. A ticklish client has trouble lying still and relaxing during the hands-on parts of the examination. Try to combat this using a controlled hands-on technique and by placing the client's hand under your own for a few moments at the beginning of palpation. Finally, warm hands are essential for the abdominal examination. Cold hands cause the client to tense the abdominal muscles. Rubbing them together or holding them under warm water just before the hands-on examination may be helpful.

Preparing the Client

Ask the client to empty the bladder before beginning the examination to eliminate bladder distention and interference with an accurate examination. Instruct the client to remove clothes and to put on a gown. Help the client to lie supine with the arms folded across the chest or resting by the sides (Fig. 22-6).

➤ **Clinical Tip** • *Raising arms above the head or folding them behind the head will tense the abdominal muscles.*

A flat pillow may be placed under the client's head for comfort. Slightly flex the client's legs by placing a pillow or rolled blanket under the client's knees to help relax the abdominal muscles. Drape the client with sheets so the abdomen is visible from the lower rib cage to the pubic area.

Instruct the client to breathe through the mouth and to take slow, deep breaths; this promotes relaxation. Before touching

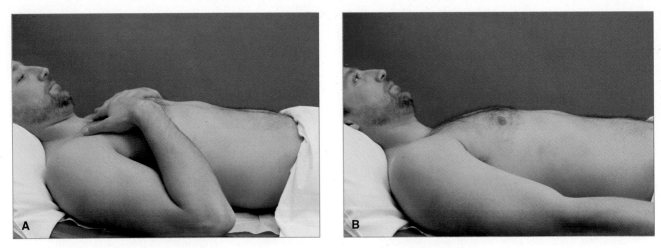

Figure 22-6 Two positions are appropriate for the abdominal assessment. The client may lie supine with hands resting on the center of the chest (**A**) or with arms resting comfortably at the sides (**B**). These positions best promote relaxation of the abdominal muscles.

the abdomen, ask the client about painful or tender areas. These areas should always be assessed at the end of the examination. Reassure the client that you will forewarn her when you will examine these areas. Approach the client with slow, gentle, and fluid movements.

Equipment

- Small pillow or rolled blanket
- Centimeter ruler
- Stethoscope (warm the diaphragm and bell)
- Marking pen

Physical Assessment

The examination evaluates the following abdominal structures in the abdominal quadrants: skin, stomach, bowel, spleen, liver, kidneys, aorta, and bladder. Remember to auscultate after inspection and before percussion and, finally, to palpate. Common abnormal findings include abdominal edema, or swelling, signifying ascites; abdominal masses signifying abnormal growths or constipation; unusual pulsations such as those seen with an aneurysm of the abdominal aorta; and pain associated with appendicitis.

(text continues on page 446)

PHYSICAL ASSESSMENT

Assessment Procedure	Normal Findings	Abnormal Findings
Inspection		
Observe the coloration of the skin.	Abdominal skin may be paler than the general skin tone because this skin is so seldom exposed to the natural elements.	Purple discoloration at the flanks (Grey Turner sign) indicates bleeding within the abdominal wall, possibly from trauma to the kidneys, pancreas, or duodenum or from pancreatitis.
		The yellow hue of jaundice may be more apparent on the abdomen.
		Pale, taut skin may be seen with ascites (significant abdominal swelling indicating fluid accumulation in the abdominal cavity).
		Redness may indicate inflammation.
		Bruises or areas of local discoloration are also abnormal.

continued

Assessment Procedure	Normal Findings	Abnormal Findings
Note the vascularity of the abdominal skin.	Scattered fine veins may be visible. Blood in the veins located above the umbilicus flows toward the head; blood in the veins located below the umbilicus flows toward the lower body. Dilated superficial capillaries without a pattern may be seen in older clients. They are more visible in sunlight.	Dilated veins may be seen with cirrhosis of the liver, obstruction of the inferior vena cava, portal hypertension, or ascites. Dilated surface arterioles and capillaries with a central star (spider angioma) may be seen with liver disease or portal hypertension.
Note any striae.	Old, silvery, white striae or stretch marks from past pregnancies or weight gain are normal.	Dark bluish-pink striae are associated with Cushing's syndrome. Striae may also be caused by ascites, which stretches the skin. Ascites usually results from liver failure or liver disease.
Inspect for scars. Ask about the source of a scar, and use a centimeter ruler to measure the scar's length. Document the location by quadrant and reference lines, shape, length, and any specific characteristics (e.g., 3-cm vertical scar in **RLQ** 4 cm below the umbilicus and 5 cm left of the midline). With experience, many examiners can estimate the length of a scar visually without a ruler.	Pale, smooth, minimally raised old scars may be seen. ➤ **Clinical Tip** • Scarring should be an alert for possible internal adhesions.	Nonhealing scars, redness, inflammation. Deep, irregular scars may result from burns. Keloids (excess scar tissue) result from trauma or surgery and are more common in African Americans and Asians (Fig. 22-7).
Assess for lesions and rashes.	Abdomen is free of lesions or rashes. Flat or raised brown moles, however, are normal and may be apparent.	Changes in moles including size, color, and border symmetry. Any bleeding moles or petechiae (reddish or purple lesions) may also be abnormal (see Chapter 13).
Inspect the umbilicus. Note the color of the umbilical area.	Umbilical skin tones are similar to surrounding abdominal skin tones or even pinkish.	Bluish or purple discoloration around the umbilicus (Cullen's sign) indicates intra-abdominal bleeding.
Observe umbilical location.	Umbilicus is midline at lateral line.	A deviated umbilicus may be caused by pressure from a mass, enlarged organs, hernia, fluid, or scar tissue.

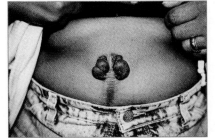

Figure 22-7 Keloid beyond the border of surgical scar.

continued

PHYSICAL ASSESSMENT *Continued*

Assessment Procedure	Normal Findings	Abnormal Findings
Assess contour of umbilicus.	It is recessed (inverted) or protruding no more than 0.5 cm and is round or conical.	An everted umbilicus is seen with abdominal distention (see Abnormal Findings 22-1). An enlarged, everted umbilicus suggests umbilical hernia (see Abnormal Findings 22-2).
Inspect abdominal contour. Look across the abdomen at eye level from the client's side (Fig. 22-8), from behind the client's head, and from the foot of the bed. Measure abdominal girth as indicated (Assessment Tool 22-2).	Abdomen is flat, rounded, or scaphoid (usually seen in thin adults) (Fig. 22-9). Abdomen should be evenly rounded.	A generalized protuberant or distended abdomen may be due to obesity, air (gas), or fluid accumulation (see Abnormal Findings 22-1). Distention below the umbilicus may be due to a full bladder, uterine enlargement, or an ovarian tumor or cyst. Distention of the upper abdomen may be seen with masses of the pancreas or gastric dilation. ➤ **Clinical Tip** • *The major causes of abdominal distention are sometimes referred to as the "6 Fs": Fat, feces, fetus, fibroids, flatulence, and fluid (Abnormal Findings 22-1).* A scaphoid (sunken) abdomen may be seen with severe weight loss or cachexia related to starvation or terminal illness.

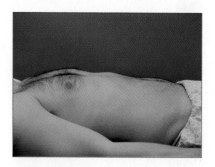

Figure 22-8 View abdominal contour from the client's side. Many abdomens are more or less flat; and many are round, scaphoid, or distended.

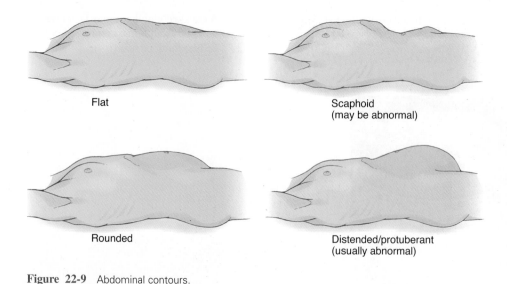

Flat

Scaphoid (may be abnormal)

Rounded

Distended/protuberant (usually abnormal)

Figure 22-9 Abdominal contours.

continued

ASSESSMENT TOOL 22-2   Measuring Abdominal Girth

In clients with abdominal distention, abdominal girth (circumference) should be assessed periodically (daily in hospital, during a doctor's office visit, with home nursing visits) to evaluate the progress or treatment of distention. Waist circumference measurement is also recommended in screening for cardiovascular risk factors.* To facilitate accurate assessment and interpretation, the following guidelines are recommended:

1. Measure abdominal girth at the same time of day, ideally in the morning just after voiding, or at a designated time for bedridden clients or those with indwelling catheters.
2. The ideal position for the client is standing; otherwise, the client should be in the supine position. The client's head may be slightly elevated (for orthopneic clients). The client should be in the same position for all measurements.

3. Use a disposable or easily cleaned tape measure. If a tape measure is not available, use a strip of cloth or gauze, then measure the gauze with a cloth tape measure or yardstick.
4. Place the tape measure behind the client and measure at the umbilicus. **Use the umbilicus as a starting point when measuring abdominal girth, especially when distention is apparent.**
5. Record the distance in designated units (inches or centimeters).
6. Take all future measurements from the same location. Marking the abdomen with a ballpoint pen can help you identify the measuring site. As a courtesy, the nurse needs to explain the purpose of the marking pen and ask the patient not to wash the mark off until it is no longer needed.

*Central obesity risk is defined as a waist circumference greater than 40 in (102 cm) in men and greater than 35 in (88 cm) in women. Central obesity is correlated with metabolic syndrome and increased risk for coronary heart disease (NCEP 2002).

Assessment Procedure	Normal Findings	Abnormal Findings
Assess abdominal symmetry. Look at the client's abdomen as she lies in a relaxed supine position.	Abdomen is symmetric.	Asymmetry may be seen with organ enlargement, large masses, hernia, diastasis recti, or bowel obstruction.
To further assess the abdomen for herniation or diastasis recti or to differentiate a mass within the abdominal wall from one below it, ask the client to raise the head.	Abdomen does not bulge when client raises head.	A hernia (protrusion of the bowel through the abdominal wall) is seen as a bulging in the abdominal wall. Diastasis recti appears as a bulging between a vertical midline separation of the abdominis rectus muscles. This condition is of little significance. An incisional hernia may occur when a defect develops in the abdominal muscles because of a surgical incision. A mass within the abdominal wall is more prominent when the head is raised, whereas a mass below the abdominal wall is obscured (Abnormal Findings 22-2).
Inspect abdominal movement when the client breathes (respiratory movements).	Abdominal respiratory movement may be seen, especially in male clients.	Diminished abdominal respiration or change to thoracic breathing in male clients may reflect peritoneal irritation.
Observe aortic pulsations.	A slight pulsation of the abdominal aorta, which is visible in the epigastrium, extends full length in thin people.	Vigorous, wide, exaggerated pulsations may be seen with abdominal aortic aneurysm.
Observe for peristaltic waves.	Normally peristaltic waves are not seen although they may be visible in very thin people as slight ripples on the abdominal wall.	Peristaltic waves are increased and progress in a ripple-like fashion from the **LUQ** to the **RLQ** with intestinal obstruction (especially small intestine). In addition, abdominal distention typically is present with intestinal wall obstruction.

continued

PHYSICAL ASSESSMENT Continued

Assessment Procedure	Normal Findings	Abnormal Findings
Auscultation		

Auscultate for bowel sounds. Use the diaphragm of the stethoscope and make sure that it is warm before you place it on the client's abdomen.

Apply light pressure or simply rest the stethoscope on a tender abdomen. Begin in the **RLQ** and proceed clockwise, covering all quadrants.

> ➤ *Clinical Tip* • Bowel sounds may be more active over the ileocecal valve in the **RLQ**.

Confirm bowel sounds in each quadrant. Listen for up to 5 minutes (minimum of 1 minute per quadrant) to confirm the absence of bowel sounds.

> ➤ *Clinical Tip* • Bowel sounds normally occur every 5 to 15 seconds. An easy way to remember is to equate one bowel sound to one breath sound.

Note the intensity, pitch, and frequency of the sounds.

A series of intermittent, soft clicks and gurgles are heard at a rate of 5 to 30 per minute. Hyperactive bowel sounds that may be heard normally are the loud, prolonged gurgles characteristic of stomach growling. These hyperactive bowel sounds are called "borborygmi."

> ➤ *Clinical Tip* • Postoperatively, bowel sounds resume gradually depending on the type of surgery. The small intestine functions normally in the first few hours postoperatively; stomach emptying takes 24 to 48 hours to recover; and the colon requires 3 to 5 days to recover propulsive activity.

Hypoactive bowel sounds indicate diminished bowel motility. Common causes include abdominal surgery or late bowel obstruction.

Hyperactive bowel sounds indicate increased bowel motility. Common causes include diarrhea, gastroenteritis, or early bowel obstruction.

Decreased or absent bowel sounds signify the absence of bowel motility, which constitutes an emergency requiring immediate referral.

Absent bowel sounds may be associated with peritonitis or paralytic ileus. High-pitched tinkling and rushes of high-pitched sounds with abdominal cramping usually indicate obstruction.

> ➤ *Clinical Tip* • The increasing pitch of bowel sounds is most diagnostic of obstruction because it signifies intestinal distention.

Auscultate for vascular sounds. Use the bell of the stethoscope to listen for bruits (low-pitched, murmurlike sound) over the abdominal aorta and renal, iliac, and femoral arteries (Fig. 22-10).

> ➤ *Clinical Tip* • Auscultating for vascular sounds is especially important if the client has hypertension or if you suspect arterial insufficiency to the legs.

Bruits are not normally heard over abdominal aorta or renal, iliac, or femoral arteries. However, bruits confined to systole may be normal in some clients depending on other differentiating factors.

A bruit with both systolic and diastolic components occurs when blood flow in an artery is turbulent or obstructed. This usually indicates aneurysm or arterial stenosis. If the client has hypertension and you auscultate a renal artery bruit with both systolic and diastolic components, suspect renal artery stenosis as the cause.

Using the bell of the stethoscope, listen for a venous hum in the epigastric and umbilical areas.

Venous hum is not normally heard over the epigastric and umbilical areas.

Venous hums are rare. However, an accentuated venous hum heard in the epigastric or umbilical areas suggests increased collateral circulation between the portal and systemic venous systems, as in cirrhosis of the liver.

Auscultate for a friction rub over the liver and spleen. Listen over the right and left lower rib cage with the diaphragm of the stethoscope.

No friction rub over liver or spleen is present.

Friction rubs are rare. If heard, they have a high-pitched, rough, grating sound produced when the large surface area of the liver or spleen rubs the peritoneum. They are heard in association with respiration.

A friction rub heard over the lower right costal area is associated with hepatic abscess or metastases.

continued

Assessment Procedure	Normal Findings	Abnormal Findings

A rub heard at the anterior axillary line in the lower left costal area is associated with splenic infarction, abscess, infection, or tumor.

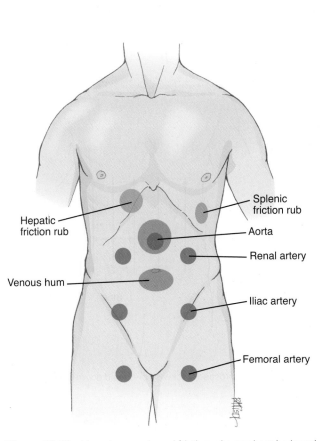

Figure 22-10 Vascular sounds and friction rubs can best be heard over these areas.

Hepatic friction rub

Splenic friction rub

Aorta

Renal artery

Venous hum

Iliac artery

Femoral artery

Percussion

Percuss for tone. Lightly and systematically percuss all quadrants. Two sequences are illustrated in Figure 22-11.

Generalized tympany predominates over the abdomen because of air in the stomach and intestines. Normal dullness is heard over the liver and spleen.

Dullness may also be elicited over a nonevacuated descending colon (Fig. 22-12).

Accentuated tympany or hyperresonance is heard over a gaseous distended abdomen.

An enlarged area of dullness is heard over an enlarged liver or spleen.

Abnormal dullness is heard over a distended bladder, large masses, or ascites.

If you suspect ascites, perform the shifting dullness and fluid wave tests. These special techniques are described later.

➤ *Clinical Tip* • *If you cannot find the lower border of the liver, keep in mind that the lower border of liver dullness may be difficult to estimate when obscured by intestinal gas.*

Percuss the span or height of the liver by determining its lower and upper borders.

The lower border of liver dullness is located at the costal margin to 1 to 2 cm below.

continued

PHYSICAL ASSESSMENT *Continued*

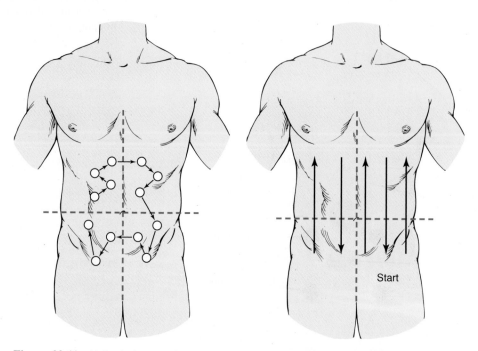

Figure 22-11   Abdominal percussion sequences may proceed clockwise or up and down over the abdomen.

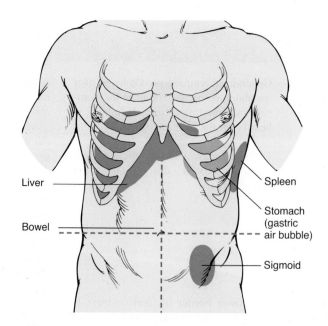

Figure 22-12   Normal percussion findings. Blue indicates dullness. Orange indicates tympany.

continued

Assessment Procedure	Normal Findings	Abnormal Findings
To assess the lower border, begin in the **RLQ** at the mid-clavicular line (MCL) and percuss upward (Fig. 22-13). Note the change from tympany to dullness. Mark this point: It is the lower border of liver dullness. To assess the descent of the liver, ask the client to take a deep breath and hold; then repeat the procedure. Remind the client to exhale after percussing.	On deep inspiration, the lower border of liver dullness may descend from 1 to 4 cm below the costal margin.	
To assess the upper border, percuss over the upper right chest at the MCL and percuss downward, noting the change from lung resonance to liver dullness. Mark this point: It is the upper border of liver dullness.	The upper border of liver dullness is located between the left fifth and seventh intercostal spaces.	The upper border of liver dullness may be difficult to estimate if obscured by pleural fluid of lung consolidation.
Measure the distance between the two marks: this is the span of the liver (Fig. 22-14).	The normal liver span at the MCL is 6 to 12 cm (greater in men and taller clients, less in shorter clients). Normally liver size decreases after age 50.	Hepatomegaly, a liver span that exceeds normal limits (enlarged), is characteristic of liver tumors, cirrhosis, abscess, and vascular engorgement. Atrophy of the liver is indicated by a decreased span. A liver in a lower position than normal may be caused by emphysema, whereas a liver in a higher position than normal may be caused by an abdominal mass, ascites, or a paralyzed diaphragm. A liver in a lower or higher position should have a normal span (Abnormal Findings 22-3).

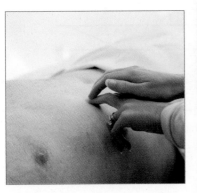

Figure 22-13 Begin liver percussion in the **RLQ** and percuss upward toward the chest (© B. Proud).

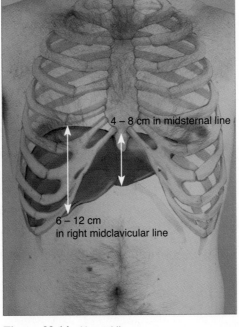

4 – 8 cm in midsternal line

6 – 12 cm in right midclavicular line

Figure 22-14 Normal liver span.

continued

PHYSICAL ASSESSMENT *Continued*

Assessment Procedure	Normal Findings	Abnormal Findings
Repeat percussion of the liver at the midsternal line (MSL).	The normal liver span at the MSL is 4 to 8 cm.	An enlarged liver may be roughly estimated (not accurately) when more intense sounds outline a liver span or borders outside the normal range.
If you cannot accurately percuss the liver borders, perform the scratch test (Fig. 22-15). Auscultate over the liver and, starting in the **RLQ**, scratch lightly over the abdomen, progressing upward toward the liver.	The sound produced by scratching becomes more intense over the liver.	
Percuss the spleen. Begin posterior to the left mid-axillary line (MAL), and percuss downward, noting the change from lung resonance to splenic dullness. ➤ *Clinical Tip • Results of splenic percussion may be obscured by air in the stomach or bowel.*	The spleen is an oval area of dullness approximately 7 cm wide near the left tenth rib and slightly posterior to the MAL.	Splenomegaly is characterized by an area of dullness greater than 7 cm wide. The enlargement may result from traumatic injury, portal hypertension, and mononucleosis.
A second method for detecting splenic enlargement is to percuss the last left interspace at the anterior axillary line (AAL) while the client takes a deep breath (Fig. 22-16). ➤ *Clinical Tip • Other sources of dullness (e.g., full stomach or feces in the colon) must be ruled out before confirming splenomegaly.*	Normally tympany (or resonance) is heard at the last left interspace.	On inspiration, dullness at the last left interspace at the AAL suggests an enlarged spleen (see Abnormal Findings 22-3).

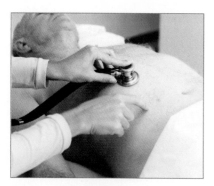

Figure 22-15 The scratch test.

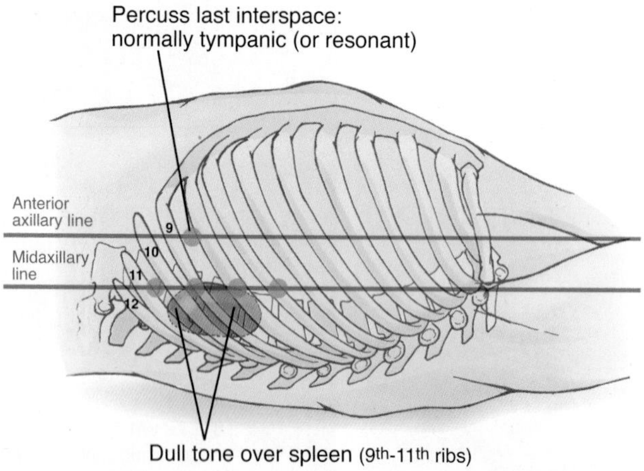

Percuss last interspace:
normally tympanic (or resonant)

Anterior
axillary line

Midaxillary
line

9
10
11
12

Dull tone over spleen (9th-11th ribs)

Figure 22-16 Last left interspace at the anterior axillary line.

continued

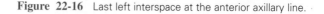

Assessment Procedure	Normal Findings	Abnormal Findings
Perform blunt percussion on the liver and the kidneys. This is to assess for tenderness in difficult-to-palpate structures. Percuss the liver by placing your left hand flat against the lower right anterior rib cage. Use the ulnar side of your right fist to strike your left hand.	Normally no tenderness is elicited.	Tenderness elicited over the liver may be associated with inflammation or infection (e.g., hepatitis or cholecystitis).
Perform blunt percussion on the kidneys at the costovertebral angles (CVA) over the twelfth rib (Fig. 22-17). ➤ **Clinical Tip** • *This technique requires that the client sit with his or her back to you. Therefore, it may be best to incorporate blunt percussion of the kidneys with your thoracic assessment because the client will already be in this position.*	Normally no tenderness or pain is elicited or reported by the client. The examiner senses only a dull thud.	Tenderness or sharp pain elicited over the CVA suggests kidney infection (pyelonephritis), renal calculi, or hydronephrosis.
Perform light palpation. Display 22-2 provides considerations for palpation. Light palpation is used to identify areas of tenderness and muscular resistance. Using the fingertips, begin palpation in a nontender quadrant, and compress to a depth of 1 cm in a dipping motion. Then gently lift the fingers and move to the next area (Fig. 22-18). To minimize the client's voluntary guarding (a tensing or rigidity of the abdominal muscles usually involving the entire abdomen), see Display 22-2. Keep in mind that the rectus abdominis muscle relaxes on expiration.	Abdomen is nontender and soft. There is no guarding.	Involuntary reflex guarding is serious and reflects peritoneal irritation. The abdomen is rigid and the rectus muscle fails to relax with palpation when the client exhales. It can involve all or part of the abdomen but is usually seen on the side (i.e., right vs. left rather than upper or lower) because of nerve tract patterns. Right-sided guarding may be due to cholecystitis.

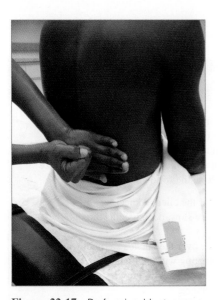

Figure 22-17 Performing blunt percussion over the kidney.

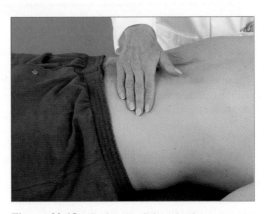

Figure 22-18 Performing light palpation.

continued

PHYSICAL ASSESSMENT Continued

Assessment Procedure	Normal Findings	Abnormal Findings
Deeply palpate all quadrants to delineate abdominal organs and detect subtle masses. Using the palmar surface of the fingers, compress to a maximum depth (5 to 6 cm). Perform bimanual palpation if you encounter resistance or to assess deeper structures (Fig. 22-19).	Normal (mild) tenderness is possible over the xiphoid, aorta, cecum, sigmoid colon, and ovaries with deep palpation.	Severe tenderness or pain may be related to trauma, peritonitis, infection, tumors, or enlarged or diseased organs.
Palpate for masses. Note their location, size (cm), shape, consistency, demarcation, pulsatility, tenderness, and mobility. Do not confuse a mass with a normally palpated organ or structure (Fig. 22-20).	No palpable masses are present.	A mass detected in any quadrant may be due to a tumor, cyst, abscess, enlarged organ, aneurysm, or adhesions.
Palpate the umbilicus and surrounding area for swellings, bulges, or masses.	Umbilicus and surrounding area are free of swellings, bulges, or masses.	A soft center of the umbilicus can be a potential for herniation. Palpation of a hard nodule in or around the umbilicus may indicate metastatic nodes from an occult gastrointestinal cancer.
Palpate the aorta. Use your thumb and first finger or use two hands and palpate deeply in the epigastrium, slightly to the left of midline (Fig. 22-21). Assess the pulsation of the abdominal aorta. If the client is older than age 50 or has hypertension, assess the width of the aorta.	The normal aorta is approximately 2.5 to 3.0 cm wide with a moderately strong and regular pulse. Possibly mild tenderness may be elicited.	A wide, bounding pulse may be felt with an abdominal aortic aneurysm. A prominent, laterally pulsating mass above the umbilicus with an accompanying audible bruit strongly suggests an aortic aneurysm (see Abnormal Findings 22-3).

DISPLAY 22-2   **Considerations for Palpating the Abdomen**

- Avoid touching tender or painful areas until last, and reassure the client of your intentions.
- Perform light palpation before deep palpation to detect tenderness and superficial masses.
- Keep in mind that the normal abdomen may be tender, especially in the areas over the xiphoid process, liver, aorta, lower pole of the kidney, gas-filled cecum, sigmoid colon, and ovaries.
- Overcome ticklishness and minimize voluntary guarding by asking the client to perform self-palpation. Place your hands over the client's. After a while, let your fingers glide slowly onto the abdomen while still resting mostly on the client's fingers. The same can be done by using a warm stethoscope

as a palpating instrument, again letting your fingers drift over the edge of the diaphragm and palpate without promoting a ticklish response.
- Work with the client to promote relaxation and minimize voluntary guarding. Use the following techniques:

  - Place a pillow under the client's knees.
  - Ask the client to take slow, deep breaths through the mouth
  - Apply light pressure over the client's sternum with your left hand while palpating with the right. This encourages the client to relax the abdominal muscles during breathing against sternal resistance.

continued

Assessment Procedure	Normal Findings	Abnormal Findings

➤ **Clinical Tip** • *Do not palpate a pulsating midline mass; it may be a dissecting aneurysm that can rupture from the pressure of palpation. Also avoid deep palpation over tender organs as in the case of polycystic kidneys, Wilms' tumor, transplantation, or suspected splenic trauma.*

Palpate the liver. Note consistency and tenderness. To palpate *bimanually,* stand at the client's right side and place your left hand under the client's back at the level of the eleventh to twelfth ribs. Lay your right hand parallel to the right costal margin (your fingertips should point toward the client's head). Ask the client to inhale then compress upward and inward with your fingers (Fig. 22-22).

To palpate by *hooking,* stand to the right of the client's chest. Curl (hook) the fingers of both hands over the edge of the right costal margin. Ask the client to take a deep breath and gently but firmly pull inward and upward with your fingers (Fig. 22-23).

The liver is usually not palpable, although it may be felt in some thin clients. If the lower edge is felt, it should be firm, smooth, and even. Mild tenderness may be normal.

A hard, firm liver may indicate cancer. Nodularity may occur with tumors, metastatic cancer, late cirrhosis, or syphilis. Tenderness may be from vascular engorgement (e.g., congestive heart failure), acute hepatitis, or abscess.

A liver more than 1 to 3 cm below the costal margin is considered enlarged (unless pressed down by the diaphragm).

Enlargement may be due to hepatitis, liver tumors, cirrhosis, and vascular engorgement.

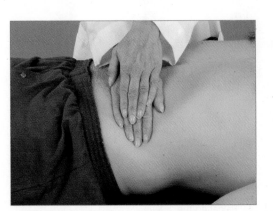

Figure 22-19 Performing deep bimanual palpation.

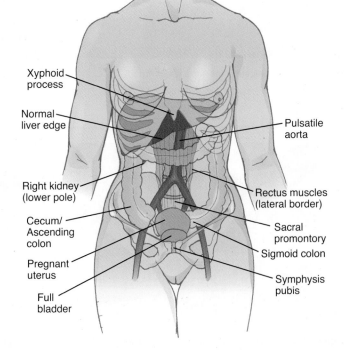

Figure 22-20 Normally palpable structures in the abdomen.

Xyphoid process

Normal liver edge

Pulsatile aorta

Right kidney (lower pole)

Rectus muscles (lateral border)

Cecum/ Ascending colon

Sacral promontory

Pregnant uterus

Sigmoid colon

Full bladder

Symphysis pubis

continued

PHYSICAL ASSESSMENT *Continued*

Assessment Procedure	Normal Findings	Abnormal Findings
Palpate the spleen. Stand at the client's right side, reach over the abdomen with your left arm, and place your hand under the posterior lower ribs. Pull up gently. Place your right hand below the left costal margin with the fingers pointing toward the client's head. Ask the client to inhale and press inward and upward as you provide support with your other hand (Fig. 22-24). Alternatively asking the client to turn onto the right side may facilitate splenic palpation by moving the spleen downward and forward (Fig. 22-25). Document the size of the spleen in centimeters below the left costal margin. Also note consistency and tenderness.	The spleen is seldom palpable at the left costal margin; rarely, the tip is palpable in the presence of a low, flat diaphragm (e.g., chronic obstructive lung disease) or with deep diaphragmatic descent on inspiration. If the edge of the spleen can be palpated, it should be soft and nontender.	A palpable spleen suggests enlargement (up to three times the normal size), which may result from trauma, mononucleosis, chronic blood disorders, and cancers. The splenic notch may be felt, which is an indication of splenic enlargement. ➤ *Clinical Tip* • Caution: *To avoid traumatizing and possibly rupturing the organ, be gentle when palpating an enlarged spleen.* The spleen feels soft with a rounded edge when it is enlarged from infection. It feels firm with a sharp edge when it is enlarged from chronic disease.

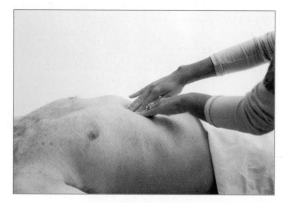

Figure 22-21   Palpating the aorta (© B. Proud).

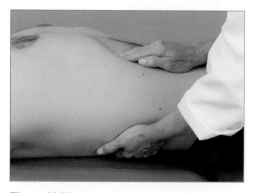

Figure 22-22   Bimanual technique for liver palpation.

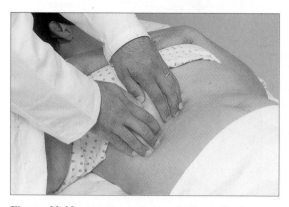

Figure 22-23   Hooking technique for liver palpation.

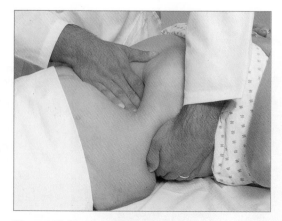

Figure 22-24   Palpating the spleen.

continued

Assessment Procedure	Normal Findings	Abnormal Findings

> ➤ **Clinical Tip •** *Be sure to palpate with your fingers below the costal margin so you do not miss the lower edge of an enlarged spleen.*

Palpate the kidneys. To palpate the right kidney, support the right posterior flank with your left hand and place your right hand in the **RUQ** just below the costal margin at the MCL.

To capture the kidney, ask the client to inhale. Then compress your fingers deeply during peak inspiration. Ask the client to exhale and hold the breath briefly. Gradually release the pressure of your right hand. If you have captured the kidney, you will feel it slip beneath your fingers. To palpate the left kidney, reverse the procedure (Fig. 22-26).

The kidneys are normally not palpable. Sometimes the lower pole of the right kidney may be palpable by the capture method because of its lower position. If palpated, it should feel firm, smooth, and rounded. The kidney may or may not be slightly tender.

Tenderness accompanied by peritoneal inflammation or capsular stretching is associated with splenic enlargement.

An enlarged kidney may be due to a cyst, tumor, or hydronephrosis. It can be differentiated from splenomegaly by its smooth rather than sharp edge, absence of a notch, and overlying tympany on percussion (see Abnormal Findings 22-3).

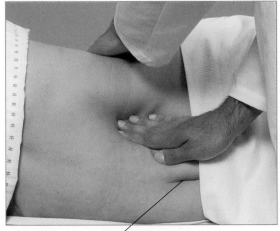

Umbilicus

Figure 22-25 Palpating the spleen with the client in side-lying position.

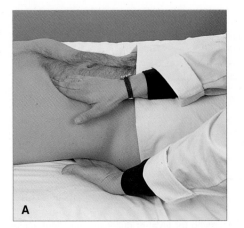

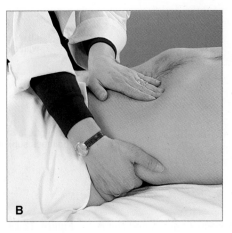

A   B

Figure 22-26 Palpating the right kidney (**A**) and the left kidney (**B**).

continued

PHYSICAL ASSESSMENT *Continued*

Assessment Procedure	Normal Findings	Abnormal Findings
Palpate the urinary bladder. Palpate for a distended bladder when the client's history or other findings warrant (e.g., dull percussion noted over the symphysis pubis). Begin at the symphysis pubis and move upward and outward to estimate bladder borders (Fig. 22-27).	Normally the bladder is not palpable.	A distended bladder is palpated as a smooth, round, and somewhat firm mass extending as far as the umbilicus. It may be further validated by dull percussion tones.

Special Abdominal Tests

Tests for Ascites

Test for shifting dullness. If you suspect that the client has ascites because of a distended abdomen or bulging flanks, perform this special percussion technique. The client should remain supine. Percuss the flanks from the bed upward toward the umbilicus. Note the change from dullness to tympany and mark this point. Now help the client turn onto his or her side. Percuss the abdomen from the bed upward. Mark the level where dullness changes to tympany (Fig. 22-28).	The borders between tympany and dullness remain relatively constant throughout position changes.	When ascites is present and the client is supine, the fluid assumes a dependent position and produces a dull percussion tone around the flanks. Air rises to the top and tympany is percussed around the umbilicus. When the client turns onto one side and ascites is present, the fluid assumes a dependent position and air rises to the top. There is a marked increase in the height of the dullness. This test is not always reliable and definitive testing by ultrasound is necessary.

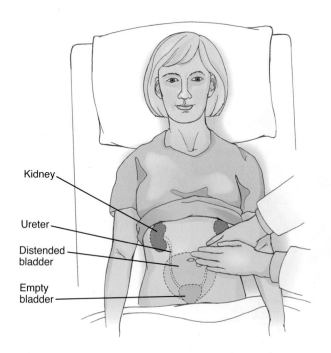

Figure 22-27 Palpating distended bladder (*Larger dotted line is area of distention*).

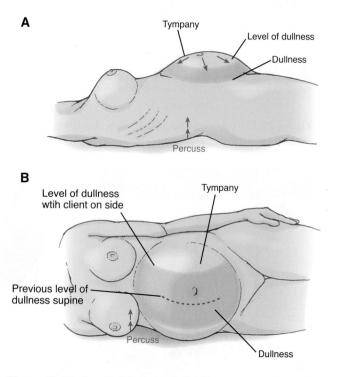

Figure 22-28 Percussing for level of dullness with client supine (**A**) and lying on the side (**B**).

continued

Assessment Procedure	Normal Findings	Abnormal Findings
Perform the fluid wave test. A second special technique to detect ascites is the fluid wave test. The client should remain supine. You will need assistance with this test. Ask the client or an assistant to place the ulnar side of the hand and the lateral side of the forearm firmly along the midline of the abdomen. Firmly place the palmar surface of your fingers and hand against one side of the client's abdomen. Use your other hand to tap the opposite side of the abdominal wall (Fig. 22-29).	No fluid wave is transmitted.	Movement of a fluid wave against the resting hand suggests large amounts of fluid are present (ascites). Because this test is not completely reliable, definitive testing by ultrasound is needed.
Use ballottement technique. Ballottement is a palpation technique performed to identify a mass or enlarged organ within an ascitic abdomen. Ballottement can be performed two different ways: single-handed or bimanually (Fig. 22-30). *Single-Hand Method:* Using a tapping or bouncing motion of the fingerpads over the abdominal wall, feel for a floating mass. *Bimanual Method:* Place one hand under the flank (receiving/feeling hand) and push the anterior abdominal wall with the other hand.	No palpable mass or masses are present.	In the client with ascites, you can feel a freely movable mass moving upward (floats). It can be felt at the fingertips. A floating mass can be palpated for size.

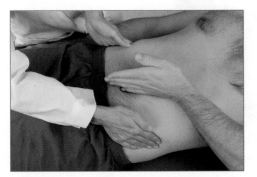

Figure 22-29 Performing fluid wave test.

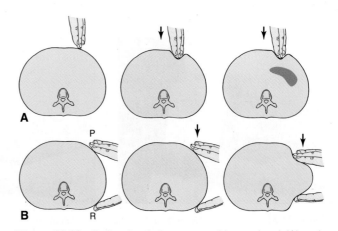

Figure 22-30 Performing ballottement with one hand (**A**) and bimanually (**B**).

continued

PHYSICAL ASSESSMENT Continued

Assessment Procedure	Normal Findings	Abnormal Findings
Tests for Appendicitis **Assess for rebound tenderness and Rovsing's Sign.** Abdominal pain and tenderness may indicate peritoneal irritation. To assess this possibility, test for rebound tenderness. Palpate deeply in the abdomen where the client has pain then suddenly release pressure (Fig. 22-31). Listen and watch for the client's expression of pain. Ask the client to describe which hurt more—the pressing in or the releasing—and where on the abdomen the pain occurred. ➤ *Clinical Tip • Test for rebound tenderness should always be performed at the end of the examination because a positive response produces pain and muscle spasm that can interfere with the remaining examination.*	No rebound tenderness is present.	The client has rebound tenderness when he or she perceives sharp, stabbing pain as the examiner releases pressure from the abdomen (Blumberg's sign). It suggests peritoneal irritation (as from appendicitis). If the client feels pain at an area other than where you were assessing for rebound tenderness, consider that area as the source of the pain (see test for referred rebound tenderness, below).
Test for referred rebound tenderness. Palpate deeply in the **LLQ** and, quickly release pressure.	No rebound pain is elicited.	Pain in the **RLQ** during pressure in the **LLQ** is a positive Rovsing's sign. It suggests acute appendicitis. ➤ *Clinical Tip • Avoid continued palpation when test findings are positive for appendicitis because of the danger of rupturing the appendix.*
Assess for Psoas sign. Raise the client's right leg from the hip and place your hand on the lower thigh. Ask the client to try to keep the leg elevated as you apply pressure downward against the lower thigh (Fig. 22-32).	No abdominal pain is present.	Pain in the **RLQ** (Psoas sign) is associated with irritation of the iliopsoas muscle due to an appendicitis (an inflamed appendix).

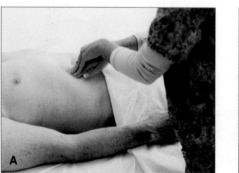 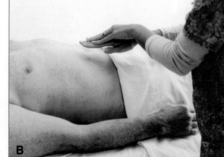

Figure 22-31 Assessing for rebound tenderness: palpating deeply (**A**); releasing pressure rapidly (**B**).

continued

Assessment Procedure	Normal Findings	Abnormal Findings
Assess for Obturator sign. Support the client's right knee and ankle. Flex the hip and knee and rotate the leg internally and externally (Fig. 22-33).	No abdominal pain in present.	Pain in the **RLQ** indicates irritation of the obturator muscle due to appendicitis or a perforated appendix.
Perform hypersensitivity test. Stroke the abdomen with a sharp object (e.g., broken cotton tipped applicator or tongue blade) or grasp a fold of skin with your thumb and index finger and quickly let go. Do this several times along the abdominal wall.	The client feels no pain and no exaggerated sensation.	Pain or an exaggerated sensation felt in the **RLQ** is a positive skin hypersensitivity test and may indicate appendicitis.
Test for Cholecystitis **Assess RUQ pain or tenderness, which may signal cholecystitis (inflammation of the gallbladder).** Press your fingertips under the liver border at the right costal margin and ask the client to inhale deeply.	No increase in pain is present.	Accentuated sharp pain that causes the client to hold his or her breath (inspiratory arrest) is a positive Murphy's sign and is associated with acute cholecystitis.

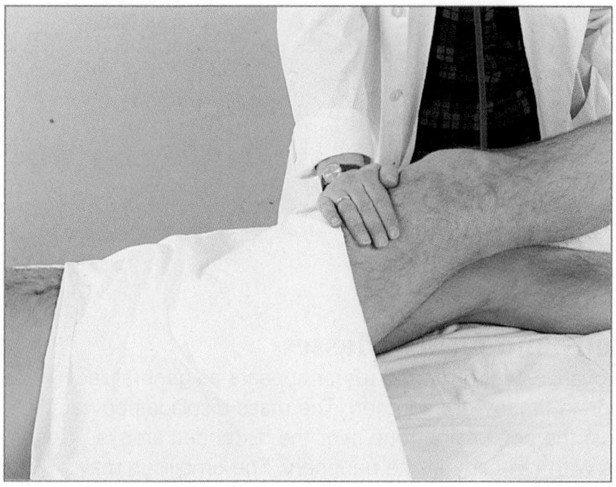

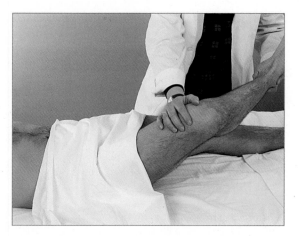

Figure 22-32 Testing for psoas sign (© B. Proud).

Figure 22-33 Testing for obturator sign (© B. Proud).

Abnormal Findings 22-1  **Abdominal Distention**

With the exception of pregnancy, abdominal distention is usually considered an abnormal finding. Percussion may help determine the cause.

Pregnancy (Normal Finding)
Pregnancy is included here so the examiner may differentiate it from abnormal findings.
It causes a generalized protuberant abdomen, protruberant umbilicus, a fetal heart beat that can be heard on auscultation, percussable tympany over the intestines, and dullness over the uterus.

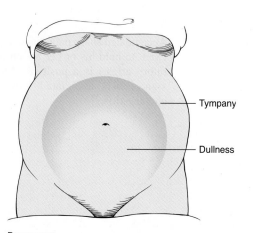

— Tympany

— Dullness

Pregnancy.

Feces
Hard stools in the colon appear as a localized distention. Percussion over the area discloses dullness.

— Dullness over feces

Feces.

Fat
Obesity accounts for most uniformly protuberant abdomens. The abdominal wall is thick and tympany is the percussion tone elicited. The umbilicus usually appears sunken.

Fat.

Fibroids and Other Masses
A large ovarian cyst or fibroid tumor appears as generalized distention in the lower abdomen. The mass displaces bowel, and, thus, the percussion tone over the distended area is dullness with tympany at the periphery. The umbilicus may be everted.

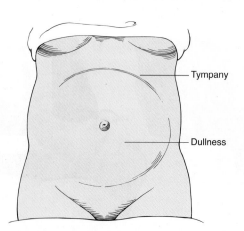

— Tympany

— Dullness

Fibrosis and masses.

continued

Abnormal Findings 22-1 — Abdominal Distention *Continued*

Flatus

The abdomen distended with gas may appear as a generalized protuberance (as shown), or it may appear more localized. Tympany is the percussion tone over the area.

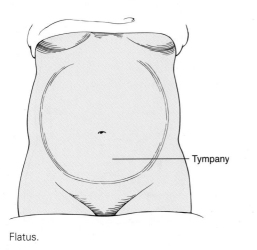

Flatus.

Ascitic Fluid

Fluid in the abdomen causes generalized protuberance, bulging flanks, and an everted umbilicus. Percussion reveals dullness over fluid (bottom of abdomen and flanks) and tympany over intestines (top of abdomen).

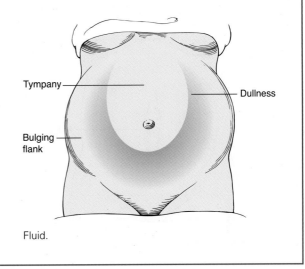

Fluid.

Abnormal Findings 22-2 — Abdominal Bulges

Umbilical Hernia

An umbilical hernia results from the bowel protruding through a weakness in the umbilical ring. This condition occurs more frequently in infants, but it also occurs in adults.

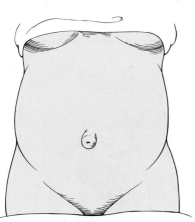

Umbilical hernia.

Epigastric Hernia

An epigastric hernia occurs when bowel protrudes through a weakness in the linea alba. The small bulge appears midline between the xiphoid process and the umbilicus. It may be discovered only on palpation.

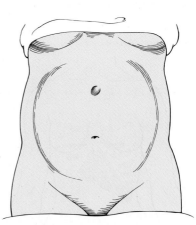

Epigastric hernia.

continued on page 444

Abnormal Findings 22-2 **Abdominal Bulges** *Continued*

Diastasis Recti

Diastasis recti occurs when bowel protrudes through a separation between the two rectus abdominis muscles. It appears as a midline ridge. The bulge may appear only when client raises head or coughs. The condition is of little significance.

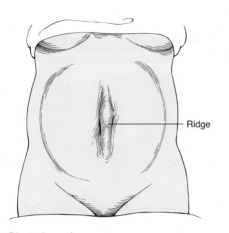

Diastasis recti.

Incisional Hernia

An incisional hernia occurs when bowel protrudes through a defect or weakness resulting from a surgical incision. It appears as a bulge near a surgical scar on the abdomen.

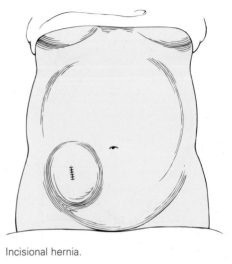

Incisional hernia.

Abnormal Findings 22-3 **Enlarged Abdominal Organs and Other Abnormalities**

Enlarged Liver

An enlarged liver (hepatomegaly) is defined as a span greater than 12 cm at the midclavicular (MCL) and greater than 8 cm at the midsternal line (MSL). An enlarged nontender liver suggests cirrhosis. An enlarged tender liver suggests congestive heart failure, acute hepatitis, or abscess.

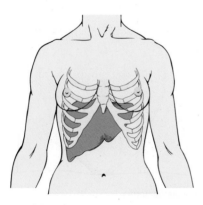

Enlarged liver.

Enlarged Nodular Liver

An enlarged firm, hard, nodular liver suggests cancer. Other causes may be late cirrhosis or syphilis.

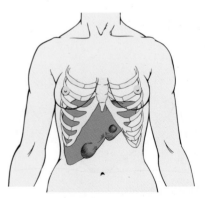

Enlarged nodular liver.

continued

Abnormal Findings 22-3

Enlarged Abdominal Organs and Other Abnormalities *Continued*

Liver Higher Than Normal

A liver that is in a higher position than normal span may be caused by an abdominal mass, ascites, or a paralyzed diaphragm.

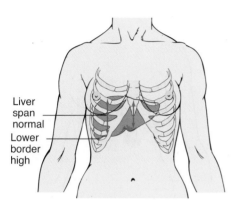

Liver higher than normal.

Enlarged Spleen

An enlarged spleen (splenomegaly) is defined by an area of dullness exceeding 7 cm. When enlarged, the spleen progresses downward and in toward the midline.

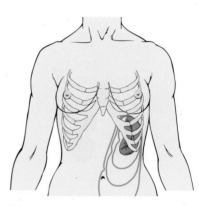

Enlarged spleen.

Liver Lower Than Normal

A liver in a lower position than normal with a normal span may be caused by emphysema because the diaphragm is low.

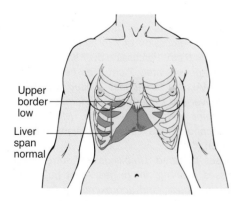

Liver lower than normal.

Aortic Aneurysm

A prominent, laterally pulsating mass above the umbilicus strongly suggests an aortic aneurysm. It is accompanied by a bruit and a wide, bounding pulse.

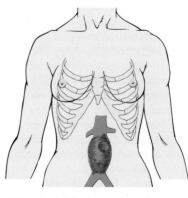

Aortic aneurysm.

continued on page 446

Abnormal Findings 22-3

Enlarged Abdominal Organs and Other Abnormalities *Continued*

Enlarged Kidney

An enlarged kidney may be due to a cyst, tumor, or hydronephrosis. It may be differentiated from an enlarged spleen by its smooth rather than sharp edge, the absence of a notch, and tympany on percussion.

Enlarged Gallbladder

An extremely tender, enlarged gallbladder suggests acute cholecystitis. A positive findings is Murphy's sign (sharp pain that causes the client to hold the breath).

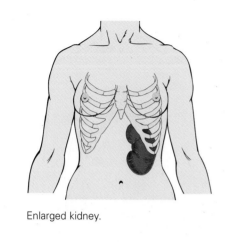

Enlarged kidney.

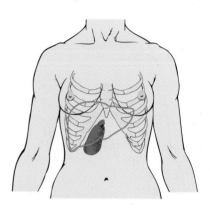

Enlarged gallbladder.

VALIDATING AND DOCUMENTING FINDINGS

Validate the abdominal assessment data you have collected. This is necessary to verify that the data are reliable and accurate. Document the assessment data following the health care facility or agency policy.

Sample Subjective Data

A 44-year-old male client denies pain in abdomen, indigestion, nausea, vomiting, constipation, and diarrhea. He says that he has had no change in his usual bowel habits and denies yellowing of skin, itching, dark urine, or clay-colored stools. Client states he has never had ulcers, gastroesophageal reflux, inflammatory or obstructive bowel disease, pancreatitis, gallbladder or liver disease, diverticulosis, or appendicitis. He did have one urinary tract infection 3 years ago but has had no other problems since that time. He never had viral hepatitis and denies known exposure. Client denies abdominal surgery or trauma to the abdomen. He does not take prescribed or over-the-counter medications except for an occasional ibuprofen for headache. He denies any family history of colon, stomach, pancreatic, liver, kidney, or bladder cancer; liver disease; gallbladder disease; or kidney disease. Client tries to follow a low-fat, high-carbohydrate, moderated protein diet and drinks a lot of fluids daily. He has approximately two alcoholic drinks per week, runs 3 days a week, and bikes 2 days a week. He reports a moderate amount of stress from work but copes with it through exercise and spending time with his wife and children.

Sample Objective Data

Skin of abdomen is free of striae, scars, lesions, or rashes. Umbilicus is midline and recessed with no bulging. Abdomen is flat and symmetric with no bulges or lumps. No bulges noted when client raises head. Slight respiratory movements and aortic pulsations noted. No peristaltic waves seen. Soft clicks and gurgles heard at a rate of 15 per minute. No bruits, venous hums, or friction rubs auscultated.

Percussion reveals generalized tympany over all four quadrants with dullness over the liver, spleen, and descending colon. Percussion of liver span reveals MCL = 8 cm and MSL = 6 cm. Percussion over spleen discloses a dull oval area approximately 7 cm wide near left tenth rib posterior to MAL. No tenderness elicited with blunt percussion over liver and kidneys. No tenderness or guarding in any quadrant with light palpation. Mild tenderness elicited over xiphoid, aorta, cecum, and sigmoid colon with deep palpation.

No masses palpated. Umbilicus and surrounding area free of masses, swelling, and bulges. Aortic pulsation moderately strong, regular, and approximately 3.0 cm wide. Liver, spleen, kidneys, and urinary bladder not palpable. Test for shifting dullness reveals constant borders between tympany and dullness throughout position changes. No fluid wave transmitted during fluid wave test. No mass palpated during ballottement test. All test findings for appendicitis are negative as is test finding for cholecystitis.

Analysis of Data

DIAGNOSTIC REASONING: POSSIBLE CONCLUSIONS

After collecting assessment data, you will need to analyze the data using diagnostic reasoning skills. Listed below are some possible conclusions that may be drawn after assessment of the client's abdomen.

Selected Nursing Diagnoses

After collecting subjective and objective data pertaining to the abdomen, you will need to identify abnormals and cluster the data to reveal any significant patterns or abnormalities. These data will then be used to make clinical judgments (nursing diagnoses: wellness, risk, or actual) about the status of the client's abdomen. Following is a listing of selected nursing diagnoses that you may identify when analyzing data for this part of the assessment.

Wellness Diagnoses

- Readiness for enhanced nutritional status
- Readiness for enhanced bowel elimination pattern
- Readiness for enhanced bladder elimination pattern
- Health-Seeking Behavior: Requests information on ways to improve nutritional status

Risk Diagnoses

- Risk for Fluid Volume Deficit related to excessive nausea and vomiting or diarrhea
- Risk for Impaired Skin Integrity related to fluid volume deficit secondary to decreased fluid intake, nausea, vomiting, diarrhea, fecal or urinary incontinence, or ostomy drainage
- Risk for Impaired Oral Mucous Membranes related to fluid volume deficit secondary to nausea, vomiting, diarrhea, or gastrointestinal intubation
- Risk for Urinary Infection related to urinary stasis and decreased fluid intake
- Risk for Imbalanced Nutrition: Less Than Body Requirements related to lack of dietary information or inadequate intake of nutrients secondary to values or religious beliefs or eating disorders

Actual Diagnoses

- Imbalanced Nutrition: Less Than Body Requirements related to malabsorption, decreased appetite, frequent nausea, and vomiting
- Imbalanced Nutrition: More Than Body Requirements related to intake that exceeds caloric needs
- Ineffective Sexuality Patterns related to fear of rejection by partner secondary to offensive odor and drainage from colostomy or ileostomy
- Grieving related to change in manner of bowel elimination
- Disturbed Body Image related to change in abdominal appearance secondary to presence of stoma
- Diarrhea related to malabsorption and chronic irritable bowel syndrome or medications
- Constipation related to decreased fluid intake, decreased dietary fiber, decreased physical activity, bedrest, or medications
- Perceived Constipation related to decrease in usual pattern and frequency of bowel elimination
- Bowel Incontinence related to muscular or neurologic dysfunction secondary to age, disease, or trauma
- Ineffective Health Maintenance related to chronic or inappropriate use of laxatives or enemas
- Disturbed Self-Concept related to obesity and difficulty losing weight
- Disturbed Self-Concept related to loss of bowel or bladder control
- Activity Intolerance related to fecal or urinary incontinence
- Anxiety related to fear of fecal or urinary incontinence
- Social Isolation related to anxiety and fear of fecal or urinary incontinence
- Pain: Abdominal (referred, distention, or surgical incision)
- Impaired Urinary Elimination related to catheterization secondary to obstruction, trauma, infection, neurologic disorders, or surgical intervention
- Urinary Retention related to obstruction of part of the urinary tract or malfunctioning of drainage devices (catheters) and need to learn bladder emptying techniques
- Impaired Patterns of Urinary Elimination related to bladder infection
- Functional Incontinence related to age-related urgency and inability to reach toilet in time secondary to decreased bladder tone and inability to recognize "need-to-void cues"
- Reflex Urinary Incontinence related to lack of knowledge of ways to trigger a more predictable voiding schedule
- Stress Incontinence related to knowledge deficit of pelvic floor muscle exercises
- Total Incontinence related to need for bladder retraining program
- Urge Incontinence related to need for knowledge of preventive measures secondary to infection, trauma, or neurogenic problems

Selected Collaborative Problems

After grouping the data, certain collaborative problems may emerge. Remember that collaborative problems differ from nursing diagnoses in that they cannot be prevented by nursing interventions. However, these physiologic complications of medical conditions can be detected and monitored by the nurse. In addition, the nurse can use physician- and nurse-prescribed interventions to minimize the complications of these problems. The nurse may also have to refer the client in such situations for further treatment of the problem. Following is a list of collaborative problems that may be identified when assessing the abdomen. These problems are worded as Risk for Complications (or RC), followed by the problem.

- RC: Peritonitis
- RC: Ileus
- RC: Afferent loop syndrome
- RC: Early dumping syndrome
- RC: Late dumping syndrome
- RC: Malabsorption syndrome
- RC: Intestinal bleeding
- RC: Renal calculi
- RC: Abscess formation

- RC: Bowel obstruction
- RC: Toxic megacolon
- RC: Mesenteric thrombosis
- RC: Obstruction of bile flow
- RC: Fistula formation
- RC: Hyponatremia/hypernatremia
- RC: Hypokalemia/hyperkalemia
- RC: Hypoglycemia/hyperglycemia
- RC: Hypocalcemia/hypercalcemia
- RC: Metabolic acidosis
- RC: Uremic syndrome
- RC: Stomal changes

- RC: Urinary obstruction
- RC: Hypertension
- RC: Gastroesophageal reflux disease
- RC: Peptic ulcer disease
- RC: Hepatic failure
- RC: Pancreatitis

Medical Problems

After grouping the data, it may become apparent that the client has signs and symptoms that may require medical diagnosis and treatment. Referral to a primary care provider is necessary.

CASE STUDY

The case study presents assessment data for a specific client. It is followed by an analysis of the data to arrive at specific conclusions. The study guide/lab manual and interactive product present additional opportunities to analyze data.

Nikki Chen, a 32-year-old graduate student, comes into the clinic complaining of undifferentiated abdominal discomfort. She states that she has been "constipated for the last 4 days." She appears nervous and fidgety and, when asked, confesses that she is very anxious about her upcoming final comprehensive examinations. "Sometimes I get so tense and upset I can't calm down. I really would like some help to learn new ways to handle my stress and to be more healthy. I'm concerned that if I don't do something soon, I will have high blood pressure like my father does." She indicates that her father took up smoking in his native China before coming to America, so she doesn't know if his high blood pressure is something she could inherit or if it's the result of his smoking. "I never got involved with that bad habit!" she says. During the interview, she describes her dietary habits as terrible: She eats salty, high-fat junk food

and doesn't drink water, just "lots of regular sodas with caffeine." She comments that her mother cooks healthful meals of rice and vegetables at home but Nikki doesn't get home very often any more. "Exercise? What graduate student has time for that?"

An examination of the client's abdomen reveals a moderately rounded, slightly firm, nontender abdomen with several small (quarter-sized), round, firm masses in the **LLQ** (sigmoid colon). Bowel sounds are active, moderate-pitched gurgles in all four quadrants. The abdomen is mostly tympanic upon percussion with scattered dullness in the **LUQ**. McBurney's and Rovsing's signs are both negative for rebound tenderness. A rectal examination reveals hard stool in the ampulla.

The following concept map illustrates the diagnostic reasoning process.

Applying COLDSPA

Applying **COLDSPA** for client symptoms: "Abdominal pain."

Mnemonic	Question	Data Provided	Missing Data
Character	Describe the sign or symptom (feeling, appearance, sound, smell, or taste if applicable).	"Constipated." Undifferentiated abdominal discomfort.	"Describe the discomfort: bloating, fullness, cramping, dull or sharp pains?"
Onset	When did it begin?	Four days ago	
Location	Where is it? Does it radiate? Does it occur anywhere else?		"Point to the areas of discomfort you are having. Do you have discomfort in any other areas?"

continued

Mnemonic	Question	Data Provided	Missing Data
Duration	How long does it last? Does it recur?		"When was your last bowel movement? Describe the color and consistency of the stool. How often do you usually have a bowel movement? Describe your usual bowel habits (frequency, regularity, character of stools, discomfort)."
Severity	How bad is it? or How much does it bother you?	"I'm very anxious about my upcoming final college exam; I get so upset and tense that I cannot calm down."	
Pattern	What makes it better or worse?	Client eats salty, high fat junk food and seldom drinks water, but rather lots of regular soda with caffeine. Unable to exercise with busy schedule.	
Associated factors/How it **A**ffects the client	What other symptoms occur with it? How does it affect you?	Client fears high blood pressure like her father because she does not know how to handle stress.	

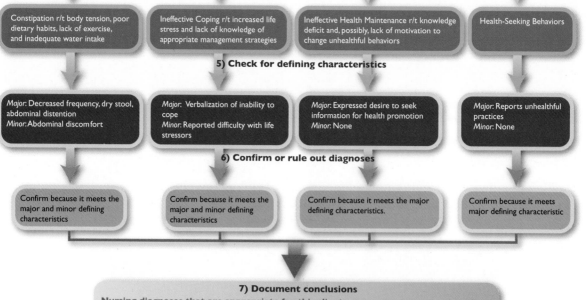

1) Identify abnormal data and client strengths

Subjective Data

- Complains of undifferentiated abdominal discomfort
- Reports constipation for the last 4 days
- Feels very anxious about upcoming final comprehensive examinations
- Gets tense and upset and cannot calm self
- Wants help learning new ways to handle stress and to be more healthy
- Voices concern that she will have high blood pressure like father who smokes
- Denies a smoking habit
- Describes diet as terrible: salty, high-fat junk food
- Doesn't drink water, just lots of sodas with caffeine
- Says mother prepares healthful meals, but client rarely eats at home
- Has no time for exercise

Objective Data

- Nervous and fidgety
- Moderately rounded, slightly firm, nontender abdomen
- Several small, quarter-sized, round, firm masses palpated in the sigmoid colon
- Bowel sound active with moderately pitched gurgles in all quadrants
- Abdomen mostly tympanic on percussion, scattered dullness in the LUQ
- Examination discloses no McBurney's or Rovsing's signs
- Rectal examination findings include hard stool in the ampulla

2) Identify cue clusters

- Complains of undifferentiated abdominal discomfort
- Constipated for the last 4 days
- Very anxious about examinations
- Gets tense and upset
- Eats salty, high-fat junk food
- Doesn't drink water; does drink lots of caffeinated sodas
- No time for exercise
- Moderately rounded, slightly firm abdomen, not tender to palpation
- Several small, round, firm masses in sigmoid colon
- Abdomen tympanic on percussion
- Negative McBurney's and Rovsing's signs
- Hard stool in the ampulla

- Anxious about final examinations
- Gets tense and upset; unable to calm self
- Wants to learn new ways to handle stress and to be healthier
- Describes dietary habits as terrible: high-fat junk food
- Doesn't drink water, just "lots of sugary, caffeinated sodas"
- No time for exercise

3) Draw inferences

Data strongly suggest constipation, probably as a result of poorly managed stress, lack of exercise, inadequate water intake

Able to identify unhealthful behaviors and inadequate coping strategies, but does not verbalize that she knows how to manage her stressors

Client appears to be seeking help for her current problems of constipation and unmanaged stress, but she is also taking this opportunity to get more information about ways to promote health

4) List possible nursing diagnoses

Constipation r/t body tension, poor dietary habits, lack of exercise, and inadequate water intake

Ineffective Coping r/t increased life stress and lack of knowledge of appropriate management strategies

Ineffective Health Maintenance r/t knowledge deficit and, possibly, lack of motivation to change unhealthful behaviors

Health-Seeking Behaviors

5) Check for defining characteristics

Major: Decreased frequency, dry stool, abdominal distention
Minor: Abdominal discomfort

Major: Verbalization of inability to cope
Minor: Reported difficulty with life stressors

Major: Expressed desire to seek information for health promotion
Minor: None

Major: Reports unhealthful practices
Minor: None

6) Confirm or rule out diagnoses

Confirm because it meets the major and minor defining characteristics

Confirm because it meets the major and minor defining characteristics

Confirm because it meets the major defining characteristics.

Confirm because it meets major defining characteristic

7) Document conclusions

Nursing diagnoses that are appropriate for this client:
- Constipation r/t body tension, lack of exercise, and inadequate water intake
- Ineffective Individual Coping r/t increased life stress and lack of knowledge of appropriate management strategies
- Ineffective Health Maintenance r/t knowledge deficit and possibly lack of motivation to change unhealthful behaviors
- Health-Seeking Behaviors
Because there is no medical diagnosis, there are no collaborative problems at this time

References and Selected Readings

Amelia, E. (2004). Presentation of illness in older adults. *American Journal of Nursing, 104*(10), 44–52.

Cook, K. (2005). Evaluating acute abdominal pain in adults. *Journal of the American Academy of Physician Assistants, 18*(3), 22.

Dagiely, S. (2006). An algorithm for triaging commonly missed causes of acute abdominal pain. *Journal of Emergency Nursing, 32*(1), 91–93.

Expert Panel. (2002, 2004). *Detection, evaluation and treatment of high blood cholesterol in adults* (Adult treatment Panel 111). National Cholesterol Education Program (NCEP). National Heart, Lung, and Blood Institute, National Institutes of Health. (NIH Publication No. 02-5212, September 2002).

Flaser, M. H. (2006). Acute abdominal pain. *The Medical Clinics of North America, 90*(3), 481–503.

Gerhardt, R. T. (2005). Derivation of a clinical guideline for assessment of nonspecific abdominal pain: The guideline for abdominal pain in the ED setting (GAPEDS) phase 1 study. *The American Journal of Emergency Medicine, 23*(6), 709–717.

Hepburn, M., Dooley, D., Fraser, S., Purcell, B., Ferguson, T., & Horvath, L. (2004). An examination of the transmissibility and clinical utility of auscultation of bowel sounds in all four abdominal quadrants. *Journal of Clinical Gastroenterology, 38*(3), 298–299.

Hibbert, F. (2007). Physical assessment in gastroenterology. *Gastrointestinal Nursing, 5*(8), 35–37.

Katz, S. K., Gordon, K. B., & Roenigk, H. H. (1996). The cutaneous manifestations of gastrointestinal disease. *Primary Care: Gastroenterology, 23*(3), 32–49.

Kirton, C. (1997). Assessing bowel sounds. *Nursing97, 27*(3), 64.

Lam, G. M., & Mobarhan, S. (2004). Central obesity and elevated liver enzymes. *Nutrition Review, 62*(10), 394–399.

Lyon, C., & Clark, D. C. (2006). Diagnosis of acute abdominal pain in older patients. *American Family Physician, 74*(9), 1537–1544.

Miller, S., & Alpert, P. (2006). Abdominal pain. *Nurse Practitioner, 31*(7), 38–47.

Movius, M. (2006). What's casing that gut pain? *R N, 69*(7), 25–29.

O'Hanlon-Nicholas, T. (1998). Basic assessment series: Gastrointestinal system. *American Journal of Nursing, 98*(4), 48–53.

Okosun, I. S., Chandra, K. M., Boev, A., Boltri, J. M., Choi, S. T., Parish, D. C., & Dev, G. E. (2004). Abdominal adiposity in U.S. adults: Prevalence and trends, 1960–2000. *Preventive Medicine, 39*(1), 197–206.

Scorza, K., Williams, A., Phillips, J. D., & Shaw, J. (2007). Evaluation of nausea and vomiting. *American Family Physician, 76*(1), 76–84.

Weight control information network (NIDDK). (June 2004). Weight and waist measurement: Tools for adults. *Guidelines on Overweight and Obesity: Electronic Textbook,* NIH Publication No. 04-5283. http://www.nhlbi.nih.gov/guidelines/obesity/

Promote Health—Gallbladder Cancer

American Cancer Society (ACS). (2008). *Gallbladder cancer.* ACS Gallbladder Cancer Resource Center. Available at http://www.cancer.org

Lowenfels, A. B., Maisonneuve, P., Boyle, P., & Zatonski, W. (1999). Epidemiology of gallbladder cancer. *Hepatogastroenterology, 46*(27), 1529–1532.

Mayo Clinic. (2007). Gallbladder cancer. Available at http://mayoclinic.com

Overfield, T. (1995). *Biological variation in health and illness: Race, age, and sex difference* (2nd ed.). Boca Raton, FL: CRC Press.

Promote Health—Peptic Ulcer Disease

Carson-DeWitt, R. (2007). Conditions InDepth: Peptic ulcer disease. Available at http://www.bidmc.org/YourHealth

Structure and Function

To perform an adequate assessment of the female genitalia, the nurse needs to have a basic understanding of the structure and function of the female reproductive system. This will guide the physical examination and readily assist in identifying abnormalities. The female genitalia consist of external structures and internal structures.

EXTERNAL GENITALIA

The external genitalia include those structures that can be readily identified through inspection (Fig. 23-1). The area is sometimes referred to as the **vulva** *or pudendum* and extends from the mons pubis to the anal opening. The **mons pubis** is the fat pad located over the symphysis pubis. The normal adult mons pubis is covered with pubic hair in a triangular pattern. It functions to absorb force and to protect the symphysis pubis during coitus. The **labia majora** are two folds of skin that extend posteriorly and inferiorly from the mons pubis to the perineum. The skin folds are composed of adipose tissue, sebaceous glands, and sweat glands. The outer surface of the labia majora is covered with pubic hair in the adult, whereas the inner surface is pink, smooth, and moist.

Inside the labia majora are the thinner skin folds of the **labia minora.** These folds join anteriorly at the clitoris and form a *prepuce* or hood; posteriorly the two folds join to form the **frenulum.** Compared with the labia majora, the labia minora are hairless and usually darker pink. They contain numerous sebaceous glands that promote lubrication and maintain a moist environment in the vaginal area. The **clitoris** is located at the anterior end of the labia minora. It is a small, cylindrical mass of erectile tissue and nerves with three parts: the *glans,* the *corpus,* and the *crura.* The glans is the visible rounded portion of the clitoris. The corpus is the body, and the crura are two bands of fibrous tissue that attach the clitoris to the pelvic bone. The clitoris is similar to the male penis and contains many blood vessels that become engorged during sexual arousal.

The skin folds of the labia majora and labia minora form a boat-shaped area or fossa called the **vestibule.** The vestibule contains several openings. Located between the clitoris and the vaginal orifice is the **urethral meatus.** The openings of **Skene's glands** are located on either side of the urethral opening. They are usually not visible. These small glands are often referred to as the **lesser vestibular glands.** Skene's glands secrete mucus that lubricates and maintains a moist vaginal environment.

Below the urethral meatus is the **vaginal orifice.** This is the external opening of the vagina and has either a slitlike or irregular circular structure, depending on the configuration of a **hymen.** The hymen is a fold of membranous tissue that covers part of the vagina. On either side of and slightly posterior to the vaginal orifice (between the vaginal orifice and the labia minora) are the openings to **Bartholin's glands.** Through the openings, the glands secrete mucus, which lubricates the area during sexual intercourse. These small glands are often referred to as the *greater vestibular glands.* The glands and the openings are not visible to the naked eye.

INTERNAL GENITALIA

The internal genital structures function as the female reproductive organs (Fig. 23-2). They include the vagina, the uterus, the cervix, the fallopian tubes, and the ovaries. The **vagina,** a muscular, tubular organ, extends up and slightly back toward the rectum from the vaginal orifice (external opening) to the cervix. It lies between the rectum posteriorly and the urethra and bladder anteriorly and is approximately 10 cm long. The vagina performs many functions. It allows the passage of menstrual flow, it receives the penis during sexual intercourse, and it serves as the lower portion of the birth canal during delivery.

The **vaginal wall** comprises four layers. The outer layer is composed of pink squamous epithelium and connective tissue. It is under the direct influence of the hormone estrogen and contains many mucus-producing cells. This outer layer of epithelium lies in transverse folds called *rugae.* These transverse folds allow the vagina to expand during intercourse; they also facilitate vaginal delivery of a fetus. The second layer is the submucosal layer. It contains the blood vessels, nerves, and lymphatic channels. The third layer is composed of smooth muscle, and the fourth layer consists of connective tissue and the vascular network. The normal vaginal environment is acidic (pH of 3.8 to 4.2). This environment is maintained because the vaginal flora is composed of Doderlein's bacilli, and the bacilli act on glycogen to produce lactic acid. This acidic environment helps to prevent vaginal infection.

In the upper end of the vagina, the **cervix** dips down and forms a circular recess that gives rise to areas known as the

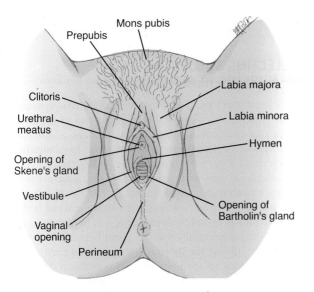

Figure 23-1 External genitalia.

anterior and posterior fornices. The *cervix* (or neck of the uterus) separates the upper end of the vagina from the isthmus of the uterus. The junction of the isthmus and the cervix forms the **internal os,** and the junction of the cervix and the vagina forms the **external os** or ectocervix. The "os" refers to the opening in the center of the cervix.

➤ **Clinical Tip** • *A woman who is nulliparous (having borne no offspring) has a small, round opening that appears as a depression on examination. A woman who has had her cervix dilated during childbirth has a slitlike external os.*

The cervix is composed of smooth muscle, muscle fibers, and connective tissue. Two types of epithelium cover the external os or ectocervix—pink squamous epithelium (which lines the vaginal walls) and red, rough-looking columnar epithelium (which lines the endocervical canal). The columnar epithelium may be visible around the os. The point where the two types of epithelium meet is called the *squamocolumnar junction.* The squamocolumnar junction migrates toward the cervical os with maturation or with increased estrogen levels. This migration creates an area known as the transformational zone. The transformational zone is important: 1) 90% of the neoplasms of the lower genital track originate in this area so 2) this is the area from which cells are obtained for cervical cytology or the Papanicolaou smear (Pap test). The cervix functions to allow the entrance of sperm into the uterus and to allow the passage of menstrual flow. It also secretes mucus and prevents the entrance of vaginal bacteria. During childbirth, the cervix can stretch to allow the passage of the fetus.

The **uterus** is a pear-shaped muscular organ that has two components: the *corpus,* or body, and the *cervix,* or neck (discussed previously). The corpus of the uterus is divided into the fundus (upper portion), the body (central portion), and the isthmus (narrow lower portion). The uterus is usually situated in a forward position above the bladder at approximately a 45-degree angle to the vagina when standing (anteverted and anteflexed position). The normal-sized uterus is approximately 7.5 cm long, 5 cm wide, and 2.5 cm thick. The uterus is movable.

The **endometrium,** the myometrium, and the *peritoneum* are the three layers of the uterine wall. The endometrium is the inner mucosal layer. The endometrium is composed of epithelium, connective tissue, and a vascular network; the thickness of this tissue is influenced by estrogen and progesterone. Uterine glands contained within the endometrium secrete an

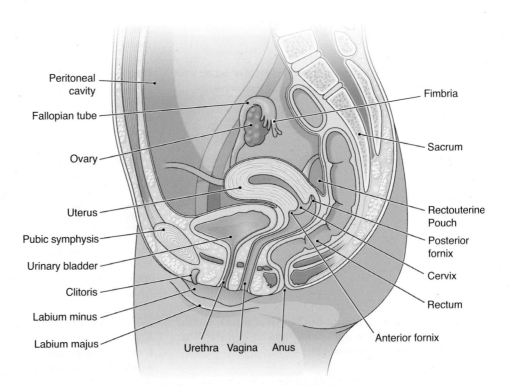

Figure 23-2 Female reproductive system (saggital section). This view shows the relationship of the reproductive organs to each other and to other structures in the pelvic cavity.

alkaline substance that keeps the uterine cavity moist. A portion of the endometrium sheds during menses and childbirth. The myometrium is the middle layer of the uterus. It is composed of three layers of smooth muscle fibers that surround blood vessels. This layer functions to expel the products of conception. The peritoneum is the outer uterine layer that covers the uterus and separates it from the abdominal cavity. The peritoneum forms anterior and posterior pouches around the uterus. The posterior pouch is called the **recto-uterine pouch** or the **cul-de-sac of Douglas.**

The **ovaries** are a pair of small, oval-shaped organs. Each is approximately 3 cm long, 2 cm wide, and 1 cm deep; each is situated on a lateral aspect of the pelvic cavity. The ovaries are connected to the uterus by the ovarian ligament. The ovary functions to develop and release ova and to produce hormones such as estrogen, progesterone, and testosterone. The **ovum** travels from the ovary to the uterus through the **fallopian tubes.** These 8- to 12-cm long tubes begin near the ovaries and enter the uterus just beneath the fundus. The end of the tube near the ovary has fringelike extensions called **fimbriae.** The ovaries, fallopian tubes, and supporting ovarian ligaments are referred to as the **adnexa** (Latin for appendages).

Nursing Assessment

COLLECTING SUBJECTIVE DATA: THE NURSING HEALTH HISTORY

When interview topics turn to the reproductive system and female genitalia, keep in mind the sensitivities of the client as well as your own feelings regarding body image, fear of cancer, sexuality, and the like. Western culture tends to emphasize the importance of a woman's reproductive ability, thereby entwining self-esteem and body image with the female sex role. Anxiety, embarrassment, and fear may affect the client's ability to discuss problems and ask questions. Because some problems can be serious or even life-threatening, it is important to establish a trusting relationship with the client because the information gathered during the subjective examination may suggest a problem or point to the possibility of a problem developing. Cancer of the cervix, for example, is associated with a high mortality rate but related risk factors are highly modifiable and cure rates are high as well in disease that is discovered early.

(text continues on page 460)

HISTORY OF PRESENT HEALTH CONCERNS

Clients from some cultures (e.g., Islam) may accept subjective or physical assessment only by a female nurse, especially when genital and/or sexual issues are being addressed.

Question	Rationale
Menstrual cycle What was the date of your last menstrual period? Do your menstrual cycles occur on a regular schedule? How long do they last? Describe the typical amount of blood flow you have with your periods. Any clotting?	A normal menstrual cycle usually occurs approximately every 18 to 45 days. The average length of menstrual blood flow is 3 to 7 days. The absence of menstruation, excessive bleeding, or a marked change in menstrual pattern indicates a need to collect more information.
What other symptoms do you experience before or during your period (cramps, bloating, moodiness, breast tenderness)?	Headache, weight gain, mood swings, abdominal cramping, and bloating are common complaints before or during the menstrual period. Some women experience premenstrual syndrome (PMS), in which the symptoms become severe enough to impair the women's ability to function.
How old were you when you started your period?	In North America, the average age is 12.5 years. Menstruation usually begins when the woman reaches 48 kg (106 lb). *Note:* Menarche (beginning of menstruation) tends to begin earlier in women living in developed countries and later in women who live in undeveloped countries. Ages of menarche range from 10 to 16 years of age, with earlier onset in shorter and fatter girls (Anderson, Dallal, & Must, 2003; Chumlea et al., 2003). Women who are poor or from less developed countries have earlier menopause.
Have you stopped menstruating or have your periods become irregular? Do you have any spotting between periods? What symptoms have you experienced?	Irregularities or amenorrhea may be due to pregnancy, depression, ovarian tumors, ovarian cysts, autoimmune disease, and hormonal imbalances. Cessation of menstruation is termed *menopause,* see next rationale.

continued

HISTORY OF PRESENT HEALTH CONCERN *Continued*

Question	Rationale
Menopause Are you still having periods? Have your periods changed?	Menopause is a normal physiologic process that occurs in women between the ages of 40 to 58 years, with a mean age of 50. Menopause occurring before age 30 is termed *premature menopause;* menopause between ages 31 and 40 is considered early; menopause occurring in women older than age 58 years is termed *delayed menopause.* Premature and delayed menopause may be due to genetic predisposition, an endocrine disorder, or gynecologic dysfunction. Artificial or surgical menopause occurs in women who have dysfunctional ovaries or who have had their ovaries removed surgically. During the perimenopausal period, hormone levels may fluctuate, resulting in menstrual irregularities. Periods may be heavier or may become scant.
Are you experiencing any symptoms of menopause?	Hormone fluctuations impact vasomotor instability resulting in symptoms. About 60% of menopausal women experience hot flashes and night sweats. Mood swings, decreased appetite, vaginal dryness, spotting, and irregular vaginal bleeding may also occur.
Are you on a hormone replacement therapy (HRT) regimen? If so, what type, and dosage? Are you satisfied with HRT?	It is important to discuss and explain risk versus benefits of HRT.
Are you continuing to have any symptoms of menopause while taking HRT?	If vasomotor symptoms continue, the client may need to have type of HRT or dosage adjusted.
What are your concerns about going through menopause?	Menopause is a normal stage in a woman's life. Some women have mixed feelings about experiencing menopause. Some may grieve their loss of child-bearing capabilities; while others may welcome this new phase of life, as they feel relieved no longer having to be concerned about pregnancy.
Vaginal discharge, pain, masses Are you experiencing vaginal discharge that is unusual in terms of color, amount, or odor?	Vaginal discharge may be from an infection.
Do you experience pain or itching in your genital or groin area?	Complaints of pain in the area of the vulva, vagina, uterus, cervix, or ovaries may indicate infection. Itching may indicate infection or infestation. The older client is more susceptible to vaginal infection because of atrophy of the vaginal mucosa associated with aging.
Do you have any lumps, swelling, or masses in your genital area?	These findings may indicate infection, lymphedema, or cancer. Past occurrences should be monitored for recurrence.
Urination Do you have any difficulty urinating? Do you have any burning or pain with urination? Has your urine changed color or developed an odor? Have you noticed any blood in your urine?	Urinary frequency, burning, or pain (dysuria) are signs of infection (urinary tract or sexually transmitted disease), whereas hesitancy or straining could indicate blockage. Change in color and development of an abnormal odor could indicate infection.
Do you have difficulty controlling your urine?	Difficulty controlling urine (incontinence) may indicate urgency or stress incontinence. During sneezing or coughing, increased abdominal pressure causes spontaneous urination.

continued on page 456

HISTORY OF PRESENT HEALTH CONCERN *Continued*

Question	Rationale
	Urinary incontinence may develop in older women from muscle weakness or loss of urethral elasticity.
Sexual Dysfunction Do you have any problems with your sexual performance?	A broad opening question about sex allows the client to focus the interview to areas where she has concerns. Some women have difficulty achieving orgasm and may believe there is something wrong with them.
Have you recently had a change in your sexual activity pattern or libido?	A change in sexual activity or libido needs to be investigated for the cause. A woman who is dissatisfied with her sexual performance may experience a decreased libido.
	As women age, their estrogen production decreases, causing atrophy of the vaginal mucosa. These women may need to use lubrication to increase comfort during intercourse. Women experiencing surgical menopause, symptoms of which occur more abruptly, may also benefit from lubrication.
Do you experience (or have you experienced) problems with fertility?	Infertility is defined as unprotected sex for 1 year without pregnancy. Approximately 35% of infertility cases are related to female fertility factors from a variety of causes.

COLDSPA Example for Burning when Urinating

Use the **COLDSPA** mnemonic as a guideline to collect needed information for each symptom the client shares. In addition, the following questions help elicit important information.

Mnemonic	Question	Client Response Example
Character	Describe the sign or symptom (feeling, appearance, sound, smell, or taste if applicable).	"I have burning when I urinate."
Onset	When did it begin?	"Last night at about 11 PM,"
Location	Where is it? Does it radiate? Does it occur anywhere else?	"The pain is right where my urine comes out. Sometimes it cramps right above my pubic area."
Duration	How long does it last? Does it recur?	"It has not gone away since it started but it hurts even more when I go to the bathroom."
Severity	How bad is it? or How much does it bother you?	"I can't do anything it hurts so bad."
Pattern	What makes it better or worse?	"I went to the pharmacy last night and bought Azodye and it gave me some relief."
Associated factors/How it **A**ffects the client	What other symptoms occur with it? How does it affect you?	"There is blood in my urine now. I stayed home from work today because I am so miserable."

PAST HEALTH HISTORY

Question	Rationale
Describe any prior gynecologic problems you have had and the results of any treatment.	Some problems, such as cancer, may recur. Prior problems directly affect the physical assessment.

PAST HEALTH HISTORY *Continued*

Question	Rationale
When was your last pelvic examination by a health care provider? Was a Pap test performed? What was the result?	Pelvic and rectal examinations are used to detect masses, ovarian tenderness, or organ enlargement. The Pap smear is a screening test for cervical cancer. The American Cancer Society recommends an annual Pap test and pelvic examination for all women who are or who have been sexually active, or who have reached age 18 years. Once a woman has had four or more consecutive satisfactory normal annual examinations, the Pap test may be performed less frequently at the discretion of the health care provider (see Promote Health—Cervical Cancer). Screening guidelines for Cervical Cancer are given in Display 23-1.
Have you ever been diagnosed with a sexually transmitted disease (STD)? If so, what? How was it treated?	Sexually transmitted diseases, also called sexually transmitted infections (STIs), can increase the client's risk of pelvic inflammatory disease, which leads to scarring and adhesions on the fallopian tubes. Scarred fallopian tubes increase the risk for infertility and ectopic pregnancy.
Have you ever been pregnant? How many times? How many children do you have? Is there any chance that you might be pregnant now? Any miscarriages or abortions?	The female client's ability to become impregnated and carry a fetus to term is important baseline information. It is important to know if the client is pregnant in case medications or x-ray tests need to be prescribed.
Have you ever been diagnosed with diabetes?	Diabetes predisposes women to vaginal yeast infections.

continued on page 458

PROMOTE HEALTH
Cervical Cancer

Overview

Cervical cancer is the third most common cancer worldwide and second only to breast cancer in women. The global statistics show that yearly there are 466,000 new cases and approximately 232,000 women die of cervical cancer. Eighty percent of the cases occur in developing countries (Medical Journal of Australia, 2003).

Cervical cancer is a slowly progressing condition beginning in the lining of the cervix wherein gradual changes lead to a precancerous state and then possibly to cancer. The cancer may be squamous cell carcinoma (80% to 90%) or adenocarcinoma (10% to 25%), or a few rarer types. Because early cervical cancers can usually be found by Pap test and are nearly 100% curable, routine screening is recommended. The ACS (2007) recommends that all women begin yearly Pap tests about 3 years after becoming sexually active, but at least by age 21. If a woman has had three normal annual Pap test results in a row, the test may be done less often at the judgment of the woman's health care provider. After hysterectomy, more frequent Pap tests may be recommended.

According to the ACS, the vast majority of cervical cancers can be prevented. First, to prevent precancers, women can avoid risk factors. (See risk factors and risk reduction measures below.) Second, to prevent invasive cancers, women should have a Pap test to detect human papillomavirus (HPV) infection and precancers and thereby treat disease in the earliest stage possible. The ACS estimates that about 4070 women will die from cervical cancer in the US in 2009. The 5-year survival rate for cervical precancer is nearly 100%, and for cervical cancer diagnosis is between 70% and 91%.

The American Cancer Society recommends that at the time of menopause all women should be informed about the risks and symptoms of endometrial cancer, and strongly encouraged to report any unexpected bleeding or spotting to their physicians. Annual screening for endometrial cancer with endometrial biopsy beginning at age 35 should be offered to women with or at risk for hereditary nonpolyposis colon cancer (HNPCC).

Risk Factors
- HPV infection, the most important risk factor
- Females, especially from late teens to mid-thirties (although rate does not decrease as one ages)
- Multiple sexual partners, especially unprotected sex and beginning at a young age or with an uncircumcised male
- Failure to have regular Pap tests (to detect precancer)
- Cigarette smoking

continued on page 458

PROMOTE HEALTH

Cervical Cancer *Continued*

- Diet low in fruits and vegetables
- Low socioeconomic status associated with low level of preventive care
- African American or Hispanic heritage
- Multiple pregnancies
- Family history
- Overweight
- History of chlamydia infection
- History of HIV infection
- Daughter of a mother who took DES in early pregnancy to prevent miscarriage
- Use of oral contraceptives for 5 or more years
- Immunosuppression

Teach Risk Reduction Tips
- Avoid exposure to HPV:
  - Practice sexual monogamy.
  - Limit number of lifetime sexual partners.
- Follow ACS guidelines for annual Pap testing and any recommended follow-up treatment.
- Learn and practice good genital hygiene.
- Do not smoke cigarettes.
- Eat a diet rich in fruits and vegetables, especially in vitamins A, C, and folate.
- Use barrier-type contraceptives cautiously. They do not protect well from HPV.
- Talk with health care provider about HPV vaccine.
- Talk with health care provider about postmenopausal screening for endometrial cancer.

DISPLAY 23-1 | **Screening Guidelines for the Early Detection of Cervical Cancer**

Screening should begin approximately 3 years after a woman begins having vaginal intercourse, but no later than 21 years of age. Screening should be done every year with regular Pap tests or every 2 years using liquid-based tests. At or after age 30, women who have had 3 normal test results in a row may get screened every 2 to 3 years. Alternatively, cervical cancer screening with HPV DNA testing and conventional or liquid-based cytology could be performed every 3 years. However, doctors may suggest a woman get screened more often if she has certain risk factors, such as HIV infection or a weak immune system. Women aged 70 years and older who have had 3 or more consecutive normal Pap tests in the last 10 years may choose to stop cervical cancer screening. Screening after total hysterectomy (with removal of the cervix) is not necessary unless the surgery was done as a treatment for cervical cancer (American Cancer Society, 2007).

FAMILY HISTORY

Question	Rationale
Is there a history of reproductive or genital cancer in your family? What type? How is the family member related to you?	Cancer has a tendency to occur in families. In such clients, the examination can focus on areas in which risk may be present.

LIFESTYLE AND HEALTH PRACTICES

Question	Rationale
Do you smoke?	Smoking and taking oral contraceptives increase the risk of cardiovascular problems. In addition, the risk for cervical cancer increases in clients who have the human papillomavirus (a type of STD) and who smoke.

continued

LIFESTYLE AND HEALTH PRACTICES *Continued*

Question	Rationale
How many sexual partners do you have?	A client who has multiple sexual partners increases her risk of contracting STDs.
Do you use contraceptives? What kind? How often?	Minor side effects (e.g., weight gain, breast tenderness, headaches, nausea) might develop from oral contraceptives but they usually subside after the third cycle. Major side effects include thromboembolic disorders, cerebrovascular accident (CVA), and myocardial infarction (MI). Failure to use a barrier type of contraceptive (male or female condom) may increase the risk of STDs and human immunodeficiency virus (HIV) infection. Failure to use any type of contraceptive increases the risk of becoming pregnant.
Have genital problems affected the way in which you normally function?	Diseases or disorders of the genitalia may cause pain and discomfort that affect a client's ability to work, to perform normal household duties, or to care for family. In addition, normal sexual activity may be affected because of pain, embarrassment, or decreased libido. Oral contraceptives increase the glycogen content of vaginal secretions, which increases the risk of vaginal yeast infections.
What is your sexual preference?	An awareness of the client's sexual preference allows the examiner to focus the examination. If the client is homosexual, she may not have the same concerns as a heterosexual woman. If she engages in oral sex, she will need to take precautions to prevent orovaginal transmission of infection.
Do you feel comfortable communicating with your partner about your sexual likes and dislikes?	Sexual relationships are enhanced through open communication. Lack of open communication can cause problems with relationships and lead to feelings of guilt and depression.
Do you have any fears related to sex? Can you identify any stress in your current relationship that relates to sex?	Fear can inhibit performance and decrease sexual satisfaction. Stress can prevent satisfactory sex role performance.
Do you have concerns about fertility? If you have trouble with fertility, how has this affected your relationship with your partner or family?	Women often feel responsible for infertility and need to discuss their feelings. Concerns about fertility can increase stress. Problems with fertility can have a negative impact on relationships with the partner and can cause tension within a family, especially when other women in the family have children.
Do you perform monthly genital self-examinations?	Each female client should be aware of the need for monthly genital self-examination and its importance in early diagnosis and treatment of problems.
How do you feel about going through menopause?	Menopause is a normal development of aging. However, in some women the process induces fear, anxiety, or even grief. The nurse can assist the client to resolve some of these feelings.
Do you take estrogen replacement therapy?	Estrogen sometimes alleviates the symptoms of menopause. However, estrogen has been linked to some types of cancer (i.e., breast, endometrial) and, in increasing the glycogen content in vaginal secretions, predisposes clients to yeast infections.

continued on page 460

Question	Rationale
Have you ever been tested for HIV? What was the result? Why were you tested?	HIV increases the client's risk for any other infection. A high-risk exposure may require serial testing.
What do you know about toxic shock syndrome?	Toxic shock syndrome is a life-threatening infection that can be prevented by frequently changing tampons.
What do you know about STDs and their prevention?	The client's knowledge of STDs and prevention provides a basis for health education in this area.
Do you wear cotton underwear and avoid tight jeans?	Cotton allows air to circulate. Nylon and tight-fitting jeans create a moist environment, which promotes vaginal yeast infections.
After a bowel movement or urination, do you wipe from front to back?	The vaginal and urethral openings are close to the anus and are easily contaminated by *Escherichia coli* and other bacteria if care is not taken to wipe from front to back.
Do you douche frequently?	Frequent douching changes the natural flora of the vagina, predisposing the vagina to yeast infections.

COLLECTING OBJECTIVE DATA: PHYSICAL EXAMINATION

The physical examination of the female genitalia may create client anxiety. The client may be very embarrassed about exposing her genitalia and nervous that an infection or disorder will be discovered. Be sure to explain in detail what you will be doing throughout the examination and to explain the significance of each portion of the examination. Encourage the client to ask questions. Begin by sitting on a stool at the end of the examination table and draping the client so only the vulva is exposed. This helps to preserve the client's modesty. The nurse should shine the light source so it illuminates the genital area, allowing the nurse to see all structures clearly.

Preparing the Client

The client should be told ahead of time not to douche for 48 hours before a gynecologic examination. When the client arrives for the examination, ask her to urinate before the examination so she does not experience bladder discomfort. If a clean-catch urine specimen is needed, provide a container and vaginal wipes. When the client is back in the examining room, ask her to remove her underwear and bra and to put on a gown with the opening in the back. If she is also having a breast examination at this time, suggest that she leave the opening in the front—a sheet can be used for draping. Tell her that she can leave her socks on if desired because the stirrups on the examination table are metal and may be cool. The nurse should leave the room while the client changes.

After the client has changed and the nurse has returned to the room, the nurse should help the patient into the dorsal lithotomy position. This is a supine position with the feet in stirrups. The client's hips should be positioned toward the bottom of the examination table so the feet can rest comfortably in the stirrups. Ask the client not to put her hands over her head because this tightens the abdominal muscles. She should relax her arms at her sides. If possible, elevate the client's head and shoulders. This allows the nurse to maintain eye contact with the client during the examination and enables the client to see what the nurse is doing. Another technique is to offer the client a mirror so she can view the examination (Fig. 23-3). This is a good way to teach normal anatomy and to get the client more involved and interested in maintaining or improving her genital health.

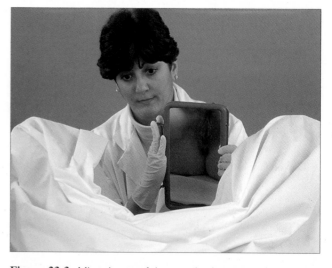

Figure 23-3 Mirror image of the examination promotes interest in gynecologic health (© B. Proud).

Equipment

Some of the following equipment is depicted in Figure 23-4.

- Stool
- Light
- Speculum
- Water-soluble lubricant
- Cotton-tipped applicators
- *Chlamydia* culture tube
- Culturette
- Test tube with water
- Sterile disposable gloves
- Ayre spatula (plastic)
- Endocervical broom
- pH paper
- Feminine napkins
- Mirror

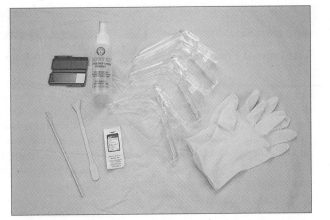

Figure 23-4 Some of the equipment needed for examining female genitalia include disposable gloves, speculums, slides and special solutions, spatulas, endocervical brooms, and other devices.

Physical Assessment

During the examination of the client, remember these key points:

- Respect the client's privacy.
- Wash hands, wear gloves, be sure equipment is between room and body temperature.

- Inspect and palpate female external and internal structures correctly.
- Use examination and laboratory equipment properly.
- Recognize the difference between common variations and abnormal findings.

(text continues on page 477)

PHYSICAL ASSESSMENT

Assessment Procedure	Normal Findings	Abnormal Findings
External Genitalia		

Inspection

Assessment Procedure	Normal Findings	Abnormal Findings
Inspect the Mons Pubis. Wash your hands and put on gloves. As you begin the examination, note the distribution of pubic hair. Also be alert for signs of infestation.	Pubic hair is distributed in an inverted triangular pattern and there are no signs of infestation. Older clients may have gray, thinning pubic hair. Some clients, particularly younger ones, shave or pluck the pubic hair. Piercings of the mons pubis are for aesthetics and do not enhance sexual pleasure.	Absence of pubic hair in the adult client is abnormal. Lice or nits (eggs) at the base of the pubic hairs indicate infestation with pediculosis pubis. This condition, commonly referred to as "crabs," is most often transmitted by sexual contact.
Observe and palpate inguinal lymph nodes.	There should be no enlargement or swelling of the lymph nodes.	Enlarged inguinal nodes may indicate a vaginal infection or may be the result of irritation from shaving pubic hairs.
Inspect the labia majora and perineum. Observe the labia majora and perineum for lesions, swelling, excoriation (Fig. 23-5).	The labia majora are equal in size and free of lesions, swelling, and excoriation. A healed tear or episiotomy scar may be visible on the perineum if the client has given birth. The perineum should be smooth.	Lesions may be from an infectious disease such as herpes or syphilis (Abnormal Findings 23-1). Excoriation and swelling may be from scratching or self-treatment of the lesions. All lesions must be evaluated and the client referred for treatment.

continued

PHYSICAL ASSESSMENT Continued

Assessment Procedure	Normal Findings	Abnormal Findings
Keep in mind the woman's childbearing status during inspection. For example, the labia of a woman who has not delivered offspring vaginally will meet in the middle. The labia of a woman who has delivered vaginally will not meet in the middle and may appear shriveled.	In pubertal rites in some cultures, the clitoris is surgically removed and the labia are sutured, leaving only a small opening for menstrual flow. Once married, the woman undergoes surgery to reopen the labia. It is increasingly common to find piercings of the labias majora and minora. Depending on placement, these may enhance sexual pleasure.	
Inspect the labia minora, clitoris, urethral meatus, and vaginal opening. Use your gloved hand to separate the labia majora and inspect for lesions, excoriation, swelling, and/or discharge (Fig. 23-6).	The labia minora appear symmetric, dark pink, and moist. The clitoris is a small mound of erectile tissue, sensitive to touch. The normal size of the clitoris varies. The urethral meatus is small and slitlike. The vaginal opening is positioned below the urethral meatus. Its size depends on sexual activity or vaginal delivery; it may be covered partially or completely by a hymen.	Asymmetric labia may indicate abscess. Lesions, swelling, bulging in the vaginal opening, and discharge are abnormal findings (see Abnormal Findings 23-1). Excoriation may result from the client scratching or self-treating a perineal irritation.
Palpation **Palpate Bartholin's glands.** If the client has labial swelling or a history of it, palpate Bartholin's glands for swelling, tenderness, and discharge (Fig. 23-7). Place your index finger in the vaginal opening and your thumb on the labia majora. With a gentle pinching motion, palpate from the inferior portion of the posterior labia majora to the anterior portion. Repeat on the opposite side.	Bartholin's glands are usually soft, nontender, and drainage free.	Swelling, pain, and discharge may result from infection and abscess (Fig. 23-8). If you detect a discharge, obtain a specimen to send to the laboratory for culture.
Palpate the urethra. If the client reports urethral symptoms or urethritis, or if you suspect inflammation of Skene's glands, insert your gloved index finger into the superior portion of the vagina and milk the urethra from the inside, pushing up and out (Fig. 23-9).	No drainage should be noted from the urethral meatus. The area is normally soft and nontender.	Drainage from the urethra indicates possible urethritis. Any discharge should be cultured. Urethritis may occur with infection with *Neisseria gonorrhoeae* or *Chlamydia trachomatis*.

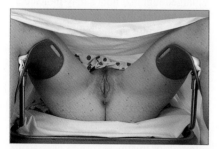

Figure 23-5 Inspecting the pubic hair, labia majora, and perineum (© B. Proud).

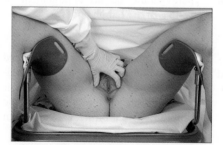

Figure 23-6 Inspecting the labia minora, clitoris, urethral orifice, and vaginal opening.

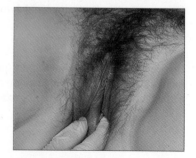

Figure 23-7 Technique for palpating Bartholin's gland.

continued

Assessment Procedure	Normal Findings	Abnormal Findings

Internal Genitalia

Inspection

Inspect the size of the vaginal opening and the angle of the vagina. Insert your gloved index finger into the vagina, noting the size of the opening. Then attempt to touch the cervix. This will help you establish the size of the speculum you need to use for the examination and the angle at which to insert it.

Next while maintaining tension, gently pull the labia majora outward. Note hymenal configuration and transections or injury.

The normal vaginal opening varies in size according to the client's age, sexual history, and whether she has given birth vaginally. The vagina is typically tilted posteriorly at a 45-degree angle.

Any loss of hymenal tissue between the 3 o'clock position and the 9 o'clock position indicates trauma (penetration by digits, penis or foreign objects) in children. See Chapter 31 for more information about sexual abuse in children. This finding is not as relevant in adults.

Inspect the vaginal musculature. Keep your index finger inserted in the client's vaginal opening. Ask the client to squeeze around your finger.

The client should be able to squeeze around the examiner's finger. Typically, the nulliparous woman can squeeze tighter than the multiparous woman.

Absent or decreased ability to squeeze the examiner's finger indicates decreased muscle tone. Decreased tone may decrease sexual satisfaction.

Use your middle and index fingers to separate the labia minora. Ask the client to bear down.

No bulging and no urinary discharge.

Bulging of the anterior wall may indicate a cystocele. Bulging of the posterior wall may indicate a rectocele. If the cervix or uterus protrudes down, the client may have uterine prolapse (see Abnormal Findings 23-1). If urine leaks out, the client may have stress incontinence.

Inspect the cervix. Follow the guidelines for using a speculum in Equipment Spotlight 23-1. With the speculum inserted in position to visualize the cervix, observe cervical color, size, and position.

The surface of the cervix is normally smooth, pink, and even. Normally, it is midline in position and projects 1 to 3 cm into the vagina. See Common Variations 23-1.

In a nonpregnant woman, a bluish cervix may indicate cyanosis; in a nonmenopausal woman, a pale cervix may indicate anemia. Redness may be from inflammation.

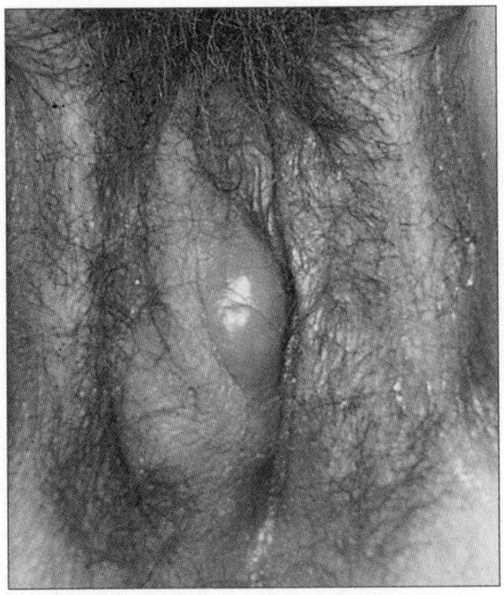

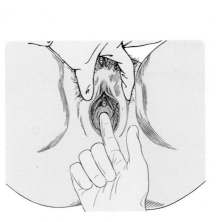

Figure 23-8 Abscess of Bartholin's gland, a painful condition and common sign of *Neisseria gonorrhoeae* infection (© 1992, National Medical Slide Bureau, CMSP).

Figure 23-9 Milking the urethra.

continued on page 465

EQUIPMENT SPOTLIGHT 23-1   **Guidelines for Using a Speculum**

1. Before using the speculum, choose the instrument that is the correct size for the client. Vaginal speculums come in two basic types:
   * *Graves speculum*—appropriate for most adult women and available in various lengths and widths.
   * *Pederson speculum*—appropriate for virgins and some postmenopausal women who have a narrow vaginal orifice. Speculums can be metal with a thumb screw that is tightened to lock the blades in place or plastic with a clip that is locked to keep the blades in place. (Plastic speculums are shown in Figure A.)

2. Encourage the client to take deep breaths and to maintain her feet in the stirrups with her knees resting in an open, relaxed fashion.

3. Place two fingers of your nondominant hand against the posterior vaginal wall and wait for relaxation to occur.

4. Insert the fingers of your nondominant hand about 2.5 cm into the vagina and spread them slightly while pushing down against the posterior vagina.

5. Lubricate the blades of the speculum with vaginal secretions from the client. Do not use commercial lubricants on the speculum. Lubricants are typically bacteriostatic and will alter vaginal pH and the cell specimens collected for cytologic, bacterial, and viral analysis.

6. Hold the speculum with two fingers around the blades and the thumb under the screw or lock. This is important for keeping the blades closed. Position the speculum so the blades are vertical.

7. Insert the speculum between your fingers into the posterior portion of the vaginal orifice at a 45-degree angle downward. When the blades pass your fingers inside the vagina, rotate the closed speculum so the blades are in a horizontal position (Figure B).

➤ *Clinical Tip • Be careful during the speculum insertion not to pinch the labia or pull the pubic hair. If the vaginal orifice seems tight or you are having trouble inserting the speculum, ask the client to bear down. This may help relax the muscles of the perineum and promote opening.*

8. Continue inserting the speculum until the base touches the fingertips inside the vagina.

9. Remove the fingers of your nondominant hand from the client's posterior vagina.

10. Press handles together (Figure C) to open blades and allow visualization of the cervix.

11. Secure the speculum in place by tightening the thumb screw or locking the plastic clip (Figure D).

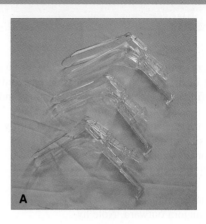

A

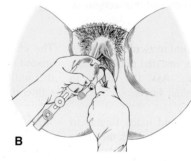

B

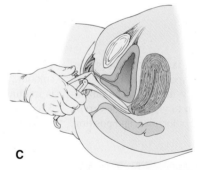

C

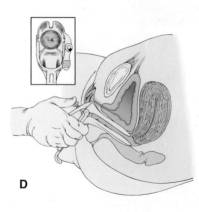

D

Assessment Procedure	Normal Findings	Abnormal Findings
Also observe the surface and the appearance of the os. Look for discharge and lesions as well. After inspecting the cervix, obtain specimens for the Pap smear and, if indicated, specimens for culture and sensitivity testing to identify possible STDs. Follow the procedure presented in Assessment Tool 23-1.	The cervical os normally appears as a small, round opening in the nulliparous women and appears slit-like in parous women (Fig. 23-10). Cervical secretions are normally clear or white and without unpleasant odor. Secretions may vary according to timing within the menstrual cycle. In pregnant clients, the cervix appears blue (Chadwick's sign). In older women, the cervix appears pale after menopause.	Cervical enlargement or projection into the vagina more than 3 cm may be from prolapse or tumor, and further evaluation is needed. Asymmetric, reddened areas, strawberry spots, and white patches are also abnormal as is colored, malodorous, or irritating discharge; a specimen should be obtained for culture. Cervical lesions may result from polyps, cancer, or infection.
Inspect the vagina. Unlock the speculum and slowly rotate and remove it. Inspect the vagina as you remove the speculum. Note the vaginal color, surface, consistency, and any discharge. If you are preparing a wet mount slide, use a cotton swab to collect the specimen of vaginal secretions from the anterior vaginal fornix or the lateral vaginal walls before you collect the specimens for the Pap or other test. Avoid the posterior fornix, which is contaminated with cervical secretions. Use part of the wet mount sample to test the pH of the vaginal secretions.	The vagina should appear pink, moist, smooth, and free of lesions and irritation. It should also be free of any colored, malodorous discharge. 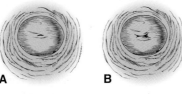 **Figure 23-10** The cervical os: **(A)** in nulliparous women; **(B)** in parous women.	Reddened areas, lesions, and colored, malodorous discharge are abnormal and may indicate vaginal infections, STDs, or cancer (Abnormal Findings 23-2 and 23-3). Altered pH may indicate infection.

Bimanual Examination

Palpation

Palpate the vaginal wall. Tell the client that you are going to do a manual examination and explain its purpose. Apply water-soluble lubricant to the gloved index and middle fingers of your dominant hand. Then stand and approach the client at the correct angle. Placing your nondominant hand on the client's lower abdomen, insert your index and middle fingers into the vaginal opening. Apply pressure to the posterior wall, and wait for the vaginal opening to relax before palpating the vaginal walls for texture and tenderness (Fig. 23-11).	The vaginal wall should feel smooth, and the client should not report any tenderness.	Tenderness or lesions may indicate infection.

Figure 23-11 Palpating the vaginal walls: Bimanual exam.

continued on page 468

ASSESSMENT TOOL 23-1   **Obtaining Tissue Specimens for Analysis**

Various laboratory tests are based on an analysis of cells obtained from tissue specimens and prepared on culture media or on slides for microscopic examination. For women especially, such tests are life-saving tools that can detect disease in early treatable stages. Some methods for obtaining tissue specimens follow:

Papanicolaou (Pap) Smear

The new standard of care for the Pap smear is liquid-based technology. The traditional Pap smear is estimated to be 80% accurate in detection of low and high grade cervical lesions of the cervix. The thin prep, or liquid-based technology has improved accuracy of findings by about 54%. The specimen for the Pap smear is obtained in the same way, but the specimen is placed in the preservative solution rather than on a slide. This solution may be used to test for Human Papilloma Virus (HPV) and to determine HPV type.

Obtaining an Ectocervical Specimen

The procedure for gathering the endocervical and ectocervical specimens is performed on nonpregnant clients. This combined procedure uses a special cytobroom to collect both endocervical and ectocervical cells.

1. Insert the cytobroom into the cervical os (Figure A).
2. Rotate the cytobroom in a full circle five times, collecting cell specimens from the squamocolumnar junction and the cervical surface.
3. Withdraw the cytobroom.
4. Swish the broom in the preservative solution by pushing the broom into the bottom of the vial 10 times, forcing the bristles apart. Swirl the broom vigorously to further release material.
5. Discard the cytobroom.
6. Tighten the cap on the preservative. This solution is sent to the laboratory.

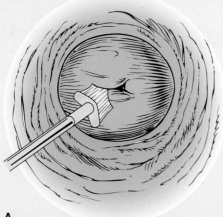

A

An alternative method for gathering the endocervical and ectocervical specimen is obtained by

1. Insert one end of plastic spatula (that is longer on the ends than in the middle) into the cervical os (Figure B).

2. Press down and rotate the spatula, scraping the cervix and the transformation zone (squamocolumnar junction) in a full circle.
3. Withdraw the spatula
4. Rinse the spatula in the preservative solution by swishing the spatula vigorously in the vial 10 times.
5. Discard the spatula.

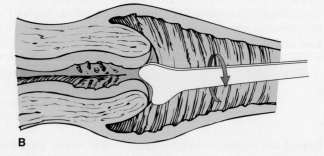

B

Obtaining an Endocervical Specimen

1. Insert the endocervical brush into the cervical os. Use the endocervical brush to increase the number of cells obtained for analysis.
2. Rotate the brush one half turn in one direction (Figure C) very gently to minimize possible bleeding.
3. Withdraw the brush.
4. Rinse the brush in the preservative solution by rotating the device in the solution 10 times while pushing against the vial wall. Swirl the brush vigorously to further release material.
5. Discard the brush.
6. Tighten the cap on the solution.
7. Record client's name and date on the vial.
8. Send vial to laboratory.

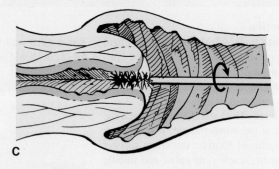

C

Vaginal Specimen

1. Moisten a cotton-tipped applicator with saline.
2. Insert the applicator into the vagina and rotate it against the vaginal wall, anterior and lateral to the cervix (Figure D).
3. Withdraw the applicator.
4. Wipe the applicator gently onto a glass slide.
5. Spray the slide with a special fixative to prevent drying (Rooney & Hopkins, 2003).

continued

ASSESSMENT TOOL 23-1 | Obtaining Tissue Specimens for Analysis *Continued*

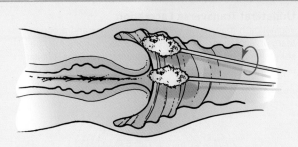

Note: Do not swab below the cervix, but to the side and above.

▶ *Clinical Tip • Do not apply great pressure when transferring the specimens onto the glass slides. Too much pressure may alter or destroy the cell structure. In addition, if you will be obtaining a specimen with the endocervical brush, do so after you obtain a tissue specimen with a spatula because bleeding may follow use of the brush.*

Culture Specimens: Gonorrhea and Chlamydia

Specimens for gonorrhea or *Chlamydia* cultures are obtained if you suspect the client has these sexually transmitted diseases. The exact procedures for gathering and preparing the specimens vary according to each laboratory's policy. General guidelines are provided below.

1. Insert a cotton-tipped applicator into the cervical os and rotate it in a full circle.
2. Leave the applicator in place for approximately 20 seconds to make sure it becomes saturated with specimen.
3. Withdraw the applicator.
4. For *Neisseria gonorrhoeae* cultures: Spread the specimen onto a special culture plate (Thayer-Martin) in a "Z" pattern while rotating the applicator, or put in a liquid medium for transport and send to the laboratory.

For *Chlamydia trachomatis* cultures: Immerse a special swab (provided with test medium) in a liquid medium and refrigerate the sample until it is transported to the laboratory.

Common Variations 23-1 | Variations of the Cervix

Certain cervical variations are common. Such variations include cervical eversion, Nabothian cysts, differently shaped cervical os (in nulliparous women and parous women), and various lacerations.

Cervical Eversion

This is a normal finding in many women and usually occurs after vaginal birth or when the woman takes oral contraceptives. The columnar epithelium from within the endocervical canal is everted and appears as a deep red, rough ring around the cervical os, surrounded by the normal pink color of the cervix.

the cervical surface. Normal odorless and nonirritating secretions may be present on pink, healthy tissue. (Irritating secretions would appear on reddened tissue.) The viscosity of these secretions ranges from thin to thick; their appearance ranges from clear to cloudy, depending on the phase of the menstrual cycle.

Nabothian cysts may occur when the everted columnar epithelium spontaneously transforms into squamous epithelium, a process called *squamous metaplasia*. Occasionally the tissue blocks endocervical glands and the cysts develop.

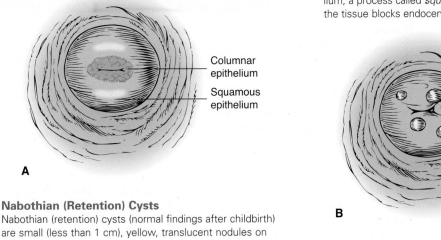

Columnar epithelium

Squamous epithelium

A

Nabothian (retention) cyst

B

Nabothian (Retention) Cysts

Nabothian (retention) cysts (normal findings after childbirth) are small (less than 1 cm), yellow, translucent nodules on

continued on page 468

Common Variations 23-1

Variations of the Cervix *Continued*

Bilateral Transverse Laceration
This drawing illustrates a type of healed laceration that may be seen in a woman who has given birth vaginally.

Unilateral Transverse Laceration
Vaginal birth may cause trauma to the cervix and produce tears or lacerations. Therefore, healed lacerations may be seen as a normal variation. This drawing illustrates a unilateral transverse laceration.

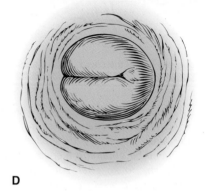

C

Stellate Laceration
This drawing illustrates a type of healed laceration that may be seen in a woman who has given birth vaginally.

D

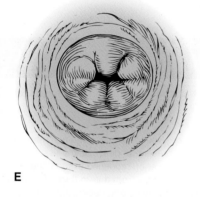

E

PHYSICAL ASSESSMENT *Continued*

Assessment Procedure	Normal Findings	Abnormal Findings
Bimanual Examination		
Palpate the cervix. Advance your fingers until they touch the cervix and run fingers around the circumference. Palpate for • Contour • Consistency • Mobility • Tenderness	The cervix should feel firm and soft (like the tip of your nose). It is rounded, and can be moved somewhat from side to side without eliciting tenderness.	A hard, immobile cervix may indicate cancer. Pain with movement of the cervix may indicate infection.
Palpate the uterus. Move your fingers intravaginally into the opening above the cervix and gently press the hand resting on the abdomen downward, squeezing the uterus between the two hands (Fig. 23-12). Note uterine size, position, shape, and consistency.	The fundus, the large upper end of the uterus, is normally round, firm, and smooth. In most women, it is at the level of the pubis; the cervix is aimed posteriorly (anteverted position). However, several other positions are considered normal (Common Variations 23-2).	An enlarged uterus above the level of the pubis is abnormal; an irregular shape suggests abnormalities such as myomas (fibroid tumors) or endometriosis (Abnormal Findings 23-4).

continued on page 470

Common Variations 23-2 | Positions of the Uterus

Anteverted

This is the most typical position of the uterus. The cervix is pointed posteriorly, and the body of the uterus is at the level of the pubis over the bladder.

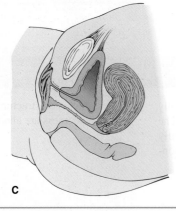

A

Midposition

This is a normal variation. The cervix is pointed slightly more anterior (compared with the anteverted position), and the body of the uterus is positioned more posterior than the anteverted position, midway between the bladder and the rectum. It may be difficult to palpate the body through the abdominal and rectal walls with the uterus in this position.

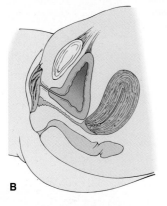

B

Anteflexed

Anteflexion is a normal variation that consists of the uterine body flexed anteriorly in relation to the cervix. The position of the cervix remains normal.

C

Retroverted Uterus

Retroversion is a normal variation that consists of the cervix and body of the uterus tilting backward. The uterine wall may not be palpable through the abdominal wall or the rectal wall in moderate retroversion. However, if the uterus is prominently retroverted, the wall may be felt through the posterior fornix or the rectal wall.

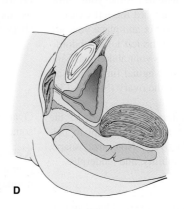

D

Retroflexed Uterus

Retroflexion is a normal variation that consists of the uterine body being flexed posteriorly in relation to the cervix. The position of the cervix remains normal. The body of the uterus may be felt through the posterior fornix or the rectal wall.

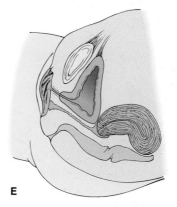

E

PHYSICAL ASSESSMENT Continued

Assessment Procedure	Normal Findings	Abnormal Findings
Attempt to bounce the uterus between your two hands to assess mobility and tenderness.	The normal uterus moves freely and is not tender.	A fixed or tender uterus may indicate fibroids, infection, or masses (see Abnormal Findings 23-4).
Palpate the ovaries. Slide your intravaginal fingers toward the left ovary in the left lateral fornix and place your abdominal hand on the left lower abdominal quadrant. Press your abdominal hand toward your intravaginal fingers and attempt to palpate the ovary (Fig. 23-13).	Ovaries are approximately $3 \times 2 \times 1$ cm (or the size of a walnut) and almond-shaped.	Enlarged size, masses, immobility, and extreme tenderness are abnormal and should be evaluated (Abnormal Findings 23-5).
Slide your intravaginal fingers to the right lateral fornix and attempt to palpate the right ovary. Note size, shape, consistency, mobility, and tenderness.	Ovaries are firm, smooth, mobile, and somewhat tender on palpation.	Large amounts of colorful, frothy, or malodorous secretions are abnormal. Ovaries that are palpable 3 to 5 years after menopause are also abnormal.
Withdraw your intravaginal hand and inspect the glove for secretions.	A clear, minimal amount of drainage appearing on the glove from the vagina is normal.	
	➤ **Clinical Tip** • *It is normal for the ovaries to be difficult or impossible to palpate in obese women, in postmenopausal women because the ovaries atrophy, or in women who are tense during the examination.*	

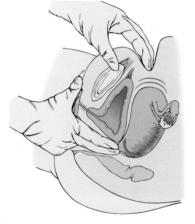

Figure 23-12 Palpating the uterus, bimanual exam.

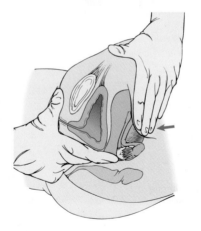

Figure 23-13 Palpating the ovaries.

Rectovaginal Examination

Explain that you are going to perform a rectovaginal examination and explain its purpose. Forewarn the client that she may feel uncomfortable as if she wants to move her bowels but that she will not. Encourage her to relax. **Change the glove** on your dominant hand and lubricate your index and middle fingers with a water-soluble lubricant.	The rectovaginal septum is normally smooth, thin, movable, and firm. The posterior uterine wall is normally smooth, firm, round, movable, and nontender.	Masses, thickened structures, immobility, and tenderness are abnormal.

continued

Assessment Procedure	Normal Findings	Abnormal Findings

Ask the client to bear down to promote relaxation of the sphincter and insert your index finger into the vaginal orifice and your middle finger into the rectum. While pushing down on the abdominal wall with your other hand, palpate the internal reproductive structures through the anterior rectal wall (Fig. 23-14). Pay particular attention to the area behind the cervix, the rectovaginal septum, the cul-de-sac, and the posterior uterine wall. Withdraw your vaginal finger and continue with the rectal examination (see Chapter 25, Anus, Rectum, and Prostate Assessment).

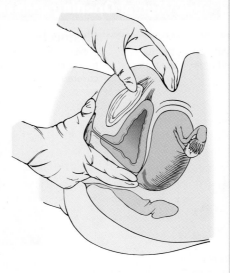

Figure 23-14 Hands positioned for recto-vaginal examination.

Abnormal Findings 23-1

Abnormalities of the External Genitalia and Vaginal Opening

When assessing the female genitalia, the nurse will see various abnormal lesions on the external genitalia as well as abnormal bulging in the vaginal opening. Some common findings appear below.

Syphilitic Chancre

Syphilitic chancres often first appear on the perianal area as silvery white papules that become superficial red ulcers. Syphilitic chancres are painless. They are sexually transmitted and usually develop at the site of initial contact with the infecting organism.

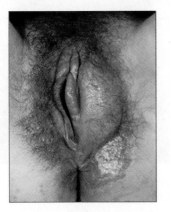

Chancre typical of syphilis. (Courtesy of Upjohn Co.)

Genital Warts

Genital warts, caused by the human papilloma virus (HPV), are moist, fleshy lesions on the labia and within the vestibule. They are painless and believed to be sexually transmitted.

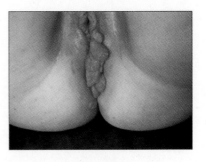

Genital warts. (Courtesy Reed & Carnrick Pharmaceuticals.)

continued on page 472

Abnormal Findings 23-1

Abnormalities of the External Genitalia and Vaginal Opening *Continued*

Genital Herpes Simplex

The initial outbreak of herpes may have many small, painful ulcers with erythematous base. Recurrent herpes lesions are usually not as extensive.

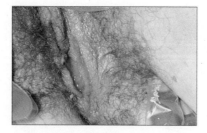

Small, painful, red-based, ulcer-like lesions of herpes simplex virus, type 2. (© 1992. Science Photo Library/CMSP.)

Cystocele

A cystocele is a bulging in the anterior vaginal wall caused by thickening of the pelvic musculature. As a result, the bladder, covered by vaginal mucosa, prolapses into the vagina.

Cystocele. (© 1995 Science Photo Library/CMSP.)

Rectocele

A rectocele is a bulging in the posterior vaginal wall caused by weakening of the pelvic musculature. Part of the rectum covered by the vaginal mucosa protrudes into the vagina.

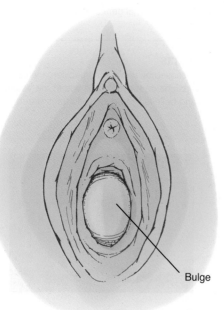

Bulge

Rectocele.

Uterine Prolapse

Uterine prolapse occurs when the uterus protrudes into the vagina. It is graded according to how far it protrudes into the vagina. In first-degree prolapse, the cervix is seen at the vaginal opening; in second-degree prolapse the uterus bulges outside of vaginal openings; in third-degree prolapse, the uterus bulges completely out of the vagina.

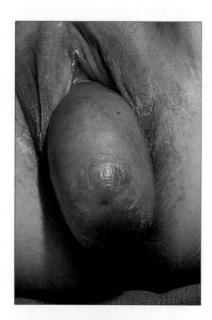

Prolapsed uterus. (© 1991, Michael English, MD/CMSP.)

Abnormal Findings 23-2 | **Abnormalities of the Cervix**

Cyanosis of the Cervix

The cervix normally appears bluish in the client who is in her first trimester of pregnancy. However, if the client is not pregnant, a bluish color to the cervix indicates venous congestion or a diminished oxygen supply to the tissues.

Cancer of the Cervix

A hardened ulcer is usually the first indication of cervical cancer, but it may not be visible on the ectocervix. In later stages, the lesion may develop into a large cauliflowerlike growth. A Pap smear is essential for diagnosis.

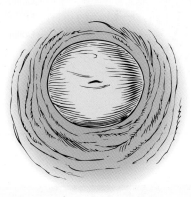

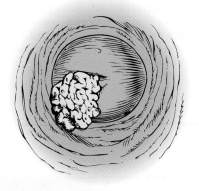

Cervical Polyp

A polyp typically develops in the endocervical canal and may protrude visibly at the cervical os. It is soft, red, and rather fragile. Cervical polyps are benign.

Cervical Erosion

This condition differs from cervical eversion in that normal tissue around the external os is inflamed and eroded, appearing reddened and rough. Erosion usually occurs with mucopurulent cervical discharge.

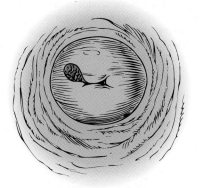

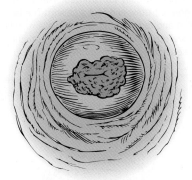

Mucopurulent Cervicitis

This condition produces a mucopurulent yellowish discharge from the external os. It usually indicates infection with *Chlamydia* or gonorrhea. However, these sexually transmitted diseases may also occur with no visible signs although the discharge may change the cervical pH (3.8–4.2).

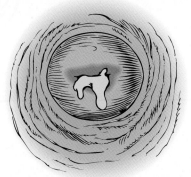

continued on page 474

Abnormal Findings 23-2   **Abnormalities of the Cervix** *Continued*

Malformations From Exposure to Diethylstilbestrol (DES)

DES, a drug used more than 50 years ago to prevent spontaneous abortion and premature labor, was learned to be terato-
genic (capable of causing malformations in the fetus). Women
who were exposed to this drug as fetuses may have cervical
abnormalities that may progress to cancer. Some abnormalities
associated with maternal DES use include columnar epithelium
that covers most or all of the ectocervix; columnar epithelium
that extends onto the vaginal wall; a circular column of tissue
that separates the cervix from the vaginal wall; transverse
ridge; and enlarged upper ectocervical lip.

Columnar
epithelium

Collar

Abnormal Findings 23-3   **Vaginitis**

In assessing female genitalia, the nurse may suspect vaginal infection from signs such as redness or lack of color, unusual
discharge and secretions, reported itching, and other typical symptoms of the kinds of vaginitis discussed below.

Trichomonas Vaginitis (Trichomoniasis)

This type of vaginal infection is caused by a protozoan organism and is usually sexually transmitted. The discharge is typically yellow-green, frothy, and foul smelling. The labia may
appear swollen and red, and the vaginal walls may be red,
rough, and covered with small red spots or petechiae. This
infection causes itching and urinary frequency in the client.
Upon testing, the pH of vaginal secretion will be greater than
4.5 (usually 7.0 or more). If a sample of vaginal secretions are
stirred into a potassium hydroxide solution (KOH prep), a foul
odor (typically known as a "+" amine) may be noted.

Atrophic Vaginitis

Atrophic vaginitis occurs after menopause when estrogen production is low. The discharge produced may be blood-tinged
and is usually minimal. The labia and vaginal mucosa appear
atrophic. The vaginal mucosa is typically pale, dry, and contains
areas of abrasion that bleed easily. Atrophic vaginitis causes
itching, burning, dryness, and painful urination.

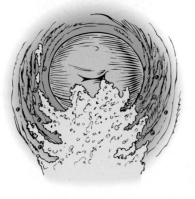

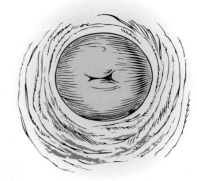

continued

Abnormal Findings 23-3   **Vaginitis** *Continued*

Candidal Vaginitis (Moniliasis)

This infection is caused by the overgrowth of yeast in the vagina. It causes a thick, white, cheesy discharge. The labia may be inflamed and swollen. The vaginal mucosa may be reddened and typically contains patches of the discharge. This infection causes intense itching and discomfort.

The pH of vaginal secretions will be <4.5 amine (vaginal secretions in KOH) is negative.

Bacterial Vaginosis

The cause of bacterial vaginosis is unknown (possibly anaerobic bacteria), but it is thought to be sexually transmitted. The discharge is thin and gray-white, has a positive amine (fishy smell), and coats the vaginal walls and ectocervix. The labia and vaginal walls usually appear normal and pH is greater than 4.5 (5.5–6.0).

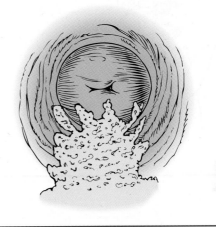

Abnormal Findings 23-4   **Uterine Enlargement**

Normal Enlargement: Pregnancy

The only uterine enlargement that is normal results from pregnancy and fetal growth. In such cases, the isthmus feels soft (Hegar's sign) on palpation, and the fundus and isthmus are compressible at between 10 and 12 weeks of pregnancy.

Uterine Fibroids (Myomas)

Uterine fibroid tumors are common and benign. They are irregular, firm nodules that are continuous with the uterine surface. They may occur as one or many and may grow quite large. The uterus will be irregularly enlarged, firm, and mobile.

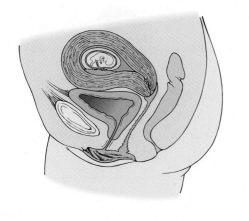

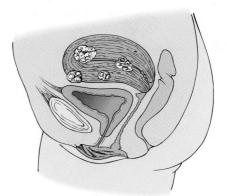

continued on page 476

Abnormal Findings 23-4   **Uterine Enlargement** *Continued*

Uterine Cancer (Cancer of the Endometrium)

The uterus may be enlarged with a malignant mass. Irregular bleeding, bleeding between periods, or postmenopausal bleeding may be the first sign of a problem.

Endometriosis

In endometriosis, the uterus is fixed and tender. Growths of endometrial tissue are usually present throughout the pelvic area and may be felt as firm, nodular masses. Pelvic pain and irregular bleeding are common.

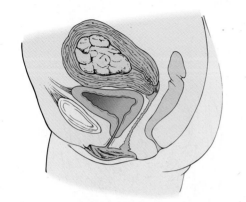

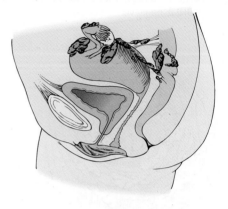

Abnormal Findings 23-5   **Adnexal Masses**

Pelvic Inflammatory Disease (PID)

PID is typically caused by infection of the fallopian tubes (salpingitis) or fallopian tubes and ovaries (salpingo-oophoritis) with a sexually transmitted disease (ie, gonorrhea, Chlamydia). It causes extremely tender and painful bilateral adnexal masses (positive chandelier sign).

Ovarian Cyst

Ovarian cysts are benign masses on the ovary. They are usually smooth, mobile, round, compressible, and nontender.

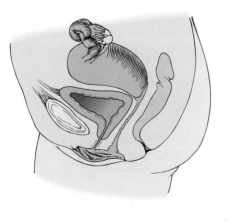

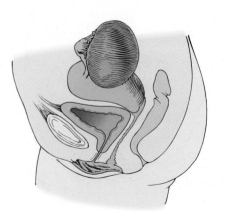

continued

Abnormal Findings 23-5   Adnexal Masses *Continued*

Ovarian Cancer

Masses that are cancerous are usually solid, irregular, non-tender, and fixed.

Ectopic Pregnancy

Ectopic pregnancy occurs when a fertilized egg attaches to the fallopian tube and begins developing instead of continuing its journey to the uterus for development. A solid, mobile, tender, and unilateral adnexal mass may be palpated if tenderness allows. The cervix and uterus will be softened, and movement of these structures will cause pain.

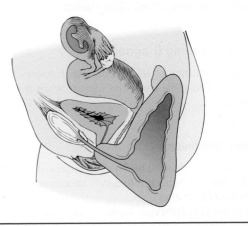

VALIDATING AND DOCUMENTING FINDINGS

Validate the female genitalia assessment data that you have collected. This is necessary to verify that the data are reliable and accurate. Document the assessment data following the health care facility or agency policy.

Sample Documentation of Subjective Data

Client states regular menstrual cycle. Last menstrual period occurred 2 weeks ago, beginning on the 10th and ending on the 13th. Experiences bloating and mild cramping with period. No vaginal discharge, pain, itching in genitalia, lumps, swelling, or masses. No difficulty urinating or controlling urine. Denies problems with sexual performance, change in sexual patterns, and decrease in sexual desire. No problems with fertility. No prior gynecologic problems.

Last pelvic examination and Pap smear 1 year ago with normal results. Denies history of sexually transmitted diseases. Gravida 2, para 1. No family history of reproductive or gynecologic cancer. Client states she does not smoke, she is married and monogamous and uses female condom for birth control. She states she is comfortable discussing sexual issues with husband. Performs monthly vulvar self-examination and is aware of risks for toxic shock syndrome. She wears tampons only during heavy flow and changes them every few hours.

Sample Documentation of Objective Data

Inspection discloses normal hair distribution, no lesions, masses, or swelling. Labia majora pink, smooth, and free of lesions, excoriation, and swelling. Labia minora dark pink, moist, and free of lesions, excoriation, swelling, and discharge. No bulging at vaginal orifice. No discharge from urethral opening.

Cervix slightly anterior, pink, smooth, slitlike os, mobile, nontender, and firm without lesions or discharge. Vaginal walls smooth and pink.

Palpation indicates firm fundus located anteriorly at level of symphysis pubis, without tenderness, lesions, or nodules. Smooth, firm, almond-shaped, mobile ovaries approximately 3 cm in size palpated bilaterally, no excessive tenderness or masses noted. No malodorous, colored vaginal discharge on gloved fingers. Routine Pap smear performed. Firm, smooth, nontender, movable posterior uterine wall and firm, smooth, thin, movable rectovaginal septum palpated during rectovaginal examination.

Analysis of Data

DIAGNOSTIC REASONING: POSSIBLE CONCLUSIONS

After collecting subjective and objective data pertaining to the female genitalia, identify abnormal findings and client strengths. Then cluster the data to reveal any significant patterns or abnormalities; these data may be used to make clinical judgments about the status of the client's genitalia.

Selected Nursing Diagnoses

Following is a listing of selected nursing diagnoses (wellness, risk, or actual) that the nurse may identify when analyzing the cue clusters.

Wellness Diagnoses

- Readiness for enhanced health management of the genitalia
- Health-Seeking Behavior: Requests information on external genitalia examination
- Health-Seeking Behavior: Requests information on ways to prevent sexually transmitted diseases
- Health-Seeking Behavior: Requests information on ways to prevent yeast infections
- Health-Seeking Behavior: Requests information on birth control
- Health-Seeking Behavior: Requests information on cessation of menses and hormone replacement therapy

Risk Diagnoses

- Risk of Ineffective Therapeutic Regimen Management (monthly external genitalia examination) related to lack of knowledge of the importance of the examination
- Risk for Infection related to unprotected sexual intercourse
- Risk for Disturbed Body Image related to perceived effects on feminine role and sexuality

Actual Diagnoses

- Fear of ovarian cancer related to high incidence of risk factors

- Ineffective Sexuality Pattern related to decreased libido
- Ineffective Therapeutic Regimen Management related to lack of knowledge of external genitalia self-examination
- Acute Pain: Dysuria related to infection
- Anticipatory Grieving related to impending loss of reproductive organs secondary to gynecologic surgery
- Ineffective Sexuality Pattern related to perceptions of effects of surgery on sexual functioning and attractiveness
- Acute Pain related to surgical incision
- Acute Pain: Dyspareunia (painful intercourse) related to inadequate vaginal lubrication

Selected Collaborative Problems

After grouping the data, certain collaborative problems may become apparent. Remember that collaborative problems differ from nursing diagnoses in that they cannot be prevented by nursing interventions. However, these physiologic complications of medical conditions can be detected and monitored by the nurse. In addition, the nurse can use physician- and nurse-prescribed interventions to minimize the complications posed by these problems. The nurse may also have to refer the client in such situations for further treatment of the problem. Following is a list of collaborative problems that may be identified when assessing the female genitalia. These problems are worded as Risk for Complications (or RC), followed by the problem.

- RC: Gonorrhea
- RC: Syphilis
- RC: *Chlamydia*
- RC: Infertility
- RC: Pregnancy
- RC: Urinary incontinence
- RC: Ovarian nodule
- RC: Abnormal Pap smear result
- RC: Vaginal bleeding

Medical Problems

After grouping the data, the client's signs and symptoms may clearly require medical diagnosis and treatment. Referral to a primary care provider is necessary, e.g., for uterine fibroids.

CASE STUDY

The case study demonstrates how to analyze female genitalia assessment data for a specific client. The critical thinking exercises included in the study guide/lab manual and interactive product that complement this text also offer opportunities to analyze assessment data.

Melinda is a 22-year-old college student who comes into the college nurse-managed clinic. She complains, "I feel like I have the flu—no energy, a headache, and fever." She reports a recent outbreak of genital lesions after a sexual encounter 10 days ago ("first and only") with a fellow student she only recently met. She denies the use of any protection or birth control, stating, "He refused to use anything and I didn't insist." She denies any problems with her menstrual cycle, no previous sexual activity, and no vaginal infections. "I have always been healthy—I don't know why I behaved so stupidly and put my health at risk." The lesions are present as vesicles and ulcerations on the external genitalia, labia, and mons, with a few vesicles extending into the perianal area. The rest of the perineal and pelvic examination is negative. Some enlarged, tender lymph nodes are noted in the inguinal areas bilaterally. Melinda's temperature by oral route is 100.6°F. When questioned, she confirms that she has a great deal of pain in the vaginal area and "urinating hurts a lot."

The following concept map illustrates the diagnostic reasoning process.

Applying COLDSPA

Applying **COLDSPA** for client symptoms: "Flu-like symptoms."

Mnemonic	Question	Data Provided	Missing Data
Character	Describe the sign or symptom (feeling, appearance, sound, smell, or taste if applicable).	"I feel like I have the flu; headache, no energy, and fever." Also reports recent outbreak of genital lesions and painful urination.	
Onset	When did it begin?	"Had unsafe sex 10 days ago"	"When did flu-like symptoms begin? When did painful urination begin?"
Location	Where is it? Does it radiate? Does it occur anywhere else?		"Describe your headaches."
Duration	How long does it last? Does it recur?		"Do your headaches come and go? Does it hurt to urinate every time?"
Severity	How bad is it? or How much does it bother you?		"Do you know what your temperature has been?"
Pattern	What makes it better or worse?		"Have you taken anything to relieve these symptoms? What aggravates your symptoms?"
Associated factors/How it **A**ffects the client	What other symptoms occur with it? How does it affect you?	Recent outbreak of genital herpes, pain in vaginal area and hurts a lot when she urinates.	"Have your symptoms restricted you from any activities that you normally perform?"

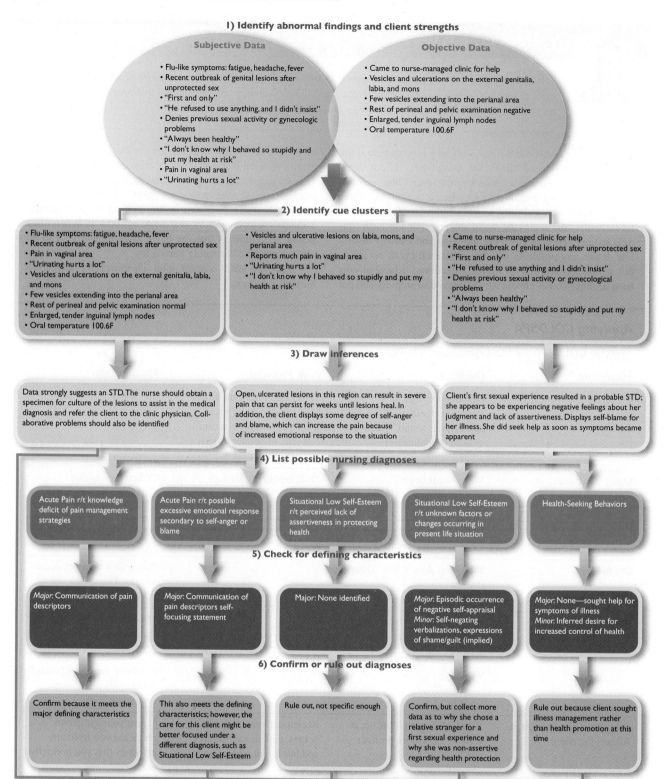

1) Identify abnormal findings and client strengths

Subjective Data

- Flu-like symptoms: fatigue, headache, fever
- Recent outbreak of genital lesions after unprotected sex
- "First and only"
- "He refused to use anything, and I didn't insist"
- Denies previous sexual activity or gynecologic problems
- "Always been healthy"
- "I don't know why I behaved so stupidly and put my health at risk"
- Pain in vaginal area
- "Urinating hurts a lot"

Objective Data

- Came to nurse-managed clinic for help
- Vesicles and ulcerations on the external genitalia, labia, and mons
- Few vesicles extending into the perianal area
- Rest of perineal and pelvic examination negative
- Enlarged, tender inguinal lymph nodes
- Oral temperature 100.6F

2) Identify cue clusters

- Flu-like symptoms: fatigue, headache, fever
- Recent outbreak of genital lesions after unprotected sex
- Pain in vaginal area
- "Urinating hurts a lot"
- Vesicles and ulcerations on the external genitalia, labia, and mons
- Few vesicles extending into the perianal area
- Rest of perineal and pelvic examination normal
- Enlarged, tender inguinal lymph nodes
- Oral temperature 100.6F

- Vesicles and ulcerative lesions on labia, mons, and perianal area
- Reports much pain in vaginal area
- "Urinating hurts a lot"
- "I don't know why I behaved so stupidly and put my health at risk"

- Came to nurse-managed clinic for help
- Recent outbreak of genital lesions after unprotected sex
- "First and only"
- "He refused to use anything and I didn't insist"
- Denies previous sexual activity or gynecological problems
- "Always been healthy"
- "I don't know why I behaved so stupidly and put my health at risk"

3) Draw inferences

Data strongly suggests an STD. The nurse should obtain a specimen for culture of the lesions to assist in the medical diagnosis and refer the client to the clinic physician. Collaborative problems should also be identified

---

Open, ulcerated lesions in this region can result in severe pain that can persist for weeks until lesions heal. In addition, the client displays some degree of self-anger and blame, which can increase the pain because of increased emotional response to the situation

---

Client's first sexual experience resulted in a probable STD; she appears to be experiencing negative feelings about her judgment and lack of assertiveness. Displays self-blame for her illness. She did seek help as soon as symptoms became apparent

4) List possible nursing diagnoses

Acute Pain r/t knowledge deficit of pain management strategies

Acute Pain r/t possible excessive emotional response secondary to self-anger or blame

Situational Low Self-Esteem r/t perceived lack of assertiveness in protecting health

Situational Low Self-Esteem r/t unknown factors or changes occurring in present life situation

Health-Seeking Behaviors

5) Check for defining characteristics

Major: Communication of pain descriptors

Major: Communication of pain descriptors self-focusing statement

Major: None identified

Major: Episodic occurrence of negative self-appraisal
Minor: Self-negating verbalizations, expressions of shame/guilt (implied)

Major: None—sought help for symptoms of illness
Minor: Inferred desire for increased control of health

6) Confirm or rule out diagnoses

Confirm because it meets the major defining characteristics

This also meets the defining characteristics; however, the care for this client might be better focused under a different diagnosis, such as Situational Low Self-Esteem

Rule out, not specific enough

Confirm, but collect more data as to why she chose a relative stranger for a first sexual experience and why she was non-assertive regarding health protection

Rule out because client sought illness management rather than health promotion at this time

7) Document conclusions

Nursing diagnoses that are appropriate for this client include:
Three diagnoses are appropriate at this time:
- Acute Pain r/t knowledge deficit of pain management strategies
- Acute Pain r/t possible excessive emotional response secondary to self-anger or blame

- Situational Low Self-Esteem r/t unknown factors or changes occurring in present life situation
In addition, an identified potential complication could be urinary retention (secondary to dysuria).
Melinda should be referred to a physician for diagnosis and treatment of her genital lesions.

References and Selected Readings

American Cancer Society. (2008). *Cancer facts & figures, 2007*. Atlanta: American Cancer Society. Available at http://www.cancer.org

Anderson, S., Dallal, G., & Must, A. (2003). Relative weight and race influence average age at menarche: Results from two nationally representative surveys of US girls studied 25 years apart. *Journal of the American Academy of Pediatrics, 111*(4), 844–850.

Apgar, B. S., & Brotzman, G. (2004). Management of cervical cytologic abnormalities. *American Family Physicians, 70*(10), 1905–1916.

Aschenbrenner, D. S. (2004). Avlimil taken for female sexual dysfunction. *American Journal of Nursing, 104*(10), 27–29.

Beals, J., & Lie, D. (2007). New guidelines for assessing gynecologic cancer predispositions. Retrieved November 1, 2007. Available at http://www.medscape.com/viewarticle/564765_print

Berman, N. (2007). Preventing cervical cancer, the age of vaccination has arrived. *Advance for Nurse Practitioner, 15*(4), 75–78, 102.

Bertrand, C. C. (2004). Evidence for practice: Oral contraception and risk of cervical cancer. *Journal of the American Academy of Nurse Practitioners, 16*(10), 455–461.

Bistoletti, P., Sennfalt, K., & Dillner, J. (2007). Cost-effectiveness of primary cytology and HPV DNA cervical screening. *International Journal of Cancer*. Retrieved October 18, 2007. Available at http://www.ncbi.nlm.gov

Blake, D. R., Weber, B. M., & Fletcher, K. E. (2004). Adolescent and young adult women's misunderstanding of the term Pap smear. *Archives of Pediatrics and Adolescent Medicine, 158*(10), 996–970.

Brown, K. (2004). Rape and sexual assault. Understanding the offense and the offender. *Advance for Nurse Practitioners, 12*(8), 69–70.

Caliendo, C., Armstrong, M., & Roberts, A. (2005). Self-reported characteristics of women and men with intimate body piercings. *Issues and innovations in nursing practice, 49*(5), 474–484.

Carrasquillo, O., & Pati, S. (2004). The role of health insurance on Pap smear and mammography utilization by immigrants living in the United States. *Preventative Medicine, 39*(5), 943–950.

Catallozzi, M., & Rudy, B. J. (2004). Lesbian, gay, bisexual, transgendered, and questioning youth: The importance of a sensitive and confidential sexual history in identifying the risk and implementing treatment for sexually transmitted infections. *Adolescent Medicine Clinics, 15*(2), 353–367.

Chumlea, W., Schubert, C., Roche, A., Kulin, H., Lee, P., Himes, J., & Sun, S. (2003). Age at menarche and racial comparison in US girls. *Journal of the American Academy of Pediatrics, 111*(1), 110–113.

Dahlberg, D. L., Lee, C., Fenlon, T., & Willoughby, D. (2004). Differential diagnosis of abdominal pain in women of childbearing age. Appendicitis or pelvic inflammatory disease? *Advance for Nurse Practitioners, 12*(1), 40–45.

D'Souza, G., Kreimer, A., Viscidi, R., Pawlita, M., Fakhry, C., Koch W., et al. (2007). Case-control study of human papillomavirus and oropharyngeal cancer. *The New England Journal of Medicine, 356*(19), 1944–1956.

Freeman, E., Samel, M., Lin, H., Gracia, C., Pien, G., Nelson, D., et al. (2007). Symptoms associated with menopausal transition and reproductive hormones in midlife women. *Obstetrics & Gynecology, 110*, 230–240.

Garcia, A. (2006). Cervical cancer. *E-medicine – Web MD*. Retrieved October 16, 2007. Available at http://www.emedicine.com/med/topic324.htm

Hall, H. I., Jamison, P. M., Coughlin, S. S., & Uhler, R. J. (2004). Breast and cervical cancer screening among Missouri Delta women. *Journal of Health Care for the Poor and Underserved, 15*(3), 375–389.

Handa, V. L., Harvey, I., Cundiff, G. W., Siddlique, S. A., & Kjerulff, K. H. (2004). Sexual function among women with urinary incontinences and pelvic organ prolapse. *American Journal of Obstetrics and Gynecology, 191*(3), 751–756.

Hartmann, U., Philippsohn, S., Heiser, K., & Ruffer-Hesse, C. (2004). Low sexual desire in midlife and older women: Personality factors, psychosocial development, present sexuality. *Menopause, 11*(6), 726–740.

Iannacchoine, M. A. (2004). The vagina dialogues: Do you douche? *American Journal of Nursing, 104*(1), 40–42, 44–45, quiz 46.

Jackson, G. (2004). Sexual dysfunction and diabetes. *International Journal of Clinical Practice, 58*(4), 358–362.

Jhala, D., & Eltoum, I. (2007). Barriers to adoption of recent technology in cervical screening. *CytoJournal, 4*, 16.

Johnson-Mallard & Lengacher, C. (2007). STI health communication intervention. *Women's Health Care, 6*(8), 27–31.

Kabat, G., Miller, A., & Rohan, T. (2007). Oral contraceptive use, hormone replacement therapy, reproductive history and risk of colorectal cancer in women. *International Journal of Cancer*. Retrieved September 10, 2007. Available at http://www3.interscience.wiley.com/cgi-bin/fulltext/116313884/HTMLSTART

Kellogg-Spadt, S., & Rejba, A. (2007). Coping with interstitial cystitis/painful bladder syndrome: Management strategies for clinician and patients. *Women's Health Care: A Practical Journal for Nurse Practitioner, 6*(8), 7–18.

Kirkland, L. (2006). New developments in the management of STDs. *The Nurse Practitioner, 31*(12), 12–23.

Liu, J., Rosee, B., Huang, X., Liao, G., Carter, J., Wu, X., & et al. (2004). Comparative analysis of characteristics of women with cervical cancer in high- versus low-incidence regions. *Gynecologic Oncology, 94*(3), 803–810.

Mandelblatt, J., Lawrence, W., Womack, S., Jacobson, D., Yi, B., Hwang, Y., et al. (2002). Benefits and costs of using HPV testing to screen for cervical cancer. *Journal of the American Medical Association, 287*(28), 2372–2381.

Marazzo, J. M., & Stine, K. (2004). Reproductive health history of lesbians: Implications for care. *American Journal of Obstetrics and Gynecology, 190*(5), 1298–1304.

McHale, M., Souther, J., Elkas, J., Monk, B., & Harrison, T. (2007). Is atypical squamous cells that cannot exclude high-grade squamous intraepithelial lesion clinically significant? *Gynecologic Oncology, 11*(2), 86–89.

Murphy, P., & Schwarz, E. (2007). NPs' cervical cancer screening practices. *Women's Health Care: A Practical Journal for Nurse Practitioners, 6*(9), 10–21.

Pitkin, J., Smetnik, V., Vadasz, P., Mustonen, M., Salminen, K., Ylikangas, S., et al. (2007). Continuous hormone replacement therapy relieves climacteric symptoms and improve health-related quality of life in early postmenopausal women. *Menopause International, 13(3),* 116–123.

Roberts, S. S. (2004). Addressing women's sexual problems. *Diabetes Forecast, 57*(9), 61–63.

Ruba, S., Schoolland, M., Allpress, S., & Sterrett, G. (2004). Adenocarcinoma in situ of the uterine cervix. *Cancer, 16*(102), 280–287.

Smith, D. (2007). Pelvic organ prolapse. *Advance for Nurse Practitioners, 15*(8), 39–42.

Sommers, M. S., & Buschur, C. (2004). Injury in women who are raped: What every critical care nurse needs to know. *Dimensions in Critical Care Nursing, 23*(2), 62–68.

ThinPrep® PapTest™ Quick Reference Guide, Broom-Like Device Protocol. (2004). http://www.fahc.org/pathology

ThinPrep® PapTest™ Quick Reference Guide, Endocervical Brush/Spatula Protocol. (2004). http://www.fahc.org/patholgy

Yilmaz, U., Kromm, B. G., & Yang, C. C. (2004). Evaluation of autonomic innervation of the clitoris and bulb. *Journal of Urology, 172*(5), 1930–1934.

Youngkin, E. Q. (2004). The myths and truths of mature intimacy: Mature guidance for nurse practitioners. *Advance for Nurse Practitioners, 12*(8), 45–48.

Promote Health—Cervical Cancer

American Cancer Society (ACS). (2009). Cervical cancer [Online]. Available at http://www.cancer.org

American Cancer Society (ACS). (2009). Cancer facts and figures [Online]. Available at http://www.cancer.org

Medical Journal of Australia (2003). Cancer screening: Can we really beat cervical cancer? [Online]. Available at http://www.mja.com/au

National Cancer Institute. (2004). SEER cancer statistics review [Online]. Available: http://www.wrongdiagnosis.com/c/cervical_cancer/prevalence

Useful Website Resources

http://cancernet.nci.nih.gov/
Website is a service of the National Cancer Institute and provides valuable cancer-related health information.

http://www.aafp.org/afp.xml
Produced by the American Academy of Family Physicians, this site strives to preserve and promote the science and art of family medicine and to ensure high-quality, cost-effective health care for patients of all ages. Online journal is available.

http://www.cancer.org
This Website, owned and copyrighted by the American Cancer Society, provides cancer information for health professionals and patients.

http://www.cdc.gov/reproductivehealth/
This site was developed by United States Department of Health and Human Services, Centers for Disease Control and Prevention, National Center for Chronic Disease Prevention and Health Promotion, Division of Reproductive Health. It features fact sheets about women's reproductive issues.

http://www.contraceptiononline.org
Baylor College of Medicine developed this online contraception resource for clinicians, researchers, and educators.

http://www.mdanderson.org
Website of M.D. Anderson Cancer Center. Contains information about cancer treatment, clinical trials, education programs and cancer prevention.

http://www.mskcc.org/mskcc/html/44.cfm
Website provides information on Memorial Sloan-Kettering Cancer Center's programs and services for research, prevention, cure, and control of cancer.

24
Male Genitalia

Structure and Function

To assess the male genitalia, a basic understanding of normal structure and function is necessary; it helps to guide the physical examination and readily assists the examiner in identifying abnormalities. Male genitalia are classified as external structures and internal structures. (*Note:* Glandular structures accessory to the male genital organs—the prostate, the seminal vesicles, and Cowper's [bulbourethral] glands—are discussed in Chapter 25.) In addition to an understanding of the male genital structures, the nurse needs to be familiar with the inguinal (or groin) structures because hernias are common in this area.

EXTERNAL GENITALIA
Penis

The external genitalia consist of the penis and the scrotum (Fig. 24-1). The penis is the male reproductive organ. Attached to the pubic arch by ligaments, the penis is freely movable. The shaft of the penis is composed of three cylindrical masses of vascular erectile tissue that are bound together by fibrous tissue—two corpora cavernosa on the dorsal side and the corpus spongiosum on the ventral side. The corpus spongiosum extends distally to form the acorn-shaped glans. The base of the glans, or corona, is somewhat larger as compared to the shaft of the penis. If the man has not been circumcised, the glans is covered by a hood-like fold of skin called the foreskin or prepuce. In the center of the corpus spongiosum is the urethra, which travels through the shaft and opens as a slit at the tip of the glans as the urethral meatus. A fold of foreskin that extends ventrally from the urethral meatus is called the frenulum. The penis has a role in both reproduction and urination.

Scrotum

The scrotum is a thin-walled sac that is suspended below the pubic bone, posterior to the penis. This darkly pigmented structure contains sweat and sebaceous glands and consists of folds of skin (rugae) and the cremaster muscle. The scrotum functions as a protective covering for the testes, epididymis, and vas deferens and helps to maintain the cooler-than-body temperature necessary for production of sperm (less than 37°C). The scrotum can maintain temperature control because the cremaster muscle is sensitive to changes in temperature. The muscle contracts when too cold, raising the scrotum and testes upward toward the body for warmth (cremasteric reflex). This accounts for the wrinkled appearance of the scrotal skin. When the temperature is warm, the muscle relaxes, lowering the scrotum and testes away from the heat of the body. When the cremaster muscle relaxes, the scrotal skin appears smooth.

INTERNAL GENITALIA
Testes

Internally the scrotal sac is divided into two portions by a septum, each portion containing one testis (testicle; see Fig. 24-1). The testes are a pair of ovoid-shaped organs, similar to the ovaries in the woman, that are approximately 3.7 to 5 cm long, 2.5 cm wide, and 2.5 cm deep. Each testis is covered by a serous membrane called the tunica vaginalis, which separates the testis from the scrotal wall. The tunica vaginalis is double layered and lubricated to protect the testes from injury. The function of the testis is to produce spermatozoa and the male sex hormone testosterone.

Spermatic Cord

The testes are suspended in the scrotum by a spermatic cord. The spermatic cord contains blood vessels, lymphatic vessels, nerves, and the vas deferens (or ductus deferens), which transports spermatozoa away from the testis. The spermatic cord on the left side is usually longer; thus the left testis hangs lower than the right testis.

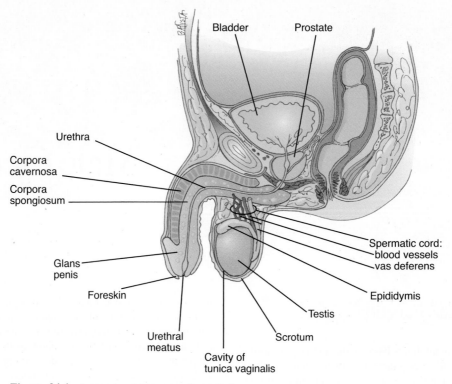

Figure 24-1 External and internal male genitalia.

The epididymis is a comma-shaped, coiled tubular structure that curves up over the upper and posterior surface of the testis.

➤ **Clinical Tip** • *While the epididymis is usually over the posterior surface of the testes, in about 6 to 7% of the male population it is located anteriorly.*

It is within the epididymis that the spermatozoa mature.

The vas deferens is a firm, muscular tube that is continuous with the lower portion of the epididymis (see Fig. 24-1). It travels up within the spermatic cord through the inguinal canal into the abdominal cavity. At this point, it separates from the spermatic cord and curves behind the bladder. It joins with the duct of the seminal vesicle and forms the ejaculatory duct. Finally, the ejaculatory duct empties into the urethra within the prostate gland.

The vas deferens provides the passage for transporting sperm from the testes to the urethra for ejaculation. Along the way, secretions from the vas deferens, seminal vesicles, prostate gland, and Cowper's or bulbourethral glands mix with the sperm and form semen.

INGUINAL AREA

When assessing the male genitalia, the nurse needs to be familiar with structures of the inguinal or groin area because hernias (protrusion of loops of bowel through weak areas of the musculature) are common in this location (Fig. 24-2). The inguinal area is contained between the anterior superior iliac spine laterally and the symphysis pubis medially.

Running diagonally between these two landmarks, just above and parallel with the inguinal ligament, is the inguinal canal. The inguinal canal is a tubelike structure (4 to 5 cm or

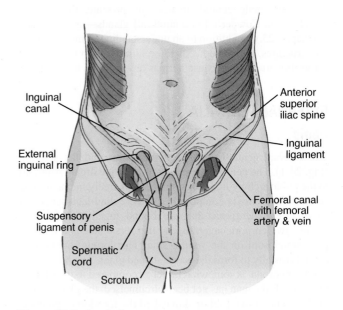

Figure 24-2 Inguinal area.

1.5 to 2 inches long in an adult) through which the vas deferens travels as it passes through the lower abdomen.

The external inguinal ring is the exterior opening of the inguinal canal and can be palpated above and lateral to the symphysis pubis. It feels triangular and slitlike. The internal inguinal ring is the internal opening of the inguinal canal. It is located 1 to 2 cm above the midpoint of the inguinal ligament and cannot be palpated. The femoral canal is another potential spot for a hernia. The femoral canal is located posterior to the inguinal canal and medial to and running parallel with the femoral artery and vein.

Health Assessment

COLLECTING SUBJECTIVE DATA: THE NURSING HEALTH HISTORY

When interviewing the male client for information regarding his genitalia, keep in mind that this may be a very sensitive topic for the client and for the examiner as well. Moreover, the examiner should be aware of his own feelings regarding body image, fear of cancer, and sexuality. Western culture emphasizes the importance of the male sex role function. Self-esteem and body image are entwined with the male sex role. Anxiety, embarrassment, and fear may influence the client's ability to discuss problems and ask questions. A trusting relationship is key to a successful interview. Keep in mind that serious or life-threatening problems may be present. Testicular cancer, for example, carries a high mortality rate, especially if not detected early. The information gathered during this portion of the health history interview provides a basis for teaching about important health screening issues such as testicular self-examination. Additionally symptoms that the client reports or hints at need to be explored in some depth with a symptom analysis.

(text continues on page 489)

HISTORY OF PRESENT HEALTH CONCERN

Question	Rationale
Pain Do you have pain in your penis, scrotum, testes, or groin?	Complaints of pain in these areas may indicate a hernia or an inflammatory process, such as epididymitis.
Lesions Have you noticed any lesions on your penis or genital area? If so, do the lesions itch, burn, or sting? Please describe the lesions.	Lesions may be a sign of a sexually transmitted disease (STD) or cancer.
Discharge Have you noticed any discharge from your penis? If so, how much? What color is it? What type of odor does it have?	Discharge may indicate an infection.
Lumps, swelling, masses Do you have any lumps, swelling, or masses in your scrotum, genital, or groin area? Have you noticed a change in the size of the scrotum?	These findings may indicate infection, hernia, or cancer. Enlargement of the scrotum may indicate hydrocele, hematocele, hernia, or cancer; the scrotum also enlarges with aging.
Do you have a heavy, dragging feeling in your scrotum?	A testicular tumor or scrotal hernia may cause a feeling of heaviness in the scrotum.
Urination Do you experience difficulty urinating (i.e., urgency, hesitancy, frequency, or difficulty starting or maintaining a stream)? How many times do you urinate during the night?	Difficulty urinating may indicate an infection or blockage including prostatic enlargement. Urinating more than one time during the night may indicate prostate abnormalities. Excessive intake of fluids may also cause nocturia.
Have you noticed any change in the color, odor, or amount of your urine?	Changes in urine color or odor may indicate an infection. Blood in the urine (hematuria) should be referred for medical investigation because this may indicate infection, benign prostatic hypertrophy (BPH), or cancer. A decrease in amount of voided urine may indicate prostate enlargement or kidney problems.
Do you experience any pain or burning when you urinate?	Painful urination may be a sign of urinary tract infection, prostatitis, or an STD, also called sexually transmitted infection (STI).

continued on page 486

HISTORY OF PRESENT HEALTH CONCERN *Continued*

Question	Rationale
Do you ever experience urinary incontinence or dribbling?	Incontinence may occur after prostatectomy. Dribbling may be a sign of overflow incontinence.
Sexual Dysfunction Have you recently had a change in your pattern of sexual activity or sexual desire?	A change in sexual activity or sexual desire (libido) needs to be investigated to determine the cause.
Do you have difficulty attaining or maintaining an erection? Do you have any problem with ejaculation? Do you have pain with ejaculation?	Erectile dysfunction occurs frequently in adult males and may be attributed to various factors or disorders (e.g., alcohol use, diabetes, depression, antihypertensive medications). Pain with ejaculation may indicate epididymitis. Erectile dysfunction increases in frequency with age.
Do you have or have you had any trouble with fertility?	About 30% of all infertility experienced by couples is due to male infertility.

COLDSPA Example for Frequent Urination

Use the **COLDSPA** mnemonic as a guideline to collect needed information for each symptom the client shares. In addition, the following questions help elicit important information.

Mnemonic	Question	Client Response Example
Character	Describe the sign or symptom (feeling, appearance, sound, smell, or taste if applicable).	"I have to get up a lot at night to urinate. I do not feel like I am emptying my bladder all the way and I have to go again about an hour later."
Onset	When did it begin?	"Gradually over the last couple of months. But it is getting worse now."
Location	Where is it? Does it radiate? Does it occur anywhere else?	(No information given)
Duration	How long does it last? Does it recur?	"It happens every night. I get up 3–4 times a night."
Severity	How bad is it? or How much does it bother you?	"My wife can't sleep at night because my getting up disturbs her. I do not want to live with this the rest of my life."
Pattern	What makes it better or worse?	"It is worse if I drink at bedtime; nothing makes it better."
Associated factors/How it **A**ffects the client	What other symptoms occur with it? How does it affect you?	"I have to strain sometimes to get my urine out and my stream is weak."

PAST HEALTH HISTORY

Question	Rationale
Describe any prior medical problems you have had, how they were treated, and the results.	Prior problems directly affect the physical assessment findings. For example, if cancer was present in the past, it may recur. Diabetes may cause impotence.

continued

PAST HEALTH HISTORY *Continued*

Question	Rationale
When was the last time you had a testicular examination by a physician? What was the result?	The American Cancer Society recommends testicular examination by a physician every 3 years for asymptomatic men ages 20 to 39 and every year for asymptomatic men age 40 years and older.
Have you ever been tested for human immunodeficiency virus (HIV), human papilloma virus, herpes simplex, chlamydia, gonorrhea, and/or trichomoniasis? What were the results? Why were you tested?	HIV increases the client's risk for other infections. A high-risk exposure may require serial testing.

FAMILY HISTORY

Question	Rationale
Is there a history of cancer in your family? What type and which family member(s)?	Cancers of the prostate and testes have a familial tendency.

LIFESTYLE AND HEALTH PRACTICES

Question	Rationale
How many sexual partners do you have?	A client with multiple sexual partners increases his risk of contracting an STD or HIV (see Promote Health—HIV/AIDS).
What kind of birth control method do you use, if any?	Vasectomy for permanent birth control results in a decreased amount of ejaculate, which concerns some men. Vasectomy affords no protection from STDs. The only type of temporary birth control method for men is the male condom. Failure to use condoms increases the client's risk for contracting and transmitting STDs and HIV and increases the female partner's risk of becoming pregnant.
Are you satisfied with your current level of activity and sexual functioning?	Pain or heaviness due to hernias may limit the ability to work or perform regular exercise. Infection may limit a client's ability to engage in sexual activity. An erectile dysfunction impedes sexual intercourse. Incontinence may affect the client's ability to work or engage in social activities.
Do you have concerns about fertility? If you experience fertility troubles, how has this affected your relationship?	Concerns about fertility can increase stress and can have a negative impact on relationships.
What is your sexual preference?	An awareness of the client's sexual preference allows the examiner to focus the examination. Acceptance of a client's sexual preference helps to put the client at ease. Therefore, the client will be more likely to talk about his special health issues or fears.
Do you have any fears related to sex? Can you identify any stress in your current relationship that relates to sex?	Fear can cause inhibition and decrease sexual satisfaction. Stress can prevent satisfactory sexual performance.

continued on page 488

LIFESTYLE AND HEALTH PRACTICES *Continued*

Question	Rationale
Do you feel comfortable communicating with your partner about your sexual likes and dislikes?	Lack of open communication can cause problems with relationships and lead to feelings of guilt and depression.
What do you know about STDs and their prevention?	The client's knowledge of STDs and their prevention provides a basis for health education in this area.
Are you currently exposed to chemicals or radiation? Have you been exposed in the past?	Exposure to radiation and certain chemicals increases the risk of developing cancer.
Describe the activity you perform in a typical day. Do you do any heavy lifting?	Strenuous activity and heavy lifting may predispose the client to development of an inguinal hernia.
Do you perform testicular self-examinations?	Male clients who do not perform testicular self-examinations need to be informed about the connection between self-examination and early interventions for abnormalities.
When was the last time you performed this examination?	Male clients should be aware of the need for a monthly testicular self-examination and its importance in the early diagnosis and treatment of testicular cancer.

PROMOTE HEALTH
HIV/AIDS

Overview

The Joint United Nations Programme on HIV/AIDS reports that globally in 2006 nearly 40 million people were estimated to be living with HIV. Also, 3 million deaths and 4.3 million new cases were estimated for 2006. In the United States, the rate of HIV infection has remained about 40,000 cases per year; however, the rates for African Americans and for women are increasing as opposed to the rate for Caucasian homosexual males. Cases in African American women now account for about 70% of new HIV cases in women.

Currently, 19% of HIV/AIDS cases occur in people who are older than 50 years of age (NIH, 2007). Diagnosed cases of AIDS in people over 50 in the United States rose twice as fast as cases in younger adults diagnosed between 1991 and 1996 (National Assessment on HIV, 2007). Nurses are often reluctant to discuss sexually related behaviors with older adults, but it is a necessary professional role.

Although transmission routes vary (male-to-male anal sex, intravenous drug use, heterosexual sex, mother-to-infant transmission, and other mechanisms of body fluid transfer), the highest incidence of HIV in the United States still occurs in men who have sex with men (MSM), followed by intravenous drug users.

Risk Factors

- Anal intercourse (especially MSM)
- Intravenous drug use (especially among people who share needles)
- Heterosexual transmission (vaginal, anal, or oral): having multiple sexual partners, bisexual partners, or partner who uses intravenous drugs (sex with any infected partner)
- Exchange of blood or body fluids through blood transfusions, needle sticks, breast-feeding by HIV infected mother, body piercing with nonsterilized instruments
- Mother-to-infant transmission during pregnancy or delivery, especially with vaginal delivery

Teach Risk Reduction Tips

Use precautions to decrease transfer of bodily fluids:

- Practice sexual abstinence.
- Use condoms.
- Double glove when handling sharp objects.
- Single glove when handling bodily secretions or objects that touch bodily secretions.
- Follow guidelines for safe handling of contaminated items.

Avoid other high-risk behaviors such as:

- Intravenous drug use (especially sharing needles)
- Sex with multiple partners
- Mixing sex and alcohol or drugs
- Anal intercourse

Openly discuss HIV risk behavior history with partner and use above precautions. Note: Nurses are often reluctant to discuss sexually related behaviors with older adults, but it is a necessary professional role.

COLLECTING OBJECTIVE DATA: PHYSICAL EXAMINATION

The purpose of examining the male genitalia is to detect abnormalities that may range from life-threatening diseases to painful conditions that interfere with normal function. Abnormalities should be detected as early as possible so the client can be referred for further testing or treatment. The physical assessment is also a good time to allow the client to demonstrate the proper techniques for testicular self-examination and to provide teaching if necessary.

The hands-on physical examination of the male genitalia may create anxiety, embarrassment, and nervousness about exposing the genitals and about what might be discovered. Ease client anxiety by explaining in detail what is going to occur and the significance of each portion of the examination while you are performing it. Also attempt to expose only those areas necessary at that point in the examination. This will help preserve the client's modesty. It is also helpful to encourage the client to ask questions during the examination.

➤ **Clinical Tip** • *Examiners and the client are often worried that the male client will have an erection during the hands-on examination. Usually the client is too nervous for this to occur. If it does occur, reassure the client that it is not unusual and continue the examination in an unhurried and unflappable manner.*

Preparing the Client

Before the examination, instruct the client to empty his bladder so he will be comfortable. If a urine specimen is necessary, provide the client with a container. If the client is not wearing an examination gown for a total physical examination, provide a drape and ask him to lower his pants and underwear. Explain to the client that he will be asked to stand (if able) for most of the examination.

Equipment

- Stool
- Gown
- Disposable gloves
- Flashlight (for possible transillumination)
- Stethoscope (for possible auscultation)

Physical Assessment

During the examination of the client, remember these key points:

- Wear disposable gloves.
- Preserve client's privacy.
- Inspect and palpate penis, scrotum, and inguinal area for inflammation, infestations, rashes, lesions, and lumps.
- During the testicular examination, describe the importance of testicular self-examination and explain how to perform the examination as you are performing it.

➤ **Clinical Tip** • *Wear gloves for every step of the male genitalia examination.*

(text continues on page 501)

PHYSICAL ASSESSMENT

Assessment Procedure	Normal Findings	Abnormal Findings
Penis		
Inspection and Palpation **Inspect the base of the penis and pubic hair.** Sit on a stool with the client facing you and standing (Fig. 24-3). Ask the client to raise his gown or drape. Note pubic hair growth pattern and any excoriation, erythema, or infestation at the base of the penis and within the pubic hair.	Pubic hair is coarser than scalp hair. The normal pubic hair pattern in adults is hair covering the entire groin area, extending to the medial thighs and up the abdomen toward the umbilicus. The base of the penis and the pubic hair are free of excoriation, erythema, and infestation (Fig. 24-4), Table 24-1.	Absence or scarcity of pubic hair may be seen in clients receiving chemotherapy. Lice or nit (eggs) infestation at the base of the penis or pubic hair is known as pediculosis pubis. This is commonly referred to as "crabs." 👓 Pubic hair may be gray and sparse in elderly clients. In addition, the penis becomes smaller and the testes hang lower in the scrotum in elderly clients.

continued

PHYSICAL ASSESSMENT *Continued*

Assessment Procedure	Normal Findings	Abnormal Findings
Inspect the skin of the shaft. Observe for rashes, lesions, or lumps.	The skin of the penis is wrinkled and hairless and is normally free of rashes, lesions, or lumps. Genital piercing is becoming more common, and nurses may see male clients with one or more piercings of the penis. Pubertal rites in some cultures include slitting the penile shaft, leaving an opening that may extend the entire length of the shaft (DeMeo, 1989).	Rashes, lesions, or lumps may indicate STD or cancer (Abnormal Findings 24-1). Drainage around piercings indicates infection.
Palpate the shaft. Palpate any abnormalities noted during inspection. Also note any hardened or tender areas.	The penis in a nonerect state is usually soft, flaccid, and nontender.	Hardness along the ventral surface may indicate cancer or a urethral stricture. Tenderness may indicate inflammation or infection.
Inspect the foreskin. Observe for color, location, and integrity of the foreskin in uncircumcised men.	The foreskin, which covers the glans in an uncircumcised male client, is intact and uniform in color with the penis.	Discoloration of the foreskin may indicate scarring or infection.

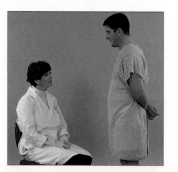

Figure 24-3 In positioning the male client for a genital examination, the examiner sits and the client stands (© B. Proud).

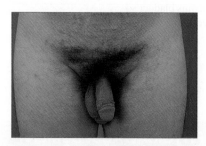

Figure 24-4 Normal appearance of external male genitalia (© B. Proud).

Table 24.1	**Tanner's Sexual Maturity Rating for Boys**		
Stage	**Pubic Hair**	**Penis**	**Testes and Scrotum**
1 (preadolescent)	None, except for fine body hair	Same size and proportions as in childhood	Same size and proportion as in childhood
2	Sparse growth, slightly curly	Slight or no enlargement	Both larger, reddened, exhibiting textural changes
3	Darker, coarse, curly, sparse hair over symphysis pubis	Larger, longer	Further enlargement
4	Coarse, curly hair that does not extend to medial thighs	Increased length and width, development of glans	Further enlargement and scrotal skin darkens
5	Adult hair in texture and quantity extends to medial aspect of thighs	Adult size and shape	Adult size and shape

Adapted from Tanner, 1962. *Growth at adolescence.* [2nd ed.]. Oxford: Blackwell Scientific Publications.

continued

Assessment Procedure	Normal Findings	Abnormal Findings
Inspect the glans. Observe for size, shape, and lesions or redness.	The glans size and shape vary, appearing rounded, broad, or even pointed. The surface of the glans is normally smooth, free of lesions, and redness.	Chancres (red, oval ulcerations) from syphilis, venereal warts, and pimple-like lesions from herpes are sometimes detected on the glans.
If the client is not circumcised, ask him to retract his foreskin, (if the client is unable to do so, the nurse may retract it) to allow observation of the glans. This may be painful.	The foreskin retracts easily. A small amount of whitish material, called smegma, normally accumulates under the foreskin.	A tight foreskin that cannot be retracted is called *phimosis*. A foreskin that once retracted cannot be returned to cover the glans is called *paraphimosis*. Chancres (red, oval ulcerations) from syphilis and venereal warts are sometimes detected under the foreskin (see Abnormal Findings 24-1).
Note the location of the urinary meatus on the glans	The urinary meatus is slit-like and normally found in the center of the glans. If pubertal mutilation has occurred, actual discharge of urine and semen will occur at the location of the shaft opening.	*Hypospadias* is displacement of the urinary meatus to the ventral surface of the penis. *Epispadias* is displacement of the urinary meatus to the dorsal surface of the penis (see Abnormal Findings 24-1).
Palpate the urethral discharge. Gently squeeze the glans between your index finger and thumb (Fig. 24-5).	The urinary meatus is normally free of discharge.	A yellow discharge is usually associated with gonorrhea. A clear or white discharge is usually associated with urethritis. All discharge should be cultured.

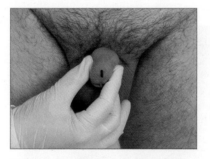

Figure 24-5 Palpating for urethral discharge (© B. Proud).

Scrotum

Inspection

Inspect the size, shape, and position. Ask the client to hold his penis out of the way. Observe for swelling, lumps, or bulges.	The scrotum varies in size (according to temperature) and shape. The scrotal sac hangs below or at the level of the penis. The left side of the scrotal sac usually hangs lower than the right side.	An enlarged scrotal sac may result from fluid (hydrocele), blood (hematocele), bowel (hernia), or tumor (cancer) (Abnormal Findings 24-2).
Inspect the scrotal skin. Observe color, integrity, and lesions or rashes. To perform an accurate inspection, you must spread out the scrotal folds (rugae) of skin (Fig. 24-6). Lift the scrotal sac to inspect the posterior skin.	Scrotal skin is thin and rugated (crinkled) with little hair dispersion. Its color is slightly darker than that of the penis. Lesions and rashes are not normally present. However, sebaceous cysts (small, yellowish, firm, nontender, benign nodules) are a normal finding.	Rashes, lesions, and inflammation are abnormal findings (Fig. 24-7).

continued

PHYSICAL ASSESSMENT *Continued*

Assessment Procedure	Normal Findings	Abnormal Findings

Palpation

Palpate the scrotal contents. Palpate each *testis* and *epididymis* between your thumb and first two fingers (Fig. 24-8). Note size, shape, consistency, nodules, and tenderness.

> ➤ *Clinical Tip* • *Do not apply too much pressure to the testes because this will cause pain.*

Palpate each *spermatic cord* and vas deferens from the epididymis to the inguinal ring. The spermatic cord will lie between your thumb and finger (Fig. 24-9). Note any nodules, swelling, or tenderness.

Testes are ovoid, approximately 3.5 to 5 cm long, 2.5 cm wide, and 2.5 cm deep, and equal bilaterally in size and shape. They are smooth, firm, rubbery, mobile, free of nodules, and rather tender to pressure. The epididymis is nontender, smooth, and softer than the testes.

Testes do not get smaller with normal aging although they may decrease in size with long-term illness.

The spermatic cord and vas deferens should feel uniform on both sides. The cord is smooth, nontender, and ropelike.

Absence of a testis suggests *cryptorchidism* (an undescended testicle). Painless nodules may indicate cancer. Tenderness and swelling may indicate acute orchitis, torsion of the spermatic cord, a strangulated hernia, or epididymitis (see Abnormal Findings 24-2). If the client has epididymitis, passive elevation of the testes may relieve the scrotal pain (Prehn's sign). If the client has a strangulated hernia, the client should be referred immediately to the physician and prepared for surgery.

Palpable, tortuous veins suggest varicocele. A beaded or thickened cord indicates infection or cysts. If you palpate a scrotal mass, have the client lie down. The mass may return to the abdomen by itself. If it does not, place your fingers above the scrotal mass. If you can get your fingers above the mass, suspect hydrocele (see Abnormal Findings 24-2). Cyst suggests hydrocele of the spermatic cord.

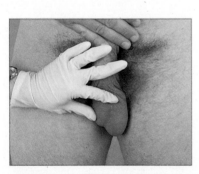

Figure 24-6 When inspecting the scrotal skin, have the client hold the penis aside while the examiner inspects (© B. Proud).

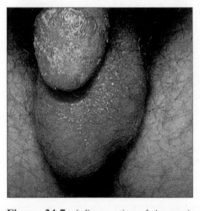

Figure 24-7 Inflammation of the penis and scrotum may be seen in Reiter's syndrome, and idiopathic inflammatory disorder affecting the skin, joints, and mucous membranes. (With permission from Goodheart, H. P. [1999]. A photoguide of common skin disorders. Baltimore: Lippincott Williams & Wilkins.)

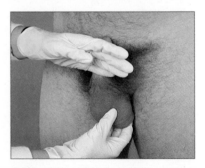

Figure 24-8 Palpating the scrotal contents (© B. Proud.).

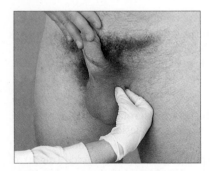

Figure 24-9 When palpating the spermatic cord, have the client hold the penis aside (© B. Proud.).

continued

Assessment Procedure	Normal Findings	Abnormal Findings
Auscultation Continue the examination of a scrotal mass by auscultating with a stethoscope.	Normal findings are not expected.	Bowel sounds may be auscultated over a hernia but will not be heard over a hydrocele.
Transillumination **Transilluminate the scrotal contents.** If an abnormal mass or swelling was noted in the scrotum, transillumination should be performed. Darken the room and shine a light from the back of the scrotum through the mass. Look for a red glow.	Normally scrotal contents do not transilluminate.	Swellings or masses that contain serous fluid—hydrocele, spermatocele—light up with a red glow. Swellings or masses that are solid or filled with blood—tumor, hernias, or varicocele—do not light up with a red glow.

Inguinal Area

Inspection **Inspect for inguinal and femoral hernia.** Inspect the inguinal and femoral areas for bulges. Ask the client to turn head and cough or to bear down as if having a bowel movement, and continue to inspect the areas.	The inguinal and femoral areas are normally free from bulges.	Bulges that appear at the external inguinal ring or at the femoral canal when the client bears down may signal a hernia (Abnormal Findings 24-3).
Palpation **Palpate for inguinal hernia and inguinal nodes.** Ask the client to shift his weight to the left for palpation of the right inguinal canal and vice versa. Place your right index finger into the client's right scrotum and press upward, invaginating the loose folds of skin (Fig. 24-10). Palpate up the spermatic cord until you reach the triangular-shaped, slitlike opening of the external inguinal ring. Try to push your finger through the opening and, if possible, continue palpating up the inguinal canal. When your finger is in the canal or at the external inguinal ring, ask the client to bear down or cough. Feel for any bulges against your finger. Then, repeat the procedure on the opposite side.	Bulging or masses are not normally palpated.	A bulge or mass may indicate a hernia.

continued

PHYSICAL ASSESSMENT *Continued*

Assessment Procedure	Normal Findings	Abnormal Findings
Palpate inguinal lymph nodes. If nodes are palpable, note size, consistency, mobility or tenderness.	No enlargement or tenderness is normal.	Enlarged or tender nodes may indicate an inflammatory process or lesion on the penis or scrotum.
Palpate for femoral hernia. Palpate on the front of the thigh in the femoral canal area (Fig. 24-11). Ask the client to bear down or cough. Feel for bulges. Repeat on the opposite thigh.	Bulges or masses are not normally palpated.	A bulge or mass may be from a hernia.
Inspect and palpate for scrotal hernia. If you discovered a mass during inspection and palpation of the scrotum and you suspect it may be a hernia, ask the client to lie down; note whether the bulge disappears. If the bulge remains, auscultate it for bowel sounds. Finally, gently palpate the mass and try to push it upward into the abdomen. ➤ **Clinical Tip** • *If the client complains of extreme tenderness or nausea, do not try to push the mass up into the abdomen.*	If the bulge disappears, no scrotal hernia is present, but the mass may result from something else and the client should be referred for further evaluation. A mass on or around the scrotum should be considered malignant until testing proves otherwise.	If the bulge disappears when the client lies down, a scrotal hernia is present. Bowel sounds auscultated over the mass indicate the presence of bowel and thus a scrotal hernia. If you cannot push the mass into the abdomen, suspect an *incarcerated hernia.* A hernia is *strangulated* when its blood supply is cut off. The client typically complains of extreme tenderness and nausea (see Abnormal Findings 24-3).

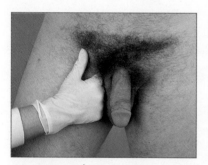

Figure 24-10 Palpating for an inguinal hernia (© B. Proud).

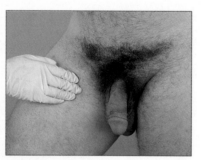

Figure 24-11 Palpating for a femoral hernia (© B. Proud).

Abnormal Findings 24-1   **Abnormalities of the Penis**

Syphilitic Chancre

- Initially a small, silvery-white papule that develops a red oval ulceration.
- Painless.
- A sign of primary syphilis (a sexually transmitted disease [STD]) that spontaneously regresses.
- May be misdiagnosed as herpes.

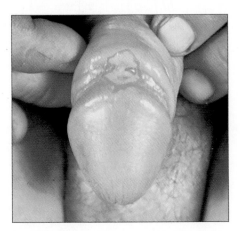

Syphilitic chancre. (Courtesy of UpJohn Co.)

Herpes Progenitalis

- Clusters of pimple-like, clear vesicles that erupt and become ulcers.
- Painful.
- Initial lesions of this STD, typically caused by HSV-1 or HSV-2, disappear, and the infection remains dormant for varying periods of time. Recurrences can be frequent or minimally episodic.

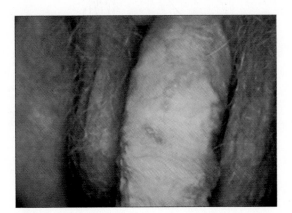

Herpes progenitalis.

Genital Warts

- Single or multiple, moist, fleshy papules.
- Painless.
- STD caused by the human papillomavirus.

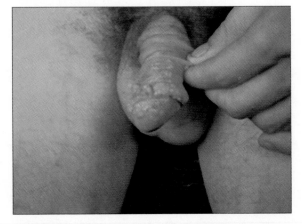

Genital warts. (Courtesy of Reed & Carnick Pharmaceuticals.)

Cancer of the Glans Penis

- Appears as hardened nodule or ulcer on the glans.
- Painless.
- Occurs primarily in uncircumcised men.

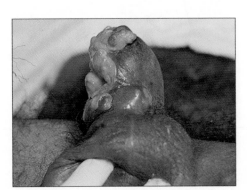

Penile carcinoma. (© 1993. Jennifer Watson-Holton/Custom Medical Stock Photo.)

continued on page 496

Abnormal Findings 24-1   **Abnormalities of the Penis** *Continued*

Phimosis

Foreskin is so tight that it cannot be retracted over the glans.

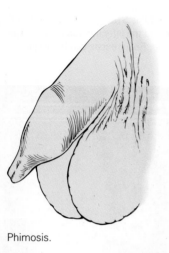

Phimosis.

Paraphimosis

Foreskin is so tight that, once retracted, it cannot be returned back over the glans.

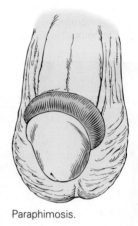

Paraphimosis.

Hypospadias

- Urethral meatus is located underneath the glans (ventral side).
- This condition is a congenital defect.
- A groove extends from the meatus to the normal location of the urethral meatus.

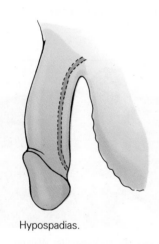

Hypospadias.

Epispadias

- The urethral meatus is located on the top of the glans (dorsal side); occurs rarely.
- This condition is a congenital defect.

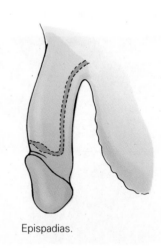

Epispadias.

Abnormal Findings 24-2   **Abnormalities of the Scrotum**

Although some scrotal abnormalities can be seen by visual inspection, most must be palpated. Some common abnormalities are described below.

Hydrocele

- Collection of serous fluid in the scrotum, outside the testes within the tunica vaginalis.
- Appears as swelling in the scrotum and is usually painless.
- Usually the examiner can get fingers above this mass during palpation.
- Will transilluminate (if there is blood in the scrotum, it will not transilluminate and is called a "hematocele").

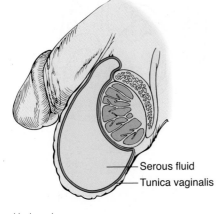

Hydrocele.

Scrotal Hernia

- A loop of bowel protrudes into the scrotum to create what is known as an indirect inguinal hernia.
- Hernia appears as swelling in the scrotum.
- Palpable as a soft mass and fingers cannot get above the mass.

Scrotal hernia.

Testicular Tumor

- Initially a small, firm, nontender nodule on the testis.
- As the tumor grows, the scrotum appears enlarged and the client complains of a heavy feeling.
- When palpated, the testis feels enlarged and smooth—tumor replaces testis.
- Will not transilluminate.

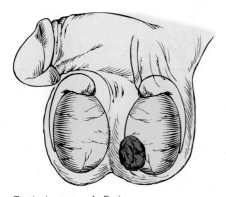

Testicular tumor A. Early

B. Late.

continued on page 498

Abnormal Findings 24-2   **Abnormalities of the Scrotum** *Continued*

Cryptorchidism

- Failure of one or both testicles to descend into scrotum.
- Scrotum appears undeveloped and testis cannot be palpated.
- Causes increased risk of testicular cancer.

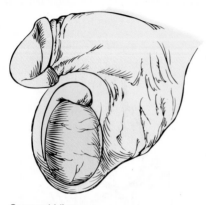

Cryptorchidism.

Epididymitis

- Infection of the epididymis.
- Client usually complains of sudden pain.
- Scrotum appears enlarged, reddened, and swollen; tender epididymis is palpated.
- Usually associated with prostatitis or bacterial infection.

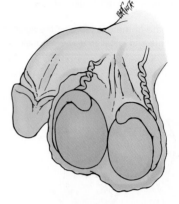

Epididymitis.

Orchitis

- Inflammation of the testes, associated frequently with mumps.
- Client complains of pain, heaviness, and fever.
- Scrotum appears enlarged and reddened.
- Swollen, tender testis is palpated. The examiner may have difficulty differentiating between testis and epididymis.

Orchitis.

Small Testes

- Small (less than 3.5 cm long), soft testes indicate atrophy. Atrophy may result from cirrhosis, hypopituitarism, estrogen administration, extended illness, or the disorder may occur after orchitis.
- Small (less than 2 cm long), firm testes may indicate Klinefelter's syndrome.

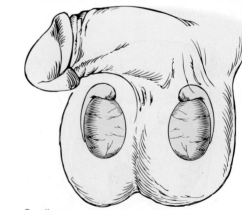

Small testes.

continued

Abnormal Findings 24-2   **Abnormalities of the Scrotum** *Continued*

Torsion of Spermatic Cord

- Very painful condition caused by twisting of spermatic cord.
- Scrotum appears enlarged and reddened.
- Palpation reveals thickened cord and swollen, tender testis that may be higher in scrotum than normal.
- This condition requires immediate referral for surgery because circulation is obstructed.

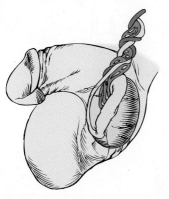

Torsion of spermatic cord.

Varicocele

- Abnormal dilation of veins in the spermatic cord.
- Client may complain of discomfort and testicular heaviness.
- Tortuous veins are palpable and feel like a soft, irregular mass or "a bag of worms," which collapses when the client is supine.
- Infertility may be associated with this condition.

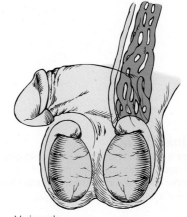

Varicocele.

Spermatocele

- Sperm-filled cystic mass located on epididymis.
- Palpable as small and nontender, and movable above the testis.
- This mass will appear on transillumination.

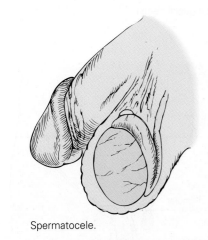

Spermatocele.

Abnormal Findings 24-3 | **Inguinal and Femoral Hernias**

Indirect Inguinal Hernia

- Bowel herniates through internal inguinal ring and remains in the inguinal canal or travels down into the scrotum (scrotal hernia).
- This is the most common type of hernia.
- It may occur in adults but is more frequent in children.

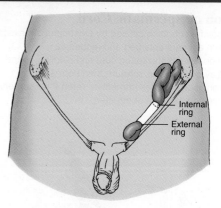

Indirect inguinal hernia.

Direct Inguinal Hernia

- Bowel herniates from behind and through the external inguinal ring. It rarely travels down into the scrotum.
- This type of hernia is less common than an indirect hernia.
- It occurs mostly in adult men older than age 40.

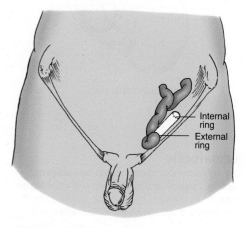

Direct inguinal hernia.

Femoral Hernia

- Bowel herniates through the femoral ring and canal. It never travels into the scrotum, and the inguinal canal is empty.
- This is the least common type of hernia.
- It occurs mostly in women.

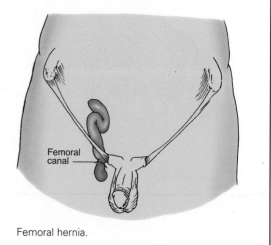

Femoral hernia.

VALIDATING AND DOCUMENTING FINDINGS

Validate the male genitalia assessment data that you have collected. This is necessary to verify that the data are reliable and accurate. Document the assessment data in accord with the health care facility or agency policy.

Sample Documentation of Subjective Data

A 35-year-old male military officer reports no current pain, lesions, discharge from penis, swelling, lumps, or heavy feeling in scrotum. States no difficulty urinating; no change in color, amount, or odor of urine; no pain when urinating; no urinary incontinence. Reports no change in sexual activity or desire, no current difficulty in attaining or maintaining an erection, and no difficulty ejaculating. Is not aware of any fertility problem. Client reports history of a right inguinal hernia 4 years ago that was surgically repaired with no complications. Last testicular examination was 3 years ago. Is tested for HIV annually as part of his military physical requirements. Reports negative results. No family history of cancer. Client states he is currently sexually monogamous with his fiancée, and he uses condoms as a backup birth control method. Denies exposure to chemicals and is very careful when he has to lift heavy items. He reports he is sexually satisfied and can talk to his fiancée about anything. He performs monthly testicular self-examinations.

Sample Documentation of Objective Data

Pubic hair growth pattern is normal for adult male; pubic hair and base of penis are free of excoriation and infestation. Circumcised penis is free of rashes, lesions, and lumps and is soft, flaccid, and nontender on palpation. Glans is rounded and free of lesions; urinary meatus is centrally located on glans; no discharge is palpated from urinary meatus. No masses or swelling noted in scrotum, and left side hangs slightly lower than right side. Skin is free of lesions and appears rugated and darkly pigmented. Two descended testes palpated. No swelling, tenderness, or masses palpated along the testicle, epididymis, or spermatic cord on either side. No bulges or masses palpated in inguinal or femoral canal.

After you have collected your assessment data, you will need to analyze the data using diagnostic reasoning skills.

Analysis of Data

DIAGNOSTIC REASONING: POSSIBLE CONCLUSIONS

After collecting subjective and objective data pertaining to the male genitalia, identify abnormal findings and client strengths. Then cluster the data to reveal any significant patterns or abnormalities. These data may then be used to make clinical judgments about the status of the male client's genitalia.

Selected Nursing Diagnoses

Following is a listing of selected nursing diagnoses (wellness, risk, or actual) that the nurse may identify when analyzing the cue clusters.

Wellness Diagnoses

- Health-Seeking Behavior: Requests information for health management of the reproductive system
- Health-Seeking Behavior: Requests information on testicular self-examination (TSE)
- Health-Seeking Behavior: Requests information on ways to prevent an STD
- Health-Seeking Behavior: Requests information on birth control
- Health-Seeking Behavior: Requests information on proper lifting techniques to prevent hernia formation

Risk Diagnoses

- Risk for Ineffective Therapeutic Regimen Management (monthly testicular self-examination, TSE) related to lack of knowledge of the importance of TSE
- Risk for Injury related to poor lifting techniques
- Risk for Infection related to unprotected sexual intercourse
- Risk for Ineffective Sexuality Pattern related to impending surgery

Actual Diagnoses

- Fear of testicular cancer related to existing risk factors
- Disturbed Body Image related to hernia repair
- Pain: Dysuria related to gonorrhea, infection, or genital reproductive surgery
- Ineffective Therapeutic Regimen Management related to lack of knowledge of testicular self-examination
- Sexual Dysfunction related to decreased libido secondary to fear of urinary incontinence, pain in surgical site, anxiety, or fear
- Sexual Dysfunction related to erectile dysfunction secondary to psychological or physiologic factors
- Sexual Dysfunction related to lack of ejaculation secondary to surgical removal of seminal vesicles and transection of the vas deferens
- Anxiety related to impending genital reproductive surgery and lack of knowledge of outcome of surgery

Selected Collaborative Problems

After grouping the data, certain collaborative problems may become apparent. Remember that collaborative problems differ from nursing diagnoses in that they cannot be prevented by nursing interventions. However, these physiologic complications of medical conditions can be detected and monitored by a nurse. In addition, the nurse can use physician- and nurse-prescribed interventions to minimize the complications of these problems. The nurse may also have to refer the client in such situations for further treatment of the problem. Following is a list of collaborative problems that may be identified when assessing the male genitalia. These problems are worded as Risk for Complications (or RC), followed by the problem.

- RC: Gonorrhea
- RC: Syphilis

- RC: Genital warts
- RC: Erectile dysfunction
- RC: Inability to ejaculate
- RC: Hernia
- RC: Hemorrhage
- RC: Urinary incontinence
- RC: Urinary retention

Medical Problems

After grouping the data, client's signs and symptoms may clearly require referral to a primary care provider for medical diagnoses (i.e., testicular cancer).

CASE STUDY

The case study demonstrates how to analyze male genitalia assessment data for a specific client. The critical thinking exercise included in the study guide/lab manual and interactive program that complement this text also offer opportunities to analyze assessment data.

Carl Weeks is a 72-year-old man who has been receiving follow-up care by the home care nurse since his discharge from the hospital 3 weeks ago during which he was treated for a diabetic coma. His diabetic status is currently stable but he complains to the home health nurse that he is having problems with urination. He states that he is "peeing often in little dribbles," has difficulty maintaining his urinary stream, and wakes up three or four times a night to void. His wife, Marie, states that neither of them is getting much sleep. She asks how she can help her husband with this problem. Mr. Weeks also reports that for the last 2 days he has had discomfort in his bladder and

burning with urination. Mrs. Weeks tells the nurse that he won't drink water and he can't have fruit juice because of his diabetes (she has heard that cranberry juice may help prevent urinary problems). On physical examination, distention is noted in the suprapubic area about 5 cm above the symphysis pubis, which is slightly tender to palpation, and a distinct area of dullness is noted in the same area. Mr. Weeks' vital signs and blood glucose level are within normal limits but his temperature is 99.2°F.

The following concept map illustrates the diagnostic reasoning process.

Applying COLDSPA

Applying **COLDSPA** for client symptoms: "Frequent urination."

Mnemonic	Question	Data Provided	Missing Data
Character	Describe the sign or symptom (feeling, appearance, sound, smell, or taste if applicable).	Client reports "peeing often in little dribbles" and difficulty maintaining urine stream	
Onset	When did it begin?		"When did the little dribbles and difficulty maintaining a stream begin?"
Location	Where is it? Does it radiate? Does it occur anywhere else?		"Point to where you feel burning and discomfort. Do you have discomfort anywhere else? Does it spread to other areas?"
Duration	How long does it last? Does it recur?		"Does this occur every time you attempt to void? Or just sometimes?"
Severity	How bad is it? or How much does it bother you?	Client reports waking up 3–4 times a night to void.	
Pattern	What makes it better or worse?		"What relieves the burning or discomfort if anything?"
Associated factors/How it **A**ffects the client	What other symptoms occur with it? How does it affect you?	For the last 2 days, "discomfort in the bladder and burning with urination."	

1) Identify abnormal findings and client strengths

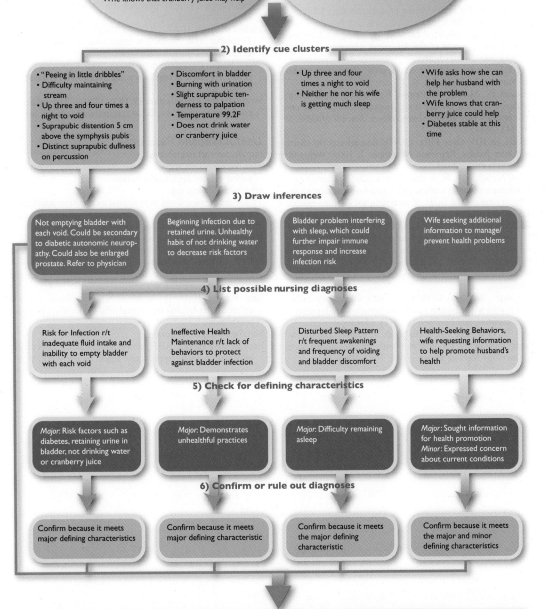

Subjective Data

- "Peeing in little dribbles"
- Has difficulty maintaining urinary stream
- Discomfort in bladder; burning with urination
- Up three and four times a night to void
- Neither he nor wife is getting much sleep
- Wife asks how to help her husband
- Mr. Weeks won't drink water
- Can't have fruit juice because of diabetes
- Wife knows that cranberry juice may help

Objective Data

- Diabetes stable at this time
- Suprapubic distention 5 cm above symphysis pubis
- Slight suprapubic tenderness to palpation
- Distinct suprapubic dullness on percussion
- Vital signs, blood glucose level within normal limits
- Temperature 99.2F

2) Identify cue clusters

- "Peeing in little dribbles"
- Difficulty maintaining stream
- Up three and four times a night to void
- Suprapubic distention 5 cm above the symphysis pubis
- Distinct suprapubic dullness on percussion

- Discomfort in bladder
- Burning with urination
- Slight suprapubic tenderness to palpation
- Temperature 99.2F
- Does not drink water or cranberry juice

- Up three and four times a night to void
- Neither he nor his wife is getting much sleep

- Wife asks how she can help her husband with the problem
- Wife knows that cranberry juice could help
- Diabetes stable at this time

3) Draw inferences

Not emptying bladder with each void. Could be secondary to diabetic autonomic neuropathy. Could also be enlarged prostate. Refer to physician

Beginning infection due to retained urine. Unhealthy habit of not drinking water to decrease risk factors

Bladder problem interfering with sleep, which could further impair immune response and increase infection risk

Wife seeking additional information to manage/prevent health problems

4) List possible nursing diagnoses

Risk for Infection r/t inadequate fluid intake and inability to empty bladder with each void

Ineffective Health Maintenance r/t lack of behaviors to protect against bladder infection

Disturbed Sleep Pattern r/t frequent awakenings and frequency of voiding and bladder discomfort

Health-Seeking Behaviors, wife requesting information to help promote husband's health

5) Check for defining characteristics

Major: Risk factors such as diabetes, retaining urine in bladder, not drinking water or cranberry juice

Major: Demonstrates unhealthful practices

Major: Difficulty remaining asleep

Major: Sought information for health promotion
Minor: Expressed concern about current conditions

6) Confirm or rule out diagnoses

Confirm because it meets major defining characteristics

Confirm because it meets major defining characteristic

Confirm because it meets the major defining characteristic

Confirm because it meets the major and minor defining characteristics

7) Document conclusions

Nursing diagnoses that are appropriate for this client include:
- Risk for Infection r/t inadequate fluid intake and inability to empty bladder with each void
- Ineffective Health Maintenance r/t lack of behaviors for preventing infection
- Disturbed Sleep Pattern r/t frequency of voiding and discomfort
- Health-Seeking Behaviors, wife seeks information regarding health promotion

Potential collaborative problems include the following:
RC: Hydronephrosis
RC: Renal failure
RC: Sepsis
Mr. Weeks should be referred to his physician for evaluation and management of causes of urinary retention and of infection.

References and Selected Readings

American Cancer Society. (2009). *Cancer facts & figures, 2009.* Atlanta: American Cancer Society. Available at http://www.cancer.org

Can testicular cancer be found early? (2009). Available at www.cancer.org

Dogra, V. & Bhatt, S. (2004). Acute painful scrotum. *Radiologic Clinics of North America, 42*(2), 349–363.

Gilchrist, K. (2004). Benign prostatic hyperplasia. *Nurse Practitioner, 19*(6), 30–37: quiz 37–39.

Hellstrom, W. (2007). Current safety and tolerability issues in men with erectile dysfunction receiving PDE5 inhibitors. *International Journal of Clinical Practice, 61*(9), 1547–1554.

Kelly, D. (2004). Male sexuality in theory and practice. *Nursing Clinics of North America, 39*(2), 341–356.

Kleier, J. A. (2004). Nurse practitioners' behavior regarding teaching testicular self examination. *Journal of the American Academy of Nurse Practitioners, 16*(5), 206–208, 210, 212.

Matthews, P. A. (2004). Getting ready for certification: obstructive uropathy. *Urological Nursing, 24*(1), 45, 61.

Naslund, M., Gilsenan, A., Midkiff, K., Brown, A., Wolford, E., & Wang, J. (2007). Prevalence of lower urinary tract symptoms and prostate enlargement in the primary care setting. *International Journal of Clinical Practice, 61*(9), 1437–1445.

National Association on HIV Over Fifty. (2007). Educational tip sheet: HIV/AIDs and Older Adults. Retrieved November 2, 1007. Web site: http://www.hivoverfifty.org/tip.html

Roobol, J., Grenabo, A., Schroder, F., & Hugosson, J. (2007). Interval cancers in prostate cancer screening: Comparing 2- and 4-year screening intervals in European randomized study of screening for prostate cancer. *Journal of the National Cancer Institute, 99*(17), 1296–1303.

Rosenberg, M., Staskin, D., Kaplan, S., MacDiarmid, S., Newman, D., & Ohl, D. (2007). A practical guide to the evaluation and treatment of male lower urinary tract symptoms in the primary care setting. *International Journal of Clinical Practice, 61*(9), 1535–1546.

Tanner, J. M. (1962). *Growth at adolescence* (2nd ed.). Oxford: Blackwell Scientific Publications.

Templeton, H., & Coates, V. (2004). Evaluation of an evidence-based education package for men with prostate cancer on hormonal manipulation therapy. *Patient Education and Counseling, 55*(1), 55–61.

Wallace, M., Bailey, D., O'Rourke, M., & Galbraith, M. (2004). The watchful waiting management option for older men with prostate cancer: State of the science. *Oncology Nursing Forum, 31*(6), 1057–1066.

Walton, J., & Sullivan, N. (2004). Men of prayer: Spirituality of men with prostate cancer: A grounded theory study. *Journal of Holistic Nursing, 22*(2), 133–151.

Promote Health—HIV/AIDS

Centers for Disease Control and Prevention (CDC). (2007). HIV/AIDS surveillance report. Available at http://www.cdc.gov/hiv

Chin, J. (ed.). (2000). *Control of communicable diseases manual* (17th ed.). Washington, DC: American Public Health Association.

DeMeo, J. (1989). The geography of genital mutilation. *The Truth Seeker.* Available at http://www.noharmm.org/geography.htm

Joint United Nations program on HIV/AIDS. (2006). Available at http://www.unaids.org

United Nations (UN). (2006). UNAIDS/WHO AIDS epidemic update: December 2006. Available at http://www.unaids.org/en/HIV_data/epi2006/default.asp

World Health Organization (WHO). (2006). Report on the global AIDS epidemic. Available at http://www.unaids.org/en/HIV_data/2006GlobalReport/default.asp

World Health Organization (WHO). (2007). The global AIDS epidemic continues to grow. Available at http://www.who.int/hiv

Useful Website Resources

http://cancernet.nci.nih.gov/

This Website is a service of the National Cancer Institute and provides cancer-related health information.

http://www.cancer.org

This website, owned and copyrighted by the American Cancer Society, provides cancer information for health professionals and patients.

http://www.cdc.gov/reproductivehealth

Site developed by United States Department of Health and Human Services, Centers for Disease Control and Prevention, National Center for Chronic Disease Prevention and Health Promotion, Division of Reproductive Health. Features factsheets about men's reproductive issues.

http://www.mdanderson.org

The Website of M. D. Anderson Cancer Center contains information about cancer treatment, clinical trials, education programs, and cancer prevention.

http://www.rhgateway.org

Reproductive Health (RH) Gateway gives quick access to relevant, accurate information about reproductive health on the World Wide Web.

Structure and Function

ANUS AND RECTUM

The **anal canal** is the final segment of the digestive system; it begins at the anal sphincter and ends at the anorectal junction (also known as the pectinate line, mucocutaneous junction, or dentate line). It measures from 2.5 cm to 4 cm long. It is lined with skin that contains no hair or sebaceous glands but does contain many somatic sensory nerves, making it susceptible to painful stimuli. The **anal opening** or anal verge can be distinguished from the perianal skin by its hairless moist appearance. The anal verge extends interiorly, overlying the external anal sphincter.

Within the anus are the two sphincters that normally hold the anal canal closed except when passing gas and feces. The **external sphincter** is composed of skeletal muscle and is under voluntary control. The **internal sphincter** is composed of smooth muscle and is under involuntary control by the autonomic nervous system. Dividing the two sphincters is the palpable intersphincteric groove. The anal canal proceeds upward toward the umbilicus. Just above the internal sphincter is the **anorectal junction,** the dividing point of the anal canal and the rectum. The rectum is lined with folds of mucosa, known as the columns of Morgagni. The anorectal junction is not palpable, but may be visualized during internal examination. The folds contain a network of arteries, veins, and visceral nerves. Between the columns are recessed areas known as anal crypts; there are 8–12 anal crypts and 5–8 papillae. If the veins in these folds undergo chronic pressure, they may become engorged with blood, forming hemorrhoids (Fig. 25-1).

The **rectum** is the lowest portion of the large intestine and is approximately 12 cm long, extending from the end of the **sigmoid colon** to the anorectal junction. It enlarges above the anorectal junction and proceeds in a posterior direction toward the hollow of the sacrum and coccyx, forming the rectal ampulla. The anal canal and rectum are at approximately right angles to each other. The inside of the rectum contains three inward foldings called the valves of Houston. The function of the valves of Houston is unclear. The lowest valve may be felt, usually on the client's left side.

The **peritoneum** lines the upper two-thirds of the anterior rectum and dips down enough so that it may be palpated where it forms the **rectovesical pouch** in men and the **rectouterine pouch** in women.

PROSTATE

The **prostate gland** is approximately 2.5 to 4 cm in diameter and surrounds the neck of the bladder and urethra and lies between these structures and the rectum in male clients. It consists of two lobes separated by a shallow groove called the median sulcus (Fig. 25-2). It secretes a thin, milky substance that promotes sperm motility and neutralizes female acidic vaginal secretions. This chestnut- or heart-shaped organ can be palpated through the anterior wall of the rectum.

 Prostatic hyperplasia, enlargement of the prostate gland, has become increasingly common in men over age 40.

Located on either side of, and above, the prostate gland are the **seminal vesicles.** These are rabbit-ear–shaped structures that produce the ejaculate that nourishes and protects sperm. They are not normally palpable. The **Cowper's or bulbourethral glands** are mucus-producing, pea-sized organs located posterior to the prostate gland. These glands surround and empty into the urethra. They are not normally palpable either.

Nursing Assessment

COLLECTING SUBJECTIVE DATA: THE NURSING HEALTH HISTORY

The data gathered during subjective assessment provide clues to the client's overall health and whether he is at risk for diseases and disorders of the anus, rectum, or prostate. The subjective assessment is a good time to teach the client about risk factors related to diseases, such as colorectal or prostate cancer, and about ways to decrease those risk factors.

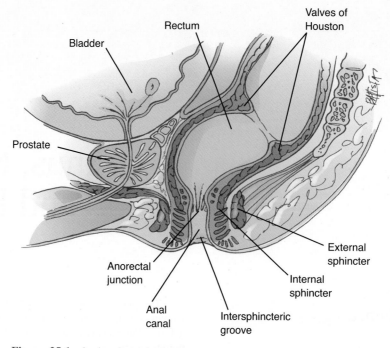

Figure 25-1   Anal and rectal structures.

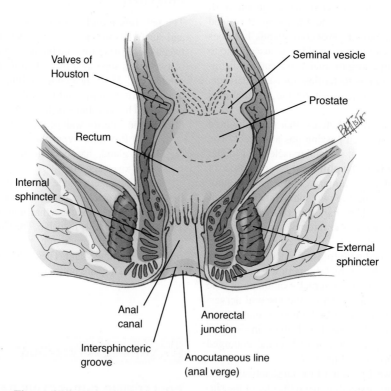

Figure 25-2   Prostate gland and nearby structures.

Collecting data about the anus, rectum, and prostate can be embarrassing for both the examiner and the client. Some questions are very personal. Therefore, it is important to ease the client's anxiety as much as possible. Ask the questions in a straightforward manner, and let the client voice any concerns throughout the assessment. In some cultural groups, only nurses of the same gender will be considered acceptable assessors of intimate body areas.

(text continues on page 511)

HISTORY OF PRESENT HEALTH CONCERN

Question	Rationale
Bowel Patterns What is your usual bowel pattern? Have you noticed any recent change in the pattern? Any pain while passing a bowel movement?	A change in bowel pattern is associated with many disorders and is one of the warning signs of cancer. A more thorough evaluation, including laboratory tests and proctosigmoidoscopy, may be necessary.
Do you experience constipation?	Constipation may indicate a bowel obstruction or the need for dietary counseling.
Do you experience diarrhea? Is the diarrhea associated with any nausea or vomiting?	Diarrhea may signal impaction or indicate the need for dietary counseling.
Do you have trouble controlling your bowels?	Fecal incontinence occurs with neurologic disorders and some gastrointestinal infections.
Stool What is the color of your stool? Hard or soft? Have you noticed any blood on or in your stool? If so, how much?	Black stools may indicate gastrointestinal bleeding or the use of iron supplements or Pepto-Bismol. Red blood in the stool is found with hemorrhoids, polyps, cancer, or colitis. Clay-colored stools result from a lack of bile pigment.
Have you noticed any mucus in your stool?	Mucus in the stool may indicate steatorrhea (excessive fat in the stool).
Itching and Pain Do you experience any itching or pain in the rectal area?	Sexually transmitted diseases, hemorrhoids, pinworms, or anal trauma may cause itching or pain (see Promote Health—Hemorrhoids).

continued on page 508

COLDSPA Example for Rectal Pain

Use the **COLDSPA** mnemonic as a guideline to collect needed information for each symptom the client shares. In addition, the following questions help elicit important information.

Mnemonic	Question	Client Response Example
Character	Describe the sign or symptom (feeling, appearance, sound, smell, or taste if applicable).	"My rectal area hurts right when I have a bowel movement and right after the bowel movement it really hurts."
Onset	When did it begin?	"About 2 weeks ago, but I thought it would go away."
Location	Where is it? Does it radiate? Does it occur anywhere else?	"I feel like I have a knot around my rectal area and I am worried about what it is."
Duration	How long does it last? Does it recur?	"Sometimes it gets better. I had this 9 months ago, but it went away. This time, after taking a long car trip and sitting for long periods, it came back and is not getting any better."
Severity	How bad is it? or How much does it bother you?	"Right now it really hurts badly. I would rate it a 9 on a scale of 1 to 10. The rectal knot is also getting bigger."
Pattern	What makes it better or worse?	"A warm bath makes it feel better for a while. Straining if I am constipated makes it worse."
Associated factors/How it **A**ffects the client	What other symptoms occur with it? How does it affect you?	"I am scared I may have cancer because of the knot down there."

PROMOTE HEALTH
Hemorrhoids

Overview

Hemorrhoids are formed when excessive pressure affects the veins in the pelvis and rectal areas. The tissues surrounding the inside of the anus fill with blood to help control bowel movements. With excessive pressure, the blood in the veins within these tissues causes veins to swell and stretch the surrounding tissue. There are many causes including straining when rushing to complete a bowel movement or with constipation or diarrhea; being overweight; the last 6 months of pregnancy and delivery; prolonged standing or sitting; liver or heart disease if blood is pooled in the abdomen or pelvis; and, rarely, tumors in the pelvic area. Hemorrhoids can occur at any age but usually occur after 30 years of age, with about 50% of people over 50 having had some hemorrhoid problems.

Risk Factors

- Poor bowel habits (rushing bowel movements with straining; not heeding the feeling of need for a bowel movement)
- Pregnancy (after 6 months and during labor)
- Inadequate fluid intake
- Inadequate fiber intake
- Prolonged standing or sitting
- Inadequate exercise

Teach Risk Reduction Tips

- Avoid constipation.
- Avoid straining with bowel movements; avoid holding breath when passing bowel movement.
- Go to the bathroom as soon as urge occurs; leave as soon as bowel movement completed.
- Eat a diet with moderate fiber intake; whole grains, raw vegetables, raw and dried fruits, legumes (beans, lentils).
- Avoid a diet high in low or no fiber foods (ice cream, soft drinks, cheese, white bread, red meat).
- Drink 8 to 10 glasses of water daily. Avoid caffeine or alcohol.
- Evaluate foods that may worsen symptoms, such as nuts, spicy foods, coffee, and alcohol.
- Consult primary health care provider for safety of taking stool softeners with bran or psyllium.
- Avoid taking laxatives (can cause diarrhea or irritate hemorrhoids).
- Get regular, moderate exercise.
- Avoid lifting heavy objects often and do not hold breath with lifting.
- When pregnant, sleep on side to reduce pressure on anal area and pelvis (WebMD, 2007).

PAST HEALTH HISTORY

Question	Rationale
Have you ever had anal or rectal trauma or surgery? Were you born with any congenital deformities of the anus or rectum? Have you had prostate surgery? Have you had hemorrhoids or surgery for hemorrhoids?	Past conditions influence the findings of physical assessment. Congenital deformities, such as imperforate anus, are often surgically repaired when the client is very young.
When was the last time you had a stool test to detect blood?	The American Cancer Society recommends a stool test every year after age 50 to detect occult blood. Clinical trials have determined that the fecal occult blood test has increased detection of both adenomatous polyps and colorectal cancer and is associated with a 15% to 33% decline in the death rate from these conditions (http://cancernet.nci.nih.gov/).
Have you ever had proctosigmoidoscopy?	A proctosigmoidoscopic examination is recommended every 3 to 5 years after age 50 based on the advice of a physician.

continued

PAST HEALTH HISTORY *Continued*

Question	*Rationale*
When was the last time you had a digital rectal examination (DRE) by a physician?	A DRE may reveal rectal masses, prostate enlargement, or prostate nodules. The American Cancer Society recommends a DRE every year after age 40.
Have you ever had blood taken for a prostate screening, which measures the level of prostate-specific antigen (PSA) in your blood? When was the test and what was the result?	PSA is a biologic marker for prostate cancer. The American Cancer Society recommends a PSA measurement yearly for men age 50 years and older (see Promote Health—Prostate Cancer).

FAMILY HISTORY

Question	*Rationale*
Is there a history of polyps, colon or rectal cancer, or prostate cancer in your family?	Colorectal and prostate cancer have a tendency to affect members of the same family.

continued on page 510

PROMOTE HEALTH
Prostate Cancer

Overview
Prostate cancer is the second leading cause of cancer death in men in the United States. (Lung cancer is first.) About 1 in 6 men are diagnosed with prostate cancer but only 3% die of the disease. Prostate cancer is slow growing and can be readily treated if found early. There is no sure way to prevent prostate cancer, but diet and lifestyle behaviors are thought to help with prevention.

Risk Factors
- Age
- Family history
- Hormones (One study shows testosterone level is highest in black males, intermediate in white males, and lowest in native Japanese males. The risks of prostate cancer in these racial groups directly parallel these androgen levels. [Ross, 1995/2006]).
- Race (in the United States, highest in African American and Afro-Caribbean men, moderate in Caucasian men, and lowest in Asian and Hispanic Americans)
- Dietary fat (especially high intake of red meat and high fat dairy products)
- Dairy and calcium intake (Some studies suggest this.)
- Cadmium exposure
- Dioxin exposure
- Multiple sex partners, especially contracting STDs
- A multi-year large scale research trial is ongoing to see if selenium or vitamin E increase or reduce risk of prostate cancer (among other cancers).

Teach Risk Reduction Tips
- Don't overeat (moderate servings and calories).
- Avoid high fat foods.
- Eat a diet rich in fruits and vegetables, high in fiber, and high in omega-3 fatty acids.
- Soy products and other legumes have phytoestrogens that may have a positive effect.
- Drink green tea daily.
- Drink no more than 2 alcoholic drinks a day (men); 1 for women.
- Get moderate exercise daily.
- Sleep in a dark room; avoid bright light at night.
- Have an annual prostate examination (including a prostate specific antigen [PSA] analysis) as recommended by a primary health care provider, especially for men 50 years and older.

LIFESTYLE AND HEALTH PRACTICES

Question	Rationale
Do you use any laxatives, stool softeners, enemas, or other bowel movement-enhancing medications?	Long-term use of these agents can alter the body's ability to regulate bowel function. Short-term use may indicate the need for dietary counseling.
Do you engage in anal sex?	Anal sex increases the risk for sexually transmitted disease, infection by human immunodeficiency virus (HIV), fissures, rectal prolapse, and hemorrhoid formation.
Do you take any medications for your prostate?	Men with benign prostatic hypertrophy (BPH) with "voiding symptoms," such as urinary urgency, may take an alpha-adrenergic blocker such as terazosin (Hytrin) or an androgen hormone inhibitor such as finasteride (Proscar).
How much high-fiber food and roughage do you consume every day? Do you eat foods high in saturated fat?	Although high-fat diets have been implicated in colon cancer (see Promote Health—Colorectal Cancer), the role of dietary fat continues to be controversial. The Nurses' Health Study indicates that the risk of colon cancer increases with the consumption of red meat and saturated and monounsaturated fats. But the Iowa Women's Health Study and a National Cancer Institute study found no such relationship. The role of dietary fiber, which was once thought to offer protection against colon cancer is also in question. Although a majority of studies conducted over the last 20 years suggest dietary fiber offers protection against colon cancer, several studies—including the Nurses' Health Study—do not support these benefits of fiber.
Do you engage in regular exercise?	Sedentary lifestyle has been linked to the development of colorectal cancer, and physical activity has been associated with a reduction in risk. The amount of exercise needed has not been established.
Do you use calcium supplements?	Some observational studies indicate that the colon cancer risk drops as calcium intake increases; others do not reflect any effect.
For postmenopausal women: Do you use hormone replacement therapy?	Studies, including a retrospective study of 400,000 women conducted by the American Cancer Society and the Nurses' Health Study, a prospective study of 120,000 women, have indicated that postmenopausal estrogen use reduces the risk of colon cancer. Further studies are needed.
Has any anal or rectal problem affected your normal activities of daily living (working or engaging in recreation)?	Some problems, such as hemorrhoids or bowel incontinence, may affect a client's ability to work or interact socially.

PROMOTE HEALTH
Colorectal Cancer

Overview

Cancer of the colon and rectum is the third most common type of cancer in men and women in Western industrialized societies. About 112,340 new cases of colon cancer and 41,420 new cases of rectal cancer were expected to be diagnosed in the United States in 2007, and about 49,960 persons were expected to die from colorectal cancer in 2008–2010. The death rate has been dropping for the last 15 years, possibly due to earlier detection and improved treatment (American Cancer Society, 2007).

Risk Factors

- Any age, but 90% occur over age 50
- Personal history of rectal or colon polyps or cancer
- Inflammatory bowel diseases
- Genetics: family history of cancer or familial colorectal cancer syndromes
- Ashkenazi Jewish descent (Eastern European); African American
- Diet mostly from animal sources (high in fat and animal protein; low in fruits, vegetables, and fiber)
- Physical inactivity
- Obesity
- Moderate to heavy alcohol consumption
- Smoking
- Diabetes mellitus
- Possibly: night shift work; other cancers and their treatment

Teach Risk Reduction Tips

- For people at average risk: Beginning at age 50, have a fecal occult blood test (FOBT) every year and a sigmoidoscopic examination every 5 years, or a colonoscopic examination every 10 years, or a double contrast barium enema every 5 to 10 years.
- For people at moderate risk, with polyps or previous cancer: Follow ACS guidelines for screening.
- For people with a personal history of polyps or with first-degree relatives who are cancer patients: Have colonoscopy at age 40 and every 5 to 10 years thereafter.
- Eat a diet high in fiber, fruit, and vegetables and low in fat and animal protein.
- Eat a half cup of raisins or three-quarters of a cup of grapes daily (tartaric acid and fiber reduce bile acids and speed food through system; Spiller et al., 2003).
- Eat foods with adequate calcium, folic acid, vitamin D, and possibly magnesium.
- Get regular exercise for at least 30 minutes most days.
- Talk to physician about the advisability of taking aspirin, nonsteroidal anti-inflammatory drugs (NSAIDs), or postmenopausal estrogen replacement therapy (ERT), all shown to be associated with decreased incidence of colorectal cancer.
- Be aware of colorectal cancer symptoms, and if they develop check with your physician. Symptoms include:

  - A change in bowel habits, such as diarrhea, constipation, or narrowing of the stool (pencil thin) that lasts for more than a few days; the feeling that you need to have a bowel movement that is not relieved by doing so
  - Rectal bleeding or blood in the stool
  - Cramping or steady abdominal pain
  - Decreased appetite
  - Weakness and fatigue
  - Jaundice (American Cancer Society, 2000)

- Limit alcohol consumption.

COLLECTING OBJECTIVE DATA: PHYSICAL EXAMINATION

A physical examination of the anus and rectum should be performed on all adult men and women. It should be performed regardless of whether the client complains of symptoms because some conditions, such as cancerous tumors, may be asymptomatic (Display 25-1). Detecting problems with the anus, rectum, or prostate is the primary objective of this examination. Early detection of a problem is one way to promote early treatment and a more positive outcome. The examiner may also use this time (especially if the examination is a well examination) to integrate teaching about ways to reduce risk factors for diseases and disorders of the anus, rectum, and prostate.

The hands-on physical examination of the anus, rectum, and prostate can cause most clients anxiety and embarrassment. It is important to proceed slowly and to explain all steps of the examination as you proceed. Use gentle movements with your finger and make sure you use adequate lubrication. Listen to and watch the client for signs of discomfort or tensing muscles. Encourage relaxation and explain each step of the examination as you proceed. If the examination is being performed as part of the comprehensive physical examination, it is best to perform the examination of the anus, rectum, and prostate at the end of the genitalia examination.

DISPLAY 25-1	**Screening Guidelines for the Early Detection of Colorectal Cancer**

Beginning at age 50, men and women should follow one of the following examination schedules:

- A fecal occult blood test (FOBT) every year
- A flexible sigmoidoscopy (FSIG) every five years
- Annual fecal occult blood test and flexible sigmoidoscopy every five years*

- A double-contrast barium enema every five years
- A colonoscopy every ten years
- People at moderate or high risk for colorectal cancer should talk with a doctor about a different testing schedule.

*Combined testing is preferred over either annual FOBT, or FSIG every 5 years alone.

American Cancer Society, 2003.

Preparing the Client

Client positioning is important for this examination, and several different positions can be assumed (Fig. 25-3). It is most logical for the female client to stay in the lithotomy position after the vaginal examination for the anus and rectum examination. Some examiners find it easiest to perform the male anus, rectum, and prostate examination while the client stands and bends over the examining table with his hips flexed.

Whichever position the examiner decides would be best for the particular client and examination, it is important to determine if the client is as comfortable as possible in that position.

The most frequently used position is the left lateral position. This position allows adequate inspection and palpation of the anus, rectum, and prostate (in men) and is usually more comfortable for the client. The client's torso and legs can be draped during the examination, which helps to lessen the feeling of vulnerability. To help the client into this position, ask

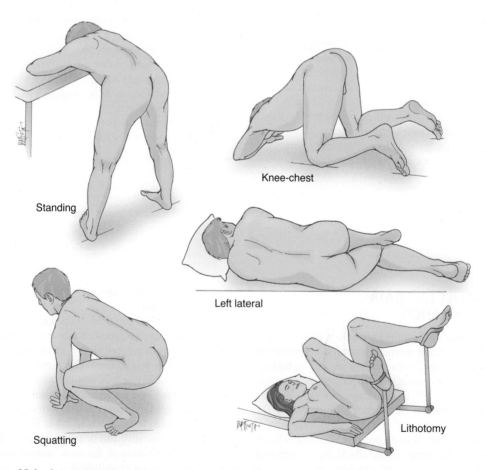

Standing

Knee-chest

Left lateral

Squatting

Lithotomy

Figure 25-3   Selected positions for anorectal examination.

him or her to lie on the left side, with the buttocks as close to the edge of the examining table as possible, and to bend the right knee. No matter which position is chosen, the examiner must realize that he or she will only be able to examine to a certain point up in the rectum using the finger. If an examination of the upper rectum and sigmoid colon is necessary, a proctosigmoidoscopy should be performed.

Equipment

- Gloves
- Water-soluble lubricant

Physical Assessment

During examination of the client, remember these key points:

- Understand the structures and functions of the anorectal region.
- Prepare the client thoroughly for the physical examination to put the client at the greatest ease.
- Perform the examination professionally and preserve the client's modesty.
- Remember to wear gloves.

(text continues on page 520)

PHYSICAL ASSESSMENT

Assessment Procedure	Normal Findings	Abnormal Findings

Anus and Rectum

Inspection

Inspect the perianal area. Spread the client's buttocks and inspect the anal opening and surrounding area (Fig. 25-4) for the following:
- Lumps
- Ulcers
- Lesions
- Rashes
- Redness
- Fissures
- Thickening of the epithelium

The anal opening should appear hairless, moist, and tightly closed. The skin around the anal opening is more coarse and more darkly pigmented. The surrounding perianal area should be free of redness, lumps, ulcers, lesions, and rashes.

Lesions may indicate sexually transmitted diseases, cancer, or hemorrhoids. A thrombosed external hemorrhoid appears swollen. It is itchy, painful, and bleeds when the client passes stool. A previously thrombosed hemorrhoid appears as a skin tag that protrudes from the anus.

A painful mass that is hardened and reddened suggests a perianal abscess. A swollen skin tag on the anal margin may indicate a fissure in the anal canal. Redness and excoriation may be from scratching an area infected by fungi or pinworms. A small opening in the skin that surrounds the anal opening may be an anorectal fistula (Abnormal Findings 25-1).

Thickening of the epithelium suggests repeated trauma from anal intercourse.

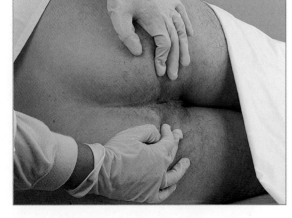

Figure 25-4 Inspecting the perianal area.

PHYSICAL ASSESSMENT *Continued*

Assessment Procedure	Normal Findings	Abnormal Findings
Ask the client to perform Valsalva's maneuver by straining or bearing down. Inspect the anal opening for any bulges or lesions.	No bulging or lesions appear.	Bulges of red mucous membrane may indicate a rectal prolapse. Hemorrhoids or an anal fissure may also be seen (see Abnormal Findings 25-1). ➤ *Clinical Tip • Document any abnormalities by noting position in relation to a face of a clock.*
Inspect the sacrococcygeal area. Inspect this area for any signs of swelling, redness, dimpling, or hair.	Area is normally smooth, and free of redness and hair.	A reddened, swollen, or dimpled area covered by a small tuft of hair located midline on the lower sacrum suggests a pilonidal cyst (see Abnormal Findings 25-1).
Palpation **Palpate the anus.** Inform the client that you are going to perform the internal examination at this point. Explain that it may feel like his or her bowels are going to move but that this will not happen. Lubricate your gloved index finger; ask the client to bear down. As the client bears down, place the pad of your index finger on the anal opening and apply slight pressure; this will cause relaxation of the sphincter. ➤ *Clinical Tip • Never use your fingertip—this causes the sphincter to tighten and, if forced into the rectum, may cause pain.*	Client's sphincter relaxes, permitting entry.	Sphincter tightens, making further examination unrealistic.
When you feel the sphincter relax, insert your finger gently with the pad facing down (Figs. 25-5 and 25-6).	Examination finger enters anus.	Examination finger cannot enter the anus. ➤ *Clinical Tip • If severe pain prevents your entrance to the anus, do not force the examination.*
If the sphincter does not relax and the client reports severe pain, spread the gluteal folds with your hands in close approximation to the anus and attempt to visualize a lesion that may be causing the pain. If tension is maintained on the gluteal folds for 60 seconds, the anus will dilate normally.		
Ask the client to tighten the external sphincter; note the tone.	The client can normally close the sphincter around the gloved finger.	Poor sphincter tone may be the result of a spinal cord injury, previous surgery, trauma, or a prolapsed rectum. Tightened sphincter tone may indicate anxiety, scarring, or inflammation.

continued

Assessment Procedure	Normal Findings	Abnormal Findings
Rotate finger to examine the muscular anal ring. Palpate for tenderness, nodules, and hardness.	The anus is normally smooth, nontender, and free of nodules and hardness.	Tenderness may indicate hemorrhoids, fistula, or fissure. Nodules may indicate polyps or cancer. Hardness may indicate scarring or cancer.
Palpate the rectum. Insert your finger further into the rectum as far as possible (Fig. 25-7). Next, turn your hand clockwise then counterclockwise. This allows palpation of as much rectal surface as possible. Note tenderness, irregularities, nodules, and hardness.	The rectal mucosa is normally soft, smooth, nontender, and free of nodules.	Hardness and irregularities may be from scarring or cancer. Nodules may indicate polyps or cancer (see Abnormal Findings 25-1).
Palpate the peritoneal cavity. This area may be palpated in men above the prostate gland in the area of the seminal vesicles on the anterior surface of the rectum. In women, this area may be palpated on the anterior rectal surface in the area of the rectouterine pouch (behind the cervix and the uterus). Note tenderness or nodules.	This area is normally smooth and nontender.	A peritoneal protrusion into the rectum, called a *rectal shelf,* (See Abnormal Findings 25-1) may indicate a cancerous lesion or peritoneal metastasis. Tenderness may indicate peritoneal inflammation.

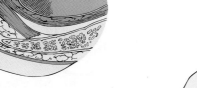

Figure 25-5 Relaxing the anal sphincter.

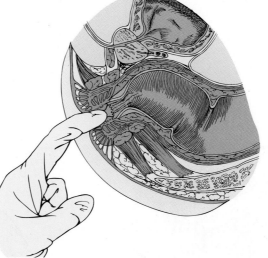

Figure 25-6 Palpating the anus.

continued

PHYSICAL ASSESSMENT *Continued*

Assessment Procedure	Normal Findings	Abnormal Findings

Prostate Gland

Palpation

In male clients, palpate the prostate. The prostate can be palpated on the anterior surface of the rectum by turning the hand fully counterclockwise so that the pad of your index finger faces toward the client's umbilicus (Fig. 25-8). Tell the client that he may feel an urge to urinate but that he will not. Move the pad of your index finger over the prostate gland, trying to feel the sulcus between the lateral lobes. Note the size, shape, and consistency of the prostate, and identify any nodules or tenderness.

> ➤ *Clinical Tip • You may need to move your body away from the client to achieve the proper angle for examination.*

The prostate is normally nontender and rubbery. It has two lateral lobes that are divided by a median sulcus. The lobes are normally smooth, 2.5 cm long, and heart-shaped.

Identify any tenderness with examination or nodules palpable.

A swollen, tender prostate may indicate acute prostatitis. An enlarged smooth, firm, slightly elastic prostate that may not have a median sulcus suggests benign prostatic hypertrophy (BPH). A hard area on the prostate or hard, fixed, irregular nodules on the prostate suggest cancer (Abnormal Findings 25-2).

Note: Palpating prostate prior to drawing a prostate specific antigen (PSA) will raise the PSA level.

Check Stool

Inspect the stool. Withdraw your gloved finger. Inspect any fecal matter on your glove. Assess the color, and test the feces for occult blood. Provide the client with a towel to wipe the anorectal area.

Stool is normally semi-solid, brown, and free of blood.

Black stool may indicate upper gastrointestinal bleeding, gray or tan stool results from the lack of bile pigment, and yellow stool suggests steatorrhea (increased fat content). Blood detected in the stool may indicate cancer of the rectum or colon. An endoscopic examination of the colon should be performed.

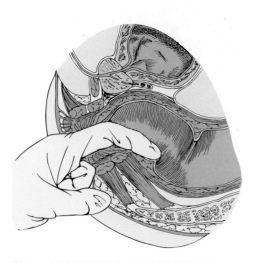

Figure 25-7 Palpating the rectal wall.

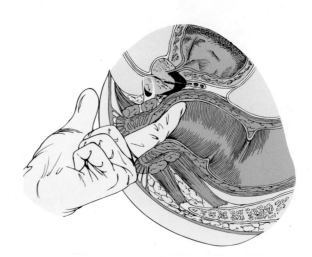

Figure 25-8 Palpating the prostate gland.

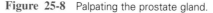

Abnormal Findings 25-1   **Abnormalities of the Anus and Rectum**

External Hemorrhoid

Hemorrhoids are usually painless papules caused by varicose veins. They can be internal or external (above or below the anorectal junction). This external hemorrhoid has become thrombosed—it contains clotted blood, is very painful and swollen, and itches and bleeds with bowel movements.

External hemorrhoid.

Perianal Abscess

Perianal abscess is a cavity of pus, caused by infection in the skin around the anal opening. It causes throbbing pain and is red, swollen, hard, and tender.

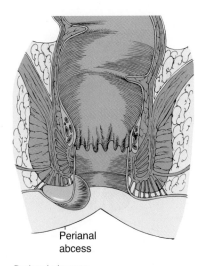

Perianal abcess.

Perianal abscess.

Anal Fissure

These splits in the tissue of the anal canal are caused by trauma. A swollen skin tag ("sentinel tag") is often present below the fissure on the anal margin. They cause intense pain, itching, and bleeding.

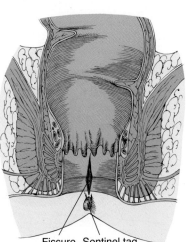

Fissure   Sentinel tag

Anal fissure.

Anorectal Fistula

This is evidenced by a small, round opening in the skin that surrounds the anal opening. It suggests an inflammatory tract from the anus or rectum out to the skin. A previous abscess may have preceded the fistula.

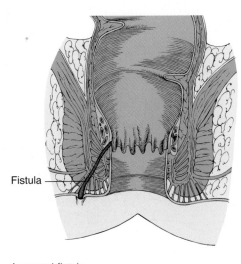

Fistula

Anorectal fistula.

continued on page 518

Rectal Prolapse

This occurs when the mucosa of the rectum protrudes out through the anal opening. It may involve only the mucosa or the mucosa and the rectal wall. It appears as a red, doughnut-like mass with radiating folds.

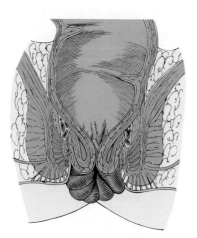

Rectal prolapse.

Pilonidal Cyst

This congenital disorder is characterized by a small dimple or cyst/sinus that contains hair. It is located midline in the sacrococcygeal area and has a palpable sinus tract.

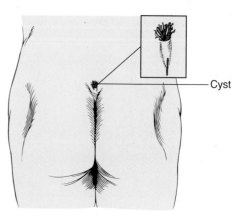

Pilonidal cyst.

Rectal Polyps

These soft structures are rather common and occur in varying size and number. There are two types: Pedunculated (on a stalk) and sessile (on the mucosal surface).

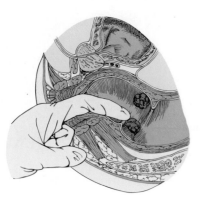

Rectal polyps.

Rectal Cancer

A rectal carcinoma is usually asymptomatic until it is quite advanced. Thus, routine rectal palpation is essential. A cancer of the rectum may feel like a firm nodule, an ulcerated nodule with rolled edges, or, as it grows, a large, irregularly shaped, fixed, hard nodule.

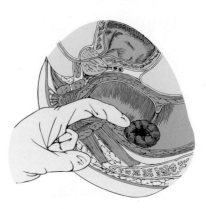

Rectal cancer.

continued

Abnormal Findings 25-1 | **Abnormalities of the Anus and Rectum** *Continued*

Rectal Shelf

If cancer metastasizes to the peritoneal cavity, it may be felt as a nodular, hard, shelflike structure that protrudes onto the anterior surface of the rectum in the area of the seminal vesicles in men and in the area of the rectouterine pouch in women.

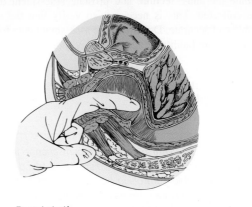

Rectal shelf.

Abnormal Findings 25-2 | **Abnormalities of the Prostate Gland**

Acute Prostatitis

The prostate is swollen, tender, firm, and warm to the touch. Prostatitis is caused by a bacterial infection.

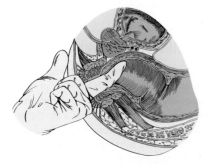

Swelling and inflammation characteristic of acute prostatitis.

Cancer of the Prostate

A hard area on the prostate or hard, fixed, irregular nodules on the prostate suggest cancer. The median sulcus may not be palpable.

Benign Prostatic Hypertrophy

The prostate is enlarged, smooth, firm, and slightly elastic. The median sulcus may not be palpable. It is common in men older than age 50 years.

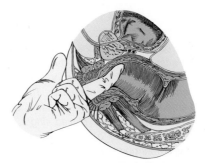

Enlargement characteristic of benign prostatic hypertrophy.

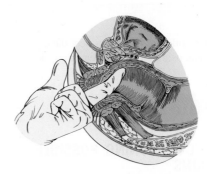

Mass characteristic of prostate cancer.

VALIDATING AND DOCUMENTING FINDINGS

Validate the anus, rectum, and prostate assessment data you have collected. This is necessary to verify that the data are reliable and accurate. Document the assessment data following the health care facility or agency policy.

Sample Documentation of Subjective Data

A 52-year-old client reports no recent change in bowel patterns, no constipation, diarrhea, or blood in stool. He has no trouble controlling his bowels and denies pain and itching in anal area. He has no history of anal or rectal surgery or trauma and no congenital deformities. He states that his last DRE, test for occult blood, and PSA screening were 1 year ago. No significant findings were reported. He says he had a proctosigmoidoscopic examination 2 years ago and the results were normal. He has no knowledge of polyps or cancer (colon, rectal, or prostate) in his family. The client explains that he seldom uses laxatives and has never used an enema. He denies engaging in anal sexual intercourse. He does not know exactly how much water and bulk he consumes but guesses a moderate to high amount.

Sample Documentation of Objective Data

Client's anal opening is hairless, moist, and closed tightly. Perianal area is free of redness, lumps, ulcers, lesions, and rashes. No bulging or lesions appear when client performs Valsalva's maneuver. The sacrococcygeal area is smooth, free of redness and hair. Client can close external sphincter around gloved finger. Anus is smooth, nontender, and free of nodules and hardness. Rectal mucosa is soft, smooth, nontender, and free of nodules. Peritoneal cavity area is smooth and nontender. Prostate gland palpated as two smooth, nontender, rubbery lobes approximately 2.5 cm long. The median sulcus is palpated between the two lobes.

After you have collected the assessment data, you will need to analyze the data, using diagnostic reasoning skills.

Analysis of Data

DIAGNOSTIC REASONING: POSSIBLE CONCLUSIONS

After collecting subjective and objective information pertaining to the anus, rectum, and prostate, identify abnormal findings and client strengths. Then cluster the data to reveal significant patterns or abnormalities; these data may be used to make clinical judgments about the status of the client's anal, rectal, and prostatic health.

Selected Nursing Diagnoses

Following is a listing of selected nursing diagnoses (wellness, risk, or actual) that you may identify when analyzing the cue clusters.

Wellness Diagnoses

- Readiness for enhanced bowel elimination pattern
- Health-Seeking Behaviors: Requests information on purpose and need for colorectal examination

Risk Diagnoses

- Risk for Ineffective Health Maintenance related to lack of knowledge of need for recommended colorectal and prostate examinations
- Risk for Impaired Skin Integrity in rectal area related to chronic irritation secondary to diarrhea

Actual Diagnoses

- Acute Pain: Rectal
- Diarrhea related to chronic inflammatory bowel disease
- Ineffective Sexuality Patterns related to feelings of loss of femininity/masculinity and sexual attractiveness secondary to chronic diarrhea or pain
- Situational Low Self-Esteem related to loss of control over bowel elimination

Selected Collaborative Problems

After grouping the data, certain collaborative problems may become apparent. Remember collaborative problems differ from nursing diagnoses in that they cannot be prevented by nursing interventions. However, the nurse can detect and monitor these physiologic complications of medical conditions. In addition, physician- and nurse-prescribed interventions can be implemented to minimize these complications. The nurse may also have to refer the client in such situations for further treatment of the problem. Following is a list of collaborative problems that may be identified when assessing the anus, rectum, and prostate. These problems are worded as Risk for Complications (or RC), followed by the problem.

- RC: Prostatic hypertrophy
- RC: Fistula
- RC: Fissure
- RC: Hemorrhoids
- RC: Rectal bleeding
- RC: Rectal abscess

Medical Problems

After grouping the data, the client's signs and symptoms, e.g., rectal prolapse and benign prostatic hypertrophy, may clearly require medical diagnosis and treatment. Referral to a primary care provider is necessary.

CASE STUDY

The case study demonstrates how to analyze anus, rectum, and prostate assessment data for a specific client. The critical thinking exercises included in the study guide/lab manual and interactive product that complement this text also offer opportunities to analyze assessment data.

George Kowalsky, 42 years old, seeks advice from the company nurse because he has been "bleeding from his rectum" and has pain and pressure in the rectal area. Mr. Kowalsky is the head accountant and tax consultant for the company. He is currently preparing for the annual audit and reports to the nurse that he is "very uptight." When questioned, he reports that he has observed small amounts of bright red blood on his stool for the last 2 days and his bowel movements have been quite painful—"like passing ground glass"—for about the last week.

He states he has had hard bowel movements for many years. He reports drinking mostly coffee—10 to 12 cups a day.

He says his meals are traditional eggs and bacon for breakfast and meat and potatoes for dinner. He doesn't much like vegetables and fruit. He doesn't eat excessively and has maintained his weight "within the chart norms" for over 20 years. He states he has used Preparation H for his "piles" for years with relief—until lately. When the anorectal area is inspected, several bluish, rounded swellings are present external to the anal sphincter and a small fissure is noted in the lining of the anus. A small amount of light red blood is visible near the anal fissure.

The following concept map illustrates the diagnostic reasoning process.

Applying COLDSPA

Applying **COLDSPA** for client symptoms: "Rectal bleeding."

Mnemonic	Question	Data Provided	Missing Data
Character	Describe the sign or symptom (feeling, appearance, sound, smell, or taste if applicable).	Client reports bleeding from rectum; has seen small amounts of bright red blood with bowel movements.	
Onset	When did it begin?	Two days ago	
Location	Where is it? Does it radiate? Does it occur anywhere else?	Client reports painful bowel movements.	
Duration	How long does it last? Does it recur?	Has occurred for the last two days.	
Severity	How bad is it? or How much does it bother you?	Bowel movements have been painful, "like passing ground glass," for the last week.	
Pattern	What makes it better or worse?	Client has used Preparation H in the past, but has not tried it recently.	
Associated factors/How it **A**ffects the client	What other symptoms occur with it? How does it affect you?	Client reports "pain and pressure in the rectal area" and states "I am very uptight." Eats a high fat meat and potato diet; does not like fruits and vegetables.	

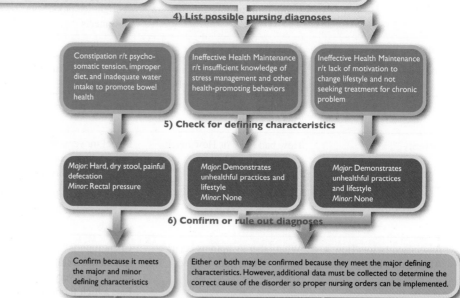

1) Identify abnormal findings and client strengths

Subjective Data

- "Bleeding from his rectum"
- Pain and pressure in the rectal area
- Observed small amounts of bright red blood on his stool for the last 2 days
- Bowel movements have been quite painful, "like passing ground glass," for about the last week
- Hard bowel movements for many years
- "Very uptight"—preparing for annual audit
- Drinks 10 to 12 cups of coffee daily
- Traditional eggs and bacon for breakfast and meat and potatoes for dinner
- Has maintained his weight "within the chart norms" for over 20 years
- Used Preparation H for relief for many years until recently

Objective Data

- Bluish, rounded swellings noted external to the anal sphincter
- Small fissure in the anal lining
- Small amount of light red blood visible near the anal fissure

2) Identify cue clusters

- Pain and pressure in the rectal area
- Observed small amounts of bright red blood on his stool for the last 2 days
- Bowel movements have been quite painful, "like passing ground glass," for about the last week
- Hard bowel movements for many years

- "Very uptight"—preparing for annual audit
- Used Preparation H for many years with relief, until lately
- Bluish, rounded swellings noted external to the anal sphincter
- Small fissure in the lining of the anus
- Small amount of light red blood visible near the anal fissure

---

- Hard bowel movements for many years
- "Very uptight"—preparing for annual audit
- Drinks 10 to 12 cups of coffee daily
- Traditional eggs and bacon for breakfast and meat and potatoes for dinner

3) Draw inferences

His history, the type of bleeding (bright, light red and on the stool), and physical findings are suggestive of hemorrhoids, which the client has self-treated with OTC medication for some time. His bleeding and increased pain could be from a recent fissure or his tension, which may cause the sphincter to tighten and possibly cut off circulation to the external varices. **Mr. K. needs to be referred to his own physican for further work-up regarding the bleeding and increased pain.** Collaborative problems should also be identified.

Apparently, Mr. Kowalsky has been living with and self-treating his bowel problem and has only sought assistance when he noted bleeding. His occupational stress and dietary habits tend to promote continuation of this problem. He does not indicate a desire to change his habits at this time.

4) List possible nursing diagnoses

Constipation r/t psycho-somatic tension, improper diet, and inadequate water intake to promote bowel health

---

Ineffective Health Maintenance r/t insufficient knowledge of stress management and other health-promoting behaviors

---

Ineffective Health Maintenance r/t lack of motivation to change lifestyle and not seeking treatment for chronic problem

5) Check for defining characteristics

Major: Hard, dry stool, painful defecation
Minor: Rectal pressure

Major: Demonstrates unhealthful practices and lifestyle
Minor: None

Major: Demonstrates unhealthful practices and lifestyle
Minor: None

6) Confirm or rule out diagnoses

Confirm because it meets the major and minor defining characteristics

---

Either or both may be confirmed because they meet the major defining characteristics. However, additional data must be collected to determine the correct cause of the disorder so proper nursing orders can be implemented.

7) Document conclusions

Nursing diagnoses that are appropriate for this client include:

- Constipation r/t psychosomatic tension, and improper diet and inadequate water intake to promote bowel health
- Ineffective Health Maintenance r/t insufficient knowledge of stress management and other health-promoting behaviors
- Ineffective Health Maintenance r/t lack of motivation to change lifestyle and not seeking treatment for chronic problem

Potential collaborative problems include:

- RC: Hemorrhage
- RC: Variceal thrombosis
- RC: Variceal strangulation

Mr. Kowalsky should be referred to a physician for evaluation and treatment of rectal bleeding and pain.

References and Selected Readings

American Cancer Society. (2008–2010). *Cancer facts & fisgures, 2008–2010.* Atlanta: American Cancer Society. Available at http://www.cancer.org

Behm, A. M., Aria, N., & Kauffman, C. L. (2004). What's your assessment? Metastatic prostate cancer. *Dermatology Nursing, 16*(1), 68–70.

Bensalah, K., Lotan, Y., Karam, J., & Shariate, S. (2007). New circulating biomarkers for prostate cancer. *Prostate Cancer and Prostatic Disease.* Retrieved November 18, 2007. Available at http://www.nature.com/pcan/journal/vaop/ncurrent/full/4501026a.html

Bharucha. A., & Fletcher, J. (2007). Recent advances in assessing anorectal structure and functions. *Gastroenterology, 133*(4), 1069–1074.

Canby-Hagino, E., Hernandez, J., Brand, T. C., Troyer, D., Higgins, B., et al. (2007). Prostate cancer risk with positive family history, normal prostate examination findings and PSA less than 4.0 ng/mL. *Urology, 70*(4), 748–752.

Carlson, S. L. (2004). Prostate disease. *RN, 67*(9), 54–59.

Corbet, M., Chambers, S. L., Shadbolt, B., Hillman, L. C., & Taupin, D. (2004). Colonoscopy screening for colorectal cancer: The outcome of two recruitment methods. *Medical Journal of Australia, 181*(8), 423–427. Available at http://www.mja.com.au/public/issues/181_08_181004/cor10265_fm.html

Engin, K., Cetin, B., Erdinc, S., Atilla, S., & Ahment, M. (2007). Association of extent and aggressiveness of inflammation with serum PSA levels and PSA density in asymptomatic patients. *Urology, 70*(4), 743–747.

Gilchrist, K. (2004). Benign prostatic hyperplasia: Is it a precursor to prostate cancer? *The Nurse Practitioner, 29*(6), 30–37.

Goldstein, S., Meslin, K., Mazza, T., Isenberg, G., Fitzgerald, J., Richards, A., et al. (2007). Stapled hemorrhoidopexy: Outcome assessment. *American Surgeon, 73*(7), 733–736.

Heo, M., Allison, D. B., & Fontaine, K. R. (2004). Overweight, obesity, and colorectal cancer screening: Disparity between men and women. *BMC Public Health, 4*(53). Available at http://www.biomedcentral.com/1471-2458/4/53

Kabat, G., Miller, A., & Rohan, T. (2007). Oral contraceptive use, hormone replacement therapy, reproductive history and risk of colorectal cancer in women. *International Journal of Cancer.* Retrieved September 10, 2007. Available at http://www3.intersciece.wiley.com

Mahon, S. M. (2004). Colorectal cancer screening: A review of the evidence. *Clinical Journal of Oncology Nursing, 8*(5), 536–540.

Naslund, M., Gilsenan, A., Midkiff, K., Brown, A., Wolford, E., & Wang, J. (2007). Prevalence of lower urinary tract symptoms and prostate enlargement in the primary care setting. *International Journal of Clinical Practice, 61*(9), 1437–1445.

Pickle, L., Yongping, H., Jemal, A., Zou, Z., Tiwari, R., Ward, E., et al. (2007). A new method of estimating United States and state-level cancer incidence counts for the current calendar year. *CA: A Cancer Journal for Clinicians, 57*(1), 30–42.

Riechers, E. A. (2004). Including partners into the diagnosis of prostate cancer: A review of the literature to provide a model of care. *Urologic Nursing, 24*(1), 22–29, 38.

Roobol, J., Grenabo, A., Schroder, F., & Hugosson, J. (2007). Interval cancers in prostate cancer screening: Comparing 2- and 4-year screening intervals in European randomized study of screening for prostate cancer. *Journal of the National Cancer Institute, 99*(17), 1296–1303.

Satish, R. (2007). Constipation: Evaluation and treatment of colonic and anorectal motility disorders. *Gastroenterology Clinics of North America, 36*, 687–711.

Schroder, F., Carter, H., Wolters, T., van den Bergh, C., Gosselaar, C., Bngma, Ch., & Roobol, M. (2007). Early detection of prostate cancer in 2007: Part 1: PSA and PSA kinetics. *European Urology.* Retrieved November 18, 2007. Available at http://www.eropeanurology.com

Sweed, M., & Vig, H. (2007). Hereditary colorectal cancer syndromes. *Advance for Nurse Practitioners, 15*(7), 49–52.

Templeton, H., & Coates, V. (2004). Evaluation of an evidence-based education package for men with prostate cancer on hormonal manipulation therapy. *Patient Education and Counseling, 55*(1), 55–61.

Wallace, M. (2003). Uncertainty and quality of life of older men who undergo watchful waiting for prostate cancer. *Oncology Nursing Forum, 30*(2), 303–309.

Wallace, M., Bailey, D., O'Rourke, M., & Galbraith, M. (2004). The watchful waiting management option for older men with prostate cancer: State of the science. *Oncology Nursing Forum, 31*(6), 1057–1066.

Weizberg, M., Gillett, B., & Sinert, R. (2007). Penile discharge as a presentation of perirectal abscess. *Journal of Emergency Medicine, 34*(1), 45–47.

Weyandt, G., & Becker, J. (2007). Initial treatment of anorectal melanoma. *American Journal of Surgery, 194*(3), 420–421.

Promote Health—Colorectal Cancer

American Cancer Society (ACS). (2007). Colon and rectum cancer. Available at http://www.cancer.org

Overfield, T. (1995). *Biologic variation in health and illness: Race, age, and sex differences* (2nd ed.). Boca Raton, FL: CRC Press.

Spiller, G., Story, J., Lodics, T., Pollack, M., Monyan, S., Butterfield, G., & Spiller M. (2003). Effects of sun-dried raisins on bile acid excretion, intestinal transit time, and fecal weight: A dose-response study. *Journal of Medicinal Food.* Available at http://www.lilbertonline.com

Promote Health—Prostate Cancer

American Cancer Society (ACS). (2008–2010). Detailed guide: Prostate cancer. Available at http://www.cancer.org/docroot/CRI/CRI_2_3x.asp?dt=36

Bright lights, big cancer. (2006). *Science News, 169*(1), 8. Available at http://www.sciencenews.org

Mayo Clinic. (2007). Prostate cancer prevention: What can you do. Available at http://www.mayoclinic.com/health/prostate-cancer-prevention/MC00027

National Cancer Institute (NCI). (2007). Risk factors for prostate cancer development. Available at http://www.cancer.gov/cancertopics/pdq/prevention/prostate/HealthProfessional/page4

National Cancer Institute (NCI). (2007). Prostate cancer: Significance. Available: http://www.cancer.gov/cancertopics/pdq/prevention/prostate/HealthProfessional/page3

National Cancer Institute (NCI). (2007). Selenium and vitamin E cancer prevention trial (SELECT). Available at http://www.cancer.gov/cancertopics/factsheet/Prevention/SELECT

Ross, R. (1995; online version 2006). Does the racial-ethnic variation in prostate cancer have a hormonal basis? *Cancer, 75*(S7), 1778–1782. Available at http://www3.interscience.wiley.com/cgi-bin/abstract/112689194/ABSTRACT/CRETRY=1&SRETRY=0

Van Howe, R. (2007). Case number and the financial impact of circumcision in reducing prostate cancer. *British Journal of Urology International, 100*(5), 1193–1194.

WebMD. (2007). More sex tied to higher prostate cancer risk. Available at http://www.webmd.com

Promote Health—Hemorrhoids

WebMD. (2007). Hemorrhoids. Available at http://www.webmd.com/a-to-z-guides/hemorrhoids

26

Musculoskeletal System

Structure and Function

The body's bones, muscles, and joints compose the musculoskeletal system. Controlled and innervated by the nervous system, the musculoskeletal system's overall purpose is to provide structure and movement for body parts.

BONES

Bones provide structure, give protection, serve as levers, store calcium, and produce blood cells. Two hundred and six (206) bones make up the **axial skeleton** (head and trunk) and the **appendicular skeleton** (extremities, shoulders, and hips; Fig. 26-1).

Composed of osseous tissue, bones can be divided into two types: **compact bone,** which is hard and dense and makes up the shaft and outer layers; and **spongy bone,** which contains numerous spaces and makes up the ends and centers of the bones. Bone tissue is formed by active cells called **osteoblasts** and broken down by cells referred to as **osteoclasts.** Bones contain red marrow that produces blood cells and yellow marrow composed mostly of fat.

The **periosteum** covers the bones and contains osteoblasts and blood vessels that promote nourishment and formation of new bone tissues. Bone shapes vary and include short bones (e.g., carpals), long bones (e.g., humerus, femur), flat bones (e.g., sternum, ribs), and bones with an irregular shape (e.g., hips, vertebrae).

SKELETAL MUSCLES

The body consists of three types of **muscles:** skeletal, smooth, and cardiac. The musculoskeletal system is made up of 650 **skeletal (voluntary) muscles,** which are under conscious control (Fig. 26-2). Made up of long muscle fibers (fasciculi) that are arranged together in bundles and joined by connective tissue, skeletal muscles attach to bones by way of strong, fibrous cords called **tendons.** Skeletal muscles assist with posture, produce body heat, and allow the body to move. Skeletal muscle movements (illustrated in Display 26-1) include

Abduction: Moving away from midline of the body

Adduction: Moving toward midline of the body

Circumduction: Circular motion

Inversion: Moving inward

Eversion: Moving outward

Extension: Straightening the extremity at the joint and increasing the angle of the joint

Hyperextension: Joint bends greater than 180 degrees

Flexion: Bending the extremity at the joint and decreasing the angle of the joint

Dorsiflexion: Toes draw upward to ankle

Plantar flexion: Toes point away from ankle

Pronation: Turning or facing downward

Supination: Turning or facing upward

Protraction: Moving forward

Retraction: Moving backward

Rotation: Turning of a bone on its own long axis

Internal Rotation: Turning of a bone toward the center of the body

External Rotation: Turning of a bone away from the center of the body

JOINTS

The **joint** (or articulation) is the place where two or more bones meet. Joints provide a variety of ranges of motion (ROM) for the body parts and may be classified as fibrous, cartilaginous, or synovial.

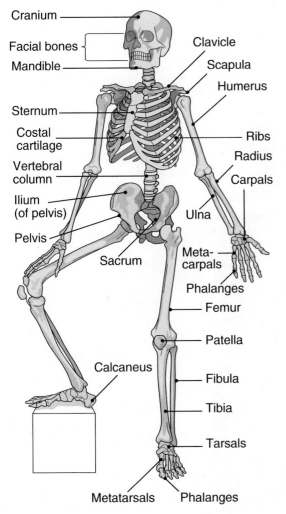

Figure 26-1   Major bones of the skeleton. The axial skeleton is shown in yellow; the appendicular, in blue.

Labels on figure:
Cranium
Facial bones
Mandible
Clavicle
Scapula
Humerus
Sternum
Costal cartilage
Ribs
Radius
Vertebral column
Carpals
Ilium (of pelvis)
Ulna
Pelvis
Sacrum
Meta-carpals
Phalanges
Femur
Patella
Calcaneus
Fibula
Tibia
Tarsals
Metatarsals
Phalanges

Fibrous joints (e.g., sutures between skull bones) are joined by fibrous connective tissue and are immovable. **Cartilaginous joints** (e.g., joints between vertebrae) are joined by cartilage. **Synovial joints** (e.g., shoulders, wrists, hips, knees, ankles; Fig. 26-3) contain a space between the bones that is filled with synovial fluid, a lubricant that promotes a sliding movement of the ends of the bones. Bones in synovial joints are joined by **ligaments,** which are strong, dense bands of fibrous connective tissue. Synovial joints are enclosed by a fibrous capsule made of connective tissue and connected to the periosteum of the bone. Articular cartilage smooths and protects the bones that articulate with each other.

Some synovial joints contain **bursae,** which are small sacs filled with synovial fluid that serve to cushion the joint. Display 26-2 reviews the appearance, characteristics, and motion of major joints.

Nursing Assessment

COLLECTING SUBJECTIVE DATA: THE NURSING HEALTH HISTORY

Assessment of the musculoskeletal system helps to evaluate the client's level of functioning with activities of daily living. This system affects the entire body, from head to toe, and greatly influences what physical activities a client can and cannot do. Only the client can give you data regarding pain, stiffness, and levels of movement and how activities of daily living are affected. In addition, information regarding the client's nutrition, activities, and exercise is a significant part of the musculoskeletal assessment. Pain or stiffness is often a chief concern with musculoskeletal problems; therefore, a pain assessment may also be needed. Always the nurse needs to remember to investigate signs and symptoms reported by the client.

Remember, too, that the neurologic system is responsible for coordinating the functions of the skeleton and muscles. Therefore, it is important to understand how these systems relate to each other and to ask questions accordingly. From this assessment, the nurse can learn the client's daily activity and exercise patterns that promote either healthy or unhealthy functioning of the musculoskeletal system. Hence, client teaching regarding exercise, diet, positioning, posture, and safety habits to promote health also becomes an essential part of this examination.

(text continues on page 535)

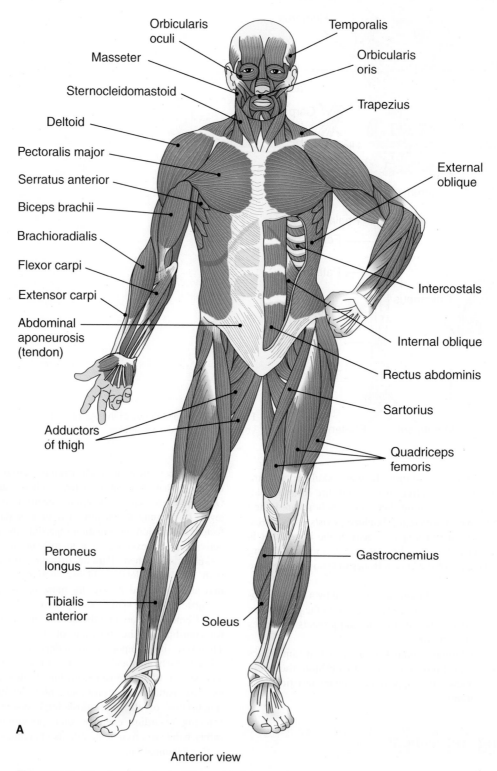

Orbicularis oculi
Temporalis
Masseter
Orbicularis oris
Sternocleidomastoid
Trapezius
Deltoid
Pectoralis major
External oblique
Serratus anterior
Biceps brachii
Brachioradialis
Flexor carpi
Intercostals
Extensor carpi
Abdominal aponeurosis (tendon)
Internal oblique
Rectus abdominis
Sartorius
Adductors of thigh
Quadriceps femoris
Peroneus longus
Gastrocnemius
Tibialis anterior
Soleus

A

Anterior view

Figure 26-2   Muscles of the body: **(A)** anterior; **(B)** posterior.

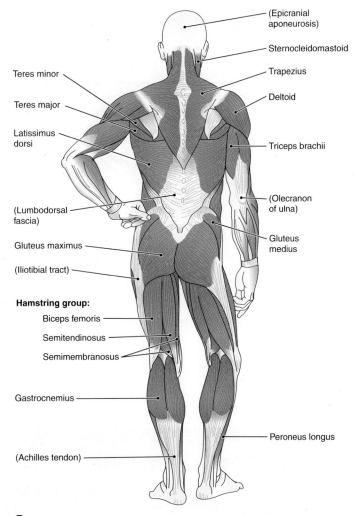

(Epicranial aponeurosis)

Sternocleidomastoid

Trapezius

Deltoid

Triceps brachii

Teres minor

Teres major

Latissimus dorsi

(Olecranon of ulna)

(Lumbodorsal fascia)

Gluteus medius

Gluteus maximus

(Iliotibial tract)

Hamstring group:

Biceps femoris

Semitendinosus

Semimembranosus

Gastrocnemius

Peroneus longus

(Achilles tendon)

Figure 26-2 *Continued* **B**

Posterior view

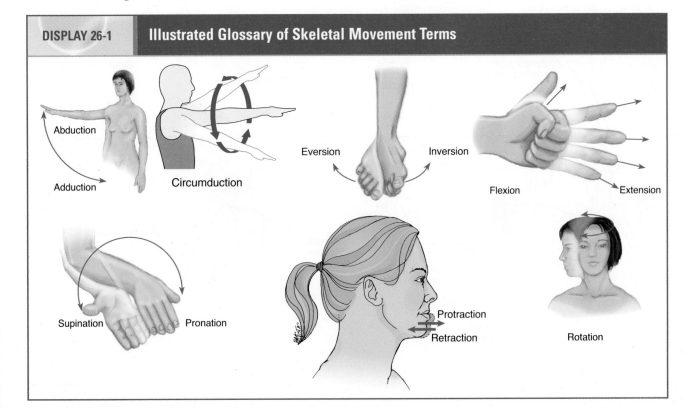

DISPLAY 26-1 **Illustrated Glossary of Skeletal Movement Terms**

Abduction

Adduction

Circumduction

Eversion

Inversion

Flexion

Extension

Supination

Pronation

Protraction

Retraction

Rotation

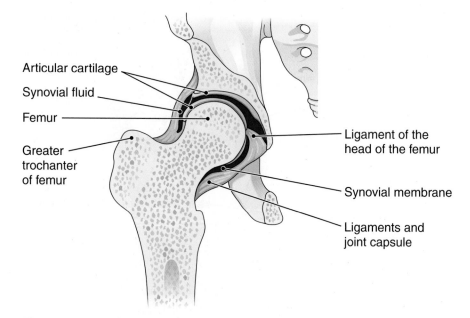

Figure 26-3   Components of synovial joints (right hip joint).

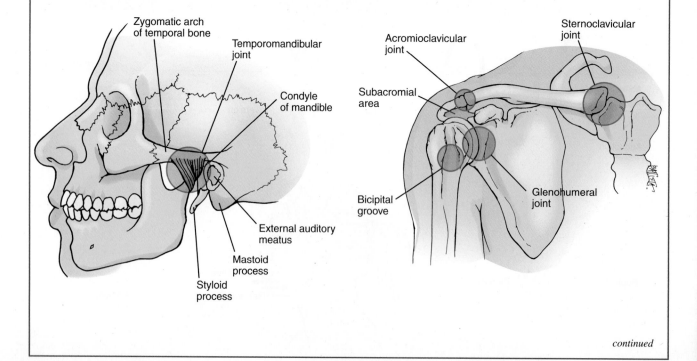

| DISPLAY 26-2 | **Understanding Major Joints** |

Temporomandibular

Articulation between the temporal bone and mandible. Motion:
- Opens and closes mouth
- Projects and retracts jaw
- Moves jaw from side to side

Sternoclavicular

Junction between the manubrium of the sternum and the clavicle; has no obvious movements.

continued

DISPLAY 26-2 | **Understanding Major Joints** *Continued*

Shoulder

Articulation of the head of the humerus in the glenoid cavity of the scapula. The acromioclavicular joint includes the clavicle and acromion process of the scapula. It contains the subacromial and subscapular bursae. Motion:

- Flexion and extension
- Abduction and adduction
- Circumduction
- Rotation (internal and external)

Elbow

Articulation between the ulna and radius of the lower arm and the humerus of the upper arm; contains a synovial membrane and several bursae. Motion:

- Flexion and extension of the forearm
- Supination and pronation of the forearm

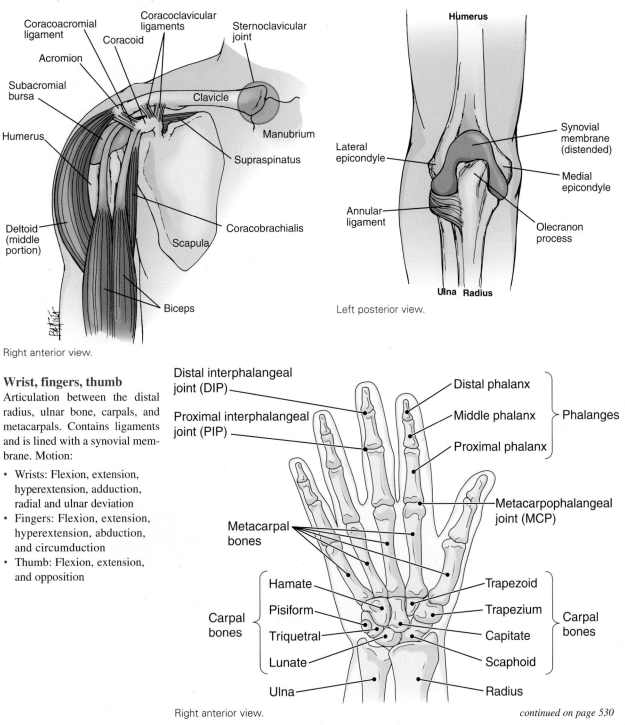

Right anterior view.

Left posterior view.

Wrist, fingers, thumb

Articulation between the distal radius, ulnar bone, carpals, and metacarpals. Contains ligaments and is lined with a synovial membrane. Motion:

- Wrists: Flexion, extension, hyperextension, adduction, radial and ulnar deviation
- Fingers: Flexion, extension, hyperextension, abduction, and circumduction
- Thumb: Flexion, extension, and opposition

Right anterior view.

continued on page 530

DISPLAY 26-2 | **Understanding Major Joints** *Continued*

Vertebrae (lateral view)

Thirty-three bones: 7 concave-shaped cervical (C), 12 convex-shaped thoracic (T), 5 concave-shaped lumbar (L), 5 sacral (S), and 3 to 4 coccygeal, connected in a vertical column. Bones are cushioned by elastic fibro-cartilaginous plates (intervertebral discs) that provide flexibility and posture to the spine. Paravertebral muscles are positioned on both sides of vertebrae. Motion:

• Flexion
• Hyperextension
• Lateral bending
• Rotation

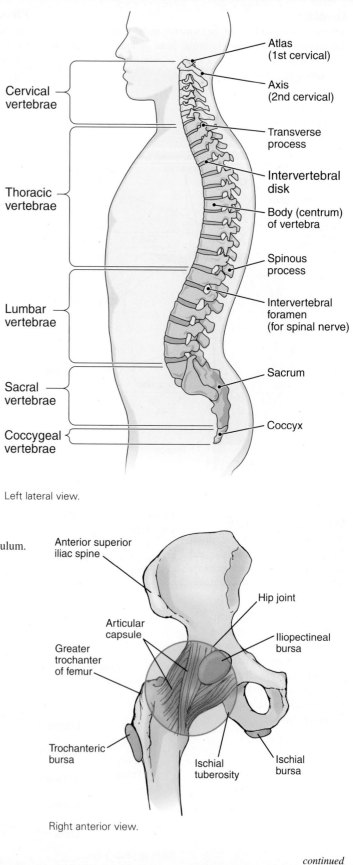

Left lateral view.

Hip

Articulation between the head of the femur and the acetabulum. Contains a fibrous capsule. Motion:

• Flexion with knee flexed and with knee extended
• Extension and hyperextension
• Circumduction
• Rotation (internal and external)
• Abduction
• Adduction

Right anterior view.

continued

Knee

Articulation of the femur, tibia, and patella; contains fibrocartilaginous discs (medial and lateral menisci) and many bursae. Motion:

- Flexion
- Extension

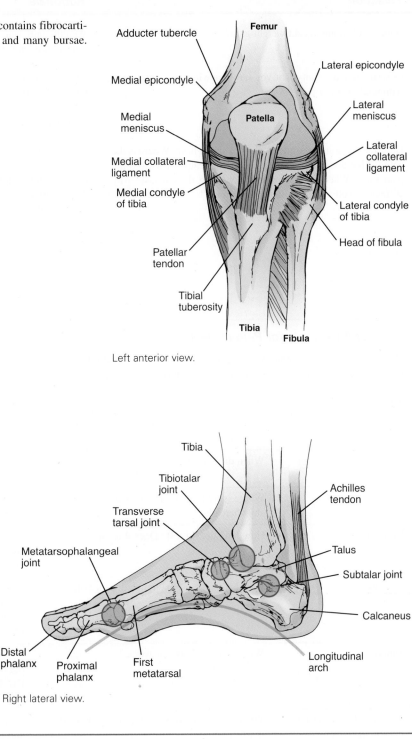

Left anterior view.

Ankle and foot

Articulation between the talus (large posterior foot tarsal), tibia, and fibula. The talus also articulates with the navicular bones. The heel (calcaneus bone) is connected to the tibia and fibula by ligaments.

- Ankle: Plantar flexion and dorsiflexion
- Foot: Inversion and eversion
- Toes: Flexion, extension, abduction, adduction

Right lateral view.

HISTORY OF PRESENT HEALTH CONCERN

Question	Rationale
Have you had any recent weight gain?	Weight gain can increase physical stress and strain on the musculoskeletal system.
Describe any difficulty that you have chewing. Is it associated with tenderness or pain?	Clients with temporomandibular joint (TMJ) dysfunction may have difficulty chewing and may describe their jaws as "getting locked or stuck." Jaw tenderness, pain, or a clicking sound may also be present with ROM.
Describe any joint, muscle, or bone pain you have. Where is the pain? What does the pain feel like (stab, ache)? When did the pain start? When does it occur? How long does it last? Any stiffness, swelling, limitation of movement?	Bone pain is often dull, deep, and throbbing. Joint or muscle pain is described as aching. Sharp, knifelike pain occurs with most fractures and increases with motion of the affected body part. Motion increases pain associated with many joint problems but decreases pain associated with rheumatoid arthritis.

continued

COLDSPA Example for Pain in Heels

Use the **COLDSPA** mnemonic as a guideline to collect needed information for each symptom the client shares. In addition, the following questions help elicit important information.

Mnemonic	Question	Client Response Example
Character	Describe the sign or symptom (feeling, appearance, sound, smell, or taste if applicable).	"I have sharp pains in my right foot, especially on the side and bottom of my heel."
Onset	When did it begin?	"I first noticed the pain about 3 months ago. It has gotten worse over the past 2 weeks."
Location	Where is it? Does it radiate? Does it occur anywhere else?	"The pain is mostly in my right heel and sometimes goes into the arch of my foot."
Duration	How long does it last? Does it recur?	"I usually notice it in the morning when I first get up. It gets a little better during the day and then I notice it in the evening again."
Severity	How bad is it? or How much does it bother you?	"It's bad enough that I can't take my daily walks. It's okay when I'm sitting but makes me hobble to the bathroom in the morning and hurts when I try to walk long distances."
Pattern	What makes it better or worse?	"Naproxen had helped some. I've tried taping the bottom of my foot, and that helps a little. I've bought shoe inserts but can't tell that they help."
Associated factors/How it **A**ffects the client	What other symptoms occur with it? How does it affect you?	"I went through menopause about a year ago and gained some weight. I think those extra 15 pounds have affected my foot. I'm discouraged because I can't walk. When I can't walk, I gain weight, and then I think my foot gets worse."

PAST HEALTH HISTORY

Question	Rationale
Describe any past problems or injuries you have had to your joints, muscles, or bones. What treatment was given? Do you have any after-effects from the injury or problem?	This information provides baseline data for the physical examination. Past injuries may affect the client's current range of motion (ROM) and level of function in affected joints and extremities. A history of recurrent fractures should raise the question of possible physical abuse. Bones lose their density with age, putting the older client at risk for bone fractures, especially of the wrists, hips, and vertebrae. Older clients who have osteomalacia or osteoporosis are at an even greater risk for fractures.
When were your last tetanus and polio immunizations?	Joint stiffening and other musculoskeletal symptoms may be a transient effect of the tetanus or polio vaccines. Joint-stiffening conditions may be misdiag nosed as arthritis, especially in the older adult.
Have you ever been diagnosed with diabetes mellitus, sickle cell anemia, systemic lupus erythematosus (SLE), or osteoporosis?	Having diabetes mellitus, sickle cell anemia, or SLE places the client at risk for development of musculoskeletal problems such as osteoporosis and osteomyelitis. Clients who are immobile or have a reduced intake of calcium and vitamin D are especially prone to development of osteoporosis. Osteoporosis is more common as a person ages because that is a time when bone resorption increases, calcium absorption decreases, and production of osteoblasts decreases as well.
For middle-aged women: Have you started menopause? Are you receiving estrogen replacement therapy?	Women who begin menarche late or begin menopause early are at greater risk for development of osteoporosis because of decreased estrogen levels, which tend to decrease the density of bone mass.

FAMILY HISTORY

Question	Rationale
Do you have a family history of rheumatoid arthritis, gout, or osteoporosis?	These conditions tend to be familial and can increase the client's risk for development of these diseases.

LIFESTYLE AND HEALTH PRACTICES

Question	Rationale
What activities do you engage in to promote the health of your muscles and bones (e.g., exercise, diet, weight reduction)?	This question provides the examiner with knowledge of how much the client understands and actively participates in trying to promote the health of the musculoskeletal system.

continued on page 534

LIFESTYLE AND HEALTH PRACTICES *Continued*

Question	*Rationale*
What medications are you taking?	Some medications can affect musculoskeletal function. Diuretics, for example, can alter electrolyte levels leading to muscle weakness. Steroids can deplete bone mass, thereby contributing to osteoporosis. Adverse reactions to HMG-CoA reductase inhibitors (statins) can include myopathy, which can cause muscle aches or weakness
Do you smoke tobacco? How much and how often?	Smoking increases the risk of osteoporosis (see Promote Health—Osteoporosis).
Do you drink alcohol or caffeinated beverages? How much and how often?	Excessive consumption of alcohol or caffeine can increase the risk of osteoporosis.
Describe your typical 24-hour diet. Are you able to consume milk or milk-containing products? Do you take any calcium supplements?	Adequate protein in the diet promotes muscle tone and bone growth; vitamin C promotes healing of tissues and bones. A calcium deficiency increases the risk of osteoporosis. A diet high in purine (e.g., liver, sardines) can trigger gouty arthritis. Between 75% and 95% of all non-Caucasian people, 60% of Mediterraneans, and 10% to 15% of Caucasians are lactose intolerant as adults (Understanding lactose intolerance, no date).
Describe your activities during a typical day. How much time do you spend in the sunlight?	A sedentary lifestyle increases the risk of osteoporosis. Prolonged immobility leads to muscle atrophy. Exposure to 20 minutes of sunlight per day promotes the production of vitamin D in the body. Vitamin D deficiency can cause osteomalacia.
Describe any routine exercise that you do.	Regular exercise promotes flexibility, bone density, and muscle tone and strength, and can help to slow the usual musculoskeletal changes (progressive loss of total bone mass and degeneration of skeletal muscle fibers) that occur with aging. Improper body positioning in contact sports results in injury to the bones, joints, or muscles.
Describe your occupation.	Certain job-related activities increase the risk for development of musculoskeletal problems. For example, incorrect body mechanics, heavy lifting, or poor posture can contribute to back problems; consistent, repetitive wrist and hand movements can lead to the development of carpal tunnel syndrome.
Describe your posture at work and at leisure. What type of shoes do you usually wear? Do you use any special footwear (i.e., orthotics)?	Poor posture, prolonged forward bending (as in sitting) or backward leaning (as in working overhead), or long-term carrying of heavy objects on the shoulders can result in back problems. Contracture of the Achilles tendon can occur with prolonged use of high-heeled shoes.
Do you have difficulty performing normal activities of daily living (bathing, dressing, grooming, eating)? Do you use assistive devices (e.g., walker, cane, braces) to promote your mobility?	Impairment of the musculoskeletal system may impair the client's ability to perform normal activities of daily living. Correct use of assistive devices can promote safety and independence. Some clients may feel embarrassed and not use their prescribed or needed assistive device.
How have your musculoskeletal problems interfered with your ability to interact or socialize with others? Have they interfered with your usual sexual activity?	Musculoskeletal problems, especially chronic ones, can disable and cripple the client, which may impair socialization and prevent the client from performing the same roles as in the past. Back problems, joint pain, or muscle stiffness may interfere with sexual activities.

continued

LIFESTYLE AND HEALTH PRACTICES *Continued*

Question	Rationale
How did you view yourself before you had this musculoskeletal problem, and how do you view yourself now?	Body image disturbances and chronic low self-esteem may occur with a disabling or crippling problem.
Has your musculoskeletal problem added stress to your life? Describe.	Musculoskeletal problems often greatly affect activities of daily living and role performance, resulting in changed relationships and increased stress.

PROMOTE HEALTH
Osteoporosis

Overview
Osteoporosis is a disease causing bones to become fragile from decalcification, producing porous bones with low bone mass. If left untreated, osteoporosis leads to broken bones. All bones can have osteoporosis, but the bones most often affected are the hips, spine, and wrists. Osteoporosis is a silent disease in that there is no pain until a bone fractures. Therefore, knowing risks and taking preventive measures is essential. Women are four times more affected than men. An estimated 44 million Americans (55%) over 50 years of age are at risk; 10 million already have osteoporosis; and 34 million are estimated to have low bone mass. Asians and non-Hispanic whites are at greatest risk, followed by Hispanics and lowest risk in African Americans, but all ethnic groups are at some level of risk.

Uncontrollable Risk Factors
- Gender: 80% women
- Age: 70 years or older (female); 80 years or older (male)
- Body size: Small-boned, thin
- Ethnicity: Caucasian and Asian at highest risk; African American and Latino at lower but significant risk
- Family history or personal history of bone fractures as an adult

Modifiable Risk Factors
- Little or no physical exercise or activity; bed rest
- Low calcium and vitamin D intake
- Anorexia nervosa
- For women: Low estrogen levels; postmenopausal woman not on estrogen replacement therapy; for men, low testosterone levels
- Smoking
- Excessive caffeine or alcohol consumption
- Medication intake (corticosteroids particularly) for chronic disorders such as rheumatoid arthritis, endocrine disorders (e.g., underactive thyroid), seizures, gastrointestinal diseases

Teach Risk Reduction Tips
- Increase physical exercise or activity, especially weight bearing (regular moderate exercise three times a week for 20 to 45 minutes each time).
- Increase calcium intake to recommended daily allowances through diet or supplements (NIH recommends 1,000–1,500 mg/day for adults).
- Get adequate vitamin D to absorb calcium (sun exposure; dietary sources include fortified milk, oily fish, liver, egg yolk).
- Avoid excessive caffeine or alcohol consumption.
- Avoid or stop smoking.
- Avoid use of steroids, glucocorticoids, and seizure medications.
- Consider risks and benefits of estrogen replacement therapy if postmenopausal or approaching menopause.
- Discuss with primary health care provider how steroids or other medications taken for chronic disorders can affect bones.
- Discuss advisability of taking bone protective medications and tests for bone density.
- If diagnosed with osteoporosis, explore ways to prevent falls.

COLLECTING OBJECTIVE DATA: PHYSICAL EXAMINATION

Physical assessment of the musculoskeletal system provides data regarding the client's posture, gait, bone structure, muscle strength, and joint mobility, as well as the client's ability to perform activities of daily living.

The physical assessment includes inspecting and palpating the joints, muscles, and bones, testing ROM, and assessing muscle strength. See Assessment Tool 26-1 for guidelines to use when performing the musculoskeletal assessment.

Preparing the Client

Because this examination is lengthy, be sure the room is at a comfortable temperature and provide rest periods as necessary. Provide adequate draping to avoid unnecessary exposure of the client yet adequate visualization of the part being examined. Explain that you will ask the client frequently to change positions and to move various body parts against resistance and gravity. Clear, simple directions need to be given throughout the examination to help the client understand how to move body parts to allow you to assess the

---

| ASSESSMENT TOOL 26-1 | Guidelines for Assessing Joints and Muscles |

The following are guidelines for assessing joints and muscle strength:

Joints

1. Inspect size, shape, color, and symmetry. Note any masses, deformities, or muscle atrophy. Compare bilateral joint findings.
2. Palpate for edema, heat, tenderness, pain, nodules, or crepitus. Compare bilateral joint findings.
3. Test each joint's range of motion (ROM). Demonstrate how to move each joint through its normal ROM, then ask the client actively to move the joint through the same motions. Compare bilateral joint findings.

 Older clients usually have slower movements, reduced flexibility, and decreased muscle strength because of age-related muscle fiber and joint degeneration, reduced elasticity of the tendons, and joint capsule calcification.

If you identify a limitation in the ROM, measure ROM with a goniometer (a device that measures movement in degrees). To do so, move the arms of the goniometer to match the angle of the joint being assessed. Then describe the limited motion of the joint in degrees: for example, "elbow flexes from 45 degrees to 90 degrees."

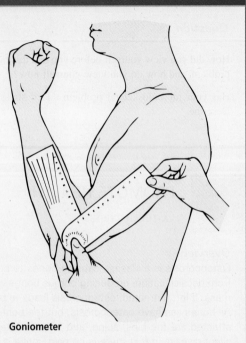

Goniometer

Muscles

1. Test muscle strength by asking the client to move each extremity through its full ROM against resistance. Do this by applying some resistance against the part being moved. Document muscle strength by using a standard scale (see Rating Scale for Muscle Strength, below). If the client cannot move the part against your resistance, ask the client to move the part against gravity. If this is not possible, then attempt passively to move the part through its full ROM. If this is not possible, then inspect and feel for a palpable contraction of the muscle while the client attempts to move it. Compare bilateral joint findings.

➤ **Clinical Tip** • *Do not force the part beyond its normal range. Stop passive motion if the client expresses discomfort or pain. Be especially cautious with the older client when testing ROM. When comparing bilateral strength, keep in mind that the client's dominant side will tend to be the stronger side.*

2. Rate muscle strength in accord with the strength table below.

Rating	Explanation	Strength Classification
5	Active motion against full resistance	Normal
4	Active motion against some resistance	Slight weakness
3	Active motion against gravity	Average weakness
2	Passive ROM (gravity removed and assisted by examiner)	Poor ROM
1	Slight flicker of contraction	Severe weakness
0	No muscular contraction	Paralysis

---

musculoskeletal system. Demonstrating to the client how to move the various body parts and providing verbal directions facilitate examination.

 Some positions required for this examination may be very uncomfortable for the older client, who may have decreased flexibility. Be sensitive to the client's needs and adapt your technique as necessary.

Equipment

- Tape measure
- Goniometer (optional)
- Skin marking pencil (optional)

Physical Assessment

- Observe gait and posture.
- Inspect joints, muscles, and extremities for size, symmetry, and color.
- Palpate joints, muscles, and extremities for tenderness, edema, heat, nodules, or crepitus.
- Test muscle strength and ROM of joints.
- Compare bilateral findings of joints and muscles.
- Perform special tests for carpal tunnel syndrome.
- Perform the "bulge," "ballottement," and McMurray's knee tests.

(text continues on page 560)

PHYSICAL ASSESSMENT

Assessment Procedure	Normal Findings	Abnormal Findings

Gait

Inspection

Observe gait. Observe the client's gait as the client enters and walks around the room. Note

- Base of support
- Weight-bearing stability
- Foot position
- Stride and length and cadence of stride
- Arm swing
- Posture

Evenly distributed weight. Client able to stand on heels and toes. Toes point straight ahead. Equal on both sides. Posture erect, movements coordinated and rhythmic, arms swing in opposition, stride length appropriate.

Uneven weight bearing is evident. Client cannot stand on heels or toes. Toes point in or out. Client limps, shuffles, propels forward, or has wide-based gait. (See Chapter 27, Nervous System, for specific abnormal gait findings.)

Assess for the risk of falling backward in the older or handicapped client by performing the "nudge test." Stand behind the client and put your arms around the client while you gently nudge the sternum.

Client does not fall backward.

Some older clients have an impaired sense of position in space, which may contribute to the risks of falling.

Falling backward easily is seen with cervical spondylosis and Parkinson's disease.

Temporomandibular Joint (TMJ)

Inspection and Palpation

Inspect and palpate the TMJ. Have the client sit; put your index and middle fingers just anterior to the external ear opening (Fig. 26-4). Ask the client to

- Open the mouth as widely as possible. (The tips of your fingers should drop into the joint spaces as the mouth opens.)
- Move the jaw from side to side.
- Protrude (push out) and retract (pull in) jaw.

Jaw moves laterally 1 to 2 cm. Snapping and clicking may be felt and heard in the normal client.

Mouth opens 1 to 2 inches (distance between upper and lower teeth).

Jaw protrudes and retracts easily. The client's mouth opens and closes smoothly.

Decreased ROM, swelling, tenderness, or crepitus may be seen in arthritis.

Decreased muscle strength with muscle and joint disease. ROM, and a clicking, popping, or grating sound may be noted with TMJ dysfunction.

Test range of motion (ROM). Ask the client to open the mouth and move the jaw laterally against resistance. Next as the client clenches the teeth, feel for the contraction of the temporal and masseter muscles to test the integrity of cranial nerve V (trigeminal nerve).

Jaw has full ROM against resistance. Contraction palpated with no pain or spasms.

Lack of full contraction with cranial nerve V lesion. Pain or spasms occur with myofacial pain syndrome.

continued

PHYSICAL ASSESSMENT *Continued*

Assessment Procedure	Normal Findings	Abnormal Findings

Sternoclavicular Joint

Inspection and Palpation

With client sitting, inspect the sternoclavicular joint for location in midline, color, swelling, and masses. Then palpate for tenderness or pain.

There is no visible bony overgrowth, swelling, or redness; joint is nontender.

Swollen, red, or enlarged joint or tender, painful joint is seen with inflammation of the joint.

Cervical, Thoracic, and Lumbar Spine

Inspection and Palpation

Observe the cervical, thoracic, and lumbar curves from the side then from behind. Have the client standing erect with the gown positioned to allow an adequate view of the spine (Fig. 26-5). Observe for symmetry, noting differences in height of the shoulders, the iliac crests and the buttock creases.

Cervical and lumbar spines are concave; thoracic spine is convex. Spine is straight (when observed from behind).

 An exaggerated thoracic curve (kyphosis) is common with aging.

Some findings that appear to be abnormalities are, in fact, variations related to culture or sex. For example, some African Americans have a large gluteal prominence, making

A flattened lumbar curvature may be seen with a herniated lumbar disc or ankylosing spondylitis. Lateral curvature of the thoracic spine with an increase in the convexity on the curved side is seen in scoliosis. An exaggerated lumbar curve (lordosis) is often seen in pregnancy or obesity (Abnormal Findings 26-1). Unequal heights of the hips suggests unequal leg lengths.

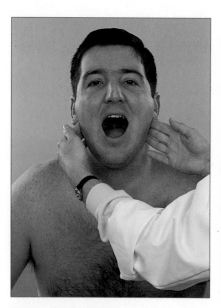

Figure 26-4 Palpating the temporomandibular joint (© B. Proud).

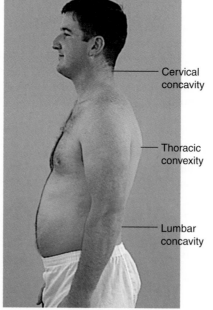

Cervical concavity

Thoracic convexity

Lumbar concavity

Figure 26-5 Normal curve of the spine (© B. Proud).

continued

Assessment Procedure	Normal Findings	Abnormal Findings
	the spine appear to have lumbar lordosis. In addition, the number of vertebrae may differ. Frequent variations from the usual 24 include women, especially African American women, who may have 23 vertebrae; and men, especially Eskimo and Indian men, with 25.	
Palpate the spinous processes and the paravertebral muscles on both sides of the spine for tenderness or pain.	Nontender spinous processes; well-developed, firm and smooth, nontender paravertebral muscles. No muscle spasm.	Compression fractures and lumbosacral muscle strain can cause pain and tenderness of the spinal processes and the paravertebral muscles.
Test ROM of the cervical spine. Test ROM of the cervical spine by asking the client to touch the chin to the chest (flexion) and to look up at the ceiling (hyperextension) (Fig. 26-6).	Flexion of the cervical spine is 45 degrees. Extension of the cervical spine is 45 degrees.	Cervical strain is the most common cause of neck pain. It is characterized by impaired ROM and neck pain from abnormalities of the soft tissue (muscles, ligaments, and nerves) due to straining or injuring the neck. Causes of strains can include sleeping in the wrong position, carrying a heavy suitcase, or being in an automobile crash.

Cervical disc degenerative disease and spinal cord tumors are associated with impaired ROM and pain that radiates to the back, shoulder, or arms. Neck pain with a loss of sensation in the legs may occur with cervical spinal cord compression.

Impaired ROM and neck pain associated with fever, chills, and headache could be indicative of a serious infection such as meningitis. |

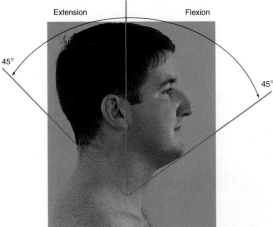

Figure 26-6 Normal range of motion of cervical spine: hyperextension-flexion (© B. Proud).

continued

PHYSICAL ASSESSMENT *Continued*

Assessment Procedure	Normal Findings	Abnormal Findings
Next test lateral bending. Ask the client to touch each ear to the shoulder on that side (Fig. 26-7).	Normally the client can bend 40 degrees to the left and 40 degrees to the right sides.	
Evaluate rotation. Ask the client to turn head to right and left (Fig. 26-8).	About 70 degrees of rotation is normal.	
Ask the client to repeat the cervical ROM movements against resistance.	Client has full ROM against resistance.	Decreased ROM against resistance is seen with joint or muscle disease.
Test ROM of the thoracic and lumbar spine. Ask the client to bend forward and touch the toes (flexion) (Fig. 26-9). Observe for symmetry of the shoulders, scapula, and hips. 👓 Similarly, ask an older client to bend forward but do not insist that he or she touches toes unless the client is comfortable with the movement.	Flexion of 75 degrees to 90 degrees, smooth movement, lumbar concavity flattens out and the spinal processes are in alignment.	Lateral curvature disappears in functional scoliosis; unilateral exaggerated thoracic convexity increases in structural scoliosis. Spinal processes are out of alignment.
Sit down behind the client, stabilize the client's pelvis with your hands, and ask the client to bend sideways (lateral bending), bend backward toward you (hyperextension), and twist the shoulders one way then the other (rotation).	Lateral bending capacity of the thoracic and lumbar should be about 35 degrees (Fig. 26-10A); hyperextension about 30 degrees; and rotation about 30 degrees (Fig. 26-10B).	Low back strain from injury to soft tissues is a common cause of impaired ROM and pain in the lumbar and thoracic regions. Other causes of impaired ROM in the lumbar and thoracic areas include osteoarthritis, ankylosing spondylitis, and congenital abnormalities that may affect the spinal vertebral spacing and mobility.

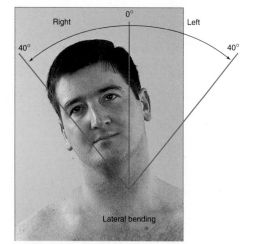

Figure 26-7 Normal range of motion of cervical spine: lateral bending (© B. Proud).

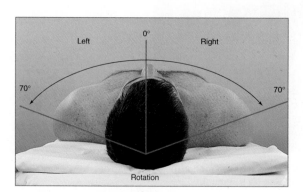

Figure 26-8 Normal range of motion of cervical spine: rotation (© B. Proud).

continued

Assessment Procedure	Normal Findings	Abnormal Findings

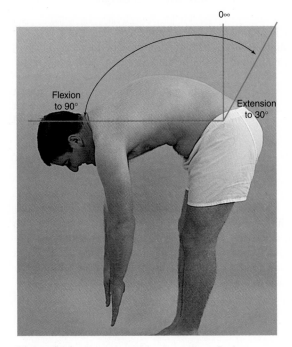

Figure 26-9 Thoracic and lumbar spines: flexion (© B. Proud).

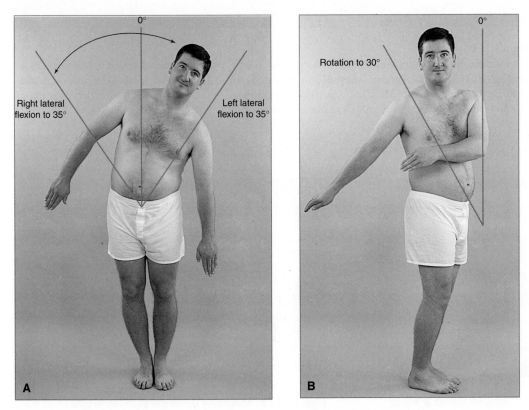

Figure 26-10 Thoracic and lumbar spines: **(A)** lateral bending; **(B)** rotation (© B. Proud).

continued

PHYSICAL ASSESSMENT *Continued*

Assessment Procedure	Normal Findings	Abnormal Findings
Test for back and leg pain. If the client has low back pain that radiates down the back, perform Lasègue's test (straight leg raising) to check a herniated nucleus pulposus. Ask the client to lie flat and raise each relaxed leg independently to the point of pain. At the point of pain, dorsiflex the client's foot (Fig. 26-11). Note the degree of elevation when pain occurs, the distribution and character of the pain, and the results from dorsiflexion of the foot.	Pain not reproduced. Patient is able to raise leg to 90 degree angle. Mild pain of the hamstring is a common finding and does not indicate sciatic pain.	Pain is reproduced. Pain that shoots and radiates down one or both legs (sciatica) below the knees may be due to a herniated intervertebral disc. Continuous, aching pain at night not relieved by rest may be from metastases. Lower back pain with tenderness and limited ROM is common in osteoporosis.
Measure leg length. If you suspect that the client has one leg longer than the other, measure them. Ask the client to lie down with legs extended. With a tape, measure the distance between the anterior superior iliac spine and the medial malleolus, crossing the tape on the medial side of the knee (true leg length) (Fig. 26-12).	Measurements are equal or within 1 cm. If the legs still look unequal, assess the apparent leg length by measuring from a nonfixed point (the umbilicus) to a fixed point (medial malleolus) on each leg.	Unequal leg lengths are associated with scoliosis. Equal true leg lengths but unequal apparent leg lengths are seen with abnormalities in the structure or position of the hips and pelvis.

Shoulders, Arms, and Elbows

Inspection and Palpation

Inspect and palpate shoulders and arms. With the client standing or sitting, inspect anteriorly and posteriorly symmetry, color, swelling, and masses.	Shoulders are symmetrically round, no redness, swelling, or deformity or heat. Muscles are fully developed. Clavicles and scapulae are even and	Flat, hollow, or less rounded shoulders are seen with dislocation. Muscle atrophy is seen with nerve or muscle damage or lack of use. Tenderness,

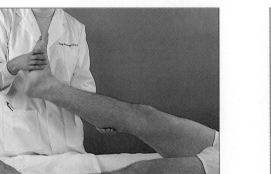

Figure 26-11 Performing Lasègue's test (© B. Proud).

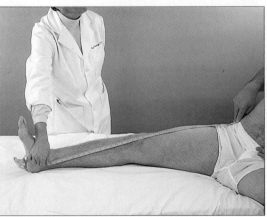

Figure 26-12 Measuring leg length (true leg length) (© B. Proud).

continued

Assessment Procedure	Normal Findings	Abnormal Findings
Palpate for tenderness, swelling, or heat. Anteriorly palpate the clavicle, acromioclavicular joint, sub acromial area, and the biceps. Posteriorly palpate the glenohumeral joint, coracoid area, trapezius muscle, and the scapular area.	symmetric. The client reports no tenderness.	swelling, and heat may be noted with shoulder strains, sprains, arthritis, bursitis, and degenerative joint disease.
Test ROM. Explain to the client that you will be assessing his range of motion (consisting of flexion, extension, adduction, abduction, and motion against resistance). Ask client to stand with both arms straight down at sides. Next ask him to move the arms forward (flexion), then backward with elbows straight (Fig. 26-13).	Extent of forward flexion should be 180 degrees; hyperextension, 50 degrees; adduction, 50 degrees; and abduction 180 degrees.	Painful and limited abduction accompanied by muscle weakness and atrophy are seen with a rotator cuff tear. Client has sharp catches of pain when bringing hands overhead when he or she has rotator cuff tendinitis. Chronic pain and severe limitation of all shoulder motions are seen with calcified tendinitis.
Then have the client bring both hands together overhead, elbows straight, followed by moving both hands in front of the body past the midline with elbows straight (this tests adduction and abduction) (Fig. 26-14).		

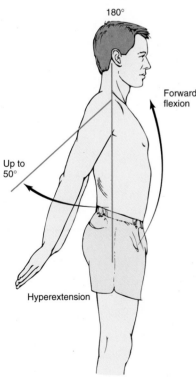

Figure 26-13 Normal range of motion of the shoulder: flexion-extension.

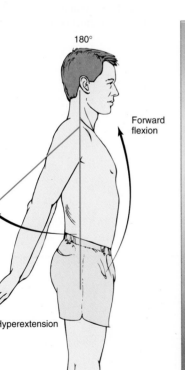

Figure 26-14 Normal range of motion of the shoulder: adduction-abduction.

continued

PHYSICAL ASSESSMENT *Continued*

Assessment Procedure	Normal Findings	Abnormal Findings
In a continuous motion, have the client bring the hands together behind the head with elbows flexed (this tests external rotation) (Fig. 26-15A) and behind the back (internal rotation) (Fig. 26-15B). Repeat these maneuvers against resistance.	Extent of external and internal rotation should be about 90 degrees, respectively. The client can flex, extend, adduct, abduct, rotate, and shrug shoulders against resistance.	Inability to shrug shoulders against resistance is seen with a lesion of cranial nerve XI (spinal accessory). Decreased muscle strength is seen with muscle or joint disease.

Elbows

Inspection and Palpation **Inspect for size, shape, deformities, redness, or swelling.** Inspect elbows in both flexed and extended positions.	Elbows are symmetric without deformities, redness, or swelling.	Redness, heat, and swelling may be seen with bursitis of the olecranon process due to trauma or arthritis.
With the elbow relaxed and flexed about 70 degrees, use your thumb and middle fingers to palpate the olecranon process and epicondyles.	Nontender; without nodules.	Firm, nontender, subcutaneous nodules may be palpated in rheumatoid arthritis or rheumatic fever. Tenderness or pain over the epicondyles may be palpated in epicondylitis (tennis elbow) due to repetitive movements of the forearm or wrists.

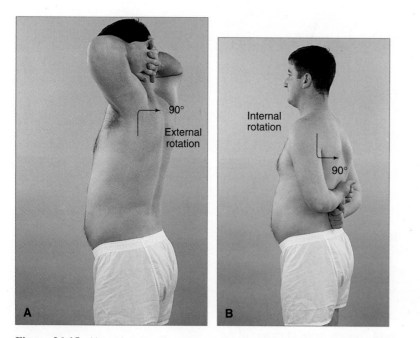

Figure 26-15 Normal range of motion of the shoulder: **(A)** external rotation; **(B)** internal rotation (© B. Proud).

continued

Assessment Procedure	Normal Findings	Abnormal Findings
Test ROM. Ask the client to perform the following movements to test ROM, flexion, extension, pronation, and supination. Flex the elbow and bring the hand to the forehead (Fig. 26-16A). Straighten the elbow. Then hold arm out, turn the palm down, then turn the palm up (Fig. 26-16B). Last have the client repeat the movements against your resistance.	Normal ranges of motion are 160 degrees of flexion; 180 degrees of extension. 90 degrees of pronation. 90 degrees of supination. Some clients may lack 5 to 10 degrees or have hyperextension. The client should have full ROM against resistance.	Decreased ROM against resistance is seen with joint or muscle disease or injury.

Wrists

Inspection and Palpation Inspect wrist size, shape, symmetry, color, and swelling. Then palpate for tenderness and nodules (Fig. 26-17).	Wrists are symmetric without redness, or swelling. They are nontender and free of nodules.	Swelling is seen with rheumatoid arthritis. Tenderness and nodules may be seen with rheumatoid arthritis. A nontender, round, enlarged, swollen, fluid-filled cyst (ganglion) may be noted on the wrists (Abnormal Findings 26-2).

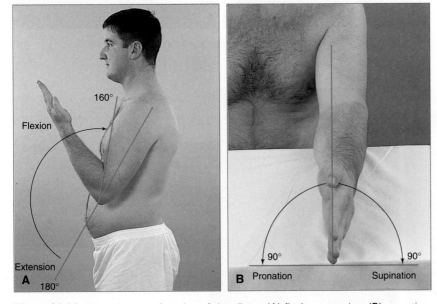

Figure 26-16   Normal range of motion of the elbow: **(A)** flexion-extension; **(B)** pronation-supination (© B. Proud).

continued

PHYSICAL ASSESSMENT *Continued*

Assessment Procedure	Normal Findings	Abnormal Findings
Palpate the anatomic snuffbox (the hollow area on the back of the wrist at the base of the fully extended thumb) (Fig. 26-18).	No tenderness palpated in anatomic snuffbox.	Snuffbox tenderness may indicate a scaphoid fracture, which is often the result of falling on an outstretched hand.
Test ROM. Ask the client to bend wrist down and back (flexion and extension) (Fig. 26-19A). Next have the client hold the wrist straight and move the hand outward and inward (deviation) (Fig. 26-19B). Repeat these maneuvers against resistance.	Normal ranges of motion are 90 degrees, flexion; 70 degrees, hyperextension; 55 degrees, ulnar deviation; and 20 degrees, radial deviation. Client should have full ROM against resistance. Unequal lengths of the ulna and radius have been found in some ethnic groups (e.g., Swedes and Chinese) (Overfield, 1995).	Ulnar deviation of the wrist and fingers with limited ROM is often seen in rheumatoid arthritis. Increased pain with extension of the wrist against resistance is seen in epicondylitis of the lateral side of the elbow. Increased pain with flexion of the wrist against resistance is seen in epicondylitis of the medial side of the elbow. Decreased muscle strength is noted with muscle and joint disease.

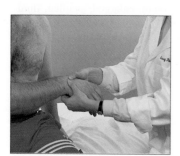

Figure 26-17 Palpating the wrists (© B. Proud).

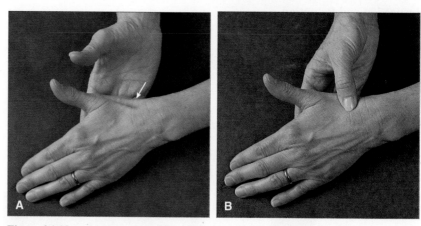

Figure 26-18 (A) Anatomic snuffbox. (B) Palpating the anatomic snuffbox.

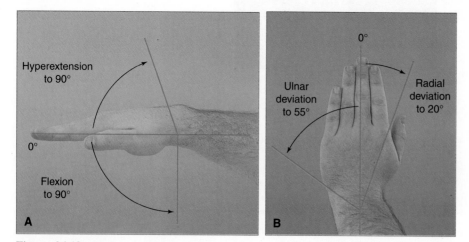

Figure 26-19 Range of motion of the wrists: (A) flexion-hyperextension; (B) radial-ulnar deviation (© B. Proud).

continued

Assessment Procedure	Normal Findings	Abnormal Findings
Test for carpal tunnel syndrome. Perform Phalen's test. Ask the client to place the backs of both hands against each other while flexing the wrists 90 degrees downward (Fig. 26-20A). Have the client hold this position for 60 seconds. Optionally test for Tinel's sign. With your finger, percuss lightly over the median nerve (located on the inner aspect of the wrist) (Fig. 26-20B).	No tingling, numbness, or pain result from Phalen's test or from Tinel's test.	After either test, client may report tingling, numbness, and pain with carpal tunnel syndrome. Median nerve entrapped in the carpal tunnel results in pain, numbness, and impaired function of the hand and fingers (Fig. 26-21).

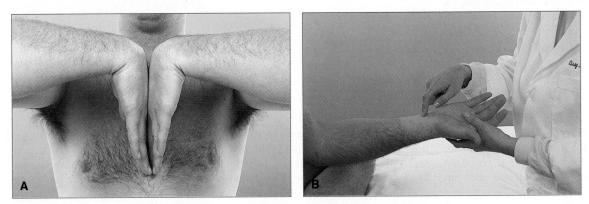

Figure 26-20   Tests for carpal tunnel syndrome: **(A)** Phalen's test; **(B)** Tinel's test (© B. Proud).

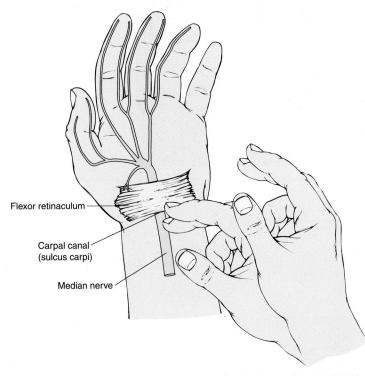

Flexor retinaculum

Carpal canal (sulcus carpi)

Median nerve

Figure 26-21   Median nerve entrapped in the carpal tunnel results in pain, numbness, and impaired function of the hand and fingers.

continued

PHYSICAL ASSESSMENT Continued

Assessment Procedure	Normal Findings	Abnormal Findings

Hands and Fingers

Inspection and Palpation

Inspect size, shape, symmetry, swelling, and color. Palpate the fingers from the distal end proximally, noting tenderness, swelling, boney prominences, nodules or crepitus of each interphalangeal joint. Assess the metacarpophalangeal joints by squeezing the hand from each side between your thumb and fingers. Palpate each metacarpal of the hand, noting tenderness and swelling.

Hands and fingers are symmetric, nontender, and without nodules. Fingers lie in straight line. No swelling or deformities. Rounded protuberance noted next to the thumb over the thenar prominence. Smaller protuberance seen adjacent to the small finger.

Swollen, stiff, tender finger joints are seen in acute rheumatoid arthritis. Boutonnière deformity and swan-neck deformity are seen in long-term rheumatoid arthritis (see Abnormal Findings 26-2). Atrophy of the thenar prominence may be evident in carpal tunnel syndrome.

In osteoarthritis, hard, painless nodules may be seen over the distal interphalangeal joints (Heberden's nodes) and over the proximal interphalangeal joints (Bouchard's nodes) (see Abnormal Findings 26-2).

Test ROM (Fig. 26-22). Ask the client to (*A*) spread the fingers apart (abduction), (*B*) make a fist (adduction), (*C*) bend the fingers down (flexion) and then up

Normal ranges are 20 degrees of abduction, full adduction of fingers (touching), 90 degrees of flexion, and 30 degrees of hyperextension. The thumb

Inability to extend the ring and little fingers is seen in Dupuytren's contracture. Painful extension of a finger may be seen in tenosynovitis (infection of the

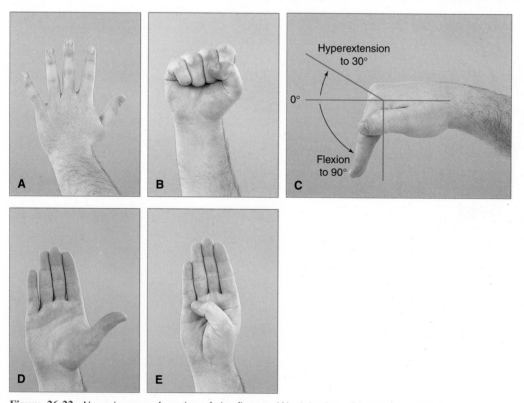

Figure 26-22 Normal range of motion of the fingers: (**A**) abduction, (**B**) adduction, (**C**) flexion-hyperextension, (**D**) thumb away from fingers, (**E**) thumb touching base of small finger (© B. Proud).

continued

Assessment Procedure	Normal Findings	Abnormal Findings
(hyperextension), (D) move the thumb away from other fingers and then (E) touch the thumb to the base of the small finger. Repeat these maneuvers against resistance.	should easily move away from other fingers and 50 degrees of thumb flexion is normal. The client normally has full ROM against resistance.	flexor tendon sheaths; see Abnormal Findings 26-2). Decreased muscle strength against resistance is associated with muscle and joint disease.

Hips

Inspection and Palpation With the client standing, inspect symmetry and shape of hips (Fig. 26-23). Palpate for stability, tenderness, and crepitus.	Buttocks are equally sized; iliac crests are symmetric in height. Hips are stable, nontender, and without crepitus.	Instability, inability to stand, and/or a deformed hip area are indicative of a fractured hip. Tenderness, edema, decreased ROM, and crepitus are seen in hip inflammation and degenerative joint disease.
Test ROM (Fig. 26-24). With the client supine, ask the client to Raise extended leg (A). Flex knee up to chest while keeping other leg extended (B).	Normal ROM: 90 degrees of hip flexion with knee straight and 120 degrees of hip flexion with the knee bent and the other leg remaining straight.	Inability to abduct hip is a common sign of hip disease.

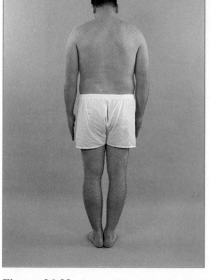

Figure 26-23 Inspecting the hips and buttocks (© B. Proud).

continued

PHYSICAL ASSESSMENT *Continued*

Assessment Procedure	Normal Findings	Abnormal Findings

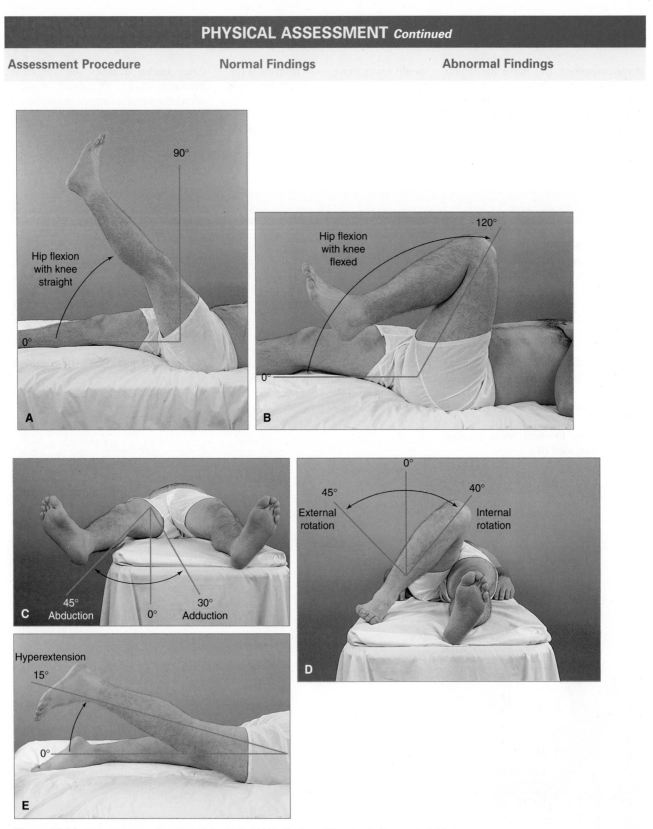

Figure 26-24   Normal range of motion of the hips: **(A)** hip flexion with extended knee straight; **(B)** hip flexion with knee bent; **(C)** abduction-adduction; **(D)** internal and external rotation; **(E)** hyperextension (© B. Proud).

continued

Assessment Procedure	Normal Findings	Abnormal Findings
➤ **Clinical Tip** • If the client has had a total hip replacement, do not test ROM unless the physician gives permission to do so. This is done to reduce the risk of dislocating the hip prosthesis.		
Move extended leg (*C*) away from midline of body as far as possible and then toward midline of body as far as possible (abduction and adduction). Bend knee and turn leg (*D*) inward (rotation) and then outward (rotation). Ask the client to lie prone (*E*) and lift extended leg off table. Alternatively, ask the client to stand and swing extended leg backward. Repeat these maneuvers against resistance.	Normal ROM: 45 degrees to 50 degrees of abduction; 20 degrees to 30 degrees of adduction. 40 degrees internal hip rotation, 45 degrees external hip rotation. 15 degrees hip hyperextension. Full ROM against resistance.	Pain and a decrease in internal hip rotation may be a sign of osteoarthritis or femoral neck stress fracture. Pain on palpation of the greater trochanter and pain as the client moves from standing to lying down may indicate bursitis of the hip. Decreased muscle strength against resistance is seen in muscle and joint disease.

Knees

Inspection and Palpation With the client supine then sitting with knees dangling, inspect for size, shape, symmetry, swelling, deformities, and alignment. Observe for quadricep muscle atrophy.	Knees symmetric, hollows present on both sides of the patella, no swelling or deformities. Lower leg in alignment with upper leg.	Knees turn in with knock knees (genu valgum) and turn out with bowed legs (genu varum). Swelling above or next to the patella may indicate fluid in the knee joint or thickening of the synovial membrane.
Palpate for tenderness, warmth, consistency, and nodules. Begin palpation 10 cm above the patella, using your fingers and thumb to move downward toward the knee (Fig. 26-25).	👓 Some older clients may have a bowlegged appearance because of decreased muscle control. Nontender and cool. Muscles firm. No nodules.	Tenderness and warmth with a boggy consistency may be symptoms of synovitis. Asymmetrical muscular development in the quadriceps may indicate atrophy.
Tests for swelling. If you notice swelling, perform the bulge test to determine if the swelling is due to accumulation of fluid or soft tissue swelling. The bulge test helps to detect small amounts of fluid in the knee. With the client in a supine position, use the ball of your hand firmly to stroke the medial side of the knee upward, three to four times,	No bulge of fluid appears on medial side of knee.	Bulge of fluid appears on medial side of knee with a small amount of joint effusion.

continued

PHYSICAL ASSESSMENT *Continued*

Assessment Procedure	Normal Findings	Abnormal Findings
to displace any accumulated fluid (Fig. 26-26A). Then press on the lateral side of the knee and look for a bulge on the medial side of the knee (Fig. 26-26B).		
Perform the ballottement test. It helps to detect large amounts of fluid in the knee. With the client in a supine position, firmly press your nondominant thumb and index finger on each side of the patella. This displaces fluid in the suprapatellar bursa located between the femur and patella. Then with your dominant fingers, push the patella down on the femur (Fig. 26-27). Feel for a fluid wave or a click.	No movement of patella noted. Patella rests firmly over femur.	Fluid wave or click palpated with large amounts of joint effusion. A positive ballottement test may be present with meniscal tears.

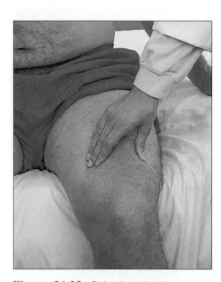

Figure 26-25 Palpating the knee area (© B. Proud).

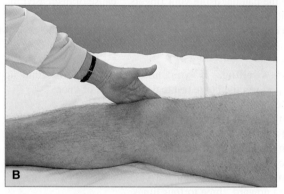

Figure 26-26 Performing the "bulge" knee test: **(A)** stroking the knee; **(B)** observing the medial side for bulging (© B. Proud).

continued

Assessment Procedure	Normal Findings	Abnormal Findings
Palpate the tibiofemoral space. As you compress the patella, slide it distally against the underlying femur. Note crepitus or pain.	There is no pain on examination. Crepitus may be present.	A patellofemoral disorder may be suspected if both crepitus and pain are present on examination.
Test ROM (Fig. 26-28). Ask the client to • Bend each knee up (flexion) toward buttocks or back. • Straighten knee (extension/hyperextension). • Walk normally. Repeat these maneuvers against resistance.	Normal ranges: 120 degrees to 130 degrees of flexion; 0 degrees of extension to 15 degrees of hyperextension. Client should have full ROM against resistance.	Osteoarthritis is characterized by a decreased ROM with synovial thickening and crepitation. Flexion contractures of the knee are characterized by an inability to extend knee fully. Decreased muscle strength against resistance is seen in muscle and joint disease.
Test for pain and injury. If the client complains of a "giving in" or "locking" of the knee, perform McMurray's test (Fig. 26-29). With the client in the supine position, ask the client to flex one knee and hip. Then place your thumb and index finger of one hand on either side of the knee. Use your other hand to hold the heel of the foot up. Rotate the lower leg and foot laterally. Slowly extend the knee, noting pain or clicking. Repeat, rotating lower leg and foot medially. Again note pain or clicking.	No pain or clicking noted.	Pain or clicking is indicative of a torn meniscus of the knee.

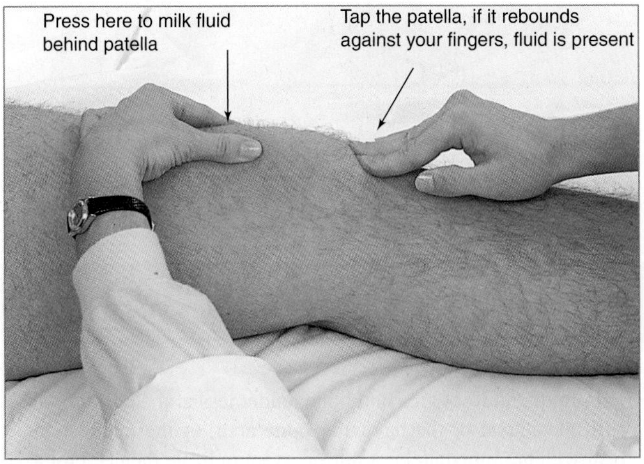

Press here to milk fluid behind patella

Tap the patella, if it rebounds against your fingers, fluid is present

Figure 26-27 Performing the "ballottement" knee test (© B. Proud).

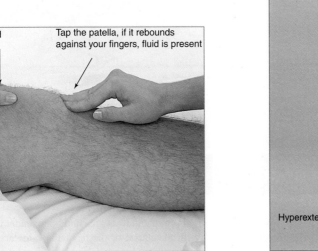

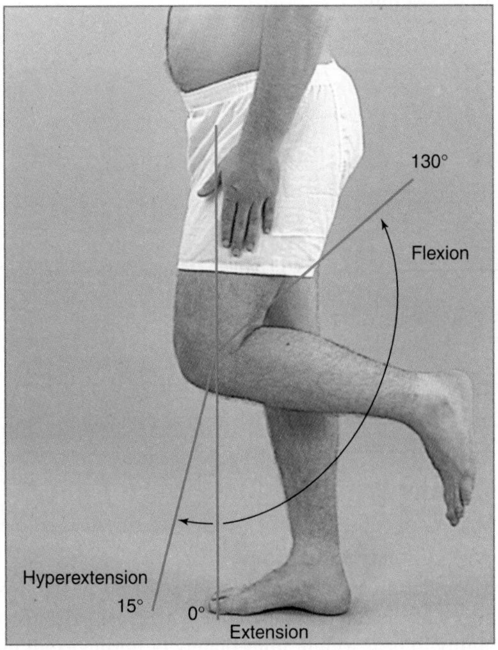

130°

Flexion

Hyperextension
15°   0°
Extension

Figure 26-28 Normal range of motion of the knee (© B. Proud).

continued

PHYSICAL ASSESSMENT Continued

Assessment Procedure	Normal Findings	Abnormal Findings

Ankles and Feet

Inspection and Palpation
With the client sitting, standing, and walking, inspect position, alignment, shape, and skin.

Toes usually point forward and lie flat; however, they may point in (pes varus) or point out (pes valgus). Toes and feet are in alignment with the lower leg. Smooth, rounded medial malleolar prominences with prominent heels and metatarsophalangeal joints. Skin is smooth and free of corns and calluses. Longitudinal arch; most of weight bearing is on foot midline.

A laterally deviated great toe with possible overlapping of the second toe and possible formation of an enlarged, painful, inflamed bursa (bunion) on the medial side is seen with hallux valgus. Common abnormalities include feet with no arches (pes planus or "flat feet"), feet with high arches (pes cavus); painful thickening of the skin over bony prominences and at pressure points (corns); nonpainful thickened skin that occurs at pressure points (calluses); and painful warts (verruca vulgaris) that often occur under a callus (plantar warts; Abnormal Findings 26-3).

Palpate ankles and feet for tenderness, heat, swelling, or nodules (Fig. 26-30). Palpate the toes from the distal end proximally, noting tenderness, swelling, boney prominences, nodules, or crepitus of each interphalangeal joint. Assess the metatarsophalangeal joints by squeezing the foot from each side with your thumb and fingers. Palpate each metatarsal, noting swelling or tenderness. Palpate the plantar area (bottom) of the foot noting pain or swelling.

No pain, heat, swelling, or nodules are noted.

Tender, painful, reddened, hot, and swollen metatarsophalangeal joint of the great toe is seen in gouty arthritis. Nodules of the posterior ankle may be palpated with rheumatoid arthritis. Pain and tenderness of the metatarsophalangeal joints are seen in inflammation of the joints, rheumatoid arthritis, and degenerative joint disease. Tenderness of the calcaneus of the bottom of the foot may indicate plantar fasciitis. Use the Ottawa ankle and foot rules (Display 26-3) to determine need for X-ray referral.

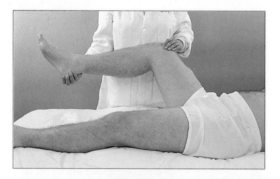

Figure 26-29 Performing McMurray's test (© B. Proud).

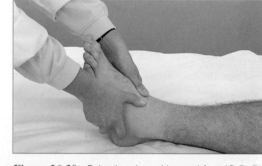

Figure 26-30 Palpating the ankles and feet (© B. Proud).

DISPLAY 26-3	Ottawa Ankle and Foot Rules

Ankle X-ray indicators
Malleolar area pain; and bone tenderness at the tips of 6 cm edges of the lateral malleolus or medial malleolus; or the inability to bear weight immediately or during exam indicate the need for an ankle x-ray.

Foot X-ray indicators
Pain in the midfoot area and bone tenderness at the base of the fifth metatarsal or the navicular bone area, or the inability to bear weight immediately or during exam indicate the need for a foot x-ray.

Adapted from Steill, I. G., Greenberg, G. H., McKnight, R. D., Nair, R. C., Mc Dowell, I., & Worthington, J. R. (1992). A study to develop clinical decision rules for the use of radiography in acute ankle injuries. *Annals of Emergency Medicine, 21*(4), 384–390.

continued

Assessment Procedure	Normal Findings	Abnormal Findings
Test ROM (Fig. 26-31). Ask the client to	Normal ranges:	Decreased strength against resistance is seen in muscle and joint disease.
Point toes upward (dorsiflexion) and then downward (plantar flexion) (*A*).	20 degrees dorsiflexion of ankle and foot; 45 degrees plantar flexion of ankle and foot.	Hyperextension of the metatarsophalangeal joint and flexion of the proximal interphalangeal joint is apparent in hammer toe (see Abnormal Findings 26-3).
Turn soles outward (eversion) and then inward (inversion) (*B*).	20 degrees of eversion; 30 degrees of inversion.	
Rotate foot outward (abduction) and then inward (adduction) (*C*).	10 degrees of abduction; 20 degrees of adduction.	Decreased strength against resistance is common in muscle and joint disease.
Turn toes under foot (flexion) and then upward (extension).	40 degrees of flexion; 40 degrees of extension.	
Repeat these maneuvers against resistance.	Client has full ROM against resistance.	

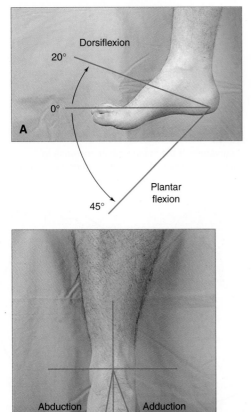

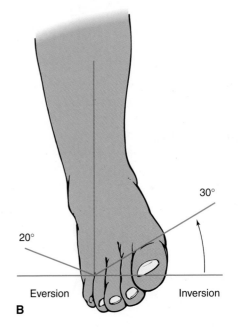

Figure 26-31 Normal range of motion of the feet and ankles: **(A)** dorsiflexion/plantar flexion; **(B)** eversion/inversion; **(C)** abduction/adduction (© B. Proud).

Abnormal Findings 26-1 | **Abnormal Spinal Curvatures**

Flattening of the lumbar curve

Flattening of the lumbar curvature may be seen with a herniated lumbar disc or ankylosing spondylitis.

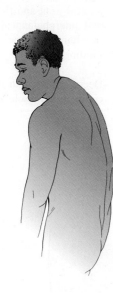

Kyphosis

A rounded thoracic convexity (kyphosis) is commonly seen in older adults.

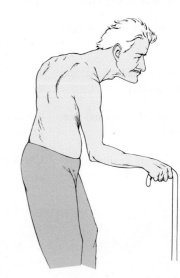

Lumbar Lordosis

An exaggerated lumbar curve (lumbar lordosis) is often seen in pregnancy or obesity.

Scoliosis

Lateral curvature of the spine with an increase in convexity on the side that is curved is seen in scoliosis.

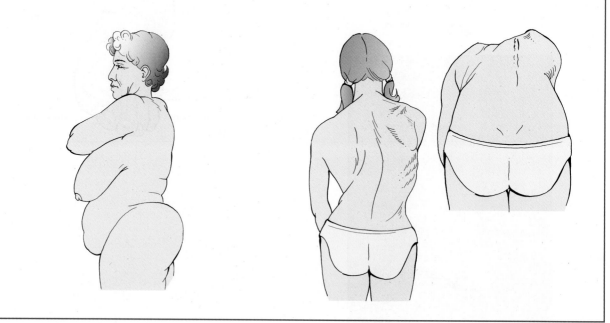

Abnormal Findings 26-2 ■ **Abnormalities Affecting the Wrists, Hands, and Fingers**

The following abnormalities are commonly associated with the upper extremities. Early detection is important because early intervention may help to preserve dexterity and daily function.

Acute Rheumatoid Arthritis

Tender, painful, swollen, stiff joints are seen in acute rheumatoid arthritis.

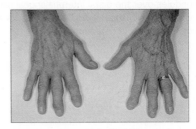

(© 1991 National Medical Slide Bank/CMSP.)

Chronic Rheumatoid Arthritis

Chronic swelling and thickening of the metacarpophalangeal and proximal interphalangeal joints, limited range of motion, and finger deviation toward the ulnar side are seen in chronic rheumatoid arthritis.

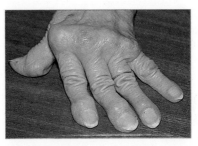

(© 1995 Science Photo Library.)

Boutonnière and Swan-Neck Deformities

Flexion of the proximal interphalangeal joint and hyperextension of the distal interphalangeal joint (boutonnière deformity) and hyperextension of the proximal interphalangeal joint with flexion of the distal interphalangeal joint (swan-neck deformity) are also common in chronic rheumatoid arthritis.

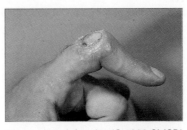

Boutonnière deformity. (© 1990 CMSP.)

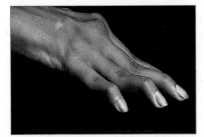

Swan neck deformity. (© 1991 National Medical Slide Bank/CMSP.)

Ganglion

Nontender, round, enlarged, swollen, fluid-filled cyst (ganglion) is commonly seen at the dorsum of the wrist.

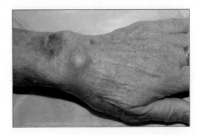

continued on page 558

Abnormal Findings 26-2   **Abnormalities Affecting the Wrists, Hands, and Fingers** *Continued*

Osteoarthritis

Hard, painless nodules over the distal interphalangeal joints (Heberden's nodes) and over the proximal interphalangeal joints (Bouchard's nodes) are seen in osteoarthritis.

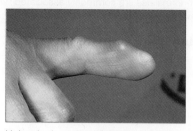

Heberden's nodes. (© 1991 National Medical Slide Bank/CMSP.)

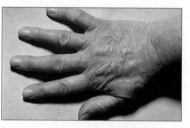

Bouchard's nodes. (© 1991 National Medical Slide Bank/CMSP.)

Tenosynovitis

Painful extension of a finger may be seen in acute tenosynovitis (infection of the flexor tendon sheathes).

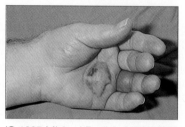

(© 1995 Michael English. MD/CMSP.)

Thenar Atrophy

Atrophy of the thenar prominence due to pressure on the median nerve is seen in carpal tunnel syndrome.

Flattened thenar eminence

Normal hypothenar eminence

The following abnormalities affect the feet and toes, typically causing discomfort and impeding mobility. Early detection and treatment can help to restore or maximize function.

Acute Gouty Arthritis

In gouty arthritis, the metatarsophalangeal joint of the great toe is tender, painful, reddened, hot, and swollen.

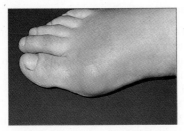

(© 1995 Science Photo Library/CMSP.)

Callus

Calluses are nonpainful, thickened skin that occur at pressure points.

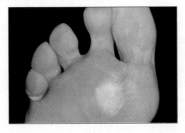

Corn

Corns are painful thickenings of the skin that occur over bony prominences and at pressure points.

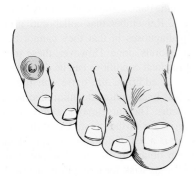

Plantar Wart

Plantar warts are painful warts (verruca vulgaris) that often occur under a callus, appearing as tiny dark spots.

Flat Feet

A flat foot (pes planus) has no arch and may cause pain and swelling of the foot surface.

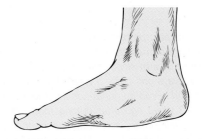

Hallux Valgus

Hallux valgus is an abnormality in which the great toe is deviated laterally and may overlap the second toe. An enlarged, painful, inflamed bursa (bunion) may form on the medial side.

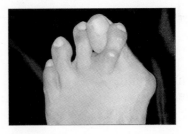

Hammer Toe

Hyperextension at the metatarsophalangeal joint with flexion at the proximal interphalangeal joint (hammer toe) commonly occurs with the second toe.

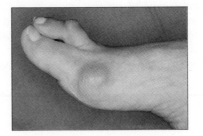

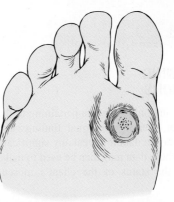

VALIDATING AND DOCUMENTING FINDINGS

Validate the musculoskeletal assessment data you have collected. This is necessary to verify that the data are reliable and accurate.

Sample Documentation of Subjective Data

No history of past problems with joints or muscles. "Broke right arm as child, had cast for 6 weeks." No problems with that arm since that time. Walks 1 mile four times a week; plays golf twice a week; likes being outside when not at work. Polio immunization as child; last tetanus immunization 3 years ago after cutting foot with garden tiller. Recalls grandmother as having rheumatoid arthritis. Does not smoke or drink alcohol. Drinks two caffeinated colas per day. Consumes food from all food groups; drinks milk daily. Client reports no recent weight gain or loss. Occupation requires long hours sitting working at a computer. Has good supportive chair. Has not had any back problems.

Sample Documentation of Objective Data

Client is 5 feet, 6 inches, weighs 140 lbs. Gait smooth, with equal stride and good base of support. Full ROM of TMJ with no pain, tenderness, clicking, or crepitus. Sternoclavicular joint midline without swelling or redness. Normal curves of cervical, thoracic, and lumbar spine. Paravertebral area nontender. Full, smooth ROM of cervical and lumbar spine. Upper and lower extremities symmetric without lesions, nodules, deformities, tenderness, or swelling. Full, smooth ROM against gravity and resistance.

Analysis of Data

DIAGNOSTIC REASONING: POSSIBLE CONCLUSIONS

After collecting subjective and objective data pertaining to the musculoskeletal assessment, identify abnormal findings and client strengths. Then cluster the data to reveal any significant patterns or abnormalities. These data may then be used to make clinical judgments about the status of the client's musculoskeletal system.

Selected Nursing Diagnoses

Following is a listing of selected nursing diagnoses (wellness, risk, or actual) that you may identify when analyzing the cue clusters.

Wellness Diagnoses

* Readiness for enhanced activity and exercise patterns

Risk Diagnoses

* Risk for Trauma related to repetitive movements of wrists or elbow with recreation or occupation
* Risk for Injury: Pathologic fractures related to osteoporosis
* Risk for Injury to joints, muscles, or bones related to environmental hazards
* Risk for Disuse Syndrome
* Risk for Urinary Tract Infection related to urine stasis secondary to immobility

Actual Diagnoses

* Impaired Physical Mobility related to impaired joint movement, decreased muscle strength, or fractured bone
* Activity Intolerance related to muscle weakness or joint pain
* Constipation related to decreased gastric motility and muscle tone secondary to immobility
* Ineffective Sexuality Pattern related to lower back pain
* Acute (or Chronic) Pain related to joint, muscle, or bone problems
* Impaired Skin Integrity related to prolonged pressure on the skin secondary to immobility
* Impaired Social Interaction related to depression or immobility
* Disturbed Body Image related to skeletal deformities

Selected Collaborative Problems

After grouping the data, certain collaborative problems may become apparent. Remember that collaborative problems differ from nursing diagnoses in that they cannot be prevented by nursing interventions alone. However, these physiologic complications of medical conditions can be detected and monitored by the nurse. In addition, the nurse can use physician- and nurse-prescribed interventions to minimize the complications of these problems. The nurse may also have to refer the client in such situations for further treatment of the problem.

Following is a list of collaborative problems that may be identified when obtaining a general impression. These problems are worded as Risk for Complications (or RC), followed by the problem.

* RC: Osteoporosis
* RC: Joint dislocation
* RC: Compartmental syndrome
* RC: Pathologic fractures

Medical Problems

After grouping the data, it may become apparent that the client's signs and symptoms clearly require medical diagnosis and treatment. Referral to a primary care provider is necessary.

CASE STUDY

The case study demonstrates how to analyze musculoskeletal assessment data for a specific client. The critical thinking exercises included in the study guide/lab manual and interactive product that complement this text also offer opportunities to analyze assessment data.

Frances Funstead has come to the occupational health nurse's office asking for help with her back problem. During the interview, she states that she has recently experienced burning in her lower back in an area just below the waist and has pain in her shoulder muscles. She denies pain in her hips and legs.

Ms. Funstead's job in the manufacturing plant requires her to stand on the assembly line where she puts together small parts from 7:00 AM to 3:00 PM. She has 30 minutes for lunch (11:00 to 11:30 AM), which she eats in the company lunchroom, and two 10-minute coffee breaks. She also states that many life changes are going on right now and she is seeking spiritual counseling in handling these. She is 55 years old and can't retire for another 7 years. Physical examination reveals rigid neck and shoulder muscles with palpable "knots," with strong shoulder shrug and neck rotation against resistance; however, neck rotation ROM is limited, with pain beyond 60-degree rotation

bilaterally. A slight right lateral spinal curvature and mild lordosis are noted from T10 to L2. Muscles in this area do not appear swollen, but the area is slightly warmer to touch than the surrounding area.

Ms. Funstead should be referred to a physician for further evaluation of possible spinal disk dislocations, arthritis, or early tumors. Depending on the findings, she should be referred to a physical therapist for muscle-strengthening exercises and instruction regarding body mechanics to prevent muscle strain. If medical evaluation indicates that this problem is a work-related disability, the nurse should refer Ms. Funstead to the appropriate person to assist with the implementation of rehabilitative measures or disability benefits.

The following concept map illustrates the diagnostic reasoning process.

Applying COLDSPA

Applying **COLDSPA** for client symptoms: "Burning in my lower back."

Mnemonic	Question	Data Provided	Missing Data
Character	Describe the sign or symptom (feeling, appearance, sound, smell, or taste if applicable).	Client reports a sensation of "burning and pain."	"Describe the type of pain you are having. Is it sharp, dull, throbbing?"
Onset	When did it begin?		"When did this burning and pain first occur?"
Location	Where is it? Does it radiate? Does it occur anywhere else?	Burning in lower back just below the waist; pain in shoulder muscles.	
Duration	How long does it last? Does it recur?		"How long does the burning and pain last?"
Severity	How bad is it? or How much does it bother you?		"Can you continue with your activities of daily living when you have this burning and pain? How does it limit your activities?"
Pattern	What makes it better or worse?		"What aggravates the burning and pain? What makes it better?"
Associated factors/How it **A**ffects the client	What other symptoms occur with it? How does it affect you?	Client stands on assembly line at work for 8 hours with one 30 minute break and two 10 minute breaks. She is going through many life changes now.	"What other symptoms do you have with this burning and pain?"

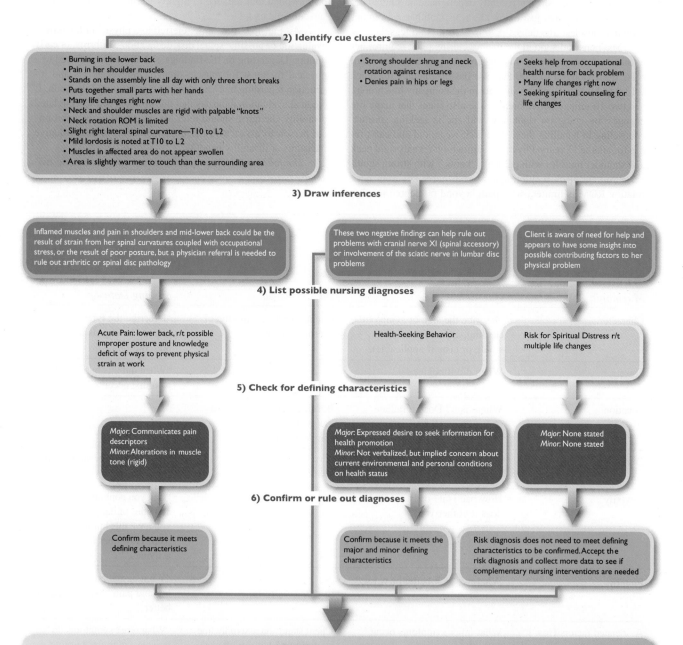

1) Identify abnormal findings and client strengths

Subjective Data

- Seeks help from nurse for back problem
- Burning in her lower back (flank)
- Pain in her shoulder muscles
- Denies pain in hips or legs
- Stands on the assembly line all day with only three short breaks
- Puts together small parts with her hands
- Many life changes right now
- 55 years old, can't retire for 7 years
- Seeking spiritual counseling for life changes

Objective Data

- Neck and shoulder muscles are rigid with palpable "knots"
- Strong shoulder shrug and neck rotation against resistance
- Neck rotation ROM is limited
- Slight right lateral spinal curvature T10 to L2
- Mild lordosis is noted at T10 to L2
- Muscles in affected area do not appear swollen
- Area is slightly warmer to touch than the surrounding area

2) Identify cue clusters

- Burning in the lower back
- Pain in her shoulder muscles
- Stands on the assembly line all day with only three short breaks
- Puts together small parts with her hands
- Many life changes right now
- Neck and shoulder muscles are rigid with palpable "knots"
- Neck rotation ROM is limited
- Slight right lateral spinal curvature—T10 to L2
- Mild lordosis is noted at T10 to L2
- Muscles in affected area do not appear swollen
- Area is slightly warmer to touch than the surrounding area

- Strong shoulder shrug and neck rotation against resistance
- Denies pain in hips or legs

- Seeks help from occupational health nurse for back problem
- Many life changes right now
- Seeking spiritual counseling for life changes

3) Draw inferences

Inflamed muscles and pain in shoulders and mid-lower back could be the result of strain from her spinal curvatures coupled with occupational stress, or the result of poor posture, but a physician referral is needed to rule out arthritic or spinal disc pathology

These two negative findings can help rule out problems with cranial nerve XI (spinal accessory) or involvement of the sciatic nerve in lumbar disc problems

Client is aware of need for help and appears to have some insight into possible contributing factors to her physical problem

4) List possible nursing diagnoses

Acute Pain: lower back, r/t possible improper posture and knowledge deficit of ways to prevent physical strain at work

Health-Seeking Behavior

Risk for Spiritual Distress r/t multiple life changes

5) Check for defining characteristics

Major: Communicates pain descriptors
Minor: Alterations in muscle tone (rigid)

Major: Expressed desire to seek information for health promotion
Minor: Not verbalized, but implied concern about current environmental and personal conditions on health status

Major: None stated
Minor: None stated

6) Confirm or rule out diagnoses

Confirm because it meets defining characteristics

Confirm because it meets the major and minor defining characteristics

Risk diagnosis does not need to meet defining characteristics to be confirmed. Accept the risk diagnosis and collect more data to see if complementary nursing interventions are needed

7) Document conclusions

Nursing diagnoses that are appropriate for this client include:
- Acute Pain: lower back, r/t possible improper posture and knowledge deficit of ways to prevent physical strain at work
- Health-Seeking Behaviors
- Risk for Spiritual Distress r/t multiple life changes

Ms. Funstead should be referred to a physician for further evaluation of possible spinal disk dislocations, arthritis, or early tumors. If medical evaluation indicates that this problem is a work-related disability, the nurse should refer Ms. Funstead to the appropriate person to assist with the implementation of rehabilitative measures or disability benefits

References and Selected Readings

Adkins III, S. B., & Figler, R. A. (2000). Hip pain in athletes. *American Family Physician, 61*(7), 2109–2118.

Adler, P. A., Roberts, B. L. (2006). The use of Tai Chi to improve health in older adults. *Orthopaedic Nurses, 25*(2), 91–92.

Altizer, L. (2003). Hand and wrist fractures. *Orthopaedic Nursing, 22*(2), 131–138.

Altizer, L. (2003). Strains and sprains. *Orthopaedic Nursing, 22*(6), 404–411.

Arcuni, S. E. (2000). Rotator cuff pathology and subacromial impingement. *The Nurse Practitioner, 25*(5), 58–78.

Azegami, M., Ohira, M., Miyoshi, K., Kobayaski, C., Hongo, M., Yanagihaski, R., & Sadoyama, T. (2007). Effect of single and multijoint lower extremity muscle strength on the functional capacity and ADL/IADL status in Japanese community-dwelling older adults. *Nursing and Health Sciences, 9*(3), 168–176.

Bonnefoy, M., Jauffret, M., & Jusot, J. F. (2007). Muscle power of lower extremities in relation to function ability and nutritional status in very elderly people. *Journal of Nutrition, Health and Aging, 11*(3), 223–228.

Cunningham, M. M., & Jillings, C. (2006). Individuals' descriptions of living with fibromyalgia. *Clinical Nursing Research, 15*(4), 258–273.

Daniels, J. M. 2nd, Zook, E. G., & Lynch, J. M. (2004). Hand and wrist injuries: Part II. Emergent evaluation. *American Family Physician, 69*(8), 1949–1956.

Dell, D. D. (2007). Getting the point about fibromyalgia. *Nursing, 37*(2), 61–64.

DiMonaco, M., Vallero, F., DiMonaco, R., Tappero, R., & Cavanna, A. (2007). Muscle mass and functional recovery in men with hip fracture. *American Journal of Physical Medicine and Rehabilitation, 86*(10), 818–825.

DiMonaco, M., Vallero, F., DiMonaco, R., Tappero, R, & Cavanna, A. (2007). Skeletal muscle mass, fat mass, and hip bone mineral density in elderly women with hip fracture. *Journal of Bone and Mineral Metabolism, 25*(4), 235–242.

Dion, L., Malouin, F., McFadyen, B., & Richards, C. I. (2003). Assessing mobility and locomotor coordination after stroke with the rise-to-walk task. *Neurorehabilitation and Neural Repair, 17*(2), 83–92.

Fiessler, F., Szues, P., Kec, R., & Richman, P. B. (2004). Can nurses appropriately interpret the Ottawa Ankle Rules? *American Journal of Emergency Medicine, 22*(3), 145–148.

Green, W. B. (Ed.). (2000). *Essentials of musculoskeletal care* (2nd ed.). Rosemont, Ill: American Academy of Orthopaedic Surgeons.

Gregory, P. L., Biswas, A. C., & Batt, M. E. (2002). Musculoskeletal problems of the chest wall in athletes. *Sports Medicine, 32*(4), 235–250.

Harnirattisai, T., Johnson, R. A., & Kawinwonggowit, V. (2006). Evaluating functional activity in older Thai adults. *Rehabilitation Nursing, 31*(3), 124–128.

Hart, E. S., Grottkau, B. E., & Albright, M. B. (2007). Slipped capital femoral epiphysis: Don't miss this pediatric hip disorder. *The Nurse Practitioner, 32*(3), 14, 16–18, 21.

Holm, G., & Moody, L. E. (2003). Carpal tunnel syndrome: Current theory, treatment, and the use of B6. *Journal of the American Academy of Nurse Practitioners, 15*(1), 18–22.

Karpas, A., Hennes, H., & Walsh-Kelly, C. M. (2002). Utilization of the Ottawa Ankle Rules by nurses in a pediatric emergency department. *Academic Emergency Medicine, 9*(2), 130–133.

Larsen, D. (2002). Assessment and management of hand and wrist fractures. *Nursing Standard, 16*(36), 45–55.

Lee, H. Y. (2006). Comparison of effects among Tai-Chi exercise, aquatic exercise, and a self-help program for patients with knee osteoarthritis. *Taehan Kanho Hakhoe Chi 26*(3), 571–580.

Lee, T. K., & Maleski, R. (2002). Physical examination of the ankle for ankle pathology. *Clinics in Podiatric Medicine and Surgery, 19*(2), 251–269.

Longley, K. (2006). Fibromyalgia: Aetiology, diagnosis, symptoms and management. *British Journal of Nursing, 15*(13), 729–733.

Lynam, L. (2006). Assessment of acute foot and ankle sprains. *Emergency Nurse, 14*(4), 24–33, quiz 34.

Mangini, M. (1998). Physical assessment of the musculoskeletal system. *Nursing Clinics of North America, 33*(4), 643–652.

Martinez-Silvestrini, J. A., Newcomer, K. L., Gay, R. E., Schaefer, M. P., Kortebein, P., & Arendt, K. W. (2005). Chronic lateral epicondylitis: comparative effectiveness of a home exercise program including stretching alone versus stretching supplemented with eccentric or concentric strengthening. *Journal of Hand Therapy, 18*(4), 411–419, quiz 240.

McCaffrey, R., & Locsin, R. (2006). The effect of music on pain and acute confusion in older adults undergoing hip and knee surgery. *Holistic Nursing Practice, 20*(5), 218–224, quiz 225–226.

Miller, N. C., & Askew, A. E. (2007). Tibia fractures: An overview of evaluation and treatment. *Orthopaedic Nursing, 26*(4), 216–223, quiz 224–225.

Muirhead, G. (2000). Diagnosing bursitis of the hip. *Patient Care, 34*(5), 196–210.

Nelson, P. J., & Tucker, S. (2006). Developing an intervention to alter catastrophizing in persons with fibromyalgia. *Orthopaedic Nursing, 25*(3), 205–214.

Padua, L., Padua, R., LoMonaco, M., Aprile, I., & Tonali, P. (1999). Multiperspective assessment of carpal tunnel syndrome: A multi-center study. Italian CTS study group. *Neurology, 58*(8), 1554–1559.

Peterson, E. L. (2007). Fibromyalgia-management of a misunderstood disorder. *Journal of American Academy of Nurse Practitioners, 19*(7), 341–348.

Phillips, G., Reibach, A. M., & Slomiany, W. P. (2004). Diagnosis and management of scaphoid fractures. *American Family Physician, 70*(5), 879–892.

Polkinghorn, B. S. (2002). A novel method for assessing elbow pain resulting from epicondylitis. *Journal of Chiropractic Medicine, 1*(3), 117–121.

Ponzer, S., Skoog, A., & Bergstrom, G. (2003). The short musculoskeletal function assessment questionnaire (SMFA). *Acta Orthopaedica Scandinavica, 74*(6), 756–763.

Quaschnick, M. S. (1996). The diagnosis and management of plantar fasciitis. *The Nurse Practitioner, 21*(4), 50–65.

Rourke, K. (2003). An orthopedic nurse practitioner's practical guide to evaluating knee injuries. *Journal of Emergency Nursing, 29*(4), 366–372.

Singh, A. S., Chin, A., Paw, M. J., Bosscher, R. J., & Van Mechelen, W. (2006). Cross-sectional relationship between physical fitness components and functional performance in older persons living in long-term care facilities. *BMC Geriatrics,* Feb 7-6:4.

Smith, D. R., Mihashi, M., Adachi, Y., Hoga, H., & Ishitake, T. (2006). A detailed analysis of musculoskeletal disorder risk factors among Japanese nurses. *Journal of Safety Research, 37*(2), 195–200.

Snider, R. K. (Ed.). (2001). *Essentials of Musculoskeletal Care* (2nd ed.). Rosemont, IL: American Academy of Orthopedic Surgeons.

_____. (1997). *Essentials of Musculoskeletal Care.* Rosemont, IL: American Academy of Orthopedic Surgeons.

Steill, I. G., & Bennett, C. (2007). Implementation of clinical decision rules in the emergency department. *Society for Academic Emergency Medicine, 14*(11), 955–959.

Steill, I. G., Greenberg, G. H., McKnight, R. D., Nair, R. C., McDowell, I., & Worthington, J. R. (1992). A study to develop clinical decision rules for the use of radiography in acute ankle injuries. *Annals of Emergency Medicine, 21*(4), 384–390.

Steill, I. G., McKnight, R. D., Greenberg, G. H., McDowell, I., Nair, R. C., Wells, G. A., et al. (1994). Implementation of the Ottawa ankle rules. *JAMA, 271*(11), 827–832.

Strand, L. I., & Solveig, L. W. (1999). The sock test for evaluating activity limitation in patients with musculoskeletal pain. *Physical Therapy, 79*(2), 136–145.

Tsai, P. & Tak, S. (2003). Disease-specific pain measures for osteoarthritis of the knee or hip. *Geriatric Nursing 24*(2), 106–109.

Visovski, C. (2006). The effects of neuromuscular alterations in elders with cancer. *Seminars in Oncology Nursing, 22*(1), 26–42.

Wexler, R. K. (1998). The injured ankle. *American Family Physician, 57*(3), 474–480.

Williams, A., Dunning, T., & Manias, E. (2007). Continuity of care and general wellbeing of patients with comorbidities requiring joint replacement. *Journal of Advanced Nursing, 57*(3), 244–256.

Woodard, T. W., & Best, T. M. (2000). The painful shoulder: Part I. Clinical evaluation. *American Family Physician, 61*(10), 3079–3088.

Promote Health—Osteoporosis

International Osteoporosis Foundation (IOF). (2001). Osteoporosis. Available at http://www.osteofound.org

National Institute of Arthritis and Musculoskeletal and Skin Diseases (NIAMS). (2007). Osteoporosis. Available at http://www.niams.nih.gov/Health_Info/Bone/Osteoporosis/default.asp

National Institutes of Health (NIH). (2001). NIH Osteoporosis and related bone disease (ORBD) national resource center. Available at http://www.osteo.org

National Osteoporosis Foundation (NOF). (2001). Prevention: Who's at risk. Available at http://nof.org

National Osteoporosis Foundation (NOF). (2007). About osteoporosis. Available at http://www.nof.org

Understanding lactose intolerance (no date). Available at http://lactoseintolerant.org/02_about.html

Useful Website Resources

American Academy of Family Physicians, http://www.aafp.org

International Osteoporosis Foundation (IOF), www.iofbonehealth.org

National Association of Orthopaedic Nurses (NAON), 401 N Michigan Avenue, Suite 2200, Chicago, IL 60611; 1-800-289-6266; http://www.orthonurse.org

National Institute of Arthritis and Musculoskeletal and Skin Diseases, Office of Communications and Public Liaison, Bldg. 31, Room 4C05, 31 Center Drive, MSC 2350, Bethesda, MD 20892-2350; 1-301-496-8190; http://www.nih.gov/niams

National Institutes of Health, http://www.nihseniorhealth.gov

Structure and Function

The very complex neurologic system is responsible for coordinating and regulating all body functions. It consists of two structural components: the central nervous system (CNS) and the peripheral nervous system.

CENTRAL NERVOUS SYSTEM

The CNS encompasses the brain and spinal cord, which are covered by meninges, three layers of connective tissue that protect and nourish the CNS. The subarachnoid space surrounds the brain and spinal cord. The subarachnoid space is filled with cerebrospinal fluid, which is formed in the ventricles of the brain and flows through the ventricles into the space. This fluid-filled space cushions the brain and spinal cords, nourishes the CNS, and removes waste materials. Electrical activity of the CNS is governed by neurons located throughout the sensory and motor neural pathways. The CNS contains upper motor neurons that influence lower motor neurons, located mostly in the peripheral nervous system.

Brain

Located in the cranial cavity, the brain has four major divisions: the cerebrum, the diencephalon, the brain stem, and the cerebellum (Fig. 27-1).

Cerebrum

The cerebrum is divided into the right and left cerebral hemispheres, which are joined by the corpus callosum—a bundle of nerve fibers responsible for communication between the hemispheres. Each hemisphere sends and receives impulses from the opposite sides of the body and consists of four lobes (frontal, parietal, temporal, and occipital). The lobes are composed of a substance known as gray matter, which mediates higher-level functions such as memory, perception, communication, and initiation of voluntary movements. Consisting of aggregations of neuronal cell bodies, gray matter rims the surfaces of the cerebral hemispheres, forming the cerebral cortex.

Table 27-1 describes the specific functions of each lobe. Damage to a lobe results in impairment of the specific function directed by that lobe.

Diencephalon

The diencephalon lies beneath the cerebral hemispheres and consists of the thalamus and hypothalamus. Most sensory impulses travel through the gray matter of the thalamus, which is responsible for screening and directing the impulses to specific areas in the cerebral cortex. The hypothalamus (which is part of the autonomic nervous system, which is a part of the peripheral nervous system) is responsible for regulating many body functions including water balance, appetite, vital signs (temperature, blood pressure, pulse, and respiratory rate), sleep cycles, pain perception, and emotional status.

Brain Stem

Located between the cerebral cortex and the spinal cord, the brain stem consists of mostly nerve fibers and has three parts: the midbrain, pons, and medulla oblongata. The midbrain serves as a relay center for ear and eye reflexes and relays impulses between the higher cerebral centers and the lower pons, medulla, cerebellum, and spinal cord. The pons links the cerebellum to the cerebrum and the midbrain to the medulla. It is responsible for various reflex actions. The medulla oblongata contains the nuclei for cranial nerves and has centers that control and regulate respiratory function, heart rate and force, and blood pressure.

Cerebellum

The cerebellum, located behind the brain stem and under the cerebrum, also has two hemispheres. Although the cerebellum does not initiate movement, its primary functions include coordination and smoothing of voluntary movements, maintenance of equilibrium, and maintenance of muscle tone.

Spinal Cord

The spinal cord (Fig. 27-2) is located in the vertebral canal and extends from the medulla oblongata to the first lumbar vertebra. (Note that the spinal cord is not as long as the vertebral canal.) The inner part of the cord has an H-shaped appearance and is made up of two pairs of columns (dorsal and ventral) consisting of gray matter. The outer part is made up of white matter and surrounds the gray matter (Fig. 27-3). The spinal cord conducts sensory impulses up ascending tracts to the brain, conducts motor impulses down descending tracts to neurons that stimulate glands and muscles throughout the body, and is responsible for simple reflex activity. Reflex activity involves

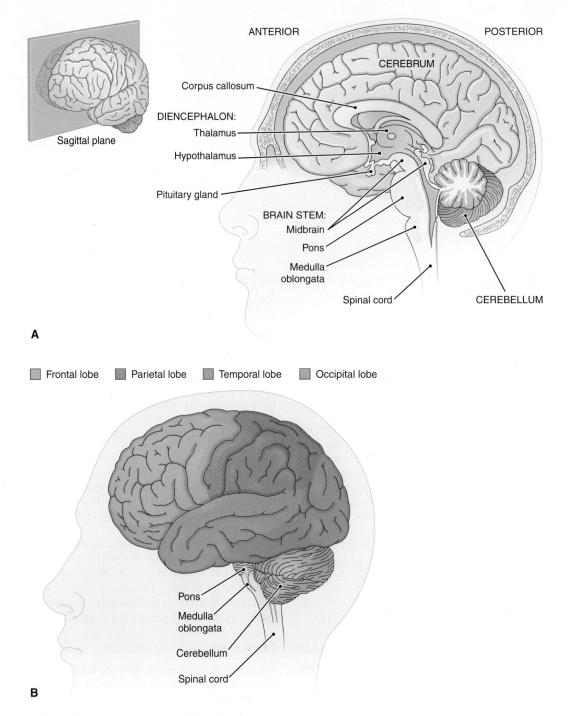

Figure 27-1 (A) Structures of the brain (sagittal section). (B) Lobes of the brain.

various neural structures. For example, the stretch reflex—the simplest type of reflex arc—involves one sensory neuron (afferent), one motor neuron (efferent), and one synapse. An example of this is the knee jerk, which is elicited by tapping the patellar tendon. More complex reflexes involve three or more neurons.

Neural Pathways

Sensory impulses travel to the brain by way of two ascending neural pathways (the spinothalamic tract and posterior columns) (Fig. 27-4). These impulses originate in the afferent fibers of the peripheral nerves and are carried through the posterior (dorsal) root into the spinal cord. Sensations of pain, temperature, and crude and light touch travel by way of the spinothalamic tract, whereas sensations of position, vibration, and fine touch travel by way of the posterior columns. Motor impulses are conducted to the muscles by two descending neural pathways: the pyramidal (corticospinal) tract and extrapyramidal tract (Fig. 27-5). The motor neurons of the pyramidal tract originate in the motor cortex and travel down to the medulla where they cross over to the opposite side then they travel down the spinal cord where they synapse with a lower motor neuron in the anterior horn of the spinal cord. These impulses are carried to muscles and produce voluntary movements that involve skill and purpose. The extrapyramidal

Table 27-1	Lobes of the Cerebral Hemispheres and Their Function
Lobe	**Function**
Frontal	Directs voluntary, skeletal actions (left side of lobe controls right side of body and right side of lobe controls left side of body). Also influences communication (talking and writing), emotions, intellect, reasoning ability, judgment, and behavior. Contains Broca's area, which is responsible for speech.
Parietal	Interprets tactile sensations, including touch, pain, temperature, shapes, and two-point discrimination.
Occipital	Influences the ability to read with understanding and is the primary visual receptor center.
Temporal	Receives and interprets impulses from the ear. Contains Wernicke's area, which is responsible for interpreting auditory stimuli.

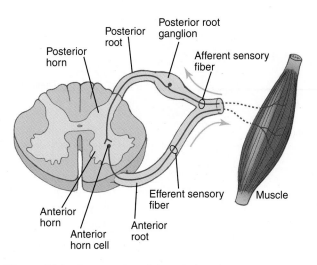

Figure 27-3 Cross-section of the spinal cord

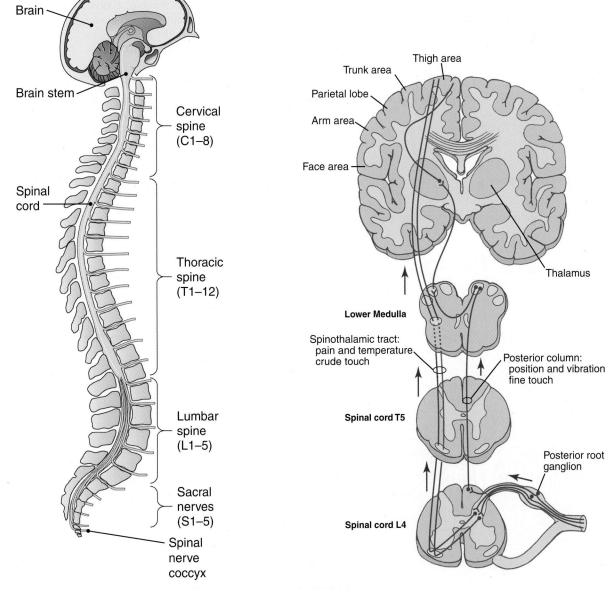

Figure 27-2 Spinal cord

Figure 27-4 Sensory (ascending) neural pathways

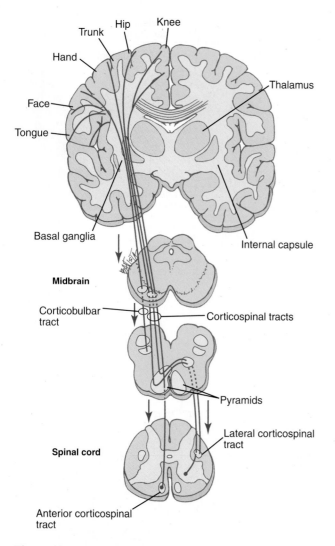

Figure 27-5   Motor (descending) neural pathways

tract motor neurons consist of those motor neurons that originate in the motor cortex, basal ganglia, brain stem, and spinal cord outside the pyramidal tract. They travel from the frontal lobe to the pons where they cross over to the opposite side and down the spinal cord where they connect with lower motor neurons that conduct impulses to the muscles. These neurons conduct impulses related to maintenance of muscle tone and body control.

PERIPHERAL NERVOUS SYSTEM

Carrying information to and from the CNS, the peripheral nervous system consists of 12 pairs of cranial nerves and 31 pairs of spinal nerves. These nerves are categorized as two types of fibers: somatic and autonomic. Somatic fibers carry CNS impulses to voluntary skeletal muscles, whereas autonomic fibers carry CNS impulses to smooth, involuntary muscles (in the heart and glands). The somatic nervous system mediates conscious, or voluntary, activities, whereas the autonomic nervous system mediates unconscious, or involuntary, activities.

Cranial Nerves

Twelve pairs of cranial nerves evolve from the brain or brain stem (Fig. 27-6) and transmit motor or sensory messages. Table 27-2 provides the number, names, type of impulse, and primary functions of the cranial nerves.

Spinal Nerves

Comprising 8 cervical, 12 thoracic, 5 lumbar, 5 sacral, and 1 coccygeal nerves, the 31 pairs of spinal nerves are named after the vertebrae below each one's exit point along the spinal cord (see Fig. 27-2). Each nerve is attached to the spinal cord by two nerve roots. The sensory (afferent) fiber enters through the dorsal (posterior) roots of the cord, whereas the motor (efferent) fiber exits through the ventral (anterior) roots of the cord. The sensory root of each spinal nerve innervates an area of the skin called a dermatome (Fig. 27-7).

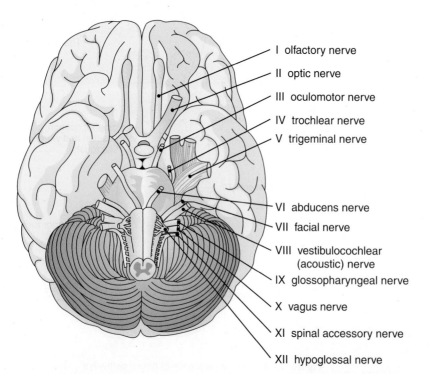

I   olfactory nerve
II   optic nerve
III   oculomotor nerve
IV   trochlear nerve
V   trigeminal nerve
VI   abducens nerve
VII   facial nerve
VIII   vestibulocochlear (acoustic) nerve
IX   glossopharyngeal nerve
X   vagus nerve
XI   spinal accessory nerve
XII   hypoglossal nerve

Figure 27-6   Cranial nerves, inferior view

Table 27.2	Cranial Nerves: Type and Function	

Cranial Nerve (Name)	Type of Impulse	Function
I (olfactory)	Sensory	Carries smell impulses from nasal mucous membrane to brain
II (optic)	Sensory	Carries visual impulses from eye to brain
III (oculomotor)	Motor	Contracts eye muscles to control eye movements (interior lateral, medial, and superior), constricts pupils, and elevates eyelids
IV (trochlear)	Motor	Contracts one eye muscle to control inferomedial eye movement
V (trigeminal)	Sensory	Carries sensory impulses of pain, touch, and temperature from the face to the brain
	Motor	Influences clenching and lateral jaw movements (biting, chewing)
VI (abducens)	Motor	Controls lateral eye movements
VII (facial)	Sensory	Contains sensory fibers for taste on anterior two thirds of tongue and stimulates secretions from salivary glands (submaxillary and sublingual) and tears from lacrimal glands
	Motor	Supplies the facial muscles and affects facial expressions (smiling, frowning, closing eyes)
VIII (acoustic, vestibulocochlear)	Sensory	Contains sensory fibers for hearing and balance
IX (glossopharyngeal)	Sensory	Contains sensory fibers for taste on posterior third of tongue and sensory fibers of the pharynx that result in the "gag reflex" when stimulated
	Motor	Provides secretory fibers to the parotid salivary glands; promotes swallowing movements
X (vagus)	Sensory	Carries sensations from the throat, larynx, heart, lungs, bronchi, gastrointestinal tract, and abdominal viscera
	Motor	Promotes swallowing, talking, and production of digestive juices
XI (spinal accessory)	Motor	Innervates neck muscles (sternocleidomastoid and trapezius) that promote movement of the shoulders and head rotation. Also promotes some movement of the larynx
XII (hypoglossal)	Motor	Innervates tongue muscles that promote the movement of food and talking

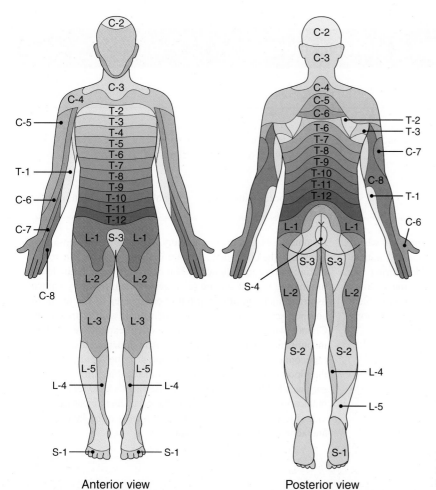

Anterior view   Posterior view

Figure 27-7 Anterior and posterior dermatomes (areas of skin innervated by spinal nerves)

AUTONOMIC NERVOUS SYSTEM

Some peripheral nerves have a special function associated with automatic activities; they are referred to as the autonomic nervous system. Autonomic nervous system impulses are carried by both cranial and spinal nerves. These impulses are carried from the CNS to the involuntary, smooth muscles that make up the walls of the heart and glands. The autonomic nervous system, which maintains the internal homeostasis of the body, incorporates the sympathetic and parasympathetic nervous systems. The sympathetic nervous system ("fight-or-flight" system) is activated during stress and elicits responses such as decreased gastric secretions, bronchiole dilatation, increased pulse rate, and pupil dilatation. These sympathetic fibers arise from the thoracolumbar level (T1 to L2) of the spinal cord. The parasympathetic nervous system functions to restore and maintain normal body functions, for example, by decreasing heart rate. The parasympathetic fibers arise from the craniosacral regions (S1 to S4 and cranial nerves III, VI, IX, and X).

Health Assessment

COLLECTING SUBJECTIVE DATA: THE NURSING HEALTH HISTORY

Problems with other body systems may affect the neurologic system, and neurologic system disorders can affect all other body systems. Regardless of the source of the neurologic problem, the client's total lifestyle and level of functioning are often affected. Because of their subjective nature, neurologic problems related to activities of daily living are typically detected through an in-depth nursing history. For example, problems with loss of concentration, loss of sensation, or dizziness are usually identified only through precise questioning during the interview with the client.

Clients who are experiencing symptoms associated with the neurologic system (such as headaches or memory loss) may be very fearful that they have a serious condition such as a metastatic brain tumor or a difficult-to-treat disease such as Alzheimer's. Fear of losing control and independence, along with threatened self-esteem or role performance, are common. The examiner needs to be sensitive to these fears and concerns because the client may decline to share important information with the examiner if these fears and concerns are not addressed.

(text continues on page 574)

HISTORY OF PRESENT HEALTH CONCERNS

Question	Rationale
Numbness and Tingling Do you experience any numbness or tingling? When and where does this occur?	Loss of sensation or tingling may occur with damage to the brain, spinal cord, or peripheral nerves.
Seizures Do you experience seizures? How often?	Seizures occur with epilepsy, metabolic disorders, head injuries, and high fevers.
Describe what happens before you have the seizure and where on your body the seizure starts. Does anything seem to initiate a seizure? Do you lose control of your bladder during the seizure? How do you feel afterward? Do you take medications for the seizures? Do you wear medical identification to alert others that you have seizures? Do you take safety precautions regarding driving or operating dangerous machinery?	In some cases, an aura (an auditory, visual, or motor sensation) forewarns the client that a seizure is about to occur. Where the seizure starts and what occurs before and after can aid in determining the type of seizure (e.g., generalized, formerly known as grand mal and affecting both hemispheres of the brain, or absence seizure, also known as petit mal) and its treatment. Clients with generalized seizures often experience bladder incontinence during the seizure. Anti-epileptic medications (anticonvulsants) must be distributed at a therapeutic level in the blood to be effective. Wearing a medical identification tag, such as a MedicAlert bracelet, and the client's knowledge of the medication regimen and the importance of safety measures provide information on the client's willingness to be involved in and adhere to the treatment plan.

continued

HISTORY OF PRESENT HEALTH CONCERNS *Continued*

Question	Rationale

Headaches

Do you experience headaches? When do they occur and what do they feel like? (See related questions in Chapter 14.)

See Chapter 14 for a description of various types of headaches. Morning headaches that subside after arising may be an early sign of increased intracranial pressure such as with a brain tumor.

Dizziness

Do you experience dizziness or lightheadedness or problems with balance or coordination? If so, how often? Does it occur with activity? Or have you experienced any falling? Do you have any clumsy movement?

Dizziness or lightheadedness may be related to carotid artery disease, cerebellar abscess, Meniere's disease, or inner ear infection. Imbalance and difficulty coordinating or controlling movements are seen in neurologic diseases involving the cerebellum, basal ganglia, extrapyramidal tracts, or the vestibular part of cranial nerve VIII (acoustic). Diminished cerebral blood flow and vestibular response may increase the risk of falls.

Senses

Have you noticed a decrease in your ability to smell or to taste?

A decrease in the ability to smell may be related to a dysfunction of cranial nerve I (olfactory) or a brain tumor. A decrease in the ability to taste may be related to dysfunction of cranial nerves VII (facial) or IX (glossopharyngeal).

 Decreased taste and scent sensation occurs normally in older adults.

Have you experienced any ringing in your ears or hearing loss?

Ringing in the ears and decreased ability to hear may occur with dysfunction of cranial nerve VIII (acoustic).

 There is a normal decrease in the older person's ability to hear.

Have you noticed any change in your vision?

Changes in vision may occur with dysfunction of cranial nerve II (optic), increased intracranial pressure, or brain tumors. Damage to cranial nerves III (oculomotor), IV (trochlear), or VI (abducens) may cause double or blurred vision. Transient blind spots may be an early sign of a cerebrovascular accident (CVA).

 There is a normal decrease in the older person's ability to see.

Difficulty Speaking

Do you have difficulty understanding when people are talking to you? Do you have difficulty making others understand you? Do you have difficulty forming words or verbally interpreting your thoughts?

Injury to the cerebral cortex can impair the ability to use or understand verbal language.

Difficulty Swallowing

Do you experience difficulty swallowing?

Difficulty swallowing may relate to CVA, Parkinson's disease, myasthenia gravis, Guillain-Barré syndrome, or dysfunction of cranial nerves IX (glossopharyngeal), X (vagus), or XII (hypoglossal).

Muscle Control

Have you lost bowel or bladder control or do you retain urine?

Loss of bowel control or urinary retention and bladder distention are seen with spinal cord injury or tumors.

continued on page 572

HISTORY OF PRESENT HEALTH CONCERNS *Continued*

Question	Rationale
Do you have muscle weakness? If so, where?	Unilateral weakness or paralysis may result from CVA, compression of the spinal cord, or nerve injury. Progressive weakness is a symptom of several nervous system diseases.
Do you experience any tremors? If so, where?	Tremors are typical in degenerative neurologic disorders, such as Parkinson's disease (three to six per second while muscles are at rest), or in cerebellar disease and multiple sclerosis (variable rate, and especially with intentional movement).
	Older adults may experience tremors with movement. Tremors may involve the hands, head (yes or no nodding), and the tongue, which may protrude back and forth. Such tremors are not associated with disease but they may cause embarrassment or emotional distress.
Memory Loss Do you experience any memory loss?	Recent memory (24-hour memory) is often impaired in amnestic disorders, Korsakoff's syndrome, delirium, and dementia. Remote memory (past dates and historical accounts) may be impaired in cerebral cortex disorders.

COLDSPA Example for Hand Numbness and Ache

Use the **COLDSPA** mnemonic as a guideline to collect needed information for each symptom the client shares. In addition, the following questions help elicit important information.

Mnemonic	Question	Client Response Example
Character	Describe the sign or symptom (feeling, appearance, sound, smell, or taste if applicable	"Numbness and aching in my right hand"
Onset	When did it begin?	"Since I started typing at my office 4 months ago"
Location	Where is it? Does it radiate? Does it occur anywhere else?	"At the center of my hand below the wrist"
Duration	How long does it last? Does it recur?	"It lasts for several hours and recurs"
Severity	How bad is it? or How much does it bother you?	"It hurts so much I cannot type for long and is beginning to affect my productivity at work"
Pattern	What makes it better or worse?	"It gets worse after I type for 10 minutes or more. It goes away when I rest it and quit typing."
Associated factors/How it **A**ffects the client	What other symptoms occur with it? How does it affect you?	"It also tingles at times."

PAST HEALTH HISTORY

Question	Rationale
Have you ever had any type of head injury with or without loss of consciousness (e.g., sports injury, auto accident, fall)? If so, describe any physical or mental changes that have occurred as a result. What type of treatment did you receive?	Head injuries, even if minor, can produce long-term neurologic deficits and affect level of functioning.
Have you ever had meningitis, encephalitis, injury to the spinal cord, or a stroke? If so, describe any physical or mental changes that have occurred as a result. What type of treatment did you receive?	These disorders can affect the long-term physical and mental status of the client.

continued

FAMILY HISTORY

Question	Rationale
Do you have a family history of high blood pressure, stroke, Alzheimer's disease, epilepsy, brain cancer, or Huntington's chorea?	These disorders may be genetic. Some tend to run in families.

LIFESTYLE AND HEALTH PRACTICES

Question	Rationale
Do you take any prescription or nonprescription medications? How much alcohol do you drink? Do you use recreational drugs such as marijuana, tranquilizers, barbiturates, or cocaine?	Prescription and nonprescription drugs can cause various neurologic symptoms such as tremors or dizziness, altered level of consciousness, decreased response times, and changes in mood and temperament.
Do you smoke?	Nicotine, which is found in cigarettes, constricts the blood vessels, which decreases blood flow to the brain. Cigarette smoking is a risk factor for CVA. See Promote Health—Cerebrovascular Accident (Stroke).
Do you wear your seat belt when riding in vehicles? Do you wear protective headgear when riding a bicycle or playing sports?	Seat belts and protective headgear can prevent head injury.
Describe your usual daily diet.	Peripheral neuropathy can result from a deficiency in niacin, folic acid, or vitamin B_{12}.
Have you ever had prolonged exposure to lead, insecticides, pollutants, or other chemicals?	Prolonged exposure to these substances can alter neurologic status.
Do you frequently lift heavy objects or perform repetitive motions?	Intervertebral disc injuries may result when heavy objects are lifted improperly. Peripheral nerve injuries can occur from repetitive movements.
Can you perform your normal activities of daily living?	Neurologic symptoms and disorders often negatively affect the ability to perform activities of daily living.
Has your neurologic problem changed the way you view yourself? Describe.	Low self-esteem and body image problems may lead to depression and changes in role functions.
Has your neurologic problem added much stress to your life? Describe.	Neurologic problems can impair ability to fulfill role responsibilities, greatly increasing stress. Stress can increase existing neurologic symptoms.

PROMOTE HEALTH
Cerebrovascular Accident (Stroke)

Overview
Cerebrovascular accident (CVA), commonly called stroke, results when the blood supply to an area of the brain is disrupted. This blood supply disruption can be caused by thrombosis, embolism, infarction, or hemorrhage. All four of these may result from underlying cerebrovascular disease.

Stroke is the leading neurologic problem in the United States and is ranked third overall in cause of death. African Americans have a higher incidence of stroke. They experience stroke at an earlier age, and they are twice as likely to die of stroke as Hispanics or whites, but Hispanics have a higher risk of CVA than whites. Strokes can also cause serious disability. Approximately 5.4 million people live with some type of disability caused by a stroke; many of them require help with their activities of daily living.

continued on page 574

PROMOTE HEALTH
Cerebrovascular Accident (Stroke) *Continued*

Risk Factors

- Older adulthood: risk doubles each decade after age 55
- Male sex (slightly higher risk)
- African American
- History of stroke or transient ischemic attack (TIA)
- Hypertension
- Smoking
- Chronic alcohol intake (more than two drinks per day)
- History of cardiovascular disease such as coronary artery disease, heart failure, rhythm abnormalities (especially atrial fibrillation), mitral valve prolapse
- Sleep apnea
- High serum levels of fibrinogen, beta-lipoproteins, cholesterol, hematocrit
- Diabetes mellitus
- Drug abuse (especially cocaine and methamphetamines)
- High-dose oral contraceptives (especially with coexisting hypertension, smoking)
- High estrogen levels
- Postmenopausal woman
- Overweight
- Sedentary lifestyle
- Newly industrializing environment
- Sickle cell anemia
- Family history of stroke

Teach Risk Reduction Tips

- Monitor blood pressure regularly; exercise regularly.
- Stop smoking, especially if taking oral contraceptives. (Quitting smoking reduces risk to non-smoker level in 5 years.)
- Limit intake of alcohol to less than three drinks per day.
- Schedule regular health care checkups.
- Adhere to a diet low in fat and cholesterol; follow cardiovascular disease risk factor modifications.
- Have regular blood tests to measure cholesterol and hematocrit levels.
- If diabetic, follow diabetes treatment plan.
- Monitor blood sugar regularly, if diabetic.
- Avoid use of drugs such as cocaine and methamphetamines.

Warning Signs of Stroke

- Sudden numbness (face, arm, leg), especially if on only one side of body
- Sudden confusion, trouble speaking or understanding speech
- Sudden vision problems in one or both eyes
- Sudden trouble walking, dizziness, loss of balance or coordination
- Sudden severe headache with no known cause

COLLECTING OBJECTIVE DATA: PHYSICAL EXAMINATION

A complete neurologic examination consists of evaluating the following five areas:

- Mental status
- Cranial nerves
- Motor and Cerebellar System
- Sensory system
- Reflexes

The examinations may be performed in an order that moves from a level of higher cerebral integration to a lower level of reflex activity.

Mental status examinations provide information about cerebral cortex function. Cerebral abnormalities disturb the client's intellectual ability, communication ability, or emotional behaviors. A mental status examination is often performed at the beginning of the head-to-toe examination because it provides clues regarding the validity of the subjective information provided by the client. For example, if the nurse finds that the client's thought processes are distorted and memory is impaired, another means of obtaining necessary subjective data must be identified (Refer to Chapter 6, Assessing Mental Status and Psychosocial Developmental Level.)

The *cranial nerve evaluation* provides information regarding the transmission of motor and sensory messages, primarily to the head and neck. Many of the cranial nerves are evaluated during the head, neck, eye, and ear examinations.

The *motor and cerebellar systems* are assessed to determine functioning of the pyramidal and extrapyramidal tracts. The cerebellar system is assessed to determine the client's level of balance and coordination. The motor system examination is usually performed during the musculoskeletal examination.

Examining the *sensory system* provides information regarding the integrity of the spinothalamic tract, posterior columns of the spinal cord, and parietal lobes of the brain, whereas testing *reflexes* provides clues to the integrity of deep and superficial reflexes. Deep reflexes depend on an intact sensory nerve, a functional synapse in the spinal cord, an intact motor nerve, a neuromuscular junction, and competent muscles. Superficial reflexes depend on skin receptors rather than muscles.

If meningitis is suspected, the examiner may try to elicit Brudzinski's and Kernig's signs, which are characteristic of meningeal irritation. Sometimes, a complete neurologic examination is unnecessary. In such cases, the nurse performs a "neuro check"—a brief screening of the client's neurologic status. A neuro check includes the following assessment points:

- Level of consciousness
- Pupillary checks
- Movement and strength of extremities
- Sensation in extremities
- Vital signs

This type of assessment is useful in an emergency situation and when frequent assessments are needed during an acute phase of illness to detect rapid changes in neurologic status. A neuro check is also useful for a client who has already had a complete neurologic examination but needs to be rechecked for changes related to therapy or other conditions.

Preparing the Client

Prepare for the neurologic examination by asking the client to remove all clothing and jewelry and to put on an examination gown. Initially have the client sit comfortably on the examination table or bed but explain to her that several different position changes are necessary throughout the different parts of the examination. Assure the client that each position will be explained before the start of the particular examination.

Explain also that the examination will take a considerable amount of time to perform and that you will provide rest periods as needed. If the client is elderly or physically weak, the examination can be divided into parts and performed over two different time periods. Explain that actions the client will be asked to perform, such as counting backward or hopping on one foot, may seem unusual but that these activities are parts of a comprehensive neurologic evaluation.

➤ **Clinical Tip** • *Demonstrate what you want the client to do—especially during the cerebellar examination, when the client will need to perform several different coordinated movements.*

Equipment

General

- Examination gloves

Cranial Nerve Examination

- Cotton-tipped applicators
- Newsprint to read
- Ophthalmoscope
- Paper clip
- Penlight
- Snellen chart

- Sterile cotton ball
- Substances to smell or taste such as soap, coffee, vanilla, salt, sugar, lemon juice
- Tongue depressor
- Tuning fork

Motor and Cerebellar Examination

- Tape measure

Sensory Examination

- Cotton ball
- Objects to feel such as a quarter or key
- Paper clip
- Test tubes containing hot and cold water
- Tuning fork (low-pitched)

Reflex Examination

- Cotton-tipped applicator
- Reflex (percussion) hammer

Physical Assessment

Prior to the examination, review these key points:

- Understand what is meant by mental status and level of consciousness.
- Know how to correctly apply and interpret mental status examinations and the Glasgow Coma Scale (GCS).
- Identify the 12 cranial nerves and their sensory and motor functions.
- Thoroughly assess movement, balance, coordination, sensation, and reflexes during physical examination.
- Know how to use a reflex hammer (Equipment Spotlight 27-1).
- Coordinate patient education—particularly in regard to risks related to stroke—with the health interview and physical examination.

(text continues on page 592)

EQUIPMENT SPOTLIGHT 27-1   **How to Use the Reflex Hammer**

The reflex (or percussion) hammer is used to elicit deep tendon reflexes. Proceed as follows to elicit a deep tendon reflex:

1. Encourage the client to relax because tenseness can inhibit a normal response.
2. Position the client properly.
3. Hold the handle of the reflex hammer between your thumb and index finger so it swings freely.
4. Palpate the tendon that you will need to strike to elicit the reflex.
5. Using a rapid wrist movement, briskly strike the tendon. Observe the response. Avoid a slow or weak movement for striking.
6. Compare the response of one side with the other.

7. To prevent pain, use the pointed end to strike a small area, and the wider, blunt (flat) end to strike a wider area or a more tender area.
8. Use a reinforcement technique, which causes other muscles to contract and thus increases reflex activity, to assist in eliciting a response if no response can be elicited.
9. For arm reflexes, ask the client to clench his or her jaw or to squeeze one thigh with the opposite hand, then immediately strike the tendon. For leg reflexes, ask the client to lock the fingers of both hands and pull them against each other, then immediately strike the tendon.

continued on page 576

EQUIPMENT SPOTLIGHT 27-1   **How to Use the Reflex Hammer** *Continued*

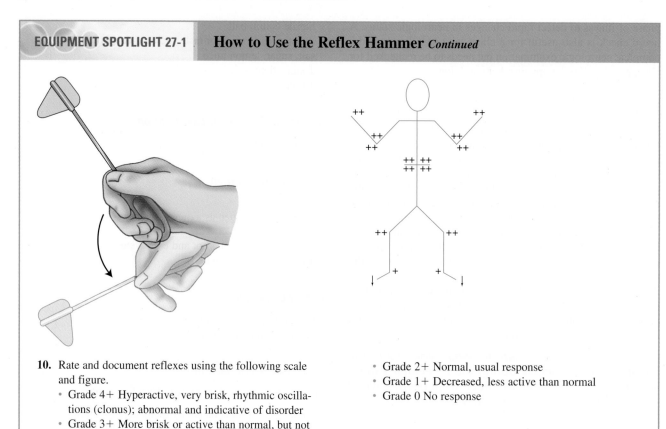

10. Rate and document reflexes using the following scale and figure.
    • Grade 4+ Hyperactive, very brisk, rhythmic oscillations (clonus); abnormal and indicative of disorder
    • Grade 3+ More brisk or active than normal, but not indicative of a disorder
    • Grade 2+ Normal, usual response
    • Grade 1+ Decreased, less active than normal
    • Grade 0 No response

PHYSICAL ASSESSMENT

Assessment Procedure	Normal Findings	Abnormal Findings

Cranial Nerves (CN)

Assessment Procedure	Normal Findings	Abnormal Findings
Test CN I (olfactory). For all assessments of the cranial nerves, have client sit in a comfortable position at your eye level. Ask the client to clear the nose to remove any mucus then to close eyes, occlude one nostril, and identify a scented object that you are holding such as soap, coffee, or vanilla (Fig. 27-8). Repeat procedure for the other nostril.	Client correctly identifies scent presented to each nostril. Some older clients' sense of smell may be decreased.	Inability to smell (neurogenic anosmia) or identify the correct scent may indicate olfactory tract lesion or tumor or lesion of the frontal lobe. Loss of smell may also be congenital or due to other causes such as nasal disease, smoking, and use of cocaine.
Test CN II (optic). Use a Snellen chart to assess vision in each eye (see Chapter 15 for additional information).	Client has 20/20 vision OD (right eye) and OS (left eye).	Abnormal findings include difficulty reading Snellen chart; missing letters, and squinting.
Ask the client to read a newspaper or magazine paragraph to assess near vision.	Client reads print at 14 inches without difficulty.	Client reads print by holding closer than 14 inches or holds print farther away as in presbyopia, which occurs with aging.

continued

Assessment Procedure	Normal Findings	Abnormal Findings
Assess visual fields of each eye by confrontation.	Full visual fields (see Chapter 15).	Loss of visual fields may be seen in retinal damage or detachment, with lesions of the optic nerve, or with lesions of the parietal cortex (see Chapter 15).
Use an ophthalmoscope to view the retina and optic disc of each eye.	Round red reflex is present, optic disc is 1.5 mm, round or slightly oval, well-defined margins, creamy pink with paler physiologic cup. Retina is pink (see Chapter 15).	Papilledema (swelling of the optic nerve) results in blurred optic disc margins and dilated, pulsating veins. Papilledema occurs with increased intracranial pressure from intracranial hemorrhage or a brain tumor. Optic atrophy occurs with brain tumors (see Chapter 15).
Assess CN III (oculomotor), IV (trochlear), and VI (abducens). Inspect margins of the eyelids of each eye.	Eyelid covers about 2 mm of the iris.	Ptosis (drooping of the eyelid) is seen with weak eye muscles such as in myasthenia gravis.
Assess extraocular movements. If nystagmus is noted, determine the direction of the fast and slow phases of movement (see Chapter 15).	Eyes move in a smooth, coordinated motion in all directions (the six cardinal fields).	Some abnormal eye movements and possible causes follow: Nystagmus: rhythmic oscillation of the eyes), *cerebellar disorders.* Limited eye movement through the six cardinal fields of gaze, *increased intracranial pressure.* Paralytic strabismus, *paralysis of the oculomotor, trochlear, or abducens nerves* (see Chapter 15).
Assess pupillary response to light (direct and indirect) and accommodation in both eyes (see Chapter 15).	Bilateral illuminated pupils constrict simultaneously. Pupil opposite the one illuminated constricts simultaneously.	Some abnormalities and their implications follow: Dilated pupil (6 to 7 mm), *oculomotor nerve paralysis.* Argyll Robertson pupils, *CNS syphilis, meningitis, brain tumor, alcoholism.* Constricted, fixed pupils, *narcotics abuse or damage to the pons.* Unilaterally dilated pupil unresponsive to light or accommodation, *damage to cranial nerve III (oculomotor).* Constricted pupil unresponsive to light or accommodation, *lesions of the sympathetic nervous system.* Bilateral muscle weakness is seen with peripheral or central nervous system dysfunction. Unilateral weakness may indicate a lesion of cranial nerve V (trigeminal).

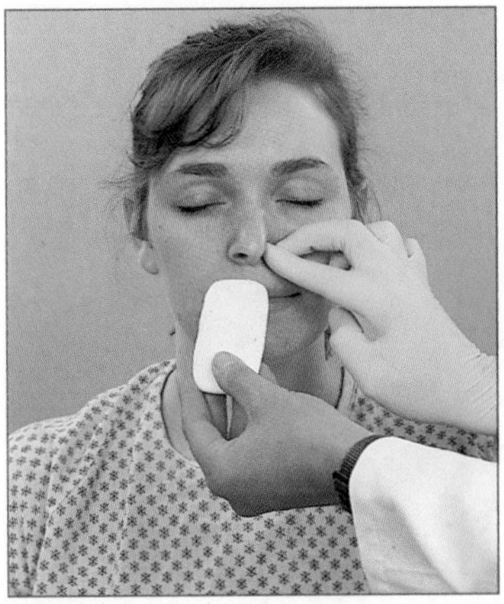

Figure 27-8   Testing cranial nerve I (© B. Proud.)

continued

PHYSICAL ASSESSMENT *Continued*

Assessment Procedure	Normal Findings	Abnormal Findings
Assess CN V (trigeminal). Test motor function. Ask the client to clench the teeth while you palpate the temporal and masseter muscles for contraction (Fig. 27-9). ➤ *Clinical Tip • This test may be difficult to perform and evaluate in the client without teeth.*	Temporal and masseter muscles contract bilaterally.	
Test sensory function. Tell the client: "I am going to touch your forehead, cheeks, and chin with the sharp or dull side of this safety pin or paper clip (a paper clip is less hazardous). Please close your eyes and tell me if you feel a sharp or dull sensation. Also tell me where you feel it" (Fig. 27-10). Vary the sharp and dull stimulus in the facial areas and compare sides. Repeat test for light touch with a wisp of cotton. ➤ *Clinical Tip • To avoid transmitting infection, use a new object with each client. Avoid "stabbing" the client with the object's sharp side.*	The client correctly identifies sharp and dull stimuli and light touch to the forehead, cheeks, and chin.	Inability to feel and correctly identify facial stimuli occurs with lesions of the trigeminal nerve or lesions in the spinothalamic tract or posterior columns.

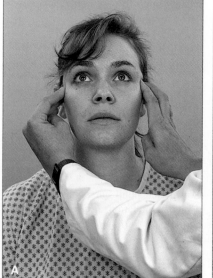
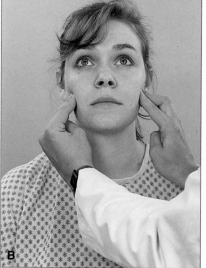

Figure 27-9 Testing motor function of cranial nerve V: **(A)** palpating temporal muscles; **(B)** palpating masseter muscles (© B. Proud.)

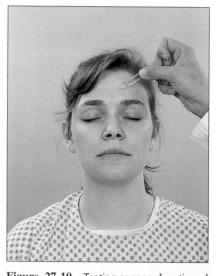

Figure 27-10 Testing sensory function of cranial nerve V: dull stimulus using a paper clip (© B. Proud).

continued

Assessment Procedure	Normal Findings	Abnormal Findings
Test corneal reflex. Ask the client to look away and up while you lightly touch the cornea with a fine wisp of cotton (Fig. 27-11). Repeat on the other side.	Eyelids blink bilaterally. ➤ *Clinical Tip • This reflex may be absent or reduced in clients who wear contact lenses.*	An absent corneal reflex may be noted with lesions of the trigeminal nerve or lesions of the motor part of cranial nerve VII (facial).
Test CN VII (facial). Test motor function. Ask the client to • Smile • Frown and wrinkle forehead (Fig. 27-12A) • Show teeth • Puff out cheeks (Fig. 27-12B) • Purse lips • Raise eyebrows • Close eyes tightly against resistance	Client smiles, frowns, wrinkles forehead, shows teeth, puffs out cheeks, purses lips, raises eyebrows, and closes eyes against resistance. Movements are symmetrical.	Inability to close eyes, wrinkle forehead, or raise forehead along with paralysis of the lower part of the face on the affected side is seen with Bell's palsy (a peripheral injury to cranial nerve VII [facial]). Paralysis of the lower part of the face on the opposite side affected may be seen with a central lesion that affects the upper motor neurons such as from CVA.
Sensory function is not routinely tested. If it is, however, touch the anterior two-thirds of the tongue with a moistened applicator dipped in salt, sugar, or lemon juice and ask the client to identify the flavor. If the client is unsuccessful, repeat the test using one of the other solutions. If needed, repeat the test using the remaining solution. ➤ *Clinical Tip • Make sure the client leaves the tongue protruded to identify the flavor. Otherwise the substance may move to the posterior third of the tongue (vagus nerve innervation). The posterior portion is tested similarly to evaluate functioning of cranial nerves IX and X. The client should rinse the mouth with water between each taste test.*	Client identifies correct flavor. 👓 In some older clients, the sense of taste may be decreased.	Inability to identify correct flavor on anterior two-thirds of the tongue suggests impairment of cranial nerve VII (facial).

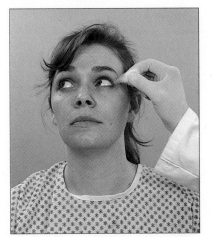

Figure 27-11 Testing corneal reflex (© B. Proud).

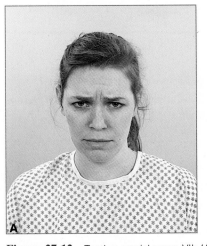
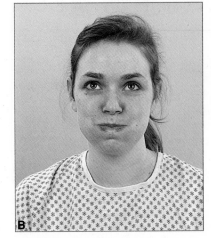

Figure 27-12 Testing cranial nerve VII: **(A)** frowning and wrinkling forehead; **(B)** puffing out cheeks (© B. Proud).

continued

PHYSICAL ASSESSMENT *Continued*

Assessment Procedure	Normal Findings	Abnormal Findings
Test CN VIII (acoustic/vestibulocochlear). Test the client's hearing ability in each ear and perform the Weber and Rinne tests to assess the cochlear (auditory) component of cranial nerve VIII (see Chapter 16, Ears, for detailed procedures). *Note:* The vestibular component, responsible for equilibrium, is not routinely tested. In comatose clients, the test is used to determine integrity of the vestibular system. (See a neurology textbook for detailed testing procedures.)	Client hears whispered words from 1 to 2 feet. *Weber test:* Vibration heard equally well in both ears. *Rinne test:* AC > BC (air conduction is twice as long as bone conduction).	Vibratory sound lateralizes to good ear in sensorineural loss. Air conduction is longer than bone conduction but not twice as long, in a sensorineural loss (see Chapter 16).
Test CN IX (glossopharyngeal) and X (vagus). Test motor function. Ask the client to open mouth wide and say "ah" while you use a tongue depressor on the client's tongue (Fig. 27-13).	Uvula and soft palate rise bilaterally and symmetrically on phonation.	Soft palate does not rise with bilateral lesions of cranial nerve X (vagus). Unilateral rising of the soft palate and deviation of the uvula to the normal side are seen with a unilateral lesion of cranial nerve X (vagus).
Test the gag reflex by touching the posterior pharynx with the tongue depressor. Warn the client that you are going to do this and that the test may feel a little uncomfortable.	Gag reflex intact. Some normal clients may have a reduced or absent gag reflex.	An absent gag reflex may be seen with lesions of cranial nerve IX (glossopharyngeal) or X (vagus).
Check the client's ability to swallow by giving the client a drink of water. Also note the client's voice quality.	Client swallows without difficulty. No hoarseness noted.	Dysphagia or hoarseness may indicate a lesion of cranial nerve IX (glossopharyngeal) or X (vagus) or other neurologic disorder.

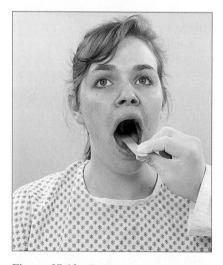

Figure 27-13 Testing cranial nerves IX and X: checking uvula rise and gag reflex (© B. Proud).

continued

Assessment Procedure	Normal Findings	Abnormal Findings
Test CN XI (spinal accessory). Ask the client to shrug the shoulders against resistance to assess the trapezius muscle (Fig. 27-14).	There is symmetric, strong contraction of the trapezius muscles.	Asymmetric muscle contraction or drooping of the shoulder may be seen with paralysis or muscle weakness due to neck injury or torticollis.
Ask the client to turn the head against resistance, first to the right then to the left, to assess the sternocleidomastoid muscle (Fig. 27-15).	There is strong contraction of sternocleidomastoid muscle on side opposite the turned face.	Atrophy with fasciculations may be seen with peripheral nerve disease.
Test CN XII (hypoglossal). To assess strength and mobility of the tongue, ask the client to protrude tongue, move it to each side against the resistance of a tongue depressor, then put it back in the mouth.	Tongue movement is symmetric and smooth and bilateral strength is apparent.	Fasciculations and atrophy of the tongue may be seen with peripheral nerve disease. Deviation to the affected side is seen with a unilateral lesion.

Motor and Cerebellar Systems

Assess condition and movement of muscles. Assess the size and symmetry of all muscle groups (see Chapter 26 for detailed procedures).	Muscles are fully developed and symmetric in size (bilateral sides may vary 1 cm from each other). Some older clients may have reduced muscle mass from degeneration of muscle fibers.	Muscle atrophy may be seen in diseases of the lower motor neurons or muscle disorders (see Chapter 26).
Assess the strength and tone of all muscle groups (see Chapter 26).	Relaxed muscles contract voluntarily and show mild, smooth resistance to passive movement. All muscle groups equally strong against resistance, without flaccidity, spasticity, or rigidity.	Soft, limp, flaccid muscles are seen with lower motor neuron involvement. Spastic muscle tone is noted with involvement of the corticospinal motor tract. Rigid muscles that resist passive movement are seen with abnormalities of the extrapyramidal tract.

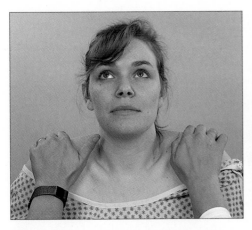

Figure 27-14 Testing cranial nerve XI: assessing strength of trapezius muscle (© B. Proud).

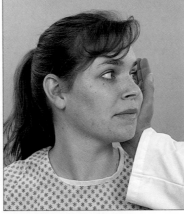

Figure 27-15 Testing cranial nerve XI: assessing strength of sternocleidomastoid muscle (© B. Proud).

continued

PHYSICAL ASSESSMENT *Continued*

Assessment Procedure	Normal Findings	Abnormal Findings
Note any unusual involuntary movements such as fasciculations, tics, or tremors.	No fasciculations, tics, or tremors are noted. Some older clients may normally have hand or head tremors or dyskinesia (repetitive movements of the lips, jaw, or tongue).	Abnormal findings include • Tic (twitch of the face, head, or shoulder) from stress or neurologic disorder • Unusual, bizarre face, tongue, jaw, or lip movements from chronic psychosis or long-term use of psychotropic drugs • Tremors (rhythmic, oscillating movements) from Parkinson's disease, cerebellar disease, multiple sclerosis (with movement), hyperthyroidism, or anxiety • Slow, twisting movements in the extremities and face from cerebral palsy • Brief, rapid, irregular, jerky movements (at rest) from Huntington's chorea
Evaluate balance. To assess gait, ask the client to walk naturally across the room. Note posture, freedom of movement, symmetry, rhythm, and balance. ➤ *Clinical Tip • It is best to assess gait when the client is not aware that you are directly observing her gait.*	Gait is steady; opposite arm swings. Some older clients may have a slow and uncertain gait. The base may become wider and shorter and the hips and knees may be flexed for a bent-forward appearance.	Gait and balance can be affected by disorders of the motor, sensory, vestibular, and cerebellar systems. Therefore, a thorough examination of all systems is necessary when an uneven or unsteady gait is noted (see Abnormal Findings 27-1 for more information about abnormal gaits).
Ask the client to walk in heel-to-toe fashion (tandem walking; Fig. 27-16), next on the heels, then on the toes. Demonstrate the walk first; then stand close by in case the client loses balance.	Client maintains balance with tandem walking. Walks on heels and toes with little difficulty. For some older clients, this examination may be very difficult.	An uncoordinated or unsteady gait that did not appear with the client's normal walking may become apparent with tandem walking or when walking on heels and toes.

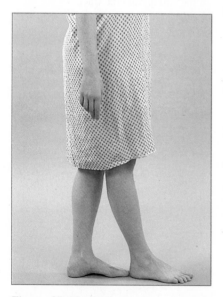

Figure 27-16 Testing balance: tandem walking (© B. Proud).

continued

Assessment Procedure	Normal Findings	Abnormal Findings
Perform the Romberg test. Ask the client to stand erect with arms at side and feet together. Note any unsteadiness or swaying. Then with the client in the same body position, ask the client to close the eyes for 20 seconds. Again note any imbalance or swaying. ➤ *Clinical Tip* • *Stand near the client to prevent a fall should she lose balance.*	Client stands erect with minimal swaying with eyes both open and closed.	Positive Romberg test: Swaying and moving feet apart to prevent fall is seen with disease of the posterior columns, vestibular dysfunction, or cerebellar disorders.
Now ask the client to stand on one foot and to bend the knee of the leg he or she is standing on (Fig. 27-17). Then ask the client to hop on that foot. Repeat on the other foot. 👓 This test is often impossible for the older adult to perform because of decreased flexibility and strength. Moreover, it is not usual to perform this test with the older adult because it puts the client at risk.	Bends knee while standing on one foot; hops on each foot without losing balance.	Inability to stand or hop on one foot is seen with muscle weakness or disease of the cerebellum.
Assess coordination. Demonstrate the finger-to-nose test to assess accuracy of movements then ask the client to extend and hold arms out to the side with eyes open. Next say "Touch the tip of your nose first with your right index finger, then with your left index finger. Repeat this three times" (Fig. 27-18). Next ask the client to repeat these movements with eyes closed.	Client touches finger to nose with smooth, accurate movements with little hesitation. ➤ *Clinical Tip* • *When assessing coordination of movements, bear in mind that normally the client's dominant side may be more coordinated than the nondominant side.*	Loss of positional sense and inability to touch tip of nose are seen with cerebellar disease.

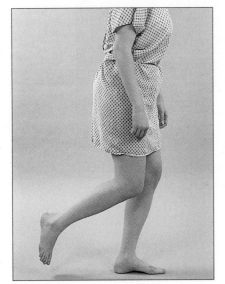

Figure 27-17 Tandem balance: standing and hopping on one foot (© B. Proud).

continued

PHYSICAL ASSESSMENT Continued

Assessment Procedure	Normal Findings	Abnormal Findings
Next assess rapid alternating movements. Have the client sit down. First ask the client to touch each finger to the thumb and to increase the speed as the client progresses. Repeat with the other side.	Client touches each finger to thumb rapidly. For some older clients, rapid alternating movements are difficult because of decreased reaction time and flexibility.	Inability to perform rapid alternating movements may be seen with cerebellar disease, upper motor neuron weakness, or extrapyramidal disease.
Next ask the client to put the palms of both hands down on both legs, then turn the palms up, then turn the palms down again (Fig. 27-19). Ask the client to increase the speed.	Client rapidly turns palms up and down.	Uncoordinated movements or tremors are abnormal findings. They are seen with cerebellar disease (dysdiadochokinesia).
Perform the heel-to-shin test. Ask the client to lie down (supine position) and to slide the heel of the right foot down the left shin (Fig. 27-20). Repeat with the other heel and shin.	Client is able to run each heel smoothly down each shin.	Deviation of heel to one side or the other may be seen in cerebellar disease.

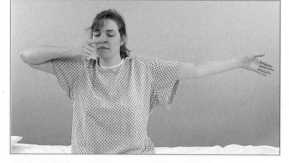

Figure 27-18 Testing coordination: finger-to-nose test (© B. Proud).

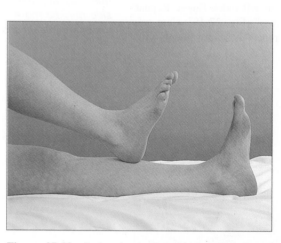

Figure 27-20 Performing heel-to-shin test (© B. Proud).

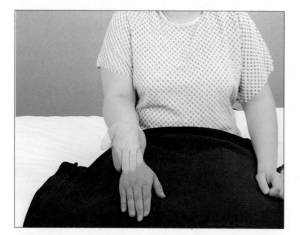

Figure 27-19 Testing rapid alternating movements: palms (© B. Proud).

continued

Assessment Procedure	Normal Findings	Abnormal Findings

Sensory System

Assess light touch, pain, and temperature sensations. For each test, ask clients to close both eyes and tell you what they feel and where they feel it. Scatter stimuli over the distal and proximal parts of all extremities and the trunk to cover most of the dermatomes. It is not necessary to cover the entire body surface unless you identify abnormal symptoms such as pain, numbness, or tingling.

To test light touch sensation, use a wisp of cotton to touch the client (Fig. 27-21).

To test pain sensation, use the blunt (Fig. 27-22A) and sharp ends (Fig. 27-22B) of a safety pin or paper clip. To test temperature sensation, use test tubes filled with hot and cold water.

➤ *Clinical Tip* • *Test temperature sensation only if abnormalities are found in the client's ability to perceive light touch and pain sensations. Temperature and pain sensations travel in the lateral spinothalamic tract, so temperature need not be tested if pain sensation is intact.*

Client correctly identifies light touch.

👓 In some older clients, light touch and pain sensations may be decreased.

Client correctly differentiates between dull and sharp sensations and hot and cold temperatures over various body parts.

Many disorders can alter a person's ability correctly to perceive sensations. These include peripheral neuropathies (due to diabetes mellitus, folic acid deficiencies, and alcoholism) and lesions of the ascending spinal cord, the brain stem, cranial nerves, and cerebral cortex.

Client reports
• Anesthesia (absence of touch sensation)
• Hypesthesia (decreased sensitivity to touch)
• Hyperesthesia (increased sensitivity to touch)
• Analgesia (absence of pain sensation)
• Hypalgesia (decreased sensitivity to pain)
• Hyperalgesia (increased sensitivity to pain)

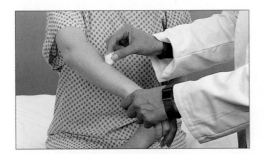

Figure 27-21 Testing light touch sensation (© B. Proud).

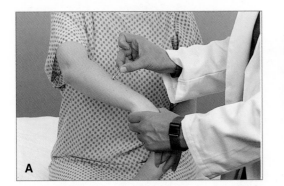
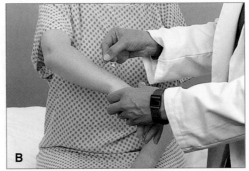

Figure 27-22 Testing pain sensation: **(A)** dull stimulus and **(B)** sharp stimulus (© B. Proud).

continued

PHYSICAL ASSESSMENT *Continued*

Assessment Procedure	Normal Findings	Abnormal Findings
Test vibratory sensation. Strike a low-pitched tuning fork on the heel of your hand and hold the base on a bony surface of the fingers or big toe (Fig. 27-23). Ask the client to indicate what he feels. Repeat on the other side. ➤ *Clinical Tip • If vibratory sensation is intact distally, then it is intact proximally.*	Client correctly identifies sensation. Vibratory sensation at the ankles usually decreases after age 70.	Inability to sense vibrations may be seen in posterior column disease or peripheral neuropathy (e.g., as seen with diabetes or chronic alcohol abuse).
Test sensitivity to position. Ask the client to close both eyes. Then move the client's toes or a finger up or down (Fig. 27-24). Ask the client to tell you the direction it is moved. Repeat on the other side. ➤ *Clinical Tip • If position sense is intact distally, then it is intact proximally.*	Client correctly identifies directions of movements. In some older clients, the sense of position of great toe may be reduced.	Inability to identify the directions of the movements may be seen in posterior column disease or peripheral neuropathy (e.g., as seen with diabetes or chronic alcohol abuse).
Assess tactile discrimination (fine touch). Remember that the client should have her eyes closed. To test stereognosis, place a familiar object such as a quarter, paperclip, or key in the client's hand and ask the client to identify it (Fig. 27-25). Repeat with another object in the other hand.	Client correctly identifies object.	Inability to correctly identify objects (astereognosis), area touched, number written in hand, discriminate between two points, or identify areas simultaneously touched may be seen in lesions of the sensory cortex.

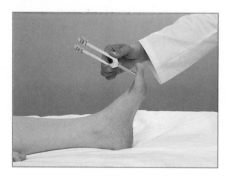

Figure 27-23 Testing vibratory sensation (© B. Proud).

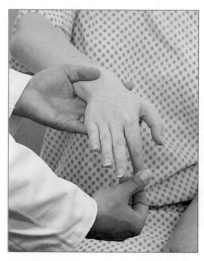

Figure 27-24 Testing position sense (© B. Proud).

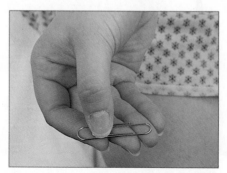

Figure 27-25 Stereognosis (© B. Proud).

continued

Assessment Procedure	Normal Findings	Abnormal Findings
To test point localization, briefly touch the client and ask the client to identify the points touched.	Client correctly identifies area touched.	Same as above.
To test graphesthesia, use a blunt instrument to write a number, such as 2, 3 or 5, on the palm of the client's hand (Fig. 27-26). Ask the client to identify the number. Repeat with another number on the other hand.	Client correctly identifies number written.	Same as above.
To test two-point discrimination, ask the client to identify the number of points felt when touched with the ends of two applicators at the same time (Fig. 27-27). Touch the client on the fingertips, forearm, dorsal hands, back, and thighs. Note the distance between the applicators.	Identifies two points on • Fingertips at 2 to 5 mm apart • Forearm at 40 mm apart • Dorsal hands at 20 to 30 mm apart • Back at 40 mm apart • Thighs at 70 mm apart	Same as above.
To test extinction, simultaneously touch the client in the same area on both sides of the body at the same point. Ask the client to identify the area touched.	Correctly identifies points touched.	Same as above.

Reflexes

Test deep tendon reflexes. Position client in a comfortable sitting position. Use the reflex hammer to elicit reflexes (see Equipment Spotlight 27-1).	Normal reflex scores range from 1+ (present but decreased) to 2+ (normal) to 3+ (increased or brisk, but not pathologic).	Absent or markedly decreased (hyporeflexia) deep tendon reflexes (rated 0) occur when a component of the lower motor neurons or reflex arc is impaired; may be seen with spinal cord injuries. Markedly hyperactive (hyperreflexia) deep tendon reflexes (rated 4+) may be seen with lesions of the upper motor neurons and when the higher cortical levels are impaired.

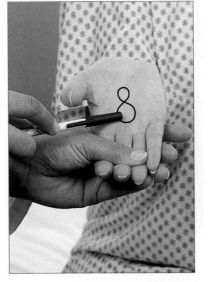

Figure 27-26 Graphesthesia (© B. Proud).

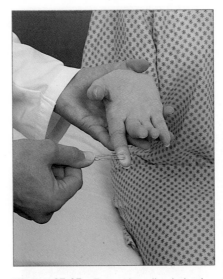

Figure 27-27 Two-point discrimination (© B. Proud).

continued

PHYSICAL ASSESSMENT Continued

Assessment Procedure	Normal Findings	Abnormal Findings
➤ *Clinical Tip • If deep tendon reflexes are diminished or absent, two reinforcement techniques may be used to enhance their response. When testing the arm reflexes, have the client clench his or her teeth. When testing the leg reflexes, have the client interlock his or her hands. Reinforcement techniques may also help the older client who has difficulty relaxing.*		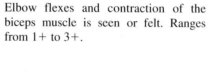 Some older clients may have decreased deep tendon reflexes because of a numeric decrease in nerve axons and increased demyelination of nerve axons. Impulse transmission also may decrease along with a delay in reaction time.
Test biceps reflex. Ask the client to partially bend arm at elbow with palm up. Place your thumb over the biceps tendon and strike your thumb with the reflex hammer (Fig. 27-28). Repeat on the other side. (This evaluates the function of spinal levels C5 and C6.)	Elbow flexes and contraction of the biceps muscle is seen or felt. Ranges from 1+ to 3+.	No response or an exaggerated response is abnormal.
Assess brachioradialis reflex. Ask the client to flex elbow with palm down and hand resting on the abdomen or lap. Tap the tendon at the radius about 2 inches above the wrist (Fig. 27-29). Repeat on other side. (This evaluates the function of spinal levels C5 and C6.)	Forearm flexes and supinates. Ranges from 1+ to 3+.	No response or an exaggerated response is abnormal.
Test triceps reflex. Ask the client to hang his or her arm freely ("limp like it is hanging from a clothesline to dry") while you support it with your nondominant hand. With the elbow flexed, tap the tendon above the olecranon process (Fig. 27-30). Repeat on the other side. (This evaluates the function of spinal levels C6, C7, and C8.)	Elbow extends, triceps contracts. Ranges from 1+ to 3+.	No response or exaggerated response.

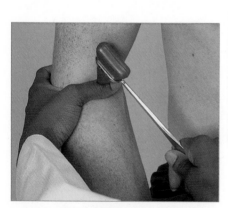

Figure 27-28 Eliciting biceps reflex.

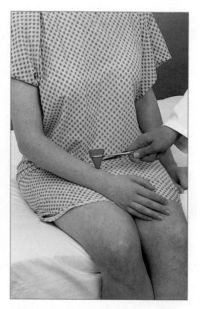

Figure 27-29 Eliciting brachioradialis reflex (© B. Proud).

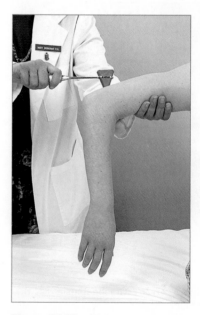

Figure 27-30 Eliciting triceps reflex (© B. Proud).

continued

Assessment Procedure	Normal Findings	Abnormal Findings
Assess patellar reflex. Ask the client to let both legs hang freely off the side of the examination table. Tap the patellar tendon, which is located just below the patella (Fig. 27-31A). Repeat on the other side. See Figure 27-31B for the client who cannot sit up. (This evaluates the function of spinal levels L2, L3, and L4.)	Knee extends, quadriceps muscle contracts. Ranges from 1+ to 3+.	No response or an exaggerated response is abnormal.
Achilles reflex. With the client's leg still hanging freely, dorsiflex the foot. Tap the Achilles tendon with the reflex hammer (Fig. 27-32A). Repeat on the other side. See Figure 27-32B for assessing the reflex in the client who cannot sit up. (This evaluates the function of spinal levels S1 and S2).	Normal response is plantar flexion of the foot. Ranges from 1+ to 3+. 👓 In some older clients, the Achilles reflex may be absent or difficult to elicit.	No response or an exaggerated response is abnormal.

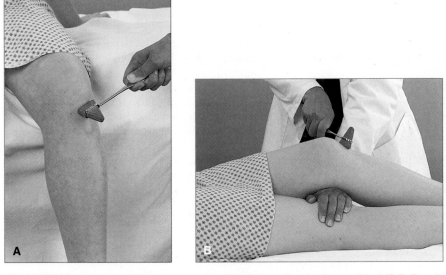

Figure 27-31 Eliciting (A) patellar reflex and (B) patellar reflex (supine position) (© B. Proud).

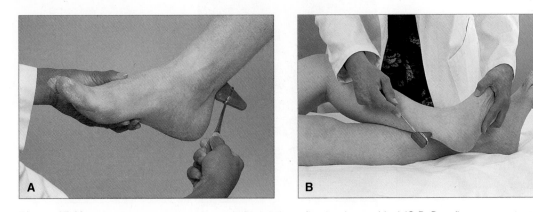

Figure 27-32 Eliciting (A) Achilles reflex and (B) Achilles reflex (supine position) (© B. Proud).

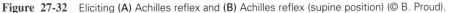

continued

PHYSICAL ASSESSMENT *Continued*

Assessment Procedure	Normal Findings	Abnormal Findings
Test ankle clonus when the other reflexes tested have been hyperactive. Place one hand under the knee to support the leg then briskly dorsiflex the foot toward the client's head (Fig. 27-33). Repeat on the other side.	No rapid contractions or oscillations (clonus) of the ankle are elicited.	Repeated rapid contractions or oscillations of the ankle and calf muscle are seen with lesions of the upper motor neurons.
Test superficial reflexes. Assess plantar reflex. ➤ *Clinical Tip • Use the handle end of the reflex hammer to elicit superficial reflexes, whose receptors are in the skin rather than the muscles.* With the end of the reflex hammer, stroke the lateral aspect of the sole from the heel to the ball of the foot, curving medially across the ball (Fig. 27-34A). Repeat on the other side. (Evaluates the function of spinal levels L4, L5, S1, and S2).	Flexion of the toes occurs (plantar response; Fig. 27-34B). 👓 In some older clients, flexion of the toes may be difficult to elicit and may be absent.	Except in infancy, extension (dorsiflexion) of the big toe and fanning of all toes (positive Babinski response) are seen with lesions of upper motor neurons. Unconscious states resulting from drug and alcohol intoxication, brain injury, or subsequent to an epileptic seizure may also cause it.
Test abdominal reflex. Lightly stroke the abdomen on each side, above and below the umbilicus. (Evaluates the function of spinal levels T8, T9, and T10 with the upper abdominal reflex and spinal levels T10, T11, and T12 with the lower abdominal reflex).	Abdominal muscles contract; umbilicus deviates toward the side being stimulated.	Superficial reflexes may be absent with lower or upper motor neuron lesions. *Caution:* The abdominal reflex may be concealed because of obesity or muscular stretching from pregnancies. This is not an abnormality.
Test cremasteric reflex in male clients. Lightly stroke the inner aspect of the upper thigh. (Evaluates the function of spinal levels T12, L1, and L2).	Scrotum elevates on stimulated side.	Absence of reflex may indicate motor neuron disorder.

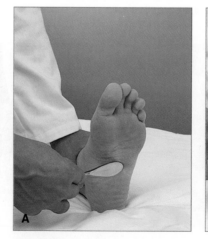

Figure 27-33 Testing for ankle clonus (© B. Proud).

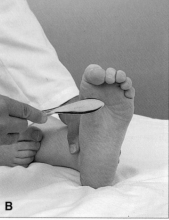

Figure 27-34 Eliciting **(A)** plantar reflex and **(B)** normal plantar response (© B. Proud).

continued

Assessment Procedure	Normal Findings	Abnormal Findings
Tests for Meningeal Irritation or Inflammation		
If you suspect the client has meningeal irritation or inflammation from infection or subarachnoid hemorrhage, assess the client's neck mobility. First make sure there is no injury to the cervical vertebrae or cervical cord. Then with the client supine, place your hands behind the patient's head and flex the neck forward until the chin touches the chest if possible.	Neck is supple; client can easily bend head and neck forward.	Pain in the neck and resistance to flexion can arise from meningeal inflammation, arthritis, or neck injury.
Test for Brudzinski's sign. As you flex the neck, watch the hips and knees in reaction to your maneuver.	Hips and knees remain relaxed and motionless.	Pain and flexion of the hips and knees are positive Brudzinski's signs and suggest meningeal inflammation.
Test for Kernig's sign. Flex the client's leg at both the hip and the knee, then straighten the knee.	No pain is felt. Discomfort behind the knee during full extension occurs in many normal people.	Pain and increased resistance to extending the knee are a positive Kernig's sign. When Kernig's sign is bilateral, the examiner suspects meningeal irritation.

Abnormal Findings 27-1 ■ Abnormal Gaits

Everyone normally walks a little bit differently from everyone else but sometimes a person's gait is distinctively abnormal suggesting that the person has a neurologic problem. Some common abnormal gaits and their causes follow:

Cerebellar Ataxia
- Wide-based, staggering, unsteady gait
- Romberg test results are positive (client cannot stand with feet together)
- Seen with cerebellar diseases or alcohol or drug intoxication

Parkinsonian Gait
- Shuffling gait, turns accomplished in very stiff manner
- Stooped-over posture with flexed hips and knees
- Typically seen in Parkinson's disease *and drug-induced parkinsonian* because of effects on the basal ganglia

Scissors Gait
- Stiff, short gait; thighs overlap each other with each step
- Seen with partial paralysis of the legs

Spastic Hemiparesis
- Flexed arm held close to body while client drags toe of leg or circles it stiffly outward and forward
- Seen with lesions of the upper motor neurons in the cortical spinal tract, such as occurs in stroke

Footdrop
- Client lifts foot and knee high with each step, then slaps the foot down hard on the ground
- Client cannot walk on heels
- Characteristic of diseases of the lower motor neurons

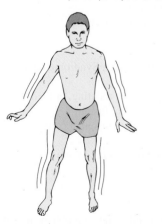

Cerebellar ataxia.

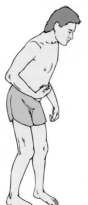

Parkinsonian gait.

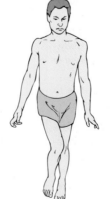

Scissors gait.

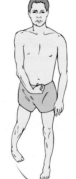

Spastic hemiparesis.

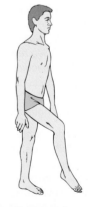

Footdrop (steppage) gait.

VALIDATING AND DOCUMENTING FINDINGS

Validate the neurologic assessment data you have collected. This is necessary to verify that the data are reliable and accurate. Document the data following the health care facility or agency policy.

> ➤ **Clinical Tip** • *When documenting your assessment findings, it is better to describe the client's response than to label the behavior.*

Sample of Subjective Data

> No history of head injury, spinal cord injury, seizures, meningitis. No dizziness, tinnitus, severe or chronic headache. No difficulty swallowing or communicating. No memory loss.

Sample of Objective Data

> *Mental Status:* Alert, oriented to person, place, day, and time. Good eye contact. Positive about daily activities and the future. Short-term and long-term memory intact. Able to follow directions, compare unlike objects, and explain simple proverbs.
>
> *Cranial Nerves:*
>
> I: Identifies correct scents.
> II: Vision 20/20 OS, 20/20 OD, full visual fields intact, red reflex present, optic disc round with well-defined borders. Retinal background pink. No hemorrhages or arteriovenous nicking noted.
> III, IV, and VI: No ptosis, full extraocular movements (EOMs), pupils equally round, react to light and accommodation (PERRLA).
> V: Temporal and masseter muscles contract bilaterally. Able to identify light, sharp, and dull touch to forehead, cheek, and chin. Corneal reflex present.
> VII: Able to smile, frown, wrinkle forehead, show teeth, puff out cheeks, purse lips, raise eyebrows, and close eyes against resistance.
> VIII: Whispered words heard bilaterally. Vibration heard equally well in both ears; air conduction (AC) greater than bone conduction (BC).
> IX and X: Uvula and soft palate rise symmetrically on phonation. Gag reflex present. Swallows without difficulty.
> XI: Equal shoulder shrug against resistance; turns head in both directions against resistance.
> XII: Protrudes tongue in midline with no tremors, able to push tongue blade to right and left without difficulty.
>
> *Motor and Cerebellar Systems:* No atrophy, tremors, weakness; full range of motion of all extremities. No fasciculations, tics, or tremors. Gait and tandem walk normal and steady. Negative Romberg test. Performs repetitive alternating movements, finger-to-nose at smooth, good pace. Runs each heel down each shin with no deviation.

> *Sensory System:* Identifies light touch, dull and sharp sensations to trunk and extremities. Vibratory sensation, stereognosis, graphesthesia, two-point discrimination intact.
>
> *Reflexes:* Reflexes 2+ bilaterally, except Achilles 1+. No ankle clonus noted. Abdominal reflex present. No Babinski's present.

Analysis of Data

DIAGNOSTIC REASONING: POSSIBLE CONCLUSIONS

After collecting subjective and objective data pertaining to the neurologic assessment, identify abnormal findings and client strengths. Then cluster the data to reveal any significant patterns or abnormalities. These data may then be used to make clinical judgments about the status of the client's neurologic health.

Selected Nursing Diagnoses

Following is a listing of selected nursing diagnoses (wellness, risk, or actual) that you may identify when analyzing the cue clusters.

Wellness Diagnoses

- Readiness for Enhanced Communication
- Readiness for Spiritual Well-being

Risk Diagnoses

- Risk for Injury related to disturbed sensory-perceptual patterns
- Risk for Aspiration related to impaired gag reflex
- Risk for Self-Directed Violence, related to depression, suicidal tendencies, developmental crisis, lack of support systems, loss of significant others, poor coping mechanisms and behaviors

Actual Diagnoses

- Disturbed Thought Processes related to abuse of alcohol or drugs, psychotic disorder, or organic brain dysfunction
- Impaired Verbal Communication related to aphasia, psychological impairment or organic brain disorder
- Acute or Chronic Confusion related to dementia, head injury, stroke, alcohol or drug abuse
- Impaired Memory related to dementia, stroke, head injury, alcohol or drug abuse
- Sexual Dysfunction
- Impaired Environmental Interpretation Syndrome related to dementia, depression, or alcoholism
- Self-Care Deficit (bathing, hygiene, toileting, or feeding) related to paralysis, weakness, or confusion
- Reflex Urinary Incontinence related to spinal cord or brain damage
- Unilateral Neglect related to poor vision on one side, trauma or neurologic disorder

Selected Collaborative Problems

After grouping the data, certain collaborative problems may become apparent. Remember that collaborative problems differ from nursing diagnoses in that they cannot be prevented with nursing interventions alone. However, these physiologic complications of medical conditions can be detected and monitored by the nurse. In addition, the nurse can use physician- and nurse-prescribed interventions to minimize the complications of these problems. The nurse may also have to refer the client in such situations for further treatment of the problem. Following is a list of collaborative problems that may be identified when assessing the neurologic system. These problems are worded as Risk for Complications (or RC), followed by the problem.

- RC: Increased intracranial pressure
- RC: Stroke
- RC: Seizures

- RC: Spinal cord compression
- RC: Meningitis
- RC: Cranial nerve impairment
- RC: Paralysis
- RC: Peripheral nerve impairment
- RC: Increased intraocular pressure
- RC: Corneal ulceration
- RC: Neuropathies

Medical Problems

After grouping the data, the client's signs and symptoms may clearly require medical diagnosis and treatment. Referral to a primary care provider is necessary.

CASE STUDY

The case study demonstrates how to analyze neurologic assessment data for a specific client. The critical thinking exercises included in the study guide/lab manual and interactive product that complement this text also offer opportunities to analyze assessment data.

Mildred Hutchinson, a 49-year-old divorced woman, had been working as an office manager at a local high school but recently she began teaching (her first love) language classes (French and German); she also is responsible for teaching two physical education (PE) classes a week.

During the interview, she tells you that she has had multiple sclerosis (MS) for over 20 years but has managed to function at a near-normal level for most of that time. "I had one severe exacerbation during my divorce, but I went into remission after about 6 months." She states that she has come to the clinic for advice about how to prevent another exacerbation. She voices her concerns: "I get so tired by the end of the week that I have difficulty maintaining urinary continence even with my medication (oxybutynin, i.e., Ditropan). I feel increasingly weak, and I get pins and needles in my legs. Also I'm not

sleeping well because spasms in my legs keep me awake." She tells you that her vision has not been affected and that, if she rests all weekend, she is "OK" by Monday morning. She goes on to say, "I have no social life, except on the telephone."

Your physical assessment reveals an alert, attractive, well-dressed, thin, middle-aged woman with mildly elevated blood pressure and pulse rate (136/92 and 98), which Ms. H. reports is usually 100/70; PERRLA; extraocular movements intact with conjugate gaze, but slight nystagmus noted when eyes are in extreme lateral positions; mental status intact; grips strong and upper extremity strength good against resistance; unable to walk heel-to-toe without some loss of balance; and 4+ patellar, Achilles, and plantar reflexes with mild clonus.

The following concept map illustrates the diagnostic reasoning process.

Applying COLDSPA

Applying **COLDSPA** for client symptoms: "Fatigue, urinary incontinence, pins and needles in legs, and insomnia"

Mnemonic	Question	Data Provided	Missing Data
Character	Describe the sign or symptom (feeling, appearance, sound, smell, or taste if applicable.)	Client reports "Fatigue, urinary incontinence, leg spasms, and insomnia" Client has had MS for over 20 years and would like to prevent an exacerbation.	
Onset	When did it begin?	With recent job change from office manager to teacher.	
Location	Where is it? Does it radiate? Does it occur anywhere else?	"It has affected my activities, rest patterns, and comfort level, but has not affected my vision."	
Duration	How long does it last? Does it recur?	"The last severe exacerbation, during my divorce, lasted 6 months before I went into remission."	"How long have you been in remission?"
Severity	How bad is it? or How much does it bother you?	"It is so bad that all I can do is rest all weekend."	
Pattern	What makes it better or worse?	"Activity and work make it worse and rest makes it better."	
Associated factors/How it **A**ffects the client	How does it affect you? What other symptoms occur with it?	"I have no social life as I have to rest all weekend after a week at work."	

1) Identify abnormal findings and client strengths

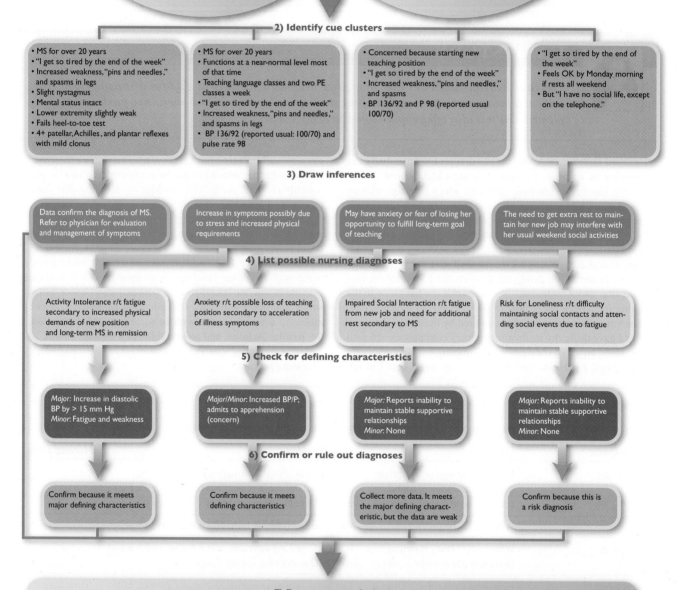

Subjective Data

- MS for more than 20 years
- Functions at a near-normal level most of that time
- One severe exacerbation during divorce
- Remission after about 6 months
- Seeking advice to prevent another exacerbation
- Concerned because starting new teaching position
- Teaching language classes and two PE classes a week
- "I get so tired by the end of the week."
- Problem maintaining urinary continence with medication
- Increased weakness and "pins and needles" in legs
- Not sleeping well because of leg spasms
- OK by Monday morning if she rests all weekend
- "But I have no social life, except on the telephone!"
- Vision not affected

Objective Data

- Thin, 49-year-old woman
- BP 136/92 (reported usual 100/70) and pulse rate 98
- PERRLA
- Extraocular movements intact with conjugate gaze, but slight nystagmus noted when eyes in extreme lateral positions
- Mental status intact
- Grips strong and upper extremity strength good against resistance
- Lower extremities show slight weakness against resistance
- Unable to walk heel-to-toe without moderate loss of balance
- 4+ patellar, Achilles, and plantar reflexes with mild clonus

2) Identify cue clusters

- MS for over 20 years
- "I get so tired by the end of the week"
- Increased weakness, "pins and needles," and spasms in legs
- Slight nystagmus
- Mental status intact
- Lower extremity slightly weak
- Fails heel-to-toe test
- 4+ patellar, Achilles, and plantar reflexes with mild clonus

---

- MS for over 20 years
- Functions at a near-normal level most of that time
- Teaching language classes and two PE classes a week
- "I get so tired by the end of the week"
- Increased weakness, "pins and needles," and spasms in legs
- BP 136/92 (reported usual: 100/70) and pulse rate 98

- Concerned because starting new teaching position
- "I get so tired by the end of the week"
- Increased weakness, "pins and needles," and spasms
- BP 136/92 and P 98 (reported usual 100/70)

- "I get so tired by the end of the week"
- Feels OK by Monday morning if rests all weekend
- But "I have no social life, except on the telephone."

3) Draw inferences

- Data confirm the diagnosis of MS. Refer to physician for evaluation and management of symptoms

- Increase in symptoms possibly due to stress and increased physical requirements

- May have anxiety or fear of losing her opportunity to fulfill long-term goal of teaching

- The need to get extra rest to maintain her new job may interfere with her usual weekend social activities

4) List possible nursing diagnoses

- Activity Intolerance r/t fatigue secondary to increased physical demands of new position and long-term MS in remission

- Anxiety r/t possible loss of teaching position secondary to acceleration of illness symptoms

- Impaired Social Interaction r/t fatigue from new job and need for additional rest secondary to MS

- Risk for Loneliness r/t difficulty maintaining social contacts and attending social events due to fatigue

5) Check for defining characteristics

- *Major:* Increase in diastolic BP by > 15 mm Hg
  Minor: Fatigue and weakness

- *Major/Minor:* Increased BP/P; admits to apprehension (concern)

- *Major:* Reports inability to maintain stable supportive relationships
  Minor: None

- *Major:* Reports inability to maintain stable supportive relationships
  Minor: None

6) Confirm or rule out diagnoses

- Confirm because it meets major defining characteristics

- Confirm because it meets defining characteristics

- Collect more data. It meets the major defining characteristic, but the data are weak

- Confirm because this is a risk diagnosis

7) Document conclusions

Nursing diagnoses that are appropriate for this client include:
- Activity Intolerance r/t fatigue secondary to increased physical demands of new position and MS in remission
- Anxiety r/t possible loss of teaching position secondary to acceleration of illness symptoms
- Risk for Loneliness r/t difficulty maintaining social contacts and attending social events due to fatigue

Potential collaborative problems include the following:
- RC: Hypertension
- RC: Urinary incontinence
- RC: Active multiple sclerosis
Ms. Hutchinson should be referred to a neurologist for evaluation of her treatment regimen

References and Selected Readings

Adams, H, P. Jr., Corbett, J. J., & DeMyer, W. E. (2005). Save time with the 5-minute neurologic exam. *Patient Care, 39*(4), 41–47.

Ajibade, B. L. (2006). Neurological assessment: A review of Glascow Coma Scale and other neurological observations. *West African Journal of Nursing, 17*(2), 153–159.

Baker, R. A. (2005). The neurological assessment of patients in vegetative and minimally conscious states. *Neuropsychological Rehabilitation, 15*(3/4), 214–223.

Beaumont, R., & Newcombe, P. (2006). Theory of mind and central coherence in adults with high-functioning autism or Asperger syndrome. *Autism: The International Journal of Research and Practice, 10*(4), 365–382.

Craig, C. L., Bauman, A., Phongsavan, P., Stephens, T., & Harris, S. J. (2006). Jolly, fit and fat: Should we be singing the "Santa too fat blues"? *CMAJ: Canadian Medical Association Journal, 175*(12), 1563–1566.

Dawes, D., Durham, L. (2007). Monitoring and recording patients' neurological observations. *Nurse Stand, 22*(10), 40–45.

Dia, D. A., & Harrington, D. (2006). Research note. What about me? Siblings of children with an anxiety disorder. *Social Work Research, 30*(3), 183–188.

Dick, J. P. (2003). The deep tendon and the abdominal reflexes. *J Neurol Neurosurg Psychiatry, 74*(2), 150–153.

Faroofqi, N., Kouyialis, A. T., & Brodbelt, A. (2006). First things first. *Lancet, 368*(9535), 617.

Fitzgerald, M. S. (2004). What nerve! Honing your skills in cranial nerve assessment. *Adv Nurse Pract, 12*(10), 21.

Fitzpatrick, T. R., Gitelson, R. J., Andereck, K. L., & Mesbur, E. S. (2005). Social support factors and health among a senior center population in southern Ontario, Canada. *Social Work in Health Care, 40*(3), 15–37.

Folstein, M., Anthony, J., Parhad, I., Duffy, B., & Gruenberg, E. (1985). The meaning of cognitive impairment in the elderly. *Journal of the American Geriatrics Society, 33*, 228–235.

Folstein, M. F., Folstein, S. E., & McHugh, P. R. (1975). Mini–Mental State: A practical method for grading the cognitive state of patients for the clinician. *Journal of Psychiatric Research, 12*(3), 89–198.

Garand, L, Mitchell, A. M., Dietrick, A., Hijjawi, S. P., & Pan, D. (2006). Suicide in older adults: Nursing assessment of suicide risk. *Issues in Mental Health Nursing, 27*(4), 335–370.

Geary, S. M. (1995). Nursing management of cranial nerve dysfunction. *Journal of Neuroscience Nursing, 27*(2), 102–108.

Greenberg, M. S. (2006). *Handbook of neurosurgery.* (6th ed.). New York: Thieme.

Idemoto, B. K. (2005). The assessment of delirium and depression in the intensive care unit. *Case Western Reserve University (Health Sciences, doctoral dissertation, 137.*

Izutsu, T., Tsutsumi, A., Islam, A. M., Kato, S., Wakai, S., & Kurita, H. (2006). Mental health, quality of life, and nutritional status of adolescents in Khaka, Bangladesh: Comparison between an urban slum and a non-slum area. *Social Science & Medicine, 63*(6), 1477–1488.

Jagoda, A., & Riggia, S. (2005). What you forgot about the neurologic exam: History, mental status, cranial nerves. *Headache & Pain: Diagnostic Challenges, Current Therapy, 16*(4), 187–194.

Krost, W. S., Mistovich, J. J., Limmer, D. D. (2006). Beyond the basics: Trauma assessment. *Emergency Medical Services, 35*(8), 71–77.

Lower, J. (2002). Facing neuro assessment fearlessly. *Nursing2002, 32*(2), 58–64.

Lemiengre, J., Nelis, T., Joosten, E., Braes, T., Foreman, M., Gastmans, C., & Lilisen, K. (2006). Detection of delirium by bedside nurses using the confusion assessment method. *Journal of the American Geriatrics Society, 54*(4), 685–689.

Limmer, D. D., Mistovich, J. J., & Krost, W. S. (2006). Beyond the basics: behavioral emergencies. *Emergency Medical Serves, 35*(10), 84–91.

McNarry, A. F., Goldhill, D. R. (2004). Simple bedside assessment of level of consciousness: Comparison of two simple assessment scales with the Glascow Coma scale. *Anaesthesia, 59*, 34–37.

Minton, M., & Hickey, J. (1999). A primer of neuroanatomy and neurophysiology. *Nursing Clinics of North America, 34*(3), 555–572.

Nair, M. (2006). Alzheimer's disease. Nursing management of the patient with Alzheimer's disease. *British Journal of Nursing, 15*(5), 258–262.

Neatherlin, J. (1999). Foundation for practice: Neuroassessment for neuroscience nurses. *Nursing Clinics of North America,34*(3), 573–592.

Parkes, J., & White Koning, M. (2006). Mental health is related to functional abilities in cerebral palsy. *Developmental Medicine & Child Neurology, 48*(supplement 107), 41.

Patal, D. R. (2006). Managing concussion in a young athlete. *Contemporary Pediatrics, 23*(11), 62–69.

Patterson, C. (2001). *Screen for cognitive impairment and dementia in the elderly.* Canadian Task Force on Preventive Health Care. Available at http://www.ctfphc.org

Ramsey–Klawsnik, H. (2006). Complexities of mental capacity. *Victimization of the Elderly and Disabled, 9*(1), 1–2, 15–16.

Stanton, K. (2007). Emergency: Communicating with ED patients who have chronic mental illnesses *American Journal of Nursing, 107*(2), 61–65.

Straus, S. H. (2007). Use of the automatic clock drawing test to rapidly screen for cognitive impairment in older adults, drivers, and the physically challenged. *Journal of the American Geriatrics Society, 55*(2), 310–311.

Takei, T., Yamashita, H., & Yoshida, K. (2006). The mental health of mothers of physically abused children: The relationship with children's behavioral problems—Report from Japan. *Child Abuse Review, 15*(3), 204–218.

Thomas, S. H., Schwamm, L. H., & Lev, M. H. (2006). Case 16–2006: A 72-year-old women admitted to the emergency department because of a sudden change in mental status. *New England Journal of Medicine, 354*(21), 2263–2271, 2305–2308.

Waterhouse, C. (2005). The Glascow Come Scale and other neurological observations. *Nurs Stand, 19*(33), 55–64.

Willette-Murphy, K., Todero, C., & Yeaworth, R. (2006). Mental health and sleep of older wife caregivers for spouses with Alzheimer's disease and related disorders. *Issues in Mental Health Nursing, 27*(8), 837–852.

Yesevage, J. (1983). Development and validation of a geriatric depression screening scale: A preliminary report. *Journal of Psychiatric Research, 17*, 38–49.

Promote Health—Cerebrovascular Accident (Stroke)

American Heart Association/American Stroke Association. Heart Disease and Stroke Statistics: 2008. Update, retrieved March, 2008. Available at http://www.strokeassociation.org

American Stroke Association. (2007). Learn about stroke. Available at http://www.strokeassociation.org

CDC, Prevalence of Stroke-United States, 2005. *JAMA,* 2007, 298, 279–281.

The Internet Stroke Center. (1997–2007). About Stroke. Available at http://www.strokecenter.org

Overfield, T. (1995). *Biologic variation in health and illness: Race, age, and sex differences* (2nd ed.). Boca Raton, FL: CRC Press.

28

Pulling It All Together

Now that you have learned how to interview a client and perform a thorough examination of every body system, you may be wondering how you will be able to complete a comprehensive assessment. While focused body systems assessments are used when a client seeks care for a particular health concern, comprehensive assessments are completed in such instances as the client's first visit to a health care provider. Thus far you have learned a systems approach and have learned about assessing specific body systems discretely. For practical reasons, a head-to-toe approach is more convenient to use when performing a total assessment. When using a head-to-toe approach, some body systems may be assessed in combination with each other. For example, when performing an eye assessment you will also be performing part of the neurological exam for cranial nerves II, III, IV, and VI, which affect vision and eye movements. When you assess the legs you will be assessing the parts of the skin (color and condition of skin on legs), peripheral vascular system (pulses, color, edema, lesions of legs), musculoskeletal system (movement, strength, and tone of legs), and neurological system (ankle and patellar reflexes, clonus). There is no one right way to integrate the entire health history and physical examination. However, it is important to stick to a routine to avoid omitting an important step that may delete significant data from your assessment.

Pulling all these skills together takes time and practice. The more you practice, the faster you will perform the assessment. To perform a complete interview and total physical examination may take up to 2 hours for the novice and only 30 minutes for the skilled practitioner. Do not get discouraged; no one becomes an expert without practice. Develop a routine that is comfortable for you and the client. It is wise to break up the assessment into parts to allow both the client and yourself short rest periods. The client's physical and mental statuses will determine how much of the total exam you may perform at one time. For example, if the client is having excruciating hip pain, an extensive assessment would need to wait until the client is more comfortable. If the client is confused, you will need to gather data from relatives or friends and proceed in a manner that does not agitate the client.

Before performing a complete assessment, you should read your state's Nurse Practice Act to find out what you can legally assess and diagnose.

Comprehensive Health Assessment

PREPARING THE CLIENT

Discuss the purpose and importance of the health history and physical assessment with your client. Acquire your client's permission to ask personal questions and to perform the various physical assessments (i.e., breast, thorax, genitourinary exam). Explain your respect for the client's privacy and for confidentiality. Respect your client's right to refuse any part of the assessment. Explain that the client will need to change into a gown for the examination.

EQUIPMENT

Display 28-1 lists the equipment needed for a very thorough assessment covering all body systems. However, the nurse rarely performs a total eye and ear examination nor does she normally perform genitalia and rectal examination. The client often sees specialists for these routine exams. The nurse, however, may have to perform these examinations when needed. Therefore, your equipment needs will be determined by the areas being assessed. In addition, modifications may be necessary when performing an assessment in a client's home. For example, use a bath scale in place of a platform scale.

COLLECTING DATA

Remember to document all your subjective and objective findings, nursing diagnoses, collaborative problems, and referrals.

Collecting Subjective Data: The Nursing Health History

While taking the nursing health history and performing the general survey and mental status examination, make sure that the room and position are comfortable for the client.

See Chapter 2, Assessment Tool 2-1, for an outline of the components of a comprehensive health history.

| DISPLAY 28-1 | Equipment for a Head-to-Toe Examination |

Assessment documentation forms
Coin or key
Cotton ball
Cover card (for eye assessment)
Gloves
Goniometer
Gown for client
Lubricating jelly
Magnifying glass
Marking pencil
Mini-Mental Status Exam (MMSE) Form
Newspaper print or Rosenbaum pocket screener
Notepad and pencil
Ophthalmoscope
Otoscope
Paper clip
Penlight
Pillows (two small pillows)

Platform scale with height attachment
Reflex hammer
Ruler with centimeter markings
Skin-fold calipers, flexible tape measure
Small cup of water for client to drink
Snellen chart
Stethoscope and sphygmomanometer
Substances for testing smell, e.g., soap and coffee
Substances for testing taste, e.g., salt, lemon, sugar, and
    pickle juice
Supplies for collecting vaginal specimen (slides, spatula,
    cotton tip applicator)
Thermometer
Tongue depressor
Tuning fork
Vaginal speculum
Watch

Collecting Objective Data: Physical Assessment

General Survey

- Observe appearance (Fig. 28-1), including
  - Overall physical and sexual development
  - Apparent age compare with stated age
  - Overall skin coloring
  - Dress, grooming, and hygiene
  - Body build as well as muscle mass and fat distribution
  - Behavior (compare with developmental stage)
- Assess the client's vital signs:
  - Temperature
  - Pulse
  - Respirations
  - Blood pressure
  - Pain (as the 5th Vital Sign)
- Take body measurements:
  - Height
  - Weight
  - Waist and hip circumference and midarm circumference
  - Triceps skin fold thickness (TSF)
- Calculate ideal body weight, body mass index, waist-to-hip ratio, mid-arm muscle area and circumference.

Mental Status Examination

- In addition to data collected about the client's appearance during the general survey, observe
  - Level of consciousness
  - Posture and body movements
  - Facial expressions
  - Speech
  - Mood, feelings, and expressions
  - Thought processes and perceptions

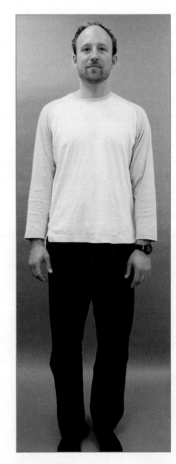

Figure 28-1 Observing overall appearance of the client.

- Assess the client's cognitive abilities (the Mini-Mental Status Exam (MMSE) may be used):
  - Orientation to person, time, and place
  - Concentration, ability to focus and follow directions
  - Recent memory of happenings today
  - Remote memory of the past
  - Recall of unrelated information in 5, 10, and 30 minute periods
  - Abstract reasoning (Explain a "Stitch in time saves nine.")
  - Judgment (What one would do in case of. . .)
  - Visual perceptual and constructional ability (draw a clock or shapes of square, etc.)

Ask the client to empty his bladder (give the client a specimen cup, if sample is needed) and change into a gown. Ask client to sit on examination table.

Skin

- As you perform each part of the head-to toe assessment, assess skin for color variations, texture, temperature, turgor, edema, and lesions.
- Teach the client skin self-examination.

Head and Face

- Inspect and palpate the head for size, shape, and configuration (Fig. 28-2).
- Note consistency, distribution, and color of hair.
- Observe face for symmetry, facial features, expressions, and skin condition.
- Check function of CN VII: Have the client smile, frown, show teeth, blow out cheeks, raise eyebrows, and tightly close eyes.
- Evaluate function CN V: Using the sharp and dull sides of a paper clip, test sensations of forehead, cheeks, and chin.
- Palpate the temporal arteries for elasticity and tenderness.
- As the client opens and closes her mouth, palpate the temporomandibular joint for tenderness, swelling, and crepitation.

Eyes

- Determine function:
  - Test vision using Snellen Chart.
  - Test visual fields.
  - Assess corneal light reflex.
  - Perform cover and position tests.
- Inspect external eye:
  - Position and alignment of the eyeball in eye socket
  - Bulbar conjunctiva and sclera
  - Palpebral conjunctiva
  - Lacrimal apparatus
  - Cornea, lens, iris, and pupil
- Test pupillary reaction to light.
- Test accommodation of pupils.
- Assess corneal reflex (CN VII—facial).
- Use the ophthalmoscope to inspect
  - Optic disc for shape, color, size, and physiologic cup
  - Retinal vessels for color and diameter and AV crossings
  - Retinal background for color and lesions
  - Fovea centralis (sharpest area of vision) and macula
  - Anterior chamber for clarity

Ears

- Inspect the auricle, tragus, and lobule for shape, position, lesions, discolorations, and discharge.
- Palpate the auricle and mastoid process for tenderness (Fig. 28-3).
- Use the otoscope to inspect
  - External auditory canal for color and cerumen (ear wax)
  - Tympanic membrane for color, shape, consistency, and landmarks
- Test hearing
  - Whisper Test
  - Weber's Test for diminished hearing in one ear
  - Rinne Test to compare bone and air conduction (tuning fork on mastoid; then in front of ear)

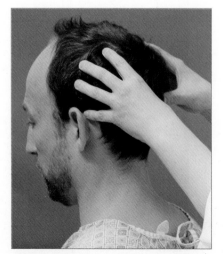

Figure 28-2 Palpating the head for shape and consistency.

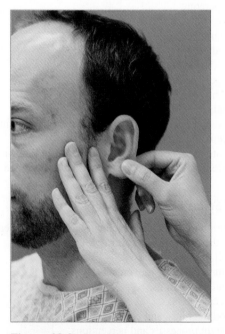

Figure 28-3 Palpating the auricle and mastoid process.

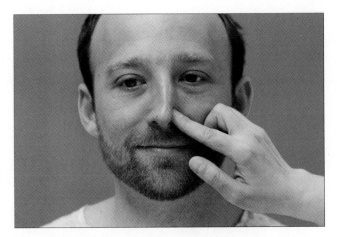

Figure 28-4 Inspecting patency of the nostrils.

Nose and Sinuses

- Inspect the external nose for color, shape, and consistency. Palpate the external nose for tenderness.
- Check patency of airflow through nostrils (occlude one nostril at a time and ask client to sniff; Fig. 28-4).
- Test CN I. Ask the client to close his eyes and smell for soap, coffee, or vanilla. (Occlude each nostril.)
- Use an otoscope with a short wide tip to inspect internal nose for color and integrity of nasal mucosa, nasal septum, and inferior and middle turbinates.
- Transilluminate maxillary sinuses with a penlight to check for fluid or pus.

Mouth and Throat

Put on gloves. Use a tongue depressor and penlight as needed.

- Inspect lips for consistency, color, and lesions.
- Inspect the teeth for number and condition.
- Check the gums and buccal mucosa for color, consistency, lesions.
- Inspect the hard (anterior) and soft (posterior) palates for color and integrity.
- Ask the client to say "aah" and observe the rise of uvula.
- Test CN X: Touch the soft palate to assess for gag reflex.
- Inspect the tonsils for color, size, lesions, and exudates.
- Inspect the tongue for color, moisture, size, and texture. Inspect the ventral surface of tongue for frenulum, color, lesions, and Wharton's Ducts.
- Palpate the tongue for lesions (Fig. 28-5).
- Test CN IX and CN X: Assess tongue strength by asking client to press tongue against tongue blade.
- Assess CN VII and CN IX: Have the patient close her eyes. Check taste by placing salt, sugar, and lemon on tongue.

Neck

- Inspect neck for appearance of lesions, masses, swelling, and symmetry.
- Test range of motion (ROM).
- Palpate the pre-auricular, post auricular, occipital, tonsillar, submandibular, and submental nodes.
- Palpate the trachea.

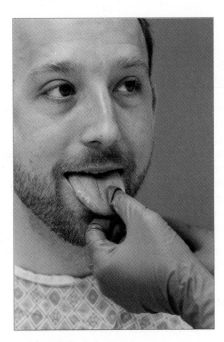

Figure 28-5 Palpating the tongue.

- Palpate the thyroid gland for size, irregularity, or masses.
- Auscultate an enlarged thyroid for bruits.
- Palpate carotid arteries and auscultate for bruits.

Arms, Hands, and Fingers

- Inspect the upper extremities for overall skin coloration, texture, moisture, masses, and lesions.
- Test function of CN XI Spinal by shoulder shrug and turning head against resistance.
- Palpate shoulders and arms for tenderness, swelling, and temperature (Fig. 28-6).
- Assess epitrochlear lymph nodes.
- Test ROM of the elbows.
- Palpate the brachial pulse.
- Palpate ulnar and radial pulses.
- Test ROM of the wrist.

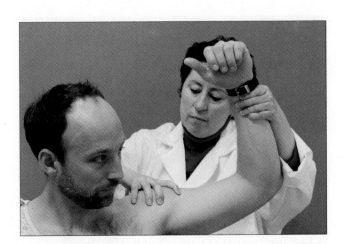

Figure 28-6 Palpating the shoulder.

- Inspect palms of hands and palpate for temperature.
- Test ROM of the fingers.
- Use a reflex hammer to test biceps, triceps, and brachioradialis reflexes.
- Test rapid alternating movements of hands.
- Ask the patient to close her eyes; test sensation:
  - Assess light touch, pain, and temperature sensation in scattered locations over hands and arms.
  - Evaluate sensitivity of position of fingers.
  - Placing a quarter or key in the client's hand to test stereognosis.
  - Assess graphesthesia by writing a number in the palm of the client's hand.
  - Assess two-point discrimination (Table 28-1) in the fingertips, forearm, and dorsal hands.

Ask client to continue sitting with arms at sides and stand behind client. Untie gown to expose posterior chest.

Posterior and Lateral Chest

- Inspect configuration and shape of scapulae and chest wall.
- Note use of accessory muscles when breathing and posture.
- Palpate for tenderness, sensation, crepitus, masses, lesions, and fremitus.
- Evaluate chest expansion at levels T9 or T10.
- Percuss for tone at posterior intercostal spaces (comparing bilaterally) (Fig. 28-7).
- Determine diaphragmatic excursion.
- Auscultate for breath sounds, adventitious sounds, and voice sounds (bronchophony, egophony, and whispered pectoriloquy) (Fig. 28-8).
- Test for two-point discrimination on the client's back.
- Ask client to lean forward and exhale; use bell of stethoscope to listen over the apex and left sternal border of the heart.

Move to front of client and expose anterior chest. Allow client to maintain modesty.

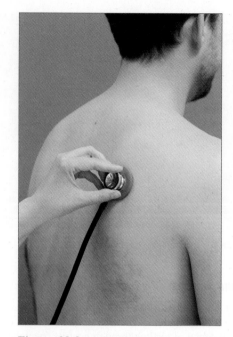

Figure 28-8 Auscultating the posterior chest for breath sounds.

Anterior Chest

- Inspect anteroposterior diameter of chest, slope of ribs, and color of chest.
- Note quality and pattern of respirations (rate, rhythm, and depth).
- Observe intercostal spaces for bulging or retractions and use of accessory muscles.
- Palpate for tenderness, sensation, masses, lesions, fremitus, and anterior chest expansion.
- Percuss for tone at apices above clavicles then at intercostals spaces (comparing bilaterally)
- Auscultate for anterior breath sounds, adventitious sounds, and voice sounds.
- Pinch skin over sternum to assess mobility (ease to pinch) and turgor (return to original shape).

Ask client to fold gown to waist and sit with arms hanging freely.

Breasts

FEMALE BREASTS

Inspect size, symmetry, color, texture, superficial venous pattern, areolas, and nipples of both breasts.

- Inspect for retractions and dimpling of nipples: Have the client raise her arms overhead, press her hands on her hips, press her hands together in front of her, and lean forward.
- Palpate axillae for rashes, infection, and anterior, central, and posterior lymph nodes.

MALE BREASTS

- Inspect for swelling, nodules, and ulcerations.
- Palpate the breast tissue and axillae.

Assist client to supine position with the head elevated to 30 to 45 degrees. Stand on client's right side.

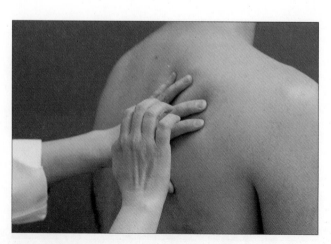

Figure 28-7 Percussing for tone.

Neck

Observe and evaluate jugular venous pressure.

Assist client to supine position (lower examination table).

Complete Examination of Female Breasts

- Palpate breasts for masses and the nipples for discharge.
- Teach breast self-examination.

Heart

- Inspect and palpate for apical impulse.
- Palpate the apex, left sternal border, and base of the heart for any abnormal pulsations.
- Auscultate over aortic area, pulmonic area, Erb's point, tricuspid area, and the mitral area (apex) for
  - Heart rate and rhythm (with diaphragm of stethoscope). If irregular, auscultate for a pulse rate deficit.
  - S_1 and S_2 (with diaphragm of stethoscope)
  - Extra heart sounds, S_3 and S_4 (with diaphragm and bell of stethoscope)
  - Murmurs (using bell and diaphragm of the stethoscope)
- Ask the client to lay on left side; use bell of stethoscope to listen to apex of the heart.

Cover chest with gown and arrange draping to expose abdomen.

Abdomen

- Inspect for
  - Overall skin color (Fig. 28-9)
  - Vascularity, striae, lesions, and rashes
  - Location, contour, and color of umbilicus
  - Symmetry and contour of abdomen
  - Aortic pulsations or peristaltic waves
- Auscultate for
  - Bowel sounds (intensity, pitch, and frequency)
  - Vascular sounds and friction rubs (over spleen, liver, aorta, iliac artery, umbilicus and femoral artery) (Fig. 28-10)
- Percuss for
  - Tone over four quadrants
  - Liver location, size, and span
  - Spleen location and size

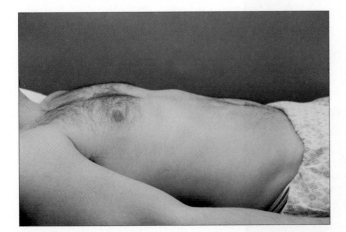

Figure 28-9 Inspecting overall skin tone/quality of the abdomen.

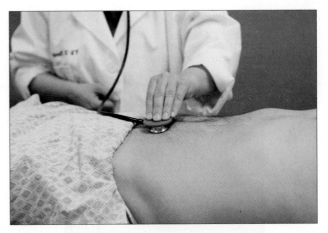

Figure 28-10 Auscultating for bruits.

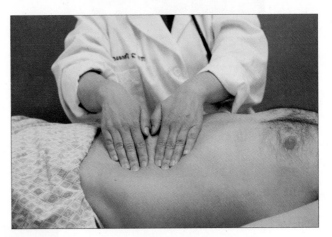

Figure 28-11 Palpating the abdomen for masses.

- Lightly palpate
  - Abdominal reflex
  - Four quadrants to identify tenderness and muscular resistance
- Deeply palpate
  - Four quadrants for masses (Fig. 28-11)
  - Aorta
  - Liver, spleen, and kidneys for enlargement or irregularities

Replace gown and position draping so lower extremities are exposed.

Legs, Feet, and Toes

- Inspect the lower extremities for overall skin coloration, texture, moisture, masses, lesions, and varicosities.
- Observe muscles of the legs and feet.
- Note hair distribution.
- Palpate joints of hips and test ROM. Palpate the femoral pulse.
- Palpate for
  - Edema, skin temperature
  - Muscle size and tone of legs and feet
- Palpate knees including popliteal pulse.
- Palpate the ankles; assess dorsalis-pedis and posterior-tibial pulses. Test ROM.

- Assess capillary refill.
- Test
  - Sensation to dull and sharp sensations
  - Two-point discrimination (on thighs)
  - Patellar reflex, Achilles reflex, and plantar reflex
  - Position sense (Fig. 28-12)
  - Vibratory sensation on bony surface of big toe

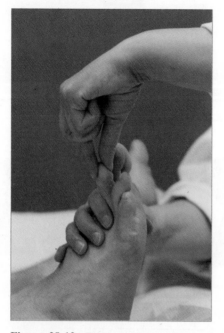

Figure 28-12 Testing position sense of the toes.

- Perform heel-to-shin test.
- As warranted, perform special tests:
  - Position change for arterial insufficiency
  - Manual compression test
  - Trendelenburg test
  - Bulge knee test
  - Ballottement test
  - McMurray's test

Secure gown and assist client to standing position.

Musculoskeletal and Neurological Systems

(Note: These systems have been assessed throughout the examination.)

- Spinal curvatures and check for scoliosis.
- Observe gait (Fig. 28-13) including base of support, weight-bearing stability, foot position, stride, arm swing, and posture.
- Observe as the client
  - Walks heel-to-toe (tandem walk)
  - Hops on one leg, then the other
  - Performs Romberg's test
  - Performs finger-to-nose test

Perform the female and male genitalia examination last, moving from the less private to more private examination for client comfort.

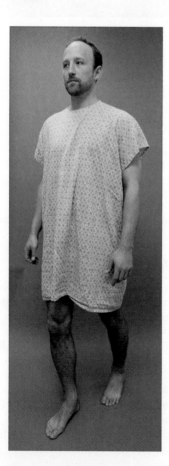

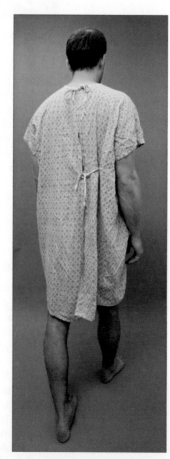

Figure 28-13 Observing gait.

Genitalia
FEMALE GENITALIA

Have female client assume the lithotomy position. Apply gloves. Apply lubricant as appropriate.

- Inspect
  - Distribution of pubic hair
  - Mons pubis, labia majora, and perineum for lesions, swelling, and excoriations
  - Labia minora, clitoris, urethral meatus and vaginal opening for lesions, swelling or discharge
- Palpate
  - Bartholin's glands, urethra, and Skene's glands
  - Size of vaginal opening and vaginal musculature
- Insert speculum and inspect
  - Cervix for lesions and discharge
  - Vagina for color, consistency, and discharge
- Obtain cytological smears and cultures.
- Perform bimanual examination; palpate
  - Cervix for contour, consistency, mobility, and tenderness
  - Uterus for size, position, shape, and consistency
  - Ovaries for size and shape

Discard gloves and apply clean gloves and lubricant.

- Perform the rectovaginal examination; palpate rectovaginal septum for tenderness, consistency, and mobility.

MALE GENITALIA AND RECTUM

Sit on a stool. Have client stand and face you with gown raised. Apply gloves.

- Inspect the penis, including
  - Base of penis and pubic hair for excoriation, erythematic, and infestation
  - Skin and shaft of penis for rashes, lesions, lumps, hardened or tender areas
  - Color, location, and integrity of foreskin in uncircumcised men
  - Glans for size, shape, lesions or redness and location of urinary meatus
- Palpate for urethral discharge by gently squeezing glans.
- Inspect scrotum, including
  - Size, shape, and position
  - Scrotal skin for color, integrity, lesions, or rashes
  - Posterior skin (by lifting scrotal sac)
- Palpate both testis and epididymis between thumb and first two fingers for size, shape, nodules, and tenderness. Palpate spermatic cord and vas deferens.
- Transilluminate scrotal contents for red glow, swelling, or masses. If a mass is found during inspection and palpation, have the client lie down and inspect and palpate for scrotal hernia.
- As client bears down, inspect for bulges in inguinal and femoral areas and palpate for femoral hernias.
- While client shifts weight to each corresponding side, palpate for inguinal hernia and
- Teach testicular self-examination.

Ask the client to remain standing and to bend over the exam table. Change gloves.

- Inspect
  - Perianal area for lump ulcers, lesions, rashes, redness, fissures, or thickening of epithelium
  - Sacrococcygeal area for swelling, redness, dimpling, or hair
- While client bears down or performs Valsalva maneuver, inspect for bulges or lesions.
- Apply lubrication and use finger to palpate
  - Anus
  - External sphincter for tenderness, nodules, and hardness
  - Rectum for tenderness, irregularities, nodules, and hardness
  - Peritoneal cavity
  - Prostate for size, shape, tenderness, and consistency
- Inspect stool for color and test feces for occult blood.

The accompanying video illustrates a head-to-toe physical examination, focusing on those assessment techniques most commonly used by the nurse. In the video, a student nurse performs the examination, demonstrating integration of the body systems and correct assessment technique.

Example of Documented Comprehensive Adult Nursing Health History and Physical Assessment

COMPLETE NURSING HEALTH HISTORY
Biographic Data

> *Client's Name (use initials):* S. L.
>
> *Data provided by:* Client
>
> *Date and Place of Birth:* 4/10/28; St. Louis, Missouri
>
> *Gender:* Female
>
> *Marital Status:* Married
>
> *Nationality, Culture, Ethnicity:* African American
>
> *Religion/Spiritual Practices:* Baptist
>
> *Who Lives With Client:* Husband
>
> *Significant Others:* Husband, two daughters, one son
>
> *Education Level:* College degree
>
> *Occupation (active/laid off/retired):* Retired elementary school teacher
>
> *Primary language (written/spoken):* English
>
> *Secondary language:* None

Reasons for Seeking Health Care Provider

Client states: "The main reason I am here today is to get a checkup, I haven't had one in 8 years. I probably should have had one sooner because I have Type 2 diabetes. I think I have it under control, but I want to make sure. Another reason I am here is because I have started to have some pain in my right hip and fingers. It is starting to really bother me, and I thought I should have it examined."

History of Present Health Concern

Client states that pain started 1 year ago and has been getting progressively worse. Says that pain is worse in morning right after getting out of bed but that it subsides in the afternoon, "after I have been moving around for several hours." Pain started gradually—client cannot think of any event that may have caused it. Client expressed that she thought it was arthritis and that it just happens when "you get old."

States pain is not aggravated by anything that she can think of but that it is relieved with exercise, warm baths, and aspirin. "I try not to let the pain affect my life—but I have trouble making the bed in the morning and I can't write letters until later in the day." Client says she is concerned about the pain getting progressively worse—"My husband and I are very self-sufficient and active; I don't want to have to cut back too much."

Past Health History

Client says she had a normal childhood—"all the childhood illnesses." Had an appendectomy at age 18 and a left arm fracture at age 20. Was hospitalized for 1 week with the birth of each child—"Can you believe I could stay in for a whole week for a normal delivery? My daughters had to leave with their babies after 24 hours!" Had a cholecystectomy at age 56 that was performed for complaint of gas pains after eating fatty foods. Satisfied with care received at local hospital. Denies food, drug, and environmental allergies.

Had polyuria and polydipsia before diagnosis of diabetes. Developed urinary tract infection (UTI) at age 60, at which time she sought medical advice and was diagnosed with Type 2 diabetes. Had a total cholesterol of 214.

Family History

Client states that there is a history of heart attack and high blood pressure in her family and that her father had Type 1 diabetes.

Review of Body Systems for Current Health Problems

Skin, Hair, Nails: Describes skin and scalp as dry. Uses lotions frequently. Denies easy bruising, pruritus, or nonhealing sores. Nails are hard and brittle. Hair is fine and soft. Denies intolerance to heat or cold.

Head and Neck: Denies neck stiffness, swelling, difficulty swallowing, sore throat, or enlarged lymph nodes. "I get a headache occasionally, but I just put a cool washcloth on my head and lie down for a bit—it usually goes away without having to take medicine."

Eyes: Has worn glasses "all my life." Cannot recall age at which they were prescribed. Prescription change from bifocals to trifocals August 1984. Complains of blurred vision without glasses. Denies diplopia, itching, excessive tearing, discharge, redness, or trauma to eyes.

Ears: Believes she is "a little slow to grasp, and I think it may be because of my hearing." Does not wear hearing aid. Cannot recall last hearing test. Denies tinnitus, pain, discharge, or trauma to ears. Does not ask for questions to be repeated.

Mouth, Throat, Nose, and Sinuses: Wears dentures. Last dental examination October 1984. Denies problems with proper fit, eating, chewing, swallowing, sore throat, sore tongue. Complains of "canker sore" if she eats strawberries. Denies difficulty with smell, pain, postnasal drip, sneezing, or frequent nosebleeds. No difficulty tasting foods.

Breasts: Denies pain, lumps, dimpling, retraction, discharge.

Thorax and Lungs: Denies chest pain, trouble breathing, coughing, or fatigue with activity.

Heart and Neck Vessels: Denies palpitations, chest pain and pressure, fatigue, or edema.

Peripheral Vascular: Denies claudication, cramping, sores on legs, or swelling/edema of legs and feet. Denies intolerance to heat or cold. States "occasionally my feet feel numb," subsides on own.

Abdomen: Denies nausea, vomiting, abdominal pain, or excessive gas. Complains of dyspepsia approximately two times per month. Voices no dislikes or food intolerances.

Genitalia: Voids four to five times per day, clear yellow urine. Denies current problem with dysuria, hematuria, polyuria, hesitancy, incontinence, or nocturia. Complains of urgency during the colder months with no increase in frequency. Age of menarche: Approximately 12 yr; age of menopause: 50 yr. States "going through my change of life wasn't difficult for me physically or emotionally." Described menstrual period as regular, lasting 4 days with moderate flow. Denies postmenopausal spotting at this time. Client is gravida 3, Para 3. No complications with pregnancy or childbirth. Has never used any form of contraception. Client states she is sexually active—"My husband and I have good relations." Denies pain, discomfort, or postcoital bleeding. Denies history of any sexually transmitted diseases. Denies problem with vaginal itching. Last Pap smear: negative in 1976.

Anus/Rectum: Soft, formed, medium brown BM every third day after Dulcolax supplement. States she becomes constipated without use of laxative. Denies mucous, bloody, or tarry stools. States discomfort with BMs starting in September 1984. When having to strain with BMs, felt "some kind of mass" prolapsing from rectum. Consulted her doctor, who explained to her "it was a piece of my colon slipping out." No surgical treatment or exercises prescribed. Gently reinserts tissue when this happens. Denies rectal bleeding, change in color, consistency, or habits.

Musculoskeletal: Pain in right hip and finger joints. Denies stiffness, joint pain, or swelling with activity—"Activity helps my hip and finger pain." Occasionally has lower back pains when carrying large amounts of food or when carrying large trays (see Activity Level under Lifestyle and Health Practices).

Neurologic: Speech clear without slur or stutter. Follows verbal cues. Expresses ideas and feelings clearly and concisely. States she has a gradual loss of memory over past 5 to 6 years. Believes long-term memory is better than short-term memory. She can recall past weekly events but has trouble recalling dates, times, and places of events. Learns best by writing information down and then reviewing it. Makes major decisions jointly with husband after prayer.

Lifestyle and Health Practices

Typical Day

A typical day for client is to arise at 6:00 AM, eat breakfast, and perform light housekeeping. Client goes to community center in early afternoon to eat lunch, quilt, and visit. Goes home around 2:00 PM. Walks about four blocks with a friend every day. Cleans own house daily for one 2-h period (includes dusting, vacuuming, washing). After walking, returns home and relaxes with crafts and visiting with husband. Attends church-related activities in the evening. Bedtime is around 10:00 PM.

Nutrition Habits and Weight Management

Client states she is on a consistent carbohydrate diet that has approximately 1600 calories/day intake. Eats breakfast of whole wheat toast, one boiled egg, orange juice, and decaffeinated coffee. Her lunch meal varies, but today she had tuna; salad with lettuce, tomatoes, and broccoli; an apple; and milk. Typical dinner includes small serving of broiled meat, green vegetables, piece of fruit, and glass of milk. Tries not to snack but will have fruit if she feels the urge. Drinks two 8-oz glasses of water a day. Drinks decaffeinated coffee—no tea or colas. Voices no food dislikes or intolerances.

Client expresses desire to maintain current weight. Weight tends to fluctuate ±5 lb/month—"I've always had to watch what I eat because I gain so easily."

Medication/Substance Use

No prescribed medications, takes the following OTC medications: ASA gr prn for "hip and finger joint pain." Takes about two times per month. Denies nausea, abdominal pains, or evidence of bleeding while taking ASA. Mylanta prn for "gas pains." Dulcolax suppository 3 times per week for past 4 years. Multivitamin 1 qd for past 4 years. Denies use of alcohol, tobacco, and illicit drugs.

Activity Level/Exercise-Fitness Plan

Client performs housekeeping for a couple of hours and walks four blocks a day. Is retired from being an elementary school teacher and part-time caterer. Volunteers to cook for church social functions. Client expresses satisfaction with activity and believes she functions above the level of the average person her age.

Sleep/Rest

Goes to bed at 10:00 PM. Denies difficulty falling asleep or sleeping. Feels well rested when she arises at 6:00 AM. Never used sleep medications. Denies orthopnea and nocturnal dyspnea. Enjoys reading one to two pages of Bible history each evening.

Self-Concept, Self-Esteem, Body Image

Describes self as normal person. Talkative, outgoing, and likes to be around people but hates noisy environments. Happy with the person she has become and states, "I can definitely live with myself." States a weakness is that she worries about "little things" more now than she used to and tends to be irritated

more easily. Client states she "feels good" about self-management of diabetes. Client rates own health as an 8 on a scale of 1 (worst) to 10 (best). Five years ago, she rated health as a 10 and predicts that 5 years in the future health will be a 6. Sees health deterioration as normal aging process and states, "I feel really good when I look at a lot of people my age with all their problems and the medicine they take."

Self-Care Responsibilities

Client seeks health care only in emergencies. Last medical examination was September 1984. Does not check own blood sugar or perform breast self-exam. Always wears seat belt, asks husband to test smoke alarm monthly, uses a sturdy step stool to reach objects out of reach.

Social Relationships

Describes relationship with other members of the church and community groups as friendly and "family-like." Has casual relationship with neighbors. Visits community center every day to socialize, attends church functions several evenings a week. Walks with a friend every day.

Family Relationships

Client has been married 55 years. Describes relationship as the best part of her life right now. Two daughters live in Texas with their husbands and children. Her son and his wife and baby boy live in Minnesota. All the children and their families come home once a year, and the client and her husband visit each family once a year. She expresses desire to visit her children and grandchildren more often and states, "I wish my babies lived nearby. I love being a grandma and miss them so much." Communicates with each of them several times a month by phone. Client was the fourth of five children in her family. Had a happy childhood, describes family as close and loving—"my daddy was very strict though."

Education and Work

Client went to college to be a teacher. Taught elementary school for 30 years. After her children were grown, she would work during the summer as a caterer—"I love to cook." Is retired now but still volunteers to cook for church social functions.

Stress Level and Coping Styles

States that husband's high blood pressure has never been a source of stress to her. Shares confidences with husband and with a few close friends. Most stressful time in life was losing two brothers and a sister, all in 1982. States that with support of husband, children, and church, she handled it "better than most people would have." States she prays and eats when under stress. Cannot identify any major stresses that have occurred in the last year.

Environmental Hazards

Is not aware of any environmental hazards in area where she lives.

Developmental Level

Integrity Versus Despair

Describes childhood as a very happy time for her. Becomes excited and smiles as she relates stories of her childhood on the farm. States she was an average child and ran and played like all the others. Companions were brothers and sisters. Has been married for 55 years. Describes relationship with husband as close and sharing. Taught elementary school for 30 years and catered in the summers for several years. Lived in a large house until 1976. Currently lives in small two-bedroom bungalow. Active in church and society. Volunteers at church functions. States she enjoys being retired and lives a "comfortable" life. Does not voice financial concerns. Has begun to write will and distribute personal heirlooms to children and grandchildren. States she is not afraid of death and wishes to have the "business part taken care of" in order to enjoy the rest of her life together with her husband.

PHYSICAL ASSESSMENT
General Survey

Ht: 5 foot 4 inches; Wt: 145 lb; Radial pulse: 71; Resp: 16; B/P: R arm—120/72, L arm—120/72; Temp: 98.6. Client alert and cooperative. Sitting comfortably on table with arms crossed and shoulder slightly slouched forward. Smiling with mild anxiety. Dress is neat and clean. Walks steadily with posture slightly stooped.

> *Mental Status Examination:* Pleasant and friendly. Appropriately dressed for weather with matching colors and patterns. Clothes neat and clean. Facial expressions symmetric and correlate with mood and topic discussed. Speech clear and appropriate. Follows through with train of thought. Carefully chooses words to convey feelings and ideas. Oriented to person, place, time, and events. Remains attentive and able to focus on examination during entire interaction. Short-term memory intact, long-term memory before 1980 unclear—especially cannot recall dates and sequencing of events. General information questions answered correctly 100% of the time. Vocabulary suitable to educational level. Explains proverb accurately. Gives semiabstract answers and enjoys joking. Is able to identify similarities 5 seconds after being asked. Answers to judgment questions in realistic manner.

Skin, Hair, Nails

> *Skin:* Light brown, warm and dry to touch. Skinfold returns to place after 1 s when lifted over clavicle. Darker "age spots" on posterior hands bilaterally in clusters of four to five and evenly distributed over lower extremities. 3-cm nodule with 2-mm macule in center noted in right axilla; indurated, nontender, and nonmobile. No evidence of vascular or purpuric lesions. No edema.

> *Hair:* Slightly curly, pulled back in a bun at nape of neck, clean, black with white and gray streaks, thin and dry in texture. No scalp lesions or flaking. Fine black hair evenly distributed over arms bilaterally and sparsely on legs bilaterally. No hair noted on axilla or on chest, back, or face.

> *Nails:* Fingernails medium length and thickness, clear. Splinter hemorrhages noted on right thumb near fingertip in midline. No clubbing or Beau's lines.

Head and Neck

Head symmetrically rounded, neck nontender with full ROM. Neck symmetric without masses, scars, pulsations. Lymph nodes nonpalpable. Trachea in midline. Thyroid nonpalpable.

Eyes

Eyes 2 cm apart without protrusion. Eyebrows sparse with equal distribution. No scalines noted. Lids light brown without ptosis, edema, or lesions, and freely closeable bilaterally. Lacrimal apparatus nonedematous. Sclera white without increased vascularity or lesions noted. Palpebral and bulbar conjunctiva slightly reddened without lesions noted. Iris uniformly blue. PERRLA, EOMs intact bilaterally. Peripheral vision is equal to examiner's. Visual acuity: Snellen chart—with glasses off vision is 20/70 OD, OS; with glasses on vision is 20/20 OD, OS. Rosenbaum vision screener—with glasses off vision is blurred at 14 inches away but can identify number of fingers held up. With glasses on vision is clear at 14 inches. Funduscopic examination: Red reflex present bilaterally. Optic disk round with well-defined margins. Physiologic cup occupies disc. Arterioles smaller than venules. No AV nicking, no hemorrhages, or exudates noted. Macula not seen.

Ears

Left auricle without deformity, lumps, or lesions. Right auricle with tag at top of pinna. Auricles and mastoid processes nontender. Bilateral auditory canals contain moderate amount of dark brown cerumen. Tympanic membrane difficult to view due to wax. Whisper test: Client identifies one out of two words in four attempts. Weber test: No lateralization of sound to either ear. Rinne test: AC is greater than BC in both ears.

Mouth, Throat, Nose, and Sinuses

Lips moist, no lesions or ulcerations. Buccal mucosa pink and moist with patchy areas of dark pigment on ventral surface of tongue, gums, and floor of mouth. No ulcers or nodules. Gums pink and moist without inflammation, bleeding, or discoloration. Hard and soft palates smooth without lesions or masses. Tongue midline when protruded, no lesions, or masses. No lesions, discolorations, or ulcerations on floor of mouth, oral mucosa, or gums. Uvula in midline and elevates on phonation. Tonsils present without exudate, edema, ulcers, or enlargement. External structure without deformity, asymmetry, or inflammation. Nares patent. Turbinates and middle meatus pale pink, without swelling, exudate, lesions, or bleeding. Nasal septum midline without bleeding, perforation, or deviation. Frontal and maxillary sinuses nontender.

Thorax and Lung

Skin light brown without scars, pulsations, or lesions. No hair noted. Thorax expands evenly bilaterally without retractions or bulging. Slope of ribs = 40 degrees. No use of auxiliary respiratory muscles and no nasal flaring. Mild kyphosis. Respirations even, unlabored, and regular (16/min). No cough noted. No tenderness, crepitus, or masses. Tactile fremitus decreases below T5 bilaterally posteriorly, and 4th ICS anteriorly bilaterally. Thorax resonance throughout. Diaphragmatic excursion: Left—on inspiration diaphragm descends to T11, and on expiration diaphragm ascends to T9. Right—on inspiration diaphragm descends to T12, and on expiration diaphragm ascends to T9. Vesicular breath sounds heard in all lung fields. No rales, rhonchi, friction rubs, whispered pectoriloquy, bronchophony, or egophony noted.

Breasts

Breasts moderate size, round, and symmetrical bilaterally. Skin light brown with dark brown areola. No dimpling or retraction. Free movement in all positions. Engorged vein noted running across UOQ to areola in right breast. Nipples inverted bilaterally. No discharge expressed. No thickening or tenderness noted. Hard, immobile 2 cm round mass noted in left breast in LOQ. Client denies ever noticing this. Nontender to palpation. Lymph nodes nonpalpable. Client does not know how to do SBE.

Heart and Neck Vessels

No pulsations visible. No heaves, lifts, or vibrations. Apical Impulse: 5th ICS to LMCL. Clear, brief heart sounds throughout. Physiologic S2. No gallops, murmurs, or rubs. AP = 72/min and regular.

Abdomen

Abdomen rounded, symmetric without masses, lesions, pulsations, or peristalsis noted. Abdomen free of hair, bruising, and increased vasculature. Healed with appendectomy scar. Umbilicus in midline, without herniation, swelling or discoloration. Bowel sounds low pitched and gurgling at 22/min × 4 quads. Aortic, renal, and iliac arteries auscultated without bruit. No venous hums or friction rubs auscultated over liver or spleen. Tympany percussed over all 4 quads. 8 cm. Liver span percussed in R MCL. Area of dullness percussed at 9th ICS in left postaxillary line. No tenderness or masses noted with light and deep palpation in all 4 quadrants. Liver and spleen nonpalpable.

Genital

Labia pink with decreased elasticity and vaginal secretions. No bulging of vaginal wall, purulent foul drainage, or lesions. Skene's gland not visible. 1-cm nodule palpated in R groin.

Anus/Rectum

Anal area pink with small amount of hair. Rectal mucosa bulges with straining.

Peripheral Vascular

Arms: Equal in size and symmetry bilaterally; pale pink; warm and dry to touch without edema, bruising, or lesions noted. Radial pulses = in rate and amplitude and strong. Allen's test: right = 2-second refill, left = 2-second refill. Brachial pulses strong, equal, and even. Epitrochlear nodes nonpalpable.

Legs: Legs large in size and bilaterally symmetric. Skin intact, light brown; warm and dry to touch without edema, bruising, lesions, or increased vascularity. Superficial inguinal, horizontal, and vertical lymph nodes nonpalpable. Femoral pulses strong and equal without bruits. Popliteal pulse nonpalpable with client supine or prone. Dorsalis pedal and posterior tibial

pulses strong and equal. No edema palpable. Homans' sign negative bilaterally. No retrograde filling noted when client stands. Toenails thick and yellowed. Special maneuver for arterial insufficiency: Feet regain color after 4 seconds and veins refilled in 5 seconds.

Musculoskeletal

Posture slightly stooped with mild kyphosis. Gait steady, smooth, and coordinated with even base. Limited ROM of lateral flexion and extension of spine. Paravertebrals equal in size and strength; upper extremities and lower extremities with full ROM. Muscles moderately firm bilaterally. No deviations, inflammations, or bony deformities. Small callus on left heel. Moves upper and lower extremities freely against gravity and against resistance. Rheumatoid nodule noted on dorsal surface of left hand.

Neurologic

Cranial Nerve Examination: CN I: Correctly identifies scent. CN II: 20/70 vision OD and OS; blurred vision at 14 inches w/o glasses; full visual fields. CN III, IV, and VI: Lid covers 2 mm of iris; bilateral eye movement, bilateral pupil response. CN V: Identifies light touch and sharp touch to forehead, cheek, and chin. Bilateral corneal reflex intact. Masseter muscles contract equally and bilaterally. Jaw jerk +1. CN VII: Identifies sugar and salt on anterior 2/3 of tongue. Smiles, frowns, shows teeth, blows out cheeks, and raises eyebrows as instructed. CN VIII: Hears whispered words from 1 to 2 feet; Weber test: Vibration heard equally well in both ears; Rhine test: AC > BC. CN IX and X: Gag reflex intact, and client identifies sugar and salt on posterior of tongue. Uvula in midline and elevates on phonation. CN XI: Shrugs shoulders and moves head to right and left against resistance. CN XII: Tongue midline when protruded without fasciculations.

Table 28-1	Two Point Discrimination Findings	
Two-Point Discrimination	**Right**	**Left**
(in mm):		
Fingertips	6	6
Dorsal hand	15	15
Chest	45	49
Forearm	39	35
Back	45	45
Upper arm	40	45
Reflexes		
Biceps	2+	2+
Triceps	2+	2+
Patellar	3+	3+
Achilles	2+	2+
Abdominal	1+	1+
Babinski	negative	negative

Motor and Cerebellar Examination: Muscle tone firm at rest, abdominal muscles slightly relaxed. Muscle size adequate for age. No fasciculations or involuntary movements noted. Muscle strength moderately strong and equal bilaterally. Alternates finger to nose with eyes closed; occasionally tends to hit opposite side of nose. Rapidly opposes fingers to thumb bilaterally without difficulty. Alternates pronation and supination of hands rapidly without difficulty. Heel to shin intact bilaterally. Romberg: Minimal swaying. Tandem walk: Steady. No involuntary movements noted.

Sensory Status Examination: Superficial light and deep touch sensation intact on arms, legs, neck, chest, and back. Position sense of toes and fingers intact bilaterally. Identifies point localization correctly. Identifies coin placed in hand and number written on back correctly.

Client's Strengths

- Positive attitude and outlook on life
- Motivation to comply with prescribed diet
- Strong support systems; husband and spiritual beliefs
- No physical limitations

Nursing Diagnoses

- Risk for Altered Maintenance related to lack of knowledge concerning importance of regular medical checkups, ie: lesion in UOQ of left breast not seen by physician, no Pap smear, and no follow-up for diabetes

- Acute right hip pain
- Constipation related to lack of bowel routine and laxative overuse, and decreased daily water consumption
- Knowledge Deficit: Signs and symptoms and treatment of hyperglycemia/hypoglycemia
- Knowledge Deficit: Management and causes of constipation
- Knowledge Deficit: Self breast exam technique
- Knowledge Deficit: Self-care behaviors regarding diabetes management: Blood glucose monitoring, yearly dilated eye exam, and yearly lipid panel

Collaborative Problems

- RC: Hyperglycemia, hypoglycemia

Abbreviated Physical Assessment for the Acute Care Setting

The following is a brief "Head-to-Toe Physical Assessment Guide" that may be used to establish the client's physical status. This type of assessment is frequently used by nurses at the beginning of a hospital shift when the nurse has multiple clients to whom she will provide nursing care. Often, a total physical examination is done upon admission to the hospital by the physician or nurse practitioner. Therefore, this shorter format is more practical for ongoing client assessments.

ABBREVIATED HEAD-TO-TOE PHYSICAL ASSESSMENT

Assessment Procedure	Normal Findings	Abnormal Findings
General Survey		
Assess Level of Consciousness (LOC).	Awake, alert and oriented to person, place, and time.	If altered LOC, consider the Glascow Coma Scale.
Assess speech.	Speech clear. Makes and maintains conversation appropriately.	
Assess comfort level.	Denies c/o pain/discomfort.	If the patient reports or c/o of pain: rate the pain using the 0–10 pain scale, intervene to provide comfort measures and evaluate the effectiveness of such interventions.
Assess skin color, temperature, moisture, turgor.	Skin: pink, warm and dry. Immediate recoil noted at the clavicle.	Pale, pallor → anemia Erythema → infection Warmth → infection Increased tenting → dehydration
Eyes Assess pupils.	Pupils equal, round, react to light and accommodation (PERRLA).	Pupils unequal or non-reactive to light.

continued

Assessment Procedure	Normal Findings	Abnormal Findings
Chest		
Assess breath sounds.	Lungs: clear to auscultation (CTA) anterior and posterior (A & P), bilaterally. Respiratory rate = 18, no reports of dyspnea	Note any wheezes or crackles and identify their location (anterior or posterior, upper or lower lobes, right or left).
Assess heart sounds. Note if rhythm is irregular.	Heart: S1 and S2 present, regular rate (82) and rhythm. No S3 or S4 appreciated. No murmur, rub, or gallop (MRG).	Heart sounds irregular or irregularly irregular. Murmurs, rub, or gallop—if present.
Abdomen		
Assess contour and firmness.	Non-distended, soft, and non-tender.	Distended and firm, visible palpations.
Assess bowel sounds.	Active bowel sounds noted in all 4 quadrants (+ABS X 4Q).	Absence of bowel sounds in one or more quadrants. One must listen for 5 minutes to document absent bowel sounds. Normal bowel sounds = 5–35/minute.
Extremities		
Assess mobility of extremities, strength of extremities, and peripheral pulses.	Able to actively move all extremities. Equal strength, 5/5. Radial, dorsalis pedis and posterior tibia pulses 2+. No peripheral edema.	Unable to actively or passively move one or more extremities.
Other		
Note any wounds or lesions.	Describe: size, shape, location, color, characteristics of any drainage, type of dressing.	
Note any drains: Jackson-Pratt, Foley catheter, Hemovac, nasogastric tube.	Describe insertion site; color, consistency, and/or odor of any drainage.	
Note any venous access devices.	Describe the location, appearance, type and size of device, type of intravenous fluids and rate of infusion, and infusion device(s).	
Note any other therapies: external ice/heat devices, continuous passive motion devices, TENS unit, etc.	Describe the presence of correct functioning of any of these devices.	

Nursing Assessment of Special Groups

29

Assessing Childbearing Women

Structure and Function

The body experiences physiologic and anatomic changes during pregnancy. Most of these changes are influenced by the hormones of pregnancy, primarily estrogen and progesterone. Normal physiologic and anatomic changes during pregnancy are discussed in this chapter.

SKIN, HAIR, AND NAILS

During pregnancy, integumentary system changes occur primarily because of hormonal influences. Many of these skin, hair, and nail changes fade or completely resolve after the end of the gestation. As the pregnancy progresses, the breasts and abdomen enlarge and striae gravidarum, or stretch marks—pinkish-red streaks with slight depressions in the skin—begin to appear over the abdomen, breasts, thighs, and buttocks. These marks usually fade to a white or silvery color, but they typically never completely resolve after the pregnancy.

Hyperpigmentation also results from hormonal influences (e.g., estrogen, progesterone, and melanocyte-stimulating hormone). It is most noted on the abdomen (linea nigra, a dark line extending from the umbilicus to the mons pubis) and face (chloasma, a darkening of the skin on the face, known as the facial "mask of pregnancy"). Some women who take oral contraceptives may also have chloasma because of the hormones in the medication.

Other skin changes during pregnancy include darkening of the areolae and nipples, axillae, umbilicus, and perineum. Scars and moles may also darken from the influence of melanocyte-stimulating hormone. Vascular changes, such as spider nevi (tiny red angiomas occurring on the face, neck, chest, arms, and legs), may occur because of elevated estrogen levels. Palmar erythema (a pinkish color on the palms of the hands) may also be noted. Pruritic urticarial papules and plaques of pregnancy (PUPPP) is a skin disorder seen during the third trimester of pregnancy, characterized by erythematous papules, plaques and urticarial lesions. The rash begins on the abdomen and may soon spread to the thighs, buttocks and arms. The intense itching and rash usually resolve within weeks of delivery. Acne

vulgaris is an unpredictable response during pregnancy. Acne may worsen or improve. It consists of erythema, pustules, comedones, and/or cysts that appear on the face, back, neck, or chest. The activity of the eccrine sweat glands and the excretion rate of sebum onto the skin increase in normal pregnancy, whereas the activity of the apocrine sweat glands appears to decrease. The changes that occur in the endocrine system help to maintain optimal maternal and fetal health. Estrogen is primarily responsible for the changes that occur to the pituitary, thyroid, parathyroid, and adrenal glands. The increased production of the hormones, especially triiodothyronine (T_3) and thyroxine (T_4), increases the basal metabolic rate, cardiac output, vasodilation, heart rate, and heat intolerance. The basal metabolic rate increases up to 30% in a term pregnancy.

Growth of hair and nails also tends to increase during pregnancy. Some women note excessive oiliness or dryness of the scalp and a softening and thinning of the nails by the 6th week of gestation. Pregnancy hormones increase the growing phases of the hair follicle and decrease the resting phase of the hair follicle. During the postpartum period, hormone withdrawal increases the resting phase of the hair follicle and transient hair loss is noticed and commonly peaks at 3 to 4 months postpartum. This loss is normally resolved within 9 months to 1 year of delivery.

Hirsutism of the face, abdomen and back may also be experienced during the second and third trimesters of pregnancy. Hormonal changes (androgens) cause this hair growth, which may improve after delivery.

EARS AND HEARING

Pregnant women may report a decrease in hearing, a sense of fullness in the ears, or earaches because of the increased vascularity of the tympanic membrane and blockage of the eustachian tubes.

MOUTH, THROAT, NOSE, AND SINUS

Some women may note changes in their gums during pregnancy. Gingival bleeding when brushing the teeth and hypertrophy are common. Occasionally epulis, which are small, irritating nodules of the gums, develop. These nodules usually resolve on their own. Occasionally the lesion may need to be surgically excised if the nodule bleeds excessively.

Vocal changes may be noted because of the edema of the larynx. Nasal "stuffiness" and epistaxis are also common during pregnancy because of the estrogen-induced edema and vascular congestion of the nasal mucosa and sinuses.

THORAX AND LUNGS

As the pregnancy progresses, progesterone influences the relaxation of the ligaments and joints. This relaxation allows the rib cage to flare, thus increasing the anteroposterior and transverse diameters. This accommodation is necessary as the pregnancy progresses and the enlarging uterus pushes up on the diaphragm. The client's respiratory pattern changes from abdominal to costal. Shortness of breath is a common complaint during the last trimester. The client may be more aware of her breathing pattern and of deep respirations and more frequent sighing. Oxygen requirements increase during pregnancy because of the additional cellular growth of the body and the fetus. Pulmonary requirements increase, with the tidal volume increasing by 30% to 40%. All of these changes are normal and are to be expected during the last trimester.

BREASTS

Soon after conception, the surge of estrogen and progesterone begins, causing notable changes in the mammary glands (Fig. 29-1). Breast changes noted by many women include

- Tingling sensations and tenderness
- Enlargement of breast and nipple
- Hyperpigmentation of areola and nipple
- Enlargement of Montgomery tubercles
- Prominence of superficial veins
- Development of striae
- Expression of colostrum in the second and third trimester

HEART

Significant cardiovascular changes occur during pregnancy. One of the most dynamic changes is the increase in cardiac output and maternal blood volume by approximately 40% to 50%. Because the heart is required to pump much harder, it actually increases in size. Its position is rotated up and to the left approximately 1 to 1.5 cm. The heart rate may increase by 10 to 15 beats/min and systolic murmurs may be heard.

PERIPHERAL VASCULAR SYSTEM

With the dynamic increase in maternal blood volume, a physiologic anemia (pseudoanemia) commonly develops. This anemia results primarily from the disproportionate increase in blood volume compared to the increased red blood cell (RBC) production. Plasma volume increases 40% to 50% and RBC volume increases 18% to 30% by 30 to 34 weeks' gestation.

As the plasma blood volume increases, the blood vessels must accommodate for this volume, so progesterone acts on the

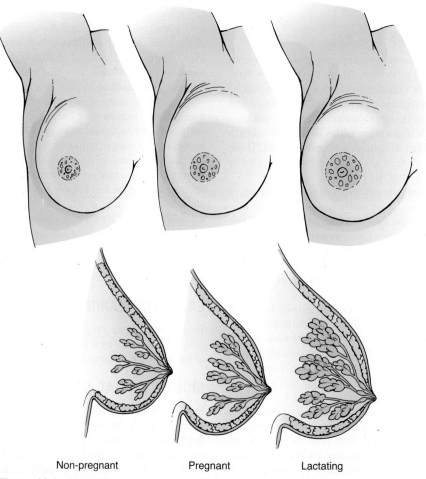

Non-pregnant   Pregnant   Lactating

Figure 29-1   Breast changes during pregnancy.

vessels to make them relax and dilate. Clients often complain of feeling dizzy and lightheaded beginning with the second trimester. These effects peak at approximately 32 to 34 weeks. As the pregnancy progresses, the arterial blood pressure stabilizes and symptoms begin to resolve. Prepregnant values return in the third trimester.

Other changes that occur during pregnancy include dependent edema and varicosities. Two-thirds of all pregnant women have swelling of the lower extremities in the third trimester. Swelling is usually noted late in the day after standing for long periods. Fluid retention is caused by the increased hormones of pregnancy, increased hydrophilicity of the intracellular connective tissue, and the increased venous pressure in the lower extremities. As the expanding uterus applies pressure on the femoral venous area, femoral venous pressure increases. This uterine pressure restricts the venous blood flow return, causing stagnation of the blood in the lower extremities and resulting in dependent edema. Varicose veins in the lower extremities, vulva, and rectum are also common during pregnancy. Pregnant women are also more prone to development of thrombophlebitis because of the hypercoagulable state of pregnancy. Women who are placed on bedrest during pregnancy are at a very high risk for development of thrombophlebitis.

ABDOMEN

During pregnancy, the abdominal muscles stretch as the uterus enlarges. These muscles, known as the rectus abdominis muscles, may stretch to the point that permanent separation occurs. This condition is known as *diastasis recti abdominis*. Four paired ligaments (broad ligaments, uterosacral ligaments, cardinal ligaments, round ligaments) support the uterus and keep it in position in the pelvic cavity (Fig. 29-2). As the uterus

enlarges, the client may complain of lower pelvic discomfort, which quite commonly results from stretching the ligaments, especially the round ligaments.

In the abdomen, the expanding uterus exerts pressure on the bladder, kidney, and ureters (especially on the right side), predisposing the client to kidney infection. Urinary frequency is a common complaint in the first and third trimesters. The applied pressure on the kidneys and ureters causes decreased flow and stagnation of the urine. As a result, physiologic hydronephrosis and hydroureter occur. During the second trimester, bladder pressure subsides and urinary frequency is relieved by the uterus enlarging and being lifted out of the pelvic area.

The enlarging uterus also applies pressure and displaces the small intestine. This pressure along with the secretion of progesterone decreases gastric motility. Gastric tone is decreased and the smooth muscles relax, decreasing emptying time of the stomach. Constipation results from these physiologic events. Heartburn, which may also result, may also be related to the decreased gastrointestinal motility and displacement of the stomach. This causes reflux of stomach acid into the esophagus. Progesterone secretion also relaxes the smooth muscles of the gallbladder; as a result, gallstone formation may occur because of the prolonged emptying time of the gallbladder.

Other gastrointestinal symptoms include ptyalism and pica. Ptyalism, excessive salivation may occur in the first trimester. Pica, a craving for or ingestion of non-nutritional substances such as dirt or clay, is seen in all socioeconomic classes and cultures. Pica can be a major concern if the craving interferes with proper nutrition during pregnancy.

Carbohydrate metabolism is also altered during pregnancy. Glucose use increases, leading to decreased maternal glucose levels. The rise in serum levels of estrogen, progesterone, and

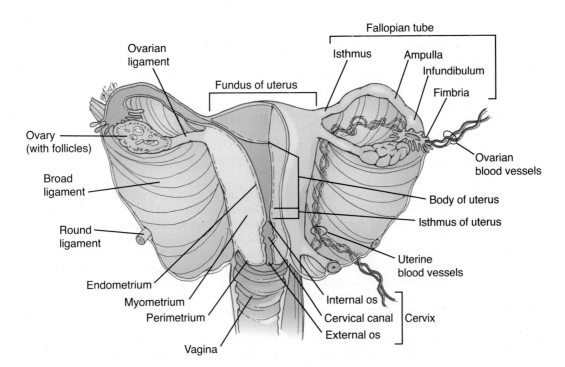

Figure 29-2 Anterior cross-section of the female reproductive structures.

other hormones stimulates beta-cell hypertrophy and hyperplasia, and insulin secretion increases. Glycogen is stored, and gluconeogenesis is reduced. In addition, the mother's body tissues develop an increased sensitivity to insulin, thus decreasing the mother's need. As a result, maternal hypoglycemia leads to hypoinsulinemia and increased rates of ketosis. Some well-controlled insulin-dependent diabetic clients have frequent episodes of hypoglycemia in the first trimester. This buildup of insulin ensures an adequate supply of glucose, because the glucose is preferentially shunted to the fetus.

In contrast during the second half of pregnancy, tissue sensitivity to insulin progressively decreases, producing hyperglycemia and hyperinsulinemia. Insulin resistance becomes maximal in the latter half of the pregnancy.

GENITALIA

Before conception, the uterus is a small, pear-shaped organ that weighs approximately 44 g. Its cavity can hold approximately 10 mL of fluid. Pregnancy changes this organ, giving it the capacity of weighing approximately 1,000 g and potentially holding approximately 5 L of amniotic fluid. This dynamic change is mainly due to the hypertrophy of preexisting myometrial cells and the hyperplasia of new cells. Estrogen and the growing fetus are primarily responsible for this growth. Once conception occurs, the uterus prepares itself for the pregnancy: ovulation ceases, the uterine endometrium thickens, and the number and size of uterine blood vessels increase.

With fetal growth, the uterus continues to expand throughout the pregnancy. At approximately 10 to 12 weeks' gestation, the uterus should be palpated at the top of the symphysis pubis. At 16 weeks' gestation, the top of the uterus, known as the fundus, should reach halfway between the symphysis pubis and the umbilicus. At 20 weeks' gestation, the fundus should be at the level of the umbilicus. For the rest of the pregnancy, the uterus grows approximately 1 cm/week, so the fundal height should equal the number of weeks pregnant (e.g., at 25 weeks' gestation, the fundal height should measure 25 cm). This formula is known as McDonald's rule. It can be calculated by taking the fundal height in centimeters and multiplying it by 8/7. With a full-term pregnancy, the fundus should reach the xiphoid process. The fundal height measurement may drop the last few weeks of the pregnancy if the fetal head is engaged and descended in the maternal pelvis. This occurrence is known as *lightening*.

Near term gestation, the uterine wall begins thinning out to approximately 5 mm or less. Fetal parts are easily palpated on the external abdomen in the term pregnancy. Braxton Hicks contractions (painless, irregular contractions of the uterus) may occur sporadically in the third trimester. These contractions are normal as long as no cervical change is noted.

Normal changes in the cervix, vagina, and vulva also occur during pregnancy. Cervical softening (Goodell's sign), bluish discoloration (Chadwick's sign), and hypertrophy of the glands in the cervical canal all occur. With these glands secreting more mucus, there is an increase in vaginal discharge, which is acidic. The mucus collects in the cervix to form the mucous plug. This plug seals the endocervical canal and prevents bacteria from ascending into the uterus, thus preventing infection. The vaginal smooth muscle and connective tissue soften and expand to prepare for the passage of the fetus through the birth canal.

ANUS AND RECTUM

Constipation is a common problem during pregnancy. Progesterone decreases intestinal motility, allowing more time for nutrients to be absorbed for the mother and fetus. This also increases the absorption time for water into the circulation, taking fluid from the large intestine and contributing to hardening of the stool and decreasing the frequency of bowel movements. Iron supplementation can also contribute to constipation for those women who take additional iron. As a result, hemorrhoids (varicose veins in the rectum) may develop because of the pressure on the venous structures from straining to have a bowel movement. Vascular congestion of the pelvis also contributes to hemorrhoid development.

MUSCULOSKELETAL SYSTEM

Anatomic changes of the musculoskeletal system during pregnancy result from fetal growth, hormonal influences, and maternal weight gain. As the pregnancy progresses, uterine growth pulls the pelvis forward, which causes the spine to curve forward, creating a gradual lordosis (Fig. 29-3). The enlarging breasts influence the shoulders to droop forward. The pregnant client typically finds herself pulling her shoulders back and straightening her head and neck to accommodate for this weight. Progesterone and relaxin (nonsteroidal hormone) influence the pelvic joints and ligaments to relax. The symphysis pubis, sacroiliac and sacrococcygeal joints become more flexible during pregnancy. This flexibility allows the pelvic outlet diameter to increase slightly, which reduces the risk of trauma during childbirth. After the postpartum period, the pelvic diameter will generally remain larger than the size before childbirth.

The relaxin hormone contributes to changing the client's gait during pregnancy. The pregnant woman's gait is often described as "waddling." Gait changes are also attributed to weight gain of the uterus, fetus, and breasts. At approximately 24 weeks gestation, the woman's center of gravity and stance change, causing the woman to lean back slightly to balance herself. Backaches are common during pregnancy. Along with these changes, the woman may also see an increase in shoe size, especially in width.

NEUROLOGIC SYSTEM

Most neurologic changes that occur during pregnancy are discomforting to the client. Common neurologic complaints include

- Pain or tingling feeling in the thigh: Caused by pressure on the lateral femoral cutaneous nerve
- Carpal tunnel syndrome: Pressure on the median nerve below the carpal ligament of the wrist causes a tingling sensation in the hand. Because fluid retention occurs during pregnancy, swollen tissues compress the median nerve in the wrist and produce the tingling sensations. Pain can be reproduced by performing Tinel's sign and Phalen's test. Up and down movement of the wrist aggravates this condition.
- Leg cramps: Caused by inadequate calcium intake
- Dizziness and lightheadedness: In early pregnancy, the client may experience dizziness because of the blood

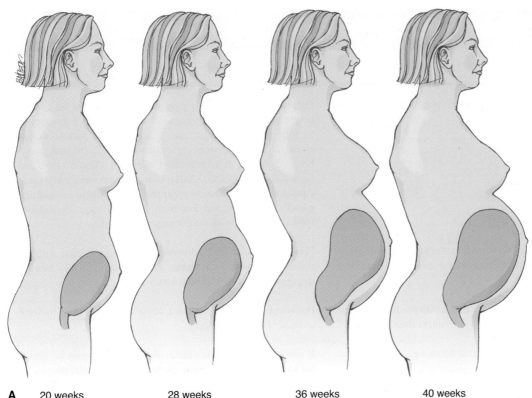

A   20 weeks   28 weeks   36 weeks   40 weeks

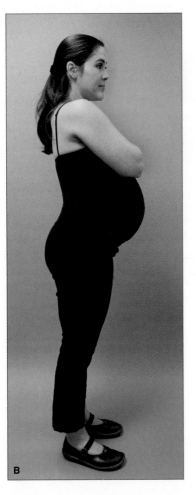

Figure 29-3 **(A)** Postural changes during pregnancy; **(B)** Lordosis in pregnant patient.

pressure slightly decreasing as a result of vasodilation and decreased vascular resistance. In later pregnancy, the client in the supine position may experience dizziness caused by the heavy uterus compressing the vena cava and aorta. This compression reduces cardiac return, cardiac output, and blood pressure. This is known as *supine hypotensive syndrome.*

Health Assessment

COLLECTING SUBJECTIVE DATA: THE NURSING HEALTH HISTORY

A complete health history is necessary to provide high-quality care for the pregnant client. If the examiner does not have access to a recent complete health history for the pregnant client, a complete health history should be performed before focusing on particular questions associated with the pregnancy, which are discussed in this section. The first prenatal visit focuses on collection of baseline data about the client and her partner and identification of risk factors.

Biographical Data

Biographical data should be included in the health history. This information may include the patient's name, birth date, address and phone number. Obtaining the patient's educational level, occupation and work status helps the staff to speak to the patient at the appropriate level for understanding. The health history should also include the patient's significant other with phone number and contact information in case of emergency.

(text continues on page 623)

HISTORY OF PRESENT HEALTH CONCERN/CURRENT HEALTH STATUS

Question	Rationale
What was your normal weight before pregnancy? Has your weight changed since a year ago?	Optimal weight gain during pregnancy depends on the client's height and weight. Recommended weight gain in pregnancy is as follows: Underweight client, 28 to 40 lb; normal weight client, 25 to 35 lb; overweight client, 15 to 25 lb; twin gestation, 35 to 45 lb (American College of Obstetricians and Gynecologists [ACOG], 2001). Low pregnant weight and inadequate weight gain during pregnancy contribute to intrauterine growth retardation and low birth weight. Figure 29-4 shows typical distribution of weight gain in pregnancy.
Is your nose often stuffed up when you don't have a cold? Have you had a fever or chills, except with a cold, since your last menstrual period?	Fetal exposure to viral illnesses has been associated with intrauterine growth retardation, developmental delay, hearing impairment, and mental retardation.
Do you have any trouble with your throat? Do you have a cough that hasn't gone away or do you have frequent chest infections?	Persistent cough and frequent chest infections may indicate pneumonia or tuberculosis.
Do you have nausea or vomiting that doesn't go away? Is your thirst greater than normal?	If proper hydration is not maintained, the client may be at risk for hyperemesis gravidarum, cholecystitis, or cholelithiasis.

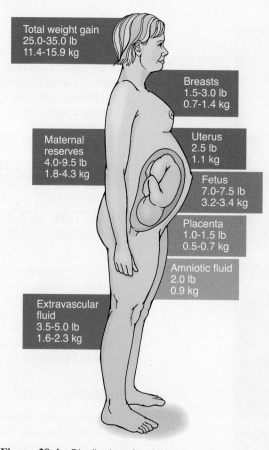

Total weight gain
25.0-35.0 lb
11.4-15.9 kg

Breasts
1.5-3.0 lb
0.7-1.4 kg

Maternal reserves
4.0-9.5 lb
1.8-4.3 kg

Uterus
2.5 lb
1.1 kg

Fetus
7.0-7.5 lb
3.2-3.4 kg

Placenta
1.0-1.5 lb
0.5-0.7 kg

Amniotic fluid
2.0 lb
0.9 kg

Extravascular fluid
3.5-5.0 lb
1.6-2.3 kg

Figure 29-4   Distribution of weight gain during pregnancy.

continued

HISTORY OF PRESENT HEALTH CONCERN/CURRENT HEALTH STATUS *Continued*

Question	Rationale
Do you ever have bloody stools? Do you have diarrhea or difficulty when trying to have a bowel movement?	Changes in stool appearance and bowel habits may indicate constipation or hemorrhoids.
Do you experience a burning sensation while urinating?	Pregnant women may have asymptomatic bacteriuria. Urinary tract infections (UTIs) need to be diagnosed and treated with antibiotics. Untreated UTIs predispose the client to complications such as preterm labor, pyelonephritis, and sepsis.
Do you have vaginal bleeding, leakage of fluid, or vaginal discharge?	Vaginal bleeding, leakage, or discharge may indicate placenta previa, membrane rupture, or vaginal infections (e.g., bacterial vaginosis, trichomoniasis, *Chlamydia*). Untreated infections can predispose the client to preterm labor or fetal infections.
Have you lost interest in eating? Do you have trouble falling asleep or staying asleep? Do you ever feel depressed or like crying for no reason? Are problems at home or work bothering you? Have you ever thought of suicide? Have you ever had professional counseling (psychiatric/psychological)?	These symptoms may indicate psychological disorders. If the client has a history of psychological disorders, be aware of these and continually monitor her for signs and symptoms. Collaboration with a psychologist or psychiatrist may be needed. If the client is on medications prescribed for psychological problems, evaluate the medications in light of their possible teratogenic effects on the fetus.
Have you noticed breast pain, lumps, or fluid leakage?	Breast pain, lumps, or fluid leakage may indicate breast disease. Colostrum secretion, however, is normal during pregnancy. Colostrum varies in color among individuals. Erythematous, painful breasts may indicate a bacterial infection.
Have you thought about breast-feeding or bottle-feeding your infant?	Discuss advantages of breast-feeding for the client and infant. Supply educational resources for the client. Be supportive of the feeding method chosen by the client.
Are there any problems or concerns you may have that we haven't discussed yet?	This question gives the client an opportunity to discuss any other concerns she may have.

continued on page 618

COLDSPA Example for Nausea

Use the **COLDSPA** mnemonic as a guideline to collect needed information for each symptom the client shares. In addition, the following questions help elicit important information.

Mnemonic	Question	Client Response Example
Character	Describe the sign or symptom (feeling, appearance, sound, smell, or taste if applicable).	"nausea; occasional small amounts of vomiting with some dry heaves"
Onset	When did it begin?	"One week ago"
Location	Where is it? Does it radiate? Does it occur anywhere else?	n/a
Duration	How long does it last? Does it recur?	"Usually all morning and seems to subside by lunch time"
Severity	How bad is it? or How much does it bother you?	"I can't eat breakfast in the morning"
Pattern	What makes it better or worse?	"Some odors like bay leaf sausage cooking makes me more nauseated"
Associated factors/How it **A**ffects the client	What other symptoms occur with it? How does it affect you?	"Some vomiting and belching and dry heaves. It is hard for me to concentrate at work."

PAST HEALTH HISTORY

Question	Rationale

List the number of times you have been pregnant, beginning with the first pregnancy.	Determine patient's gravida/para status.
	• Gravida—total number of pregnancies
	• Para—number of pregnancies that have delivered at 20 weeks gestation or greater
	  ○ **Term Gestation**—delivery of pregnancy 38–42 weeks
	  ○ **Preterm Gestation**—delivery of pregnancy after 20 weeks and before the start of 38 weeks gestation
	  ○ **Abortion**—termination of pregnancy (miscarriage) prior to the 20th week of gestation
	  ○ **Living**—number of living children
	
	Example:
	$G_{\#}P_{\text{T Pt Ab L}}$
	$G_{4}P_{2113}$
	This represents a patient who has been pregnant 4 times; 2 term deliveries, 1 preterm delivery, 1 miscarriage, and 3 children living.

Describe your previous pregnancies including child's name, birth date, birth weight, sex, gestational age, type of delivery (if cesarean section, discuss reason). Did you experience any complications (e.g., pregnancy-induced hypertension, diabetes, bleeding, depression) during any of these pregnancies?	History of previous pregnancies helps identify clients at risk for complications during current pregnancy (e.g., preterm labor, gestational diabetes).
Describe any neonatal complications such as birth defects, jaundice, infection, or any problems within the first 2 weeks of life. Describe any perinatal or neonatal losses, including when the loss occurred and the reason for the loss, if known.	Previous neonatal complications may be hereditary and may recur in future births. Knowledge of such complications helps in detecting abnormalities early.
Discuss previous abortions (elective or spontaneous) including procedures required and gestational age of fetus.	Previous history of abortions helps to identify women who have had habitual abortions and who may need medical treatment to maintain the pregnancy.
Have you ever had a hydatidiform mole (molar pregnancy)?	Molar pregnancies occur in 1 of every 1,000 pregnancies in the United States and Europe. Incidence increases with the woman's age and particularly after age 45. Recurrence of the hydatidiform mole is seen in approximately 1%–2% of cases. Due to prompt diagnosis, mortality rates have been reduced to practically zero. Nearly 20% of complete moles progress to gestational trophoblastic tumor (Cunningham et al., 2005).
Have you ever had a tubal (ectopic) pregnancy (pregnancy outside of the uterus)?	Ectopic pregnancy occurs in 1 in every 100 pregnancies in the United States. A history of previous ectopic pregnancy increases the risk of having a second ectopic pregnancy to between 7% and 15% (Cunningham et al., 2005).
Do you have regular periods? When was the first day of your last menstrual period (LMP)? Was this period longer, shorter, or normal? Have you had any bleeding or spotting since your last period? Are your periods usually regular or irregular?	Menstrual history helps to determine expected date of confinement (EDC).
Describe the most recent form of birth control used. If you've used birth control pills in the past, when did you take the last pill?	Intrauterine devices in place at the time of conception place the client at risk for an ectopic pregnancy. Birth control pills should be discontinued when pregnancy is confirmed.

continued

PAST HEALTH HISTORY *Continued*

Question	*Rationale*
Have you had any difficulty in getting pregnant for more than 1 year?	Inability to conceive after trying for more than 1 year may signal reproductive complications such as infertility.
Have you ever had any type of reproductive surgery? Have you ever had an abnormal Pap smear? Have you ever had any treatment performed on your cervix for abnormal Pap smear results? When was your last Pap test, and what were the results?	Reproductive surgery and instrumentation to the cervix place the client at risk for complications during pregnancy. Conization of the cervix places the client at risk for an incompetent cervix during pregnancy.
Do you have a history of having any type of sexually transmitted infections (STIs) such as a chlamydial infection, gonorrhea, herpes, genital warts, or syphilis? If so, describe when it occurred and the treatment. Does your partner have a history of STI? If so, when was he treated?	Early identification and treatment of STIs prevent intrauterine complications from long-term exposure to infections.
Do you have a history of any vaginal infections such as bacterial vaginosis, yeast infection, or others? If so, when did the last infection occur and what was the treatment?	Vaginal infections need treatment. During pregnancy, nonteratogenic medications, such as clindamycin (Cleocin 2%) intravaginal cream or oral tablets, may be recommended. Metronidazole may be used in the second or third trimester (ACOG, 1996).
Do you know your blood type and Rh factor? If you are Rh negative, do you know the Rh factor of your partner?	Rh-negative mothers should receive Rho immune globulin at 28 weeks' gestation and with antepartum testing (chorionic villi sampling, amniocentesis) if the partners blood type is unknown to prevent isoimmunization.
Have you ever received a blood transfusion for any reason? If so, explain reason and provide date.	Infections (hepatitis, human immunodeficiency virus [HIV]) and antibodies can be received from contaminated blood during blood transfusions, which can be detrimental to the mother and fetus. Foreign antibodies can be life threatening for the fetus. Positive antibody screens need to be followed up to identify the antibody detected in the blood. Besides Rh antibody, other antibodies include Kell, Duffy, and Lewis. Titers should be followed to prevent fetal complications.
Do you have a history of any major medical problem (e.g., heart trouble, rheumatic fever, hypertension, diabetes, lung problems, tuberculosis, asthma, trouble with nerves and/or depression, kidney disease, cancer, convulsions or epilepsy, abnormality of female organs [uterus, cervix], thyroid problems, or hearing loss in infancy)?	Identification of any medical problem is important during pregnancy because the body undergoes so many physiologic changes. Certain medical conditions put the mother at high risk for maternal or fetal complications.
Do you have diabetes?	The fetus of diabetic clients who have uncontrolled disease and high $HgbA_{1c}$ values at the time of conception have a 6% to 8% incidence of anomalies and increased risk of spontaneous abortion.
Have you had twins or multiple gestation?	Early identification of multiple gestation is important. Refer clients with multiple gestation to an obstetrician for continued care. Multiple gestation places the client in the "high risk" category during pregnancy.
Do you have a history of medication, food, or other allergies? If so, list the allergies and describe the reactions.	Identification of medication allergies is necessary to prevent complications.
Have you ever been hospitalized or had surgery (not including hospitalizations or surgery related to pregnancy)? If so, discuss the reason for the hospitalization or surgery, the date, and if the problem is resolved today.	Previous hospitalizations or surgeries must be noted to assess for potential medical complications during the pregnancy.

continued on page 620

PAST HEALTH HISTORY *Continued*

Question	Rationale
Are you currently taking any medications (either prescription or nonprescription) or have you taken any since you have become pregnant? If so, list the medication, the amount taken, the date you started taking it, and the reason for taking it.	Some medications are teratogenic to the fetus during pregnancy. All medications taken since the LMP need to be discussed with the practitioner.
Are your immunizations up to date? Have you received the influenza immunization this year?	Assessment for immunity for rubella and hepatitis B is performed at the initial OB visit along with the other prenatal labs. CDC recommends influenza vaccination for women who are pregnant during the influenza season (Lugo, 2008).
Genetic Information Will you be 35 years or older at the time the baby is born? Are you and the baby's father related to each other (e.g., cousins or other relations)?	Women who are age 35 or older at the time of delivery should be offered genetic counseling and testing. Obtain genetic information so you can assess fetal risk of abnormal karyotype or genetic disorders.
Have you had two or more pregnancies that ended in miscarriage?	A woman who has had habitual abortions needs medical evaluation for incompetent cervix, systemic lupus erythematosus, and other potential complications.
Have you ever had a child that died around the time of delivery or in the first year of life?	Death of a child in the first year of life may indicate a risk for fetal cardiac disease or other diseases. This information is necessary for assessing fetal risk for birth defects.
Do you have a child with a birth defect? Do you have any type of birth defect or inherited disease such as cleft lip or cleft palate, clubfoot, hemophilia, mental retardation, or any others? Are there any members in your family with a birth defect? What is your ethnic or racial group: Jewish, Black/African, Asian, Mediterranean (e.g., Greek, Italian), French Canadian?	Certain inherited disorders occur more often in particular ethnic groups such as Tay-Sachs disease in the Ashkenazi Jewish population.

FAMILY HISTORY

Question	Rationale
Has anyone in your family (grandparents, parents, siblings, children) had rheumatic fever or heart trouble before age 50 years?	Cardiovascular disease or heart defects may be inherited.
Has anyone in your family had lung problems, diabetes, tuberculosis, or asthma?	Pulmonary or endocrine disorders may be familial.
Has anyone in your family been diagnosed with any type of cancer? If so, what kind?	There is a genetic component associated with certain types of cancer.
Has anyone in your family been born with any birth defects, inherited diseases, blood disorders, mental retardation, or any other problems?	There is a genetic risk factor for Down's syndrome, spina bifida, brain defects, chromosome problems, anencephaly, heart defects, muscular dystrophy, cystic fibrosis, hemophilia, thalassemia, and other inherited diseases. Cystic fibrosis screening should be offered to all patients during preconceptual counseling.
For the African-American client: Is there a history of sickle cell disease?	Identification of signs and symptoms of sickle cell disease is important to assist in early interventions and treatment.

continued

LIFESTYLE AND HEALTH PRACTICES

Question	*Rationale*
Since the start of this pregnancy, have you had drinks containing alcohol almost each day or frequently?	Daily alcohol intake puts the fetus at risk for fetal alcohol syndrome.
Do you smoke? If so, how much do you smoke per day?	Maternal cigarette smoking correlates with an increased incidence of perinatal mortality, preterm delivery, premature rupture of membranes, abruptio placentae, stillbirth, and bleeding during pregnancy (Niebyl et al., 2001). Smoking is also associated with decreased fetal size, low birth weight, attention deficit hyperactivity disorder (ADHD), and behavioral and learning disorders in school (Cunningham, 2005). Women who quit smoking during the 9-month gestation quit smoking for the health of themselves and for the fetus. These women may also have a lower relapse rate of smoking again when compared to women who are not pregnant (ACOG, 1997).
Have you used cocaine, marijuana, speed, or any street drug during this pregnancy?	Women who use cocaine during pregnancy have a higher rate of spontaneous abortions and abruptio placentae. Infants exposed to these drugs in utero are shown to have poor organizational response to stimuli compared with a control group (ACOG, 2004).
Does anyone in your family consider your social habits to be a problem? Do your social habits interfere with your daily living? If so, please explain.	Women who abuse substances (e.g., alcohol, cocaine, marijuana) do not always consider their habits to be a problem. They also tend to underestimate the amount of substances used. Family members or friends may give a truer estimate of the substances abused. These habits need to be known to assist the client during pregnancy and to alert neonatal personnel after delivery to prepare for potential neonatal complications.
What is a normal daily intake of food for you? Are you on any special diet? Do you have any diet intolerances or restrictions? If so, what are they?	Maternal nutrition has a direct relationship to maternal—fetal well-being. Daily maternal caloric intake, as reflected by weight gain, has a direct relationship to birth weight. The caloric content required to supply daily energy needs and to achieve appropriate weight gain can be estimated by multiplying the client's optimal body weight (in kilograms) by 35 kcal and adding 300 kcal to the total.
Do you eat lunch meats and milk products?	Unpasteurized milk products and deli meats should be avoided or cooked well. Undercooked meats and unpasteurized milk products can cause an infection called listeriosis. Maternal infection can cause fetal infection and mortality may approach 50%. Listeria can cause neonatal sepsis or meningitis (Creasy & Resnick, 2004).
Do you currently take any vitamin supplements? If so, what are they?	The client's balanced diet should provide an appropriate supply of vitamins required for pregnancy. Routine multivitamin supplementation for clients is based solely on a needs assessment. The diet selection should be from protein-rich foods, whole-grain breads and cereals, dairy products, and fruits and vegetables. Of the minerals, only iron supplementation is recommended to maintain body stores and minimize the occurrence of iron deficiency anemia. All women of childbearing age are recommended to consume 400 μg of folic acid daily to help prevent neural tube defects in the fetus. This can be achieved by eating fruits, vegetables, and fortified cereals and/or a folic acid supplement. Women who have previously had newborns born

continued on page 622

LIFESTYLE AND HEALTH PRACTICES *Continued*

Question	*Rationale*
	with spinal cord defects can decrease the risk of neural tube defects in future pregnancies by supplementing the diet with folic acid 2 to 3 months prior to conceiving.
Activity and Exercise	
Do you exercise daily? If so, what do you do and for how long?	Daily exercise is highly recommended as long as it is tolerated well by the pregnant client. Women who are in good physical condition tend to have shorter, less difficult labors compared with women who are not physically fit.
Do you perform any type of heavy labor working? If so, please describe.	Pregnancy places a tremendous amount of stress on the body due to the physiologic changes that occur. Encourage rest periods.
Are you easily fatigued? If so, please describe. What are your normal sleeping patterns?	Sleep restores the body and assists with the energy level of the client.
Do you frequently have rest periods? If so, for how long? Has your normal routine or exercise ever had a negative impact on your previous pregnancies? If so, please discuss.	Regular and routine exercise may be continued as long as tolerated. Caution women not to start *new* forms of exercise during pregnancy.
Toxic Exposure	
Have you or your partner ever worked around chemicals or radiation? If so, please explain. Are you exposed to an excessive amount of smoke daily?	Assessment of toxic exposure can identify potential teratogens to the fetus.
Do you have a cat? If so, are you exposed to the cat litter or the cat's feces?	Education regarding proper handling of cat litter is needed because of risk of infection (toxoplasmosis). Advise clients to have other family members change cat litter. Encourage the client to wash hands well after petting cats and to wear gloves when planting in outdoor soil if cats are present in neighborhood.
Role and Relationships	
What is the highest level of education you have completed? What is your occupation or major activity?	This helps to identify environmental exposures/risks for the patient.
Discuss your feelings about this pregnancy. Is the father of the baby involved with the pregnancy? How does your partner feel about the pregnancy? To what degree do you feel that the father of the baby will be involved with the pregnancy (e.g., not involved, interested and supportive, full caretaker of the pregnancy)?	These questions identify psychosocial issues for the patient. Assess social support systems for the family.
What type of support systems do you have at home? Who is your primary support person? List the people living with you including their names, ages, relationship to you, and any health problems that they may have. Are they aware of your pregnancy?	Assessment of social structures and supportive influences is required to determine potential client needs. If additional needs are noted, contact social services for assistance.
How have you introduced this pregnancy to the siblings? What are their reactions regarding this pregnancy? Do you plan to involve the siblings in any type of education program to enhance the attachment process for the newborn?	Sibling rivalry can interfere with the bonding process between siblings. Education and preparation for the new family member (the newborn) can alleviate potential problems with sibling rivalry. Encourage siblings to attend sibling class offered at your institution.
Has anyone close to you ever threatened to hurt you? Has anyone ever hit, kicked, choked, or physically hurt you? Has anyone ever forced you to have sex?	Lack of recognition of domestic violence is one of the primary barriers to recognizing domestic violence for women. Universal screening is recommended for all women.

continued

Question	*Rationale*
What is your partner's highest level of education? What is your partner's occupation or major activity? Does your partner consume alcohol? If yes, how much alcohol does your partner use daily? List type and amount. Does your partner smoke? If yes, how often does your partner smoke? List amount and frequency. Does your partner use illicit drugs? If yes, how often does your partner use illicit drugs? List drug type, amount, and frequency.	Exploration of the partner's social or cultural habits may identify needs of the family unit.

COLLECTING OBJECTIVE DATA: PHYSICAL EXAMINATION

Preparing the Client

The nurse needs to provide a warm and comfortable environment for the physical assessment. After meeting the client, the nurse should quickly explain the sequence of events for the visit. Note that a full head-to-toe examination will be performed including a pelvic examination. Pelvic cultures obtained with this examination include a Pap smear and gonorrhea and chlamydial cultures. Explain that after the examination is complete, the client will go to the laboratory for initial prenatal blood tests including complete blood count, blood type and screen, Rh status, rubella titer, serologic test for syphilis, hepatitis B surface antigen, and sickle cell anemia screen (for clients of African ancestry). Universal screening for HIV is recommended.

The first procedure involves obtaining a clean-catch, midstream urine specimen. After the client has voided, instruct her to undress. Provide adequate gowns and cover-up drapes to ensure privacy.

Equipment

- Adequate room lighting
- Ophthalmoscope
- Otoscope
- Stethoscope
- Sphygmomanometer
- Speculum
- Light for pelvic examination
- Tape measure
- Fetal Doppler ultrasound device
- Disposable gloves
- Lubricant
- Slides
- KOH (potassium hydroxide)
- Normal saline solution
- Thin prep Pap smear test

Physical Assessment

Remember these key points during examination:

- Obtain an accurate and complete prenatal history.
- Understand and recognize cardiovascular changes of pregnancy.
- Recognize skin changes.
- Identify common complaints of pregnancy and explain what causes them.
- Correctly measure growth of uterus during pregnancy.
- Demonstrate the four Leopold's maneuvers and explain their significance.

(text continues on page 638)

PHYSICAL ASSESSMENT

Assessment Procedure	Normal Findings	Abnormal Findings
General Survey: Vital Signs, Height, and Weight		
Measure blood pressure (BP). Have the client sit on the examination table.	BP range: systolic 90–139 mmHg and diastolic 60–89 mmHg. BP decreases during the second trimester because of the relaxation effect on the blood vessels. By 32 to 34 weeks, the client's BP should be back to normal.	Elevated BP at 9 to 11 weeks may be indicative of chronic hypertension hydatidiform mole pregnancy or thyroid storm. After 20 weeks, increased BP (>140/90) may be associated with pregnancy-induced hypertension. Decreased blood pressure may indicate supine hypotensive syndrome.

continued

PHYSICAL ASSESSMENT Continued

Assessment Procedure	Normal Findings	Abnormal Findings
Measure pulse rate.	60 to 90 beats/min; may increase 10 to 15 beats/min higher than prepregnant levels	Irregularities in heart rhythm, chest pain, dyspnea, and edema may indicate cardiac disease.
Take the client's temperature.	97° to 98.6°F	An elevated temperature (above 100°) may indicate infection.
Measure height and weight (Fig. 29-5.)	Establish a baseline height and weight. The client should gain 2 to 4 lb in the first trimester and approximately 11 to 12 lb in both the second and third trimesters for a total weight gain between 25 and 35 lb.	A sudden gain exceeding 5 lb a week may be associated with pregnancy-induced hypertension and fluid retention. Weight gain <2 lb a month may indicate insufficient nourishment.
Observe behavior.	*First trimester:* Tired, ambivalent. *Second trimester:* Introspective, energetic. *Third trimester:* Restless, preparing for baby, labile moods (father may also experience these same behaviors).	Denial of pregnancy, withdrawal, depression, or psychosis may be seen in the client with psychological problems.

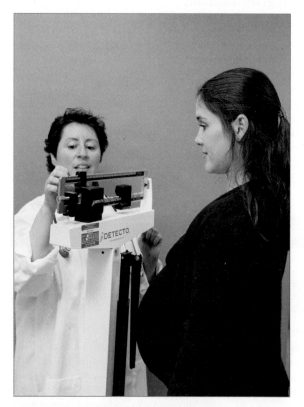

Figure 29-5   Weighing the pregnant client.

continued

Assessment Procedure	Normal Findings	Abnormal Findings
Skin, Hair, and Nails		
Inspect the skin. Note hyperpigmented areas associated with pregnancy.	Linea nigra, striae, gravidarum, chloasma, and spider nevi may be present.	Pale skin suggests anemia. Yellow discoloration suggests jaundice.
Observe skin for vascular markings associated with pregnancy.	Angiomas and palmar erythema are common.	
Inspect the hair and nails.	Hair and nails tend to increase in growth; softening and thinning are common.	
Head and Neck		
Inspection and Palpation **Inspect and palpate the neck.** Assess the anterior and posterior cervical chain lymph nodes. Also palpate the thyroid gland.	Smooth, nontender, small cervical nodes may be palpable. Slight enlargement of the thyroid may be noted during pregnancy.	Hard, tender, fixed, or prominent nodes may indicate infection or cancer. Marked enlargement of the thyroid gland indicates thyroid disease. Benign and malignant nodules as well as tenderness are noted in thyroiditis.
Eyes		
Inspection **Inspect eyes.** Examine cornea, lens, iris, and pupil. Use an ophthalmoscope to examine the fundus of the eye.	Pupils are equal and round, reactive to light and accommodate.	Narrowing of the arterioles or AV nicking may indicate hypertension.
Ears		
Inspection **Inspect the ears.**	Tympanic membranes clear: landmarks visible.	Tympanic membrane red and bulging with pus indicates infection.
Mouth, Throat, and Nose		
Inspection **Inspect the mouth.** Pay particular attention to the teeth and the gingival tissues, which may normally appear swollen and slightly reddened.	Hypertrophy of gingival tissue is common. Bleeding may occur due to brushing teeth or dental examinations.	Epulis nodules may be present (Fig. 29-6).
Inspect the throat.	Throat pink, no redness or exudate.	Throat red, exudate present, tonsillary hypertrophy indicate infection.
Inspect the nose.	Nasal mucosal swelling and redness may result from increased estrogen production. Epistaxis is a common variation because of the increased vascular supply to the nares during pregnancy.	Abnormal findings are the same as those in nonpregnant clients.

continued

PHYSICAL ASSESSMENT *Continued*

Assessment Procedure	Normal Findings	Abnormal Findings
Thorax and Lungs		
Inspect, palpate, percuss, and auscultate the chest.	Normal findings include increased anteroposterior diameter, thoracic breathing, slight hyperventilation; shortness of breath in late pregnancy. Lung sounds are clear to auscultation bilaterally.	Dyspnea, rales, rhonchi, wheezes, rubs, absence of breath sounds, and unequal breath sounds are signs of respiratory distress. Patients with a history of asthma have increased risk of perinatal morbidity mortality, and increased risk of pregnancy-induced hypertension, preterm labor, and low birth weight (Brown, 2006).
Breasts		
Inspection and Palpation **Inspect and palpate the breasts and nipples for symmetry and color (Fig. 29-7).**	Venous congestion is noted with prominence of veins. Montgomery's tubercles are prominent. Breast size is increased and nodular. Breasts are more sensitive to touch. Colostrum is excreted, especially in the third trimester. Hyperpigmentation of nipples and areolae is evident (Fig. 29-8).	Nipple inversion could be problematic for breast-feeding. Inverted nipples should be identified in the beginning of the third trimester. Breast shields can be inserted in the bra to train the nipple to turn outward. Localized redness, pain, and warmth could indicate mastitis. Bloody discharge of the nipple and retraction of the skin could indicate breast cancer.

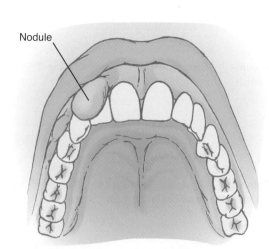

Nodule

Figure 29-6 Epulis.

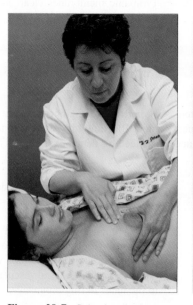

Figure 29-7 Palpating the breasts.

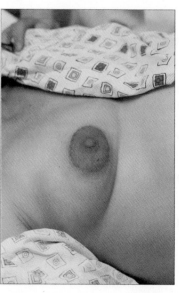

Figure 29-8 Hyperpigmentation of the nipples and areolae.

continued

Assessment Procedure	Normal Findings	Abnormal Findings
Heart		
Auscultation **Auscultate the heart.**	Normal sinus rhythm. Soft systolic murmurs are audible during pregnancy secondary to the increased blood volume.	Irregular rhythm. Progressive dyspnea, palpitations, and markedly decreased activity tolerance indicate cardiovascular disease.
Peripheral Vascular		
Inspection and Percussion **Inspect face and extremities.** Note color and edema.	During the third trimester, dependent edema is normal. Varicose veins may also appear.	Abnormal findings include calf pain, positive Homans' sign, generalized edema (or facial edema), and diminished pedal pulses. These findings may indicate thrombophlebitis. Facial edema may indicate pregnancy-induced hypertension with elevated blood pressure and weight gain.
Percuss deep tendon reflexes.	Normal reflexes 1 to 2+. Clonus is absent.	Reflexes 3 to 4+ and positive clonus require evaluation for pregnancy-induced hypertension.
Abdomen		
Inspection **Inspect the abdomen.** For this part of the examination, ask the client to recline with a pillow under her head and her knees flexed. Note striae, scars, and the shape and size of the abdomen.	Striae and linea nigra are normal. The size of the abdomen may indicate gestational age. The shape of the uterus may suggest fetal presentation and position in later pregnancy.	Scars indicate previous surgery; be careful to note cesarean section scars and location. A transverse lie may be suspected by abdominal palpation, noting enlargement of the width of the uterus.
Palpation **Palpate the abdomen.** Note organs and any masses.	The uterus is palpable beginning at 10 to 12 weeks' gestation.	Abnormal masses palpable in the abdomen may indicate uterine fibroids or hepatosplenomegaly.
Palpate for fetal movement after 24 weeks.	Fetal movement should be felt by the mother by approximately 18 to 20 weeks.	If fetal movement is not felt, the EDC may be wrong or possibly intrauterine fetal demise may have occurred.
Palpate for uterine contractions (Fig. 29-9). Note intensity, duration, and frequency of contractions.	The uterus contracts and feels firm to the examiner.	Regular contractions before 37 completed weeks' gestation may suggest preterm labor.
Palpate the abdomen. Notice the difference between the uterus at rest and during a contraction.	Intensity of contractions may be mild, moderate, or firm to palpation.	Regular contractions prior to 37 weeks' gestation suggests premature labor.

continued

PHYSICAL ASSESSMENT Continued

Assessment Procedure	Normal Findings	Abnormal Findings
Time the length of the contraction from the beginning to the end. Also note the frequency of the contractions, timing from the beginning of one contraction until the beginning of the next (Fig. 29-10).	Contraction may last 40 to 60 seconds and occur every 5 to 6 min.	Contractions lasting too long or occurring too frequently cause fetal distress.
Fundal Height **Measure fundal height.** Do this by placing one hand on each side of the abdomen and walk hands up the sides of the uterus until you feel the uterus curve; hands should meet. Take a tape measure and place the zero point on the symphysis pubis and measure to the top of the fundus (Fig. 29-11).	Uterine size should approximately equal the number of weeks of gestation (e.g., the uterus at 28 weeks' gestation should measure approximately 28 cm) (Fig. 29-12). Measurements may vary by about 2 cm and examiners' techniques may vary but measurements should be about the same.	Measurements beyond 4 cm of gestational age need to be further evaluated. Measurements greater than expected may indicate a multiple gestation, polyhydramnios (excess of amniotic fluid), fetal anomalies, or macrosomia (great increase in size similar to obesity). Measurements smaller than expected may indicate intrauterine growth retardation.

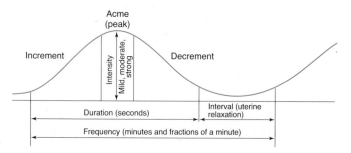

Figure 29-10 Contraction cycle.

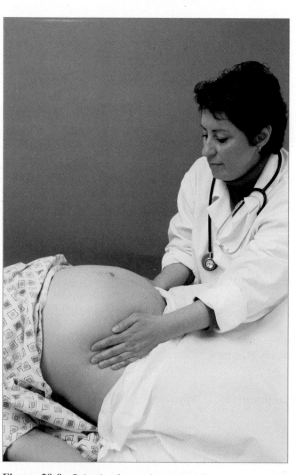

Figure 29-9 Palpating for uterine contractions.

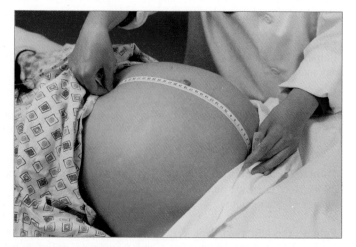

Figure 29-11 Measuring the fundal height.

continued

Assessment Procedure	Normal Findings	Abnormal Findings
Fetal Position **Using Leopold's maneuvers, palpate the fundus, lateral aspects of the abdomen, and the lower pelvic area.** Leopold's maneuvers assist in determining the fetal lie (where the fetus is lying in relation to the mother's back), presentation (the presenting part of the fetus into the maternal pelvis), size, and position (the fetal presentation in relation to the maternal pelvis).	A longitudinal lie, in which the fetal spine axis is parallel to the maternal spine axis, is the expected finding. The presentation may be cephalic, breech, or shoulder. The size of the fetus may be estimated by measuring fundal height and by palpation. Fetal positions include right occiput anterior (ROA), left occiput posterior (LOP), left sacrum anterior (LSA), and so on. (Refer to a textbook on obstetrics for further detail.)	Oblique or transverse lie needs to be noted. If vaginal delivery is expected, external version can be performed to rotate the fetus to the longitudinal lie. Breech or shoulder presentations can complicate delivery if it is expected to be vaginal.
For the first maneuver, face the client's head. Place your hands on the fundal area, expecting to palpate a soft, irregular mass in the upper quadrant of the maternal abdomen (Fig. 29-13).	The soft mass is the fetal buttocks. The fetal head feels round and hard.	

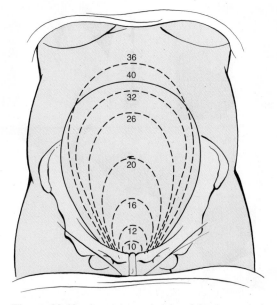

Figure 29-12 Approximate height of fundus at various weeks of gestation.

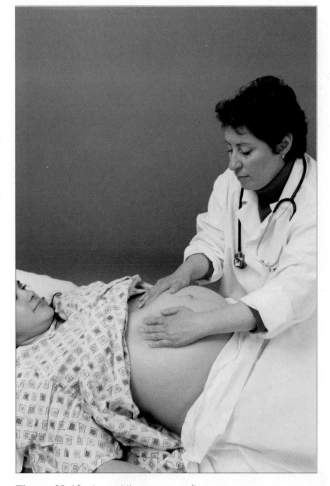

Figure 29-13 Leopold's maneuver: first maneuver.

continued

PHYSICAL ASSESSMENT *Continued*

Assessment Procedure	Normal Findings	Abnormal Findings
For the second maneuver, move your hands to the lateral sides of the abdomen (Fig. 29-14).	On one side of the abdomen, you will palpate round nodules; these are the fists and feet of the fetus. Kicking and movement are expected to be felt. The other side of the abdomen feels smooth; this is the fetus's back.	
For the third maneuver, move your hands down to the lower pelvic area and palpate the area just above the symphysis pubis to determine the presenting part. Grasp the presenting part with the thumb and third finger (Fig. 29-15).	The unengaged head is round, firm, and ballottable, whereas the buttocks are soft and irregular.	Soft, presenting part at the symphysis pubis indicates breech presentation.

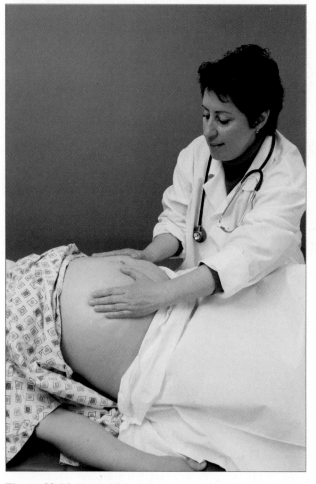

Figure 29-14   Leopold's maneuver: second maneuver.

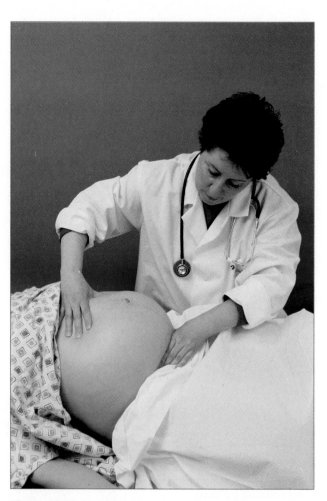

Figure 29-15   Leopold's maneuver: third maneuver.

continued

Assessment Procedure	Normal Findings	Abnormal Findings
For the fourth maneuver, face the client's feet, place your hands on the abdomen, and point your fingers toward the mother's feet. Then try to move your hands toward each other while applying downward pressure (Fig. 29-16).	If the hands move together easily, the fetal head has not descended into the maternal pelvic inlet. If the hands do not move together and stop to resistance met, the fetal head is engaged into the pelvic inlet.	

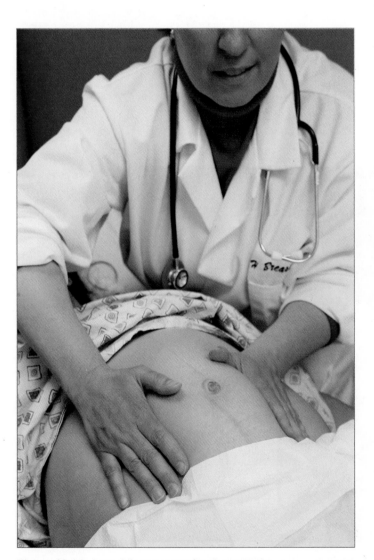

Figure 29-16   Leopold's maneuver: fourth maneuver.

continued

PHYSICAL ASSESSMENT Continued

Assessment Procedure	Normal Findings	Abnormal Findings

Fetal Heart

Determine the location, rate, and rhythm of the fetal heart. Auscultate the fetal heart rate in the left lower quadrant when the fetal back is noted on maternal left, vertex position (Fig. 29-17). When the fetal back is located elsewhere, note other locations illustrated in Display 29-1 for auscultation.

➤ **Clinical Tip** • *After assessing the fetal position, you can auscultate fetal heart tones best through the back of the fetus. A fetal Doppler ultrasound device can be used after 10 to 12 weeks' gestation to hear the fetal heartbeat. A fetoscope may also be used to hear the heartbeat after 18 weeks' gestation.*

Fetal heart rate ranges from 120 to 160 beats/min. During the third trimester, the fetal heart rate should accelerate with fetal movement.

Inability to auscultate fetal heart tones with a fetal Doppler at 12 weeks may indicate a retroverted uterus, uncertain dates, fetal demise, or false pregnancy. Fetal heart rate decelerations could indicate poor placental perfusion. In breech presentations, fetal heart rate is heard in the upper quadrant of maternal abdomen.

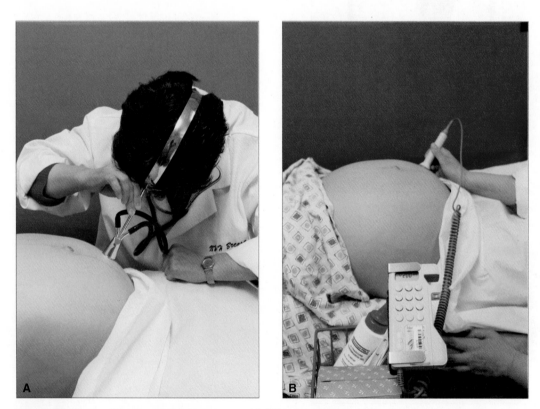

Figure 29-17 Auscultating the fetal heart rate with **(A)** a fetoscope and **(B)** a Doppler ultrasound device.

continued on page 634

DISPLAY 29-1	Where to Auscultate Fetal Heart Rate

The illustrations below represent the best locations for auscultating the fetal heart rate: Left occiput anterior (LOA), right occiput anterior (ROA), left occiput posterior (LOP), right occiput posterior (ROP), left sacrum anterior (LSA), and right sacrum posterior (RSP).

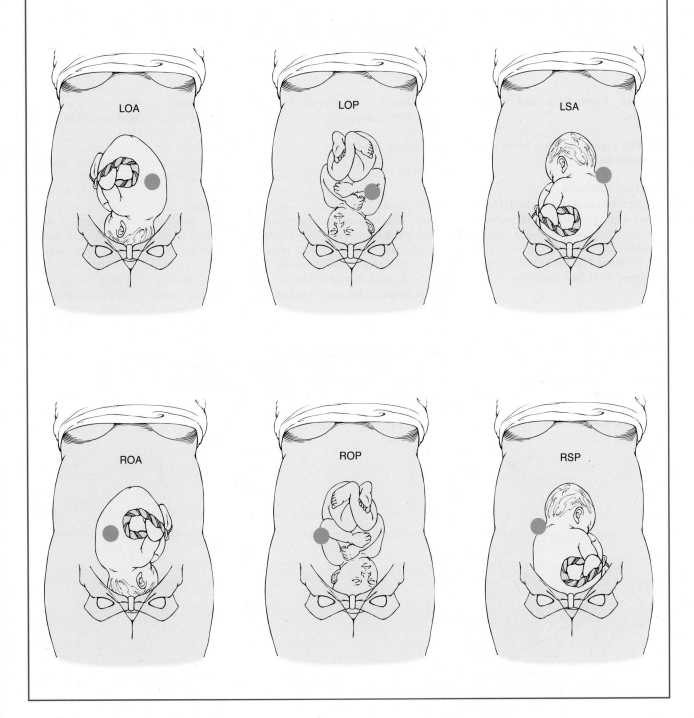

PHYSICAL ASSESSMENT *Continued*

Assessment Procedure	Normal Findings	Abnormal Findings
Genitalia		

External Genitalia

Inspect the external genitalia. Note hair distribution, color of skin, varicosities, and scars.

Normal findings include enlarged labia and clitoris, parous relaxation of the introitus, and scars from an episiotomy or perineal lacerations (in multiparous women).

Labial varicosities, which can be painful.

Palpate Bartholin's and Skene's glands.

There should be no discomfort or discharge with examination.

Discomfort and discharge noted with palpation may indicate infection.

Inspect vaginal opening for cystocele or rectocele.

No cystocele or rectocele.

Cystocele or rectocele may be more pronounced because of the muscle relaxation of pregnancy.

Internal Genitalia

Inspect internal genitalia (refer to gynecologic examination in textbook). Insert speculum into the vagina. Visualize the cervix, noting position and color. Obtain Pap smear and cultures if indicated. Withdraw speculum.

Cervix should look pink, smooth, and healthy. With pregnancy, the cervix may appear bluish (Chadwick's sign). In multiparous women, the cervical opening has a slitlike appearance known as "fish mouth." A small amount of whitish vaginal discharge (leukorrhea) is normal.

Gonorrhea infection may present with thick, purulent vaginal discharge. A thick, white, cheesy discharge presents with a yeast infection. Grayish-white vaginal discharge, positive "whiff test" (fishy odor), and clue cells positive on microscopic wet prep (epithelial cells that have been invaded by disease-causing bacteria) are evidence of bacterial vaginosis.

Perform pelvic examination. Put on gloves lubricated with water or KY jelly, gently insert fingers into the vagina, and palpate the cervix. Estimate the length of the cervix by palpating the lateral surface of the cervix from the cervical tip to the lateral fornix.

The cervix may be palpated in the posterior vaginal vault. It should be long, thick, and closed. Cervical length should be approximately 2.3 to 3 cm. Positive Hegar's sign (softening of the lower uterine segment) should be present (Fig. 29-18).

An effaced opened cervix may indicate preterm labor or an incompetent cervix if gestation is not at term (Fig. 29-19).

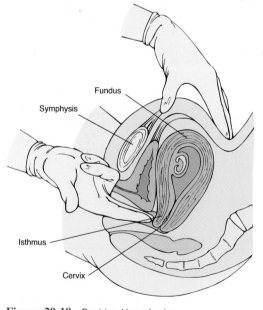

Fundus

Symphysis

Isthmus

Cervix

Figure 29-18   Positive Hegar's sign.

continued

Assessment Procedure	Normal Findings	Abnormal Findings
Feel for uterus. While leaving the fingers in the vagina, place the other hand on the abdomen and gently press down toward the internal hand until you feel the uterus between the two hands.	The uterus should feel about the size of an orange at 10 weeks (palpable at the suprapubic bone) and about the size of a grapefruit at 12 weeks.	If uterine size is not consistent with dates, consider wrong dates, uterine fibroids, or multiple gestation.
Palpate the left and right adnexa.	No masses should be palpable. Discomfort with examination is due to stretching of the round ligaments throughout the pregnancy.	Adnexal masses may indicate ectopic pregnancy (Fig. 29-20).

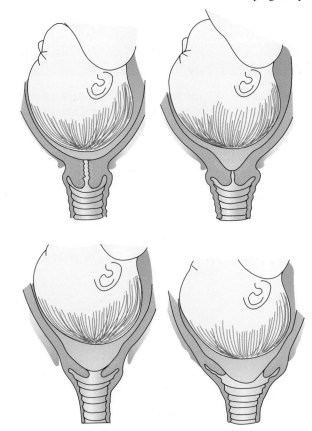

Figure 29-19 Effacement and dilation. (Top left) Before labor, 0% effacement. (Top right) Early effacement, 30%. (Bottom left) Complete effacement, 100%. (Bottom right) Complete effacement and dilation.

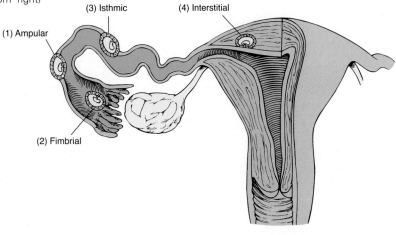

(3) Isthmic   (4) Interstitial

(1) Ampular

(2) Fimbrial

Figure 29-20 Sites of ectopic pregnancy.

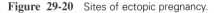

continued

PHYSICAL ASSESSMENT *Continued*

Assessment Procedure	Normal Findings	Abnormal Findings
Anus and Rectum		
Inspect the anus and rectum. Note color, varicosities, lesions, tears, or discharge.	Mucosa should be pink and intact. No varicosities, lesions, tears, or discharge present. Hemorrhoids or varicose veins may be present. Hemorrhoids usually get bigger and more uncomfortable during pregnancy. Bleeding and infection may occur.	Masses may indicate cancer.
Musculoskeletal		
Determine pelvic adequacy for a vaginal delivery by estimating the angle of the subpubic arch. Place hands as shown in Figure 29-21, noting angle between thumb and first finger.	The subpubic arch should be greater than 90 degrees.	A narrow pubic arch displaces the presenting part posteriorly and impedes the fetus from passing under the pubic arch.
Determine the height and inclination of the symphysis pubis (Fig. 29-22).	The height and inclination of the symphysis pubis should be short and gradual, respectively.	A long or steeply inclined symphysis pubis may interfere with a successful vaginal delivery.
Palpate the lateral walls of the pelvis.	Lateral walls should be straight or divergent.	Lateral walls that narrow as they approach the vagina may be problematic with vaginal delivery.

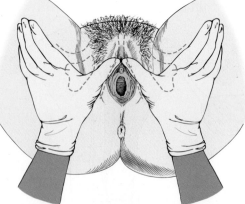

Figure 29-21 Estimating the angle of the sub-pubic arch.

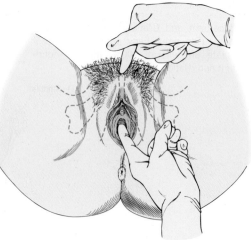

Figure 29-22 Determining the height and incline of the symphysis pubis.

continued

Assessment Procedure	Normal Findings	Abnormal Findings
Palpate the ischial spines. Sweep the finger posteriorly from one spine over to the other spine.	Ischial spines are small, not prominent. Interspinous diameter is at least 10.5 cm (Fig. 29-23).	Prominent spines. Interspinous diameter less than 10.5 cm may interfere with delivery.
Examine the sacrum and coccyx. Sweep fingers down the sacrum. Gently press back on the coccyx to determine mobility.	Gynecoid pelvis is most common. Mobile coccyx increases ease of delivery by expansion, enlarging the area in the pelvis.	Anthropoid or platypoid pelvis with an immobile coccyx may interfere with vaginal birth.
Measure the diagonal conjugate. The diagonal conjugate measures the antero-posterior diameter of the pelvic inlet through which the fetal head passes first. Measure the diagonal conjugate by pressing internal hand into the sacral promontory and up; mark the spot on your hand directly below the symphysis pubis (Fig. 29-24).	Pelvic adequacy is expected if diagonal conjugate measures 12.5 cm or greater. If the middle finger cannot reach the sacral promontory, space is considered adequate.	A diagonal conjugate measuring less than 12.5 cm may impede vaginal delivery process.
Calculate the obstetric conjugate. The obstetric conjugate is the smallest opening through which the fetal head must pass. To calculate it, subtract 1.5 cm from the diagonal conjugate measurement (Fig. 29-25).	Measurement of the obstetric conjugate should be 10.5 to 11 cm.	An obstetric conjugate measuring less than 10.5 cm may pose difficulty with vaginal delivery.
Measure the transverse diameter of the pelvic outlet. To do this, make a fist and place it between the ischial tuberosities (Fig. 29-26). ➤ *Clinical Tip • Know the measurement of your own hand to estimate the measurement of the transverse diameter at pelvic outlet.*	The measurement between ischial tuberosities is usually 10 to 11 cm.	Diameters of less than 10 cm may inhibit fetal descent toward the vagina.

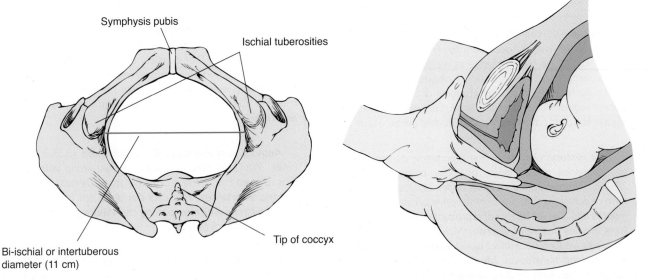

Figure 29-23 Ischial spines.

Symphysis pubis

Ischial tuberosities

Bi-ischial or intertuberous diameter (11 cm)

Tip of coccyx

Figure 29-24 Measuring the diagonal conjugate.

continued

PHYSICAL ASSESSMENT *Continued*

Assessment Procedure	Normal Findings	Abnormal Findings

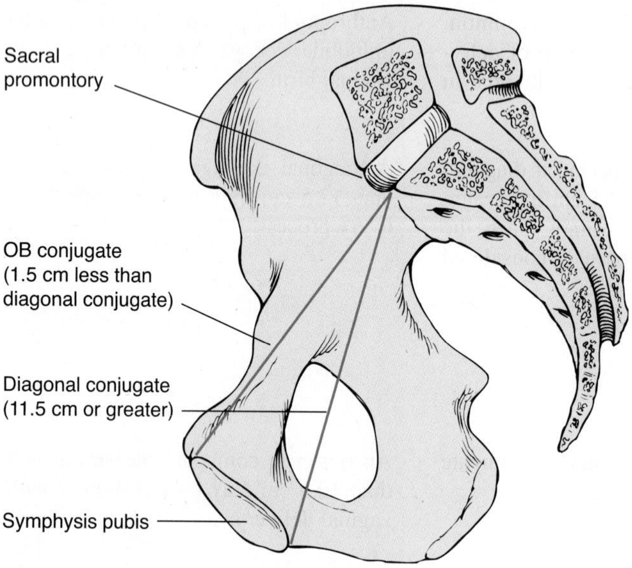

Sacral promontory

OB conjugate (1.5 cm less than diagonal conjugate)

Diagonal conjugate (11.5 cm or greater)

Symphysis pubis

Figure 29-25 Pelvic structure: Obstetric (OB) conjugate, diagonal conjugate.

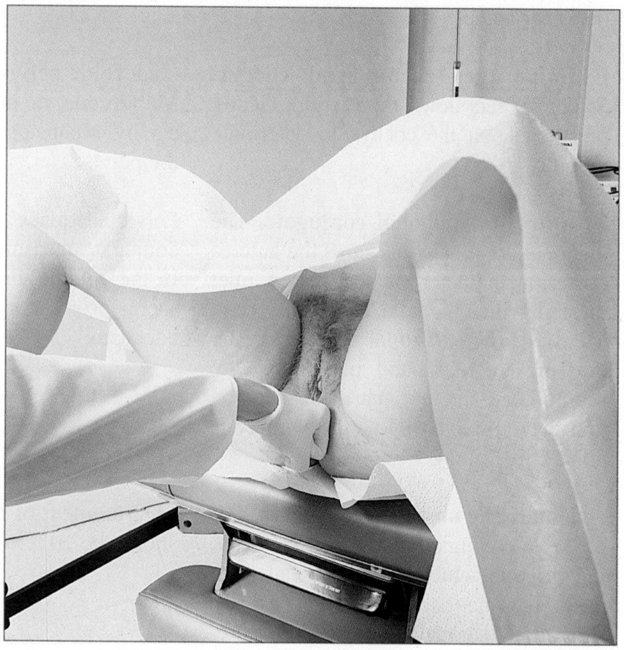

Figure 29-26 Using the fist to measure the pelvic outlet.

VALIDATING AND DOCUMENTING FINDINGS

Validate the assessment data that you have collected about the childbearing woman. This is necessary to verify that the data are reliable and accurate. Document the assessment data following the health care facility or agency policy.

Sample of Subjective Data

Client is a 25-year-old white, married, obstetric patient at 10 weeks' gestation by LMP. Prepregnancy weight 125 lb. No recent change in weight. No s/s cold or illness since LMP. Has occasional nausea and vomiting. Drinks fluids well. No change in stools or urinary pattern. Denies vaginal bleeding or discharge. Eats well. No history of psychological problems. Reports normal breast exam.

Past History: Gravida 1: first pregnancy; denies previous deliveries, miscarriages, or molar pregnancy. LMP 2/20/05. Normal period: 28-day cycle. No spotting. Last form of contraception: oral contraceptive pill; stopped pill 4 months ago. Denies history of reproductive or fertility problems. Denies history of vaginal infections or STIs; partner also negative for STIs. Patient blood type A positive; no history of blood transfusion. Medical history: unremarkable. Allergies: no known drug allergies. Surgeries: none. Hospitalizations: none. Gynecological: no problems. Pap smear: up to date; no history of abnormal pap smears.

Breast: unremarkable. Current medications: Prenatal vitamin: one daily. Father not related to client. Primigravida: no history of past pregnancies. Race: white.

Family History: No history of early deaths, diabetes, tuberculosis, asthma, cancer, birth defects, blood disorders, or mental retardation.

Lifestyle and Health Practices: No alcohol, cigarettes, or drug use since LMP. No family members consider habits a problem. Diet consists of three meals a day and snacks (primarily meats, vegetables, fruits, bread, water). Prepregnant weight is 125 lb with no significant weight changes. Current vitamins: one prenatal vitamin with folic acid daily.

Activity and Exercise: Exercises three to five times week. Walks 30 min; occasional weight lifting with aerobics. Denies heavy lifting or heavy labor. Denies exposure to toxic substances. Has cats but does not change litter. Washes hands well after petting cat. Wears gloves if working outdoors in dirt/plants.

Role and Relationships: Highest level education: M.S. Occupation: RN. Lives with husband who is delighted about pregnancy. Additional support: parents, in-laws, sister, and friends. Partner: highest level education B.S. in business administration; current occupation: CPA; non-smoker; drinks alcohol occasionally on weekends with friends; no history of illicit drug use.

Sample of Objective Data

B/P 100/60; pulse 90; temp 98.6°; height 5 feet 4 inches; weight 125 lb. Behavior: ambivalent, excited. Skin: no hyperpigmentation yet. Hair/nails: soft, smooth, clean. Neck: supple. Thyroid: no masses or enlargement noted. Ears: TM clear; landmarks visible. Mouth/throat/nose: pink, no exudate, no hypertrophy. Thorax/lungs: CTA bilaterally. Breasts: no masses palpable, no discharge, symmetric, no nipple inversion. Heart: NSR without murmur. Abdomen: soft, nontender, no hepatosplenomegaly; fundal height palpable above symphysis pubis, approx. 10 weeks' size. Fetal heart tones: audible with fetal Doppler, rate 158 b/min. Genitalia: External: no scars or varicosities; Bartholin's and Skene's glands negative; no cystocele or rectocele noted. Speculum: Chadwick's sign present; no vaginal discharge or bleeding; Pap smear performed. GC and Chlamydia cultures taken and sent to lab. Pelvic: Cervix: posterior, closed, long and thick. Uterus: approx. 10 weeks' size. No masses palpable. Adnexa: negative R and L. Anus/rectum: negative for lesions or varicosities. Peripheral vascular: Face/extremities:no edema; pink, well perfused; pulses equal bilaterally, Homans' sign negative, DTRs 1–2 +, −clonus. Pelvis: subpubic arch >90°; symphysis pubis: short, gradual inclination. Lateral walls straight. Ischial spines: blunt. Interspinous diameter >10.5 cm. Pelvis: gynecoid, coccyx mobile. Diagonal conjugate >12.5 cm. Obstetric conjugate >10.5 cm. Transverse diameter >11 cm. Assessment: Healthy obstetric physical examination. Plan: Routine obstetric care.

Analysis of Data

After collecting your assessment data, you will need to analyze the data using diagnostic reasoning skills presented in Chapter 5. In Diagnostic Reasoning: Possible Conclusions, you will see an overview of common conclusions you may reach after assessment of the childbearing woman. Also the Diagnostic Reasoning: Case Study at the end of this chapter shows you how to analyze assessment data for a *specific* childbearing client. Finally you have an extra opportunity to analyze data in the critical thinking exercise presented in the lab manual study guide available with the textbook.

DIAGNOSTIC REASONING: POSSIBLE CONCLUSIONS

Listed are some possible conclusions after assessing a childbearing woman.

Selected Nursing Diagnoses

After collecting subjective and objective data pertaining to the assessment of the childbearing woman, you will need to identify abnormalities and cluster the data to reveal any significant patterns or abnormalities. These data will then be used to make clinical judgments (nursing diagnoses: wellness, risk, or actual) about the status of the client's pregnancy. Following is a listing of selected nursing diagnoses that you may identify when analyzing data for this part of the assessment.

Wellness Diagnoses

- Opportunity for enhanced self-care during pregnancy

Risk Diagnoses

- Risk for Deficient Fluid Volume (related to excessive nausea/vomiting)
- Risk for Injury (maternal; related to elevated arterial pressure)
- Risk for Injury (fetal; related to decreased placental perfusion due to blood loss)

Actual Diagnoses

- Anxiety (related to fear of loss of pregnancy)
- Imbalanced Nutrition: Less Than Body Requirements, related to lack of knowledge of proper nutrition during pregnancy
- Disturbed Body Image, related to excessive weight gain during pregnancy

Selected Collaborative Problems

After grouping the data, certain collaborative problems may emerge. Remember that collaborative problems differ from nursing diagnoses in that they cannot be prevented with nursing interventions alone. However, these physiologic complications of medical conditions can be detected and monitored by the nurse. In addition, the nurse can use physician- and nurse-prescribed interventions to minimize the complications of these problems. The nurse may also have to refer the client in such situations for further treatment of the problem. Following is a list of collaborative problems that may be identified when assessing the childbearing woman. These problems are worded as Risk for Complications (or RC) followed by the problem.

- RC: Anemia
- RC: Advanced maternal age
- RC: Gestational diabetes

Medical Problems

After grouping the data, it may become apparent that the client has signs and symptoms that may require medical diagnosis and treatment. Referral to a primary care provider is necessary.

CASE STUDY

The case study presents assessment data for a specific client. It is followed by an analysis of the data, working out the seven key steps to arrive at specific conclusions.

Mrs. Mary Farrow is a 29-year-old Caucasian woman, gravida 3, para 2, who presents to the clinic today for her initial prenatal examination. She states that her last menstrual period (LMP) was on September 15, approximately 16 weeks ago. Because she was unable to get transportation to the clinic, she did not come in for prenatal care earlier in this pregnancy. "I do know how important early prenatal care is, but I just couldn't get here. And I feel good—no problems so far." Mrs. Farrow lives with her husband and two sons in a two-bedroom trailer on land owned by her in-laws. She states that her in-laws are very supportive and help out during tough times by not charging rent. Her husband works full time at a fast-food chain restaurant but is looking for a job that pays more money. It is often hard for them to meet their financial responsibilities; however, they believe it is important for her to stay home with the children so she does not contribute financially. She reports that, in general, she encourages healthful practices for herself and family, but because her husband gets a discount on food and soda from his work, they don't eat as well as she knows they should. "But I am eating less so I don't gain so much weight this time."

Mrs. Farrow's past medical history is unremarkable; her two pregnancies were term gestations and deliveries were vaginal. However, during the last pregnancy, she was diagnosed with pregnancy-induced hypertension and gestational diabetes, and labor was induced at 38 weeks' gestation. She states that she gained 60 lb with that pregnancy and that her son weighed 9 lb, 2 oz.

Your physical assessment of Mrs. Farrow reveals BP 100/60 right arm, sitting; pulse rate 86, regular and strong; respirations 18, regular and moderately shallow; temperature 36.7 degrees centigrade. Her apical beat is also 86 and strong; heart sounds: S_1 and S_2 with no murmurs or clicks. Skin is warm and dry, slightly pale with light pink nail beds, pale palpebral conjunctiva and oral mucous membranes. Abdomen moderately rounded with striae; fundal height 20 cm; fetal heart rate 158 per Doppler, right lower quadrant. Current weight 138 lb at 5 feet 9 inches tall, 2 lb less than her stated usual weight. Lab values show hemoglobin (Hgb) 10.2 g/dL; hematocrit (Hct) 29.9%; red blood cell (RBC) count $3.20 \times 10^{-6}/mm^3$. The remainder of the blood values is within normal limits. Urinalysis results are negative for protein and glucose.

The following concept map illustrates the diagnostic reasoning process.

Applying COLDSPA

Applying **COLDSPA** for client symptoms: "29 year old woman G3 P2; LMP 16 weeks ago."

Mnemonic	Question	Data Provided	Missing Data
Character	Describe the sign or symptom (feeling, appearance, sound, smell, or taste if applicable).	Client says she feels good but has no transportation to get to clinic for prenatal care during the last 16 weeks	"How did you get to the clinic today?"
Onset	When did it begin?	During the client's last pregnancy, she gained 60 pounds and her son weighed 9lb.2oz. at birth. She tries to eat healthy, but says her husband brings home free "fast food" often.	
Location	Where is it? Does it radiate? Does it occur anywhere else?		
Duration	How long does it last? Does it recur?		"What is your typical fluid and food intake at this time? Are you taking any prenatal vitamins? What proteins do you typically eat?"

continued

Mnemonic	Question	Data Provided	Missing Data
Severity	How bad is it? or How much does it bother you?	Client is 5′9″ and weighs 138 lbs; 2 pounds less than normal stated weight. Oral mucous membranes and conjunctiva are pale.	
Pattern	What makes it better or worse?	During her last pregnancy, the client was diagnosed with pregnancy-induced hypertension and gestational diabetes. Labor was induced at 38 weeks.	
Associated factors/How it **A**ffects the client	What other symptoms occur with it? How does it affect you?	The client has financial concerns; her husband works at a fast food chain and is looking for a better paying job.	What prenatal resources does the client qualify for and which ones has the client used in the past?

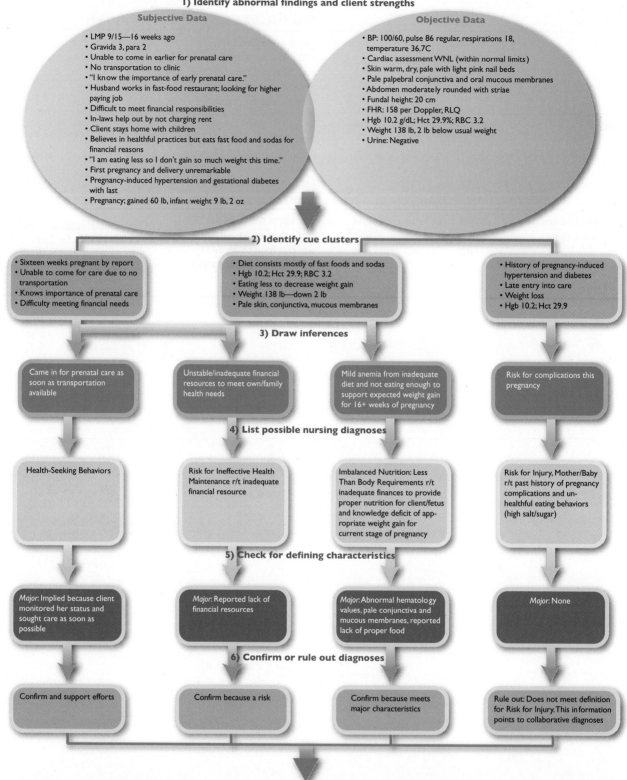

1) Identify abnormal findings and client strengths

Subjective Data
- LMP 9/15—16 weeks ago
- Gravida 3, para 2
- Unable to come in earlier for prenatal care
- No transportation to clinic
- "I know the importance of early prenatal care."
- Husband works in fast-food restaurant; looking for higher paying job
- Difficult to meet financial responsibilities
- In-laws help out by not charging rent
- Client stays home with children
- Believes in healthful practices but eats fast food and sodas for financial reasons
- "I am eating less so I don't gain so much weight this time."
- First pregnancy and delivery unremarkable
- Pregnancy-induced hypertension and gestational diabetes with last
- Pregnancy; gained 60 lb, infant weight 9 lb, 2 oz

Objective Data
- BP: 100/60, pulse 86 regular, respirations 18, temperature 36.7C
- Cardiac assessment WNL (within normal limits)
- Skin warm, dry, pale with light pink nail beds
- Pale palpebral conjunctiva and oral mucous membranes
- Abdomen moderately rounded with striae
- Fundal height: 20 cm
- FHR: 158 per Doppler, RLQ
- Hgb 10.2 g/dL; Hct 29.9%; RBC 3.2
- Weight 138 lb, 2 lb below usual weight
- Urine: Negative

2) Identify cue clusters

- Sixteen weeks pregnant by report
- Unable to come for care due to no transportation
- Knows importance of prenatal care
- Difficulty meeting financial needs

- Diet consists mostly of fast foods and sodas
- Hgb 10.2; Hct 29.9; RBC 3.2
- Eating less to decrease weight gain
- Weight 138 lb—down 2 lb
- Pale skin, conjunctiva, mucous membranes

- History of pregnancy-induced hypertension and diabetes
- Late entry into care
- Weight loss
- Hgb 10.2; Hct 29.9

3) Draw inferences

Came in for prenatal care as soon as transportation available

Unstable/inadequate financial resources to meet own/family health needs

Mild anemia from inadequate diet and not eating enough to support expected weight gain for 16+ weeks of pregnancy

Risk for complications this pregnancy

4) List possible nursing diagnoses

Health-Seeking Behaviors

Risk for Ineffective Health Maintenance r/t inadequate financial resource

Imbalanced Nutrition: Less Than Body Requirements r/t inadequate finances to provide proper nutrition for client/fetus and knowledge deficit of appropriate weight gain for current stage of pregnancy

Risk for Injury, Mother/Baby r/t past history of pregnancy complications and unhealthful eating behaviors (high salt/sugar)

5) Check for defining characteristics

Major: Implied because client monitored her status and sought care as soon as possible

Major: Reported lack of financial resources

Major: Abnormal hematology values, pale conjunctiva and mucous membranes, reported lack of proper food

Major: None

6) Confirm or rule out diagnoses

Confirm and support efforts

Confirm because a risk

Confirm because meets major characteristics

Rule out: Does not meet definition for Risk for Injury. This information points to collaborative diagnoses

7) Document conclusions

Nursing diagnoses that are appropriate for this client include:
- Health-Seeking Behavior
- Risk for Ineffective Health Maintenance r/t inadequate financial resources
- Risk for Interrupted Family Coping r/t inadequate resources
- Imbalanced Nutrition: Less Than Body Requirements r/t inadequate finances to provide proper nutrition and knowledge deficit of appropriate weight gain for current stage of pregnancy

Potential collaborative problems include the following:
- RC: Pregnancy-induced hypertension
- RC: Fetal compromise
- RC: Multiple gestation
- RC: Hyperglycemia
- RC: Fetal abnormality

References and Selected Readings

Albrecht, S., Maloni, J., Thomas, K., Jones, R., Halleran, J., & Osborne, J. (2004). Smoking Cessation Counseling for pregnant women who smoke. Scientific Basis for Practice for AWHONN's Success Project. *JOGNN, 33*(3), 298–305.

Bowen, A., & Mubajarine, N. (2006). Prevalence of Antenatal Depression in Women Enrolled in an Outreach Program Canad. *JOGNN, July/August 35(14),* 491–498.

Brown, W. (2006). Pharmacological Management of Asthma during Pregnancy. *Women's Health in Primary Care. May/June,* 23–28.

Buist, A., Morse, C., & Durkin, S. (2003). Men's Adjustment to Fatherhood. Implications for Obstetric Health Care. *JOGNN, 32(2),* 172–180.

Case, A., Ramadhani, T., Canfield, M., Beverly, L., & Wood, R. (2007). Folic Acid Supplementation Among Diabetic, Overweight, or Obese Women of Childbearing Age. *JOGNN, 36(4),* 335–341.

Cunnigham, E., Levano, K., Bloom, S., et al. (2005). *Williams Obstetrics.* (22nd ed.). New York: McGraw-Hill.

Dunn, L., & Oths, K. (2004). Prenatal Predictors of Intimate Partner Abuse. *JOGNN, 33(1),* 54–63.

George, T., Shefer, A. M., Ricket, D., David, F., Stevenson, J., & Fishbein, D. (2007). A status report from 1996–2004: are more effective immunization interventions being used in the women, infants, and children (WIC) program? *Maternal and Child Health Journal, July 11 (4),* 327–333.

Harner, H. (2004). Domestic Violence and Trauma Care in Teenage Pregnancy: Does Paternal Age make a Difference. *JOGNN 33(3),* 312–319.

Johnson, T., Mulder, P., Strube, K. (2007). Mother-Infant Breastfeeding Progress Tool: A guide for Education and Support of Breastfeeding Dyad. *JOGNN 36(4),* 319–327.

Lindgren, K. (2005). Testing the Health Practices in Pregnancy. Questionnaire-II. *JOGNN 34(4),* 465–473.

Lugo, N. (2008). Responding to Patient's Concerns: Influenza Immunization in Pregnancy. *The American Journal for Nurse Practitioners. July/August 12, (7–8),* 8–11.

McKinney, E. S., James, S. R., Murray, S. S., Ashwill, J. W. (2005). *Maternal-Child Nursing.* (2nd ed.). St. Louis, MO: Elsevier Inc.

Palmer, L, & Carter, E. (2006). Deciding when it's Labor: the experience of women who have received antepartum care at home for preterm labor. *JOGNN, July/August 35(4),* 509–515.

Sandelowski, M., & Barroso, J. (2005). The travesty of choosing after positive prenatal diagnosis. *JOGNN 34(3),* 307–318.

Shieh, C., & Kravitz, M. (2006). Severity of Drug Use, Initiation of Prenatal Care and Maternal-Fetal Attachment in pregnant Marijuana and Cocaine/Heroin Users. *JOGNN. July/August 35(4),* 499–508.

30

Assessing Newborns and Infants

Structure and Function

A newborn, or neonate, is the term used to describe a child from birth to 28-days-old. An infant refers to a child between the ages of 28 days and 1 year.

SKIN, HAIR, AND NAILS

At birth, the newborn's skin is smooth and thin. It may appear ruddy because of visible blood circulation through the newborn's thin layer of subcutaneous fat. This thin layer of fat, combined with the skin's inability to contract and shiver, results in ineffective temperature regulation. The skin may appear mottled on the trunk, arms, or legs. The dermis and epidermis are thin and loosely bound together. This increases the skin's susceptibility to infection and irritation and creates a poor barrier, resulting in fluid loss. When the newborn's body temperature drops, the hands and/or feet may appear blue (acrocyanosis). Vernix caseosa may be visible on the skin. It appears as a thick, cheesy, white substance on the skin and is especially prevalent in skin folds. This is normal and usually absorbs into the skin.

After birth, the newborn's sebaceous glands are active because of high levels of maternal androgen. Milia develop when these glands become plugged. Eccrine glands function at birth, creating palmar sweating, which is helpful when assessing pain. Apocrine glands stay small and nonfunctional until puberty.

The fine, downy hairs called lanugo, which appear on the newborn's body, shoulders, and/or back at birth, develop in the fetus at 3 months gestation and disappear within the first 2 weeks of life. Scalp hair-follicle growth phases occur concurrently at birth but are disrupted during early infancy. This may result in overgrowth or alopecia (hair loss).

Nails are usually present at birth. Missing or short nails usually signify prematurity, and long nails usually signify postmaturity. Nails are usually pink, convex, and smooth throughout childhood and adolescence.

HEAD AND NECK

Head growth predominates during the fetal period. At birth, the head circumference is greater (by 2 cm) than that of the chest. The cranial bones are soft and separated by the coronal, lambdoid, and sagittal sutures, which intersect at the anterior and posterior fontanelle (Fig. 30-1). Ossification begins in infancy and continues into adulthood.

The newborn's skull is typically asymmetric (plagiocephaly) because of molding that occurs as the newborn passes through the birth canal. The skull molds easily during birth, allowing for overlapping of the cranial bones.

The posterior fontanelle usually measures 1 to 2 cm at birth and usually closes at 2 months. The anterior fontanelle usually measures 4 to 6 cm at birth and closes between 12 and 18 months.

> ➤ **Clinical Tip** • *A full anterior fontanelle may be palpable when the newborn cries.*

Visible pulsations may also appear, representing the peripheral pulse. The sutures and fontanelles allow the skull to expand to accommodate brain growth. Brain growth is reflected by head circumference (occipital—frontal circumference), which increases six times as much during the first year as it does the second. Half of postnatal brain growth is achieved within the first year of life.

The neck is usually short during infancy (lengthening at about age 3 or 4 years). Lymphoid tissue is well developed at birth and reaches adult size by age 6 years.

EYES

Eye structure and function are not fully developed at birth. The iris shows little pigment, and the pupils are small. The macula, which is absent at birth, develops at 4 months and is mature by 8 months. Pupillary reflex is poor at birth and improves at 5 months of age. The sclera is clear. Small subconjunctival hemorrhages are normal after birth. Peripheral vision is developed, but central vision is not. The newborn is farsighted and has a visual acuity of 20/200. At 4 months, an infant can fixate on a singular

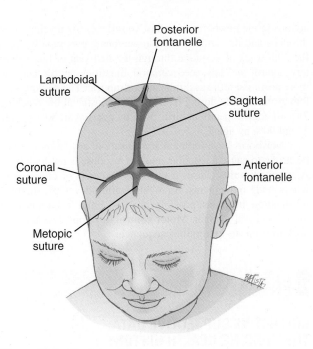

Posterior
fontanelle

Lambdoidal
suture

Sagittal
suture

Coronal
suture

Anterior
fontanelle

Metopic
suture

Figure 30-1 The infant head.

object with both eyes simultaneously (binocularity). Tearing and voluntary control over eye muscles begin at 2 to 3 months; by 4 months, infants establish binocular vision and focus on a single image with both eyes simultaneously. These functions are better developed by 9 months. Newborns cannot distinguish between colors; this ability develops by 8 months.

EARS

The inner ear develops during the first trimester of gestation. Therefore, maternal problems during this time, such as rubella, may impair hearing. Newborns can hear loud sounds at 90 decibels and react with the startle reflex. They respond to low-frequency sounds, such as a heartbeat or a lullaby, by decreasing crying and motor movement. They react to high-frequency sounds with an alerting reaction. In infants, the external auditory canal curves upward and is short and straight. Therefore, the pinna must be pulled down and back to perform the otoscopic examination. The eustachian tube is wider, shorter, and more horizontal, increasing the possibility of infection rising from the pharynx.

MOUTH, THROAT, NOSE, AND SINUS

Saliva is minimal at birth but drooling is evident by 3 months because of the increased secretion of saliva. Drooling persists for a few months until the infant learns to swallow the saliva. Drooling does not signify tooth eruption. The development of both temporary (deciduous) and permanent teeth begins in utero. Deciduous tooth eruption takes place between the ages of 6 and 24 months.

The tonsils and adenoids are small in relation to body size and hard to see at birth. The pharynx is best seen when the newborn is crying.

Newborns are obligatory nose breathers and, therefore, have significant distress when their nasal passages are ob-

structed. The maxillary and ethmoid sinuses are present at birth but they are small and cannot be examined until they develop.

THORAX AND LUNGS

At term gestation, the fetal lungs should be developed and the alveoli should be collapsed. Gas exchange is performed by the placenta. Immediately after birth, the lungs aerate; blood flows through them more vigorously, causing greater expansion and relaxation of the pulmonary arteries. The decrease in pulmonary pressure closes the foramen ovale, increasing oxygen tension and closing the ductus arteriosus. The lungs continue to develop after birth, and new alveoli form until about 8 years of age.

BREASTS

Ventral epidermal ridges (milk lines), which run from the axilla to the medial thigh, are present during gestation. True breasts develop along the thoracic ridge; the other breasts along the milk line atrophy. Occasionally a supernumerary nipple persists along the ridge track. At birth, lactiferous ducts are present in the nipple but there are no alveoli. Although the newborn's breasts may be temporarily enlarged from the effects of maternal estrogen, they are usually flat and remain so until puberty.

HEART

Because oxygenation takes place in the placenta in fetal circulation, the lungs are bypassed and arterial blood is returned to the right side of the heart. Blood is shunted through the foramen ovale and ductus arteriosus into the left side of the heart and out the aorta. At birth, lung aeration causes circulatory changes. The foramen ovale closes within the first hour because of the newly created low pressure in the right side of the heart, and the ductus arteriosus closes about 10 to 15 hours after birth.

When listening to the heart in the infant, systolic murmurs may be audible due to the transition from intrauterine to extrauterine life. This murmur generally resolves within 24 to 48 hours after birth. The pulse rate is usually between 120 to 160 b/minute. The rate decreases as the child ages, having a normal heart rate of 120 to 160 at birth and declining to approximately 120s at 6 months of age and down to 110s from 6 months to 1 year old. The heart should be auscultated at approximately the 4th intercostal margin to the left of the midclavicular line. The heart lays more horizontal in the chest and may seem enlarged with percussion. Heart sounds are also more audible in the newborn secondary to the thin subcutaneous layer of skin on the newborn.

PERIPHERAL VASCULAR SYSTEM

The skin should appear pink and well perfused. The hands and feet may appear blue at times (acrocyanosis) which is normal, especially when the newborn is cold. With warming the extremities, skin color should return to pink normal color. If the infant does not respond to this technique, consider a congenital heart defect in the newborn.

Pulses should be audible at the 4th intercostal space. Pulses should be felt in extremities, assessing the radial, brachial, and femoral pulses bilaterally. Weakness or absence of femoral pulses may indicate coarctation of the aorta. Bounding pulses can be seen with patent ductus arteriosus.

ABDOMEN

The umbilical cord is prominent in the newborn and contains two arteries and one vein. The umbilicus consists of two parts: the amniotic portion and the cutaneous portion. The amniotic portion is covered with a gel-like substance and dries up and falls off within 2 weeks of life. The cutaneous portion is covered with skin and draws back to become flush with the abdominal wall.

The abdomen of infants is cylindrical. Peristaltic waves may be visible in infants and may be indicative of a disease or disorder.

The newborn's liver is palpable at 0.5 to 2.5 cm below the right costal margin, thereby occupying proportionately more space than at any other time after birth. In infants and small children, the liver is palpable at 1 to 2 cm below the right costal margin, indicative of a disease or disorder. Kidney development is not complete until 1 year of age.

Bladder capacity increases with age; the bladder is considered an abdominal organ in infants because it is located between the symphysis pubis and the umbilicus (higher than in adults).

GENITALIA

In male infants the testes develop prenatally and drop into the scrotum during month 8 of gestation. Each testis measures about 1 cm wide and 1.5 to 2 cm long.

At birth, female genitalia may be engorged. Mucoid or bloody discharge may be noted because of the influence of maternal hormones. The genitalia return to normal size in a few weeks and remain small until puberty.

ANUS, RECTUM, AND PROSTATE

Meconium is passed during the first 24 hours of life, signifying anal patency. Stools are passed by reflex, and anal sphincter control is not reached until 1.5 to 2 years of age after the nerves supplying the area have become fully myelinated. Meconium not passed within 24 hours of birth could signify a problem. In boys, the prostate gland is underdeveloped and not palpable.

MUSCULOSKELETAL SYSTEM

At birth the newborn should have full range of motion of all extremities. Many newborns have feet that may appear deformed in position due to the intrauterine position of extremities. The feet should turn to the normal position with ease by the examiner.

The hips should also be checked for dislocation and ease of movement by performing Ortolani test and Barlow's sign.

The newborn vertebral column differs in contour from the normal adult vertebral column. The spine has a single C-shaped curve at birth. By 3 to 4 months, the anterior curve in the cervical region develops from the infant raising its head when prone.

NEUROLOGIC SYSTEM

The neurologic system is not fully developed at birth. Motor control is maintained by the spinal cord and medulla, and most actions in the newborn are primitive reflexes. As myelinization develops and the number of brain neurons grows rapidly, from the 30th week of gestation through the first year of life, voluntary control and advanced cerebral functions appear and the more primitive reflexes diminish or disappear. The nervous system grows rapidly during fetal and early postnatal life reaching 25% of adult capacity at birth, 50% by age 1 year, 80% by age 3, and 90% by age 7.

Newborns have rudimentary sensation; any stimulus must be strong to cause a reaction, and the response is not localized. A strong stimulus causes a vigorous response of crying with whole-body movements. As myelinization develops, stimulus localization becomes possible and the child responds in a more localized manner. Motor control develops in a head-to-neck to trunk-to-extremities sequence.

Health Assessment

COLLECTIVE SUBJECTIVE DATA: THE NURSING HEALTH HISTORY

Interviewing Parents

The initial assessment of the newborn occurs immediately after delivery. Therefore, parent interviewing is not performed. However, the nurse needs to get a complete maternal history of the mother before and during pregnancy. Delivery record information is also imperative for the initial newborn assessment. This information is usually obtained from the maternal hospital chart.

For assessment following this time period, the nurse interviews the parent(s).

Subjective assessment of the infant encompasses interviewing and compiling a complete nursing history from the parents or the primary care taker. The nurse should use a friendly, nonjudgemental approach when interviewing the family. Portray proficiency and competence when talking with the parents. Explain the purpose of the interview and clarify any misunderstandings during this time. Explain the importance of getting accurate information about the infant to ensure that the correct diagnosis and treatment are provided for the infant. Realize that common behaviors of the family may not be portrayed at this setting. The unfamiliar setting and concerns for the infant, especially if the infant is ill, may cause the parents to be very nervous and anxious during the interview. Providing a safe, relaxed environment will help the parents to be calm and be able to answer questions accurately.

Cultural variations may also exist with the family. The nurse should provide a nonjudgemental environment, using active listening skills and providing empathy as appropriate.

Nurses should also be aware of barriers to effective nurse–parent communication. These include time constraints, frequent interruptions, lack of privacy and language differences as well as provider callousness and cultural insensitivity. Make every effort to prevent these barriers. Providing enough time for the interview, keeping interruptions to a minimum, maintaining patient privacy, and using interpreters when language barriers exist will help with obtaining accurate information regarding the newborn's history.

(text continues on page 651)

BIOGRAPHIC DATA

Question	Rationale
What is the child's name? Nickname? What are the parents' or caregivers' names?	Knowing personal information about the child and caregivers helps to establish rapport with child and family.
Who is the child's primary health care provider, and when was the child's last well-child care appointment?	This determines the child's access to health care. It tells the nurse where to find the client's previous medical information/record.
Where does the child live? (Address)	In addition, assess the family's living conditions.
Do the parents and child live in the same residence? Are the child's parents married, single, divorced, homosexual? Who else lives in this residence? What are the parents' ages?	This indicates the availability of potential caregivers and support people for the client. It also helps to define familial relationships.
What is the child's age? What is the child's date of birth?	This provides a reference for assessing the child's developmental level.
Is the child adopted, foster, natural?	Certain health problems run in families. It is helpful to know the child's genetic relationship with the parents.
What is the child's ethic origin? Religion?	This information helps the nurse to examine special needs and beliefs that may affect the client or family's health care.
What do the child's parents do for a living?	This provides insight into the economic status of the family.

HISTORY OF PRESENT HEALTH CONCERN/CURRENT HEALTH STATUS

Elicit the reason for seeking care and ask questions about the child's current health status. During the first year of life, many visits to the health care provider will be well visits (check-ups).

Question	Rationale
Describe the child's general state of health. Does the child have a chronic illness?	Obtaining baseline information about the client helps to identify important areas of assessment.
Does the child have any allergies? If so, what is the specific allergen? How does the child react to it?	This identifies allergens and helps the nurse plan to prevent exposure.
What prescriptions, over-the-counter medications, devices, and treatments, and home or folk remedies is the child taking? Please provide the name of the drug, dosage, frequency, and reason it is administered.	It is always important to know what medications a client is taking, especially young clients.

continued on page 648

COLDSPA Example for Inability to Breast Feed

If there is a health concern, use the **COLDSPA** mnemonic as a guideline to collect needed information for each symptom the client shares.

Mnemonic	Question	Client Response Example
Character	Describe the sign or symptom (feeling, appearance, sound, smell, or taste if applicable).	Inability to nurse
Onset	When did it begin?	"The first time I tried to nurse my infant."
Location	Where is it? Does it radiate? Does it occur anywhere else?	"I tried both breasts."
Duration	How long does it last? Does it recur?	"I have tried with to breast feed with the nurse's help three times already."
Severity	How bad is it? or How much does it bother you?	"I am really worried because this is the best way to bond with my baby and I want him to have the immunity from my milk."
Pattern	What makes it better or worse?	"I've tried all positions and nothing works."
Associated factors/How it **A**ffects the client	What other symptoms occur with it? How does it affect you?	"I'm very stressed about being unable to breast feed."

PAST HEALTH HISTORY

Question	Rationale
Ask about the pregnancy:	
Was the pregnancy planned? How did you feel when you found out you were pregnant?	The caregiver's answer may provide insight into her feelings about the child.
When did you first receive prenatal care? How was your general health during pregnancy?	Prenatal information helps to identify potential health problems for the child.
Did you have any problems with your pregnancy?	
Did you have any accidents during this pregnancy?	
Did you take any medications during pregnancy?	Certain medications should not be taken during pregnancy and may be harmful to the child.
Did you use any tobacco, alcohol, or drugs during this pregnancy?	Smoking, alcohol, and drug use may cause complications or anomalies with the fetus.
Ask about delivery of the child:	Delivery details and complications are pertinent for assessing fetal injury and potential risk for infection.
Where was the child born?	
What type of delivery did you have?	
Were there any problems during the delivery? Did you have any vaginal infections at time of delivery?	
What was the child's Apgar score?	
What were the child's weight, length, and head circumference? Did the child have any problems after birth (e.g., feeding, jaundice)?	
Ask about past illnesses or injuries:	Previous illnesses and hospitalizations may affect the present examination.
Has the child ever been hospitalized?	
Has the child ever had any major illnesses?	
What immunizations has the child received thus far? Has your child had any reactions to immunizations?	This helps identify risk for infection and/or potential reactions to immunizations.

continued

FAMILY HISTORY

Question	Rationale
Please list any chronic health conditions in the family.	Certain conditions tend to run in families and increase the client's risk for such condition.
Please list the age and cause of death for blood relatives.	This helps to identify risk factors.
Does the child have family members with communicable diseases?	This also helps to identify risk factors.

REVIEW OF SYSTEMS

Question	Rationale
Skin, Hair, Nails	
Has your child had any changes in hair texture?	Changes may indicate an underlying problem.
Does your child exhibit scaling on her scalp?	Cradle cap is a common problem.
Has your child been exposed to any contagious disease such as measles, chickenpox, lice, ringworm, scabies and the like?	This helps to identify risks for health problems.
Has your child ever had any rashes or sores? Does your child have diaper rash?	Diaper rash is a common finding in infants.
Has your child had any excessive bruising or burns?	This helps to assess for child abuse. Excessive bruising or burns suggest abuse.
Does your child have any birthmarks?	Birthmarks are normal findings.
Head and Neck	
Has your child ever had a head injury?	Head injuries may cause neurological problems.
Did the fontanelles close on schedule? Does the child have head control? If so, at what age did this occur?	These questions assess normal growth and development.
Eyes and Vision	
Does your infant have any unusual eye movements? Does your infant/child excessively cross eyes?	This helps to determine eye and vision development.
Does your infant blink when necessary?	Absent blinking is abnormal.
Is your infant able to focus on moving objects?	By one month, the infant should be able to follow a moving object or light.
Has your infant ever had cloudiness in the eyeball?	Cloudiness of the eyeball may indicate the presence of cataracts.
Ears and Hearing	
Does your child appear to be paying attention when you speak? (Infants should respond to the human voice.) Does the child respond to loud noise?	Infants who do not respond to the human voice or loud voices may have a hearing loss.
Has your child had frequent ear infections? Tubes in ears?	Frequent otitis media is a risk factor for hearing loss.
Does anyone in the child's home smoke?	Smoking increases the risk of otitis media.

continued on page 650

REVIEW OF SYSTEMS *Continued*

Question	Rationale
Mouth, Throat, Nose, and Sinuses	
Does your child have any teeth?	No teeth by age one is a variation of normal.
Does your child attend day care?	Attending day care increases risk of upper respiratory infections (through exposure to other children).
Thorax and Lungs	
Has your child ever had cough, wheezing, shortness or breath, nocturnal dyspnea; if so, when does it occur? Has your child had frequent or severe colds?	Positive answers to any of these questions may indicate upper respiratory disorders.
Heart and Neck Vessels	
Does your infant become fatigued or short of breath during feedings?	Infants who fatigue easily with feedings may have congenital heart defect or disorder.
Peripheral Vascular System	
Does your child ever experience bluing of the extremities? Do our child's hands and/or feet get unusually cold?	These questions assess vascular supply and perfusion.
Abdomen	
Are you breast or bottle feeding? What foods does the infant eat?	Feeding patterns help the nurse to assess nutrition and gastrointestinal function.
Has your child ever had any excessive vomiting? Abdominal pain? Please describe.	Excessive vomiting may indicate neurological disorder.
Genitalia	
How often does your child urinate? How many wet diapers do you change per day?	The caregiver's answer helps the nurse to assess the genitourinary system.
Is the child prone to frequent diaper rash.	Diaper rash (irritant contact dermatitis) is common in infants.
Anus and Rectum	
How often does your child have bowel movement? What does it look like?	These questions help to assess gastrointestinal function.
Is there any history of bleeding, constipation, diarrhea, or hemorrhoids?	
Musculoskeletal System	
Has your child ever had limited range of motion, joint pain, stiffness, paralysis?	These questions assess musculoskeletal development.
Has your child ever had any fractures? Have you noticed any bone deformities?	Frequent fractures may indicate child abuse.
Neurologic System	
Has your child ever had a seizure?	Seizures indicate a neurologic or other systemic disorder.
Has your child ever experienced any problems with motor coordination?	If the child is not meeting developmental landmarks, it may indicate an underlying problem.

Growth and Development

Growth and development of the newborn/infant may be assessed using the Denver Developmental Screening Test (see Assessment Tool 30-1). This test is used to guide the nurse to the appropriate developmental milestones for the child's gross motor, language, fine motor, and personal social development.

Motor Development

GROSS MOTOR

Newborns can turn their heads from side to side when prone unless they are lying on a soft surface. This inability to turn their head while lying on a soft surface makes suffocation a real concern. By 3 to 4 months, there is almost no head lag and the infant may push up to prone position. Infants roll from front to back at 5 months and sit unsupported by 6 to 7 months. They pull to stand by 9 months, cruise by 10 months, and walk when hand-held by 12 months. Figure 30-2 displays gross motor development of the infant.

FINE MOTOR

The grasp reflex is present at birth and strengthens at 1 month. This reflex fades at 3 months, at which time an infant can actively hold a rattle. Five-month-old infants can grasp voluntarily, and 7-month-old infants can hand-to-hand transfer. The pincer grasp develops by 9 months, and 12-month-old infants will attempt to build a two-block tower.

Sensory Perception (Vision, Hearing, and Other Senses)

VISUAL

The newborn's visual impressions are unfocused, and the ability to distinguish between colors is not developed until approximately 8 months of age. Therefore, stimuli should be bright, simple, moving, and, preferably black and white (e.g., a mobile that consists of black and white circles and cubes; Fig. 30-3).

AUDITORY

Newborns can distinguish sounds and turn toward voices and other noises. They may be very familiar with their mother's voice, and other sounds gradually gain significance when associated with pleasure.

OLFACTORY

Smell is fully developed at birth, and a 2-week-old infant can differentiate the smell of his or her mother's milk and parents' body odors.

TACTILE

Touch is well developed at birth, especially the lips and tongue. Touch should be used frequently because infants enjoy rocking, warmth, and cuddling. Infants normally attend to the human voice; therefore, question parents as to whether their child appears to be paying attention when they speak.

Cognitive and Language Development (Piaget)

The sensorimotor stage, from birth to around 18 months, involves the development of intellect and knowledge of the environment gained through the senses. During this stage, development progresses from reflexive activity to purposeful acts. At the completion of this stage, the infant achieves a sense of object permanence (retains a mental image of an absent object; sees self as separate from others). An emerging sense of body image parallels sensorimotor development.

Crying is the first means of communication, and parents can usually differentiate cries. Cooing begins by 1 to 2 months, laughing and babbling by 3 to 4 months, and consonant sounds by 3 to 4 months. The infant begins to imitate sounds by 6 months. Combined syllables ("mama") are vocalized by 8 months, and the infant understands "no-no" by 9 months. "Mama" and "dada" are said with meaning by 10 months, and the infant says a total of 2 to 4 words with meaning by 12 months.

Moral Development (Kolberg)

Although Kolberg's theory of moral development begins with toddlerhood, infants cannot be overlooked. Child moral development begins with the value and belief system of the parents and the infant's own development of trust. Parental discipline patterns may start with the young infant in the form of interventions for crying behaviors. Stern discipline and withholding love and affection may affect infant moral development. Love and affection are the building blocks of an infant's developing sense of trust (Fig. 30-4).

Psychosocial Development (Erikson)

The crisis faced by an infant (birth to 1 year) is termed trust versus mistrust. In this stage, the infant's significant other is the "caretaking" person. Developing a sense of trust in caregivers and the environment is a central focus for an infant. This sense of trust forms the foundation for all future psychosocial tasks. The quality of the caregiver—child relationship is a crucial factor in the infant's development of trust. An infant who receives attentive care learns that life is predictable and that his or her needs will be met promptly; this fosters trust. In contrast, an infant experiencing consistently delayed needs gratification develops a sense of uncertainty, leading to mistrust of caregivers and the environment. An infant commonly seeks comfort from a security blanket or other object such as a favorite stuffed animal.

Psychosexual Development (Freud)

In the *oral stage* of development, from birth to 18 months, the erogenous zone is the mouth, and sexual activity takes the form of sucking, swallowing, chewing, and biting. In this stage, the infant meets the world by crying, tasting, eating, and early vocalization; biting, to gain a sense of having a hold on and having greater control of the environment; and grasping and touching to explore texture variations in the environment.

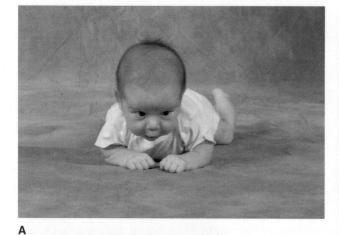

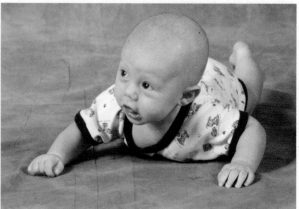

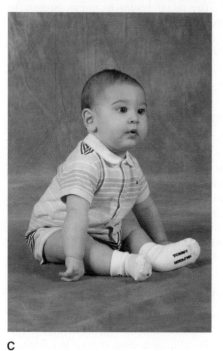

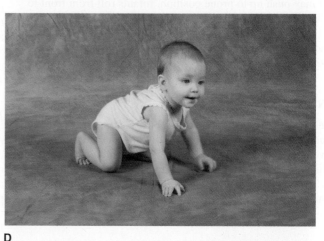

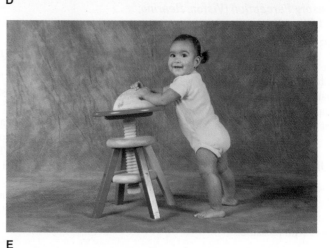

Figure 30-2 Growth and development of the infant. **(A)** At 4 weeks, this infant turns head when lying in a prone position. **(B)** At 12 weeks, this infant pushes up from a prone position. **(C)** At 21 weeks, this infant sits up but tilts forward for balance. **(D)** At 30 weeks, this infant is crawling around and on the go. **(E)** At 43 weeks, this infant is getting ready to walk.

Lifestyle and Health Practices

Normal Nutritional Requirements

Breast milk is the most desirable complete food for the first 6 months of a child's life. However, commercially prepared, iron-fortified formula is an acceptable alternative. Formula intake varies per infant. Most infants take 100 cal/kg body weight/day. This amount of formula should be offered to the infant every 3 to 4 h, approximately four to six times a day. Solids are not recommended before 4 months of age due to the

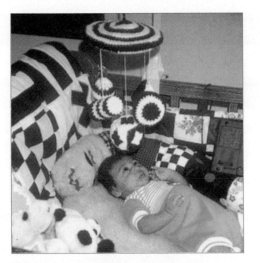

Figure 30-3 A black-and-white mobile is a good visual stimulus for an infant (courtesy of S. Ludington).

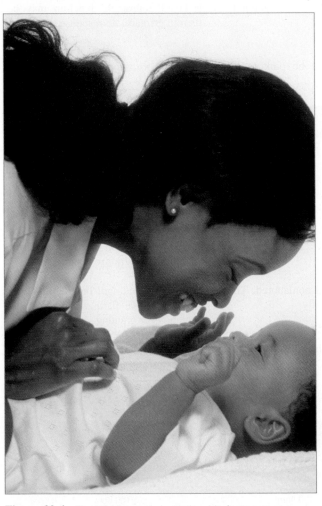

Figure 30-4 The infant-caregiver relationship fosters trust.

presence of the protrusion or sucking reflexes and the immaturity of the gastrointestinal tract and the immune system. Infant rice cereal is usually the initial solid food given because it is easy to digest, contains iron, and rarely triggers allergy.

Additional foods usually include other cereals followed by fruits and vegetables and finally meats. Juices may be offered at 6 months of age. Finger foods are introduced at 8 or 9 months. Weaning from breast or bottle to cup should be gradual. The desire to imitate at 8 to 9 months increases the success of weaning. Honey should be discouraged during the first year of life because it may cause infant botulism.

Normal Sleep Requirements and Patterns

Sleep patterns vary among infants. During the first month, most infants sleep when not eating. By 3 to 4 months, most infants sleep 9 to 11 hours at night. By 12 months, most infants take morning and afternoon naps. Bedtime rituals should begin in infancy to prepare the infant for sleep and prevent future sleep problems. Because of the possibility of SIDS (sudden infant death syndrome), it is suggested that young infants sleep in the supine or side-lying position.

COLLECTING OBJECTIVE DATA: PHYSICAL EXAMINATION

Preparing the Client

Make sure the caregiver understands the examination process. Describe what will be performed and how it will be performed. Explain that the Denver Development Examination assesses normal development milestones. Encourage the caregiver to ask questions during the examination. For most of the examination, the child should be unclothed.

Equipment

- Denver Development Kit
- Measuring tape
- Ophthalmoscope
- Otoscope
- Scale
- Stethoscope
- Thermometer

Physical Assessment

Initial Assessment

Immediately after birth, the newborn should be evaluated while the infant is supine under a radiant warmer.

Subsequent Assessment

After the initial newborn assessment, the child will be assessed using the following physical assessment guide.

(text continues on page 683)

INITIAL NEWBORN ASSESSMENT

Assessment Procedure	Normal Findings	Abnormal Findings
Apgar Score		
Assign Apgar scores at 1 and at 5 minutes after delivery. The Apgar Score is an assessment of infant's ability to adapt to extrauterine life. Assess the following:	The score is 8 to 10. See Table 30-1 for Apgar scoring.	A score of less than 8 may indicate poor transition from intrauterine to extrauterine life.
Auscultate apical pulse.	The pulse is less than 100 bpm.	Pulse is greater the 100 bpm, indicating bradycardia. Absent heartbeat indicates fetal demise.
Inspect chest and abdomen for respiratory effort.	The newborn is crying.	The newborn has absent, slow, or irregular respirations.
Inspect muscle tone by extending legs and arms. Observe degree of flexion and resistance in extremities.	The extremities are flexed, and you note active movement.	Delayed neurologic function may be seen in grimace, no response.
Inspect body and extremities for skin color.	The full body should be pink (acrocyanosis).	The newborn is cyanotic, pale.
Vital signs		
Monitor axillary temperature (Fig. 30-5).	Temperature is 97.5 to 99°F (36.4 to 37.2°C).	A temperature of less than 97.5°F (36.4°C) indicates hypothermia, which may suggest sepsis.
		A temperature of greater than 99°F (37.2°C) indicates hyperthermia. (Consider infection or improper monitoring of temperature probe).
Inspect and auscultate lung sounds.	Breathing is easy and nonlabored. The lungs are clear bilaterally.	Abnormal findings include labored breathing, nasal flaring, rhonchi, rales, retractions or grunting.
Monitor respiratory rate.	Rate is 30 to 60 breaths/min.	A rate less than 30 or greater than 60 breaths/min is seen with respiratory distress.

Table 30-1 · APGAR Scoring

	Scores 0	Scores 1	Scores 2
Heart rate	Absent	<100 bpm	>100 bpm
Respiratory rate	Absent	Slow, irregular	Good lusty cry
Reflex irritability	No response	Grimace, some motion	Cry, cough
Muscle tone	Flaccid, limp	Flexion of extremities	Active flexion
Color	Cyanotic, pale	Pink body, acrocyanosis	Pink body, pink extremities

continued

Assessment Procedure	Normal Findings	Abnormal Findings
Auscultate apical pulse.	Pulse is regular and within a range of 120 to 140 beats/min while at rest. The rate may rise to 180 beats/min when crying or or fall to 100 beats/min when sleeping.	Pulse is irregular or the rate is above 180 beats/min while crying; below 100 beats/min while sleeping may indicate cardiac abnormalities.

Measurements

Weigh the newborn using a newborn scale (Fig. 30-6). The child should be unclothed.	The newborn weighs between 2500 to 4000 g.	Weight is less than 2500 g or greater than 4000 g.
Measure length (Fig. 30-7).	The newborn is 44 to 55 cm.	Length is less than 44 or greater than 55 cm.
Measure head circumference (Fig. 30-8). (See instructions below under Subsequent Assessment.)	Circumference is 33 to 35.5 cm.	Circumference is less than 33 cm or greater than 35.5 cm. This may indicate microcephaly, improper brain growth, premature closing of the sutures, intrauterine infection, or chromosomal defect.
Measure chest circumference. Place tape measure at nipple line and wrap around infant.	Circumference is 30 to 33 cm (1 to 2 cm less than head).	Circumference is less than 29 cm or greater than 34 cm.

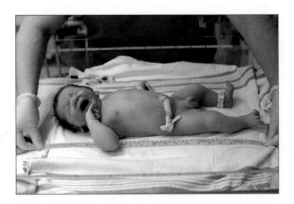

Figure 30-5 Measuring the newborn's axillary temperature.

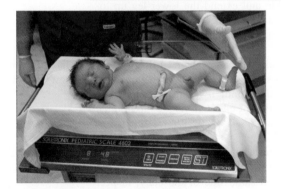

Figure 30-6 Weighing the newborn.

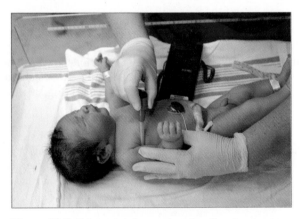

Figure 30-7 Measuring the length of the newborn.

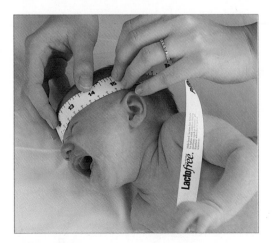

Figure 30-8 Measuring the circumference of an infant's head (© B. Proud).

continued

INITIAL NEWBORN ASSESSMENT *Continued*

Assessment Procedure	Normal Findings	Abnormal Findings
Gestational Age		

Assess gestational age within four hours after birth to identify any potential age-related problems that may occur within the next few hours. This exam requires assessing the newborn's neuromuscular and physical maturity. Use the Ballard Scale to rate.

To assess neuromuscular maturity (with the newborn in supine position):

Assessment Procedure	Normal Findings	Abnormal Findings
Inspect posture (with the newborn undisturbed).	Arms and legs are flexed.	In premature children, the newborn's arms and legs may be limp and extend away from the body.
Assess for square window sign. Bend wrist toward ventral forearm until resistance is met. Measure angle.	Angle is 0 to 30° (Fig. 30-9).	Premature newborns may have a square window measurement of less than 30°.
Test arm recoil. Bilaterally flex elbows up.	Elbow angle is less than 90° and the arm rapidly recoils to a flexed state.	In premature children, elbow angle may be greater than 110° and delayed recoil may be seen.
Assess popliteal angle. Flex thigh on top of the abdomen; push behind the ankle and extend the lower leg up towards the head until resistance is met. Measure the angle behind the knee.	The angle should be less than 100°.	Premature children may have a popliteal angle of greater than 100°.
Assess for Scarf sign. Lift the arm across the chest toward the opposite shoulder until resistance is met; note location of elbow in relation to midline of chest.	Elbow position is less than midline of chest (Fig. 30-10).	In premature children, elbow position is at midline of chest or greater (toward opposite shoulder) (Fig. 30-10).
Perform heel to ear test. Keeping buttocks flat on the bed, pull leg toward ear on same side of the body; inspect popliteal angle and proximity of heel to ear.	Popliteal angle is less than 90°; heel is distal from ear.	In premature infants, popliteal angle may be greater than 90°, and the heel may be proximal to ear.

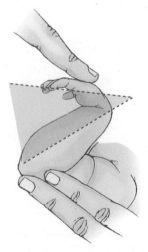

A   **B**

Figure 30-9 Square window sign: **(A)** term infant **(B)** preterm infant.

continued

Assessment Procedure	Normal Findings	Abnormal Findings
To assess for physical maturity:		
Inspect skin.	Inspection reveals parchment, few or no vessels on the abdomen, and crackling, especially in the ankle area.	Inspection reveals translucent, visible veins; rash; leathery, wrinkled skin that is seen in most postmature children.
Inspect for lanugo.	Normally there is thinning and balding on the back, shoulders, and knees.	In premature children, abundant amounts of fine hair may be seen on the face.
Inspect the plantar surface of the feet for creases.	There are creases on the anterior two thirds or entire sole.	Transverse crease on sole only, no creases, or fewer creases indicate prematurity.
Inspect and palpate breast bud tissue with middle finger and forefinger; measure bud in millimeters.	The areola is raised and full.	In premature infants, there may be an absence of breast tissue and a bud less than 3 mm.
Observe ear cartilage in upper pinna for curving. Fold pinna down toward side of the head and release; note recoil of the ear.	Normally you find a well-curved pinna, well-formed cartilage, and instant recoil.	With prematurity, you may find a slightly curved pinna and slow recoil.
Inspect the genitals. *Male:* Assess scrotum for rugae and palpate position of testes.	*Male:* There are deep rugae; testes are positioned down in scrotal sac.	*Male:* There is decreased presence of rugae; testes are positioned in upper inguinal canal.
Female: Inspect labia majora, labia minora, and clitoris.	*Female:* Labia majora cover labia minora and clitoris.	*Female:* In prematurity, labia majora and labia minora are equally prominent and clitoris is prominent.
Determine score rating: Use Figure 30-11. Mark the boxes that most closely represent each observation.	Score totals 35 to 45.	Score totals less than 35 or greater than 45.

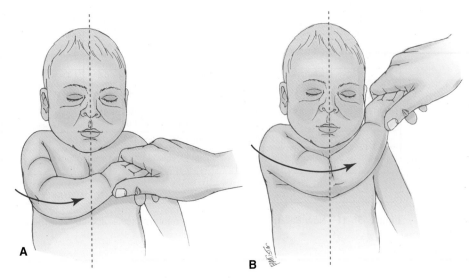

Figure 30-10 Scarf sign: **(A)** term infant; **(B)** preterm infant.

continued

INITIAL NEWBORN ASSESSMENT *Continued*

Assessment Procedure	Normal Findings	Abnormal Findings
Newborn Reflexes		
Assess newborn reflexes. See Display 30-1 for techniques.	See Display 30-1.	See Display 30-1.

NEUROMUSCULAR MATURITY

NEUROMUSCULAR MATURITY SIGN	SCORE							RECORD SCORE HERE
	−1	0	1	2	3	4	5	
POSTURE								
SQUARE WINDOW (Wrist)	>90°	90°	60°	45°	30°	0°		
ARM RECOIL		180°	140°–180°	110°–140°	90°–110°	<90°		
POPLITEAL ANGLE	180°	160°	140°	120°	100°	90°	<90°	
SCARF SIGN								
HEEL TO EAR								
						TOTAL NEUROMUSCULAR MATURITY SCORE		

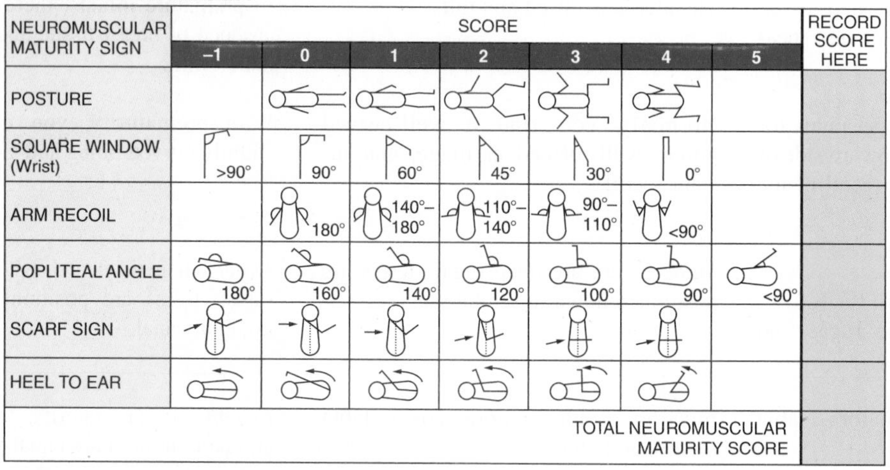

PHYSICAL MATURITY

PHYSICAL MATURITY SIGN	SCORE							RECORD SCORE HERE
	−1	0	1	2	3	4	5	
SKIN	sticky, friable, transparent	gelatinous, red, translucent	smooth, pink, visible veins	superficial peeling and/or rash, few veins	cracking pale areas, rare veins	parchment, deep cracking, no vessels	leathery, cracked, wrinkled	
LANUGO	none	sparse	abundant	thinning	bald areas	mostly bald		
PLANTAR SURFACE	heel-toe 40–50 mm:−1 <40 mm:−2	>50 mm no crease	faint red marks	anterior transverse crease only	creases ant. 2/3	creases over entire sole		
BREAST	impercep-tible	barely perceptible	flat areola no bud	stippled areola 1–2 mm bud	raised areola 3–4 mm bud	full areola 5–10 mm bud		
EYE-EAR	lids fused loosely: −1 tightly: −2	lids open pinna flat stays folded	sl. curved pinna; soft; slow recoil	well-curved pinna; soft but ready recoil	formed and firm instant recoil	thick cartilage, ear stiff		
GENITALS (Male)	scrotum flat, smooth	scrotum empty, faint rugae	testes in upper canal, rare rugae	testes descending, few rugae	testes down, good rugae	testes pendulous, deep rugae		
GENITALS (Female)	clitoris prominent and labia flat	prominent clitoris and small labia minora	prominent clitoris and enlarging minora	majora and minora equally prominent	majora large, minora small	majora cover clitoris and minora		
						TOTAL PHYSICAL MATURITY SCORE		

SCORE
Neuromuscular _____
Physical _____
Total _____

MATURITY RATING

Score	Weeks
−10	20
−5	22
0	24
5	26
10	28
15	30
20	32
25	34
30	36
35	38
40	40
45	42
50	44

GESTATIONAL AGE (weeks)
By dates _____
By ultrasound _____
By exam _____

Figure 30-11 New Ballard scale. Used to rate neuromuscular and physical maturity of gestational age.

DISPLAY 30-1   **Newborn Reflexes: Differentiating Normal and Abnormal Findings**

The reflexes illustrated and described below are the most commonly tested newborn reflexes. These reflexes are present in all normal newborns, and most disappear within a few months after birth. Therefore, absence of a reflex at birth or persistence of a reflex past a certain age may indicate a problem with central nervous system function.

Rooting Reflex
To elicit the rooting reflex, touch the newborn's upper or lower lip or cheek with a gloved finger or sterile nipple. The newborn will move the head toward the stimulated area and open the mouth.

Disappearance of Reflex
The rooting reflex disappears by 3 to 4 months.

Abnormal Findings
Absence of a rooting indicates serious CNS disease.

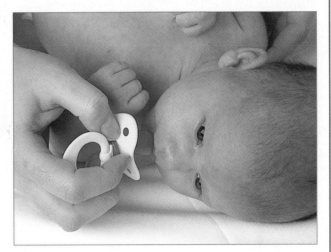

Sucking Reflex
Place a gloved finger or nipple in the newborn's mouth, and note the strength of the sucking response. (A diminished response is normal in a recently fed newborn.)

Disappearance of Reflex
This reflex disappears at 10 to 12 months.

Abnormal Findings
A weak or absent sucking reflex may indicate a neurologic disorder, prematurity, or CNS depression caused by maternal drug use or medication during pregnancy.

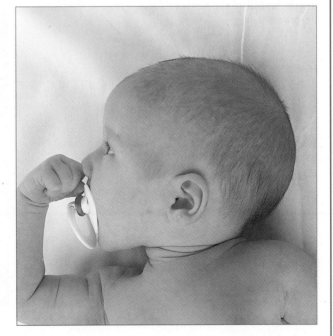

continued on page 660

Palmar Grasp Reflex

Press your fingers against the palmar surface of the newborn's hand from the ulnar side. The grasp should be strong—you may even be able to pull the newborn to a sitting position.

Disappearance of Reflex

This reflex disappears at 3 to 4 months.

Abnormal Findings

A diminished response usually indicates prematurity; no response suggests neurologic deficit; asymmetric grasp suggests fracture of the humerus or peripheral nerve damage. If this reflex persists past 4 months, cerebral dysfunction may be present.

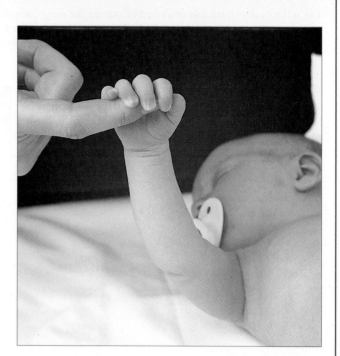

Plantar Grasp Reflex

Touch the ball of the newborn's foot. The toes should curl downward tightly.

Disappearance of Reflex

This reflex disappears at 8 to 10 months.

Abnormal Findings

A diminished response usually indicates prematurity; no response suggests neurologic deficit.

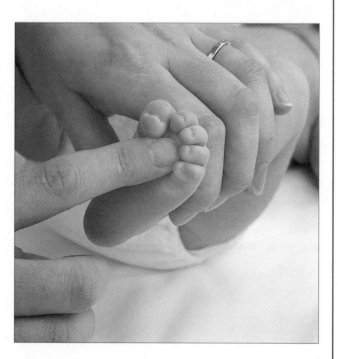

continued

Tonic Neck Reflex

The newborn should be supine. Turn the head to one side with newborn's jaw at the shoulder. The tonic neck reflex is present when the arm and leg on the side to which the head is turned extend and the opposite arm and leg flex. This reflex usually does not appear until 2 months of age.

Disappearance of Reflex

This reflex disappears by 4 to 6 months. The reflex may not occur every time that the examiner tries to elicit it, in which case, repeat stimulus of turning head to one side to re-elicit the response.

Abnormal Findings

If this reflex persists until later in infancy, brain damage is usually present.

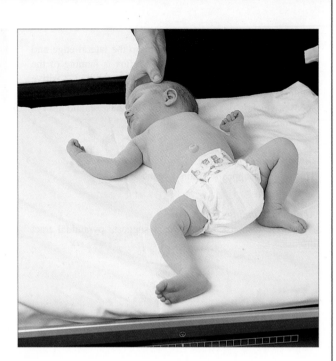

Moro (or Startle) Reflex

The Moro reflex is a response to sudden stimulation or an abrupt change in position. This reflex can be elicited by using either one of the following two methods:

1. Hold the infant with the head supported and rapidly lower the whole body a few inches.
2. Place the infant in the supine position on a flat, soft surface. Hit the surface with your hand or startle the infant in some way.

The reflex is manifested by the infant slightly flexing and abducting the legs, laterally extending and abducting the arms, forming a "C" with thumb and forefinger, and fanning the other fingers. This is immediately followed by anterior flexion and adduction of the arms. All movements should be symmetric.

Disappearance of Reflex

This reflex disappears by 3 months.

Abnormal Findings

An asymmetric response suggests injury of the part that responds more slowly. Absence of a response suggests CNS injury. If the reflex was elicited at birth and disappears later, cerebral edema or intracranial hemorrhage is suspected. Persistence of the response after 4 months suggests CNS injury.

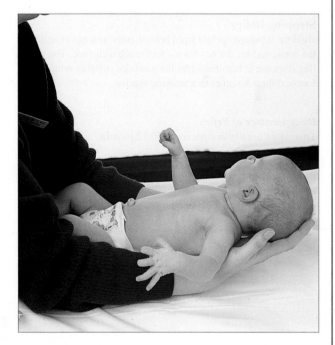

continued on page 662

Babinski Reflex

Hold the newborn's foot and stroke up the lateral edge and across the ball. A positive Babinski reflex is fanning of the toes. Many normal newborns will not exhibit a positive Babinski reflex; instead, they will exhibit the normal adult response, which is flexion of the toes. Response should always be symmetric bilaterally.

Disappearance of Reflex

This reflex disappears within 2 years.

Abnormal Findings

A positive response after 2 years suggests pyramidal tract disease.

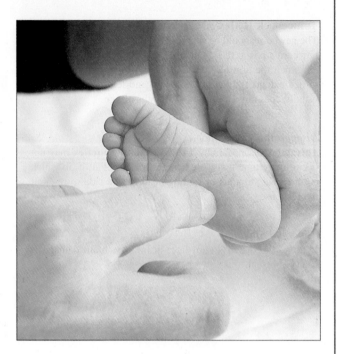

Stepping Reflex

Hold the newborn upright from behind, provide support under the arms, and let the newborn's feet touch a surface. The reflex response is manifested by the newborn stepping with one foot and then the other in a walking motion.

Disappearance of Reflex

This reflex usually disappears within 2 months.

Abnormal Findings

An asymmetric response may indicate injury of the leg, CNS damage, or peripheral nerve injury.

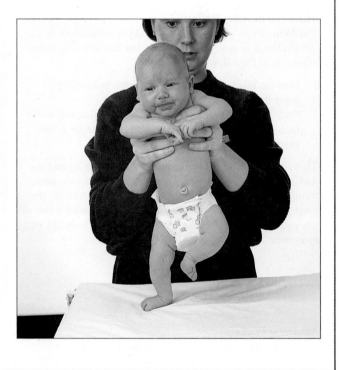

SUBSEQUENT PHYSICAL ASSESSMENT

Assessment Procedure	Normal Findings	Abnormal Findings
General Appearance and Behavior		
Observe general appearance. Observe hygiene. Note interaction with parents and yourself (and siblings if present). Note also facies (facial expressions) and posture.	Child appears stated age; is clean, has no unusual body odor, and clothing is in good condition and appropriate for climate. Child is alert, active, responds appropriately to stress of the situation. Child is appropriately interactive for age, seeks comfort from parent; appears happy. Newborn's arms and legs are in flexed position.	Note any facies that indicate acute illness, respiratory distress. Flaccidity or rigidity in newborn may be from neurologic damage, sepsis, or pain. Poor hygiene and clothes may indicate neglect, poverty. Child does not appear stated age (mental retardation, abuse, neglect).
Developmental Assessment		
Screen for cognitive, language, social, and gross and fine motor developmental delays in the beginning of the physical assessment in infants. Assessment Tool 30-1 presents the DDST II and directions for its use.	Child meets normal parameters for age. See information contained in subjective data section.	Child lags in earlier stages.
Vital Signs		
Assess temperature. Use rectal, axillary, skin, or tympanic route when assessing the temperature of an infant. The rectal temperature is most accurate. To take a rectal temperature in a newborn, lay the child supine and lift lower legs up into the air, bending the legs at the hips. Insert lubricated rectal thermometer no more than 2 cm into rectum. Temperature registers in 3 to 5 min on a rectal thermometer. Axillary and/or tympanic temperature may also be used. For axillary temperature, place the thermometer under axilla, holding arm close to chest for approximately 3 to 5 minutes. For tympanic temperature, use digital tympanic thermometer as directed in manufacturer's instructions.	Temperature is 99.4°F (because of excess heat production).	Temperature may be altered by exercise, stress, crying, environment, diurnal variation (highest between 4 and 6 PM). Both hyperthermic and hypothermic conditions are noted in children.

continued on page 666

ASSESSMENT TOOL 30-1   Using the Denver Developmental Screening Test

The following is an example of the Denver Developmental Screening Test (DDST), which assesses a child's gross motor, language, fine motor, and personal social development according to the child's age. Testing kits, test forms, and reference manuals (which must be used to ensure accuracy in administering the test) may be ordered from Denver Developmental Materials Inc., P.O. Box 6919, Denver, CO 80206-0919. (Reprinted with permission from William K. Frankenburg, M.D.).

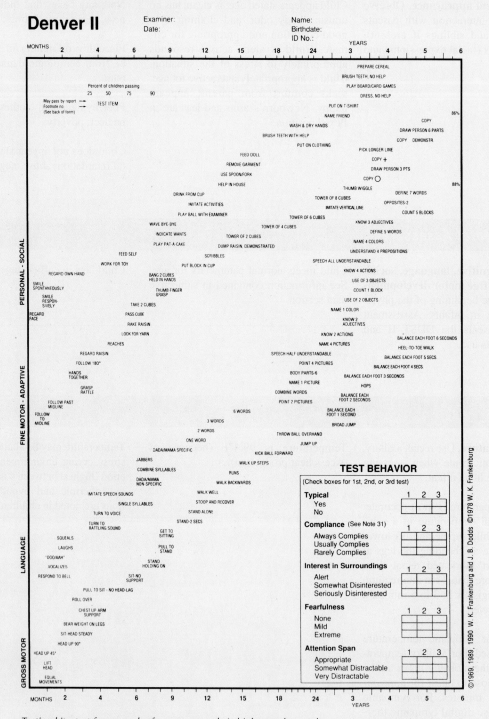

Testing kits, test forms, and reference manuals (which must be used to ensure accuracy in administration of the test) for the DDST may be ordered from Denver Developmental Materials Incorporated, P.O. Box 6919, Denver, CO 80206-0919. (Reprinted with permission from William K. Frankenburg, M.D.)

continued

ASSESSMENT TOOL 30-1 | **Using the Denver Developmental Screening Test** *Continued*

DIRECTIONS FOR ADMINISTRATION

1. Try to get child to smile by smiling, talking or waving. Do not touch him/her.
2. Child must stare at hand several seconds.
3. Parent may help guide toothbrush and put toothpaste on brush.
4. Child does not have to be able to tie shoes or button/zip in the back.
5. Move yarn slowly in an arc from one side to the other, about 8" above child's face.
6. Pass if child grasps rattle when it is touched to the backs or tips of fingers.
7. Pass if child tries to see where yarn went. Yarn should be dropped quickly from sight from tester's hand without arm movement.
8. Child must transfer cube from hand to hand without help of body, mouth, or table.
9. Pass if child picks up raisin with any part of thumb and finger.
10. Line can vary only 30 degrees or less from tester's line. /
11. Make a fist with thumb pointing upward and wiggle only the thumb. Pass if child imitates and does not move any fingers other than the thumb.

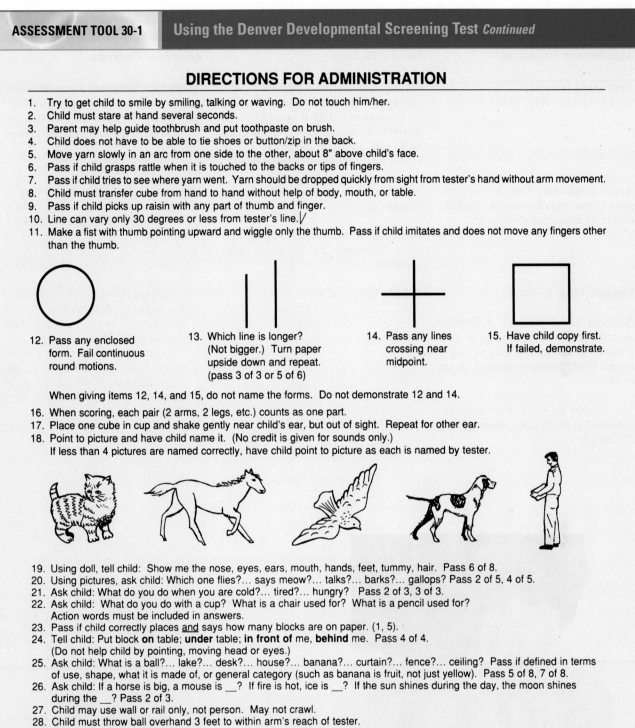

12. Pass any enclosed form. Fail continuous round motions.
13. Which line is longer? (Not bigger.) Turn paper upside down and repeat. (pass 3 of 3 or 5 of 6)
14. Pass any lines crossing near midpoint.
15. Have child copy first. If failed, demonstrate.

When giving items 12, 14, and 15, do not name the forms. Do not demonstrate 12 and 14.

16. When scoring, each pair (2 arms, 2 legs, etc.) counts as one part.
17. Place one cube in cup and shake gently near child's ear, but out of sight. Repeat for other ear.
18. Point to picture and have child name it. (No credit is given for sounds only.)
    If less than 4 pictures are named correctly, have child point to picture as each is named by tester.

19. Using doll, tell child: Show me the nose, eyes, ears, mouth, hands, feet, tummy, hair. Pass 6 of 8.
20. Using pictures, ask child: Which one flies?... says meow?... talks?... barks?... gallops? Pass 2 of 5, 4 of 5.
21. Ask child: What do you do when you are cold?... tired?... hungry? Pass 2 of 3, 3 of 3.
22. Ask child: What do you do with a cup? What is a chair used for? What is a pencil used for?
    Action words must be included in answers.
23. Pass if child correctly places <u>and</u> says how many blocks are on paper. (1, 5).
24. Tell child: Put block **on** table; **under** table; **in front of** me, **behind** me. Pass 4 of 4.
    (Do not help child by pointing, moving head or eyes.)
25. Ask child: What is a ball?... lake?... desk?... house?... banana?... curtain?... fence?... ceiling? Pass if defined in terms of use, shape, what it is made of, or general category (such as banana is fruit, not just yellow). Pass 5 of 8, 7 of 8.
26. Ask child: If a horse is big, a mouse is __? If fire is hot, ice is __? If the sun shines during the day, the moon shines during the __? Pass 2 of 3.
27. Child may use wall or rail only, not person. May not crawl.
28. Child must throw ball overhand 3 feet to within arm's reach of tester.
29. Child must perform standing broad jump over width of test sheet (8 1/2 inches).
30. Tell child to walk forward, ⚬◌⚬◌⚬◌➤ heel within 1 inch of toe. Tester may demonstrate.
    Child must walk 4 consecutive steps.
31. In the second year, half of normal children are non-compliant.

OBSERVATIONS:

SUBSEQUENT PHYSICAL ASSESSMENT *Continued*

Assessment Procedure	Normal Findings	Abnormal Findings
Note apical pulse rate. Count the pulse for a full minute (Fig. 30-12).	Awake and resting rates vary with the age of the child. For a newborn to 1 month-old child it should be 120 to 160 beats/minute. Rate decrease gradually with age. At 6 months to 1 year, rate is approximately 110 beats/minute.	Pulse may be altered by medications, activity, and pain as well as pathologic conditions. Bradycardia (<100 beats/min) in an infant is usually an ominous finding.
Assess respiratory rate. Measure respiratory rate and character in infants by observing abdominal movements.	Neonates: Rate is 30 to 60 breaths/minute. Breathing is unlabored; lung sounds clear. Newborns are obligatory nose breathers.	Respiratory rate and character may be altered by medications, positioning, fever, activity as well as pathologic conditions.
Evaluate blood pressure. Newborn blood pressure: A Doppler stethoscope should be used or an electronic Dynamap machine may be used to record blood pressure readings in the newborn. ➤ **Clinical Tip** • *The child should not be crying as this can elevate blood pressure.*	Specific to age and size.	➤ **Clinical Tip** • *If the blood pressure reading is too high for age, the cuff may be too small; it should cover two-thirds of the child's upper arm. If the blood pressure reading is too low for age, the cuff may be too large. Chapter 8 explains how to take a blood pressure reading.*

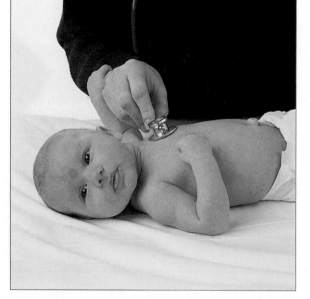

Figure 30-12 Auscultating apical pulse rate in the infant (© B. Proud).

continued

Assessment Procedure	Normal Findings	Abnormal Findings

Measurements

Measure height.

Determine height by measuring the recumbent length. Fully extend the body, holding the head in midline and gently grasping the knees and pushing them downward until the legs are fully extended and touching the table (Fig. 30-13). If using a measuring board, place the head at the top of the board and the heels firmly at the bottom. Without a board, use paper under the child and mark the paper at the top of the head and bottom of the heels. Then measure the distance between the two points. Plot height measurement on an age- and gender-appropriate growth chart.

Measure weight. Measure weight on an appropriately sized beam scale with nondetectable weights. Weigh an infant lying or sitting on a scale that measures to the nearest 0.5 oz or 10 g (Fig. 30-14). Weigh an infant naked. Plot weight measurement on age- and gender-appropriate growth chart.

See Appendix F for growth charts.

Asian and black newborns are smaller than Caucasian newborns. Asian children are smaller at all ages.

See the growth charts in Appendix F for normal findings.

Significant deviation from normal in the growth charts would be considered abnormal.

Deviation from the wide range of normal weights is abnormal. See Appendix F and compare differences.

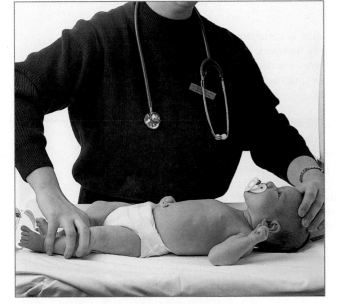

Figure 30-13 Positioning for measuring an infant.

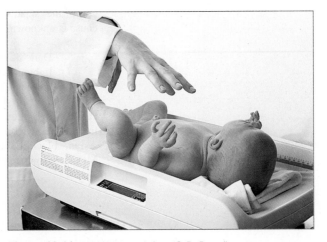

Figure 30-14 Weighing an infant (© B. Proud).

continued

SUBSEQUENT PHYSICAL ASSESSMENT *Continued*

Assessment Procedure	Normal Findings	Abnormal Findings
Determine head circumference. Measure head circumference (HC) or occipital frontal circumference (OFC) at every physical examination for infants and toddlers younger than 2 years and older children when conditions warrant. Plot the measurement on standardized growth charts specific for gender from birth to 36 months.	HC (OFC) measurement should fall between the 5th and 95th percentiles and should be comparable to the child's height and weight percentiles.	HC (OFC) not within the normal percentiles may indicate pathology. Those greater than 95% may indicate macrocephaly. Those under the 5th percentile may indicate microcephaly.

Skin, Hair, and Nails

Assess for skin color, odor, and lesions.	Skin color ranges from pale white with pink, yellow, brown, or olive tones to dark brown or black. No strong odor should be evident, and the skin should be lesion free. Skin should be soft, warm, slightly moist with good turgor and without edema or lesions. Common newborn skin variations include • Physiologic jaundice • Birthmarks • Milia (Fig. 30-15) • Erythema toxicum (Fig. 30-15) • Telangiectatic nevi (stork bites) (Fig. 30-15) Another common variation is harlequin sign (one side of the body turns red; the other side is pale). There is a distinct color line separation at midline. The cause is unknown. Dark-skinned newborns have lighter skin color than their parents. Their color darkens with age. Bluish pigmented areas called Mongolian spots (Fig. 30-15) may be noted on the sacral areas of Asian, black, Native American, and Mexican-American infants.	Yellow skin may indicate jaundice or passage of meconium in utero secondary to fetal distress. Jaundice within 24 hours after birth is pathologic and may indicate hemolytic disease of the newborn. Blue skin suggests cyanosis, pallor suggests anemia, and redness suggests fever, irritation.

continued

Assessment Procedure	Normal Findings	Abnormal Findings
Palpate for texture, temperature, moisture, turgor, and edema.	Skin is warm and slightly moist. Vernix caseosa (cheesy, white substance that is found on the skin, especially in skin folds) is a common finding; it eventually absorbs into the skin.	Ecchymoses in various stages or in unusual locations or circular burn areas suggest child abuse although bruising or burning may also be from cultural practices such as *cupping* or *coining*. Petechiae, lesions, or rashes may indicate serious disorders.
Inspect and palpate hair. Observe for distribution, characteristics, and presence of any unusual hair on body.	Hair is normally lustrous, silky, strong, and elastic. Fine, downy hair covers the body. African-American children usually have hair that is curlier and coarser than white children.	Dirty, matted hair may indicate neglect. Tufts of hair over spine may indicate spina bifida occulta.
Inspect and palpate nails. Note color, texture, shape, and condition of nails.	Dark-skinned children have deeper nail pigment. Nails extend to end of fingers or beyond; are well-formed.	Blue nailbeds indicate cyanosis. Yellow nailbeds indicate jaundice. Blue-black nailbeds suggest a nailbed hemorrhage.

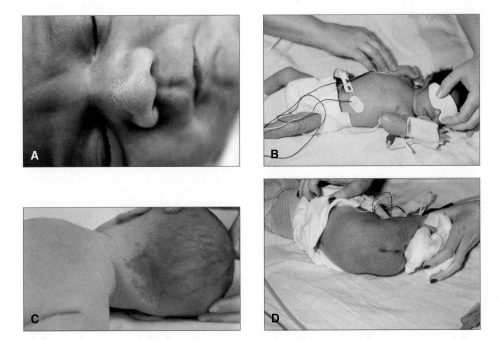

Figure 30-15 Common skin variations found in newborns: **(A)** milia; **(B)** erythema toxicum; **(C)** telangiectatic nevi; **(D)** Mongolian spot.

continued

SUBSEQUENT PHYSICAL ASSESSMENT *Continued*

Assessment Procedure	Normal Findings	Abnormal Findings

Head, Neck, and Cervical Lymph Nodes

Inspect and palpate the head. Note shape and symmetry. In newborns, inspect and palpate the condition of fontanelles and sutures (Fig. 30-16).

Head is normocephalic and symmetric. In newborns, the head may be oddly shaped from molding (overriding of the sutures) during vaginal birth. The diamond-shaped anterior fontanelle measures about 4 to 5 cm at its widest part; it usually closes by 12 to 18 months. The triangular posterior fontanelle measures about 0.5 to 1 cm at its widest part and it should close at 2 months of age.

A very large head is found with hydrocephalus.

An oddly shaped head is found with premature closure of sutures (possibly genetic). One-sided flattening of the head suggests prolonged positioning on one side.

A third fontanelle between the anterior and posterior fontanelle is seen with Down's syndrome.

Premature closure of sutures (craniosynostosis) may result in caput succedaneum (edema from trauma), which crosses the suture line, and cephalohematoma (bleeding into the periosteal space), which does not extend across the suture line (Fig. 30-17). Craniotabes may result from osteoporosis of the outer skull bone. Palpating too firmly with the thumb or forefinger over the temporoparietal area will leave an indentation of the bone.

Bulging fontanelle indicates increased cranial pressure. Microcephaly is seen with infants who have been exposed to congenital infections.

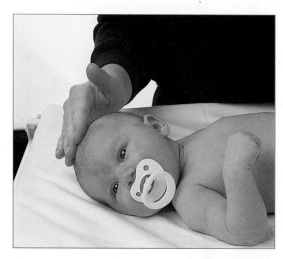

Figure 30-16   Palpating the anterior fontanel (© B. Proud).

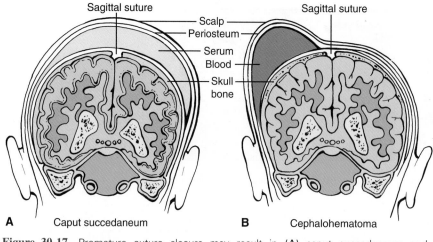

A   Caput succedaneum   **B**   Cephalohematoma

Figure 30-17   Premature suture closure may result in **(A)** caput succedaneum and **(B)** cephalohematoma.

continued

Assessment Procedure	Normal Findings	Abnormal Findings
Test head control, head posture, range of motion.	Full range of motion—up, down, and sideways—is normal. **Infant should have head control at 4 months.**	Hyperextension is seen with opisthotonos or significant meningeal irritation. Limited range of motion may indicate torticollis (wryneck).
Inspect and palpate the face. Note appearance, symmetry, and movement. Palpate the parotid glands for swelling.	Face is normally proportionate and symmetric. Movements are equal bilaterally. Parotid glands are normal size.	Unusual proportions (short palpebral fissures, thin lips, and wide and flat philtrum, which is the groove above the upper lip) may be hereditary or they may indicate specific syndromes such as Down's syndrome and fetal alcohol syndrome. Unequal movement may indicate facial nerve paralysis. Abnormal facies may indicate chromosomal anomaly.
Inspect and palpate the neck. Palpate the thyroid gland and the trachea. Also inspect and palpate the cervical lymph nodes for swelling, mobility, temperature, and tenderness. ➤ *Clinical Tip • The thyroid is very difficult to palpate in an infant because of the short, thick neck.*	The neck is usually short with skin folds between the head and shoulder during infancy. The isthmus is the only portion of the thyroid that should be palpable. The trachea is midline. Lymph nodes are usually nonpalpable in infants. Clavicles are symmetrical and intact.	Implications of some abnormal findings include the following: Short, webbed neck suggests anomalies or syndromes such as Down's syndrome. Distended neck veins may indicate difficulty breathing. Enlarged thyroid or palpable masses suggest a pathologic process. Shift in tracheal position from midline suggests a serious lung problem (e.g., foreign body or tumor). Crepitus when clavicle palpated along with decreased movement in arm of that side may indicate fractured clavicle.

Eyes

Inspect the external eye. Note the position, slant, and epicanthal folds of the external eye.	Inner canthus distance approximately 2.5 cm, horizontal slant, no epicanthal folds. Outer canthus aligns with tips of the pinnas. 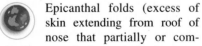 Epicanthal folds (excess of skin extending from roof of nose that partially or completely covers the inner canthus) are normal findings in Asian children, whose eyes also slant upward.	Wide-set position (hypertelorism), upward slant, and thick epicanthal folds suggest Down syndrome. "Sun-setting" appearance (upper lid covers part of the iris) suggests hydrocephalus.
Observe eyelid placement, swelling, discharge, and lesions.	Eyelids have transient edema, absence of tears.	Eyelid inflammation may result from infection. Swelling, erythema, or purulent discharge may indicate infection or blocked tear ducts.

continued

SUBSEQUENT PHYSICAL ASSESSMENT *Continued*

Assessment Procedure	Normal Findings	Abnormal Findings
		Purulent discharge seen with sexually transmitted infections (gonorrhea, chlamydia).
Inspect the sclera and conjunctiva for color, discharge, lesions, redness, and lacerations.	Sclera and conjunctiva are clear and free of discharge, lesions, redness, or lacerations. Small subconjunctival hemorrhages may be seen in newborns.	Yellow sclera suggests jaundice, blue sclera may indicate osteogenesis imperfecta ("brittle bone disease").
Observe the iris and the pupils.	Typically the iris is blue in light-skinned infants and brown in dark-skinned infants; permanent color develops within 9 months. Brushfield's spots (white flecks on the periphery of the iris) may be normal in some infants. Pupils are equal, round, and reactive to light and accommodation (PERRLA).	Brushfield's spots may indicate Down syndrome. Sluggish pupils indicate a neurologic problem. Miosis (constriction) indicates iritis or narcotic use or abuse. Mydriasis (pupillary dilation) indicates emotional factors (fear), trauma, or certain drug use.
Finally inspect the eyebrows and eyelashes.	Eyebrows should be symmetric in shape and movement. They should not meet midline. Eyelashes should be evenly distributed and curled outward.	Sparseness of eyebrows or lashes could indicate skin disease.
Perform visual acuity tests. Assess visual acuity by observing infants inability to gaze at object.	Visual acuity is difficult to test in infants; it is usually tested by observing the infant's ability to fix on and follow objects. Normal visual acuity is as follows: Birth: 20/100 to 20/400 1 year: 20/200 By 4 weeks of age, child should be able to fixate on objects. By 6 to 8 weeks, eyes should follow a moving object. By 3 months, the child is able to follow and reach for an object.	Children with a one-line difference between eyes should be referred. Abnormal findings include congenital defects such as cataracts.
Perform extraocular muscle tests. Hirschberg test: Shine light directly at the cornea while the child looks straight ahead.	In the Hirschberg test, the light reflects symmetrically in the center of both pupils. Light causes pupils to vasoconstrict bilaterally and blink reflex occurs. Blink reflex also occurs as an object is brought towards the eyes.	Unequal alignment of light on the pupils in the Hirschberg test signals strabismus.
Perform ophthalmoscopic examination. The procedure is the same as for adults. Distraction is preferred over the use of restraint, which is likely to result in crying and closed eyes. Careful ophthalmoscopic examination of newborns is difficult without the use of mydriatic medications.	Red reflex is present. This reflex rules out most serious defects of the cornea, aqueous chamber, lens, and vitreous humor. When visualized, the optic disc appears similar to an adult's. A newborn's optic discs are pale; peripheral vessels are not well developed.	Absence of the red reflex indicates cataracts. Papilledema is unusual in children of this age owing to the ability of the fontanelles and sutures to open during increased intracranial pressure. Disc blurring and hemorrhages should be reported immediately.

continued

Assessment Procedure	Normal Findings	Abnormal Findings

Ears

Assessment Procedure	Normal Findings	Abnormal Findings
Inspect external ears. Note placement, discharge, or lesions of the ears.	Top of pinna should cross the eye-occiput line and be within a 10-degree angle of a perpendicular line drawn from the eye-occiput line to the lobe. No unusual structure or markings should appear on the pinna.	Low-set ears with an alignment greater than a 10-degree angle (Fig. 30-18) suggest retardation or congenital syndromes. Abnormal shape may suggest renal disease process, which may be hereditary. Preauricular skin tags or sinuses suggest other anomalies of ears or the renal system.
Inspect internal ear. The internal ear examination requires using an otoscope. The nurse should always hold the otoscope in a manner that allows for rapid removal if the child moves. Have the caregiver hold and restrain the child. Because an infant's external canal is short and straight, pull the pinna down and back (Fig. 30-19).	No excessive cerumen, discharge, lesions, excoriations, or foreign body in external canal. Amniotic fluid/vernix may be present in canal of ear of newborn. Tympanic membrane is pearly gray to light pink with normal landmarks. Tympanic membranes redden bilaterally when child is crying or febrile.	Presence of foreign bodies or cerumen impaction. Purulent discharge may indicate otitis externa or presence of foreign body. Purulent, serous discharge suggests otitis media. Bloody discharge suggests trauma, and clear discharge may indicate cerebrospinal fluid leak. Perforated tympanic membrane may also be noted.
Assess the mobility of the tympanic membrane by pneumatic otoscopy. This consists of creating pressure against the tympanic membrane using air. To do this, you need to create a seal in the external canal and direct a puff of air against the tympanic membrane. Create the seal by using the largest speculum that will comfortably insert into the ear canal. Cover the tip with rubber for a better and more comfortable seal. Attach a pneumatic bulb to the otoscope and squeeze the bulb lightly to direct air against the tympanic membrane.	Tympanic membrane is mobile; moves inward with positive pressure (squeeze of bulb) and outward with negative pressure (release of bulb).	Immobility indicates fluid behind tympanic membrane.

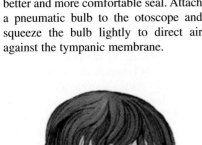
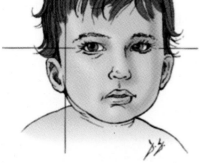

Figure 30-18 Low-set ears with alignment greater than 10-degree angle.

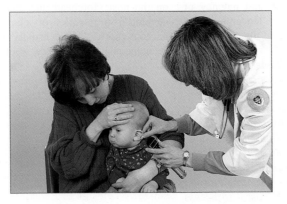

Figure 30-19 To examine the ears of an infant, restrain the child and pull the pinna down and back (© B. Proud).

continued

SUBSEQUENT PHYSICAL ASSESSMENT *Continued*

Assessment Procedure	Normal Findings	Abnormal Findings
Hearing acuity. In the infant, test hearing acuity by noting the reaction to noise. Stand approximately 12 inches from the infant and create a loud noise (e.g., clap hands, shake/squeeze a noisy toy). Routine newborn hearing screening is performed in most newborn nurseries 24 to 48 hours after birth or prior to discharge.	A newborn will exhibit the startle (Moro) reflex and blink eyes (acoustic blink reflex) in response to noise. Older infant will turn head.	No reactions to noise may indicate a hearing deficit. Audiometry results outside normal range suggest hearing deficit.

Mouth, Throat, Nose, and Sinuses

Inspection

Inspect mouth and throat. Note the condition of the lips, palates, tongue, and buccal mucosa.	Epstein's pearls, small yellow-white retention cysts on the hard palate and gums, are common in newborns and usually disappear in the first weeks of life. In infants, a sucking tubercle (pad) from the friction of sucking may be evident in the middle of the upper lip.	Cleft lip and/or palate are congenital abnormalities.
Observe the condition of the gums. When teeth appear, count teeth and note location.	Gums appear pink and moist. Teeth may begin erupting at 4 to 6 months. Teeth develop in sequential order. By 10 months, most infants have two upper and two lower central incisors.	Abnormal findings include lesion and edema.
Note the condition of the throat and tonsils. Also observe the insertion and ending point of the frenulum.	Tonsils are not visible in newborns. As the infant gets older, it is possible but still difficult to see tonsils.	Extension of the frenulum to the tip of tongue may interfere with extension of the tongue, which causes speech difficulties.
Inspect nose and sinuses. To inspect the nose and sinuses, avoid using the nasal speculum in infants and young children. Instead push up the tip of the nose and shine the light into each nostril. Observe the structure and patency of the nares, discharge, tenderness, and any color or swelling of the turbinates.	Nose is midline in face, septum is straight, and nares are patent. No discharge or tenderness is present. Turbinates are pink and free of edema. Milia are small, white papules found on the nose, forehead and chin. They develop from retention of sebum in sebaceous pores. They usually resolve spontaneously within a few weeks.	Choanal atresia is blockage of the posterior nares in the newborn. If the blockage is bilateral, the newborn is at risk for acute respiratory distress. Immediate referral is necessary. Deviated septum may be congenital or caused by injury. Foul discharge from one nostril may indicate a foreign body.
➤ *Clinical Tip • Infants are obligatory nose breathers. Consequently obstructed nasal passages may precipitate serious health conditions, making it very important to assess the patency of the nares in the newborn. If, after suctioning fluid and mucus from the nares, you suspect obstruction, insert a small-lumen catheter into each nostril to assess patency.*		

continued

Assessment Procedure	Normal Findings	Abnormal Findings

Thorax

Inspection

Inspect the shape of the thorax.

Infant's thorax is smooth, rounded, and symmetric.

Abnormal shapes of the thorax include pectus excavatum and pectus corinatum.

Observe respiratory effort, keeping in mind newborns and young infants are obligatory nose breathers.

Respirations should be unlabored and regular in all ages except for immediate newborn period when respirations are irregular (see "Vital Signs" section). Some newborns, especially the premature, have periodic irregular breathing, sometimes with apnea (episodes when breathing stops) lasting a few seconds. This is a normal finding if bradycardia does not accompany irregular breathing.

Retractions (suprasternal, sternal, substernal, intercostal) and grunting suggest increased inspiratory effort, which may be due to airway obstruction. Periods of apnea that last longer than 20 s and are accompanied by bradycardia may be a sign of a cardiovascular or CNS disease.

Nasal flaring, tachypnea, seesaw movement of chest indicate respiratory distress.

Percussion and Auscultation

Percuss the chest. During percussion of the lungs, note tone elicited.

Hyperresonance is the normal tone elicited in infants because of thinness of the chest wall.

A dull tone may indicate a mass, fluid, or consolidation.

Auscultate for breath sounds and adventitious sounds. If a newborn lung sounds seem noisy, auscultate the upper nostrils.

Breath sounds may seem louder and harsher in young children because of their thin chest walls. No adventitious sounds should be heard although transmitted upper airway sounds may be heard on auscultation of thorax.

Diminished breath sounds suggest respiratory disorders such as pneumonia or atelectasis. Stridor (inspiratory wheeze) is a high-pitched, piercing sound that indicates a narrowing of the upper tracheobronchial tree. Expiratory wheezes indicate narrowing in the lower tracheobronchial tree. Rhonchi and rales (crackles) may indicate a number of respiratory diseases such as pneumonia, bronchitis, or bronchiolitis.

Breasts

Inspection and Palpation

Inspect and palpate breasts. Note shape, symmetry, color, tenderness, discharge, lesions, and masses.

Newborns may have enlarged and engorged breasts with a white liquid discharge resulting from the influence of maternal hormones (Fig. 30-20). This condition resolves spontaneously within days.

A palpable mass of the breast in abnormal. The newborn or infant may have extra nipples noted on the chest or abdomen called supernumerary nipples.

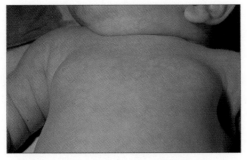

Figure 30-20 The enlarged breasts of this newborn are normal and result from the influence of maternal hormones (© 1994 Science Photo Library/CMSP).

continued

SUBSEQUENT PHYSICAL ASSESSMENT *Continued*

Assessment Procedure	Normal Findings	Abnormal Findings
Heart		
Inspection and Palpation **Inspect and palpate the precordium.** Note lifts, heaves, apical impulse (Fig. 30-21).	The apical pulse is at the 4th intercostal space (ICS) until the age of 7 years, when it drops to the 5th. It is to the left of the midclavicular line (MCL) until age 4.	A systolic heave may indicate right ventricular enlargement. Apical impulse that is not in proper location for age may indicate cardiomyopathy, pneumothorax, or diaphragmatic hernia.
Auscultation **Auscultate heart sounds.** Listen to the heart. Note rate and rhythm of apical impulse, S_1, S_2, extra heart sounds, and murmurs. Keep in mind that sinus arrhythmia is normal in infants. Heart sounds are louder, higher pitched, and of shorter duration in infants. A split S_2 at the apex occurs normally in some infants and S_3 is a normal heart sound in some children. A venous hum also may be normally heard in children.	Normal heart rates are cited in the "Vital Signs" section above. Innocent murmurs, which are common throughout childhood, are classified as systolic; short duration; no transmission to other areas; grade III or less; loudest in pulmonic area (base of heart); low-pitched, musical, or groaning quality that varies in intensity in relation to position, respiration, activity, fever, and anemia. No other associated signs of heart disease should be found.	Murmurs that do not fit the criteria for innocent murmurs may indicate a disease or disorder. Extra heart sounds and variations in pulse rate and rhythm also suggest pathologic processes.
Abdomen		
Inspection **Inspect the shape of the abdomen.**	In infants, the abdomen is prominent in supine position.	A scaphoid (boat-shaped; i.e., sunken with prominent rib cage) abdomen may result from malnutrition or dehydration. Distended abdomen may indicate pyloric stenosis.

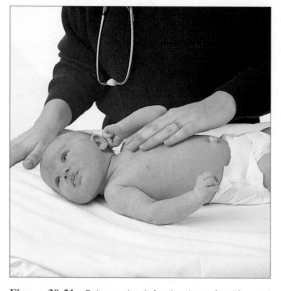

Figure 30-21 Palpate the infant's chest for lifts and heaves (© B. Proud).

continued

Assessment Procedure	Normal Findings	Abnormal Findings
Inspect umbilicus. Note color, discharge, evident herniation of the umbilicus.	Umbilicus is pink, no discharge, odor, redness, or herniation. Cord should demonstrate three vessels (two arteries and one vein). Remnant of cord should appear dried 24 to 48 hours after birth.	Inflammation, discharge, and redness of umbilicus suggest infection. Diastasis recti (separation of the abdominal muscles) is seen as midline protrusion from the xiphoid to the umbilicus or pubis symphysis. This condition is secondary to immature musculature of abdominal muscles and usually has little significance. As the muscles strengthen, the separation resolves on its own. A bulge at the umbilicus suggests an umbilical hernia (Fig. 30-22), which may be seen in newborns; many disappear by the age of 1 year. Abnormal insertion of cord, discolored cord, or two-vessel cord could indicate genetic abnormalities; however, these are also seen in newborns without abnormalities. Umbilical hernias are seen more frequently in African American children.

Auscultation

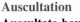

Auscultate bowel sounds. Follow auscultation guidelines for adult clients provided in Chapter 22.	Normal bowel sounds occur every 10 to 30 s. They sound like clicks, gurgles, or growls.	Marked peristaltic waves almost always indicate a pathologic process such as pyloric stenosis.

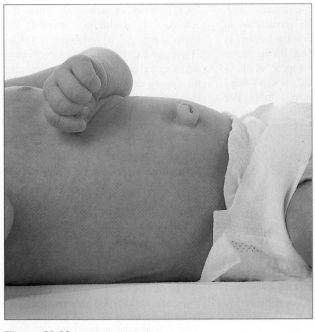

Figure 30-22 Umbilical hernia.

continued

SUBSEQUENT PHYSICAL ASSESSMENT *Continued*

Assessment Procedure	Normal Findings	Abnormal Findings
Palpation **Palpate for masses and tenderness.** Palpate abdomen for softness or hardness.	Abdomen is soft to palpation and without masses or tenderness.	A rigid abdomen is almost always an emergent problem. Masses or tenderness warrants further investigation. Hirschsprung's disease could also be considered, especially with suprapubic mass palpable.
Palpate liver. Palpate the liver the same as you would for adults (see Chapter 22).	Liver is usually palpable 1 to 2 cm below the right costal margin in young children. The liver is hard to palpate in the newborn.	An enlarged liver with a firm edge that is palpated more than 2 cm below the right costal margin usually indicates a pathologic process.
Palpate spleen. Palpate the spleen the same as you would for adults.	Spleen tip may be palpable during inspiration. The spleen is difficult to palpate in the newborn.	Enlarged spleen is usually indicative of a pathologic process.
Palpate kidneys. Palpate the kidneys the same as you would for adults.	The tip of the right kidney may be palpable during inspiration.	Enlarged kidneys are usually indicative of a pathologic process.
Palpate bladder. Palpate the bladder the same as you would for adults.	Bladder may be slightly palpable in infants and small children.	An enlarged bladder is usually due to urinary retention but may be due to a mass.

Male Genitalia

Inspection and Palpation **Inspect penis and urinary meatus.** Inspect the genitalia, observing size for age and any lesions.	Penis is normal size for age, and no lesions are seen. Diaper rash, however, is a common finding in infants (Fig. 30-23). The foreskin is retractable in uncircumcised child. Urinary meatus is at tip of glans penis and has no discharge or redness. Penis may appear small in large for gestational age (LGA) boys because of overlapping skin folds. For circumcised boys, the site is dry with minimal swelling and drainage.	An unretractable foreskin in a child older than 3 months suggests phimosis. Paraphimosis is indicated when the foreskin is tightened around the glans penis in a retracted position. Hypospadias, urinary meatus on ventral surface of glans, and epispadias, urinary meatus on dorsal surface of glans, are congenital disorders (see Chapter 24).
Inspect and palpate scrotum and testes. To rule out cryptorchidism, it is important to palpate for testes in the scrotum in infants. ► *Clinical Tip • When palpating the testicles in the infant, you must keep the cremasteric reflex in mind. This reflex pulls the testicles up into the inguinal canal and abdomen and is elicited in response to touch, cold, or emotional factors.*	Scrotum is free of lesions. Testes are palpable in scrotum with the left testicle usually lower than the right. Testes are equal in size, smooth, mobile, and free of masses. If a testicle is missing from the scrotal sac but the scrotal sac appears well developed, suspect physiologic cryptorchidism. The testis has originally descended into the scrotum but has moved back up into the inguinal canal because of the cremasteric reflex and the small size of the testis. You should be able to milk the testis down	Absent testicle(s) and atrophic scrotum suggest true cryptorchidism (undescended testicles). This suggests that the testicle(s) never descended. This condition occurs more frequently in preterm than term infants because testes descend at 8 months of gestation. It can lead to testicular atrophy and infertility, and increases the risk for testicular cancer. Hydroceles are common in infants. They are fluid-filled masses that can be transilluminated (see Chapter 24, Abnormal Findings 24-2). They usually

continued

Assessment Procedure	Normal Findings	Abnormal Findings
	into the scrotum from the inguinal canal. This normal condition subsides at puberty.	resolve spontaneously. A scrotal hernia is usually caused by an indirect inguinal hernia that has descended into the scrotum. It can usually be pushed back into the inguinal canal. This mass will not transilluminate.
Inspect and palpate inguinal area for hernias. Observe for any bulge in the inguinal area. Using your pinky finger, palpate up the inguinal canal to the external inguinal ring if a hernia is suspected.	No inguinal hernias are present.	A bulge in the inguinal area or palpation of a mass in the inguinal canal suggests an inguinal hernia. Indirect inguinal hernias occur most frequently in children (see Chapter 24).

Female Genitalia

Inspection **Inspect external genitalia.** Note labia majora, labia minora, vaginal orifice, urinary meatus, and clitoris.	Labia majora and minora are pink and moist. Newborn's genitalia may appear prominent because of influence of maternal hormones. Bruises and swelling may be caused by breech vaginal delivery.	Enlarged clitoris in newborn combined with fusion of the posterior labia majora suggests ambiguous genitalia.

Anus and Rectum

Inspection **Inspect the anus.** The anus should be inspected in infants. Spread the buttocks with gloved hands; note patency of anal opening, presence of any lesions and fissures, and condition and color of perianal skin.	The anal opening should be visible, moist. Perianal skin should be smooth and free of lesions. Perianal skin tags may be noted. Meconium passed within 24 to 48 hours after birth.	Imperforate anus (no anal opening) should be referred. Pustules may indicate secondary infection of diaper rash. No passage of stool could indicate no patency of anus or cystic fibrosis.
Palpation Palpate rectum. This internal examination is not routinely performed in infants.		

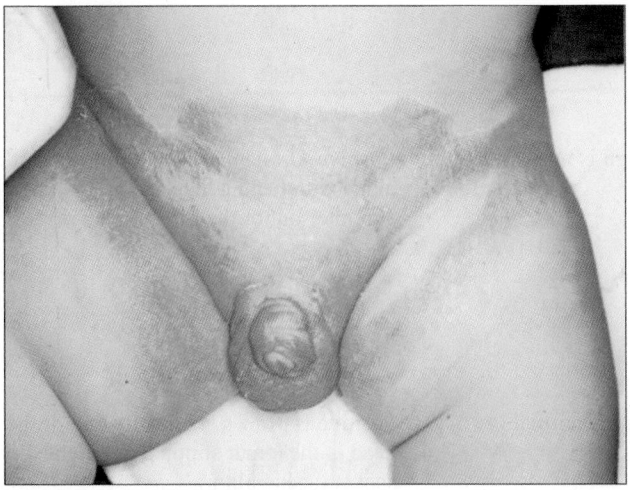

Figure 30-23 Diaper rash, a common finding in infants (© Princess Margaret Rose Orthopedic Hospital/Science Photo Library/CMSP).

continued

SUBSEQUENT PHYSICAL ASSESSMENT *Continued*

Assessment Procedure	Normal Findings	Abnormal Findings

Musculoskeletal

Inspection

Assess arms, hands, feet and legs. Note symmetry, shape, movement, and positioning of the feet and legs. Perform neurovascular assessment.

> ➤ *Clinical Tip • If the client is a newborn, keep in mind that the feet may retain their intrauterine position and appear deformed (positioned outward or inward from normal right angle to the leg). This is normal if the foot easily returns to its normal position with manipulation (either scratch along the lateral edge of the affected foot or gently push the forefoot into its normal position).*

Feet and legs are symmetric in size, shape, and movement. Extremities should be warm and mobile with adequate capillary refill. All pulses (radial, brachial, femoral, popliteal, pedal) should be strong and equal bilaterally. This is an inward (pointing toward center of the body) positioning of the forefoot with the heel in normal straight position; it resolves spontaneously. Tibial torsion, also common in infants and toddlers, consists of twisting of the tibia inward or outward on its long axis, and is usually caused by intrauterine positioning; this typically corrects itself by the time the child is 2 years old.

Short, broad extremities, hyperextensible joints, and palmar simian crease may indicate Down's syndrome. Polydactyly (extra digits) and syndactyly (webbing) are sometimes found in children with mental retardation. Absent femoral pulses may indicate coarctation of the aorta. Neurovascular deficit in children is usually secondary to trauma (e.g., fracture).

Fixed-position (true) deformities do not return to normal position with manipulation. Metatarsus varus is inversion (a turning inward that elevates the medial margin) and adduction of the forefoot.

Talipes varus is adduction of the forefoot and inversion of the entire foot.

Talipes equinovarus (clubfoot) is indicated if foot is fixed in the following position: adduction of forefoot, inversion of entire foot, and equinus (pointing downward) position of entire foot.

Assess for congenital hip dysplasia. Assessing for hip dysplasia is an important aspect of the physical examination for infants. The assessment should be performed at each visit until the child is about 1 year old. (Several tests are described below.)

Begin by assessing the symmetry of the gluteal folds. Also assess hip abduction using the maneuvers below.

Equal gluteal folds and full hip abduction are normal findings.

Unequal gluteal folds and limited hip abduction are signs of congenital hip dysplasia.

Perform Ortolani's maneuver to test for congenital hip dysplasia (Fig. 30-24). With the infant supine, flex infant's knees while holding your thumbs on midthigh and your fingers over the greater trochanters; abduct the legs, moving the knees outward and down toward the table.

Negative Ortolani's sign is normal.

Positive Ortolani's sign: A click heard along with feeling the head of the femur slip in or out of the hip.

Perform Barlow's maneuvers (Fig. 30-25). With the infant supine, flex the infant's knees while holding your thumbs on midthigh and your fingers over the greater trochanters; adduct legs until thumbs touch.

Negative Barlow's sign is normal.

Positive Barlow's sign: A feeling of the head of the femur slipping out of the hip socket (acetabulum).

continued

Assessment Procedure	Normal Findings	Abnormal Findings
Assess spinal alignment. Observe spine and posture.	In newborns, the spine is flexible with convex dorsal and sacral curves. In infants younger than 3 months, the spine is rounded (Fig. 30-26). The newborn's spine is flexed.	In newborns, flaccid or rigid posture is considered abnormal. In older infants and children, abnormal posture suggests neuromuscular disorders such as cerebral palsy.

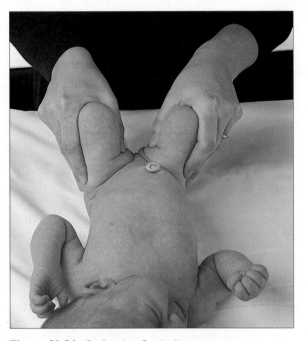

Figure 30-24 Performing Ortolani's maneuver.

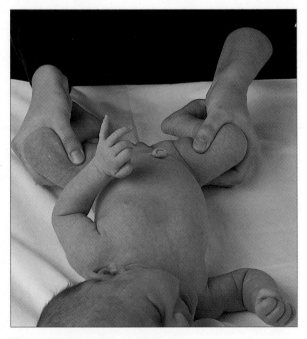

Figure 30-25 Performing Barlow's maneuver.

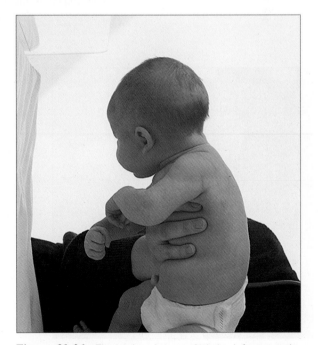

Figure 30-26 The spine is rounded in infants under 3 months old.

continued

SUBSEQUENT PHYSICAL ASSESSMENT *Continued*

Assessment Procedure	Normal Findings	Abnormal Findings
Assess joints. Note range of motion, swelling, redness, and tenderness.	Full range of motion and no swelling, redness, or tenderness.	Limited range of motion, swelling, redness, and tenderness indicate problems ranging from mild injuries to serious disorders.
Assess muscles. Note size and strength. (For example, can the infant bear weight on her legs?)	Muscle size and strength should be adequate for the particular age and should be equal bilaterally.	Inadequate muscle size and strength for the particular age indicate neuromuscular disorders such as muscular dystrophy.
Neurologic System **Assess the newborn's cry, responsiveness, and adaptation.**	The newborn cries are lusty and strong; responds appropriately to stimuli and quiets to soothing when held in the *en face* position (Fig. 30-27). Infantile reflexes are present when appropriate and are symmetric.	Inappropriate response to stimuli suggests CNS disorders or problems. An inability to quiet to soothing and gaze aversion is seen in "cocaine babies." Infantile reflexes present when inappropriate, absent, or asymmetric may indicate a CNS problem.
Test deep tendon and superficial reflexes.	The Babinski response is normal in children younger than 2 years (this response usually disappears between 2 and 24 months), and triceps reflex is absent until age 6. Ankle clonus (rapid, rhythmic plantar flexion) in response to eliciting ankle reflex is common in newborns.	Absence or marked intensity of these reflexes, asymmetry, and presence of Babinski response after age 2 years may demonstrate pathology.
Test motor function. See Denver Developmental Screening Tool for exam (Assessment Tool 30-1).	Gross and fine motor skills should be appropriate for the child's developmental age. Head control should be acquired by 4 months of age. Hand preference is developed during the preschool years.	Gross and fine motor skills that are inappropriate for developmental age and lack of head control by age 6 months may indicate cerebral palsy. Hand preference that is not developed during preschool years may indicate paresis on opposite side.

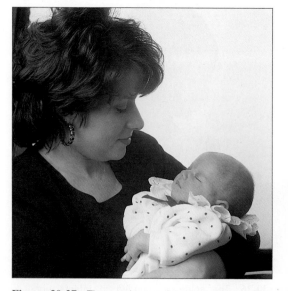

Figure 30-27 The newborn quiets to soothing when held *en face.*

VALIDATING AND DOCUMENTING FINDINGS

Validate the assessment data you have collected. This is necessary to verify that the data are reliable and accurate. Document the assessment data following the health care facility or agency policy.

Sample of Subjective Data

J.M. is a 4-month-old male in for well-child visit. Primary caregiver is mother. Father works in sales. Mother remains at home with child. She reports the child is healthy and happy. Child pushes himself up when in prone position. Responds to mother's voice. Sleeps through the night. Child breast feeds. Mother reports no problems with feeding. Stools normal and regular. Immunizations are up-to-date.

Sample of Objective Data

Child weighs 15 lbs 2 oz and is 63 cm long. Temp 99.5°F. Pulse, normal and regular. HC 42 cm. Skin, soft and warm; no lesions present. Head symmetric. Child holds head erect and midline. Mouth free of lesions. Nose free of obstruction. Eye placement normal. Infant follows object with eyes. Red reflex present. Ears aligned and symmetrical. Internal ears free of discharge or lesions. Respirations even and unlabored. Breath sounds clear bilaterally. S_1 and S_2 auscultated and normal. No herniation of umbilicus. Bowel sounds normal. Genitalia appropriate size for age; no lesions. Testes palpable, equal in size, smooth, and mobile. Anus free of lesions and hemorrhoids. Negative Ortolani's sign and Barlow's maneuver. Full ROM in joints.

Analysis of Data

After collecting subjective and objective data, identify abnormal findings and client strengths. Then cluster the data to reveal any significant patterns or abnormalities. These data may then be used to make clinical judgments about the health status of the neonate or infant.

DIAGNOSTIC REASONING: POSSIBLE CONCLUSIONS

The following is a listing of selected nursing diagnoses that you may identify when analyzing data for this assessment.

Selected Nursing Diagnoses

Wellness Diagnoses

- Effective Breastfeeding

Risk Diagnoses

- Risk for Impaired Parent/Infant Attachment
- Risk for Delayed Development
- Risk for Disproportionate Growth
- Risk for Disorganized Infant Behavior

Actual Diagnoses

- Ineffective Breastfeeding related to poor infant sucking reflex
- Delayed Growth and Development related to inadequate caretaking
- Disorganized Infant Behavior related to malnutrition
- Ineffective Infant Feeding Pattern

Selected Collaborative Problems

After grouping the data, it may become apparent that certain collaborative problems emerge. Remember that collaborative problems differ from nursing diagnoses in that they cannot be prevented with nursing interventions alone. However, these physiologic complications of medical conditions can be detected and monitored by the nurse. In addition, the nurse can use physician- and nurse-prescribed interventions to minimize the complications of these problems. The nurse may also have to refer the client in such situations for further treatment of the problem. Following is a list of collaborative problems seen more frequently in the newborn or infant. However, other collaborative problems seen in the adult are also seen in pediatric clients. These problems are worded as Risk for Complications (or RC) followed by the problem.

- RC: Severe malnutrition/dehydration
- RC: Delayed growth
- RC: Failure to thrive
- RC: Respiratory distress
- RC: Permanently deformed femoral head
- RC: Hydrocephalus/shunt infections

Medical Problems

After grouping the data, the client's signs and symptoms may clearly require medical diagnosis and treatment. Referral to a primary care provider is necessary.

CASE STUDY

The case study demonstrates how to analyze assessment data for a specific pediatric client. The critical thinking exercises included in the study guide/lab manual and interactive product that complement this text also offer opportunities to analyze assessment data.

Six-month old Lee Simpson has right congenital hip dysplasia. After a trial with a Pavlik harness, she has been placed in a hip spica cast. The cast has just been applied.

Following cast application, you visit with Lee and her mother. Mrs. Simpson tells you that she is anxious to bring Lee home and asks "What type of special care will she need?" Mrs. Simpson also summarizes the type of care provided to Lee while she had the Pavlik harness.

Mrs. Simpson says that her child responds well to her voice. She informs you that Lee is generally content, eats well (bottle), and sleeps through the night. You notice mother is attentive to child during the interview.

While assessing Lee, you note she is fussy and seems uncomfortable. The skin around her cast is slightly red; there is no edema.

The following concept map illustrates the diagnostic reasoning process.

Applying COLDSPA

Applying **COLDSPA** for: Six-month-old infant with right congenital hip dysplasia. Mother reports she is anxious about the special care needed while the infant is in a spica cast. Note that when assessing an infant, you are really assessing the mother and infant as a pair.

Mnemonic	Question	Data Provided	Missing Data
Character	Describe the sign or symptom (feeling, appearance, sound, smell, or taste if applicable).	Mother is anxious about not knowing what special care her infant with congenital hip dysplasia will need while in a spica cast.	
Onset	When did it begin?	After a trial with a Pavlik harness, the child needed a spica cast, which has just been applied. The child is now fussy and seems uncomfortable.	
Location	Where is it? Does it radiate? Does it occur anywhere else?	Skin around cast is red with no edema.	What is the extent of the redness? Is there any rash? Is the redness getting worse? Does the child have any redness anywhere else where clothing restricts the skin?
Duration	How long does it last? Does it recur?		"Has the child had skin irritations in the past? Describe. What was done to treat previous skin irritations? Did it help?"
Severity	How bad is it? or How much does it bother you?		How does the mother respond to the current fussiness of the child?
Pattern	What makes it better or worse?		"What usually helps the child to feel better when fussy?"
Associated factors/How it **A**ffects the client	What other symptoms occur with it? How does it affect you?	Mother is attentive to child and reports that the child responds to her voice, is generally content, and eats and sleeps well.	How does mother respond to directions given to her to care for her infant in the spica cast?

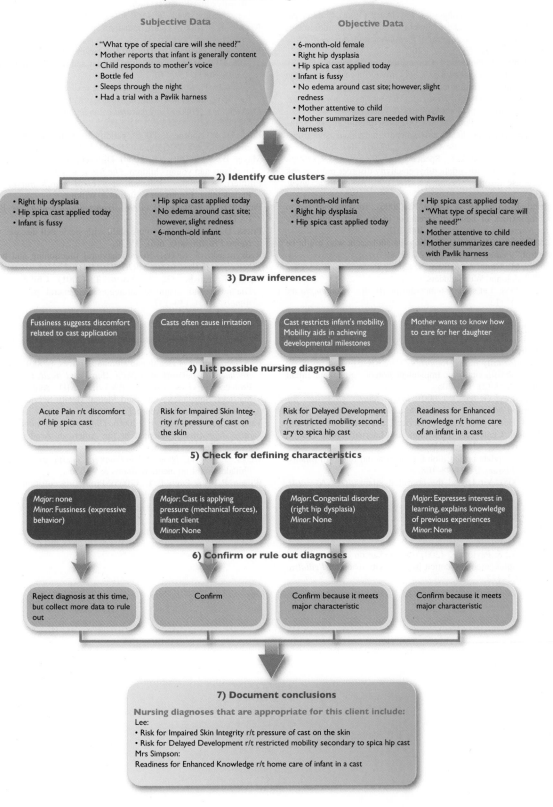

1) Identify abnormal findings and client strengths

Subjective Data
- "What type of special care will she need?"
- Mother reports that infant is generally content
- Child responds to mother's voice
- Bottle fed
- Sleeps through the night
- Had a trial with a Pavlik harness

Objective Data
- 6-month-old female
- Right hip dysplasia
- Hip spica cast applied today
- Infant is fussy
- No edema around cast site; however, slight redness
- Mother attentive to child
- Mother summarizes care needed with Pavlik harness

2) Identify cue clusters

- Right hip dysplasia
- Hip spica cast applied today
- Infant is fussy

- Hip spica cast applied today
- No edema around cast site; however, slight redness
- 6-month-old infant

- 6-month-old infant
- Right hip dysplasia
- Hip spica cast applied today

- Hip spica cast applied today
- "What type of special care will she need?"
- Mother attentive to child
- Mother summarizes care needed with Pavlik harness

3) Draw inferences

Fussiness suggests discomfort related to cast application

Casts often cause irritation

Cast restricts infant's mobility. Mobility aids in achieving developmental milestones

Mother wants to know how to care for her daughter

4) List possible nursing diagnoses

Acute Pain r/t discomfort of hip spica cast

Risk for Impaired Skin Integrity r/t pressure of cast on the skin

Risk for Delayed Development r/t restricted mobility secondary to spica hip cast

Readiness for Enhanced Knowledge r/t home care of an infant in a cast

5) Check for defining characteristics

Major: none
Minor: Fussiness (expressive behavior)

Major: Cast is applying pressure (mechanical forces), infant client
Minor: None

Major: Congenital disorder (right hip dysplasia)
Minor: None

Major: Expresses interest in learning, explains knowledge of previous experiences
Minor: None

6) Confirm or rule out diagnoses

Reject diagnosis at this time, but collect more data to rule out

Confirm

Confirm because it meets major characteristic

Confirm because it meets major characteristic

7) Document conclusions

Nursing diagnoses that are appropriate for this client include:
Lee:
- Risk for Impaired Skin Integrity r/t pressure of cast on the skin
- Risk for Delayed Development r/t restricted mobility secondary to spica hip cast
Mrs Simpson:
Readiness for Enhanced Knowledge r/t home care of infant in a cast

References and Selected Readings

American Academy of Child & Adolescent Psychiatry. (1998). Practice parameters for the assessment and treatment of children and adolescents with substance use disorders. *Journal of the American Academy of Child & Adolescent Psychiatry, 37*(1), 122–126.

American Academy of Pediatrics, Committee on Nutrition. (1998). *Pediatric Nutrition Handbook* (4th ed.). Elk Grove Village, IL: American Academy of Pediatrics, Committee on Nutrition.

Andrews, M., & Boyle, J. (1999). *Transcultural concepts in nursing care.* (3rd ed.). Philadelphia: Lippincott Williams & Wilkins.

Barr, S. I., Murphy, S. P., & Poos, M. I. (2002). Interpreting and using the dietary reference intakes in dietary assessment of individuals and group. *Journal of the American Dietetic Association, 102*(6), 780–789.

Biederman, J., Wilens, T., Mick, E., Spencer, T., & Faraone, S. V. (1999). Pharmacotherapy of attention-deficit/hyperactivity disorder reduces risk for substance use disorder. *Pediatrics, 104,* e20. Available at www.pediatrics.org

Blood-Siegfried, J., Lider, H., & Deary, K. (2006). To screen or not to screen: Complexities of newborn screening in the 21st century. *The Journal for Nurse Practitioners, 2*(5), 300–307.

Brown, R., & Friedman, S. (2001). Treating the adolescent who might be "out of control." *Pediatric Annals, 30*(2), 81–86.

Burns, C., Brady, M., Dunn, A., & Starr, N. (2000). *Pediatric primary care* (2nd ed.). Philadelphia: WB Saunders.

Carey, W. B. (1998). Let's give temperament its due. *Contemporary Pediatrics, 15,* 91–113.

Cash, J. C., & Glass, C. A. (2000). *Family practice guidelines.* Philadelphia: Lippincott Williams & Wilkins.

Centers for Disease Control and Prevention. (1998, April 3). Recommendations to prevent and control iron deficiency in the U. S. *Morbidity and Mortality Weekly Report, 47* (No. RR–3).

Gallo, A. (2003). The fifth vital sign: Implementation of the neonatal infant pail scale. *JOGNN, 32*(2), 199–206.

Green, M., & Palfrey, G. (eds.). (2000). *Bright futures guidelines for health supervision of infants, children and adolescents* (2nd ed.). U. S. Department of Health and Human Services, Maternal Child Health Bureau, National Center for Education in Maternal Child Health, Georgetown University, Arlington, VA.

Gregory, K. (2005). Update on nutrition for preterm and full-term infants. *JOGNN, Clinical Issues, 34*(1), 98–108.

Henderson, A. (2005). Vit D and the breastfed infant. *JOGNN, 34(4),* 367–372.

Hoekelman, R. A. (Ed.). (1997). *Pediatric primary care.* (3rd ed.). St. Louis: C. V. Mosby.

Huff, R., & Kline, M. (1999). *Promoting health in multicultural populations.* Thousand Oaks, CA: Sage.

Hunt, R., Paguin, A., & Payton, K. (2001). An update on assessment and treatment of complex attention–deficit hyperactivity disorder. *Pediatric Annals, 30(3),* 162–172.

Johnson, T. S., Mulder, P. J., & Strube, K. (2007). Mother–infant Breastfeeding Progress Tool: A guide for education and support of the breastfeeding dyad. *JOGNN, 36(4),* 319–327.

Kenny, K. (2000). Heart murmurs in children. *Advance for Nurse Practitioners, 8(9),* 26–31.

Leonard, H., Freeman, J., Garcia, A., Garvey, M., Snider, L., & Sweden, S. (2001). Obsessive-compulsive disorder and related conditions. *Pediatric Annals, 30*(3), 154–161.

Loewenson, P., & Blum, R. (2001). The resilient adolescent: Implications for the pediatrician. *Pediatric Annals, 30*(2), 76–80.

Luckmann, J. (2000). *Transcultural communication in health care.* Albany, NY: Delmar.

Lund, D., & Osborne, J. (2006). Validity and reliability of the neonatal skin condition score. *JOGNN, 33*(3), 320–327.

Mayer, B. W., & Burns, P. (2000). Differential diagnosis of abuse injuries in infants and young children. *The Nurse Practitioner, 25(10),* 15–35.

Pillitteri, A. (2002). *Maternal and child health nursing.* (4th ed.). Philadelphia: Lippincott Williams & Wilkins.

Purnell, L., & Paulanka, B. (1998). *Transcultural health care.* Philadelphia: FA Davis.

Priess, D. J. (1998). The young child with sickle cell disease. *Advance for Nurse Practitioners, 6*(6), 33–39.

Radzyminski, S. (2005). Neurobehavioral functioning and breastfeeding behaviors in the newborn. *JOGNN, 34*(4), 335–341.

Shoaf, T., Emslie, G., & Mayers, T. (2001). Childhood depression: Diagnosis and treatment strategies in general pediatrics. *Pediatric Annals, 30*(3), 130–137.

Tanner, J. M. (1962). *Growth at adolescence.* (2nd ed.). Oxford: Blackwell Science Publications.

Thureen, P., Deacon, J., Hernandez, J., & Hall, D. (2005). *Assessment and care of the well newborn.* St. Louis, MO: Elsevier.

U. S. Department of Health and Human Services. (2000). *Substance abuse treatment of persons with child abuse and neglect issues:* Treatment Protocol Services, No. 36. Rockville, MD: Author, Public Health Services, Substance Abuse and Mental Health Services Administration Center for Substance Abuse Treatment.

Varley, C., & McCauley, E. (2000). *Diagnosis and management of pediatric depression.* Presented at the American Academy of Pediatrics Annual Meeting, October 28, 2000.

Weber, J. (2001). *Nurse's handbook of health assessment.* (4th ed.). Philadelphia: Lippincott Williams & Wilkins.

Wilson, P. R., & Pugh, L. C. (2005). Promoting nutrition in breastfeeding women. *JOGNN, Clinical Issues, 34*(1), 120–124.

Wong, D. L. (2003). *Wong's nursing care of infants and children.* (7th ed.). St. Louis: Mosby.

Wrightson, A. S. (2007). Universal newborn hearing screening. *American Family Physician, 75*(9), AARP.org/afp/200705011349.

31

Assessing Children and Adolescents

Structure and Function

SKIN, HAIR, AND NAILS

During early childhood, the skin develops a tighter bond with the dermis, making it more resistant to infection, irritation, and fluid loss. Skin color appears pink and evenly distributed and may include normal variations such as freckles. The texture is smooth because the skin has not had years of exposure to the environment and because the hair is less coarse than in adulthood. The sebaceous glands and eccrine glands are minimally active with the eccrine glands producing little sweat.

During the toddler years, scalp hair grows coarser, thicker, and darker and usually loses curliness. Fine hair becomes visible on the distal portions of the upper and lower extremities.

As the child ages, skin structure and function remain stable until puberty, when adrenarche (adrenocortical maturation) signals the onset of increased sebum production from the sebaceous glands, a process that continues until late adolescence. Sebum is involved in the development of acne. The apocrine glands also respond more to emotional stimulation and heat, with the end result being body odor.

HEAD AND NECK

During infancy, body growth predominates and the head grows proportionately to body size, reaching 90% of its full adult size by age 6 years. Facial bone growth is variable, especially for the nasal and jaw bones. During the toddler years, the nasal bridge is low and the mandible and maxilla are small, making the face seem small compared with the whole skull. During the school-age years, the face grows proportionately faster than the rest of the cranium, and secondary teeth appear too large for the face. In adolescence, the nose and thyroid cartilage enlarge in boys. Lymph tissue is well developed at birth and continues to grow rapidly until age 10 or 11 years, exceeding adult

size before puberty, after which the tissue atrophies and stabilizes to adult dimensions by the end of adolescence.

EYES

During childhood, the eyes are less spherical than adult eyes. In addition, children remain farsighted until age 6 or 7 years, when they achieve a visual acuity of 20/20.

EARS

As the child grows, the inner ear matures. In older children, the eustachian tube lengthens but it may become occluded from growth of lymphatic tissue, specifically the adenoids. The canal shortens and straightens as the child ages, and the pinna can be pulled up and back as in the adult.

MOUTH, NOSE, THROAT AND SINUSES

Children have 20 deciduous teeth, which are lost between the ages of 6 and 12 years. Permanent teeth begin forming in the jaw by age 6 months and begin to replace temporary teeth at age 6 years, usually starting with the central incisors. Permanent teeth appear earlier in African Americans than in Caucasians and in girls before boys.

Nasal cartilage grows during adolescence with the secondary sex characteristics. Growth starts at age 12 or 13 years and reaches full size by 16 years in girls and 18 years in boys. The maxillary and ethmoid sinuses are present at birth, but they are small and cannot be examined until they develop, when the child is much older. The frontal sinuses develop around age 7 to 8 years, and the sphenoid sinuses develop after puberty.

The tonsils and adenoids rapidly grow, reaching maximum development by age 10 to 12 years. At this point, they may be about twice their adult size. However, as with other lymphoid tissue, they atrophy to stable adult dimensions by the end of adolescence.

THORAX AND LUNGS

The lungs continue to develop after birth and new alveoli form until about 8 years of age. Thus, in a child with pulmonary damage or disease at birth, pulmonary tissue may regenerate and the lungs can eventually attain normal respiratory function. The child will have 300 million alveoli by adolescence.

The chest wall is thin with very little musculature. The ribs are soft and pliable with the xiphoid process movable. The airways of children are also smaller and narrower than in adults; therefore, children are at risk for airway obstruction from edema and infections in the lungs. A child's respiratory rate is much faster than an adult's rate: children younger than 7 years old tend to be abdominal breathers. In children between 8 and 10 years old, respiratory rates lower and breathing becomes thoracic like the adult's.

BREASTS

In girls, breast growth is stimulated by estrogen at the onset of puberty. Between 8 and 13 years of age, thelarche may occur and breasts continue to develop in stages (Table 31-1). Breasts enlarge primarily as a result of fat deposits. However, the duct system also grows and branches, and masses of small cells develop at the duct endings. These masses are potential alveoli. Tenderness and asymmetric development are common, and anticipatory guidance and reassurance are needed. Gynecomastia, enlargement of breast tissue in boys, may be noted in some male adolescents. This is related to pubertal changes and is usually temporary. However, use of marijuana and anabolic steroids are two of several external causes of gynecomastia.

HEART

In children, the heart is positioned more horizontally in the chest. The apical impulse is felt at the fourth intercostal space left of the midclavicular line in young children. By the time the child is 7 years old, the apical pulse reaches the fifth intercostal space and the midclavicular line. Heart sounds are louder, higher pitched, and of shorter duration in children. Physiologic splitting of the second sound, which widens with inspiration, may be heard in the second left intercostal space. A third heart sound (S_3) may be heard at the apex and is present in one-third of all children. Sinus arrhythmia is normal and reaches its greatest degree during adolescence. Some children may have physiologic murmurs that do not indicate disease. The heart rate decreases as the child gets older, usually dropping to about 85 beats/min by 8 years of age. Athletic adolescents may have even lower heart rates.

ABDOMEN

The abdomen of small children is cylindrical, prominent in the standing position, and flat when supine. The abdomen of toddlers appears prominent and gives the child what is popularly called a pot-belly appearance. The contours of the abdomen change to adult shapes during adolescence. Peristaltic waves

Table 31-1	Tanner's Sexual Maturity Rating: Female Breast Development

Developmental Stage		Illustration
Stage 1	Prepubertal: Elevation of nipple only	
Stage 2	Breast bud stage; elevation of breast and nipple as small mound, enlargement of areolar diameter	
Stage 3	Enlargement of the breasts and areola with no separation of contours	
Stage 4	Projection of areola and nipple to form secondary mound above level of breast	
Stage 5	Adult configuration; projection of nipple only, areola receded into contour of breast	

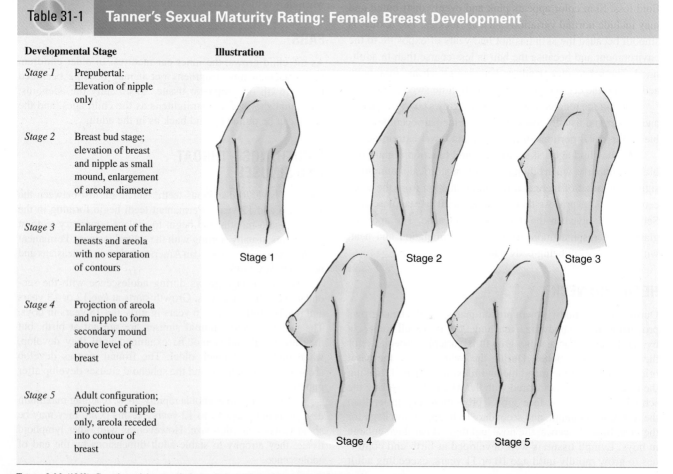

Stage 1   Stage 2   Stage 3

Stage 4   Stage 5

Tanner, J. M. (1962). Growth at adolesence (2nd ed.). Oxford: Blackwell Scientific Publications.

may be visible in thin children; they may also be indicative of a disease or disorder.

The tip of the right kidney may be felt in young children, especially during inspiration.

In small children, the liver is palpable at 1 to 2 cm below the right costal margin. The spleen may be palpable below the left costal margin at 1 to 2 cm. Often in older children, these structures are not palpable.

GENITALIA

Male genitalia generally develop over a 2 to 5 year period, beginning from preadolescence to adulthood. In the adolescent male enlargement of the testes is an early sign of puberty, occurring between the ages of 9.5 and 13.5 years. Pubic hair signifies the onset of puberty in boys. Pubic hair development and penile enlargement are concurrent with testicular growth (Table 31-2). Axillary hair development occurs late in puberty. It follows definitive penile and testicular enlargement in boys. Facial hair in boys also develops at this time. The onset of spontaneous nocturnal emission of seminal fluid is a sign of puberty similar to menarche in females. During puberty, the prostate gland grows rapidly to twice its prepubertal size under the influence of androgens.

In female adolescents puberty is the time that estrogen stimulates the development of the reproductive tract and secondary sex characteristics. The external genitalia increase in size and sensitivity, whereas the internal reproductive organs increase in weight and mass. Pubic hair begins growing early in puberty (2 to 6 months after thelarche [breast development]) and follows a distinct pattern (Table 31-3). Axillary hair development precedes menarche (first menstrual period) in girls. Menarche takes place in the latter half of puberty after breast and pubic hair begin to develop. Menarche typically begins 2.5 years after the onset of puberty. The menstrual cycle is usually irregular during the first 2 years because of physiologic anovulation.

ANUS AND RECTUM

The anus and rectum appear and function like those in the adult.

MUSCULOSKELETAL SYSTEM

The skeleton of small children is made chiefly of cartilage, accounting for the relative softness and malleability of the bones and the relative ease with which certain deformities can be corrected. Bone formation occurs by ossification, beginning during the gestational period and continuing throughout childhood. Bones grow rapidly during infancy. As children grow into adolescence, they will experience a skeletal growth spurt, usually seen in correlation with Tanner's stage 2 for girls and Tanner's stage 3 for boys. Skeletal growth continues throughout Tanner's stage 5 for both sexes.

Bone growth occurs in two dimensions: diameter and length. Growth in diameter takes place predominantly in children and adolescents and slows as the person ages because of the predominance of bone breakdown over bone formation. Growth in length takes place at the epiphyseal plates, vascular areas of active cell division. Bones increase in circumference and length under the influence of hormones, primarily pituitary growth hormone and thyroid hormone.

Muscle growth is related to growth of the underlying bone. Individual fibers, ligaments, and tendons grow throughout childhood. Bone and muscle development is influenced by use of the extremities. If extremities are not used, minimal growth of the muscle will occur. Walking and weight-bearing activities stimulate bone and muscle growth.

The anterior curve in the lumbar region of the vertebral column develops between ages 12 and 18 months, when the toddler starts to stand erect and walk.

Muscle growth contributes significantly to weight gain in the child. Individual fibers grow throughout childhood, and growth is considerable during the adolescent growth spurt, which usually peaks at 12 years in girls and 14 years in boys.

NEUROLOGIC SYSTEM

Motor control develops in a head-to-neck to trunk-to-extremities sequence. Development takes place in an orderly progression, but each child develops at his or her own pace. The norms demonstrate wide variation among individuals as well as within a single individual under different circumstances.

Health Assessment

COLLECTING SUBJECTIVE DATA: THE NURSING HEALTH HISTORY

The complete pediatric nursing history is one of the most crucial components of child health care. Many of the materials and questions are unique to this population. The nursing history interview usually provides an opportunity to observe the caregiver—or parent—child interaction and to participate in early detection of health problems and prevention of future difficulties.

Nurses must have the communication skills needed to elicit data about the child and family within a framework that incorporates biographic data, current health status, past history, family history, a review of each body system, knowledge of growth and development, and lifestyle and health practices–related information. It is important to keep in mind that data collected in one category may have relevance to another category. For example, data collected about the condition of the child's skin, hair, and nails may indicate a problem in the area of nutrition.

Because infants and children are uniquely different from adults, a separate subjective assessment that focuses on questions suited for this population is vital. Subjective assessment of children encompasses interviewing and compiling a complete nursing history. General interviewing techniques used for the adult are used in the pediatric setting. However, in pediatrics, someone other than the client, usually the parent, gives the history. Thus, the interview becomes the onset of a relational triad between the nurse, the child or adolescent, and the parents. Nurses establish a comfortable, yet professional, rapport that forms the foundation for the ongoing therapeutic relationship. Nurses accomplish this by developing communication and interviewing skills that incorporate the needs of both the parent and child or adolescent, treating both as equal partners.

(text continues on page 692)

Table 31-2 Tanner's Sexual Maturity Rating: Male Genitalia and Pubic Hair

Developmental Stage	Illustration
Stage 1 Genitalia: Prepubertal Pubic Hair: Prepubertal: No pubic hair; fine vellus hair	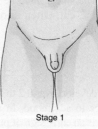 Stage 1
Stage 2 Genitalia: Initial enlargement of scrotum and testes with rugation and reddening of the scrotum Pubic Hair: Sparse, long, straight, downy hair	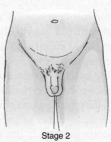 Stage 2
Stage 3 Genitalia: Elongation of the penis; testes and scrotum further enlarge Pubic Hair: Darker, coarser, curly; sparse over entire pubis	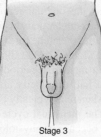 Stage 3
Stage 4 Genitalia: Increase in size and width of penis and the development of the glans; scrotum darkens Pubic Hair: Dark, curly, and abundant in pubic area; no growth on thighs or up toward umbilicus	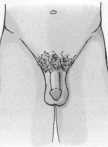 Stage 4
Stage 5 Genitalia: Adult configuration Pubic Hair: Adult pattern (growth up toward umbilicus may not be seen); growth continues until mid-20s	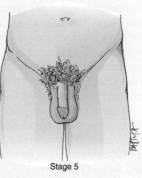 Stage 5

Tanner, J. M. (1962). Growth at adolesence (2nd ed.). Oxford: Blackwell Scientific Publications.

Table 31-3	Tanner's Sexual Maturity Rating: Female Pubic Hair

Developmental Stage	Illustration
Stage 1 Prepubertal: No pubic hair; fine vellus hair	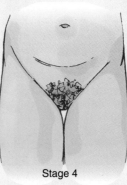 Stage 1
Stage 2 Sparse, long, straight, downy hair	Stage 2
Stage 3 Darker, coarser, curly; sparse over mons pubis	Stage 3
Stage 4 Dark, curly, and abundant on mons pubis; no growth on medial thighs	Stage 4

continued on page 692

Table 31-3	Tanner's Sexual Maturity Rating: Female Pubic Hair *Continued*

Developmental Stage	Illustration
Stage 5 Adult pattern of inverse triangle; growth on medial thighs	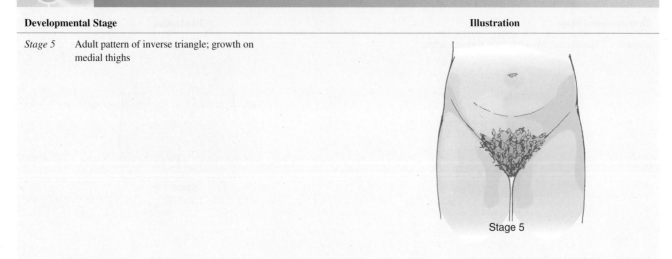 Stage 5

Tanner, J. M. (1962). Growth at adolesence (2nd ed.). Oxford: Blackwell Scientific Publications.

Interviewing

Interviewing Parents

The parental interview entails more than just fact gathering. The tone of future contacts is established as parents begin to develop a trusting relationship with the nurse (Fig. 31-1). Parents expect health professionals to be sources of information and education, and they assess professional competence during the initial contact. Therefore, it is important that the nurse use a friendly, nonjudgmental approach while demonstrating proficiency as a practitioner. Rarely is the interview just data gathering; it is also a forum for rapport building, explaining, and health teaching.

INTRODUCTORY STAGE

As with all clients, the nurse—parent relationship begins with the introduction, when nurses explain their roles and the purpose of the interview. Clarification and consistency are crucial from the start because parents may be anxious about the

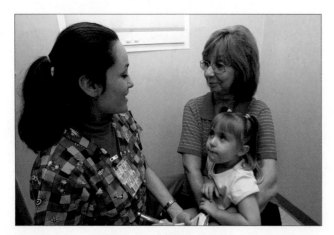

Figure 31-1 Developing a trusting relationship with the parent(s) is an essential aspect of the interview process.

child's condition or uncomfortable about their roles, especially if the setting is a hospital. Anxiety may be overt or masked, even demonstrated by negative behaviors such as hostility.

Cultural variations may also affect parental reactions and response. Active listening facilitates the use of leads and better enables nurses to keep the interview focused on specific concerns. It also allows nurses to uncover clues that further the interview, to seek validation of perceptions and responses that may have alternate meanings, and to provide reassurance for both the expressed and hidden concerns that parents may be experiencing.

ENCOURAGING TALK

By encouraging parents to talk, you can identify information that affects all aspects of a child's life. Some parents take the lead without prompting (e.g., "He's been pulling up his legs like he's in pain"). Others offer vague concerns (e.g., ". . . she's just not acting right") and need more direction. However, all have significant information about their child. You can further encourage verbalization through communication techniques such as open-ended questioning ("How does Sarah behave when she isn't acting just right?") and focus directing ("When does Darryl have the pain?"). Communication skills allow nurses to elicit information in all patient groups, even in the most difficult situations.

The atmosphere should create an exchange of information rather than one directed solely by the nurse. Nurses use problem solving, collaboration, and anticipatory guidance. For example, ask the parent, "What do you see as the problem?" Once the problem is identified, lead the parent through the problem-solving process to arrive at a solution. Parents should also be asked what they found to be effective or ineffective in managing their child's problems. Anticipatory guidance promotes an exchange because parents can better participate in discussions of their child's future developmental trends.

Be aware of the barriers to effective nurse—parent communication. These include time constraints, frequent interruptions, lack of privacy, and language differences as well as provider callousness and cultural insensitivity. Make every effort possible to avoid these barriers. Allow adequate time and privacy for every interview and keep interruptions at a minimum. Interpreters can assist when language differences are present.

Nurses should always display a warm, professional manner when interacting with clients and families, and they should be sensitive to cultural differences displayed in values, beliefs, and customs.

Interviewing Children and Adolescents

As noted earlier, the child or adolescent and parent are treated as equal partners in the health care triad. Include the child in the introductory stage of the interview and observe for signs of readiness to evaluate the level of participation. Readiness evaluation includes questioning the parents about how the child copes with stressful situations and what the child has been told about this particular health encounter.

COMMUNICATION TECHNIQUES

Direct communication, such as open-ended and closed-ended questions, age-appropriate humor, and dialogue strategies, is usually more beneficial when used with indirect communication techniques including sentence completion, mutual story telling, and using drawings, play (the universal language of children), and magic.

Play as Communication

Nurses should talk to the child at eye level (be aware of cultural variations in eye contact) and actively engage children through play and verbalization. Play is one of the most valuable communication techniques when working with children; it allows for the discovery of important cues to children's development and illness behaviors. Rushing creates anxiety; therefore, time should be taken to listen and to allow children to feel comfortable. Privacy and confidentiality are important in pediatric nursing, especially when assessing the adolescent. Children or adolescents may be anxious, fearful, or embarrassed. Their emotions should be respected.

The interview process and assessment procedures should be explained in clear and honest terms. Directions should be stated in a positive manner, and choices should be offered only when available and appropriate. Honest praise is used to reinforce positive behaviors; gratuitous praise is quickly recognized by children and may decrease the child's trust in the nurse.

Touch

Touch is a powerful communication tool. However, the child may find touch intrusive if the nurse has not yet begun to formulate a relationship with the child. Cultural taboos may also prohibit touch. Therefore, it is prudent to communicate with the child at a "safe distance" until the relationship begins to form.

DEVELOPMENTAL CONSIDERATIONS

Nurses should also be familiar with developmentally oriented approaches to interviewing children. Display 31-1 presents specific developmentally oriented approaches that may be used in interviewing children and adolescents.

These approaches are important to know because barriers can exist when communicating with children. For example, some nurses overestimate the understanding abilities of young children and underestimate those of older children and adolescents. This creates frustration for all involved. Nurses need to be habitually aware of children's cognitive status when interacting with them. Another barrier develops when the child is excluded altogether. Children and adolescents can be eager participants and should be treated as such.

Finally, although many children are eager participants, others need encouragement, especially toddlers and preschoolers who may react with crying and lack of cooperation.

Nurses should avoid power struggles and instead rely on empathy, developmental strategies, parental assistance, and a good sense of humor.

ADOLESCENT CONCERNS

Adolescents are neither children nor adults and, therefore, should be treated accordingly. Privacy is essential as are respect and confidentiality. General health issues may or may not be discussed with the parent present. However, sensitive issues, such as sex, sexuality, drugs, and alcohol, are best handled without parental presence. Trust and genuineness are important; nurses should not "talk down" to adolescents or mimic their language style. The approach should be as a professional, not as a peer, parent, or big sister or brother (Fig. 31-2). Use open-ended and specific questions to avoid "yes/no" answers; use silence sparingly because it may be viewed as threatening to this age group. Be aware of your own nonverbal and facial expressions. Delicate issues should be approached with sensitivity and a nonjudgmental, matter-of-fact manner to keep them from appearing to be focal points. History taking provides an excellent opportunity for health teaching with adolescents, who are eager to learn about their ever-changing bodies. Questions should be encouraged and answered throughout the history.

Biographic Data

Gathering this type of information is a good way to begin the health history. It consists of general, easy-to-answer information that puts the parent and child at ease. It also can provide the

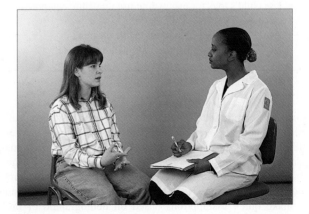

Figure 31-2 Handle sensitive issues with adolescents by establishing trust and genuineness (© B. Proud).

DISPLAY 31-1	Age-Specific Interview Techniques

Each child responds differently during the assessment interview according to his or her developmental status, severity and perception of illness, experience with health care, intrusiveness of procedures, and the child's own uniqueness. The following are some guidelines for adapting the interview techniques to the child's status.

Toddlers: Sensorimotor to Preoperational Stages

Trial and error experimentation and relentless exploration are typical in the early toddler stage; later, the toddler uses representational thought in intellectual development. Children under 5 years of age are egocentric. Toddler's attention span ranges between 5 and 10 minutes.

- Encourage parental presence.
- Provide careful and simple explanations just before procedure.
- Use play as a communication technique.
- Tell child it is okay to cry.
- Encourage expression through toys.
- Use simple terminology; child's receptive language is more advanced than his or her expressive language.
- Allow child to be close to parent—be alert for separation anxiety.
- Acknowledge child's favorite toy or a unique characteristic about the child.

Preschoolers: Preoperational Stage

Preschoolers progress from making simple classifications and associating one event with a simultaneous one to classifying and quantifying and exhibiting intuitive thought processes. A preschooler's attention span ranges between 10 and 15 minutes. Preschoolers use magical thinking.

- Explain why things are as they are, simply.
- Validate child's perceptions.
- Avoid threatening words.
- Use simple visual aids.
- Involve child in teaching by doing something (handling equipment).
- Allow child to ask questions.
- Use child's toys for expression; use miniature equipment on toys.
- Avoid using words that have double meaning.
- Explain sensations that the child will experience.

- Answer "why" questions with simple explanations.
- Be direct and concrete; do not use analogies, abstractions, or words with more than one meaning; avoid slang (such as "laugh your head off"—preschoolers interpret literally).
- Ask simple questions.
- Allow child to manipulate equipment.
- Use the child's active imagination—use toys, puppets, and play.

School-Age Children: Operational Stage

Egocentric thinking progresses to objective thinking in school-age children who begin using inductive reasoning, logical operations, and reversible concrete thought. A school-age child's attention span ranges between 30 and 45 minutes. Use books and other visual aids to advance the assessment interview.

- Remember to remain concrete (ie, avoid abstractions).
- Use group discussion to educate children among their peers; also use games.
- Provide health teaching; perform demonstrations.
- Give more responsibility to child.
- School-age children like explanations and need assistance in vocalizing their needs.
- Allow children to engage in discussions.

Adolescents: Formal Operations Stage

Abstract thought develops, as does thinking beyond the present and forming theories about everything.

- Give adolescents control whenever possible.
- Use scientific explanations and make expectations clear.
- Explore expected parental level of involvement before initiating it.
- Involve adolescents in planning.
- Clearly explain how body will be affected.
- Anticipate feelings of anger and grief.
- Use peers with common situation to help with teaching.
- Encourage expression of ideas and feelings.
- Maintain confidentiality; facilitate trust.
- Give adolescents your undivided attention.
- Make expectations clear.
- Ask to speak to adolescent alone.
- Encourage open and honest communication.
- Be nonjudgmental; respect views, differences, and feelings.
- Ask open-ended questions.

---

nurse with important clues that can benefit the rest of the subjective examination. For example, discovering that a 5-year-old child lives in the city with his 40-year-old professional parents and no brothers or sisters may give the nurse clues about his developmental level, activity, relationships, and socioeconomic status. However, the nurse must be careful not to make quick assumptions based on demographic or biographic data.

These types of questions are often asked on a form that the parent fills out before the assessment. However, the nurse should go over the form with the parent and child (if feasible) at the beginning of the assessment. Typical data include the following:

(text continues on page 709)

BIOGRAPHICAL DATA

Question	Rationale
What is the child's name? Nickname? What are the parents' or caregivers' names?	Knowing personal information about the child and caregivers helps to establish rapport with child and family.
Who is the child's primary health care provider, and when was the child's last well-child care appointment? (Table 31-4 provides guidelines for primary health care provider visits developed by the Committee on Practice and Ambulatory Medicine and the American Academy of Pediatrics [AAP]).	This determines the child's access to health care. It tells the nurse where to find the client's previous medical information/record.
Where does the child live? (Address) Do the parents and child live in the same residence? Who else lives in this residence? Are the child's parents married, single, divorced, homosexual? What are the parents' ages?	This provides insight into living conditions and family dynamics, which contribute to the child's health.
What is the child's age? What is the child's date of birth?	This provides a reference for assessing the child's developmental level.
Is the child adopted, foster, natural?	Certain health problems run in families. It is helpful to know the child's genetic relationship with the parents.
What is the child's ethic origin? Religion?	This information helps the nurse to examine special needs and beliefs that may affect the client or family's health care.
What do the child's parents do for a living?	This provides insight into the economic status of the family.

HISTORY OF PRESENT HEALTH CONCERN/CURRENT HEALTH STATUS

As with adults, it is important to obtain information regarding the child's current status of health. Nurses should ask the parent, and child if possible, to describe the child's general state of health and compare it with how it was 1 and 5 years ago (if age appropriate). If the answer is "good," ask what "good" means to them. "Good" could mean "only one cold this year" for a generally healthy child or "only two hospitalizations this year" for a child with a chronic illness such as cystic fibrosis.

Current health status also includes information regarding chronic illnesses and allergies. Chronic illness, such as asthma, or disability, such as cerebral palsy, must be established early in the history to allow for better assessment and teaching strategies. Allergies are very common during childhood. Nurses need to ask what the specific allergen is and how the child reacts to it. Some parents consider medication side effects to be allergic responses (e.g., diarrhea that is common after antibiotic use) and need information to differentiate side effects from actual allergies.

Finally nurses must ask for complete medication and treatment information. This includes prescription and over-the-counter medications, devices and treatments (e.g., hot/cold compresses, respiratory therapy, assistive devices, such as orthopedic braces), and home or folk remedies. The child may be taking a combination of medications that are incompatible or a folk remedy that is harmful (e.g., azaron, used in Mexico for digestive problems, contains lead). As with adults, children's medication information should include the name of the drug, dosage, frequency, and the reason why the medication is administered.

The purpose of asking about the child's current health status is to determine why the child was brought in for an examination. For some examinations, the child and parents may have no symptoms to report. In this case, the parent and child should be asked to describe the general state of the child's health.

If there is a perceived problem with the child's health or if the child or parent notices symptoms, the same focus questions that are asked for each body system for the adult client are used for the child (e.g., location, intensity, duration). However, for the child, it is important to ask both the parent and the child (if possible) to get the most accurate information. Conflicting information may clue

continued on page 698

Table 31-4 Recommendations for Preventive Pediatric Health Care

Each child and family is unique; therefore, these **Recommendations for Preventive Pediatric Health Care** are designed for the care of children who are receiving competent parenting, have no manifestations of any important health problems, and are growing and developing in satisfactory fashion. **Additional visits may become necessary** if circumstances suggest variations from normal.

*Column groups: **Infancy** = Prenatal–9 mo; **Early Childhood** = 12 m–4 y*

Age[a]	Prenatal[b]	Newborn[c]	3–5 d[d]	By 1 mo	2 mo	4 mo	6 mo	9 mo	12 m	15 mo	18 mo	24 mo	30 mo	3 y	4 y
HISTORY															
Initial/interval	•	•	•	•	•	•	•	•	•	•	•	•	•	•	•
MEASUREMENTS															
Length/height and weight		•	•	•	•	•	•	•	•	•	•	•	•	•	•
Head circumference		•	•	•	•	•	•	•	•	•	•	•			
Weight for length		•	•	•	•	•	•	•	•	•	•	•			
Body mass index												•	•	•	•
Blood pressure[e]		★	★	★	★	★	★	★	★	★	★	★	★		
SENSORY SCREENING															
Vision[f]		★	★	★	★	★	★	★	★	★	★	★	★		
Hearing	•[g]	★	★	★	★	★	★	★	★	★	★	★	★	★	
DEVELOPMENTAL/ BEHAVIORAL ASSESSMENT															
Developmental screening[h]								•			•		•		
Autism screening[i]											•	•			
Developmental surveillance[h]		•		•	•	•	•		•	•		•		•	•
Psychosocial/behavioral assessment		•	•	•	•	•	•	•	•	•	•	•	•	•	•
Alcohol and drug use assessment															
PHYSICAL EXAMINATION[j]		•	•	•	•	•	•	•	•	•	•	•	•	•	•
PROCEDURES[k]															
Newborn metabolic/hemoglobin screening[l]		←		•	→										
Immunization[m]		•	•	•	•	•	•	•	•	•	•	•	•	•	•
Hematocrit or hemoglobin[n]						★			•		★	★		★	★
Lead screening[o]							★	★	•or★[p]		★	•or★[p]		★	★
Tuberculin test[q]				★				★	★		★	★		★	★
Dyslipidemia screening[r]												★			★
STI screening[s]															
Cervical dysplasia screening[t]															
ORAL HEALTH[u]									★		★	•or★[u]	•or★[u]	•or★[u]	•[v]
ANTICIPATORY GUIDANCE[w]	•	•	•	•	•	•	•	•	•	•	•	•	•	•	•

[a] If a child comes under care for the first time at any point on the schedule, or if any items are not accomplished at the suggested age, the schedule should be brought up to date at the earliest possible time.

[b] A prenatal visit is recommended for parents who are at high risk, for first-time parents, and for those who request a conference. The prenatal visit should include anticipatory guidance, pertinent medical history, and a discussion of benefits of breastfeeding and planned method of feeding per AAP statement "The Prenatal Visit" (2001) [URL: http://aappolicy.aappublications.org/cgi/content/full/pediatrics;107/6/1456].

[c] Every infant should have a newborn evaluation after birth, breastfeeding encouraged, and instruction and support offered.

[d] Every infant should have an evaluation within 3 to 5 days of birth and within 48 to 72 hours after discharge from the hospital, to include evaluation for feeding and jaundice. Breastfeeding infants should receive formal breastfeeding evaluation, encouragement, and instruction as recommended in AAP statement "Breastfeeding and the Use of Human Milk" (2005) [URL: http://aappolicy.aappublications.org/cgi/content/full/pediatrics;115/2/496]. For newborns discharged in less than 48 hours after delivery, the infant must be examined within 48 hours of discharge per AAP statement "Hospital Stay for Healthy Term Newborns" (2004) [URL: http://aappolicy.aappublications.org/cgi/content/full/pediatrics;113/5/1434].

[e] Blood pressure measurement in infants and children with specific risk conditions should be performed at visits before age 3 years.

[f] If the patient is uncooperative, rescreen within 6 months per AAP statement "Eye Examination and Vision Screening in Infants, Children, and Young Adults" (1996) [URL: http://aappolicy.aappublications.org/cgi/reprint/pediatrics;98/1/153.pdf].

[g] All newborns should be screened per AAP statement "Year 2000 Position Statement: Principles and Guidelines for Early Hearing Detection and Intervention Programs" (2000) [URL: http://aappolicy.aappublications.org/cgi/content/full/pediatrics;106/4/798]. Joint Committee on Infant Hearing. Year 2007 position statement: principles and guidelines for early hearing detection and intervention programs. Pediatrics. 2007;120:898–921.

[h] AAP Council on Children With Disabilities, AAP Section on Developmental Behavioral Pediatrics, AAP Bright Futures Steering Committee, AAP Medical Home Initiatives for Children With Special Needs Project Advisory Committee. Identifying infants and young children with developmental disorders in the medical home: analgorithm for developmental surveillance and screening. Pediatrics. 2006;118:405–420 [URL: http://aappolicy.aappublications.org/cgi/content/full/pediatrics;118/1/405].

[i] Gupta VB, Hyman SL, Johnson CP, et al. Identifying children with autism early? Pediatrics. 2007;119:152–153 [URL: http://pediatrics.aappublications.org/cgi/content/full/119/1/152].

[j] At each visit, age-appropriate physical examination is essential, with infant totally unclothed, older child undressed and suitably draped.

[k] These may be modified, depending on entry point into schedule and individual need.

[l] Newborn metabolic and hemoglobinopathy screening should be done according to state law. Results should be reviewed at visits and appropriate retesting or referral done as needed.

• = to be performed   ★ = risk assessment to be performed, with appropriate action to follow,

Developmental, psychosocial, and chronic disease issues for children and adolescents may require frequent counseling and treatment visits separate from preventive care visits.

These guidelines represent a consensus by the American Academy of Pediatrics (AAP) and Bright Futures. The AAP continues to emphasize the great importance of **continuity of care** in comprehensive health supervision and the need to avoid **fragmentation of care**.

Middle Childhood						Adolescence										
5 y	6 y	7 y	8 y	9 y	10 y	11 y	12 y	13 y	14 y	15 y	16 y	17 y	18 y	19 y	20 y	21 y
•	•	•	•	•	•	•	•	•	•	•	•	•	•	•	•	•
•	•	•	•	•	•	•	•	•	•	•	•	•	•	•	•	•
•	•	•	•	•	•	•	•	•	•	•	•	•	•	•	•	•
•	•	•	•	•	•	•	•	•	•	•	•	•	•		•	•
•	•	★	•	★	•	★	•	★	★	•	★	★	•	★	★	★
•	•	★	•	★	•	★	★	★	★	★	★	★	★	★	★	★
•	•	•	•	•	•	•	•	•	•	•	•	•	•	•	•	•
•	•	•	•	•	•	•	•	•	•	•	•	•	•	•	•	•
						★	★	★	★	★	★	★	★	★	★	★
•	•	•	•	•	•	•	•	•	•	•	•	•	•	•	•	•
•	•	•	•	•	•	•	•	•	•	•	•	•	•	•	•	•
★	★	★	★	★	★	★	★	★	★	★	★	★	★	★	★	★
★	★															
★	★	★	★	★	★	★	★	★	★	★	★	★	★	★	★	★
	★		★		★	★	★	★	★	★	★	★	←		•	→
						★	★	★	★	★	★	★	★	★	★	★
						★	★	★	★	★	★	★	★	★	★	★
	•[v]															
•	•	•	•	•	•	•	•	•	•	•	•	•	•	•	•	•

[m] Schedules per the Committee on Infectious Diseases, published annually in the January issue of *Pediatrics*. Every visit should be an opportunity to update and complete a child's immunizations.

[n] See AAP *Pediatric Nutrition Handbook*, 5th Edition (2003) for a discussion of universal and selective screening options. See also Recommendations to prevent and control iron deficiency in the United States. *MMWR Recomm Rep.* 1998;47(RR-3):1–36.

[o] For children at risk of lead exposure, consult the AAP statement "Lead Exposure in Children: Prevention, Detection, and Management" (2005) [URL: http://aappolicy.aappublications.org/cgi/content/full/pediatrics;116/4/1036]. Additionally, screening should be done in accordance with state law where applicable.

[p] Perform risk assessments or screens as appropriate, based on universal screening requirements for patients with Medicaid or high prevalence areas.

[q] Tuberculosis testing per recommendations of the Committee on Infectious Diseases, published in the current edition of *Red Book: Report of the Committee on Infectious Diseases*. Testing should be done on recognition of high-risk factors.

[r] "Third Report of the National Cholesterol Education Program (NCEP) Expert Panel on Detection, Evaluation, and Treatment of High Blood Cholesterol in Adults (Adult Treatment Panel III) Final Report" (2002) [URL: http://circ.ahajournals.org/cgi/content/full/106/25/3143] and "The Expert Committee Recommendations on the Assessment, Prevention, and Treatment of Child and Adolescent Overweight and Obesity." Supplement to *Pediatrics*. In press.

[s] All sexually active patients should be screened for sexually transmitted infections (STIs).

[t] All sexually active girls should have screening for cervical dysplasia as part of a pelvic examination beginning within 3 years of onset of sexual activity or age 21 (whichever comes first).

[u] Referral to dental home, if available. Otherwise, administer oral health risk assessment. If the primary water source is deficient in fluoride, consider oral fluoride supplementation.

[v] At the visits for 3 years and 6 years of age, it should be determined whether the patient has a dental home. If the patient does not have a dental home, a referral should be made to one. If the primary water source is deficient in fluoride, consider oral fluoride supplementation.

[w] Refer to the specific guidance by age as listed in Bright Futures Guidelines. (Hagan JF, Shaw JS, Duncan PM, eds. *Bright Futures: Guidelines for Health Supervision of Infants, Children, and Adolescents*. 3rd ed. Elk Grove Village, IL: American Academy of Pediatrics; 2008.)

if positive ←——— • ———→ = range during which a service may be provided, with the symbol indicating the preferred age

HISTORY OF PRESENT HEALTH CONCERN/CURRENT HEALTH STATUS *Continued*

the nurse in to other areas that may need to be assessed. When asking the child about symptoms, the following techniques are usually helpful:

- Ask the child to point with one finger to where the pain or symptom is located.
- Use a pain scale developed for children such as the FACES Pain Rating Scale characters ranging from a happy face signifying no pain to a tearful face signifying the worst pain); the Oucher scale (six photographs of children's faces ranging from "no hurt" to "biggest hurt you could ever have;" also comes with scale from 0 to 100); or a numeric scale (straight line with numbers from 0 to 10 representing no pain to worst pain). Figure 31-3 illustrates the FACES and numeric pain-rating scales.

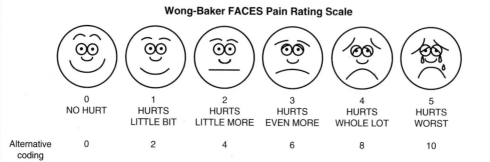

Wong-Baker FACES Pain Rating Scale

0 NO HURT	1 HURTS LITTLE BIT	2 HURTS LITTLE MORE	3 HURTS EVEN MORE	4 HURTS WHOLE LOT	5 HURTS WORST

Alternative coding: 0   2   4   6   8   10

Explain to the person that each face is for a person who feels happy because he has no pain (hurt) or sad because he has some or a lot of pain. Face 0 is very happy because he doesn't hurt at all. Face 1 hurts just a little bit. Face 2 hurts a little more. Face 3 hurts even more. Face 4 hurts a whole lot. Face 5 hurts as much as you can imagine, although you don't have to be crying to feel this bad. Ask the person to choose the face that best describes how he is feeling.

Rating scale is recommended for persons age 3 years and older.

Brief word instructions: Point to each face using the words to describe the pain intensity. Ask the child to choose face that best describes own pain and record the appropriate number.

Figure 31-3 Pain rating scales: Numerical scale and FACES pain rating scale. (From Hockenberry M. J., Wilson D. (2009). *Wong's essentials of pediatric nursing.* (8th ed.). St. Louis: Mosby. Used with permission. Copyright Mosby.)

continued

COLDSPA Example

Use the **COLDSPA** mnemonic as a guideline to collect needed information for each symptom the client shares. In addition, the following questions help elicit important information.

Assessment of a 9-year-old child.

Mnemonic	*Question*	*Client Response Example*
Character	Describe the sign or symptom (feeling, appearance, sound, smell, or taste if applicable).	"My ear hurts."
Onset	When did it begin?	"Yesterday."
Location	Where is it? Does it radiate? Does it occur anywhere else?	"Inside my right ear and down to my jaw."
Duration	How long does it last? Does it recur?	"It hurts all the time."
Severity	How bad is it? or How much does it bother you?	"Really bad." Client gives the pain a rating of 8 on a scale of 1–10.
Pattern	What makes it better or worse?	"Tylenol and heat made it a little better."
Associated factors/How it **A**ffects the client	What other symptoms occur with it? How does it affect you?	"My head hurts and my nose is stuffy. I keep coughing. I can't sleep and I can't think in school either because I feel bad all over."

Question	Rationale
Describe the child's general state of health.	Obtaining baseline information about the client helps to identify important areas of assessment.
Does the child have a chronic illness?	Chronic illnesses may explain or affect assessment findings.
Does the child have any allergies? If so, what is the specific allergen? How does the child react to it?	This identifies allergens and helps the nurse plan to prevent exposure.
What prescriptions, over-the-counter medications, devices, and treatments, and home or folk remedies is the child taking? Please provide the name of the drug, dosage, frequency, and reason it is administered.	It is always important to know what medications a client is taking, especially young clients.

PAST HEALTH HISTORY

Past history is important information to collect when assessing children. Certain problems and conditions can be associated with a difficult birth experience, whether the child was immunized, genetic conditions acquired from parents, and the like. Obviously, most of this information must come from the birth parent. If the child is a foster child or adopted, some of the information may be obtained from hospital records.

Question	Rationale
Sample nursing history questions include	
Was this child's pregnancy planned? How did you feel when you found out you were pregnant?	The caregiver's answer may provide insight into her feelings about the child.
When did you first receive prenatal care? How was your general health during pregnancy?	Prenatal information helps to identify potential health problems for the child.
Did you have any problems with your pregnancy?	Certain medications should not be taken during pregnancy and may be harmful to the child.
Did you have any accidents during this pregnancy?	Smoking, alcohol, and drug use may cause complications or anomalies with the fetus.
Did you take any medications during pregnancy?	
Did you use any tobacco, alcohol, or drugs during this pregnancy?	
Ask about delivery of the child:	Delivery details and complications are pertinent for assessing fetal injury and potential risk for infection.
Where was the child born?	
What type of delivery did you have?	
Were there any problems during the delivery? Did you have any vaginal infections at time of delivery?	
What was the child's Apgar score?	
What were the child's weight, height, and head circumference? Did the child have any problems after birth (e.g., feeding, jaundice)?	
Ask about past illnesses or injuries:	Previous illnesses and hospitalizations may affect the present examination.
Has the child ever been hospitalized?	
Has the child ever had any major illnesses?	
Has the child ever experienced any major injuries?	
What immunizations has the child received thus far (Tables 31-5, 31-6, and 31-7)? Has your child had any reactions to immunizations?	This helps to identify risk for infection and/or potential reactions to immunizations.

continued on page 704

Table 31-5 — Recommended Immunization Schedule for Persons Aged 0–6 Years—United States—2008

For those who fall behind or start late, see the catch-up schedule

Vaccine ▼ Age ▶	Birth	1 month	2 months	4 months	6 months	12 months	15 months	18 months	19–23 months	2–3 years	4–6 years
Hepatitis B[1]	HepB	HepB	HepB	see footnote1	HepB	HepB	HepB	HepB			
Rotavirus[2]			Rota	Rota	Rota						
Diphtheria, Tetanus, Pertussis[3]			DTaP	DTaP	DTaP	see footnote3	DTaP	DTaP			DTaP
Haemophilus influenzae type b[4]			Hib	Hib	Hib[4]	Hib	Hib				
Pneumococcal[5]			PCV	PCV	PCV	PCV	PCV			PPV	
Inactivated Poliovirus			IPV	IPV	IPV	IPV	IPV	IPV			IPV
Influenza[6]					Influenza (Yearly)	Influenza (Yearly)	Influenza (Yearly)	Influenza (Yearly)	Influenza (Yearly)	Influenza (Yearly)	Influenza (Yearly)
Measles, Mumps, Rubella[7]						MMR	MMR				MMR
Varicella[8]						Varicella	Varicella				Varicella
Hepatitis A[9]						HepA (2 doses)	HepA (2 doses)	HepA (2 doses)		HepA Series	
Meningococcal[10]										MCV4	MCV4

Range of recommended ages

Certain high-risk groups

This schedule indicates the recommended ages for routine administration of currently licensed childhood vaccines, as of December 1, 2007, for children aged 0 through 6 years. Additional information is available at www.cdc.gov/vaccines/recs/schedules. Any dose not administered at the recommended age should be administered at any subsequent visit, when indicated and feasible. Additional vaccines may be licensed and recommended during the year. Licensed combination vaccines may be used whenever any components of the combination are indicated and other components of the vaccine are not contraindicated and if approved by the Food and Drug Administration for that dose of the series. Providers should consult the respective Advisory Committee on Immunization Practices statement for detailed recommendations, including for **high-risk conditions:** http://www.cdc.gov/vaccines/pubs/ACIP-list.htm. Clinically significant adverse events that follow immunization should be reported to the Vaccine Adverse Event Reporting System (VAERS). Guidance about how to obtain and complete a VAERS form is available at www.vaers.hhs.gov or by telephone, 800-822-7967.

1. Hepatitis B vaccine (HepB). *(Minimum age: birth)*
At birth:
- Administer monovalent HepB to all newborns prior to hospital discharge.
- If mother is hepatitis B surface antigen (HBsAg) positive, administer HepB and 0.5 mL of hepatitis B immune globulin (HBIG) within 12 hours of birth.
- If mother's HBsAg status is unknown, administer HepB within 12 hours of birth. Determine the HBsAg status as soon as possible and if HBsAg positive, administer HBIG (no later than age 1 week).
- If mother is HBsAg negative, the birth dose can be delayed, in rare cases, with a provider's order and a copy of the mother's negative HBsAg laboratory report in the infant's medical record.

After the birth dose:
- The HepB series should be completed with either monovalent HepB or a combination vaccine containing HepB. The second dose should be administered at age 1–2 months. The final dose should be administered no earlier than age 24 weeks. Infants born to HBsAg-positive mothers should be tested for HBsAg and antibody to HBsAg after completion of at least 3 doses of a licensed HepB series, at age 9–18 months (generally at the next well-child visit).

4-month dose:
- It is permissible to administer 4 doses of HepB when combination vaccines are administered after the birth dose. If monovalent HepB is used for doses after the birth dose, a dose at age 4 months is not needed.

2. Rotavirus vaccine (Rota). *(Minimum age: 6 weeks)*
- Administer the first dose at age 6–12 weeks.
- Do not start the series later than age 12 weeks.
- Administer the final dose in the series by age 32 weeks. Do not administer any dose later than age 32 weeks.
- Data on safety and efficacy outside of these age ranges are insufficient.

3. Diphtheria and tetanus toxoids and acellular pertussis vaccine (DTaP). *(Minimum age: 6 weeks)*
- The fourth dose of DTaP may be administered as early as age 12 months, provided 6 months have elapsed since the third dose.
- Administer the final dose in the series at age 4–6 years.

4. *Haemophilus influenzae* type b conjugate vaccine (Hib). *(Minimum age: 6 weeks)*
- If PRP-OMP (PedvaxHIB® or ComVax® [Merck]) is administered at ages 2 and 4 months, a dose at age 6 months is not required.
- TriHIBit® (DTaP/Hib) combination products should not be used for primary immunization but can be used as boosters following any Hib vaccine in children age 12 months or older.

5. Pneumococcal vaccine. *(Minimum age: 6 weeks for pneumococcal conjugate vaccine [PCV]; 2 years for pneumococcal polysaccharide vaccine [PPV])*
- Administer one dose of PCV to all healthy children aged 24–59 months having any incomplete schedule.
- Administer PPV to children aged 2 years and older with underlying medical conditions.

6. Influenza vaccine. *(Minimum age: 6 months for trivalent inactivated influenza vaccine [TIV]; 2 years for live, attenuated influenza vaccine [LAIV])*
- Administer annually to children aged 6–59 months and to all eligible close contacts of children aged 0–59 months.
- Administer annually to children 5 years of age and older with certain risk factors, to other persons (including household members) in close contact with persons in groups at higher risk, and to any child whose parents request vaccination.
- For healthy persons (those who do not have underlying medical conditions that predispose them to influenza complications) ages 2–49 years, either LAIV or TIV may be used.
- Children receiving TIV should receive 0.25 mL if age 6–35 months or 0.5 mL if age 3 years or older.
- Administer 2 doses (separated by 4 weeks or longer) to children younger than 9 years who are receiving influenza vaccine for the first time or who were vaccinated for the first time last season but only received one dose.

7. Measles, mumps, and rubella vaccine (MMR). *(Minimum age: 12 months)*
- Administer the second dose of MMR at age 4–6 years. MMR may be administered before age 4–6 years, provided 4 weeks or more have elapsed since the first dose.

8. Varicella vaccine. *(Minimum age: 12 months)*
- Administer second dose at age 4–6 years; may be administered 3 months or more after first dose.
- Do not repeat second dose if administered 28 days or more after first dose.

9. Hepatitis A vaccine (HepA). *(Minimum age: 12 months)*
- Administer to all children aged 1 year (i.e., aged 12–23 months). Administer the 2 doses in the series at least 6 months apart.
- Children not fully vaccinated by age 2 years can be vaccinated at subsequent visits.
- HepA is recommended for certain other groups of children, including in areas where vaccination programs target older children.

10. Meningococcal vaccine. *(Minimum age: 2 years for meningococcal conjugate vaccine (MCV4) and for meningococcal polysaccharide vaccine (MPSV4))*
- Administer MCV4 to children aged 2–10 years with terminal complement deficiencies or anatomic or functional asplenia and certain other high-risk groups. MPSV4 is also acceptable.
- Administer MCV4 to persons who received MPSV4 3 or more years previously and remain at increased risk for meningococcal disease.

The Recommended Immunization Schedules for Persons Aged 0–18 Years are approved by the Advisory Committee on Immunization Practices (www.cdc.gov/vaccines/recs/acip), the American Academy of Pediatrics (http://www.aap.org), and the American Academy of Family Physicians (http://www.aafp.org).

DEPARTMENT OF HEALTH AND HUMAN SERVICES • CENTERS FOR DISEASE CONTROL AND PREVENTION • SAFER • HEALTHIER • PEOPLE™

Table 31-6 Recommended Immunization Schedule for Persons Aged 7–18 Years—United States—2008

For those who fall behind or start late, see the green bars and the catch-up schedule

Vaccine ▼ Age ►	7–10 years	11–12 years	13–18 years
Diphtheria, Tetanus, Pertussis[1]	see footnote 1	Tdap	Tdap
Human Papillomavirus[2]	see footnote 2	HPV (3 doses)	HPV Series
Meningococcal[3]	MCV4	MCV4	MCV4
Pneumococcal[4]	PPV		
Influenza[5]	Influenza (Yearly)		
Hepatitis A[6]	HepA Series		
Hepatitis B[7]	HepB Series		
Inactivated Poliovirus[8]	IPV Series		
Measles, Mumps, Rubella[9]	MMR Series		
Varicella[10]	Varicella Series		

Range of recommended ages

Catch-up immunization

Certain high-risk groups

This schedule indicates the recommended ages for routine administration of currently licensed childhood vaccines, as of December 1, 2007, for children aged 7–18 years. Additional information is available at www.cdc.gov/vaccines/recs/schedules. Any dose not administered at the recommended age should be administered at any subsequent visit, when indicated and feasible. Additional vaccines may be licensed and recommended during the year. Licensed combination vaccines may be used whenever any components of the combination are indicated and other components of the vaccine are not contraindicated and if approved by the Food and Drug Administration for that dose of the series. Providers should consult the respective Advisory Committee on Immunization Practices statement for detailed recommendations, including for **high risk conditions:** http://www.cdc.gov/vaccines/pubs/ACIP-list.htm. Clinically significant adverse events that follow immunization should be reported to the Vaccine Adverse Event Reporting System (VAERS). Guidance about how to obtain and complete a VAERS form is available at www.vaers.hhs.gov or by telephone, 800-822-7967.

1. Tetanus and diphtheria toxoids and acellular pertussis vaccine (Tdap).
(Minimum age: 10 years for BOOSTRIX® and 11 years for ADACEL™)
- Administer at age 11–12 years for those who have completed the recommended childhood DTP/DTaP vaccination series and have not received a tetanus and diphtheria toxoids (Td) booster dose.
- 13–18-year-olds who missed the 11–12 year Tdap or received Td only are encouraged to receive one dose of Tdap 5 years after the last Td/DTaP dose.

2. Human papillomavirus vaccine (HPV). *(Minimum age: 9 years)*
- Administer the first dose of the HPV vaccine series to females at age 11–12 years.
- Administer the second dose 2 months after the first dose and the third dose 6 months after the first dose.
- Administer the HPV vaccine series to females at age 13–18 years if not previously vaccinated.

3. Meningococcal vaccine.
- Administer MCV4 at age 11–12 years and at age 13–18 years if not previously vaccinated. MPSV4 is an acceptable alternative.
- Administer MCV4 to previously unvaccinated college freshmen living in dormitories.
- MCV4 is recommended for children aged 2–10 years with terminal complement deficiencies or anatomic or functional asplenia and certain other high-risk groups.
- Persons who received MPSV4 3 or more years previously and remain at increased risk for meningococcal disease should be vaccinated with MCV4.

4. Pneumococcal polysaccharide vaccine (PPV).
- Administer PPV to certain high-risk groups.

5. Influenza vaccine.
- Administer annually to all close contacts of children aged 0–59 months.
- Administer annually to persons with certain risk factors, health-care workers, and other persons (including household members) in close contact with persons in groups at higher risk.

- Administer 2 doses (separated by 4 weeks or longer) to children younger than 9 years who are receiving influenza vaccine for the first time or who were vaccinated for the first time last season but only received one dose.
- For healthy nonpregnant persons (those who do not have underlying medical conditions that predispose them to influenza complications) ages 2–49 years, either LAIV or TIV may be used.

6. Hepatitis A vaccine (HepA).
- Administer the 2 doses in the series at least 6 months apart.
- HepA is recommended for certain other groups of children, including in areas where vaccination programs target older children.

7. Hepatitis B vaccine (HepB).
- Administer the 3-dose series to those who were not previously vaccinated.
- A 2-dose series of Recombivax HB® is licensed for children aged 11–15 years.

8. Inactivated poliovirus vaccine (IPV).
- For children who received an all-IPV or all-oral poliovirus (OPV) series, a fourth dose is not necessary if the third dose was administered at age 4 years or older.
- If both OPV and IPV were administered as part of a series, a total of 4 doses should be administered, regardless of the child's current age.

9. Measles, mumps, and rubella vaccine (MMR).
- If not previously vaccinated, administer 2 doses of MMR during any visit, with 4 or more weeks between the doses.

10. Varicella vaccine.
- Administer 2 doses of varicella vaccine to persons younger than 13 years of age at least 3 months apart. Do not repeat the second dose if administered 28 or more days following the first dose.
- Administer 2 doses of varicella vaccine to persons aged 13 years or older at least 4 weeks apart.

The Recommended Immunization Schedules for Persons Aged 0–18 Years are approved by the Advisory Committee on Immunization Practices (www.cdc.gov/vaccines/recs/acip), the American Academy of Pediatrics (http://www.aap.org), and the American Academy of Family Physicians (http://www.aafp.org).

DEPARTMENT OF HEALTH AND HUMAN SERVICES • CENTERS FOR DISEASE CONTROL AND PREVENTION
SAFER • HEALTHIER • PEOPLE™

Table 31-7   Catch-Up Immunization Schedule for Persons Aged 4 Months–18 Years Who Start Late or Who Are More than 1 Month Behind—United States—2008

The table below provides catch-up schedules and minimum intervals between doses for children whose vaccinations have been delayed. A vaccine series does not need to be restarted, regardless of the time that has elapsed between doses. Use the section appropriate for the child's age.

CATCH-UP SCHEDULE FOR PERSONS AGED 4 MONTHS–6 YEARS

Vaccine	Minimum Age for Dose 1	Minimum Interval Between Doses			
		Dose 1 to Dose 2	Dose 2 to Dose 3	Dose 3 to Dose 4	Dose 4 to Dose 5
Hepatitis B[1]	Birth	4 weeks	8 weeks (and 16 weeks after first dose)		
Rotavirus[2]	6 wks	4 weeks	4 weeks		
Diphtheria, Tetanus, Pertussis[3]	6 wks	4 weeks	4 weeks	6 months	6 months[3]
Haemophilus influenzae type b[4]	6 wks	4 weeks: if first dose administered at younger than 12 months of age 8 weeks (as final dose): if first dose administered at age 12–14 months No further doses needed if first dose administered at 15 months of age or older	4 weeks[4]: if current age is younger than 12 months 8 weeks (as final dose)[4]: if current age is 12 months or older and second dose administered at younger than 15 months of age No further doses needed if previous dose administered at age 15 months or older	8 weeks (as final dose): This dose only necessary for children aged 12 months–5 years who received 3 doses before age 12 months	
Pneumococcal[5]	6 wks	4 weeks: if first dose administered at younger than 12 months of age 8 weeks (as final dose): if first dose administered at age 12 months or older or current age 24–59 months No further doses needed for healthy children if first dose administered at age 24 months or older	4 weeks: if current age is younger than 12 months 8 weeks (as final dose): if current age is 12 months or older No further doses needed for healthy children if previous dose administered at age 24 months or older	8 weeks (as final dose): This dose only necessary for children aged 12 months–5 years who received 3 doses before age 12 months	
Inactivated Poliovirus[6]	6 wks	4 weeks	4 weeks	4 weeks[6]	
Measles, Mumps, Rubella[7]	12 mos	4 weeks			
Varicella[8]	12 mos	3 months			
Hepatitis A[9]	12 mos	6 months			

CATCH-UP SCHEDULE FOR PERSONS AGED 7–18 YEARS

Vaccine	Minimum Age for Dose 1	Dose 1 to Dose 2	Dose 2 to Dose 3	Dose 3 to Dose 4	Dose 4 to Dose 5
Tetanus, Diphtheria/Tetanus, Diphtheria, Pertussis[10]	7 yrs[10]	4 weeks	4 weeks: if first dose administered at younger than 12 months of age	6 months: if first dose administered at younger than 12 months of age	

continued

Table 31-7 Catch-Up Immunization Schedule for Persons Aged 4 Months–18 Years Who Start Late or Who Are More than 1 Month Behind—United States—2008 *Continued*

CATCH-UP SCHEDULE FOR PERSONS AGED 7–18 YEARS

Vaccine	Minimum Age for Dose 1	Minimum Interval Between Doses: Dose 1 to Dose 2	Dose 2 to Dose 3	Dose 3 to Dose 4	Dose 4 to Dose 5
			6 months: if first dose administered at age 12 months or older		
Human Papillomavirus[11]	9 yrs	4 weeks	12 weeks (and 24 weeks after the first dose)		
Hepatitis A[9]	12 mos	6 months			
Hepatitis B[1]	Birth	4 weeks	8 weeks (and 16 weeks after first dose)		
Inactivated Poliovirus[6]	6 wks	4 weeks	4 weeks	4 weeks[6]	
Measles, Mumps, Rubella[7]	12 mos	4 weeks			
Varicella[8]	12 mos	4 weeks: if first dose administered at age 13 years or older 3 months: if first dose administered at younger than 13 years of age			

1. Hepatitis B vaccine (HepB).
- Administer the 3-dose series to those who were not previously vaccinated.
- A 2-dose series of Recombivax HB® is licensed for children aged 11–15 years.

2. Rotavirus vaccine (Rota).
- Do not start the series later than age 12 weeks.
- Administer the final dose in the series by age 32 weeks.
- Do not administer a dose later than age 32 weeks.
- Data on safety and efficacy outside of these age ranges are insufficient.

3. Diphtheria and tetanus toxoids and acellular pertussis vaccine (DTaP).
- The fifth dose is not necessary if the fourth dose was administered at age 4 years or older.
- DTaP is not indicated for persons aged 7 years or older.

4. *Haemophilus influenzae* type b conjugate vaccine (Hib).
- Vaccine is not generally recommended for children aged 5 years or older.
- If current age is younger than 12 months and the first 2 doses were PRP-OMP (PedvaxHIB® or ComVax® [Merck]), the third (and final) dose should be administered at age 12–15 months and at least 8 weeks after the second dose.
- If first dose was administered at age 7–11 months, administer 2 doses separated by 4 weeks plus a booster at age 12–15 months.

5. Pneumococcal conjugate vaccine (PCV).
- Administer one dose of PCV to all healthy children aged 24–59 months having any incomplete schedule.
- For children with underlying medical conditions, administer 2 doses of PCV at least 8 weeks apart if previously received less than 3 doses, or 1 dose of PCV if previously received 3 doses.

6. Inactivated poliovirus vaccine (IPV).
- For children who received an all-IPV or all-oral poliovirus (OPV) series, a fourth dose is not necessary if third dose was administered at age 4 years or older.
- If both OPV and IPV were administered as part of a series, a total of 4 doses should be administered, regardless of the child's current age.
- IPV is not routinely recommended for persons aged 18 years and older.

7. Measles, mumps, and rubella vaccine (MMR).
- The second dose of MMR is recommended routinely at age 4–6 years but may be administered earlier if desired.
- If not previously vaccinated, administer 2 doses of MMR during any visit with 4 or more weeks between the doses.

8. Varicella vaccine.
- The second dose of varicella vaccine is recommended routinely at age 4–6 years but may be administered earlier if desired.
- Do not repeat the second dose in persons younger than 13 years of age if administered 28 or more days after the first dose.

9. Hepatitis A vaccine (HepA).
- HepA is recommended for certain groups of children, including in areas where vaccination programs target older children. See *MMWR* 2006;55(No. RR-7):1–23.

10. Tetanus and diphtheria toxoids vaccine (Td) and tetanus and diphtheria toxoids and acellular pertussis vaccine (Tdap).
- Tdap should be substituted for a single dose of Td in the primary catch-up series or as a booster if age appropriate; use Td for other doses.
- A 5-year interval from the last Td dose is encouraged when Tdap is used as a booster dose. A booster (fourth) dose is needed if any of the previous doses were administered at younger than 12 months of age. Refer to ACIP recommendations for further information. See *MMWR* 2006;55(No. RR-3).

11. Human papillomavirus vaccine (HPV).
- Administer the HPV vaccine series to females at age 13–18 years if not previously vaccinated.

Information about reporting reactions after immunization is available online at http://www.vaers.hhs.gov or by telephone via the 24-hour national toll-free information line 800-822-7967. Suspected cases of vaccine-preventable diseases should be reported to the state or local health department. Additional information, including precautions and contraindications for immunization, is available from the National Center for Immunization and Respiratory Diseases at http://www.cdc.gov/vaccines or telephone, 800-CDC-INFO (800-232-4636).

DEPARTMENT OF HEALTH AND HUMAN SERVICES • CENTERS FOR DISEASE CONTROL AND PREVENTION • SAFER • HEALTHIER • PEOPLE

FAMILY HISTORY

The questions asked about family history for the child are basically the same types of questions that are asked of the adult client (e.g., whether certain diseases/conditions run in the family, the age and cause of death for blood relatives, and family members with communicable diseases). This is an area of the subjective assessment in which the nurse focuses primarily on the parent for the necessary information. An exception might be if the child is older and knows a great deal about his or her family history. As with the past history information, if the child is adopted or a foster child, family history information may not be known. An important reason for collecting these data is to implement preventive teaching at a young age.

Question	Rationale
Do certain diseases/conditions run in the family?	Certain conditions tend to run in families and increase the client's risk for such condition.
Please list the ages and causes of death for blood relatives.	This helps to identify risk factors.
Does the child have family members with communicable diseases?	This also helps to identify risk factors.

REVIEW OF SYSTEMS

It is essential that pertinent subjective data be collected for each body system. Many of the questions for each body system asked of the adult are asked of the parent or child.

The additional nursing history questions listed in the following sections for each system are of special concern in children.

Skin, Hair, Nails

Has your child had any changes in hair texture?	Changes may indicate an underlying problem.
Does your child complain of scalp itching?	Itching may indicate lice, seborrhea, allergies, or ringworm.
Have you noticed any changes in your child's nails? Color? Cracking? Shape? Lines?	Changes may indicate an underlying problem.
Has your child been exposed to any contagious disease such as measles, chickenpox, lice, ringworm, scabies and the like?	These communicable diseases are common in childhood.
Has your child ever had any rashes or sores? Acne?	Rashes may represent a number of diseases/disorders. Acne is a common problem for adolescents. They often have a hard time talking about it but they want treatment.
Has your child had any excessive bruising or burns?	This helps to assess for child abuse. Excessive bruising or burns suggest abuse.
Does your child use any cosmetics? Have tattoos? Have any pierced body parts?	This provides insight into personal habits.
Does your child have any birthmarks?	This helps to identify any lesions and lets the examiner know to assess areas for changes.

continued

REVIEW OF SYSTEMS *Continued*

Question	*Rationale*
Head and Neck	
Has your child ever had a head injury?	Head injuries may cause neurological problems.
Does your child experience headaches? How frequently?	Many neurologic disorders cause headaches.
Has your child ever had swollen neck glands for any significant length of time?	This may indicate an underlying disorder.
Has your child ever experienced any neck stiffness?	Stiffness may indicate disorders such as meningitis.
Eyes	
Does your child excessively cross eyes?	Eye crossing may indicate visual or neurologic problems.
Does your child frequently rub his or her eyes or blink repeatedly?	This could indicate visual problems.
Does your child strain/squint to see distant objects?	These suggest visual problems.
Has your child's vision been tested?	Children require regular vision screening.
Does your child wear glasses or contact lenses? Does she wear them when needed? Do the glasses help your child to see better?	This helps to gauge usage and if the prescription needs to be reassessed.
Ears	
Does your child appear to be paying attention when you speak?	Children should respond. A child who often appears to not be paying attention may have a hearing deficit or neurological disorder.
Does your child speak? At what age did talking start?	It is important to assess developmental milestones.
Does your child or adolescent listen to loud music?	This is common behavior among adolescents and usually does not indicate hearing deficit. However, it can lead to a hearing deficit. Preventative education may be needed.
Does your child use a hearing aid? If so, has it improved the child's ability to interact and understand others.	This helps to evaluate the effectiveness of the hearing aid.
Has your child had frequent ear infections? Tubes in ears?	Frequent ear infections may contribute to hearing loss.
How frequently does your child have his or her hearing tested?	Screening for hearing deficits should be done regularly.
Mouth, Throat, Nose, and Sinuses	
Has your child ever had any difficulty swallowing or chewing?	Difficulty may indicate a mechanical/neurological disorder.
Has your child ever had strep throat, tonsillitis, or any other mouth or throat infections? Does your child get frequent oral lesions?	Past infections may affect current condition.
When did your child's teeth erupt? When did the child lose her baby teeth? When did adult teeth erupt?	See Chapter 30 for a schedule for teeth eruption.

continued on page 706

REVIEW OF SYSTEMS *Continued*

Question	Rationale
Does your child have any dental problems? Does he visit the dentist regularly? Does he wear any dental appliances?	Children should visit the dentist twice a year. If child has frequent dental problems, provide education about dental care and preventive care.
Does your child experience nosebleeds?	Nosebleeds may occur with allergies, trauma, nose-picking, or foreign bodies.
Does your child have any sinus problems?	Sinus pain may indicate allergies or infection.

Thorax and Lungs

Question	Rationale
Has your child ever had cough, wheezing, shortness or breath, nocturnal dyspnea; if so, when does it occur?	Many respiratory problems, such as asthma and bronchitis, are frequently seen in children. They may affect current health status.
Has your child received the influenza vaccine?	American Academy of Pediatrics (AAP) recommends children who are 6 months old and older with high risk health conditions receive influenza immunization annually (AAP, 2008).
Does your child smoke? When did the child start smoking? How much does he smoke?	Smoking increases the risk for many diseases, including lung cancer. Provide appropriate client teaching.
Is your child exposed to second-hand smoke? (Adolescents and older school-age children should be asked about smoking, including smokeless tobacco, in private.)	Respiratory infections are more common in children exposed to second-hand smoke.

Breasts and Lymphatics

Question	Rationale
Has your daughter started developing breasts (thelarche)? If so, when did development start?	This helps to determine the child's sexual development stage.
Have you noticed any abnormal breast development in your son or young daughter?	Gynecomastia is enlargement of breast tissue in males. It is a normal finding during puberty.

Heart and Neck Vessels

Question	Rationale
Has your child ever experienced chest pain, heart murmurs, congenital heart disease, or hypertension?	All of these symptoms indicate possible cardiac problems.
Has your child ever complained of fatigue? Does your child have difficulty keeping up with peers when running or exercising?	Fatigue may result from decreased cardiac output. Heart problems may impede the child's ability to perform physical activities.
Has your child ever fainted?	Children who faint should be screened for cardiac problems.
Has your child ever turned "blue" during activity?	This may suggest cardiac arrhythmia.
Do you believe that your child is meeting the normal growth requirements for his or her age?	Children with congenital heart disease may grow and develop more slowly than other children.

Peripheral Vascular System

Question	Rationale
Does your child ever experience bluing of the extremities? Do our child's hands and/or feet get unusually cold?	Cyanosis and/or coldness in the extremities suggests vascular problems.
Has your child ever had problems with blood clots?	A history of blood clots increases the risk of recurrence.

continued

Question	Rationale
Abdomen	
Has your child ever had any excessive vomiting? Abdominal pain? Please describe.	Excessive vomiting may be associated with gastrointestinal problems. Abdominal pain may accompany many disorders/problems.
Does your child have any digestive problems (i.e., irritable bowel, constipation)?	Bowel problems should be explored further.
Has your child ever experienced any trauma to the abdomen?	Trauma may result in injuries or contribute to disorders.
Does your child have any hernias?	
Genitalia and Sexuality	
How often does your child urinate? How many wet diapers do you change per day?	This helps to determine nutritional habits, e.g., is the child receiving enough fluids?
At what age was your child toilet (bladder) trained? Night?	This helps to determine whether and when child reaches developmental milestones.
Does your child ever wet his or her pants?	If there is a history of enuresis, obtain routine that family follows to deal with problem.
Is there any history of frequency, burning, pain during urination?	These genitourinary problems should be further explored.
Do you have any concerns about your child related to masturbation, asking/answering questions about sex, not respecting other's privacy, or wanting too much privacy?	This helps to assess the child's sexual development.
Has anyone ever touched your child in a way that made him or her feel uncomfortable? (Make sure to ask the parent and child this question.)	It is important to screen for sexual abuse.
Has child started puberty, thelarche, menarche?	See Tables 31-1, 31-2, and 31-3 for Tanner's stages of sexual development.
Has the child started having wet dreams (nocturnal emissions)?	Pubescent clients should be reassured that nocturnal emissions are normal.
Who is/are the source(s) of sex/AIDS education? Questions to the adolescent about sexuality and reproductive issues should be asked privately. Gynecologists recommend that the first visit to the gynecologist be between the ages of 13 to 15 years for health screening, guidance and preventive services (ACOG, 2004).	This helps to determine the child's need for sexual education.
Do you know how to perform breast self-examination or testicular self-examination?	Self-examination is an important screening tool and should be taught.
Ask about menstruation: How old were you when you started menstruating? When was your last menstrual period? What is your menstrual cycle schedule? Has it always been this way?	This assesses the client's development and gynecological needs.

continued on page 708

Question	Rationale
What is your bleeding like? Light, moderate, heavy?	
Do you experience any cramps? Tell me about them?	
Do you experience any other physical or emotional discomfort associated with menstruation?	
Do you use tampons? How frequently do you change them?	
Assess sexual history:	A careful sexual history should be taken for all sexually active clients.
What was your age at first intercourse?	
Have you received information regarding the Human Papillomavirus vaccine that can reduce the incidence of cervical cancer? Have you received the vaccine?	All girls and women 9–25 years of age who have not previously been immunized should receive the 3 doses of the Quadrivalent Human Papillomavirus vaccine (HPV), administered intramuscular at 0, 2, and 6 months. HPV vaccine is not recommended during pregnancy (AAP, Committee on Infectious Diseases, 2007). The vaccine prevents development of the 4 types of HPV (6, 11, 16, and 18) that are responsible for 70% of cervical cancer (16 & 18) and 90% of genital warts (6 & 11). Prevention is most effective if the vaccine is administered between 9 and 15 years of age and prior to the first sexual intercourse (AAP, 2007).
Have you ever had a pap smear? Do you experience any discomfort/pain with intercourse?	The American Cancer Society recommends a first pap smear for cervical cancer should be performed no later than 3 years after their first intercourse or no later than 21 years of age (ACOG, 2004).
How many sexual partners do you have/have you had?	
What type of contraception do you use and how do you use it? Do you use condoms? How do you use them?	Contraceptive education (preventive education) should be provided.
Have you ever had a sexually transmitted disease?	
Were you ever pregnant? What was the result of that pregnancy?	
Have you had or considered having a gynecologic examination?	This examination should be performed for all sexually active adolescent girls and is suggested as a routine examination for those older than 21 years of age (ACOG, 2004).
Anus and Rectum	
How often does your child have bowel movement? What does it look like?	This helps to assess the child's nutritional intake and gastrointestinal function.
At what age was your child toilet trained (bowel)?	This helps to determine whether and when child reaches developmental milestones.
Does your child ever soil his or her pants?	With a history of encopresis, obtain the routine that the family follows to deal with problem.
Is there any history of bleeding, constipation, diarrhea, rectal itching, or hemorrhoids?	Hemorrhoids are very unusual in children, unless chronically constipated. They may indicate an intraabdominal mass or child abuse (sodomy).
Musculoskeletal System	
Has your child ever had limited range of motion, joint pain, stiffness, paralysis? Have you noticed any bone deformity?	A positive history of any of these requires further investigation.

continued

REVIEW OF SYSTEMS *Continued*

Question	Rationale
Has your child ever had any fractures?	Frequent fractures may suggest a disorder of the musculoskeletal system or child abuse.
Has your child ever used any corrective devices (orthopedic shoes, scoliosis brace)?	This should be noted as it may affect/explain findings during the physical examination.
Describe your child's posture?	Children, especially females, should be screened for scoliosis.
Is your child involved in any sports? What type of protective gear do they use?	Provide appropriate client teaching about safety and protective gear as needed.
Neurologic System Does your child have any learning disabilities? Does your child have any attention problems at home or at school?	Learning disabilities may hinder a child's performance at school and/or indicate a neurological disorder.
Has your child ever experienced any problems with memory?	Memory problems may indicate neurological disorders.
Has your child ever had a seizure?	Seizures may indicate a neurological or cardiovascular disorder.
Has your child ever had a head injury?	Head trauma may cause intracranial bleeding or other injuries.
Has your child ever experienced any problems with motor coordination?	Uncoordinated movements or difficulty with coordination may indicate neurological disorders.

Growth and Development

Nurses must possess a baseline knowledge of the fundamental principles of growth and development as well as strategies for assessment and client teaching. Several theories exist regarding the various stages and phases of development. It is suggested that nurses review the basic principles of the major theorists, such as Erikson and Piaget, to refresh their frames of reference. Information about these theorists is readily accessible in any basic or developmental psychology text. The Denver Developmental Screening Test is also available for guidance when assessing the child's motor, language, and social development at the particular age (see Chapter 30, Assessment Tool 30-1).

Growth Patterns

Appendix F includes pediatric growth charts.

TODDLERS

Height and weight increase in a steplike rather than a linear fashion, reflecting the growth spurts and lags characteristic of toddlerhood. The toddler's characteristic protruding abdomen results from underdeveloped abdominal muscles. Bow-leggedness typically persists through toddlerhood because the leg muscles must bear the weight of the relatively large trunk. The height at age 2 years approximately equals one-half of the child's adult height. The child's birth weight quadruples by age 2.5 years. HC equals chest circumference by 1 to 2 years. Total increase in HC in the second year of life is 2.5 cm, and the rate then increases slowly at 0.5 inch per year until age 5 years. Primary dentition (20 deciduous teeth) is completed by 2.5 years.

PRESCHOOLERS

Preschoolers are generally slender, graceful, and agile. The average 4-year-old child is 101.25 cm tall and weighs 16.8 kg (37 lb).

SCHOOL-AGE CHILDREN

During the school-age period, girls often grow faster than boys and commonly surpass boys in height and weight. During preadolescence extending from about age 10 to 13, children commonly experience rapid and uneven growth compared with age mates. The average 6-year-old child is 112.5 cm tall and weighs 21 kg (46 lb), whereas the average 12-year-old child is 147.5 cm tall and weighs 40 kg (88 lb). Beginning around age 6, permanent teeth erupt and deciduous teeth are gradually lost. Caries, malocclusion, and periodontal disease become evident.

ADOLESCENTS

From 20% to 25% of adult height is achieved in adolescence. Girls grow 5 to 20 cm until about age 16 or 17. Boys grow 10 to 30 cm until about 18 or 20 years of age. From 30% to 50% of adult weight is achieved during adolescence (see Appendix F). Adolescence encompasses puberty—the period during which primary and secondary sex characteristics begin to develop and reach maturity. In girls, puberty begins between the ages of 8 and 14 years and is completed within 3 years. In boys, puberty begins between the ages of 9 and 16 years and is completed by age 18 or 19. During adolescence, hormonal influence causes important developmental changes.

Body mass reaches adult size, sebaceous glands become active, and eccrine sweat glands become fully functional. Apocrine sweat glands develop, and hair grows in the axillae, areola of the breast, and genital and anal regions. Body hair assumes characteristic distribution patterns and texture changes (see Tables 31-1, 31-2, and 31-3).

During puberty, girls experience growth in height, weight, breast development, and pelvic girth with expansion of uterine tissue. Menarche typically occurs about 2.5 years after onset of puberty. Boys experience increases in height, weight, muscle mass, and penis and testicle size. Facial and body hair growth and voice deepening also occur. The onset of spontaneous nocturnal emissions of seminal fluid is an overt sign of puberty, analogous to menarche in girls. Sexual development is evaluated by noting the specific stages that take place in boys and girls.

Motor Development

TODDLERS

Motor development should be evaluated at well-child visits. Using the Denver Developmental Tool can assist the nurse in noting the developmental milestones of the child at the particular age.

The major gross motor skill is locomotion. At 15 months, toddlers walk without help (Fig. 31-4). At 18 months, they walk upstairs with one hand held. At 24 months, toddlers walk up and down stairs one step at a time. At 30 months, they jump with both feet.

Fifteen-month-old toddlers can build a two-block tower and scribble spontaneously. At 18 months, they can build a three- to four-block tower. Toddlers at 24 months imitate a vertical stroke; at 30 months, they build an eight-block tower and copy a cross.

Sample questions for toddlerhood include

- When did your child first walk?
- Can your toddler walk up and down steps?
- Can your toddler jump with both feet?
- Does your toddler spontaneously scribble?

PRESCHOOLERS

At 3 years old, children can ride a tricycle (Fig. 31-5), go upstairs using alternate feet, stand on one foot for a few seconds, and broad jump. Four-year-old children can skip, hop on one foot, catch a ball, and go downstairs using alternate feet. At

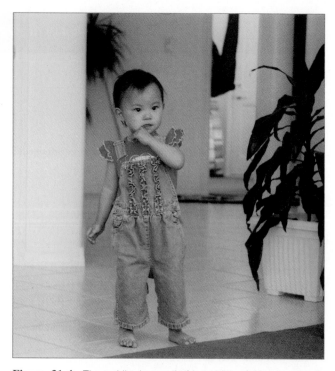

Figure 31-4   The toddler is proud of her ability to stand and walk without help.

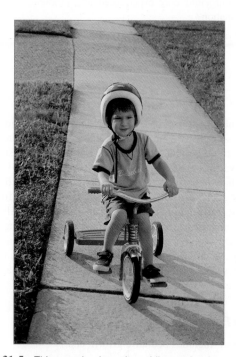

Figure 31-5   This preschooler enjoys riding a tricycle.

5 years, children can skip on alternate feet, throw and catch a ball, jump rope, and balance on alternate feet with eyes closed.

Three-year-old children can build a tower of up to 10 blocks, build three-block bridges, copy a circle, and imitate a cross. At 4 years old, children can lace shoes, copy a square shape, trace a diamond shape, and add three parts to a stick figure. A five-year-old child can tie shoelaces, use scissors well, copy diamond and triangle shapes, add seven to nine parts to a stick figure, and print a few letters and numbers and her or his first name.

Sample questions for preschoolers include

• Can your preschooler run, hop, and skip?
• Can your preschooler lace shoes?
• Can your preschooler write his or her first name?

SCHOOL-AGE CHILDREN

Skills acquired during the school years include bicycling, rollerskating, rollerblading, and skateboarding. Running and jumping improve progressively, and swimming is added to the child's repertoire.

Printing skills develop in the early school years; script skills in later years. School-age children also develop greater dexterity and competence for crafts (Fig. 31-6), video games, and computers.

Sample questions for school-age children include

• Can your school-age child ride a bicycle?
• Can your school-age child write script?

ADOLESCENTS

Gross motor skills have reached adult levels, and fine motor skills continue to be refined.

Sample questions for the adolescent include

• Does your adolescent have a job, hobby, or interest that involves hand skills? If so, how is his or her performance?
• Does you adolescent participate in sports?

Sensory Perception
TODDLERS

Toddlers' visual acuity and depth perception improve, and they are able to recall visual images. Toddlers begin learning the

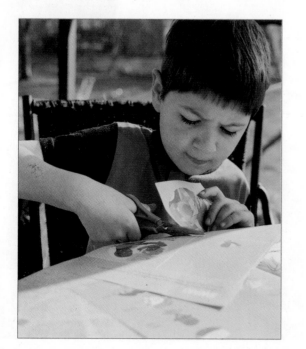

Figure 31-6 This 6-year-old enjoys cutting shapes with safety scissors.

ability to listen and comprehend. As every parent knows, listening is different from hearing. This ability includes attending to what is heard, discriminating sound qualities, creating cognitive associations with previous learning, and remembering. The olfactory and gustatory senses are influenced by voluntary control and are associated with other sensory and motor areas. Therefore, toddlers refuse to eat anything that looks unpleasant to them. Children also begin to learn conditioned reactions to odors at this age.

PRESCHOOLERS

Color and depth perception become fully developed. Preschoolers may be aware of visual difficulties. Hearing reaches its maximum level and listening further develops. Preschoolers usually enjoy vision and hearing testing.

SCHOOL-AGE CHILDREN

Visual capacity reaches adult level (20/20) by age 6 or 7 years. Hearing acuity is almost complete.

ADOLESCENTS

All senses have reached their mature capacity by adolescence.

Sample questions to assess for vision problems include

Does your child frequently rub his eyes?

Does your child become irritable with close work?

Does your child blink repeatedly?

Does your child ever appear cross-eyed?

Does your child strain to see distant objects or sit close to the TV?

Does your child reverse letters or numbers?

Does your child ever complain of headache?

Sample questions to assess for hearing deficits include:

Does your child respond to verbal commands? (Remember that we can only test hearing, not listening.)

Does your child sit too close to the TV?

Does your adolescent blast the stereo? (This may not indicate a hearing deficit, as it is typical behavior; however, it can lead to hearing deficit.)

Does your child have any speech difficulties?

Sample questions to assess sense of smell and taste include:

Does your child ever complain of having difficulty with his sense of smell?

Does your child experience difficulty with taste?

Cognitive and Language and Development
TODDLERS

The sensorimotor phase (between ages 12 and 24 months) involves two substages in toddlerhood: tertiary circular reactions (age 12 to 18 months) involving trial-and-error experimentation and relentless exploration and mental combinations (age 18 to 24 months) during which the toddler begins to devise new means for accomplishing tasks through mental calculations. Toddlers go through a preconceptual substage of the preoperational phase typical of preschoolers. During this time, the child uses representational thought to recall the past, represent the present, and anticipate the future. As toddlers get older, they begin to enter the preoperational phase. This phase is described in the following section on preschoolers.

At 15 months, toddlers use expressive jargon. At 2 years, they say 300 words and use 2-to 3-word phrases and pronouns. At 2.5 years, toddlers give their first and last names and use plurals.

Sample nursing history questions for toddlers include

- Can your toddler name some body parts?
- Can your toddler state first and last name?
- Does your toddler imitate adults?
- Does your toddler put two words together to form sentence? (e.g., "me go")?

PRESCHOOLERS

This stage of preoperational thought (age 2 to 7 years) consists of two phases. In the preconceptual phase, extending from age 2 to 4, the child forms concepts that are not as complete or logical as an adult's; makes simple classifications; associates one event with a simultaneous one (transductive reasoning); and exhibits egocentric thinking.

In the intuitive phase extending from age 4 to 7, the child becomes capable of classifying, quantifying, and relating objects but remains unaware of the principles behind these operations; exhibits intuitive thought processes (is aware that something is right but cannot say why); is unable to see viewpoint of others; and uses many words appropriately but without a real knowledge of their meaning. Preschoolers exhibit magical thinking and believe that thoughts are all-powerful. They may feel guilty and responsible for bad thoughts, which, at times, may coincide with the occurrence of a wished event (e.g., wishing a sibling were dead and the sibling suddenly needs to be hospitalized.).

Three-year-old children can say 900 words, 3- to 4-word sentences, and can talk incessantly. Four-year-old children can say 1,500 words, tell exaggerated stories, and sing simple songs. This is also the peak age for "why" questions. Five-year-old children can say 2,100 words, and they know four or more colors, the names of the days of the week, and the months.

Sample questions for preschoolers include

- Does your preschooler tell fantasy stories or have an imaginary friend?
- Does your preschooler have an invisible friend?
- Can your preschooler make simple classifications? (e.g., dogs and cats)?
- Is your preschooler "chatty"? Does your preschooler frequently ask "why?"
- Can your preschooler name at least four colors?

SCHOOL-AGE CHILDREN

A child aged 7 to 11 years is in the stage of concrete operations marked by inductive reasoning, logical operations, and reversible concrete thought. Specific characteristics of this stage include movement from egocentric to objective thinking:

seeing another's point of view; seeking validation and asking questions; focusing on immediate physical reality with inability to transcend the here and now; difficulty dealing with remote, future, or hypothetical matters; development of various mental classifying and ordering activities; and development of the principle of conservation of volume, weight, mass, and numbers. Typical activities of a child at this stage may include collecting and sorting objects (e.g., baseball cards, dolls, marbles); ordering items according to size, shape, weight, and other criteria; and considering options and variables when problem solving. Electronic games (X-Box, PlayStation) are popular with this age group.

Children develop formal adult articulation patterns by age 7 to 9. They learn that words can be arranged in terms of structure. The ability to read is one of the most significant skills learned during these years (Fig. 31-7).

Sample questions for school-age children include

- Can your school-age child see another's point of view?
- Does your school-age child collect things? (e.g., baseball cards, dolls)?
- Does your school-age child try to solve problems?
- How well does your school-age child do in school? Also ask school-age child and compare the answers.
- How well does your school-age child read?

ADOLESCENTS

In the development of formal operations, which commonly occurs from ages 11 to 15 years, the adolescent develops abstract

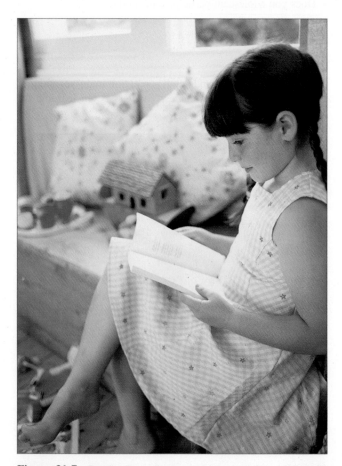

Figure 31-7 Reading is a milestone achievement for a school-age child.

reasoning. This period consists of three substages:

Substage 1: The adolescent sees relationships involving the inverse of the reciprocal.

Substage 2: The adolescent develops the ability to order triads of propositions or relationships.

Substage 3: The adolescent develops the capacity for true formal thought.

In true formal thought, the adolescent thinks beyond the present and forms theories about everything, delighting especially in considerations of "that which is not." However, adolescents in this age group do not have futuristic thoughts. They do not relate current events "here and now" to long-term results (2 years from now). An example of this includes teenagers who are sexually active and who may not consider the consequences of sexual activity (pregnancy and parenthood).

Sample nursing history questions for adolescents include

- Do you consider your adolescent to be a problem solver?
- How well does your adolescent do in school? Also ask the adolescent and compare the responses.

Moral Development (Kolberg)

TODDLER

A toddler is typically at the first substage of the preconventional stage involving punishment and obedience orientation in which he or she makes judgments on the basis of avoiding punishment or obtaining a reward. Discipline patterns affect a toddler's moral development. For example, physical punishment and withholding privileges tend to give the toddler a negative view of morals; withholding love and affection as punishment leads to feelings of guilt in the toddler. Appropriate disciplinary actions include providing simple explanations about why certain behaviors are unacceptable, praising appropriate behavior, and using distraction when the toddler is headed for danger.

PRESCHOOLER

A preschooler is in the preconventional stage of moral development, which extends to 10 years. In this phase, conscience emerges, and the emphasis is on external control. The child's moral standards are those of others, and he or she observes them either to avoid punishment or reap rewards.

SCHOOL-AGE CHILD

A child at the conventional level of the role conformity stage (generally age 10 to 13 years) has an increased desire to please others. The child observes and, to some extent, externalizes the standards of others. The child wants to be considered "good" by those people whose opinion matters to him or her.

ADOLESCENT

Development of the postconventional level of morality occurs at about age 13, marked by the development of an individual conscience and a defined set of moral values. For the first time, the adolescent can acknowledge a conflict between two socially accepted standards and try to decide between them. Control of conduct is now internal, both in standards observed and in reasoning about right or wrong.

Sample nursing history questions for toddlerhood through adolescence include

- Does your child understand the difference between right and wrong?
- Do you discuss family values with your child?
- Do you have family rules? How are they implemented?
- How are disciplinary measures handled?
- Has your child ever had any problems with lying, cheating, or stealing?
- Has your child ever required disciplinary action at school?
- Has your child ever violated the law?

Psychosocial Development (Erikson)

TODDLER

Erikson terms the psychosocial crises facing a child between ages 1 and 3 years *autonomy versus shame and doubt*. The psychosocial theme is "to hold on; to let go." The toddler has developed a sense of trust and is ready to give up dependence to assert his or her budding sense of control, independence, and autonomy (Fig. 31-8). The toddler begins to master the following:

- Individuation—differentiation of self from others
- Separation from parent(s)
- Control over bodily functions
- Communication with words
- Acquisition of socially acceptable behavior
- Egocentric interactions with others

The toddler has learned that his or her parents are predictable and reliable. The toddler begins to learn that his or her own behavior has a predictable, reliable effect on others. The toddler learns to wait longer for needs gratification. The toddler often uses "no" even when he or she means "yes." This is done to assert independence (negativistic behavior). A sense of shame and doubt can develop if the toddler is kept dependent in areas where he or she is capable of using newly acquired skills or if made to feel inadequate when attempting new skills. A toddler often continues to seek a familiar security object, such as a blanket, during times of stress.

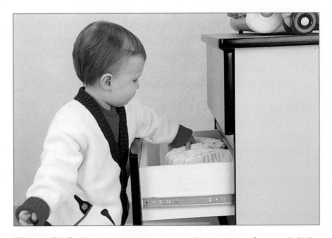

Figure 31-8 Toddlers love to assert their sense of control, independence, and autonomy.

Sample questions for the toddler include

- Does your toddler try to do things for himself or herself (e.g., feed, dress)?
- Does your toddler have temper tantrums? How are they handled?
- Does your toddler frequently use the word "no"?
- At what age was your toddler completely toilet trained?
- Does your toddler actively explore the environment?

PRESCHOOLER

Between ages 3 and 6 years, a child faces a psychosocial crisis that Erikson terms *initiative versus guilt*. The child's significant other is the family. At this age, the child has normally mastered a sense of autonomy and moves on to master a sense of initiative. A preschooler is an energetic, enthusiastic, and intrusive learner with an active imagination. Conscience (an inner voice that warns and threatens) begins to develop. The child explores the physical world with all his or her senses and powers. Development of a sense of guilt occurs when the child is made to feel that his or her imagination and activities are unacceptable. Guilt, anxiety, and fear result when the child's thoughts and activities clash with parental expectations. A preschooler begins to use simple reasoning and can tolerate longer periods of delayed gratification.

Sample questions for the preschooler include

- Does your preschooler have an active imagination?
- Does your preschooler imitate adult activities?
- Does your preschooler engage in fantasy play?
- Does your preschooler frequently ask questions?
- Does your preschooler enjoy new activities?

SCHOOL-AGE CHILD

Erikson terms the psychosocial crisis faced by a child aged 6 to 12 years *industry versus inferiority*. During this period, the child's radius of significant others expands to include school and instructive adults. A school-age child normally has mastered the first three developmental tasks—trust, autonomy, and initiative—and now focuses on mastering industry. A child's sense of industry grows out of a desire for real achievement. The child engages in tasks and activities that he or she can carry through to completion. The child learns rules and how to compete with others and to cooperate to achieve goals. Social relationships with others become increasingly important sources of support. The child can develop a sense of inferiority stemming from unrealistic expectations or a sense of failing to meet standards set for him or her by others. Because the child feels inadequate, his or her self-esteem sags.

Sample questions for the school-age child include

- What are your school-age child's interests/hobbies?
- Does your school-age child interact well with teachers, peers?
- Does your school-age child enjoy accomplishments?
- Does your school-age child shame self for failures?
- What is your school-age child's favorite activity?

ADOLESCENT

Erikson terms the psychosocial crisis faced by adolescents (aged 13 to 18 years) *identity versus role diffusion*. For an adolescent, the radius of significant others is the peer group. To an adolescent, development of who he or she is and where he or she is going becomes a central focus. The adolescent continues to redefine his or her self-concept and the roles that he or she can play with certainty. As rapid physical changes occur, adolescents must reintegrate previous trust in their body, themselves, and how they appear to others. The inability to develop a sense of who he or she is and what he or she can become results in role diffusion and inability to solve core conflicts.

Sample questions for adolescents include

- Does your adolescent have a peer group?
- Does your adolescent have a best friend?
- Does your adolescent exhibit rebellious behavior at home?
- How does your adolescent see self as fitting in with peers?
- What does your adolescent want to do with her life?

Psychosexual Development (Freud)

It is suggested that children of all ages be questioned about sexual abuse. This may be elicited by asking, "Has anyone ever touched you where or when you did not want to be touched?"

TODDLER

In the *anal stage,* typically extending from age 8 months to 4 years, the erogenous zone is the anus and buttocks and sexual activity centers on the expulsion and retention of body waste. In this stage, the child's focus shifts from the mouth to the anal area with emphasis on bowel control as he or she gains neuromuscular control over the anal sphincter. The toddler experiences both satisfaction and frustration as he or she gains control over withholding and expelling, containing and releasing. The conflict between "holding on" and "letting go" gradually resolves as bowel training progresses; resolution occurs once control is firmly established. Toilet training is a major task of toddlerhood (Fig. 31-9). Readiness is not usual until 18 to 24 months of age. Bowel training occurs before bladder;

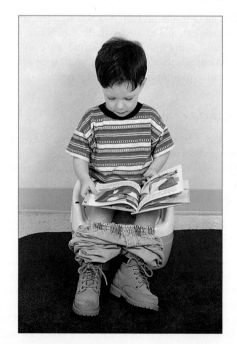

Figure 31-9 Toilet training is a major task of toddlerhood.

night bladder training usually does not occur until 3 to 5 years of age. Masturbation can occur from body exploration. Toddlers learn words associated with anatomy and elimination and can distinguish the sexes.

Sample questions for the toddler include

• Does your toddler have any problems with toilet training?
• Does your toddler masturbate?

PRESCHOOLER

In the *phallic stage* extending from about 3 to 7 years of age, the child's pleasure centers on the genitalia and masturbation. Many preschoolers masturbate for physiologic pleasure. The Oedipal stage occurs, marked by jealousy and rivalry toward the same-sex parent and love of the opposite-sex parent. The Oedipal stage typically resolves in the late preschool period with a strong identification with the same-sex parent. Sexual identity is developed during this time. Modesty may become a concern, and the preschooler may have fears of castration. Because preschoolers are keen observers but poor interpreters, the child may recognize but not understand sexual activity. Before answering a child's questions about sex, parents should clarify what the child is really asking and what the child already thinks about the specific subject. Questions about sex should be answered simply and honestly, providing only the information that the child requests; additional details can come later.

Sample questions for the preschooler include

• Does your preschooler masturbate?
• Does your preschooler know what sex he or she is?
• Has your preschooler asked questions about sex, childbirth, and the like?

SCHOOL-AGE CHILD

The *latency period,* extending from about 5 to 12 years, represents a stage of relative sexual indifference before puberty and adolescence. During this period, development of self-esteem is closely linked with a developing sense of industry in gaining a concept of one's value and worth. Preadolescence begins near the end of the school-age years and discrepancies in growth and maturation between the sexes become apparent. A school age child has acquired much of his or her knowledge of and many of his or her attitudes toward sex at a very early age. During the school-age years, the child refines this knowledge and these attitudes. Questions about sex require honest answers based on the child's level of understanding.

Sample questions for the school age child include

• Does your school-age child interact with same-sex peers?
• What has your school-age child been told about puberty and sex?

ADOLESCENT

In the *genital stage,* which extends from about age 12 to 20 years, an adolescent focuses on the genitals as an erogenous zone and engages in masturbation and sexual relations with others. During this period of renewed sexual drive, an adolescent experiences conflict between his or her own needs for sexual satisfaction and society's expectations for control of sexual expression. Core concerns of adolescents include body image development and acceptance by the opposite sex. Relationships

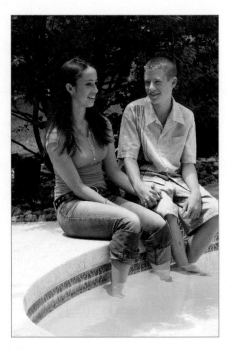

Figure 31-10 During adolescence, relationships with the opposite sex are important stepping stones to adulthood.

with the opposite sex are important (Fig. 31-10). Adolescents engage in sexual activity for pleasure, to satisfy drives and curiosity, as a conquest, for affection, and because of peer pressure. Teaching about sexual function, begun during the school years, should expand to cover more in-depth information on the physical, hormonal, and emotional changes of puberty. An adolescent needs accurate, complete information on sexuality and cultural and moral values. Information must include how pregnancy occurs; methods of preventing pregnancy stressing that male and female partners both are responsible for contraception; and transmission of and protection against sexually transmitted diseases, especially acquired immunodeficiency syndrome (AIDS) and hepatitis.

A full, confidential sexual/sexuality history should be obtained from adolescents. This history includes questioning previously noted in the reproductive review of systems as well as

• What is your sexual preference?
• How do you feel about becoming a man/woman?

Lifestyle and Health Practices
Normal Nutritional Requirements

Proper nutrition is necessary for childhood growth and development. Food and feeding are important parts of growing up with needs and desires changing as the child grows (Fig. 31-11). Table 31-8 provides several nutritional requirements for each age group.

General overviews for each phase of nutritional follow.

TODDLERS

Growth rate slows dramatically during the toddler years, thus decreasing the need for calories, protein, and fluid.

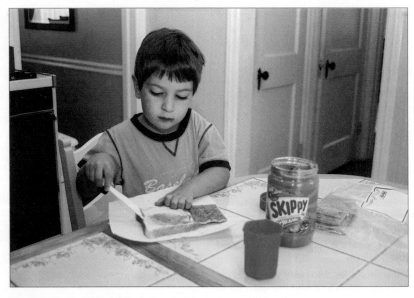

Figure 31-11   This toddler enjoys helping prepare his lunch.

Table 31-8	How Food Label Reference Values (DV) Compare to the Nutritional Recommendations for Children

		Nutrient Recommendations by Age (DRI)*				
Nutrient	DV	2–3 years	4–8 years	9–13 years	14–18 yr girls	14–18 yr boys
Protein (grams)	50	13	19	34	46	52
Iron (mg)	18	7	10	8	15	11
Calcium (mg)	1000	500	800	1300	1300	1300
Vitamin A (IU)	5000	1000	1333	2000	2333	3000
Vitamin C (mg)	60	15	25	45	65	75
Fiber (g)	23	14–19	19–23	23–28 (girls) 25–31 (boys)	23	31–34
Sodium (mg)	2400	1000–1500	1200–1900	1500–2200	1500–2300	1500–2300
Cholesterol (mg)	300	<300 for over age 2	<300	<300	<300	<300
Total Fat (g)**	65	33–54 (30–35% of calories)	39–62 (25–35% of calories)	62–85 (25–35% calories)	55–78 (25–35% calories)	61–95 (25–35% of calories)
Saturated Fat (g)**	20	12–16 (>age 2) (<10% calories)	16 to 18 (<10% calories)	girls: 18–22 boys: 20–24 (<10% calories)	22 (<10% calories)	24–27 (<10% calories)
Calories***	2000	1000–1400 (2–3 years)	1400–1600	girls: 1600–2000 boys: 1800–2200	2000	2200–2400

Baylor College of Medicine. (2007). How food label reference values (DV) compare to the nutritional recommendations for children. Available at http://www.bcm.edu.

Starting at about 12 months, most toddlers are eating the same foods as the rest of the family. At 18 months, many toddlers experience physiologic anorexia and become picky eaters. They experience food jags and eat large amounts one day and very little the next. They like to feed themselves and prefer small portions of appetizing foods. Frequent, nutritious snacks can replace a meal. Food should not be used as a reward or a punishment. Milk should be limited to no more than 1 quart per day to ensure intake and absorption of iron-enriched foods to prevent anemia. Recommendations for screening for anemia should be based on age, sex, and risk of anemia.

PRESCHOOLERS

Requirements are similar to those of the toddler. Three- and four-year-old children may still be unable to sit with family during meals. Four-year-old children are picky eaters. Five-year-old children are influenced by food habits of others. A 5-year-old child tends to be focused on the "social" aspects of eating: table conversation, manners, willingness to try new foods, and help with meal preparation and cleanup.

SCHOOL-AGE CHILDREN

A school-age child's daily caloric requirements diminish in relation to body size. Caregivers should continue to stress the need for a balanced diet from the food pyramid because resources are being stored for the increased growth needs of adolescence. The child is exposed to broader eating experiences in the school lunchroom; he or she may still be a "picky" eater but should be more willing to try new foods. Children may trade, sell, or throw away home-packed school lunches. At home, the child should eat what the family eats; the patterns that develop now stay with the child into adulthood.

ADOLESCENTS

An adolescent's daily intake should be balanced among the foods in the pyramid; average daily caloric intake requirements vary with sex and age, as noted in Table 31-8. Adolescents typically eat whatever they have at break activities; readily available nutritious snacks provide good insurance for a balanced diet. Milk (calcium) and protein are needed in quantity to aid in bone and muscle growth. Maintaining adequate quality and quantity of daily intake may be difficult because of factors such as busy schedule, influence of peers, and easy availability of fast foods. Family eating patterns established during the school years continue to influence an adolescent's food selection. Female adolescents are very prone to negative dieting behaviors. Common dietary deficiencies include iron, folate, and zinc.

Sample nursing history questions for toddlerhood to adolescence include

- What does your child eat in a typical day?
- Is your child on any special type of diet? If so, what for?
- What types of food does your child like/dislike most?

- Does your child have any feeding problems?
- Is your child allergic to any foods? If so, how does your child react to those foods?
- Does your child take any vitamin or mineral supplements?
- How much fluid does your child drink per day?
- Is your water fluorinated? If not, does your child take supplements?
- Has your child had any recent weight gain or loss?

These questions should be also asked directly of adolescents when parents are not present:

- Does your child have any concerns with body image?
- Has your child been on any self-imposed diet?
- How often does your child weigh himself or herself?
- Has your child ever used any of the following methods for weight loss: self-induced vomiting? Laxatives? Diuretics? Excessive exercise? Fasting?

Normal Activity and Exercise

Activity and exercise are important components of a child's life and, therefore, should be assessed when a complete subjective examination is being performed. Play, activity, and exercise patterns can give the nurse valuable clues about the overall health of a child. Display 31-2 describes play characteristics across childhood. This assessment also allows the examiner to provide health promotion teaching.

Sample nursing history questions for toddlerhood to adolescence include

- What is your child's activity like during a typical 24-hour day (including activities of daily living, play, and school)?
- What are your child's favorite activities and toys?
- How many hours of television or video games does your child watch per day? What is his or her favorite programs/movies? Do you discuss TV shows/movies with your child?
- Are there any restrictions on TV watching (content, hours, relationship to chores/homework)?
- What chores does your child do at home (school-age child/adolescent)?
- Does the older child/adolescent work outside the home? What does he or she do?
- How many hours does he or she work during the school year?
- Does the work interfere with school or social life?
- Why does the child work?
- Does your child have any problems that restrict physical activity?
- Does your child require any special devices to manage with activities of daily living/play?
- At what age did your child first walk?
- Can your child keep up with his or her peers?
- Does your child have any hobbies/interests (ages 6 and older)?
- What sports does your child participate in?

(text continues on page 719)

DISPLAY 31-2	Characteristics of Play Among Children

Toddlers

Toddlers engage in parallel play—they play alongside, not with, others. Imitation is one of the most common forms of play and locomotion skills can be enhanced with push-pull toys. Toddlers change toys frequently because of short attention spans.

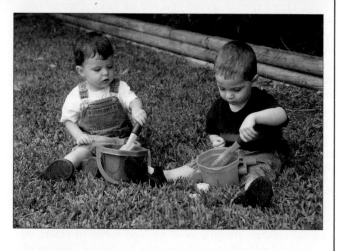

Preschoolers

Typical preschool play is associative—interactive and cooperative with sharing. Preschoolers need contact with age mates. Activities, such as jumping, running and climbing, promote growth and motor skills. Preschoolers are at a typical age for imaginary playmates. Imitative, imaginative, and dramatic play are important. TV and video games should only be a part of the child's play and parents should monitor content and amount of time spent in use. Associative play materials include dress-up clothes and dolls, housekeeping toys, play tents, puppets, and doctor and nurse kits. Curious and active preschoolers need adult supervision, especially near bodies of water and gym sets.

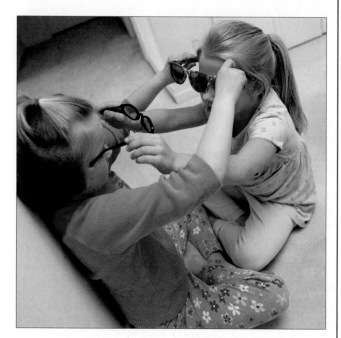

School-Age Children

Play becomes more competitive and complex during the school-age period. Characteristic activities include joining team sports, secret clubs, and "gangs"; scouting or like activities; working complex puzzles, collecting, playing quiet board games, reading, and hero worshiping. Rules and rituals are important aspects of play and games.

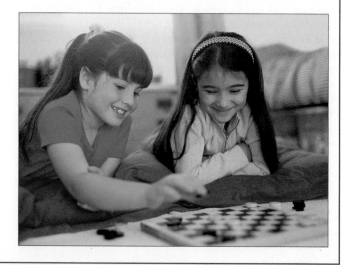

Normal Sleep Requirements and Patterns

Sleep is an integral part of health assessment. Lack of sleep can affect all areas of health including cognitive, physical, and emotional health. Children require varying amounts of sleep based primarily on their age. They also have varying sleep habits that correlate with their developmental status.

TODDLERS

Total sleep requirements decrease during the second year and average about 12 hours per day. Most toddlers nap once a day until the end of the second or third year. Sleep problems are common and may be due to fears of separation. Bedtime rituals and transitional objects, such as a blanket or stuffed toy, are helpful.

PRESCHOOLERS

The average preschooler sleeps 11 to 13 hours per day. Preschoolers typically need an afternoon nap until age 5, when most begin kindergarten. Bedtime rituals persist and sleep problems are common. These include nightmares, night terrors, difficulty settling in after a busy day, and stretching bedtime rituals to delay sleep. Continuing reassuring bedtime rituals with relaxation time before bedtime should help the child settle in. The daytime nap may be eliminated if it seems to interfere with nighttime sleep. For many preschoolers, a security object and night light continue to help relieve anxiety/fears at bedtime (Fig. 31-12).

SCHOOL-AGE CHILDREN

School-age children's individual sleep requirements vary but typically range from 8 to 9.5 h per night. Because the growth rate has slowed, children actually need less sleep now than during adolescence. The child's bedtime can be later than during the preschool period but should be firmly established and adhered to on school nights. Reading before bedtime may facilitate sleep and set up a positive bedtime pattern. Children may be unaware of fatigue, and, if allowed to remain up, they will be tired the next day.

ADOLESCENTS

During adolescence, rapid growth, overexertion in activities, and a tendency to stay up late commonly interfere with sleep and rest requirements. In an attempt to "catch up" on missed sleep, many adolescents sleep late at every opportunity. Each adolescent is unique in the number of sleep hours required to stay healthy and rested.

Sample nursing history questions for toddlerhood to adolescence include

- Where does child sleep; what type of bed?
- With whom does the child sleep?
- Does child use a sleep aid (blanket, toy, night light, medication, beverage)?
- Does the child have a bedtime ritual?
- What time does child go to bed at night?

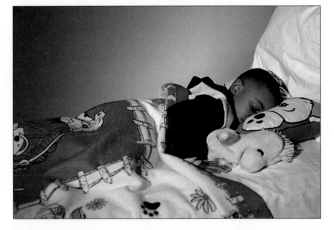

Figure 31-12 A security object, such as a favorite toy, can help a preschooler to sleep (© B. Proud).

- What time does child get up in the morning?
- Does child sleep through the night?
- Does child require feeding at night, and, if so, what and how is it administered (bottle caries)?
- What is child's nap schedule, and how long does child sleep for naps?
- Is the child's sleep restful or restless; any snoring or breathing problems?
- Does the child sleepwalk or -talk?
- Does the child have nightmares or night terrors?
- If the child has sleep problems, what do you do for them?

Socioeconomic Situation

A family's socioeconomic situation greatly affects all aspects of a child's life including development, nutrition, and overall health and functioning. Low socioeconomic status has the greatest adverse effect on health, and many children in this country live below the poverty level. Therefore, it is critical to obtain this assessment to initiate intervention strategies at the earliest opportunity.

Sample nursing history questions for infancy to adolescence include

- Does the child have health care insurance?
- Would you seek more medical assistance (e.g., in the way of preventive screenings, checkups, sick visits, medication requests, eyeglass prescriptions) for your child if you had the money to do so?
- Do you have any financial difficulties with which you need assistance?
- How would you describe the family's living conditions?

Relationship and Role Development

The development of relationships and a role within groups is a crucial aspect of childhood. The ability of children to establish high-quality relationships and form specific roles in the early years significantly determines their ability to form high-quality relationships and roles when adulthood is reached.

Culture is an important factor in a person's relationship and role development. Things to consider include whether the child's culture/ethnicity is a minority within the major cultural group; the traditional role of children in the particular child's culture; and whether there is male or female dominance in the particular culture. Another major influence on the child's development of relationships and roles is the structure of the family. Various family structures include two-parent families, single-parent families, blended families, homosexual parent families, families with an adopted child, or families with a foster child.

Early intervention in and early prevention of poor relationships between the child and his or her caregivers, siblings, peers, and influential adults outside the immediate family are vital. Therefore, assessment of this aspect of a child's life is extremely important. It is important to ask the parent or caregiver as well as the child questions because they may have differing views concerning the nature of the child's relationships.

Sample nursing history questions for toddlerhood to adolescence (specifically geared to parent or caregiver) include

- What is your family structure?
- With what culture or ethnic group does your family identify?
- How would you describe your family support system?
- Who is child's primary caretaker (especially for smaller children, not in school)?
- What is the child's role in the family?
- What are the family occupations and schedules?
- How much time do you spend with children and what activities do you participate in when you are together?
- Have there been any changes in family lately—divorce, birth, deaths, moves?
- How does child get along with parents, siblings, extended family, teachers, and peers?
- Discuss your child's circle of friends.
- What disciplinary measures do you use?

Sample nursing history questions for toddlerhood to adolescence (specifically geared to child and/or adolescent) include

- How do you get along with your parents? brothers? sisters?
- What activities does the family do together?
- What chores do you do around the house?
- What would you consider your role in the family?
- What are the names of your family members and friends?
- Do you have a best friend?
- What do you like best about family/friends?
- What do you dislike about family/friends?
- What do you do/share with your friends?
- Do your parents know your friends? Do they like them?
- Do you get along with the other kids at school?
- Do you get along with your teacher(s)?

Self-Esteem and Self-Concept Development

Childhood is the time when an individual develops the self-esteem and self-concept that shapes him or her in adult life (Table 31-9). Therefore, an assessment of this nature is crucial to provide health promotion teaching, prevent future problems, and intervene with current problems. This is a good time to ask questions regarding the child's values and beliefs because these areas tend greatly to influence a person's self-concept. This assessment requires that the same questions be asked of both the parent and the child, because their opinions

may be significantly different. Reassure the parent and child that all answers discussed will be kept confidential.

Sample nursing history questions for toddler to adolescence include (also ask these questions directly to the child; these questions are given in italics)

- How would you describe your child? *How would you describe yourself?*
- What does your child do best? *What do you do best?*
- In what areas does your child need improvement? *In what areas do you think you need improvement?*
- Is your child ever overly concerned about his or her weight? *Do you like your present weight? What would you like to weigh?*
- Are culture and religion important factors in your home? *Are culture and religion important to you?*
- In what religion is the child being reared? *What religion are you?*
- How does your child define right and wrong? *How would you decide if something were right or wrong?*
- What are your family values? *What values are important to you?*
- What are the child's goals in life? *What are your goals in life?*

Coping and Stress Management

Childhood is full of stressors and fears, including the developmental crises of transition to each life stage and common childhood fears such as the dark and being left alone (Tables 31-10 and 31-11). The ways in which children cope with stress and fear can affect their development and how they will handle subsequent life events. Coping mechanisms vary depending on developmental level, resources, situation, style, and previous experience with stressful events (Table 31-12). The ability of a child to cope is often influenced by individual

Table 31-9	Self-Concept Development
Toddler/Preschoolers	Greater sense of independence
Schoolagers	More aware of differences, norms, and morals; sensitive to social pressures
Adolescents	Self-concept crystallizes in later adolescence when child focuses on physical and emotional changes and peer acceptance

Table 31-10	Stressors in Children
Young children	Change in daily structure New sibling Separation
Older children	Starting school Long vacations Moving Change in family structure (remarriage) Christmas
Adolescents	Pregnancy Peer loss Breakup with boy/girl friend
All children	Parental loss (divorce, death, jail)

Table 31-11	Common Childhood Fears
Infants	Loud noises; falling and sudden movements in the environment; stranger anxiety begins around age 6 months
Toddlers	Loss of parents—separation anxiety; stranger anxiety; loud noises; going to sleep; large animals; certain people (doctor, Santa Claus); certain places (doctor's office); large objects or machines
Preschoolers	The dark; being left alone, especially at bedtime; animals (particularly large dogs); ghosts and other supernatural beings; body mutilation; pain; objects and people associated with painful experiences
Schoolagers	Failure at school; bullies; intimidating teachers; supernatural beings; storms; staying alone; scary things in TV and movies; consequences related to unattractive appearance; death
Adolescents	Relationships with people of the opposite sex; homosexual tendencies; ability to assume adult roles; drugs; AIDS; divorce; gossip; public speaking; plane and car crashes; death

Table 31-12	Coping Mechanisms in Children
Infants	Restlessness, rocking, playing with toys, crying, thumb sucking, sleeping
Toddlers/Preschoolers	Asking questions, wanting order, holding favorite toy, learning by trial and error, tantrums, aggression, thumb sucking, withdrawal, regression
Schoolagers	Trying problem solving; communicating, fantasizing, acting out situations, quiet, denial, regression, reaction formation
Adolescents	Problem solving, philosophical discussions, conforming with peers, asserting control, acting out, using drugs/alcohol, denial, projection, rationalization, intellectualization

temperament. Temperament involves the child's style of emotional and behavioral responses across situations. Temperament is biologic in origin; however, it is influenced by environmental characteristics and patterned by the society. This is significant because short- and long-term psychosocial adjustments are shaped by the goodness of fit between the child's temperament and the social environment.

Sample nursing history questions for infancy to adolescence include (questions asked of a child appear in italic print)

- What does your child do when he or she gets angry/frustrated? *What do you do when you get angry or frustrated?*
- What does your child do when he or she gets tired? *What do you do when you get tired?*
- When your child has a tantrum, how do you handle it?
- What things make your child scared? *What things scare you?*
- What does he or she do when scared? *What do you do when you're scared?*
- What kinds of things does your child worry about? *What kinds of things do you worry about?*

- When your child has a problem, what does he or she do? *When you have a problem, what do you do?*
- Have there been any big problems or changes in your family lately? *Have there been any big problems or changes in your family lately?*
- Is there a problem with alcohol or drugs? *Do you use tobacco, alcohol, or drugs?*
- Has your child ever run away from home? *Have you ever run away from home?*
- How does your child react when needs are not met immediately, and what do you do about it? *What do you do when you are sad? What do you do when you are angry?*
- Is your child "accident prone," and why do you think he or she is? *Did you ever think about hurting yourself? Did you ever think about killing yourself?* (Display 31-3)

COLLECTING OBJECTIVE DATA: PHYSICAL EXAMINATION

Preparing the Client

In most cases, physical assessment involves a head-to-toe examination that encompasses each body system. When examining children, the sequence should be altered to accommodate the child's developmental needs. Less threatening and least intrusive procedures, such as general inspection and heart and lung auscultation, should be completed first to secure the child's trust. Explain what you will be doing and what the child can expect to feel; allow the child to manipulate the equipment before it is used. Try to perform examination in a comfortable, nonthreatening area. The temperature should be warm, the room well lit, and all threatening instruments out of the child's view. The room should contain age-appropriate diversions such as toys and cartoons for younger children and posters for adolescents. If the child is uncooperative, first assess the reason (usually fear) then intervene appropriately. If still unsuccessful, involve parents, use a firm approach, and complete the examination as quickly but completely as possible. Involve the child in the physical examination at all times unless it is stressful for him or her.

Equipment

- Denver Developmental Kit
- Ophthalmoscope
- Otoscope with nasal speculum
- Scale/stadiometer
- Snellen Eye Chart
- Stethoscope

Physical Assessment

- Recognize how techniques and demeanor for interviewing and examining children differ among the age groups and from those used for interviewing and examining adults. Display 31-4 gives developmental approaches to the physical examination.
- Evaluate growth and development patterns according to the different pediatric age groups and across body systems.
- Recognize children who are difficult to examine because of anxiety or fear.
- Develop forms of age-appropriate "play" to distract less cooperative children so physical examination can be completed.

DISPLAY 31-3	Suicide Assessment: Risks and Signs

Suicide is a leading killer of young people, particularly teenagers. The nurse can be instrumental in detecting signs of impending suicide and possibly, intervening to prevent it. During the nursing assessment, several interviewing methods and questions may help uncover a young client's suicidal thoughts.

- Ask if the child ever thought of hurting or killing self (hurting is different from killing).
- If the answer is "yes," ask the child when he or she thought of killing self.
- Ask how the child planned to do it.
- Ask if the child ever tried to kill himself or herself before and if any help was received after the incident.
- Ask if the child believes that there are any other options besides suicide to resolve problems.

Children and adolescents who verbalize planned, lethal means to commit suicide, and who feel that they do not have any other options, are at extremely high risk of carrying out their plan—especially if they have attempted suicide in the past. Some risk factors and warning signs of potential suicide include the following:

Risk Factors
- Previous attempt
- Suicide of family member or close friend
- History of abuse, neglect, or psychiatric hospitalization
- Persistent depression
- Mental disorder (voices tell child to kill self)
- Substance abuse
- Difficult home situation
- Incarceration
- Few social opportunities; isolated
- Firearms in the home

Warning Signs
- Seems preoccupied with death themes, as in books, music, art, films, or TV shows
- Gives away valued possessions
- Talks about death, especially own
- Acts recklessly or adopts antisocial behavior
- Experiences rapid change in school performance
- Has episode of sudden cheerfulness after being depressed
- Exhibits dramatic change in everyday behaviors, such as sleeping and eating
- Smokes continuously (chain smoking)
- Expresses sense of worthlessness or hopelessness

DISPLAY 31-4	Developmental Approaches to the Physical Assessment

Children in each age group respond differently to the hands-on physical assessment; however, the following guidelines should be kept in mind:

Toddlers
Allow toddler to sit on parent's lap; enlist parent's aid; use play; praise cooperation.

Preschoolers
Use story telling; use doll and puppet play; give choices when able.

Schoolagers
Maintain privacy; use gown; explain procedures and equipment; teach about their bodies.

Adolescents
Ensure privacy and confidentiality; provide option of having parent present or not; emphasize normality; provide health teaching.

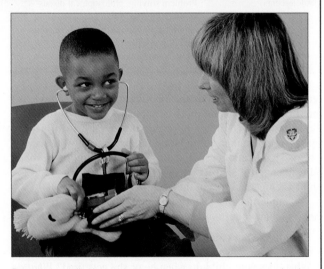

Puppet or doll play is a great way to prepare a preschooler for physical examination. (© B. Proud.)

PHYSICAL ASSESSMENT

Assessment Procedure	Normal Findings	Abnormal Findings

General Appearance and Behavior

Note overall appearance. Observe hygiene, interaction with parents and yourself (and siblings if present). Note also facies (facial expressions), posture, nutritional status, speech, attention span, and level of cooperation.

> **Clinical Tip** • *Behavioral observation is one of the most important assessments to make with children because alterations usually signify health problems.*

Child appears stated age, is clean, appears well nourished, and has no unusual body odor. Clothing is in good condition and appropriate for climate.

Child is alert, active, responds appropriately to stress of the situation, and maintains eye contact. Child is appropriately interactive for age, seeks comfort from parent; appears happy or appropriately anxious because of examination. Child is attentive and speech is appropriate for age, follows age-appropriate commands, and is reasonably cooperative. Toddler is lordotic when standing; preschooler is slightly bowlegged; older child demonstrates straight and well-balanced posture.

Lack of eye contact indicates many things including anxiety or significant psychosocial problems.

 Lack of eye contact is normal for certain cultural groups such as Asians and Native Americans.

Deviations from normal that can be discerned from a child's appearance or behavior are listed below.

Certain faces may indicate fear, anxiety, anger, allergies, acute illness, pain, mental deficiency, or respiratory distress.

A child's posture or movement may indicate pain, low self-esteem, rejection, depression, hostility or aggression.

Hygiene gives insight into neglect, poverty, mental illness or retardation, knowledge deficit regarding hygiene (e.g., teen parent).

Abnormal behavior may suggest neurologic problems (head trauma, cranial lesions), metabolic problems (diabetic ketoacidosis), psychiatric disorders, or psychosocial problems.

Abnormal development (child does not appear stated age) may indicate mental retardation, abuse, neglect, or psychiatric disorders.

Developmental Assessment

Screen for cognitive, language, social, and gross and fine motor developmental delays in the beginning of the physical assessment for preschoolers. Use a standardized assessment tool such as the Draw a Person, Revised Prescreening Developmental Questionnaire, or the Denver Developmental Screening Test II (DDST). In Chapter 30, Assessment Tool 30-1 presents the DDST II and directions for its use.

Child meets normal parameters for age.

Child lags in earlier stages.

continued

PHYSICAL ASSESSMENT *Continued*

Assessment Procedure	Normal Findings	Abnormal Findings

Vital Signs

Assess temperature. Use rectal, axillary, skin, or tympanic route when assessing the temperature. For children older than 4 years of age, the oral route can be used in addition to the other routes.

To take a rectal temperature in a toddler, lay the child supine and lift lower legs up into the air, bending the legs at the hips. Insert lubricated rectal thermometer no more than 2 cm into rectum. Temperature registers in 3 to 5 min on a rectal thermometer. Lay a school-age child on the stomach on a table. Maintain firm hold on child's hips so child does not raise buttocks up during the procedure. Separate buttocks with thumb and forefinger of nondominant hand and insert thermometer. Axillary and/or tympanic temperature may also be used; however, these methods are less accurate and less reliable than the rectal temperature.

See Chapter 7 for other temperature techniques.

Temperature is 98.6°F.

➤ **Clinical Tip** • *Use the rectal route only when absolutely necessary because of increased discomfort in older children. Rectal temperatures are also contraindicated in certain circumstances, such as perforated anus.*

Temperature may be altered by exercise, stress, crying, environment, diurnal variation (highest between 4 and 6 PM). Both hyperthermic and hypothermic conditions are noted in children.

Assess pulse rate. Count the pulse for a full minute. Children younger than 2 years should have apical pulse measured. Radial pulses may be taken in children over 2 years old (Fig. 31-13).

Awake and resting rates vary with the age of the child:

3 mo–2 y: 80–150
2–10 y: 70–110
10 y–adult: 55–90

Athletic adolescents tend to have lower pulse rates.

Pulse may be altered by apprehension or anxiety, medications, activity, and pain, as well as pathologic conditions.

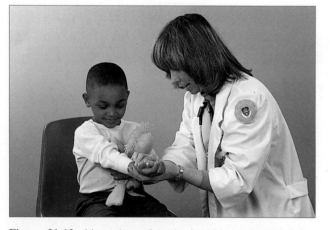

Figure 31-13 Measuring radial pulse in child over 2 years (© B. Proud).

continued

Assessment Procedure	Normal Findings	Abnormal Findings
Assess respiratory rate. Monitor respirations in children older than 1 year the same as for adults.	Normal ranges are as follows: 6 mo–2 y: 20–30 3–10 y: 20–28 10–18 y: 12–20	Respiratory rate and character may be altered by medications, positioning, fever, activity, and anxiety or fear as well as pathologic conditions.
Evaluate blood pressure. Blood pressure should be measured annually in children 3 years and older, and in all ages when conditions warrant it. The appropriate cuff width is 50% to 75% of the upper arm (Fig. 31-14). The length should encircle the circumference without overlapping. A small diaphragm should be used for the stethoscope. If for some reason the arm cannot be used, a measurement can be taken on the thigh. If children younger than 3 years old require a blood pressure reading, a Doppler stethoscope should be used.	Normal ranges are as follows: *Systolic:* 1–7 years = age in years + 90 8–18 years = (2 × age in years) + 90 *Diastolic:* 1–5 years = 56 6–18 years = age in years + 52 (see also Table 31-13)	Systolic and diastolic BP above 95th percentiles for age and sex after three readings is considered high blood pressure. ➤ *Clinical Tip • If the blood pressure reading is too high for age, the cuff may be too small; it should cover two thirds of the child's upper arm. If the blood pressure reading is too low for age, the cuff may be too large. Chapter 7 explains how to take a blood pressure reading.*

Measurements

Measure height. In a child younger than 2 years, determine height by measuring the recumbent length. Fully extend the body, holding the head in midline and gently grasping the knees and pushing them downward until the legs are fully extended and touching the table. If using a measuring board, place the head at the top of the board and the heels firmly at the bottom. Without a board, use paper	See the growth charts in Appendix F for normal findings. Asian children are smaller at all ages.	Significant deviation from normal in the growth charts would be considered abnormal.

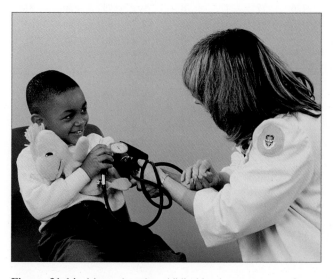

Figure 31-14 Measuring the child's blood pressure requires a cuff that is appropriately sized (© B. Proud).

continued on page 728

Table 31-13 — Blood Pressure Levels for the 90th and 95th Percentiles of Blood Pressure for Girls and Boys, Ages 1 to 17

Age	BP Percentile[a]	Systolic BP (mmHg), by Height Percentile from Standard Growth Curves							Diastolic BP (mmHg), by Height Percentile from Standard Growth Curves						
		5%	10%	25%	50%	75%	90%	95%	5%	10%	25%	50%	75%	90%	95%
Girls															
1	90th	97	98	99	100	102	103	104	53	53	53	54	55	56	56
	95th	101	102	103	104	105	107	107	57	57	57	58	59	60	60
2	90th	99	99	100	102	103	104	105	57	57	58	58	59	60	61
	95th	102	103	104	105	107	108	109	61	61	62	62	63	64	65
3	90th	100	100	102	103	104	105	106	61	61	61	62	63	63	64
	95th	104	104	105	107	108	109	110	65	65	65	66	67	67	68
4	90th	101	102	103	104	106	107	108	63	63	64	65	65	66	67
	95th	105	106	107	108	109	111	111	67	67	68	69	69	70	71
5	90th	103	103	104	106	107	108	109	65	66	66	67	68	68	69
	95th	107	107	108	110	111	112	113	69	70	70	71	72	72	73
6	90th	104	105	106	107	109	110	111	67	67	68	69	69	70	71
	95th	108	109	110	111	112	114	114	71	71	72	73	73	74	75
7	90th	106	107	108	109	110	112	112	69	69	69	70	71	72	72
	95th	110	110	112	113	114	115	116	73	73	73	74	75	76	76
8	90th	108	109	110	111	112	113	114	70	70	71	71	72	73	74
	95th	112	112	113	115	116	117	118	74	74	75	75	76	77	78
9	90th	110	110	112	113	114	115	116	71	72	72	73	74	74	75
	95th	114	114	115	117	118	119	120	75	76	76	77	78	78	79
10	90th	112	112	114	115	116	117	118	73	73	73	74	75	76	76
	95th	116	116	117	119	120	121	122	77	77	77	78	79	80	80
11	90th	114	114	116	117	118	119	120	74	74	75	75	76	77	77
	95th	118	118	119	121	122	123	124	78	78	79	79	80	81	81
12	90th	116	116	118	119	120	121	122	75	75	76	76	77	78	78
	95th	120	120	121	123	124	125	126	79	79	80	80	81	82	82
13	90th	118	118	119	121	122	123	124	76	76	77	78	78	79	80
	95th	121	122	123	125	126	127	128	80	80	81	82	82	83	84
14	90th	119	120	121	122	124	125	126	77	77	78	79	79	80	81
	95th	123	124	125	126	128	129	130	81	81	82	83	83	84	85
15	90th	121	121	122	124	125	126	127	78	78	79	79	80	81	82
	95th	124	125	126	128	129	130	131	82	82	83	83	84	85	86
16	90th	122	122	123	125	126	127	128	79	79	79	80	81	82	82
	95th	125	126	127	128	130	131	132	83	83	83	84	85	86	86
17	90th	122	123	124	125	126	128	128	79	79	79	80	81	82	82
	95th	126	126	127	129	130	131	132	83	83	83	84	85	86	86

continued

| Table 31-13 | Blood Pressure Levels for the 90th and 95th Percentiles of Blood Pressure for Girls and Boys, Ages 1 to 17 *Continued* | | | | | | | | | | | | | |

		Systolic BP (mmHg), by Height Percentile from Standard Growth Curves							Diastolic BP (mmHg), by Height Percentile from Standard Growth Curves						
Age	BP Percentile[a]	5%	10%	25%	50%	75%	90%	95%	5%	10%	25%	50%	75%	90%	95%
Boys															
1	90th	94	95	97	98	100	102	102	50	51	52	53	54	54	55
	95th	98	99	101	102	104	106	106	55	55	56	57	58	59	59
2	90th	98	99	100	102	104	105	106	55	55	56	57	58	59	59
	95th	101	102	104	106	108	109	110	59	59	60	61	62	63	63
3	90th	100	101	103	105	107	108	109	59	59	60	61	62	63	63
	95th	104	105	107	109	111	112	113	63	63	64	65	66	67	67
4	90th	102	103	105	107	109	110	111	62	62	63	64	65	66	66
	95th	106	107	109	111	113	114	115	66	67	67	68	69	70	71
5	90th	104	105	106	108	110	112	112	65	65	66	67	68	69	69
	95th	108	109	110	112	114	115	116	69	70	70	71	72	73	74
6	90th	105	106	108	110	111	113	114	67	68	69	70	70	71	72
	95th	109	110	112	114	115	117	117	72	72	73	74	75	76	76
7	90th	106	107	109	111	113	114	115	69	70	71	72	72	73	74
	95th	110	111	113	115	116	118	119	74	74	75	76	77	78	78
8	90th	107	108	110	112	114	115	116	71	71	72	73	74	75	75
	95th	111	112	114	116	118	119	120	75	76	76	77	78	79	80
9	90th	109	110	112	113	115	117	117	72	73	73	74	75	76	77
	95th	113	114	116	117	119	121	121	76	77	78	79	80	80	81
10	90th	110	112	113	115	117	118	119	73	74	74	75	76	77	78
	95th	114	115	117	119	121	122	123	77	78	79	80	80	81	82
11	90th	112	113	115	117	119	120	121	74	74	75	76	77	78	78
	95th	116	117	119	121	123	124	125	78	79	79	80	81	82	83
12	90th	115	116	117	119	121	123	123	75	75	76	77	78	78	79
	95th	119	120	121	123	125	126	127	79	79	80	81	82	83	83
13	90th	117	118	120	122	124	125	126	75	76	76	77	78	79	80
	95th	121	122	124	126	128	129	130	79	80	81	82	83	83	84
14	90th	120	121	123	125	126	128	128	76	76	77	78	79	80	80
	95th	124	125	127	128	130	132	132	80	81	81	82	83	84	85
15	90th	123	124	125	127	129	131	131	77	77	78	79	80	81	81
	95th	127	128	129	131	133	134	135	81	82	83	83	84	85	86
16	90th	125	126	128	130	132	133	134	79	79	80	81	82	82	83
	95th	129	130	132	134	136	137	138	83	83	84	85	86	87	87
17	90th	128	129	131	133	134	136	136	81	81	82	83	84	85	85
	95th	132	133	135	136	138	140	140	85	85	86	87	88	89	89

Source: Reprinted from National High Blood Pressure Education Program Working Group on Hypertension Control in Children and Adolescents. www.cdc.gov.
[a] Blood pressure percentile determined by a single measurement.

PHYSICAL ASSESSMENT *Continued*

Assessment Procedure	Normal Findings	Abnormal Findings
under the child and mark the paper at the top of the head and bottom of the heels. Then measure the distance between the two points. Determine an older child's height by having the shoeless child stand as straight as possible with head midline and vision line parallel between the ceiling and floor (Fig. 31-15). Child's back, buttocks, and back of heels should be against the wall; measure height with a stadiometer. Plot height measurement on an age- and gender-appropriate growth chart (birth to 36 months and 2 to 20 years).		
Measure weight on an appropriately sized beam scale with nondetectable weights. Weigh a small child lying or sitting on a scale that measures to the nearest 0.5 oz or 10 g. Weigh an older child standing on a scale that measures to the nearest 0.25 lb or 100 g. Weigh an older child in underpants or light gown to respect modesty. Plot weight measurement on age- and gender-appropriate growth chart (birth to 36 months and 2 to 20 years).	See Appendix F for normal findings.	Deviation from the wide range of normal weights is abnormal. See the growth charts in Appendix F and compare differences.
Measure head circumference (HC) or occipital frontal circumference (OFC) at every physical examination for toddlers younger than 2 years and older children when conditions warrant. Plot the measurement on standardized growth charts specific for gender.	HC (OFC) measurement should fall between the 5th and 95th percentiles and should be comparable to the child's height and weight percentiles.	HC (OFC) not within the normal percentiles may indicate pathology. Those greater than 95% may indicate macrocephaly. Those under the 5th percentile may indicate microcephaly. Increased HC (OFC) in children older than 3 years may indicate separation of cranial sutures due to increased intracranial pressure.

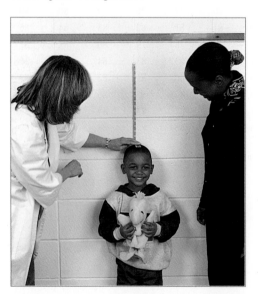

Figure 31-15 Measuring the height of a preschooler (© B. Proud).

continued

Assessment Procedure	Normal Findings	Abnormal Findings

Skin, Hair, and Nail

Inspection and Palpation

Assessment Procedure	Normal Findings	Abnormal Findings
Observe skin color, odor, and lesions.	Skin color ranges from pale white with pink, yellow, brown, or olive tones to dark brown or black. No strong odor should be evident, and the skin should be lesion free. Normal skin variations (Common Variations 31-1) include • Port wine stains • Hemangiomas • Café-au-lait spots (are normal in small numbers)	Yellow skin may indicate jaundice or intake of too many yellow vegetables in infants (sclera is white in the latter). Blue skin suggests cyanosis, pallor suggests anemia, and redness suggests fever, irritation, or allergies. Body piercing may be cultural or a fad, but excessive piercing may indicate underlying self-abusive tendencies. If tattoos appear to be "homemade," consider the possibility of contamination with hepatitis B virus or HIV from infected needles. Urine odor suggests incontinence, dirty diaper, or uremia. Salty sweat may indicate cystic fibrosis (a parent may report that the child's skin tastes salty when the parent kisses the child). Ecchymoses in various stages or in unusual locations or circular burn areas suggest child abuse although bruising or burning may also be from cultural practices such as *cupping* or *coining*. Petechiae, lesions, or rashes may indicate serious disorders. Greater than six café-au-lait spots may indicate neurovascular disease.
Palpate for texture, temperature, moisture, turgor, and edema.	Skin should be soft, warm, slightly moist with good turgor and without edema. Skin should be soft and elastic, with no tenting when tested for turgor.	Excessive dryness suggests poor nutrition, excessive bathing, or an endocrine disorder. Flaking or scaling suggests eczema or fungal infections. Poor skin turgor indicates dehydration or malnutrition, edema suggests renal or cardiac disorders; periorbital edema may indicate pathology but may also be due to recent crying, sleeping, or allergies. Russell's sign (abrasion or scarring on joints of index and middle finger) suggests self-induced vomiting. Bite marks may indicate child abuse or self-abusive behavior (psychiatric disorders, mental retardation).
Inspect and palpate hair. Observe for distribution, characteristics, infestation, and presence of any unusual hair on body.	Hair is normally lustrous, silky, strong, and elastic. Fine, downy hair covers the body. Adolescents may display a variety of hair styles to assert independence and group conformity.	Dirty, matted hair may indicate neglect. Dull, dry, brittle hair may indicate poor nutrition, hypothyroidism, excessive use of chemical hair products (teens).

continued on page 731

Common Variations 31-1   **Common Skin Variations in Children**

Port-Wine Stain
This birthmark consisting of capillaries is dark red or bluish and darkens with exertion or temperature exposure. It appears as a large, irregular, macular patch on the scalp or face. Unlike a hemangioma, this birthmark does not fade with time.

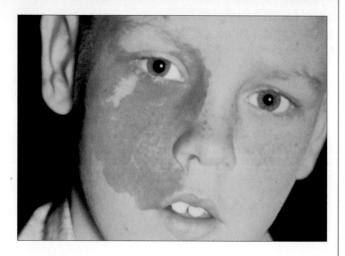

Café au Lait Spot
This birthmark is a light brown, round or oval patch. If there are more than six separate, large (>1.5 cm) patches, an inherited neurocutaneous disease may be present.

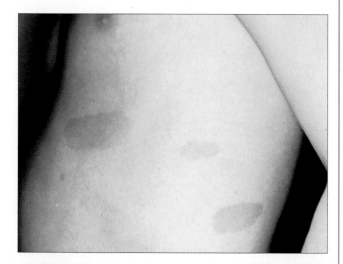

Hemangioma
This skin variation is caused by an increased amount of blood vessels in the dermis.

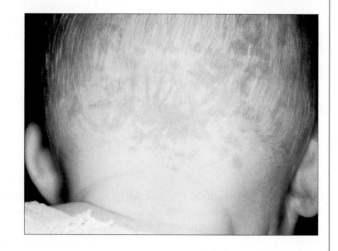

Assessment Procedure	Normal Findings	Abnormal Findings
	African-American children usually have hair that is curlier and coarser than white children.	Grayish, translucent flakes that adhere to hair shaft suggest lice (ova, nits).
		Grayish or brown oval bodies suggest ticks.
		Balding (alopecia) suggests neglect, trichotillomania (hair pulling), skin diseases, or chemotherapy.
		Tufts of hair over the spine may indicate spina bifida occulta.
		Coarse body hair in a prepubertal child or older girl may be from endocrine disorder.
		Pubic hair in child younger than 8 years may indicate precocious adrenarche or precocious puberty.
Inspect and palpate nails. Note color, texture, shape, and condition of nails.	Nails should be clean and groomed. Adolescents may color or pierce nails. Pink undertones should be seen. Dark-skinned children have deeper nail pigment.	Blue nailbeds indicate cyanosis. Yellow nailbeds suggest jaundice. Blue-black nailbeds are found with nailbed hemorrhage. White color suggests fungal infection. Scaly lesions also indicate fungal infections, especially in adolescents who use artificial nails.
		Short, ragged nails are common with nail biting; dirty, uncut nails suggest poor hygiene. Concave shape, "spoon nails" (koilonychia) indicate iron deficiency anemia. Clubbing indicates chronic cyanosis.
		Macerated thumb tip is found with thumb sucking.
		Inflammation at the nail base indicates paronychia.

Head, Neck, and Cervical Lymph Nodes

Inspection and Palpation **Inspect and palpate the head.** Note shape and symmetry.	Head is normocephalic and symmetric.	Very large head is hydrocephalus. Oddly shaped head suggests premature closure of sutures (possibly genetic).
		Third fontanelle located between the anterior and posterior fontanelle indicates Down's syndrome.

continued

PHYSICAL ASSESSMENT Continued

Assessment Procedure	Normal Findings	Abnormal Findings
		Craniotabes—from osteoporosis of the outer skull bone. Palpating too firmly with the thumb or forefinger over the temporoparietal area will leave an indentation of the bone.
Test head control, head posture, and range of motion.	Full range of motion—up, down, and sideways—is normal.	Hyperextension suggests opisthotonos or significant meningeal irritation.
		Limited range of motion suggests torticollis (wryneck).
Inspect and palpate the face. Note appearance, symmetry, and movement (have child make faces). Palpate the parotid glands for swelling.	Face is normally proportionate and symmetric. Movements are equal bilaterally. Parotid glands are normal size. ➤ *Clinical Tip • Some adolescents may appear to have unusual skin tones or markings from applying makeup as a form of self-expression.*	Unusual proportions (short palpebral fissures, thin lips, and wide and flat philtrum, which is the groove above the upper lip) may be hereditary or they may indicate specific syndromes, such as Down's syndrome (Fig. 31-16) and fetal alcohol syndrome. Other findings may indicate the following: Unequal movement—facial nerve paralysis Enlarged parotid gland—mumps or bulimia Abnormal facies—chromosomal anomaly Crease across nose, shiners (dark circles under eyes), and mouth agape—allergies (allergic facies)

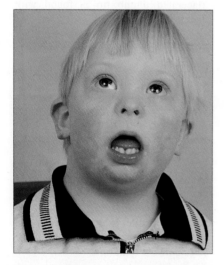

Figure 31-16 Down's syndrome results from a genetic abnormality (© B. Proud).

continued

Assessment Procedure	Normal Findings	Abnormal Findings
Inspect and palpate the neck. Palpate the thyroid gland and the trachea. Also inspect and palpate the cervical lymph nodes for swelling, mobility, temperature, and tenderness (Fig. 31-17).	The isthmus is the only portion of the thyroid that should be palpable. The trachea is midline. Lymph nodes are usually nonpalpable in adolescents. "Shotty" lymph nodes (small, nontender, mobile) are commonly palpated in children between the ages of 3 and 12 years.	Implications of some abnormal findings include the following: Short, webbed neck—anomalies or syndromes Distended neck veins—difficulty breathing Enlarged thyroid or palpable masses—pathologic processes Shift in tracheal position from midline—serious lung problem (e.g., foreign body or tumor) Enlarged firm lymph nodes—Hodgkin's disease or HIV infection Enlarged, warm, and tender lymph nodes—lymphadenitis or infection in the head and neck area that is drained by the affected node

Mouth, Throat, and Sinuses

Inspection

Note the condition of the lips, palates, tongue, and buccal mucosa (Fig. 31-18).	Lips, tongue and buccal mucosa appear pink and moist. No lesions are present.	Dry lips may indicate mouth breathing or dehydration. Stomatitis suggests infection or immunodeficiency. Koplik's spots (tiny white spots on red bases) on the buccal mucosa may be a prodromal sign of measles. Cleft lip and/or palate are congenital abnormalities (Fig. 31-19).

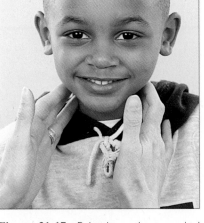

Figure 31-17 Palpating the cervical lymph nodes (© B. Proud).

continued

PHYSICAL ASSESSMENT *Continued*

Assessment Procedure	Normal Findings	Abnormal Findings
Observe the condition of the teeth and gums.	Deciduous teeth begin to develop between 4 and 6 months; all 20 erupt by 36 months; teeth begin to fall out around 6 years, when permanent tooth eruption begins and progresses until all 32 have erupted.	Dental caries may herald "bottle caries syndrome." Enamel erosion may indicate bulimia.
Note the condition of the throat and tonsils. Also observe the insertion and ending point of the frenulum.	Tonsils are are easily seen by age 6 when they increase to adult dimensions. They reach maximum size (about twice adult size) between ages 10 and 12. A trophy to stable adult dimensions usually occurs by the end of adolescence.	Tonsillar or pharyngeal inflammation suggests infection. Extension of the frenulum to the tip of tongue may interfere with extension of the tongue, which causes speech difficulties.
Inspect nose and sinuses. To inspect the nose and sinuses, avoid using the nasal speculum in young children. Instead, push up the tip of the nose and shine the light into each nostril. Observe the structure and patency of the nares, discharge, tenderness, and any color or swelling of the turbinates.	Nose is midline in face, septum is straight, and nares are patent. No discharge or tenderness is present. Turbinates are pink and free of edema.	Deviated septum may be congenital or caused by injury. Foul discharge from one nostril may indicate a foreign body. Pale, boggy nasal mucosa with or without possible polyps suggests allergic rhinitis. Nasal polyps are also seen in children with cystic fibrosis.
Palpation **Palpate the sinuses in older children if sinusitis is suspected.** The sinuses of young children are not palpable.	No tenderness palpated over sinuses.	Tender sinuses suggest sinusitis.

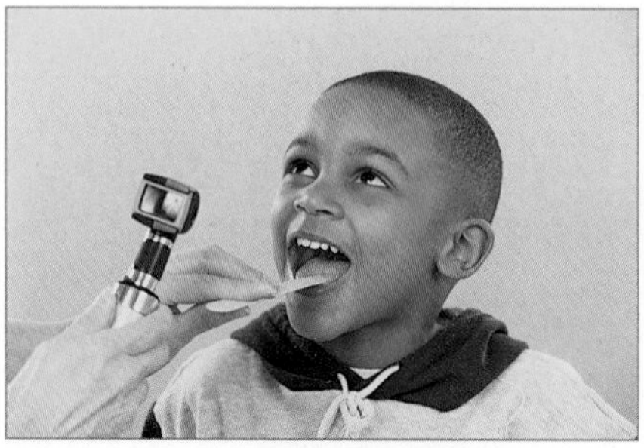

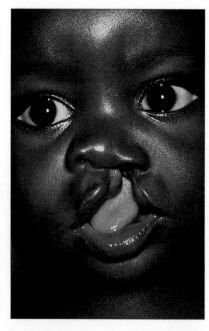

Figure 31-18 Inspecting the mouth (© B. Proud).

Figure 31-19 Cleft lip (© 1991 National Medical Slide Bank/CMSP).

continued

Assessment Procedure	Normal Findings	Abnormal Findings

Eyes

Inspection

Inspect the external eye. Note the position, slant, and epicanthal folds of the external eye.

Inner canthus distance approximately 2.5 cm, horizontal slant, no epicanthal folds. Outer canthus aligns with tips of the pinnas (Fig. 31-20).

Epicanthal folds (excess of skin extending from roof of nose that partially or completely covers the inner canthus) are normal findings in Asian children, whose eyes also slant upward.

Wide-set position (hypertelorism), upward slant, and thick epicanthal folds suggest Down syndrome. "Sun-setting" appearance (upper lid covers part of the iris) suggests hydrocephalus.

Observe eyelid placement, swelling, discharge, and lesions.

No swelling, discharge, or lesions of eyelids.

Eyelid inflammation may result from blepharitis, hordeolum, or dacryocystis (inflammation or blockage of lacrimal sac or duct). Ptosis (drooping eyelids) suggests oculomotor nerve palsy, congenital syndrome, or a familial trait. A painful, edematous, erythematous area on eyelid may be a hordeolum (style). A nodular, nontender lesion on the eyelid may be a chalazion (cyst). Swelling, erythema, or purulent discharge may indicate infection or blocked tear ducts. Sunken area around eyelids may indicate dehydration. Periorbital edema suggests fluid retention.

Inspect the sclera and conjunctiva for color, discharge, lesions, redness, and lacerations.

Sclera and conjunctiva are clear and free of discharge, lesions, redness, or lacerations.

Yellow sclera suggests jaundice, blue sclera may indicate osteogenesis imperfecta ("brittle bone disease"), and redness may indicate conjunctivitis.

Observe the iris and the pupils.

Pupils are equal, round, and reactive to light and accommodation (PERRLA).

Brushfield's spots may indicate Down syndrome. Sluggish pupils indicate a neurologic problem. Miosis (constriction) indicates iritis or narcotic use or abuse. Mydriasis (pupillary dilation) indicates emotional factors (fear), trauma, or certain drug use.

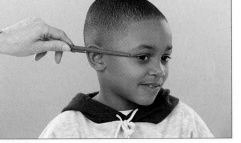

Figure 31-20 Outer canthus is in alignment with the tip of the pinna (© B. Proud).

continued

PHYSICAL ASSESSMENT *Continued*

Assessment Procedure	Normal Findings	Abnormal Findings
Finally inspect the eyebrows and eyelashes.	Eyebrows should be symmetric in shape and movement. They should not meet midline. Eyelashes should be evenly distributed and curled outward.	Sparseness of eyebrows or lashes could indicate skin disease or deliberate pulling out of hairs (usually due to anxiety or habit). Corneal abrasions are common during childhood and may not be easily visible to the naked eye.
Perform visual acuity tests. Use the following diagnostic tools to perform visual acuity testing: Snellen letter chart Snellen symbol chart (E chart; used for preschoolers) Blackbird Preschool Vision Screening Test (uses modified E that resembles a bird and a story to engage children's attention) Faye symbol chart (uses pictures) ➤ ***Clinical Tip*** • *Fatigue, anxiety, hunger, and distractions interfere with vision testing. Testing should precede procedures that create discomfort.*	Normal visual acuity is as follows: 1 year—20/200 2 years—20/70 5 years—20/30 6 years—20/20 Children should be able to differentiate colors by age 5.	Children with a one-line difference between eyes should be referred. Children should also be referred for abnormal visual acuity or inability to distinguish colors. Visual impairment can indicate congenital defects (cataracts), malignant tumors, chronic disease (diabetes), drugs, trauma, enzyme deficiencies, or refractive errors (myopia, hyperopia, astigmatism).
Perform extraocular muscle tests.	In the cover test, the eyes remain focused.	Eye movement is present during the cover test; this may indicate strabismus.
Cover test: Have the child cover one eye and look at an interesting object (Fig. 31-21). Observe the uncovered eye for any movement. When the child is focused on the object, remove the cover and observe that eye for movement.	In the Hirschberg test, the light reflects symmetrically in the center of both pupils.	Unequal alignment of light on the pupils in the Hirschberg test signals strabismus.

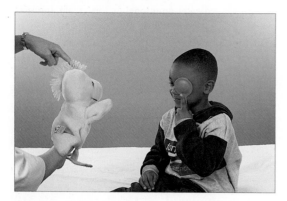

Figure 31-21   Performing the cover test (© B. Proud).

continued

Assessment Procedure	Normal Findings	Abnormal Findings
Hirschberg test: Shine light directly at the cornea while the child looks straight ahead. ➤ *Clinical Tip • Use a toy, a puppet, and the parent to focus the child's eyes. Older children, including adolescents, focus better if they are given something to focus on instead of being told to "look straight ahead."*		
Inspect the internal eye. Perform ophthalmoscopic examination. The procedure is the same as for adults. Distraction is preferred over the use of restraint, which is likely to result in crying and closed eyes. Careful ophthalmoscopic examination of newborns is difficult without the use of mydriatic medications.	Red reflex is present. This reflex rules out most serious defects of the cornea, aqueous chamber, lens, and vitreous humor. When visualized, the optic disc appears similar to an adult's.	Absence of the red reflex indicates cataracts. Papilledema is unusual in children under 3 years of age owing to the ability of the fontanelles and sutures to open during increased intracranial pressure. Disc blurring and hemorrhages should be reported immediately.

Ears

Assessment Procedure	Normal Findings	Abnormal Findings
Inspect external ears. Note placement, discharge, or lesions of the ears.	Top of pinna should cross the eye-occiput line and be within a 10-degree angle of a perpendicular line drawn from the eye-occiput line to the lobe. No unusual structure or markings should appear on the pinna.	Low-set ears with an alignment greater than a 10-degree angle suggest mental retardation or congenital syndromes. Abnormal shape may suggest renal disease process, which may be hereditary. Preauricular skin tags or sinuses suggest other anomalies of ears or the renal system.
Inspect internal ear. The internal ear examination requires using an otoscope and, for toddlers, restraint by (1) having a parent hold the seated child in the lap while holding the child's hands with one hand and the child's head sideways against chest (as shown) or (2) laying the child supine, with the parent holding the child's arms up over head. Then the nurse can gently but firmly hold child's head to the side. Regardless of technique used, the nurse should always hold the otoscope in a manner that allows for rapid removal if the child moves. Because an infant's external canal is short and straight, pull the pinna down and back. Because an older child's canal shortens and becomes less straight, like the adult's, gently pull the pinna up and back.	No excessive cerumen, discharge, lesions, excoriations, or foreign body are in external canal. Tympanic membrane is pearly gray to light pink with normal landmarks. Tympanic membranes redden bilaterally when child is crying or febrile.	Presence of foreign bodies or cerumen impaction. Purulent discharge may indicate otitis externa or presence of foreign body. Purulent, serous discharge suggests otitis media. Bloody discharge suggests trauma, and clear discharge may indicate cerebrospinal fluid leak. Perforated tympanic membrane may also be noted.
Assess the mobility of the tympanic membrane by pneumatic otoscopy. This consists of creating pressure against the tympanic membrane using air. To do this, you need to create a seal in the	Tympanic membrane is mobile; moves inward with positive pressure (squeeze of bulb) and outward with negative pressure (release of bulb).	Immobility suggests chronic (serous) otitis media; decreased mobility may occur with acute otitis media.

continued

PHYSICAL ASSESSMENT Continued

Assessment Procedure	Normal Findings	Abnormal Findings
external canal and direct a puff of air against the tympanic membrane. Create the seal by using the largest speculum that will comfortably insert into the ear canal. Cover the tip with rubber for a better and more comfortable seal. Attach a pneumatic bulb to the otoscope and squeeze the bulb lightly to direct air against the tympanic membrane.		
Test hearing acuity. Test acuity initially by whispering questions from a distance of approximately 8 feet. If hearing deficit is suspected, complete audiometric testing should be performed. Audiometry measures the threshold of hearing for frequencies and loudness. In addition, all children should have audiometric testing performed before entering school.	Answers whispered questions. Audiometry results are within normal ranges.	Failure to respond to whispered questions may indicate hearing deficit. Audiometry results outside normal range suggest hearing deficit.

Thorax and Lungs

Inspection Inspect the shape of the thorax.	By age 5 to 6 years, the thoracic diameter reaches the adult 1:2 or 5:7 ratio (anteroposterior to transverse).	Abnormal shapes of the thorax include pectus excavatum and pectus corinatum.
Children under 7 years old are abdominal breathers.	Respirations should be unlabored and regular in all ages. Respirations should be 2 years to 10 years: 20–28 breaths per minute 10 years to 18 years: 12–20 breaths per minute	Retractions (suprasternal, sternal, substernal, intercostal) and grunting suggest increased inspiratory effort, which may be due to asthma, atelectasis, pneumonia, or airway obstruction. Periods of apnea that last longer than 20 s and are accompanied by bradycardia may be a sign of a cardiovascular or CNS disease.
Percussion and Auscultation **Percuss and auscultate the lungs.** During percussion of the lungs, note tone elicited.	Hyperresonance is the normal tone elicited in young children because of thinness of the chest wall. This diminishes as the child ages and the chest wall develops.	A dull tone may indicate a mass, fluid, or consolidation.
Auscultate for breath sounds and adventitious sounds. If a toddler's lung sounds seem noisy, auscultate the upper nostrils. Toddlers with an upper respiratory infection may transmit noisy breathing from the upper nostrils to the upper lobes of the lungs. Encourage deep breathing in children; try one of the following techniques: blow out light on otoscope (Fig. 31-22), blow cotton ball in air, blow pinwheel, "race" paper off table.	Breath sounds may seem louder and harsher in young children because of their thin chest wall. No adventitious sounds should be heard, although transmitted upper airway sounds may be heard on auscultation of thorax.	Diminished breath sounds suggest respiratory disorders such as pneumonia or atelectasis. Stridor (inspiratory wheeze) is a high-pitched, piercing sound that indicates a narrowing of the upper tracheobronchial tree. Expiratory wheezes indicate narrowing in the lower tracheobronchial tree. Rhonchi and rales (crackles) may indicate a number of respiratory diseases such as pneumonia, bronchitis, or bronchiolitis.

continued

Assessment Procedure	Normal Findings	Abnormal Findings
Breasts		
Inspect and palpate breasts. Note shape, symmetry, color, tenderness, discharge, lesions, and masses.	Breasts are flat and symmetric in prepubertal children. Obese children may appear to have breast tissue.	Redness, edema, and tenderness indicate mastitis. Enlargement in adolescent boys suggests gynecomastia. Masses in the adolescent female breast usually indicate cysts or trauma.
Assess stage of breast/sexual development of girl client. Teach breast self-exam to adolescents.	See Tanner's sexual maturity rating in Table 31-1.	Breast development before age 8 may indicate precocious puberty or thelarche. Lack of breast development after age 13 may indicate delayed puberty and/or a pathologic process.
Heart		
Inspection and Palpation **Inspect and palpate the precordium.** Note lifts and heaves. Palpate apical impulse (Fig. 31-23).	The apical pulse is at the 4th intercostal space (ICS) until the age of 7 years, when it drops to the 5th. It is to the left of the midclavicular line (MCL) until age 4, at the MCL between ages 4 and 6, and to the right at age 7.	A systolic heave may indicate right ventricular enlargement. Apical impulse that is not in proper location for age may indicate cardiomyopathy, pneumothorax, or diaphragmatic hernia.

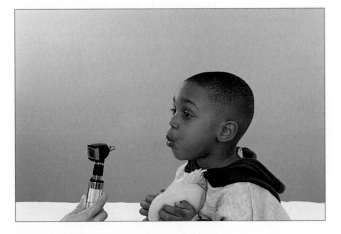

Figure 31-22 To encourage deep breathing, ask a child to blow out the light on an otoscope or a penlight (© B. Proud).

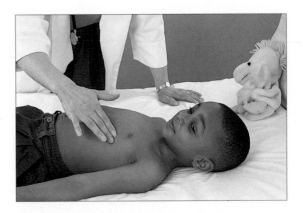

Figure 31-23 To palpate a preschooler's apical pulse, place your hand at the 4th intercostal space to the left of the midclavicular line (© B. Proud).

continued

PHYSICAL ASSESSMENT *Continued*

Assessment Procedure	Normal Findings	Abnormal Findings
Auscultation		
Auscultate heart sounds. Listen to the heart. Note rate and rhythm of apical impulse, S_1, S_2, extra heart sounds, and murmurs. ➤ *Clinical Tip • Keep in mind that sinus arrhythmia is normal in young children. Heart sounds are louder, higher pitched, and of shorter duration in children. A split S2 at the apex occurs normally in some children, and S3 is a normal heart sound in some children. A venous hum also may be normally heard in children.*	Normal heart rates are cited in the "Vital Signs" section above. Innocent murmurs, which are common throughout childhood, are classified as systolic; short duration; no transmission to other areas; grade III or less; loudest in pulmonic area (base of heart); low-pitched, musical, or groaning quality that varies in intensity in relation to position, respiration, activity, fever, and anemia. No other associated signs of heart disease.	Murmurs that do not fit the criteria for innocent murmurs may indicate a disease or disorder. Extra heart sounds and variations in pulse rate and rhythm also suggest pathologic processes.

Abdomen

Inspection		
Inspect the shape of the abdomen.	In children up to 4 years of age, the abdomen is prominent in standing and supine positions. After age 4, the abdomen appears slightly prominent when standing, but flat when supine until puberty.	A scaphoid (boat-shaped; i.e, sunken with prominent rib cage) abdomen may result from malnutrition or dehydration.
Inspect umbilicus. Note color, discharge, evident herniation of the umbilicus.	Umbilicus is pink, no discharge, odor, redness or herniation.	Inflammation, discharge, and redness of umbilicus suggest infection. Diastasis recti (separation of the abdominal muscles) is seen as midline protrusion from the xiphoid to the umbilicus or pubis symphysis. This condition is secondary to immature musculature of abdominal muscles and usually has little significance. As the muscles strengthen, the separation resolves on its own. A bulge at the umbilicus suggests an umbilical hernia, which may be seen in newborns; many disappear by the age of 1 year, and most by 4 or 5 years of age. Umbilical hernias are seen more frequently in African American children.

continued

Assessment Procedure	Normal Findings	Abnormal Findings
Auscultation **Auscultate bowel sounds.** Follow auscultation guidelines for adult clients provided in Chapter 22.	Normal bowel sounds occur every 10 to 30 s. They sound like clicks, gurgles, or growls.	Marked peristaltic waves almost always indicate a pathologic process such as pyloric stenosis.
Palpation **Palpate for masses and tenderness.** Palpate abdomen for softness or hardness. ➤ *Clinical Tip* • *To decrease ticklishness, have the child help by placing his or her hand under yours, using age-appropriate distraction techniques, and maintaining conversation focused on something other than the examination (Fig. 31-24).*	Abdomen is soft to palpation and without masses or tenderness.	A rigid abdomen is almost always an emergent problem. Masses or tenderness warrants further investigation.
Palpate liver. Palpate the liver the same as you would for adults (see Chapter 22).	Liver is usually palpable 1 to 2 cm below the right costal margin in young children.	An enlarged liver with a firm edge that is palpated more than 2 cm below the right costal margin usually indicates a pathologic process.
Palpate spleen. Palpate the spleen the same as you would for adults.	Spleen tip may be palpable during inspiration.	Enlarged spleen is usually indicative of a pathologic process.
Palpate kidneys. Palpate the kidneys the same as you would for adults.	The tip of the right kidney may be palpable during inspiration.	Enlarged kidneys are usually indicative of a pathologic process.
Palpate bladder. Palpate the bladder the same as you would for adults.	Bladder may be slightly palpable in small children.	An enlarged bladder is usually due to urinary retention but may be due to a mass.

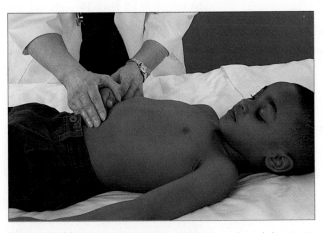

Figure 31-24 Let a child help palpate his or her abdomen to decrease ticklishness (© B. Proud).

continued

PHYSICAL ASSESSMENT *Continued*

Male Genitalia

Inspect penis and urinary meatus. Inspect the genitalia observing size for age and any lesions.

➤ *Clinical Tip • Use distraction or teaching (such as testicular self-examination) when examining the genitalia in older children and adolescents to decrease embarrassment.*

Penis is normal size for age, and no lesions are seen. The foreskin is retractable in uncircumcised child. Urinary meatus is at tip of glans penis and has no discharge or redness. Penis may appear small in obese boys because of overlapping skin folds.

An unretractable foreskin in a child older than 3 months suggests phimosis. Paraphimosis is indicated when the foreskin is tightened around the glans penis in a retracted position. Hypospadias, urinary meatus on ventral surface of glans, and epispadias, urinary meatus on dorsal surface of glans, are congenital disorders (see Abnormal Findings 24-1). Discharge, redness, or lacerations may indicate abuse in young children but may occur from infections or foreign body. Discharge in adolescents may be due to sexually transmitted disease, infection, or irritation.

Inspect and palpate scrotum and testes. To rule out cryptorchidism, it is important to palpate for testes in the scrotum in infants and young boys.

➤ *Clinical Tip • When palpating the testicles in the infant and young boy, you must keep the cremasteric reflex in mind. This reflex pulls the testicles up into the inguinal canal and abdomen and is elicited in response to touch, cold, or emotional factors. Have young boys sit with knees flexed and abducted. This lessens the cremasteric reflex and enables you to examine the testicles.*

Scrotum is free of lesions. Testes are palpable in scrotum, with the left testicle usually lower than the right. Testes are equal in size, smooth, mobile, and free of masses. If a testicle is missing from the scrotal sac but the scrotal sac appears well developed, suspect physiologic cryptorchidism. The testis has originally descended into the scrotum but has moved back up into the inguinal canal because of the cremasteric reflex and the small size of the testis. You should be able to milk the testis down into the scrotum from the inguinal canal. This normal condition subsides at puberty.

Absent testicle(s) and atrophic scrotum suggest true cryptorchidism (undescended testicles; see Chapter 6). This suggests that the testicle(s) never descended. This condition occurs more frequently in preterm than term infants because testes descend at 8 months of gestation. It can lead to testicular atrophy and infertility, and increases the risk for testicular cancer. Hydroceles are common in infants. They are fluid-filled masses that can be transilluminated (see Abnormal Findings 24-2). They usually resolve spontaneously. A scrotal hernia is usually caused by an indirect inguinal hernia that has descended into the scrotum. It can usually be pushed back into the inguinal canal. This mass will not transilluminate. A painless nodule on the testis may indicate testicular cancer, which appears most frequently in males aged 15 to 34 years; therefore, testicular self-examination (TSE) should be taught to all boys 14 years old and older.

Inspect and palpate inguinal area for hernias. Observe for any bulge in the inguinal area. Ask the child to bear down or try to lift something heavy to elicit a possible hernia. Using your pinky finger, palpate up the inguinal canal to the external inguinal ring if a hernia is suspected.

No inguinal hernias are present.

A bulge in the inguinal area or palpation of a mass in the inguinal canal suggests an inguinal hernia. Indirect inguinal hernias occur most frequently in children (see Chapter 24).

continued

Assessment Procedure	Normal Findings	Abnormal Findings
Assess sexual development. Note pubic hair pattern, and size and development of penis and scrotum.	See Tanner's sexual maturity ratings in Table 31-2.	Pubic hair growth, enlargement of the penis to adolescent or adult size, and enlarged testes in a boy less than 8 years of age suggest precocious puberty.

Female Genitalia

Inspect external genitalia. Note labia majora, labia minora, vaginal orifice, urinary meatus, and clitoris. ➤ *Clinical Tip • Have female children assist with genitalia examination by using their hands to spread the labia. This helps to decrease any stress and embarrassment.*	Labia majora and minora are pink and moist. Young girls have flattened majora, thin minora, small clitoris, and thin hymen. Starting at school age, the labia become fuller and the hymen thickens. This progresses until puberty when the genitalia develop adult characteristics. No discharge from vagina or meatus; no redness or edema present normally.	Partial or complete labia minora adhesions are sometimes seen in girls younger than 4 years of age. Referral is necessary to disintegrate the thin, membranous adhesion. An imperforate hymen (no central orifice) is sometimes seen and is not significant unless it persists until puberty and causes problems with menstruation. Discharge from vagina or urinary meatus, redness, edema, or lacerations may suggest abuse in the young child. However, infections or a foreign body in the vagina may cause these symptoms. Discharge in adolescents suggests sexually transmitted disease, infection, or irritation.
Inspect internal genitalia. An internal genitalia examination is not routinely performed in the child although it may be called for if infection, bleeding, a foreign body, disease, or sexual abuse is suspected. A pediatric specialist should perform the examination. An internal genital examination consisting of both the speculum and bimanual examinations is recommended for all sexually active adolescents and/or virgins starting at 18 years of age. In addition, an internal examination is indicated in the adolescent who has nonmenstrual bleeding or discharge. The procedure is the same as for the adult. Time and care must be taken for adequate teaching and reassurance.	See Chapter 23 for normal findings.	See Chapter 23 for abnormal findings.

continued

PHYSICAL ASSESSMENT *Continued*

Assessment Procedure	Normal Findings	Abnormal Findings
Assess sexual development. Note pubic hair pattern.	See Tanner's sexual maturity ratings in Table 31-2 and 31-3 for normal findings.	Growth of pubic hair in young girls (<8 years of age) suggests precocious puberty. Unusual pubic hair distribution in pubertal girls may indicate a disorder. For example, a male pattern of hair growth may suggest polycystic ovary disease.

Anus and Rectum

Inspection and Palpation

Inspect the anus. The anus should be inspected in children and adolescents. Perform quickly at the end of the genitalia examination to limit embarrassment in the older child and adolescent. Spread the buttocks with gloved hands, and note patency of anal opening, presence of any lesions and fissures, and condition and color of perianal skin.	The anal opening should be visible, moist, and hairless. No hemorrhoids or lesions. Perianal skin should be smooth and free of lesions. A mild diaper rash (red papules) may be seen in infants. Perianal skin tags may be noted.	Imperforate anus (no anal opening) should be referred. Hemorrhoids are unusual in children and could be due to chronic constipation, but may be caused by sexual abuse or abdominal pressure from lesion. Bleeding and pain often indicate tears or fissures in the anus, which often cause constipation because of pain of passing stool. Pustules may indicate secondary infection of diaper rash. A dark ring around the anus may indicate heavy metal poisoning. Lacerations, purulent discharge, or extreme apprehension during examination may indicate physical or sexual abuse. Diaper rashes with more than mild red/pink papules suggest problems such as seborrhea, diaper dermatitis, and monilial infection.
Palpate rectum. This internal examination is not routinely performed in children or adolescents. However, it should be performed if symptoms suggest a problem. The child should be in a supine position with the legs flexed. Provide reassurance throughout the examination. If the child is old enough, ask him or her to bear down. This helps to relax the sphincter. Slowly insert a gloved, lubricated finger (the pinky finger may be used for comfort, but the index finger is more sensitive) into the anal opening, aiming the finger toward the umbilicus.	Prostate gland is nonpalpable in young boys. Bimanual rectoabdominal exam in girls may reveal small midline mass (cervix).	If other masses are palpated, they are considered abnormal; no other structures are palpable until adolescence.

Musculoskeletal

Inspection

Assess feet and legs. Note symmetry, shape, movement, and positioning of the feet and legs. Perform neurovascular assessment.	Feet and legs are symmetric in size, shape, movement, and positioning (Fig. 31-25). Extremities should be warm, and mobile with adequate capillary refill. All	Short, broad extremities, hyperextensible joints, and palmar simian crease may indicate Down syndrome. Polydactyly (extra digits) and syndactyly (webbing)

continued

Assessment Procedure	Normal Findings	Abnormal Findings
	pulses (radial, brachial, femoral, popliteal, pedal) should be strong and equal bilaterally. A common finding in children (up to 2 or 3 years old) is metatarsus adductus deformity. This is an inward positioning of the forefoot with the heel in normal straight position, and it resolves spontaneously. Tibial torsion, also common in infants and toddlers, consists of twisting of the tibia inward or outward on its long axis, is usually caused by intrauterine positioning, and typically corrects itself by the time the child is 2 years old.	are sometimes found in children with mental retardation. Neurovascular deficit in children is usually secondary to trauma (e.g., fracture). Fixed-position (true) deformities do not return to normal position with manipulation. Metatarsus varus is inversion (a turning inward that elevates the medial margin) and adduction of the forefoot. Talipes varus is adduction of the forefoot and inversion of the entire foot. Talipes equinovarus (clubfoot) is indicated if foot is fixed in the following position: adduction of forefoot, inversion of entire foot, and equinus (pointing downward) position of entire foot (Fig. 31-26).
Assess spinal alignment. Observe spine and posture. Assess for scoliosis (Fig. 31-27).	By 12 to 18 months, the lumbar curve develops. Toddlers display lordotic posture. Findings in older children and adolescents are similar to those in adults.	Kyphosis may result from poor posture or from pathologic conditions. Scoliosis usually is idiopathic and is more common in adolescent girls. Abnormal posture suggests neuromuscular disorders such as cerebral palsy (Fig. 31-28). Extremities that are asymmetric in size, shape, and movement indicate scoliosis or hip disease.

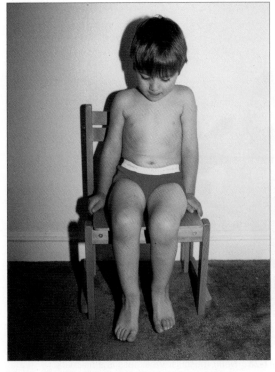

Figure 31-25 Normally positioned feet and legs.

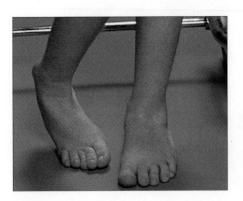

Figure 31-26 Talipes equinovarus, also called clubfoot (© 1995 Science Photo Library/CMSP).

continued

PHYSICAL ASSESSMENT *Continued*

Assessment Procedure	Normal Findings	Abnormal Findings
Assess gait. Observe gait initially when the child enters the exam room. This enables you to observe the child when he or she is unaware of being observed and gait is most natural. Later have the child walk to and from the parent (the child should be barefoot), and observe gait.	Toddlers have a wide-based gait and are usually bow-legged (genu varum). Children aged 2 to 7 are usually knock-kneed (genu valgum). (See Fig. 31-29.) Gait in older children is the same as in adults.	"Toeing in" or "toeing out" indicates problems such as tibial torsion or club-foot. Limping may indicate congenital hip dysplasia (toddlers); synovitis (preschoolers); Legg-Calvé-Perthes disease (school-age children); slipped capital femoral epiphysis, scoliosis (adolescents). When child is wearing shoes, limping usually suggests poorly fitting shoes or presence of a pebble. Many abnormal gaits are noted in cerebral palsy.
Assess joints. Note range of motion, swelling, redness, and tenderness.	Full range of motion and no swelling, redness, or tenderness.	Limited range of motion, swelling, redness, and tenderness indicate problems ranging from mild injuries to serious disorders, such as rheumatoid arthritis.
Assess muscles. Note size and strength.	Muscle size and strength should be adequate for the particular age and should be equal bilaterally.	Inadequate muscle size and strength for the particular age indicate neuromuscular disorders such as muscular dystrophy.

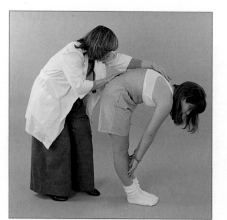

Figure 31-27 Assessing spinal curvature for scoliosis (© B. Proud).

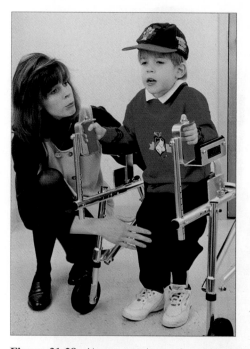

Figure 31-28 Neuromuscular weakness is a hallmark of cerebral palsy.

continued

Assessment Procedure	Normal Findings	Abnormal Findings

Neurologic

Inspection

Much of the neurologic examination of children older than age 2 years is performed in much the same way as for adults.

> **Clinical Tip** • As with adults, integrate the neurologic assessment into the overall assessment, observing the child first in the natural state, then purposefully. Playing games such as "Simon Says" can help elicit responses from young children.

Test cerebral function. Assess level of consciousness, behavior, adaptation, and speech.

The child should be alert and active, respond appropriately, and relate well to the parent and the nurse. Increased independence will be demonstrated with age. By age 3 years, speech should be easily understood.

Abnormal findings include altered level of consciousness and inappropriate responses. Maladaptation is displayed by an inability to relate well to parent and nurse, lack of independence with age, inappropriate responses to commands, hyperactivity, and poor attention span. Although physiologic dysfluency is normal in preschoolers, unintelligible speech by age 3 years, prolonged stuttering, slurring, and lisping indicate speech disorders or neurologic problems. Slurring may also be indicative of substance abuse, drug toxicity, or conditions such as diabetic ketoacidosis.

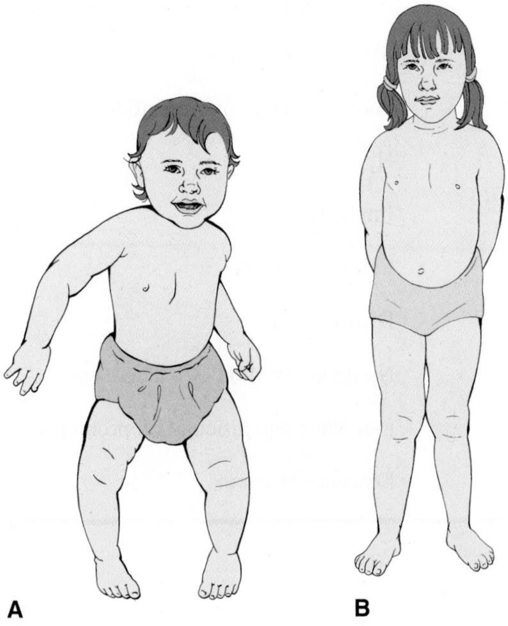

Figure 31-29 (A) Genu varum (bow legs); (B) genu valgum (knock knees).

continued

PHYSICAL ASSESSMENT *Continued*

Assessment Procedure	Normal Findings	Abnormal Findings
Test cranial nerve function. Test cranial nerve function in young people the same way as for adults when possible.	Normal findings are the same as for adults.	Alterations in cranial nerve function demonstrate problem or pathologic process.
Test deep tendon and superficial reflexes. Test deep tendon and superficial reflexes in young people the same way as for adults. Display 30-1 addresses reflex testing in newborns.	Normal findings are the same as for adults, except the Babinski response is normal in children younger than 2 years (this response usually disappears between 2 and 24 months), and triceps reflex is absent until age 6.	Absence or marked intensity of these reflexes, asymmetry, and presence of Babinski response after age 2 years may demonstrate pathology. Sustained (continuous) ankle clonus is abnormal and suggests CNS disease.
Test balance and coordination. Balance and coordination in a child are tested in much the same way as for an adult. Have the child hop, skip, and jump, when appropriate for developmental age.	School-age children and adolescents should be able to perform most balance and coordination tests.	Abnormal findings include unstable gait, lack of coordination of movements, and positive Romberg. These may indicate a number of problems, including CNS disease and neuromuscular disorders.
Test sensory function. Same as for adults, when possible.	Sensitivity to touch and discrimination should be present. The thresholds of touch, pain, and temperature are higher in older children.	Absent or decreased sensitivity to touch and two-point discrimination may indicate paresthesia.
Test motor function. Tests for motor function in children are similar to tests for adults. Also watch for hand preference.	Gross and fine motor skills should be appropriate for the child's developmental age. Hand preference is developed during the preschool years.	Gross and fine motor skills that are inappropriate for developmental age and lack of head control by age 6 months may indicate cerebral palsy. Hand preference that is not developed during preschool years may indicate paresis on opposite side.
Observe for "soft signs." Soft signs of neurologic problems are controversial, because these signs do not always indicate a pathologic process.	Soft signs disappear with age.	Soft signs include but are not limited to

Short attention span

Poor coordination of position

Hypoactivity

Impulsiveness

Labile emotions

Distractibility

No demonstration of handedness

Language and articulation problems

Learning problems |

VALIDATING AND DOCUMENTING FINDINGS

Documentation for children and adolescents is the same as that for adults. Nurses document what they observed, palpated, percussed, and auscultated. Descriptions should be objective, accurate, and concise, yet comprehensive. Terms such as *good,* *poor,* and *normal* should be avoided. Phrases and standardized abbreviations are preferable to full sentences, and a sequential manner should be followed.

Sample of Subjective Data

Caucasian female, age 13 months. Visiting for well-child care. Current health and illness status: Has been well since last health care visit at age 9 months; no current problems, health concerns, or medications. Past Health History: Birth FTNSVD (full-term, normal, spontaneous delivery), BW (birth weight) 7 lb; no problems. Otitis media at age 6 months. Allergies (and reaction to same): None. Immunization status: UTD (up to date).

Growth and developmental milestones: Sat at 6-1/2 months; walked at 11 months; first word ("dada") at 8 months. Habits: None.

ROS: General: Well child, three "colds" in first year; Integument: No lesions, bruising; Head: No trauma, headaches; Eyes: Visual acuity, no problems by history; last eye exam (N/A [nonapplicable]); no drainage, infections; Ears: Hearing acuity, no problems by history; last hearing exam (N/A); no drainage; history of (h/o) otitis media at 6 months treated with amoxicillin); Nose: No bleeding, congestion, discharge; Mouth: No lesions, soreness; no tooth eruption, last dental exam (N/A); Throat: No sore throats, hoarseness, difficulty swallowing; Neck: No stiffness, tenderness; Chest: No pain, cough, wheezing, shortness of breath, asthma, infections; Breasts: No thelarche, lesions, discharge; Cardiovascular: No history of murmurs, exercise tolerance, dizziness, palpitations, congenital defects; Gastrointestinal: Appetite excellent; bowel habits (one soft, brown BM/day); no food intolerances, nausea, vomiting, pain, history of parasites; Genitourinary: No urgency, frequency, discharge, urinary tract infections; Gynecologic: No discharge; Musculoskeletal: No pain, swelling, fractures, mobility problems; Neurologic: No tremors, unusual movements, seizures; Lymphatic: No pain, swelling or tenderness, enlargement of spleen or liver; Endocrine/metabolic: Growth patterns follow 50%; no polyuria, polydipsia, polyphagia.

Psychiatric history: No developmental disorder. Family history: Diabetes (maternal grandmother); hypertension (paternal grandfather). Nutritional history: Drinks three 8-oz bottles of whole milk/day; eats three meals consisting of mixture of baby and table foods. Likes finger foods; hates strained meats and string beans. No problems with feeding, feeds self with much assistance, uses spoon and cup. Takes multivitamin daily.

Determine the quantity and the types of food or formula ingested daily: use 24-h recall, food diary for 3 days (2 weekdays and 1 weekend day), or food frequency record.

Sleep history: Bedtime is 8 PM, awakens at 6 AM. Takes two brief naps/day. Sleeps with favorite blanket, "Kermie."

Psychosocial history: Lives with single mother, age 35 years. Mother is vice president at major company; mother completed graduate school. Cultural background is Italian/Irish; religion, Protestant. Mother has no contact with child's father but does have strong network of friends and family members. No financial difficulties. Attends day care while mother works. Plays with dolls and push toys; mother very safety conscious of toys and uses car seat. Discipline: Mother uses distraction and reinforces word "no." No history of domestic violence; no guns in household

Developmental History: Cognitive: Likes to put things in her mouth to explore them; likes to feel different textures. Knows her name and can point to five body parts. Searches for hidden objects. Language: Knows 10 words, including "no." Gross motor: Walks without help, starting to climb. Fine motor: Right-handed, builds two-block tower

Sample of Objective Data

General appearance: Alert, active, well-developed, well-nourished 1-year-old girl, in no acute distress.

Vital signs: BP 90/50; P 100; T 98.6. Wt: 21 lb. (50%); Ht: 29 in (50%); HC 45 cm (50%).

Skin: Pink, moist, appropriate turgor, no lesions; hair curly with normal distribution; nails pink and hard

Head and neck: Normocephalic, fontanelles not palpable, neck supple, no lymph nodes palpable

Mouth, throat, nose, and sinus: Pharynx clear, no adenopathy, nares patent, turbinates pink with scant clear discharge

Eyes and ears: Sclera clear, pupils equally round, react to light and accommodation (PERRLA), external ear canal free of cerumen impaction, foreign body, discharge, tympanic membrane pink with regular rhythm, no murmurs auscultated

Abdomen: Soft, no masses or organomegaly

Genitalia and rectum: Tanner's 1, no discharge or lesions

Musculoskeletal: Spine straight, no tufts or dimples, FROM, adequate muscle strength and tone

Neurologic: Cranial nerves II to XII intact, deep tendon reflexes 2+, no Babinski, sensitive to touch, coordination, gross and fine motor movement appropriate for age.

Thorax and lungs: Thorax round and symmetric, hyperresonance percussed over lung fields

Heart: 100 beats/min

Analysis of Data

DIAGNOSTIC REASONING: POSSIBLE CONCLUSIONS

After collecting subjective and objective data pertaining to children and adolescents, identify abnormal findings and client's strengths. Then cluster the data to reveal any significant patterns or abnormalities. These data may then be used to make clinical judgments about the status of the child or adolescent.

Selected Nursing Diagnoses

Following is a listing of selected nursing diagnoses (wellness, risk, or actual) that you may identify when analyzing the cue clusters.

Wellness Diagnoses

- Readiness for enhanced knowledge of eye care during the growing years
- Readiness for enhanced nutritional metabolic pattern of child
- Readiness for enhanced sexual function

Risk Diagnoses

- Risk for Impaired Skin Integrity: "diaper rash" to parental knowledge deficit of skin care for diapered infant or child
- Risk for Injury related to open fontanelles
- Risk for Injury to teeth related to developmental age and play activities
- Risk for Injury related to insertion of foreign bodies into nasal cavity
- Risk for Injury related to attempts to insert foreign objects into ear
- Risk for Aspiration related to improper feeding and small size of stomach in newborns
- Risk for Impaired Urinary Elimination related to parental knowledge deficit of toilet-training techniques
- Risk for Injury related to premature physical developmental level

- Risk for Imbalanced Nutrition: Less Than Body Requirements

Actual Diagnoses

- Impaired Skin Integrity: Acne related to developmental changes
- Ineffective Health Maintenance related to lack of proper mouth care
- Ineffective Airway Clearance related to bronchospasm and increased pulmonary secretions
- Deficient Fluid Volume related to vomiting or diarrhea
- Imbalanced Nutrition: More Than Body Requirements

Selected Collaborative Problems

After grouping the data, it may become apparent that certain collaborative problems emerge. Remember that collaborative problems differ from nursing diagnoses in that they cannot be prevented with nursing interventions alone. However, these physiologic complications of medical conditions can be detected and monitored by the nurse. In addition, the nurse can use physician- and nurse-prescribed interventions to minimize the complications of these problems. The nurse may also have to refer the client in such situations for further treatment of the problem. Following is a list of collaborative problems seen more frequently in the pediatric client. However, other collaborative problems seen in the adult are also seen in pediatric clients. These problems are worded as Risk for Complications (or RC), followed by the problem.

- RC: Severe malnutrition/dehydration
- RC: Delayed growth
- RC: Failure to thrive
- RC: Respiratory distress
- RC: Permanently deformed femoral head
- RC: Hydrocephalus/shunt infections

Medical Problems

After grouping the data, the client's signs and symptoms may clearly require medical diagnosis and treatment. Referral to a primary care provider is necessary.

CASE STUDY

The case study demonstrates how to analyze children and adolescent assessment for a specific client. The critical thinking exercises included in the study guide/lab manual and interactive product that complement this text also offer opportunities to analyze assessment data.

Mrs. Carter brings 2½-year-old Michael to the pediatrician's office because he has "been irritable and feverish since last night." Further history reveals that Michael also had a runny nose and cough for 2 days and that his appetite and fluid intake have decreased since the fever started. Michael is otherwise healthy; this is his first episodic illness. His physical examination reveals slight, irritable, 2½-year-old boy, pulling at ears,

temperature of 102°F; nasal congestion with clear discharge, tympanic membranes red and bulging bilaterally, pharynx slightly red without exudates, chest clear, abdomen soft without hepatosplenomegaly (HSM), and no meningeal signs.

The pediatrician diagnoses an upper respiratory infection (URI) and bilateral otitis media (BOM) and orders amoxicillin 250 mg tid for 10 days. You, the office nurse, are to

continued

perform the parent teaching for Michael's home care. During your discussion with Mrs. Carter, she tells you that she is concerned that Michael is jealous of his new baby sister because he has occasional tantrums when she holds the baby. She is also concerned about Michael's development because he recently started to refuse using the potty, a skill that is newly acquired. Mrs. Carter is very attentive to both the new baby and Michael throughout the interview, and she asks you for suggestions in how to help Michael cope with the new arrival. While doing so, she points out that her husband has been extra attentive to Michael since his sister was born.

The following concept map illustrates the diagnostic reasoning process.

Applying COLDSPA

Applying **COLDSPA** for client symptoms: "Male 2½-year-old irritable and feverish."

Mnemonic	Question	Data Provided	Missing Data
Character	Describe the sign or symptom (feeling, appearance, sound, smell, or taste if applicable).	"Irritable and feverish."	"Describe the child's irritable behaviors. How high was the temperature? Did the child have chills?"
Onset	When did it begin?	"Last night."	
Location	Where is it? Does it radiate? Does it occur anywhere else?	Nasal congestion with clear discharge; red, bulging bilateral tympanic membranes.	
Duration	How long does it last? Does it recur?	Runny nose and cough for 2 days.	
Severity	How bad is it? or How much does it bother you?	Child pulling at ears and has temperature of 102°F.	
Pattern	What makes it better or worse?	Father gives extra attention to child.	Has the child been given any medications? If so, what type, dose, frequency, and affects on fever and irritability? How long has the child's father been giving extra attention to his son? How does the child respond to this?
Associated factors/How it **A**ffects the client	What other symptoms occur with it? How does it affect you?	Child has had a poor appetite and decreased fluid intake since the onset of the fever; throws temper tantrums when mother holds his new baby sister; refuses to use the potty, a newly acquired skill.	"Describe the child's fluid and food intake during the last 2 days as compared to typical intake prior to irritability and fever. Have temper tantrums worsened since runny nose and cough began? How long has the child been introduced to the new potty?"

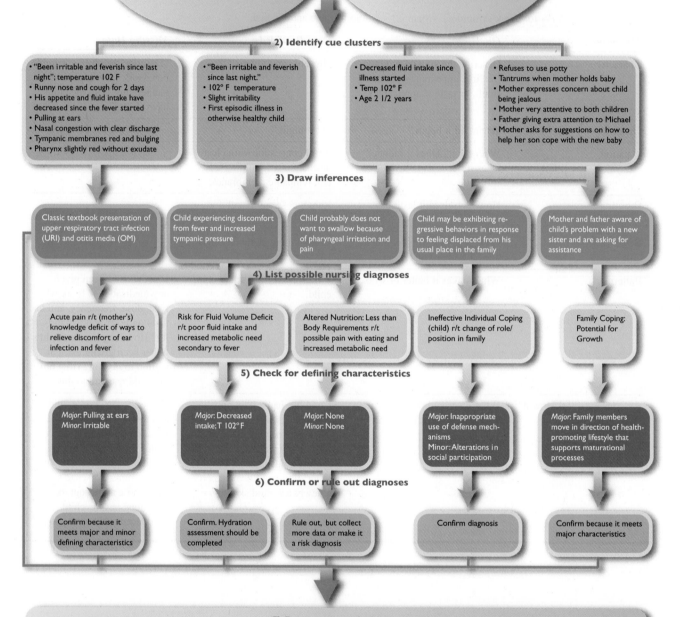

1) Identify abnormal findings and client strengths

Subjective Data
- "Been irritable and feverish since last night"
- Runny nose and cough for 2 days
- His appetite and fluids intake have decreased
- Michael is otherwise healthy; this is his first episodic illness
- [Mother] concerned that Michael is jealous of new baby; he has occasional tantrums when she holds the baby
- [Mother] concerned about Michael's development because he recently started to refuse using the potty
- [Mother] asks you for suggestions in how to help
- Father extra attentive to Michael

Objective Data
- 2 1/2 years old
- Slight irritability
- Pulling at ears
- Temperature of 102°F
- Nasal congestion with clear discharge
- Tympanic membranes red and bulging
- Pharynx slightly red without exudate
- Mrs. Carter is very attentive to both the new baby and Michael throughout the interview

2) Identify cue clusters

- "Been irritable and feverish since last night"; temperature 102 F
- Runny nose and cough for 2 days
- His appetite and fluid intake have decreased since the fever started
- Pulling at ears
- Nasal congestion with clear discharge
- Tympanic membranes red and bulging
- Pharynx slightly red without exudate

- "Been irritable and feverish since last night."
- 102° F temperature
- Slight irritability
- First episodic illness in otherwise healthy child

- Decreased fluid intake since illness started
- Temp 102° F
- Age 2 1/2 years

- Refuses to use potty
- Tantrums when mother holds baby
- Mother expresses concern about child being jealous
- Mother very attentive to both children
- Father giving extra attention to Michael
- Mother asks for suggestions on how to help her son cope with the new baby

3) Draw inferences

- Classic textbook presentation of upper respiratory tract infection (URI) and otitis media (OM)

- Child experiencing discomfort from fever and increased tympanic pressure

- Child probably does not want to swallow because of pharyngeal irritation and pain

- Child may be exhibiting regressive behaviors in response to feeling displaced from his usual place in the family

- Mother and father aware of child's problem with a new sister and are asking for assistance

4) List possible nursing diagnoses

- Acute pain r/t (mother's) knowledge deficit of ways to relieve discomfort of ear infection and fever

- Risk for Fluid Volume Deficit r/t poor fluid intake and increased metabolic need secondary to fever

- Altered Nutrition: Less than Body Requirements r/t possible pain with eating and increased metabolic need

- Ineffective Individual Coping (child) r/t change of role/position in family

- Family Coping: Potential for Growth

5) Check for defining characteristics

- *Major:* Pulling at ears
  Minor: Irritable

- *Major:* Decreased intake; T 102°F

- *Major:* None
  Minor: None

- *Major:* Inappropriate use of defense mechanisms
  Minor: Alterations in social participation

- *Major:* Family members move in direction of health-promoting lifestyle that supports maturational processes

6) Confirm or rule out diagnoses

- Confirm because it meets major and minor defining characteristics

- Confirm. Hydration assessment should be completed

- Rule out, but collect more data or make it a risk diagnosis

- Confirm diagnosis

- Confirm because it meets major characteristics

7) Document conclusions

Nursing diagnoses that are appropriate for this client include:
- Acute Pain r/t (mother's) knowledge deficit of ways to relieve the discomforts of ear infection and fever
- Risk for Fluid Volume Deficit r/t decreased fluid intake secondary to sore throat and increased metabolic need secondary to fever
- Ineffective Individual Coping (child) r/t change of role and position in family
- Family Coping: Potential for Growth

Potential collaborative problems include the following:
- RC: Hyperthermia
- RC: Impairment of hearing
- RC: Pneumonia
Michael should return for follow-up with his pediatrician in 10 to 14 days to check for resolution of his upper respiratory infection and otitis media

References and Selected Readings

ACOG Committee on Adolescent Health Care. (2004). *Compendium of selected publications 2005. Sexually transmitted diseases in adolescents.* Committee Opinion. Number 301, 161–167.

ACOG Committee on Adolescent Health Care. (2004). *Compendium of selected publications 2005. Cervical cancer screening in adolescents.* Committee Opinion, Number 300, 24–28.

American Academy of Pediatrics, Committee on Infectious Diseases. (2007–2008). Prevention of Influenza: Recommendations for Influenza Immunization of Children. *Pediatrics, 121*(4), April 2008. Available at http://www.pediatrics.aappublications.org/cgi/content/full/121/4/e1016/maxtoshow+&HITS=10/ Accessed 9-7-08.

Barr, S. I., Murphy, S. P., & Poos, M. I. (2002). Interpreting and using the dietary reference intakes in dietary assessment of individuals and group. *Journal of the American Dietetic Association, 102*(6), 780–789.

Bright Futures, 3rd ed. (2003). *American Academy of Pediatrics.* Elk Grove Village, IL.

Centers for Disease Control and Prevention. (2007) Quadrivalent human papillomavirus vaccine. Recommendations of the Advisory Committee on Immunization Practices (ACIP). *MMWR,* Early Release. *56,* 1–24.

Glass, N., Fredland, N., Campbell, J., Yonas, M., Sharps, P., & Kub, J. (2003). Adolescent dating violence: Prevalence, risk factors and health outcomes and implications for clinical outcomes. *JOGNN, 32*(2), 227–238.

Hauenstein, E. (2003). Depression in adolescence. *JOGNN, 32*(2), 239–249.

Gregory, K. (2005). Update on nutrition for preterm and full-term infants. *Journal of Obstetric, Gynecologic, and Neonatal Nursing Clinical Issues, 34*(1), 98–108.

Task Force on Newborn and Infant Hearing. (2000). Principles and guidelines for early hearing detection and intervention program. Year 2000 position statement. *Pediatrics, 106*(4), 798–817.

Wilson, P. R., & Pugh, L. C. (2005). Promoting nutrition in breastfeeding women. *JOGNN, Clinical Issues, 34*(1), 120–124.

Wong, D. L. (2003). *Wong's nursing care of infants and children.* (7th ed.). St. Louis, MO: Mosby.

32

Assessing Frail Elderly Clients

Challenges and Approaches

Common physical findings in elderly clients have been identified throughout the preceding body system chapters. It is not, however, the physiologic changes of aging alone that warrant a special approach to assessment of the elderly client. Many older adults are healthy, active, and independent despite these normal physical changes in their bodies. It is, rather, the tendency that advancing age has to place a person at greater risk for chronic illness and disability that has led to using the term *frail elderly.* The term describes the vulnerability of the "old-old" (generally mid-eighties, nineties, and centenarians) to be in poorer health, to have more chronic disabilities, and to function less independently. Nearly 20% of those 64 to 74 years old have limitations on activity because of chronic conditions. Disability takes a much heavier toll on the very old, with nearly 75% of those over age 80 reporting at least one disability. Over one-half have one or more severe disabilities and 35% report needing assistance as a result of disability (Administration on Aging, 2003). Loss of physiological reserve is the main reason that older persons are more likely to be sick and disabled. The average 85-year-old is living with almost 50% less cellular function in organ systems throughout his body. On a daily basis, he may have no ill effects from this loss of reserve. However, if this 85-year-old is living with a chronic problem such as diabetes and then becomes suddenly sick with what is usually a very treatable problem in a younger person (such as a bladder infection), this loss of reserve can have dramatic consequences.

Assessment Modifications for the Frail Elderly

When the physiology of advanced age is combined with co-morbidity, assessment is complicated. In fact, the signs and symptoms of illness often present differently in the oldest-old. Adverse events (AE) or adverse drug effects (ADE) in this population often include falls, confusion, incontinence, generalized weakness, and lethargy. These complications are also referred to as geriatric syndromes and are more common signs and symptoms of illness in the very old than are the more common manifestations of illness in younger adults such as fever, pain, and abnormal lab values. The population at greatest risk for developing atypical presentation is the very elderly who also have cognitive or functional impairment, have multiple co-morbidities, and are being treated with multiple medications (Micelli, 2007).

Knowing the older person's usual daily pattern and functional level is the best baseline against which to compare assessment data. For example, new onset incontinence for the 92-year-old resident of an assisted living facility who still drives her own car should not be viewed as a normal consequence of aging. The incontinence could be the result of an infection or worsening heart failure. A more subtle presentation of these same problems could be signaled by complete incontinence in a 92-year-old man with severe cognitive impairment who until very recently had only occasional incontinence. Clearly, the key to recognizing pathology and illness in the very old is in knowing the person's baseline functional status and recognizing a deviation from it.

COLLECTING SUBJECTIVE DATA: THE NURSING HEALTH HISTORY

Adapting Interview Techniques

In today's youth-oriented culture, it is not uncommon to think of physical frailty as a serious problem. If older people experience some degree of declining health, fear of increasing dependency may be paramount in their minds. Many elderly clients approach clinicians with hesitation because they have known friends and family members who have become sicker or died as a result of intervention. They may also be reluctant to admit health problems because they fear being admitted to a hospital or nursing home. It is essential that the nurse adapt routine interviewing techniques from the perspective that, regardless of the extent of disability and illness being experienced by the older adult, there is always something positive that the older person is doing. Otherwise, the client couldn't have lived to advanced age! For example, it is important to look for good nutritional habits as well as to identify which foods are to be avoided or to focus on everyday activities that keep an older person ambulatory just as it is important to identify risk factors for falls. The nurse needs to acknowledge the older client's accomplishments that have made life meaningful.

Determining Functional Status

Functional assessment is an evaluation of the person's ability to carry out the basic self-care activities of daily living (ADLs) such as bathing, eating, grooming, and toileting. There are many tools available for measuring ability to perform ADLs. One commonly used tool is the Katz Activities of Daily Living (Assessment Tool 32-1), which includes those activities necessary for well-being as an individual in a society. These activities, known as Instrumental Activities of Daily Living (Assessment Tool 32-2), focus primarily on household chores (such as cooking, cleaning, laundry), mobility-related activities (such as shopping and transportation), and cognitive abilities (such as money management, using the telephone, and making decisions affecting basic safety and social needs). Functional ability is determined by the dynamic interplay of the frail elder's physiologic status, emotional and cognitive statuses, and the physical, interpersonal, and social environments. A major purpose of assessing the frail elderly person is to correctly identify and describe the client's ability to perform activities of daily living.

Atypical Presentations of Acute Illness

Symptoms of disease and disability in the very old frequently manifest as incontinence, falls, weakness and lethargy, confusion, changes in sleep or level of alertness, and loss of appetite or weight loss. Not only do these syndromes describe the common and most recognizable ways in which disease often presents itself in the frail elderly, they also describe the consequences of physiologic stress. For example, incontinence and confusion are often signs of infection in the frail elderly person. The incontinence and confusion can easily lead to a fall when the older person attempts to walk to the bathroom, but on the way experiences lightheadedness caused by dehydration and postural hypotension. The fall may result in a hip fracture and immobility, which may lead to a pressure ulcer, urinary tract infection, and delirium. This type of cascade of unfortunate events often leads a frail but independent elder living at home to dependence and disability.

Risk screening tools, such as SPICES (see Display 32-1), may be used to monitor the population of high-risk frail aged for some of the more common nonspecific indicators of disease. Because the oldest-old have the highest prevalence of

---

ASSESSMENT TOOL 32-1	Katz Activities of Daily Living

Activities Points (1 or 0)	Independence: (1 Point) NO supervision, direction or personal assistance	Dependence: (0 Points) WITH supervision, direction, personal assistance or total care
Bathing Points: _____	(1 POINT) Bathes self completely or needs help in bathing only a single part of the body such as the back, genital area or disabled extremity.	(0 POINTS) Needs help with bathing more than one part of the body getting in or out of the tub or shower. Requires total bathing.
Dressing Points: _____	(1 POINT) Gets clothes from closets and drawers and puts on clothes and outer garments complete with fasteners. May have help tying shoes.	(0 POINTS) Needs help with dressing self or needs to be completely dressed.
Toileting Points: _____	(1 POINT) Goes to toilet, gets on and off, arranges clothes, cleans genital area without help.	(0 POINTS) Needs help transferring to the toilet, cleaning self or uses bedpan or commode.
Transferring Points: _____	(1 POINT) Moves in and out of bed or chair unassisted. Mechanical transferring aides are acceptable.	(0 POINTS) Needs help in moving from bed to chair or requires a complete transfer.
Continence Points: _____	(1 POINT) Exercises complete self control over urination and defecation.	(0 POINTS) Is partially or totally incontinent of bowel or bladder.
Feeding Points: _____	(1 POINT) Gets food from plate into mouth without help. Preparation of food may be done by another person.	(0 POINTS) Needs partial or total help with feeding or requires parenteral feeding.
Total Points = _____	6 = High *(patient independent)*	0 = Low *(patient very dependent)*

Adapted with permission from Gerontological Society of America. Katz, S., Down, T. D., Cash, H. R., & Grotz, R. C. (1970). Progress in the development of the index of ADL. *Gerontologist, 10,* 20–30.

ASSESSMENT TOOL 32-2	Lawton Scale for Instrumental Activities of Daily Living (IADL)

Instructions: Start by asking the patient to describe her/his functioning in each category; then complement the description with specific questions as needed.

Ability to Telephone

1. Operates telephone on own initiative: looks up and dials numbers, etc.
2. Answers telephone and dials a few well-known numbers.
3. Answers telephone but does not dial.
4. Does not use telephone at all.

Shopping

1. Takes care of all shopping needs independently.
2. Shops independently for small purchases.
3. Needs to be accompanied on any shopping trip.
4. Completely unable to shop.

Food Preparation

1. Plans, prepares, and serves adequate meals independently.
2. Prepares adequate meals if supplied with ingredients.
3. Heats and serves prepared meals, or prepares meals but does not maintain adequate diet.
4. Needs to have meals prepared and served.

Housekeeping

1. Maintains house alone or with occasional assistance (e.g., heavy work done by domestic help).
2. Performs light daily tasks such as dishwashing and bedmaking.
3. Performs light daily tasks but cannot maintain acceptable level of cleanliness.
4. Needs help with all home maintenance tasks.
5. Does not participate in any housekeeping tasks.

Laundry

1. Does personal laundry completely.
2. Launders small items; rinses socks, stockings, and so on.
3. All laundry must be done by others.

Mode of Transportation

1. Travels independently on public transportation, or drives own car.
2. Arranges own travel via taxi, but does not otherwise use public transportation.
3. Travels on public transportation when assisted or accompanied by another.
4. Travel is limited to taxi, automobile, or ambulette, with assistance.
5. Does not travel at all.

Responsibility for Own Medication

1. Is responsible for taking medication in correct dosages at correct time.
2. Takes responsibility if medication is prepared in advance, in separated dosages.
3. Is not capable of dispensing own medication.

Ability to Handle Finances

1. Manages financial matters independently (budgets, writes checks, pays rent and bills, goes to bank); collects and keeps track of income.
2. Manages day-to-day purchases but needs help with banking, major purchases, controlled spending, and so on.
3. Incapable of handling money.

Scoring: Circle one number for each domain. Total the numbers circled. Total score can range from 8–28. The lower the score, the more independence. Scores are only good for individual patients. Useful to see score comparison over time.

M. P. Lawton. (1971). Functional assessment of elderly people. *Journal of the American Geriatrics Society,* 9(6), 465–481. Reprinted by permission of Blackwell Science, Inc.

DISPLAY 32-1	Common Problems in the Elderly Warranting Further Investigation as Identified by the Acronym "SPICES"

- **S**kin impairment
- **P**oor nutrition
- **I**ncontinence
- **C**ognitive impairment
- **E**vidence of falls or functional decline
- **S**leep disturbances (Francis, Fletcher & Simon, 1998)

chronic illness and comorbidity, one disease may mask the symptoms of another. For example, the fatigue and dyspnea of severe congestive heart failure may mask the anemia caused by a duodenal ulcer. A severe illness is more likely to affect multiple organ systems as the body's reserves and ability to respond to physiologic stress are impaired. For instance, pneumonia will typically precipitate congestive heart failure.

To complicate the assessment process even more, medications often result in significant adverse effects rather than improving the symptoms in the frail elderly. Often a drug is used to treat the adverse drug effect and the problems spiral into a nearly indecipherable multiplicity of symptoms. The adapted Beers' Criteria (HCFA Guidelines for Potentially Inappropriate Medication in the Elderly) identifies medications noted by experts to have potential risks that outweigh potential benefits of the drug for persons older than 65 years of age, regardless of their level of frailty (Molony, 2002).

Thus, collection of subjective data from the frail elderly must take into consideration the more common ways in which diseases and disorders present in elderly people (Amella, 2004). Information regarding falls, weakness, incontinence, confusion, sleep difficulties, and loss of appetite is essential. Finally, the client's family social and economic resources and/or environment must be assessed to determine any relationship to the client's symptoms. For example, isolation, physical barriers, or neglect may precipitate physiologic and functional decline.

(text continues on page 766)

BIOGRAPHIC DATA

Cultural norms were not always as informal as they are today. Many of the elderly grew up when older people were not addressed by their first names except by those very close to them. One should always begin the interview by addressing an older person as "Mr.," "Mrs.," or "Ms.," or with an appropriate title such as "Reverend" or "Doctor." In general, younger people today are more likely to feel comfortable sharing personal information with regard to finances, personal likes and dislikes, and feelings than are older adults. Many older people are also aware of their vulnerability with regard to scams and fraud. Thus, they are reluctant (for good reasons) to give out personal information. An important maxim of geriatric care is: "Collect no more information than is essential for optimal care." If the individual is cognitively impaired, a trusted caregiver may need to be involved in the history. Being sensitive to the older person's need to be respected and acknowledged is essential.

HISTORY OF PRESENT HEALTH CONCERN/CURRENT HEALTH STATUS

Question	Rationale
Mental Status Have you noticed any changes in your ability to concentrate or think clearly enough to keep up with your daily activities? If so, about when did this begin and describe what you have noticed? ➤ *Clinical Tip • If the older person is too lethargic, agitated, or medically unstable to respond, family or professional caregivers should be queried with regard to how current cognition and behavior compares with the client's prior level of function. If the client appears to be excessively distracted during the interview or has revealed multiple inconsistencies or the inability to describe daily activities or to answer specific questions, it is generally advisable to speak with a family member/caregiver when the client is not present about noted changes in cognition or behavior.*	A common symptom of acute illness in the frail elderly is a sudden deterioration of cognition. The aging brain is more easily affected by pathology because it is especially vulnerable to deficits in oxygenation and nutrition. Changes in cognition that have occurred suddenly and recently (e.g. past few days or within past week or two) must ALWAYS be assumed to be the result of a disease or illness and must be thoroughly assessed and appropriately referred for treatment. Although intellectual capacity does not diminish with advancing age, the brain as it ages does become more susceptible to injury. When such a change in cognition develops over a short period of time and is characterized by a change in level of alertness, ranging from extreme lethargy to agitation, it is called delirium. (See Display 32-2.) Delirious people may continuously shift attention from one stimulus to another. Their speech is often difficult to understand because they shift abruptly and inappropriately from one thought to another. It is usually difficult to hold a conversation with a delirious person. Disorientation is more often to time and place rather than to self and delusions and hallucinations may occur.
The Saint Louis University Mental Status (SLUMS) and the Confusion Assessment Method (CAM) are valid Mental Status Examination Tools (Assessment Tool 6-1) for identifying those at risk for developing an acute change in mental status or monitoring progress of mental status.	A common symptom of acute illness in the frail elderly is a sudden deterioration of cognition. The aging brain is more easily affected by pathology because it is especially vulnerable to deficits in oxygenation and nutrition. If assaults to the brain are not reversed quickly enough, irreversible brain tissue damage can ensue. Thus, what was incorrectly diagnosed initially as dementia can actually become that with lack of proper assessment and treatment. Changes in cognition that have occurred suddenly and recently (e.g. past few days or within past week or two) must ALWAYS be

continued on page 758

HISTORY OF PRESENT HEALTH CONCERN/CURRENT HEALTH STATUS *Continued*

Question	*Rationale*
	assumed to be the result of a disease or illness and must be thoroughly assessed and appropriately referred for treatment.
Do you believe that you have more problems with memory than most? Do you believe that life is empty? Have you recently had to drop many of your activities and interests?	Depression is not more common in old age. However, symptoms of depression in the elderly more commonly manifest as changes in cognition (memory deficits, paranoia, and agitation) and physical symptoms (muscle aches, joint pains, gastrointestinal disturbances, headache, and weight loss) than they do in younger adults. Depression in the elderly has even been called "pseudodementia." It can also be a symptom of certain physical disorders, especially endocrine disorders such as hypothyroidism, pancreatic and adrenal disorders, and cancers of all types. Certain antihypertensives, antianxiety drugs, and hormones may also precipitate depressive symptoms.
Open-ended questions usually yield the most beneficial information when screening for depression in the elderly. However, when time is limited or whenever warning signs are noted, a screening instrument such as the short version of the Geriatric Depression Scale (Yesavage & Brink, 1983) should be used for further validation. (See Self Assessment 32-1.)	When more than five questions are answered as indicated on the tool, a high probability of depressive symptoms exists. The purpose of a screening tool is not to confirm a diagnosis but rather to point out the need for a more in-depth assessment or referral.
Are you concerned about changes in your memory? Are you bothered by anger or inability to control your frustrations with day-by-day living?	By age 85, nearly half the population will be exhibiting signs of the most common type of dementia, Alzheimer's disease (AD). Dementia is a broad diagnostic category that includes multiple physical disorders characterized by alterations in memory, abstract thinking, judgment, and perception. Unlike delirium, dementias are characterized by gradual decline in cognitive function to the extent that daily functions are affected (ADLs or IADLs) usually over months or years. Although memory impairment is generally characterized as the key diagnostic criteria for AD, the earliest signs may more often be behavioral and characterized by irritability, aggression or angry outbursts, suspiciousness, or even withdrawal.

continued

COLDSPA Example Adapted to Frail Elderly

Use the **COLDSPA** mnemonic as a guideline to collect needed information for each symptom the client shares. In addition, the following questions help elicit important information.

Mnemonic	*Question*
Character	Describe the sign or symptom. How does it feel, look, sound, smell, and so forth?
Onset	When did it begin? Did the onset occur shortly after taking a new medication? Is the onset associated with a certain activity or time of day?
Location	Where is it? Does it radiate?
Duration	How long does it last? Does it recur?
Severity	How bad is it? Does it affect functional ability to perform ADLs or instrumental activities of daily life (IADLS)?
Pattern	What makes it better? What makes it worse? Does the pattern fit disease geriatric syndrome?
Associated factors/How it **A**ffects the client	What other symptoms occur with it? What other data would be useful in solving the answer to the presenting problem?

HISTORY OF PRESENT HEALTH CONCERN/CURRENT HEALTH STATUS *Continued*

Question	Rationale
Falls Do you ever need to grab onto something because you feel like you're going to stumble or fall? Have you ever used anything to steady yourself when you're walking?	Risk factor assessment for falls is important because the fall can be a symptom of another problem needing attention. A fall can be the symptom of a treatable medical condition, the result of an adverse response to a medication, or a problem associated with chronic illness and frailty. The nurse must be sensitive to an older person's fears and anxieties. Loved ones are also concerned with the safety threat imposed by falls and the possible guilt associated with not being available at the time that a fall occurs. Although the fear of falling is a realistic and common fear, the need to stay active both before and after a fall is even greater. Falling is not a normal part of aging. Limitations in activity are not the appropriate response to a positive fall assessment. The risk of falling can be minimized by a comprehensive assessment followed by appropriate medical, exercise, and adaptive environmental interventions.
Have you had any recent falls? What were you doing? Where did it occur? What other kinds of feelings or symptoms did you have when you fell (i.e. headache, confusion)? Do you ever feel lightheaded or dizzy when you get up from a chair or a bed?	The history should determine the circumstances surrounding any previous falls of the past 3 months to determine if a pattern exists. The pattern and circumstances surrounding the fall can provide valuable clues with regard to the physical, medication, or environmental basis for the fall. For example, falls occurring with standing up and associated with dizziness may point to orthostatic hypotension and an adverse reaction to medication. If the client reports tripping or slipping in the absence of stiffness

continued on page 760

DISPLAY 32-2 | **Causes of Delirium and Dementia**

Various disease states, some diagnosed and some undetected, may contribute to delirium or dementia or both in frail elderly clients.

Disorders Contributing to Delirium
- Brain tumors
- Dehydration
- Toxic drug levels or interactions
- Infections
- Electrolyte imbalances
- Liver or kidney disease
- Hypoxia secondary to respiratory or circulatory disorders
- Hyperthermia or hypothermia
- Metabolic disorders (especially thyroid and blood glucose abnormalities)
- Nutritional deficiencies (especially folate, vitamin B_{12}, and iron deficiencies)

Disorders Contributing to Dementia
Infections
- Creutzfeldt-Jakob disease
- Human immunodeficiency virus (HIV)
- Syphilis

Degenerative Neurologic Disorders
- Alzheimer's disease
- Pick's disease
- Huntington's disease
- Parkinson's disease

Vascular Disorders
- Ministrokes
- Cardiovascular accidents (CVA)

Structural and Traumatic Disorders
- Normal pressure hydrocephalus
- Subdural hematoma
- Head injury
- Tumors

Adapted from Johnson, B. P. 2005. The elderly. In N. C. Frisch & L. E. Frisch (Eds). *Psychiatric mental health nursing.* Albany, NY: Delmar Publishers.

HISTORY OF PRESENT HEALTH CONCERN/CURRENT HEALTH STATUS *Continued*

Question	Rationale
	or weakness and any symptoms, an environmental basis such as shoes or floors with a slick surface or loose carpeting or rugs may be suspected.
Do you have any difficulty when getting up out of bed or from sitting in a chair? Does stiffness and soreness inhibit your ability to move about? Do you ever feel like your legs are going to "give way" or that they are weak? If so, describe. What is your usual daily pattern of activity? Exercise routine?	Clients may benefit from exercises to improve flexibility, fitness, and endurance and to delay functional decline. Exercises can benefit even those who have led sedentary lifestyles or who already have some functional deficits.
Do you have any discomfort in your legs with activity? Would you describe the discomfort as pain, cramping, aching, fatigue, or weakness in the calf? Do your hips, thighs, and/or buttocks hurt with ambulation? If so, how far can you walk before the pain occurs? Does the pain go away with rest?	These symptoms are commonly associated with intermittent claudication, a circulatory disorder affecting the peripheral blood vessels of the leg. Symptoms are usually bilateral and progressive.

continued

SELF ASSESSMENT 32-1	**Assessing Geriatric Depression**

Choose the best answer for how you felt over the past week

1. Are you basically satisfied with your life?	yes/no
2. Have you dropped many of your activities and interests?	yes/no
3. Do you feel that your life is empty?	yes/no
4. Do you often get bored?	yes/no
5. Are you hopeful about the future?	yes/no
6. Are you bothered by thoughts you can't get out of your head?	yes/no
7. Are you in good spirits most of the time?	yes/no
8. Are you afraid that something bad is going to happen to you?	yes/no
9. Do you feel happy most of the time?	yes/no
10. Do you often feel helpless?	yes/no
11. Do you often get restless and fidgety?	yes/no
12. Do you prefer to stay at home, rather than going out and doing new things?	yes/no
13. Do you frequently worry about the future?	yes/no
14. Do you feel you have more problems with memory than most?	yes/no
15. Do you think it is wonderful to be alive now?	yes/no
16. Do you often feel downhearted and blue?	yes/no
17. Do you feel pretty worthless the way you are now?	yes/no
18. Do you worry a lot about the past?	yes/no
19. Do you find life very exciting?	yes/no
20. Is it hard for you to get started on new projects?	yes/no
21. Do you feel full of energy?	yes/no
22. Do you feel that your situation is hopeless?	yes/no
23. Do you think that most people are better off than you are?	yes/no
24. Do you frequently get upset over little things?	yes/no
25. Do you frequently feel like crying?	yes/no
26. Do you have trouble concentrating?	yes/no
27. Do you enjoy getting up in the morning?	yes/no
28. Do you prefer to avoid social gatherings?	yes/no
29. Is it easy for you to make decisions?	yes/no
30. Is your mind as clear as it used to be?	yes/no

For scoring, reverse the answers for Nos. 1, 5, 7, 9, 15, 19, 21, 27, 29, and 30, then count the total number of "yes" answers.

Scoring: 0–10 = within normal range; 11 or higher = possible indication of depression.

Brink, T. A., et al. (1982). Screening tests for geriatric depression. *Clinical Gerontologist,* 1, 37–44.

HISTORY OF PRESENT HEALTH CONCERN/CURRENT HEALTH STATUS *Continued*

Question	*Rationale*

Weakness: Fatigue and Dyspnea

How has your energy level changed in the last few days or weeks? How does it affect your daily activities such as cooking, household chores, or activities outside the home (e.g. shopping, social, church)? When is your energy at its lowest level? When does it seem to be at its best?

> ➤ *Clinical Tip* • *When an older person complains of weakness and fatigue, anemia must always be ruled out. Anemia is always a symptom of an underlying pathology. A few common causes in the elderly are gastrointestinal bleeding and nutritional deficiencies (especially B$_{12}$, folate, and iron). Anticoagulants and NSAIDS increase the risk of GI bleeding.*

Self-reported fatigue and weakness, as well as a decline in physical activity and appetite, are common elements of frailty syndrome. The progression of the weakness and how it relates to ADLs and IADLs provides clues as to possible etiologies. For example, a sudden and severe fatigue that affects self-care activities such as bathing and dressing may be more likely to have an acute cause such as infection, myocardial infarction, or a dysrhythmia such as atrial fibrillation. Diminishing energy over months or weeks is more likely to indicate a more insidious pathology such as a slow gastrointestinal bleed, arthritis and pain, or even depression.

Weakness: Nutrition and Hydration

Do you ever experience shortness of breath? If so, is it related to activity? (Specific questions about endurance, stair climbing, or activities of daily living are necessary for quantifying the extent of the problem.) Does it occur at rest or when lying down? How many pillows do you use? Any pain with breathing?

Dyspnea is a frequently reported symptom associated with common illnesses among elderly clients, including COPD, asthma, lung cancer, and heart failure. Older adults with chronic respiratory or cardiac problems who experience some constant degree of dyspnea are unlikely to seek care or note dyspnea unless there is a change in functional capabilities.

Do you seem to be breathing faster? Sweating? Do you experience anorexia (loss of appetite) or fatigue?

In the frail elder, an increase in respirations, sweating, or overall malaise may be the only indication of a respiratory problem (Kennedy-Malone et al., 2000).

Do you have a recurrent cough? Does it ever have blood in it? Do you use tobacco or have you in the past?

A recurrent cough, fatigue, weight loss, shortness of breath, and productive cough (sometimes blood-tinged) are hallmarks of lung cancer (second most common type of cancer in men over age 75, with incidence rising in women).

Have you experienced any change in your appetite in the past 6 months? If yes, when did you first notice a decline in appetite? Did you have any other health problem at about this same time? Did you start taking any new medication at this time?

A loss of appetite is a nearly universal cofactor of both physical and mental diseases in the elderly.

Can you describe what you eat in an average day? (Compile a 24-hour food and fluid diary noting food preferences and cravings, vitamin and food supplement intake, and dietary restrictions (e.g., salt). On a day when your appetite is less, how would your eating habits change?

A sudden loss of appetite is most often a symptom of disease or an adverse medication effect. Because the aged body is housing a "smaller engine," the minimum caloric intake does decrease in old age. Even healthy older adults consume only an estimated 1,200 to 1,600 calories per day. This has led to the general consensus that older adults need nutrient-dense foods to ingest enough essential nutrients. A 3-day food diary, with 1 day being a weekend day, is the most reliable method of obtaining a diet history.

A screening tool (Self Assessment 32-2) may be helpful in identifying those at risk for being malnourished.

Do you limit the kind or amount of food you eat because of problems with your teeth or dentures (e.g., biting apples or chewing meat)? An oral health assessment tool (Assessment Tool 32-3) may help to detect problems.

Oral health is a vital component of good nutrition, socialization, and a positive self-concept. Untreated oral health problems are a common cause of discomfort that may interfere with chewing and digestion.

Do you ever feel like you're choking when you drink water or feel like food is catching in your throat?

Dysphagia is a frequent problem associated with neurological conditions as well as when food is not sufficiently chewed or

continued on page 762

HISTORY OF PRESENT HEALTH CONCERN/CURRENT HEALTH STATUS *Continued*

Question	*Rationale*
	there is insufficient saliva to mix with food. Dysphagia increases risk of choking, aspiration, dehydration, and malnutrition.
	Signs and symptoms of dysphagia range from weak or hoarse voice, pocketing of food, coughing after food or fluids to drooling.
How much fluid do you think you drink each day?	Fluid intake of fewer than 1,500 mL daily (excluding caffeine-containing beverages) is a possible indicator of dehydration. Fluid requirements for older persons without cardiac or renal disease are approximately 30 ml/kg of body weight per day. Loss of appetite almost always coexists with inadequate hydration. Decreased thirst sensation is common with aging. And decreased mobility makes it less possible for the frail elderly person to respond to an already diminished sense of thirst. Drug use may contribute to dehydration as well. For example, diuretics are widely used in treating cardiovascular and renal disease as are fluid restrictions.
Have you experienced weight loss or changes in your health along with your cough?	Weight loss, night sweats, or changes in respiratory status, such as coughing, may be signs of tuberculosis (TB). Debilitated elderly people are at increased risk of TB. In addition, glucocorticosteroid therapy and nutritional deficiencies depress the immune system, thereby exacerbating the chances of reactivating a dormant TB infection.

continued

SELF ASSESSMENT 32-2   NSI Checklist to Determine Your Nutritional Health

The older adult fills out the following questions, which have associated points.

	Yes
I have an illness or condition that made me change the kind or amount of food I eat.	2
I eat fewer than two meals/day.	3
I eat few fruits or vegetables, or milk products.	2
I have three or more drinks of beer, liquor, or wine almost everyday.	2
I have tooth or mouth problems that make it hard for me to eat.	2
I don't always have enough money to buy the food I need.	4
I eat alone most of the time.	1
I take three or more different prescribed or OTC drugs a day.	1
Without wanting to, I have lost or gained 10 pounds in the last 6 months.	2
I am not always physically able to shop, cook, or feed myself.	2

Total Nutritional Score _____

Scoring:

0–2 indicates good nutrition
3–5 indicates moderate risk
6 or more indicates high nutritional risk

White, J. V., Ham, R. J., Lipschitz, D. A., Dwyer, J. T., & Wellman, N. S. (1991). Consensus of the Nutrition Screening Initiative: Risk factors and indicators of poor nutritional status in older Americans. *Journal of the American Dietetic Society,* 91, 783–787 (used with permission).

HISTORY OF PRESENT HEALTH CONCERN/CURRENT HEALTH STATUS *Continued*

Question	*Rationale*
Have you received the pneumococcal vaccine within the past 6 years? Do you get annual flu vaccines?	Pneumonia is the most common cause of infection-related deaths in the elderly. The pneumovax is recommended once a lifetime for those over age 65 and every 6 years for high-risk patients. Debilitated and institutionalized elders are particularly at risk for serious influenza-related illness.
Urinary Incontinence Explain to the client that many illnesses and medications can cause problems with urine control. This is not normal just because one is getting older, but it is a common problem. Do you ever have any urine leakage or problems controlling your urine flow?	(Between 8 and 38% of older adults living at home are incontinent (Anger, Saigal, & Litwin, 2006). The incidence of UI is higher for elderly who are institutionalized and cognitively impaired. Incidence of new-onset incontinence among hospitalized elderly has been reported at 35% to 45% (Kresevic, 1997; Palmer, Baumgarten, Langenber, & Carson, 2002). Loss of

continued on page 764

ASSESSMENT TOOL 32-3 — The Geriatric Oral Health Assessment Index

Indicate, in the past three months, how often you feel the way described in each of the following statements. Circle one answer for each.

	1	2	3	4	5
1. How often did you limit the kind or amounts of food you eat because of problems with your teeth or dentures?	Always	Often	Sometimes	Seldom	Never
2. How often did you have trouble biting or chewing any kinds of food such as firm meat or apples?	Always	Often	Sometimes	Seldom	Never
3. How often were you able to swallow comfortably?*	Always	Often	Sometimes	Seldom	Never
4. How often have your teeth or dentures prevented you from speaking the way you wanted?	Always	Often	Sometimes	Seldom	Never
5. How often were you able to eat anything without feeling discomfort?*	Always	Often	Sometimes	Seldom	Never
6. How often did you limit contacts with people because of the condition of your teeth or dentures?	Always	Often	Sometimes	Seldom	Never
7. How often were you pleased or happy with the looks of your teeth and gums or dentures?*	Always	Often	Sometimes	Seldom	Never
8. How often did you use medication to relieve pain or discomfort from around your mouth?	Always	Often	Sometimes	Seldom	Never
9. How often were you worried or concerned about the problems with your teeth, gums or dentures?	Always	Often	Sometimes	Seldom	Never
10. How often did you feel nervous or self-conscious because of problems with your teeth, gums or dentures?	Always	Often	Sometimes	Seldom	Never
11. How often did you feel uncomfortable eating in front of people because of problems with your teeth or dentures?	Always	Often	Sometimes	Seldom	Never
12. How often were your teeth or gums sensitive to hot, cold or sweets?	Always	Often	Sometimes	Seldom	Never

Total Score: _____

*Items 3, 5, 7 are reverse scored with a "1" for never and a "5" for always. All other items are a "1" for always.

Source: Hartford Institute for Geriatric Nursing, Division of Nursing, New York University (used with permission).

HISTORY OF PRESENT HEALTH CONCERN/CURRENT HEALTH STATUS *Continued*

Question	*Rationale*
	bladder function or control can be an embarrassing and demeaning problem. Unfortunately, many older adults believe that problems with bladder control are a normal and expected part of aging. Yet this is not an expected part of aging. Incontinence is often associated with chronic conditions such as stroke, multiple sclerosis, prostatitis, and urinary tract infection. It may also be the result of a fecal impaction, constipation, an adverse drug effect, or urinary tract infection (UTI).
(Male) Do you have difficulty starting a stream of urine? Frequency? Nighttime frequency? Dribbling? If yes, do you ever take any cold or sinus medications or medication to help you sleep?	Benign prostatic hypertrophy occurs in 80% of men over age 70 from exposure to androgen hormones. It may result in urinary frequency, difficulty starting a stream of urine, nocturia, and urinary retention with overflow incontinence and an increased risk of urinary tract infections. Over-the-counter drugs with anticholinergic side effects (e.g. cold/sinus preparations and sleep medications) may contribute to urinary retention or add to obstructive symptoms.
How long has the leakage (or use client's descriptive words) been going on? Has it ever suddenly gotten worse?	Any new onset of incontinence or exacerbation may indicate an infection. In the hospitalized elder, UTI ranks high as a suspected cause for any new onset of incontinence. UTI is the most common hospital-acquired bacterial infection. UTI must also be a concern for elders at home or in long-term care because it is the most frequent source of bacteremia for these people. A UTI is particularly perplexing in elderly clients because it presents in such an atypical way (i.e., without fever, or elevation in white blood cell counts, or dysuria, or urinary frequency). Even more common symptoms of a UTI in the frail elderly person may be confusion, lethargy, anorexia, and nocturia.
What activities are associated with your loss of urine control?	The client's activities during an episode of incontinence may help to determine the type of incontinence and, therefore, its treatment. See Display 32-3 for a description of the kinds of urinary incontinence.
Bowel Elimination Do you have any problems with bowel elimination?	As people age, GI motility decreases because of a loss of muscle tone and atrophy. Dehydration, immobility, and poor intake exacerbate the likelihood of constipation. Adequate fluid intake, dietary fiber, and moderate exercise are key factors in maintaining efficient elimination.
Have you had a change in bowel habits recently? Have you ever had blood in your stools? Have you had your stools tested for blood? What medications do you take?	The guaiac stool test to detect occult blood is a common test administered to detect abnormalities of the GI tract. Clients with a past history of polyps, adenomas, and inflammatory bowel disease are at increased risk for colorectal cancer in old age. Warning signs include rectal bleeding, unexplained weight loss, and a change in bowel habits. NSAIDs, such as aspirin and naproxen, corticosteroids, and anticoagulants such as warfarin may promote GI bleeding.
Pain Assessment Do you have pain, discomfort, aching, or soreness? If so, is the discomfort worse with activity? Relieved by rest? Do you have problems with grasping, reaching, or activities that use your hands, arms, back, or legs?	Functional limitations and pain are common consequences of inflammatory joint disease in the frail elderly person The combination of pain and functional impairment may predispose the client to social isolation and depression.

continued

HISTORY OF PRESENT HEALTH CONCERN/CURRENT HEALTH STATUS *Continued*

Question	*Rationale*
Pain scales used with adults are also usually valid in evaluating pain in an elderly client except in the more severe stages of dementia. For those with moderate levels of dementia but who are still able to verbalize, short and frequent questioning about pain using words such as "hurting," "soreness," "aching," or "uncomfortable" may be useful. For nonverbal demented individuals, behaviors such as grimacing, striking out, and moaning should be routinely evaluated to identify pain as well as to evaluate the degree to which the pain is being relieved (Display 32-4). Many of the behaviors commonly labeled as "aggressive" or "combative" are the result of untreated pain (Douzijian, Wilson, Shultz, Berger, Tapnio, & Blanton, 2002).	As many as 50% of community dwelling older people suffer from persistent pain and up to 80% of nursing home residents have substantiated pain that is undertreated (Flaherty, 2007). Pain can lead quickly to a downward cascade of anxiety, depression, isolation, and functional decline. Acute pain frequently manifests as confusion.

DISPLAY 32-3 **Understanding Urinary Incontinence: Assessment and Intervention**

Types of Incontinence

The signs and symptoms associated with the involuntary loss of urine have been clustered into three categories: urge, stress, and overflow incontinence. Any one or a combination of all three types may be present in an individual. Voiding diaries are useful for determining the type of incontinence that is occurring based on the amount, timing, and associated symptoms of incontinent episodes.

Voiding Diary

Time	Drinks		Voiding	
	Kind	How much	How many times	How much
6–7 AM	coffee	2 cups	I	medium
7–8 AM	orange juice	1 glass	II	lots
8–9 AM	———	———	I ———	little
9–10 AM	———	———	———	———
10–11 AM	water	1 glass	I	medium

Time	Leaks/Accidents	Strength of urge	Activity at the time of leak
6–7 AM		strong	no leak
7–8 AM		strong	
8–9 AM	I		frying eggs
9–10 AM			
10–11 AM			

Urge Incontinence

Urge incontinence is the involuntary loss of urine associated with an abrupt and strong desire to void. It is frequently caused by a neurologic disorder such as a cerebrovascular accident (CVA) or multiple sclerosis (MS), which impairs the ability of the bladder or urinary sphincter to contract and relax.

Stress Incontinence

Stress incontinence is the involuntary loss of urine during coughing, sneezing, laughing, or other physical activities that increase abdominal pressure. In women, stress incontinence may result from weakened and relaxed muscles from the combined effects of aging superimposed on the effects of childbirth.

continued on page 766

DISPLAY 32-3 | **Understanding Urinary Incontinence: Assessment and Intervention** *Continued*

Note: Atrophic vaginitis from estrogen deficiency usually results in symptoms of urge incontinence as well as stress incontinence (mixed incontinence).

Overflow Incontinence

Overflow incontinence is the involuntary loss of urine associated with overdistention of the bladder. Prostatic hypertrophy is a common cause in men, and diabetic neuropathy is a common cause in both sexes.

Functional Incontinence

Functional incontinence is the inability to get to the bathroom in time or to understand the cues to void due to problems with mobility or cognition.

Steps of Assessment

The nursing assessment varies somewhat depending on the client's general health status and whether the problem is an acute or chronic one. In general, however, a comprehensive nursing assessment can be described as a five-step process that includes screening for an infection with a urinalysis, obtaining a voiding diary, evaluating functional status, compiling a health history, and performing a physical examination. Key features within the five steps follow:

- Record all incontinent and continent episodes for 3 days in a voiding diary.
- Review medication for any newly prescribed drugs that may be triggering incontinence. Follow up with physician regarding need to discontinue therapy or change medication.
- Rule out constipation or fecal impaction as a source of urinary incontinence. If client has had no bowel movement within last 3 days or is oozing stool continuously, check for impaction by digital examination or abdominal palpation. Problem should be treated if identified.
- Assess functional status along with signs and symptoms as they relate to incontinence. Contributors to incontinence may include immobility, insufficient fluid intake, and confusion. Accompanying signs and symptoms include polyuria, nocturia, dysuria, hesitancy, poor or interrupted urine stream, straining, suprapubic or perineal pain, urgency and characteristics of incontinent episodes (precipitated by walking, coughing, getting in and out of bed and so forth).
- Consult physician regarding physical examination and need to measure postvoid residual volume by straight catheterization (particularly if client dribbles, reports urgency, has difficulty starting stream). Components of the physical examination include direct observation of urine loss using a cough stress test; abdominal, rectal, genital and pelvic examination; and identification of neurologic abnormalities. Abdominal and vaginal examinations are performed to detect prolapse or a palpable bladder after micturition.

Interventions

The physician is responsible for identifying and treating the conditions causing reversible or chronic incontinence. A physical therapist may play a role in identifying specific activities that are associated with incontinent episodes. Either a nurse or physical therapist may be involved in teaching Kegel exercises to help relieve stress incontinence. When functional incontinence and urgency have been identified, the expertise of an occupational therapist in appropriate dressing and undressing and for choosing incontinence aids may be beneficial.

DISPLAY 32-4 | **Indicators of Pain in the Cognitively Impaired**

- Medical diagnoses known to commonly cause pain such as arthritis, osteoporosis, fractures, cancer, and history of back pain
- Pain history and use of analgesics
- Family or professional caregiver reports of possible pain
- Behavioral patterns of aggressiveness or resisting care
- Rubbing on specific areas of body
- Vocalizations, such as moaning (yelling, or increases in the loudness of existing vocalizations)

COLLECTING OBJECTIVE DATA: PHYSICAL EXAMINATION

There is often a fine line between deterioration of function from aging and deterioration from disease. For this reason, it is crucial to integrate the subjective, functional, and physical assessments. The significance of a physical finding is often determined by the effect it has on the person's level of comfort and ability to function. A medical pathology should be suspected whenever any physical or functional change has occurred suddenly (days to weeks).

An efficient and effective way to determine the significance of physical findings in an older person is to collect subjective data while you are conducting a physical examination. Because medication is often a primary method of treating disease in this country and polypharmacy is such a common occurrence in the elderly, sudden changes or abnormalities noted in the physical examination must always be analyzed for the possibility of being the result of an adverse drug effect. Because many diseases have a "silent" presentation in the elderly, an in-depth, comprehensive physical examination is especially important to detect and treat disease in a timely way.

Preparing the Client

The nurse needs to examine one's own attitudes or stereotypical assumptions of the elderly client. It is essential that the nurse also be sensitive to the client's need for privacy as well as his or her wishes for a caregiver to remain in the room during all or parts of the assessment.

The examination of a frail elderly adult usually takes longer than that of a younger adult because of the chronic conditions, disabilities, and ensuing discomfort that many frail elderly people experience. It is best to limit the length of the examination. This may mean that a complete assessment may require several sessions over a period of time. The client may feel less hurried if paperwork, such as a health questionnaire, can be completed at home either by the client alone or with the help of a caregiver. Some modifications and techniques appropriate for an examination of the frail elderly person include:

- Keep the temperature of the examination room warmer than may be comfortable for younger adults.
- Eliminate background noise as much as possible.
- When interacting with an elderly client, remember that it may be more acceptable to be more formal than informal. For example, address the client by first name only if the client specifically requests that you do so.
- Keep your voice volume down even if you anticipate the client has difficulty hearing. Speaking clearly and at a moderate pace is more beneficial in cases of hearing loss. Remember to face the client when speaking with him or her.
- Do not assume that the client cannot answer questions if he or she has a cognitive impairment. However, if the impairment has significantly impaired function or verbal expression, give only one-step directions and avoid questions that require two responses. The cognitively impaired elderly person with few remaining verbal abilities may have no or only minimal loss of the ability to comprehend nonverbal cues.
- If you need to question caregivers or collateral sources to validate or clarify information, avoid consulting them in the presence of the client.
- Elderly people with physical disabilities may need assistance with dressing and with parts repositioning during the examination. Allow additional time in deference to the client's need for independence as well as your need to know how much the client can do independently.

Equipment

In addition to the equipment needed for performing a complete adult physical examination, the following items will be needed for assessing the functional capacity of the frail elderly adult:

- Newspaper or book and lamp light for vision testing
- Lemon slice or mint for sense of smell test
- Pudding or food of pudding consistency and spoon for swallowing examination (A teacup with water to swallow may also be used.)
- Food and fluid diary sheets or forms
- Two or three pillows for client comfort and positioning
- Straight-backed chair for "Get Up and Go" test

(text continues on page 788)

PHYSICAL ASSESSMENT

Assessment Procedure	Normal Findings or Variations	Abnormal Findings
Measure and record the client's height and weight, noting weight changes and problems with swallowing or chewing. Review laboratory test values (complete blood count, and vitamin B$_{12}$, cholesterol, albumin, and prealbumin levels). ➤ **Clinical Tip** • *Suspect drug toxicity in clients taking medications such as digoxin, theophylline, quinidine, or antibiotics if client reports nausea or diarrhea.*	Antral cells and intestinal villi atrophy, and gastric production of hydrochloric acid decreases with age. Chronic diseases such as cancer and arthritis are associated with increases in inflammatory chemicals that can cause anorexia and fatigue. A certain degree of anorexia also always accompanies pain—especially chronic pain. (See Chapter 8 for a discussion of pain assessment.) Toxic levels of drugs must always be suspected when appetite loss is sudden and severe. The ability to smell and taste decreases with age which can also diminish appetite. Medications can also decrease sense of smell and taste in older people.	Indicators of malnutrition include: Client weighs less than 80% ideal body weight. Client has had 10% loss in body weight over past 6 months or 5% loss in body weight over past month. Hemoglobin level is lower than 12 g/dL. Hematocrit is lower than 35. Vitamin B$_{12}$ level is lower than 100 µg/ml. Indicators of poor nutritional status include: Serum cholesterol level lower than 160 mg/dL Serum albumin level lower than 3.5 g/dL Serum prealbumin levels (used to monitor improvement of nutritional status) that do not increase 1 mg/dL/day

continued

PHYSICAL ASSESSMENT Continued

Assessment Procedure	Normal Findings or Variations	Abnormal Findings
Because muscle mass decreases and fatty tissues increase, the elderly client is at increased risk for dehydration. Evaluate hydration status as you would nutritional status. Begin with accurate serial measurements of weight, careful review of laboratory test findings (serial serum sodium level, hematocrit, osmolality, BUN level, and urine-specific gravity), and a 2- to 3-day diary of fluid intake and output.	Normal findings include stable weight and stable mental status. ➤ *Clinical Tip* • *Increases over time in laboratory values are usually indicators of deteriorating hydration (even though values may be within normal limits).*	Sudden weight loss; fever; dry, warm skin; furrowed, swollen, and red tongue; decreased urine output; lethargy and weakness are all signs of dehydration. An acute change in mental status (particularly confusion), tachycardia, and hypotension may indicate severe dehydration, which may be precipitated by certain medications such as diuretics, laxatives, tricyclic antidepressants, or lithium.

Assessment Procedure	Normal Findings	Abnormal Findings

Skin and Hair

Inspection and Palpation **Inspect and palpate skin lesions.** Wear gloves when palpating lesions. Note whether lesions are flat or raised, palpable or nonpalpable. Also note color, size, and exudates, if any. Despite decrease in total number of melanocytes, hyperpigmentation occurs in sun-exposed skin (neck, face, & arms). Although dermatologic lesions are common, many are benign. The combination of environmental exposure and diminished immunity increases risk of skin cancer and cutaneous infections such as ringworm, Candidal infections of mouth, vagina, and nail beds. This risk is increased by predisposing conditions such as Diabetes mellitus, malnutrition, steroid, or antibiotic use.	Normal findings include the following: Lentigenes: Hyperpigmentation in sun-exposed areas appear as brown, pigmented, round or rectangular patches (Fig. 32-1). Often called liver spots. Venous lakes: Reddish vascular lesions on ears or other facial areas resulting from dilation of small, red blood vessels. Skin tags: Acrochordons, flesh-colored pedunculated lesions. Seborrheic keratoses: Tan, brown, or reddish, flat lesions commonly found on fair-skinned persons in sun-exposed areas. Cherry angiomas: Small, round, red spots. Senile purpura: Vivid purple patches (lesion should not blanch to touch).	Abnormal findings include: Irregularly shaped lesion or scaly, elevated lesion (squamous cell carcinoma) Actinic keratoses, round or irregularly shaped tan, scaly lesions that may bleed or be inflamed (premalignancy). Waxy or raised lesion, especially on sun-exposed (basal cell carcinoma) Herpes zoster vesicles (shingles) draining clear fluid or pustules atop an erythematous base following a clear linear pattern and accompanied by pain. More than half of elderly with shingles will have neuralgia that persists after resolution of the skin lesions. Pinpoint-sized, red-purple, nonblanchable petecchia (common sign of platelet deficiency) Large bruises may result from anticoagulant therapy, a fall, renal or liver failure, or elder abuse.
Note color, texture, integrity, and moisture of skin and sensitivity to heat or cold.	Somewhat transparent, pale, skin with an overall decrease in body hair on lower extremities. Dry skin is common.	Torn skin (possibly the result of abrasive tape used to hold bandages or tubes in place)
Elastic collagen is gradually replaced with more fibrous tissue and loss of subcutaneous tissue. Decreased vascularity and diminished neurological response to temperature changes and atrophy of eccrine sweat glands	Skin may wrinkle and tent when pinched. *Note:* Pinching skin is not an accurate test of turgor in the elderly.	Extremely thin, fragile skin (friable skin) with excessive purpura (possibly from corticosteroid use) Dry, warm skin, furrowed tongue, and sunken eyes from dehydration (especially when the client has decreased

continued

Assessment Procedure	Normal Findings	Abnormal Findings
increases risk of hyperthermia and hypothermia. ➤ *Clinical Tip • Room humidifiers, avoidance of harsh deodorants or soaps, and use of lanolin-containing products after bathing (while skin is still moist) may help to relieve effects of dry skin.*		urinary output, increased serum sodium, BUN and creatinine levels, increased osmolality, and hematocrit values, tachycardia; and mental confusion). Sudden heat or cold intolerance could be signs of thyroid dysfunction.
Inspect and palpate hair and scalp.	Loss of pigmentation causes graying of scalp, axillary, and pubic hair. Mild hair growth on upper lip of women may appear as result of decreased estrogen to testosterone ratio. Toenails usually thicken while fingernails often become thinner. Both usually become yellowish and dull.	Patchy or asymmetric hair loss is abnormal.

Head and Neck

Inspection **Inspect head and neck for symmetry and movement. Observe facial expression (Fig. 32-2).**	Atrophy of face and neck muscles Reduced range of motion of head and neck Shortening of neck due to vertebral degeneration and development of "buffalo hump" at top of cervical vertebrae	Abnormalities include: Asymmetry of mouth or eyes possibly from Bell's palsy or CVA Marked limitation of movement or crepitation in back of neck from cervical arthritis Involuntary facial or head movements from an extrapyramidal disorder such as Parkinson's disease or some medications Reported episodic, unilateral, shocklike or burning pain of the face or continuous pain, which may be postherpetic or caused by a dental caries or abscess. *Note:* In cognitively impaired elders, sleep disturbances or agitation may be the only sign of neuropathic pain.

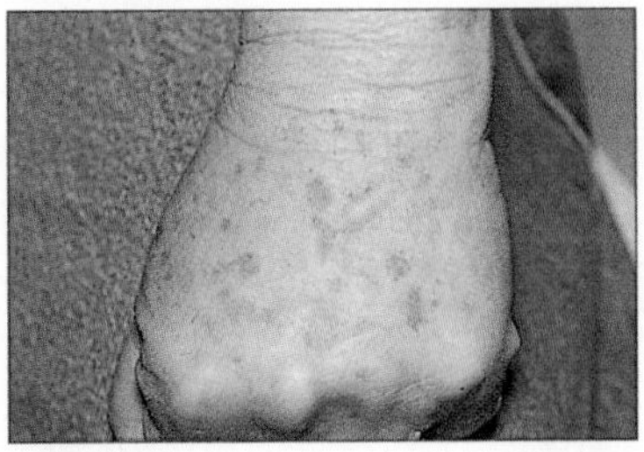

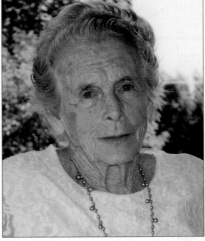

Figure 32-1 Solar lentigines are very common on aging skin.

Figure 32-2 Observe facial expression.

continued

PHYSICAL ASSESSMENT *Continued*

Assessment Procedure	Normal Findings	Abnormal Findings
Mouth and Throat		
Inspection **Inspect the gums and buccal mucosa for color and consistency.**	Slight decrease in saliva production	Saliva-depressing medications include antihistamines, antipsychotics, antihypertensives, and any drug with anticholinergic side effects may promote dental caries and increase risk of pneumonia.
If the client is wearing dentures, inspect them for fit. Then ask the client to remove them for the rest of the oral examination.	Resorption of gum ridge commonly results in poorly fitting dentures. Tooth surfaces may be worn from prolonged use.	Loose-fitting dentures or inability to close mouth completely may also be the result of a significant weight gain or loss. Foul-smelling breath may indicate periodontal disease. Whitish or yellow-tinged patches in mouth or throat may be candidiasis from use of steroid inhalers or antibiotics.
Examine the tongue. Observe symmetry and size.	Tongue pink and moist	A swollen, red, and painful tongue may indicate vitamin B or riboflavin deficiency.
Observe the client swallowing food or fluids (Fig. 32-3). ➤ *Clinical Tip* • *Help the client who reports dysphagia to lean slightly forward with the chin tucked in toward the neck when swallowing and offer food of pudding consistency to minimize the risk of aspiration.*	Mild decrease in swallowing ability	Coughing, drooling, pocketing, or spitting out food after intake are all possible signs of dysphagia. A drooping mouth, chronic congestion, or a weak or hoarse voice (especially after eating or drinking) also suggests dysphagia. Observed swallowing difficulties in which case a nutritional assessment should be completed and the client referred for a barium swallow examination.
Depress the posterior third of the tongue, and note gag reflex.	Gag reflex may be slightly sluggish.	Absence of a gag reflex may be the result of a neurologic disorder and indicates the need to be alert for signs of aspiration pneumonia.

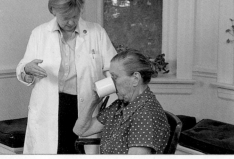

Figure 32-3 Assessing for swallowing problems (© B. Proud).

continued

Assessment Procedure	Normal Findings	Abnormal Findings

Nose and Sinuses

Inspection

Inspect the nose for color and consistency.

Nose and nasal passages are not inflamed, and skin and mucous membranes are intact. Nose may seem more prominent on face because of loss of subcutaneous fat. Nasal hairs are coarser.

Edema, redness, swelling, or clear drainage, which may indicate allergies or rhinitis.

> *Clinical Tip* • *Relocation into a newly constructed residential or long-term care facility should be investigated further as a possible cause of allergic or non-allergic rhinitis. New carpet, cabinetry of fiberboard, and paint fumes can elicit a nonallergic vasomotor response as well as an allergic one.*

Evaluate the sense of smell. Have the client close the eyes and smell a common substance, such as mint, lemon, or soap (Fig. 32-4).

> *Clinical Tip* • *Alert clients with diminished smell to the importance of smoke alarms and routine inspections of stoves and furnaces.*

Slightly diminished sense of smell and ability to detect odors

Client cannot identify strong odor. This may cause a decrease in appetite and may be a safety concern.

Test nasal patency by asking the client to breathe while blocking one nostril at a time (Fig. 32-5).

Breathes with reasonable ease

Client reports feeling of inadequate breath intake, which may result from nasal polyps, a deviated septum, or allergic or infectious rhinitis or sinusitis.

Palpation

Palpate the frontal and maxillary sinuses for consistency and to elicit possible pain.

> *Clinical Tip* • *Elderly clients with nasogastric feeding tubes are at increased risk for sinusitis related to the obstruction.*

No lesions or pain

Client reports pain and dryness; inflammation is evident.

> *Clinical Tip* • *Elderly clients may self-treat sinus pain and/or nasal congestion with decongestants and antihistamines, which may further dry the nasal passages and prevent normal sinus drainage. These drugs*

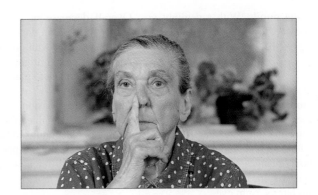

Figure 32-4 Assessing sense of smell (© B. Proud).　　**Figure 32-5** Testing nasal patency (© B. Proud).

continued

PHYSICAL ASSESSMENT *Continued*

Assessment Procedure	Normal Findings	Abnormal Findings
		may also aggravate hypertension (in clients taking antihypertensive drugs) and exacerbate cardiac dysrhythmias. In clients taking antibiotics for sinusitis, watch for adverse effects on renal function. Because antibiotics also may kill normal bacteria, watch for signs of candidal or Clostridium difficile infection in the GI tract, mouth, or vagina.

Eyes and Vision

Inspection

Assessment Procedure	Normal Findings	Abnormal Findings
Inspect eyes, eyelids, eyelashes, and conjunctiva. Also observe eye and conjunctiva for dryness, redness, tearing, or increased sensitivity to light and wind.	Skin around the eyes becomes thin, and wrinkles appear normally with age. Stretched skin in eyelid may produce feeling of heaviness and a tired feeling. In lower eyelid, "bags" form. Excessive stretching of lower eyelid may cause it to droop downward, which keeps it from shutting completely and can cause dryness, redness, or sensitivity to light and wind. Eyes are described as irritated or having a "scratchy sensation."	A turning in of the lower eyelid (entropion) is more common and causes the eyelashes to touch the conjunctiva and cornea. Severe entropion may result in an ulcerous corneal infection. Abnormalities in blinking may result from Parkinson's disease; dull or blank staring may be a sign of hypothyroidism.
Inspect the cornea and lens. Also ask the client when he or she last had an eye and vision examination. ➤ *Clinical Tip* • *To detect glaucoma, tonometry should be performed every 1 to 2 years on everyone older than 35. Elevated intraocular pressure indicates the need for referral to an ophthalmologist and confirmation with applanation tonometry.*	An arcus senilis, a cloudy or grayish ring around the iris, and decreased pigment in iris are age-related changes. The lens loses elasticity, which results in decreased ability to change shape (presbyopia). A loss of transparency in the crystalline lens of the eyes is a natural part of aging process. Exposure to sunlight, smoking, and inherited tendencies increases risk.	Cataracts most commonly affect people after age 55 and result in a yellowish or brownish discoloration of the lens. Common symptoms include painless blurring of vision, glare and halos around lights, poor night vision, colors that look dull or brownish. Location and extent of cloudiness determine degree to which a person's vision is affected. A thickening of the bulbar conjunctiva that grows over the cornea (called pterygium) may interfere with vision.
Inspect the pupils. With a penlight or similar device, test pupillary reaction to light (Fig. 32-6).	Overall decrease in size of pupil and ability to dilate in dark and constrict in light may occur with advanced age; this results in poorer night vision and decreased tolerance to glare.	An irregularly shaped pupil may indicate removal of a cataract. Asymmetric response may be due to a neurologic condition.
Test vision. Ask the client to read from a newspaper or magazine. Use only room lighting for the initial reading. Use task lighting for a second reading (Fig. 32-7). Ask about changes in vision, trouble with night vision, or differences in vision with left vs. right eye.	Impaired near vision is indicative of presbyopia (farsightedness), a common finding in older adults. Also common are slight decreases in peripheral vision and difficulty in differentiating blues from greens.	A significant decrease in central vision, to the extent needed for activities of daily living, may signal a cataract in one or both eyes. *Macular degeneration* (thin membrane in the center of the retina) is suspected if the client has difficulty in seeing with

continued

Assessment Procedure	Normal Findings	Abnormal Findings
	➤ **Clinical Tip** • *Older adults generally require two to three times more diffuse and task lighting.*	one eye (Abnormal Findings 32.1). The disorder almost always becomes bilateral. Related abnormal findings include blurry words in the center of the page or door frames that don't appear straight. This condition should be referred and evaluated.
Also ask client about small specks or "clouds" that move across the field of vision.	With aging, tiny clumps of gel may develop within the eye. These are referred to as "floaters." They should occur occasionally and not increase significantly in frequency.	A noticeable loss of vision—including cloudiness, distortion of familiar objects, and occasionally blind spots or floaters—is a common symptom of diabetic retinopathy. New floaters, an increase in frequency of floaters associated with flashes of light may be a sign of retinal detachment. This requires immediate referral to prevent blindness (Abnormal Findings 32-1).

Ears and Hearing

Inspection

Inspect the external ear. Observe shape, color, and hair growth. Also look for lesions or drainage.	Hairs may become coarser and thicker in the external ear, especially in men. Earlobes may elongate and penna increases in length and width.	Inflammation, drainage, or swelling may be from infection.
Perform an otoscopic examination to determine quantity, color, and consistency of cerumen.	Cerumen production decreases leading to dryness and tendency toward accumulation.	Hard, dark brown cerumen signals impaction of the auditory canal, which commonly causes a conductive hearing loss. A darkened hole in the tympanic membrane or patches indicates perforation or scarring of the tympanic membrane.
Perform the *voice–whisper test,* a functional examination to detect obvious (conversational) hearing loss. Instruct the client to put a hand over one ear and to repeat the sentence you say. Stand approximately 2 feet away from the	The inability to hear high-frequency sounds (presbycusis) or to discriminate a variety of simultaneous sounds and soft consonant sounds or background noises is due to degeneration of hair cells of inner ear.	Inability to hear the whispered sentence indicates a hearing deficiency and the need to refer the client to an audiologist for testing.

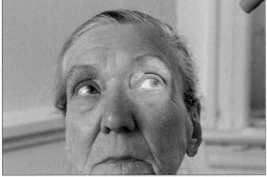

Figure 32-6   Testing pupillary reaction (© B. Proud).

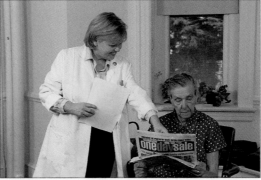

Figure 32-7   Reading with room lighting (© B. Proud).

continued

PHYSICAL ASSESSMENT *Continued*

Assessment Procedure	Normal Findings	Abnormal Findings
client and whisper a sentence (Fig. 32-8).	➤ *Clinical Tip • Assess hearing acuity before as well as after the otoscopic examination, if cerumen is removed during the examination. If you are facing the client, hold your hand close to your mouth so the client cannot read your lips.*	➤ *Clinical Tip • Raising one's voice to someone with presbycusis usually only makes it more difficult for them to hear. Speaking more slowly will usually lower the frequency and be more therapeutic.*

Thorax and Lungs

Inspection

Inspect shape of thorax. Note respiratory rate, rhythm, and quality of breathing.

Decreased elasticity of alveoli causes lungs to recoil less during expiration and loss of resilience that holds thorax in a contracted position, loss of skeletal muscle strength in thorax and abdomen, decreased vital capacity, increased residual volume, and slight barrel chest.

Increased reliance on diaphragmatic breathing and increased work of breathing.

Respiratory rate exceeding 25 breaths/ min may signal a pulmonary infection along with increased sputum production, confusion, loss of appetite, and hypotension (McGann, 2000).

Respiratory rate of less than 16 breaths/ min may be a sign of neurologic impairment, which may lead to aspiration pneumonia. Significant loss of aerobic capacity and dyspnea with exertion is usually due to disease, exposure over a lifetime to pollutants, smoke, or severe or prolonged lack of exercise.

Percussion

Percuss lung tones as you would in a younger adult.

Resonant, except in the presence of structural changes such as kyphosis or a slight barrel chest, when hyperresonance may occur.

Consolidation of infection will cause dullness to percussion; alveolar retention of air, as occurs in emphysema, results in hyperresonance.

Note: Supine positioning, shallow breathing, and poor dental hygiene increase the risk of pulmonary infection. Pneumonia is the most common cause of infection-related deaths in the elderly and is called the "silent killer." It seldom presents as the classic triad of cough, fever, and pleuritic pain. Instead, subtle changes such as an increase in respiratory rate and sputum production, confusion, loss of appetite, and hypotension are more likely to be the presenting symptoms (Fitzpatrick, Fulmer, Wallace, & Flaherty, 2000).

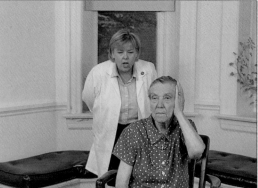

Figure 32-8 Assessing hearing with the voice-whisper test (© B. Proud).

continued

Assessment Procedure	Normal Findings	Abnormal Findings
Auscultation **Auscultate lung sounds as you would in a younger adult.**	Vesicular sounds should be heard over all areas of air exchange. However, because lung expansion may be diminished, it may be necessary to emphasize taking deep breaths with the mouth open during the exam. This may be very difficult for those with dementia.	Breath sounds may be distant over areas affected by kyphosis or the barrel chest of aging. Rales and rhonchi are heard only with diseases, such as pulmonary edema, pneumonia, or restrictive disorders. Diminished breath sounds, wheezes, crackles, rhonchi that do not clear with cough, and egophony are common signs of consolidation caused by pneumonia.

Heart and Blood Vessels

Blood Pressure **Take blood pressure to detect actual or potential orthostatic hypotension and, therefore, the risk for falling.** Measure pressure with the client in lying, sitting, and standing positions. Also measure pulse rate. Have the client lie down for 5 minutes; take the pulse and blood pressure; at 1 minute, take blood pressure and pulse after client is sitting and again at 1 minute after client stands (Fig. 32-9). If dizziness occurs, instruct client to sit a few minutes before attempting to stand up from a supine or reclining position.	An elderly person's baroreceptor response to positional changes is slightly less efficient. A slight decrease in blood pressure may occur. Blood pressure increases as elasticity decreases in arteries with proportionately greater increase in systolic pressure, resulting in a widening of pulse pressure. ➤ *Clinical Tip* • *Any client with blood pressure exceeding 160/90 mm Hg should be referred to the health care provider for follow-up.*	A greater than 10 mm Hg drop in systolic or diastolic pressure and an increase in heart rate of 20 beats or more per minute indicate orthostatic hypotension. A serious consequence is the potential for lightheadedness and dizziness, which may precipitate hip fracture or head trauma from a fall. ➤ *Clinical Tip* • *Some sources of orthostatic hypotension include medications, such as antihypertensives, diuretics, and drugs with anticholinergic side effects (anxiolytics, antipsychotics, hypnotics, tricyclic antidepressants, and antihistamines).* A sudden and increasingly widened pulse pressure, especially in combination with other neurologic abnormalities and a change in mental status, is a classic sign of increased intracranial

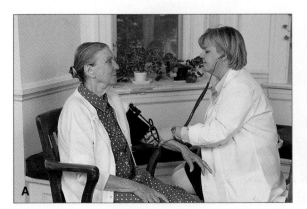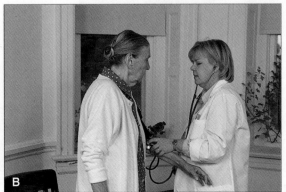

Figure 32-9   Assessing blood pressure (© B. Proud).

continued

PHYSICAL ASSESSMENT *Continued*

Assessment Procedure	Normal Findings	Abnormal Findings
		pressure (which in elderly clients may be due to a hemorrhagic stroke or hematoma).

Exercise Tolerance

Measure activity tolerance. Evaluate, either by reviewing results of stress testing or by observing the client's ability to move from a sitting to a standing position (Fig. 32-10) or to flex and extend fingers rapidly.

> ➤ *Clinical Tip • Poor lower body strength, especially in the ankles, may impair the ability of the frail elderly person to rise from a chair to a standing position. Poor upper body strength, especially in the shoulders, may impede the ability to push up from a bed or chair or to extend and flex fingers.*

The maximal heart rate with exercise is less than in a younger person. The heart rate will also take longer to return to its pre-exercise rate.

Rise in pulse rate should be no greater than 10 to 20 beats/min. The pulse rate should return to the baseline rate within 2 minutes.

A rise in pulse rate greater than 20 beats/min and a rate that does not return to baseline within 2 minutes is an indicator of exercise intolerance. Cardiac dysrhythmias as determined by stress testing are also indicative of exercise intolerance.

Pulses

Determine adequacy of blood flow by palpating the arterial pulses in all locations (carotid, brachial, radial, femoral, popliteal, posterior tibial, and dorsalis pedis) for strength and quality (Fig. 32-11).

> ➤ *Clinical Tip • Palpate carotid arteries gently and one side at a time to avoid stimulating vagal receptors in the neck, dislodging existing plaque, or causing syncope or a stroke.*

Proximal pulses may be easier to palpate due to loss of supporting surrounding tissue. However, distal lower extremity pulses may be more difficult to feel or even nonpalpable. The dorsalis pedis pulse is absent in approximately 20% of older persons (Mezey, Rauckorst & Stokes, 1993, p. 90).

Insufficient or absent pulses are a likely indication of arterial insufficiency. Partially obstructed blood flow increases the risk of ulcers and infection; completely obstructed blood flow is a medical emergency requiring immediate intervention to prevent gangrene and possible amputation.

Arteries and Veins

Auscultate the carotid, abdominal, and femoral arteries (Fig. 32-12).

No unusual sounds should be heard.

A bruit is abnormal, and the client needs a prompt referral for further care

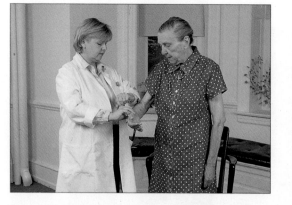

Figure 32-10 Assessing heart rate after the client rises from a sitting position provides clues to his or her tolerance of physical exertion (© B. Proud).

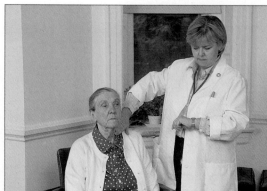

Figure 32-11 Palpating the carotid artery to assess blood flow (© B. Proud).

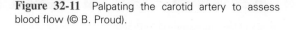

continued

Assessment Procedure	Normal Findings	Abnormal Findings
Evaluate arterial and venous sufficiency of extremities. Elevate the legs above the level of the heart and observe color, temperature, size of the legs, and skin integrity.	Hair loss with advanced age (cannot be used singly as an indicator of arterial insufficiency).	because of the high risk of CVA from a carotid embolism or an abdominal or femoral aneurysm. Leg pain associated with walking, burning or cramping, duskiness or mottling when the leg is in a dependent position; paleness with elevation; cool, thin, shiny skin; thickened, brittle nails; and diminished pulses are signs of arterial insufficiency.
Inspect and palpate veins while client is standing.	Prominent, bulging veins are common. Varicosities are considered a problem only if ulcerations, signs of thrombophlebitis, or cords, are present. Cords are nontender; palpable veins having a rubber tubing consistency.	Unilateral warmth, tenderness, and swelling may be indications of thrombophlebitis.

Heart

Assessment Procedure	Normal Findings	Abnormal Findings
Inspect and palpate the precordium.	The precordium is still, not visible, and without thrills, heaves, palpable pulsations (noted exception may be the apex of the heart if close to the surface).	Heaves are felt with an enlarged right or left ventricular aneurysm. Thrills indicate aortic, mitral, or pulmonic stenosis and regurgitation that may originate from rheumatic fever. Pulsations suggest an aortic or ventricular aneurysm, right ventricular enlargement, or mitral regurgitation.
Auscultate heart sounds. **The accumulation of lipofuscin, amyloid, collagen, and fats in the pacemaker cells of the heart and loss of pacemaker cells in the sinus node predispose the older adult to dysrhythmias, even in the absence of heart disease.**	A soft systolic murmur heard best at the base of the heart may result from calcification, stiffening, and dilation of the aortic and mitral valve.	Abnormal heart sounds are generally considered to be disease-related only if there is additional evidence of compromised cardiovascular function. However, any previously undetected extra heart sound warrants further investigation. S_3 and S_4 sounds may reflect the cardiac and fluid overloads of heart failure, aortic stenosis, cardiomyopathy, or myocardial infarction. ➤ *Clinical Tip • Falls, dyspnea, fatigue, and palpitations are common symptoms of dysrhythmias in the elderly.*

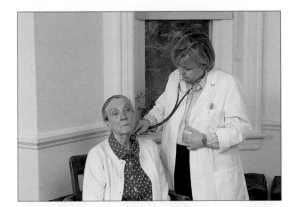

Figure 32-12 Use the bell of the stethoscope to listen for bruits (© B. Proud).

continued

PHYSICAL ASSESSMENT *Continued*

Breasts

Assessment Procedure	Normal Findings	Abnormal Findings
Inspection and Palpation **Inspect and palpate breast and axillae.** When viewing axillae and contour of breasts, assist a client with arthritis to raise the arms over the head. Do this gently and without force and only if it is not painful for the client. If the breasts are pendulous, assist the client to lean slightly so the breasts hang away from the chest wall, enabling you to best observe symmetry and form. ➤ *Clinical Tip • A greater percentage of elderly women have had radical mastectomies. If so, inquiring about pain and swelling from lymphedema is important.*	The breasts of elderly women are often described as pendulous due to the atrophy of breast tissue and supporting tissues and the forward thrust of the client brought about by kyphosis. Decreases in fat composition and increase in fibrotic tissue may make the terminal ducts feel more fibrotic and palpable as linear, spoke-like strands. Nipples may retract due to loss in musculature. Unlike nipple retraction due to a mass, nipples retracted because of aging can be everted with gentle pressure (Mezey et al., 1993).	Pain upon palpation may indicate an infectious process or cancer. Or breast tenderness, pain, or swelling may be side effects of hormone replacement therapy and an indication that a lower dosage is needed. Male breast enlargement (gynecomastia) may result from a decrease in testosterone.
Inspect skin under breasts.	Skin intact without lesions or rashes	Macerated skin under the breasts may result from perspiration or fungal infection (usually seen in an immunocompromised client).

Abdomen

Assessment Procedure	Normal Findings	Abnormal Findings
Motility **Assess GI motility and auscultate bowel sounds. Review fiber intake and laxative use.**	5 to 30 sounds/min are heard. A decrease in gastric emptying time occurs with aging and may cause early satiety. Intestinal motility is generally reduced from a general loss of muscle tone. Risk of constipation is increased by diminished physical activity, fluid intake, fiber in diet, and by certain medications such as iron or narcotics.	Absence of bowel sounds and vomiting of undigested food is abnormal. Decreased motility is exacerbated by common pathologies such as Parkinson's, stroke, and diabetes mellitus. Results in propensity for chronic constipation and diverticula. ➤ *Clinical Tip • If diverticula become infected, emergency treatment may be required to prevent perforation and sepsis.* Hiatal hernia that manifests by postprandial chest fullness, heartburn, or nausea.
Determine absorption or retention problems in elderly clients receiving enteral feedings. *Note:* An abdominal radiograph, flatplate, should be taken to check for correct placement of newly inserted nasogastric tubes.	Less than 100 mL residual is a normal finding for intermittent feedings.	More than 100 mL residual measured before a scheduled feeding is a sign of insufficient absorption and excessive retention. Abdominal distention, diarrhea, fluid overload, aspiration pneumonia, or fluid/electrolyte imbalances may indicate excessive retention although mental status changes may be the first or only sign.

continued

Assessment Procedure	Normal Findings	Abnormal Findings
Inspect and percuss abdomen in same manner as for younger adults. ➤ *Clinical Tip* • *The loss of abdominal musculature that occurs with aging may make it easier to palpate abdominal organs.* Atrophy of intestinal villi is a common aging change.	Liver, pancreas, and kidneys normally decrease in size, but the decrease is not generally appreciable upon physical examination.	Anorexia, abdominal pain and distention, impaired protein digestion, and vitamin B_{12} malabsorption suggest inflammatory gastritis or a peptic ulcer. Abdominal distention, cramping, diarrhea, and increased flatus are signs of lactose intolerance, which may occur for the first time in old age. Bruits over aorta suggest an aneurysm. If present, do not palpate because this could rupture the aneurysm. Guarding upon palpation, rebound tenderness, or a friction rub (sounds like pieces of sandpaper rubbing together) often suggests peritonitis, which could be secondary to ruptured diverticuli, tumor, or infarct.
Palpate the bladder. (Ask client to empty bladder before the examination.) If the bladder is palpable, percuss from symphysis pubis to umbilicus. If the client is incontinent, postvoid residual content may also need to be measured.	Empty bladder is not palpable or percussable.	Full bladder sounds dull. More than 100 mL drained from bladder is considered abnormal for a postvoid residual. A distended bladder with an associated small-volume urine loss may indicate overflow incontinence. (See Display 32-3.)

Genitalia

Female

Assessment Procedure	Normal Findings	Abnormal Findings
Inspect external genitalia. Assist the client into the lithotomy position. Inspect the urethral meatus and vaginal opening. ➤ *Clinical Tip* • *Arthritis may make the lithotomy position particularly uncomfortable for the elderly woman, necessitating changes. If the client has breathing difficulties, elevating the head to a semi-Fowler's position may help.*	Many atrophic changes begin in women at menopause. Pubic hair is usually sparse, and labia are flattened. Clitoris is decreased in size. The size of ovaries, uterus, and cervix also decreases.	White, glistening particles attached to pubic hair may be a sign of lice. Redness or swelling from the urethral meatus indicates a possible urinary tract infection.
Ask the client to cough while in the lithotomy position. ➤ *Clinical Tip* • *Incontinence is not a normal part of aging. If embarrassment or acceptance is preventing the client from acknowledging the problem, the genital examination may be a more acceptable time to introduce the topic.*	No leakage of urine occurs.	Leakage of urine that occurs with coughing is a sign of stress incontinence and may be due to lax pelvic muscles from childbirth, surgery, obesity, cystocele, rectocele, or a prolapsed uterus. *Note:* In noncommunicative patients, an excoriated perineum may be the result of incontinence, which warrants further investigation.

continued

PHYSICAL ASSESSMENT Continued

Assessment Procedure	Normal Findings	Abnormal Findings
Test for prolapse. Ask the client to bear down while you observe the vaginal opening.	No prolapse is evident.	A protrusion into the vaginal opening may be a cystocele, rectocele, or uterine prolapse, which is a common sequelae of relaxed pelvic musculature in older women.
Perform a pelvic examination. Put on disposable gloves and use a small speculum if the vaginal opening has narrowed with age. Use lubrication on speculum and hand because natural lubrication is decreased.	Vagina narrows and shortens. A loss of elastic tissue and vascularity in vagina results in a thin, pale epithelium. Atrophic changes are intensified by infrequent intercourse. Loss of elasticity and reduced vaginal lubrication from diminishing levels of estrogen can cause dyspareunia (painful intercourse). Sexual desire, pleasure are not necessarily diminished by these structural changes, nor do women lose capacity for orgasm with age. Because the ovaries, uterus, and cervix shrink with age, the ovaries may not be palpable.	Malignancy, vulvar dystrophies, urinary tract infections, and other infections, such as *Candida albicans,* bacterial vaginosis, gonorrhea, or *Chlamydia,* can mimic atrophic vaginitis (Kennedy-Malone et al., 2000).
Test pelvic muscle tone. Ask the woman to squeeze muscles while the examiner's finger is in the vagina. Assess perineal strength by turning fingers posterior to the perineum while the woman squeezes muscles in the vaginal area.	The vaginal wall should constrict around the examiner's finger, and the perineum should feel smooth.	If the client has a cystocele, the examiner's finger in the vagina will feel pressure from the anterior surface of the vagina. In clients with uterine prolapse, protrusion of the cervix is felt down through the vagina. A bulging of the posterior vaginal wall and part of the rectum may be felt with a rectocele.
Male **Inspect the male genital area with the client in standing position if possible.**	The decline in testosterone brings about atrophic changes. Pubic hair is thinner. Scrotal skin is slightly darker than surrounding skin and is smooth and flaccid in the older man. Penis and testicular size decreases, scrotum hangs lower.	Scrotal edema may be present with portal vein obstruction or heart failure. Lesions on the penis may be a sign of infection. Associated symptoms frequently include discharge, scrotal pain, and difficulty with urination.
Observe and palpate for inguinal swelling or bulges suggestive of hernia in the same manner as for a younger male.	No swelling or bulges are present.	Masses or bulges are abnormal, and pain may be a sign of testicular torsion. A mass may be due to a hydrocele, spermatocele, or cancer.
Auscultate the scrotum if a mass is detected; otherwise, palpate the right and left testicle using the thumb and first two fingers.	No detectable sounds or masses are present.	Bowel sounds heard over the scrotum may suggest an indirect inguinal hernia. Masses are abnormal, and the client should be referred to a specialist for follow-up examination.

continued

Assessment Procedure	Normal Findings	Abnormal Findings

Anus, Rectum, and Prostate

Inspection and Palpation
Inspect the anus and rectum.

The anus is darker than the surrounding skin.

Bluish, grapelike lumps at the anus are indicators of hemorrhoids.

Lesions, swelling, inflammation, and bleeding are abnormalities.

If hemorrhoids account for discomfort, the degree to which bleeding, swelling, or inflammation interferes with bowel activity generally determines if treatment is warranted.

Put on gloves to palpate the anus and rectum. Also palpate the prostate in the male client.

➤ *Clinical Tip • The left side-lying position with knees tucked up toward the chest is the preferred one for comfort. Pillows may be needed for positioning and client comfort.*

The prostate is normally soft or rubbery-firm and smooth, and the median sulcus is palpable. Some degree of enlargement (BPH) almost always occurs by age 85 as does a decrease in amount and viscosity of seminal fluid. Sperm count may decrease by as much as 50%. Orgasm may be briefer and time to obtain an erection may increase. These changes alone, however, do not usually result in any loss of libido or satisfaction.

Palpation of internal masses could indicate polyps, internal hemorrhoids, rectal prolapse, cancer, or fecal impaction. Obliteration of the median sulcus is felt with prostatic hyperplasia.

A hard, asymmetrically enlarged, and nodular prostate is suggestive of malignancy (Mezey et al., 1993). A tender and softer prostate is more common with prostatitis. Fever and painful urination are common with acute prostatitis. Obstructive symptoms are seen with both malignancy and infection of prostate.

Musculoskeletal System

Inspection and Palpation
Observe the client's posture and balance when standing, especially the first 3 to 5 seconds.

➤ *Clinical Tip • The ability to reach for everyday items without losing balance can be assessed by asking the client to remove an object from a shelf that is high enough to require stretching or standing on the toes and to bend down to pick up a small object, such as a pen, from the floor.*

Client stands reasonably straight with feet positioned fairly widely apart to form a firm base of support. This stance compensates for diminished sense of proprioception in lower extremities. Body usually bends forward as well.

A "humpback" curvature of the spine, called kyphosis, usually results from osteoporosis. The combination of osteoporosis, calcification of tendons and joints, and muscle atrophy makes it difficult for the frail elderly person to extend the hips and knees fully when walking. This impairs the ability to maintain balance early enough to prevent a fall.

Client cannot maintain balance without holding onto something or someone. Postural instability increases the risk of falling and immobility from the fear of falling.

Observe the client's gait by performing the timed "Get Up and Go" test (Fig. 32-13):

1. Have the client rise from a straight-backed armchair, stand momentarily, and walk about 3 m toward a wall.
2. Ask the client to turn without touching the wall and walk back to the chair; then turn around and sit down.

Widening of pelvis and narrowing of shoulders.

Client walks steadily without swaying, stumbling, or hesitating during the walk. The client does not appear to be at risk of falling. Elderly clients without impairments in gait or balance can complete the test within 10 seconds.

Shuffling gait, characterized by smaller steps and minimal lifting of the feet, increases the risk of tripping when walking on uneven or unsteady surfaces.

Abnormal findings from the timed "Get Up and Go" test include hesitancy, staggering, stumbling, and abnormal movements of the trunk and arms.

continued

PHYSICAL ASSESSMENT *Continued*

Assessment Procedure	Normal Findings	Abnormal Findings
3. Using a watch or clock with a second hand, time how long it takes the client to complete the test. 4. Score performance on a 1–5 scale: 1 = normal; 2 = very slightly abnormal; 3 = mildly abnormal; 4 = moderately abnormal; 5 = severely abnormal.		People who take more than 30 seconds to complete the test tend to be dependent in some activities of daily living such as bathing, getting in and out of bed, or climbing stairs.
Inspect the general contour of limbs, trunk, and joints. Palpate wrist and hand joints.	Enlargement of the distal, interphalangeal joints of the fingers, called Heberden's nodes, are indicators of degenerative joint disease (DJD), a common age-related condition involving joints in the hips, knees, and spine as well as the fingers (Fig. 32-14).	With accumulated damage and loss of cartilage, bony overgrowths protrude from the bone into the joint capsule, causing deformities, limited mobility, and pain. Hand deformities such as ulnar deviation, swan-neck deformity, and boutonniere deformity are of concern because of the limitations they impose on activities of daily living and related pain.

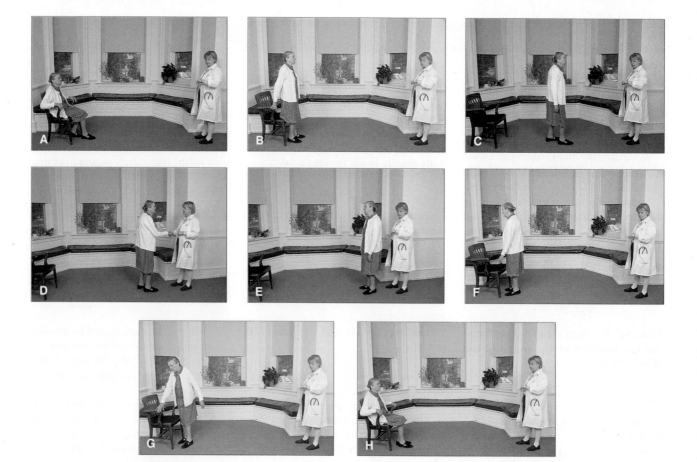

Figure 32-13 "Get up and go test" (© B. Proud).

continued

Assessment Procedure	Normal Findings	Abnormal Findings
Test range of motion. Ask client to touch each finger with the thumb of the same hand, to turn wrists up toward the ceiling and down toward the floor, to push each finger against yours while you apply resistance, and to make a fist and release it (Fig. 32-15).	There is full ROM of each joint and equal bilateral resistance	Limitations in ROM or strength may be due to degenerative disk disease (DJD), rheumatoid arthritis, or a neurologic disorder, which, if unilateral, suggests CVA. Signs of pain such as grimacing, pulling back, or verbal messages are indicators of the need to do a pain assessment. Grating, popping, crepitus, and palpation of fluid are also abnormalities. Crepitus and joint pain that is worse with activity and relieved by rest in the absence of systemic symptoms is often associated with DJD.

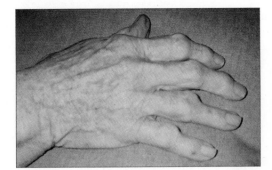

Figure 32-14 Degenerative joint disease.

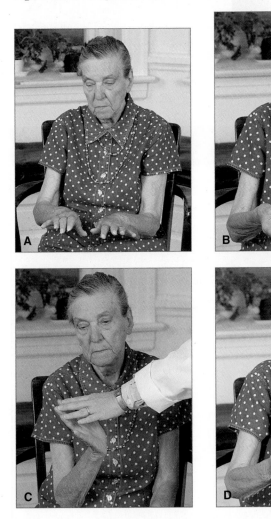

Figure 32-15 Testing range of motion (© B. Proud).

continued

PHYSICAL ASSESSMENT *Continued*

Assessment Procedure	Normal Findings	Abnormal Findings
Similarly assess ROM and strength of shoulders (left) and elbows (right) (Fig. 32-16).	There is full ROM of each joint and equal strength.	Tenderness, stiffness, and pain in the shoulders and elbows (and hips), which is aggravated by movement, are common signs associated with polymyalgia rheumatica (PMR).
Assess hip joint for strength and ROM in the same manner as for a younger adult.	Intact flexion, extension, and internal and external rotation	Hip pain that is worse with weight bearing and relieved with rest may indicate DJD. There is usually also an associated crepitation and decrease in ROM. Complaints of hip or thigh pain, external rotation and adduction of the affected leg, and an inability to bear weight are the most common signs of a hip fracture. Much less common signs may be mild discomfort and minimal shortening of the leg (Burke & Walsh, 1997).

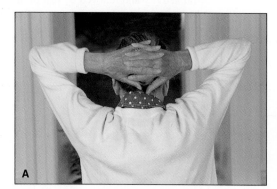
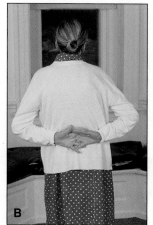

Figure 32-16   Testing range of motion. (© B. Proud.)

ASSESSMENT TOOL 32-4	Short Blessed Test

Patient: _____   DATE: _____

Age: _____

Short Blessed Test (SBT)[1]

"Now I would like to ask you some questions to check your memory and concentration. Some of them may be easy and some of them may be hard."

1. What year is it now?_____   Correct (0)   Incorrect (1)

2. What month is it now?_____   Correct (0)   Incorrect (1)

Please repeat this name and address after me:
    John Brown, 42 Market Street, Chicago
    John Brown, 42 Market Street, Chicago
    John Brown, 42 Market Street, Chicago

    (underline words repeated correctly in each trial)
    Trials to learning_____(can't do in 3 trials = C)
  Good, now remember that name and address for a few minutes.

---

[1] Katzman R., Brown T., Fuld P., Peck A., Schechter R., Schimmel, H. Validation of a short orientation-memory concentration test of cognitive impairment. Am J Psyhciatry 140:734–739, 1983.

continued on page 787

ASSESSMENT TOOL 32-4	Short Blessed Test *Continued*

3. Without looking at your watch or clock, tell me about what time it is.

    (If response is vague, prompt for specific response)

    (within 1 hour) _____

    Actual time: _____

	Correct (0)	Incorrect (1)

4. Count aloud backwards from 20 to 1

    (Mark correctly sequenced numerals)

      If subject starts counting forward or forgets the task, repeat instructions and score one error

    20 19 18 17 16 15 14 13 12 11

    10 9 8 7 6 5 4 3 2 1

    0 1 2 Errors

5. Say the months of the year in reverse order.

    If the tester needs to prompt with the last name of the month of the year, one error should be scored

    (Mark correctly sequenced months)

    D N O S A JL JN MY AP MR F J   0 1 2 Errors

6. Repeat the name and address I asked you to remember.

    (The thoroughfare term (Street) is not required)

    (John Brown, 42 Market Street, Chicago)   0 1 2 3 4 5 Errors

    _____, _____, ___, _____, _____

      Check correct items   **USE ATTACHED SCORING GRID & NORMS**

Short Blessed Test (SBT) Administration and Scoring Guidelines[2]

A spontaneous self-correction is allowed for all responses without counting as an error.

1. What is the year?

    Acceptable Response: The exact year must be given. An incomplete but correct numerical response is acceptable (e.g., 01 for 2001).

2. What is the month?

    Acceptable Response: The exact month must be given. A correct numerical answer is acceptable (e.g., 12 for December).

3. The clinician should state: "I will give you a name and address to remember for a few minutes. Listen to me say the entire name and address and then repeat it after me."

    It is important for the clinician to carefully read the phrase and give emphasis to each item of the phrase. There should be a one second delay between individual items.

    The trial phrase should be re-administered until the subject is able to repeat the entire phrase without assistance or until a maximum of three attempts. If the subject is unable to learn the phrase after three attempts, a "C" should be recorded. This indicates the subject could not learn the phrase in three tries.

    Whether or not the trial phrase is learned, the clinician should instruct "Good, now remember that name and address for a few minutes."

4. Without looking at your watch or clock, tell me about what time it is?

    This is scored as correct if the time given is within plus or minus one hour. If the subject's response is vague (e.g., "almost 1 o'clock), they should be prompted to give a more specific response.

5. Counting. The instructions should be read as written. If the subject skips a number after 20, an error should be recorded. If the subject starts counting forward during the task or forgets the task, the instructions should be repeated and one error should be recorded. The maximum number of errors is two.

[2] These guidelines and scoring rules are based on the administration experience of faculty and staff of the Memory and Aging Project, Alzheimer's Disease Research Center, Washington University School of Medicine, St. Louis (John C. Morris, MD, Director & PI; morrisj@abraxas.wustl.edu). For more information about the ADRC, please visit our website: http://alzheimer.wustl.edu or call 314-286-2881.

| ASSESSMENT TOOL 32-4 | Short Blessed Test *Continued* |

6. Months. The instructions should be read as written. To get the subject started, the examiner may state "Start with the last month of the year. The last month of the year is_____." If the subject cannot recall the last month of the year, the examiner may prompt this test with "December"; however, one error should be recorded. If the subject skips a month, an error should be recorded. If the subject starts saying the months forward upon initiation of the task, the instructions should be repeated and no error recorded. If the subject starts saying the months forward during the task or forgets the task, the instructions should be repeated and one error recorded. The maximum number of errors is two.

7. Repeat. The subject should state each item verbatim. The address number must be exact (i.e. "4200" would be considered an error for "42"). For the name of the street (i.e. Market Street), the thoroughfare term is not required to be given (ie. Leaving off "drive" or "street") or to be correct (ie. Substituting "boulevard" or lane") for the item to be scored correct.

8. The final score is a weighted sum of individual error scores. Use the table on the next page to calculate each weighted score and sum for the total.

Final SBT Score & Interpretation

Item #	Errors (0–5)	Weighting Factor	Final Item Score
1		× 4	
2		× 3	
3		× 3	
4		× 2	
5		× 2	
6		× 2	
			Sum Total = _____ *(Range 0–28)*

Interpretation

A screening test in itself is insufficient to diagnose a dementing disorder. The SBT is, however, quite sensitive to early cognitive changes associated with Alzheimer's disease. Scores in the impaired range (see below) indicate a need for further assessment. Scores in the "normal" range suggest that a dementing disorder is unlikely, but a very early disease process cannot be ruled out. More advanced assessment may be warranted in cases where other objective evidence of impairment exists.

- In the original validation sample for the SBT (Katzman et al., 1983), 90% of normal scores 6 points or less. Scores of 7 or higher would indicate a need for further evaluation to rule out a dementing disorder, such as Alzheimer's disease.
- Based on clinical research findings from the Memory and Aging Project[3], the following cut points may also be considered:
  - 0–4   Normal Cognition
  - 5–9   Questionable Impairment (evaluate for early dementing disorder)
  - 10 or more Impairment Consistent with Dementia (evaluate for dementing disorder)

---

[3] Morris J. C., Heyman A., Mohs R. C., Hughes J. P., van Belle G., Fillenbaum G., Mellits E. D., Clark C. (1989). The Consortium to Establish a Registry for Alzheimer's Disease (CERAD). Part I. Clinical and neuropsychological assessment of Alzheimer's disease. *Neurology,* 39(9): 1159–65.

Assessment Procedure	Normal Findings	Abnormal Findings
Inspect and palpate knees, ankles, and feet. Also assess comfort level particularly with movement (flexion, extension, rotation).	The common problems associated with the aged foot, such as soreness and aching, are most frequently due to improperly fitting footwear.	A great toe overriding or underlying the second toe may be halluces valgus (bunion). Other abnormal findings may be enlargement of the medial portion of the first metatarsal head and inflammation of the bursae over the medial aspect of the joint. Bunions are associated with pain and difficulty walking.
Inspect client's muscle bulk and tone.	Atrophy of the hand muscles may occur with normal aging.	Muscle atrophy can result from rheumatoid arthritis, muscle disuse, malnutrition, motor neuron disease, or diseases of the peripheral nervous system. Increased resistance to passive range of motion is a classic sign of Parkinson's disease especially in clients with bradykinesia. Decreased resistance may also suggest peripheral nervous system disease, cerebellar disease, or acute spinal cord injury.

Neurologic System

Assessment Procedure	Normal Findings	Abnormal Findings
Observe for tremors and involuntary movements.	Resting tremors increase in the aged. In the absence of an identifiable disease process, they are not considered pathologic.	The tremors of Parkinson's may occur when the client is at rest. They usually diminish with voluntary movement. They usually begin in the hand and may affect only one side of the body (especially early in the disease). The tremors are accompanied by muscle rigidity.

Sensory System

Assessment Procedure	Normal Findings	Abnormal Findings
Test sensation to pain, temperature, touch position and vibration as you would for a younger adult.	Touch and vibratory sensations may diminish normally with aging.	Unilateral sensory loss suggests a lesion in the spinal cord or higher pathways; a symmetric sensory loss suggests a neuropathy that may be associated with a condition such as diabetes.
Assess positional sense by using the Romberg test as presented in Chapter 27. The exceptions to the test are clients who must use assistive devices such as a walker.	There is minimal swaying without loss of balance.	Significant swaying with appearance of a potential fall.

Abnormal Findings 32-1   Age-Related Abnormalities of the Eye

Common age-related abnormalities of the eye include glaucoma, macular degeneration, retinal detachment, and diabetic retinopathy.

Glaucoma

The client with glaucoma is usually symptom free. In elderly people, diabetes and atherosclerosis are conditions that increase the risk of glaucoma. The disorder is caused by increased pressure that can destroy the optic nerve and cause blindness if not treated properly. An acute form of glaucoma can occur at any age and is a true medical emergency because blindness can result in a day or two without treatment. Rainbow-like halos or circles around lights, severe pain in the eyes or forehead, nausea, and blurred vision may occur with the acute form of glaucoma.

Macular Degeneration

Macular degeneration, a gradual loss of central vision, is caused by aging and thinning of the micro-thin membrane in the center of the retina called the macula. Additional risk factors include sunlight exposure, family history, and white race. Most cases begin to develop after age 50, but damage may be occurring for months to years before symptoms occur. Peripheral vision is not affected, and the condition may occur initially in only one eye. Only about 10% of all age-related macular degeneration leaks occur in the small blood vessels in the retinal pigment epithelium. This type accounts for the most serious loss of vision.

Retina Detachment

Retinal detachment occurs at a greater frequency with aging as the vitreous pulls away from its attachment to the retina at the back of the eye, causing the retina to tear in one or more places. A retinal detachment is always a serious problem. Blindness will result if the detachment is not treated.

Diabetic Retinopathy

Many older adults have diabetes, which can lead to cataracts, glaucoma, and diabetic retinopathy. Of those with diabetes mellitus, about 90% will develop diabetic retinopathy to some degree. The more serious of the two forms of the disease, proliferative diabetic retinopathy, occurs most often among those who have had diabetes for more than 25 years. People with the advanced form of the disease usually experience a noticeable loss of vision, including cloudiness, distortion of familiar objects, and, occasionally, blind spots or floaters. If not treated, diabetic retinopathy will lead to connective scar tissue, which over time can shrink, pulling on the retina and resulting in a retinal detachment. In the early stages of the milder form of the disease, background diabetic retinopathy, the person may be unaware of problems because the loss of sight is usually gradual and mainly affects peripheral vision.

VALIDATING AND DOCUMENTING FINDINGS

The prevalence of chronic conditions in the frail elderly redefines the meaning of normalcy. The ability of the elderly person to function in everyday activities, albeit with environmental and pharmacologic interventions, is a more meaningful measure of normalcy than are physical findings alone. Thus the objective and subjective data must reflect a functional and physical assessment.

Sample of Subjective Data

Health complaints or abnormalities are as likely to be the result of an adverse reaction to drug therapy as they are to a disease process. Compiling a profile of prescription and over-the-counter medications is an essential component of any assessment of the frail elderly person—whether it is being performed to treat a specific health complaint or for compiling baseline data of the client's health status.

Client is an 86-year-old female who moved to a residential care facility 2 years ago because of difficulty climbing stairs and maintaining her home of 43 years. Eats two meals a day in dining room and has had gradually improving appetite since moving into the care facility where meals are provided. Reports occasional episodes (about once every 2 to 3 weeks) of some difficulty swallowing, especially food that is dry or meat that is tough. Takes Metamucil to keep bowel movements regular and soft. Current prescription medications are Sinemet 1 tid and sodium Diuril 500 mg qd.

Has regular dental examinations and sucks on hard candy to alleviate dry mouth. Until last 5 to 10 years was 5 foot 5 inches and weighed approximately 130 lb. Denies any recent falls, syncopal episodes, or dyspnea with daily activities. However, client reports that she tries to sit for 5 to 10 minutes before standing to avoid becoming lightheaded. Client has yearly mammograms and Pap smears done. She is a breast cancer survivor and stopped taking supplemental estrogen when diagnosed and treated 20 years ago. She reports no bleeding or change in moles or skin lesions. Client receives B_{12} injections once a month and reports that she always has more energy for 2 to 3 weeks after that. Client reports that she has had to get new eyeglasses twice in the last 4 years and that she sees occasional halos around lights. She can still read the newspaper if she shines a bright light directly on it, and she enjoys quilting. Client states that she is contented with her life and keeps in touch with family and friends with frequent phone calls and occasional visits. She also has made several new friends since moving into the care facility.

Sample of Objective Data

Client is 5 foot 3 inches, 122 lb; no orthostatic BP (lying = 150/85, HR = 88; sitting = 148/84, HR = 90; standing = 148/84, HR = 90); RR = 22. Client is independent in transfers and uses a walker for ambulating. She has a pill-rolling tremor at rest. She completes the "Get Up and Go" test with no noted abnormalities. Physical examination reveals a soft systolic murmur, absent pedal pulses, and soft and nondistended abdomen. She has no pedal edema; toenails are thick and yellowish; no ulcerations or discoloration of skin on lower extremities. No abdominal or carotid bruits noted on auscultation; lungs are clear to auscultation. The client's tongue is pink and moist. Her skin is thin and transparent. Numerous moles and brown, pigmented flat lesions (lentigenes) are noted on her hands, lower arms, and neck. Her fingernails are yellowish and brittle. A yellowish discoloration is noted for the lens of both eyes. Slight accumulation of dry earwax in outer ear; tympanic membrane is pink and intact. Mini Mental Status exam is normal. Client has no noted difficulties in conversation with memory, judgment, comprehension, or word recall.

Analysis of Data

DIAGNOSTIC REASONING: POSSIBLE CONCLUSIONS

After collecting subjective and objective data pertaining to the frail elderly assessment, identify abnormal findings and client strengths. Then cluster the data to reveal any significant patterns or abnormalities. These data may then be used to make clinical judgments about the status of the client's health.

Selected Nursing Diagnoses

Following is a listing of selected nursing diagnoses (wellness, risk, or actual) that you may identify when analyzing the cue clusters.

Wellness Diagnoses

- Readiness for Enhanced Effective Caregiving

Risk Diagnoses

- Risk for Caregiver Role Strain, related to complexity of illness and lack of resources
- Risk for Ineffective Family Coping related to emotional conflicts secondary to chronic illness of parent
- Risk for Social Isolation related to inability to communicate effectively, decreased mobility, effects of chronic illness, or pain
- Risk for Imbalanced Nutrition, Less Than Body Requirements related to dysphagia, or decreased desire to eat secondary to altered level of consciousness
- Risk for Constipation related to decreased physical mobility, decreased intestinal motility, lower fluid intake, reduced fiber and bulk in diet, and effects of medications

- Risks for Impaired Skin Integrity related to loss of subcutaneous tissue, immobility, malnutrition
- Risk for Ineffective Thermoregulation related to loss of subcutaneous tissue, atrophy of eccrine sweat glands, decreased functioning of sebaceous glands
- Risk for Disturbed Sensory Perception: Visual—related to dry eyes, loss of lens transparency, slow pupil constriction; Auditory—related to presbycusis
- Risk for Impaired Gas Exchange related to diminished recoil of lungs, less elastic alveoli, and loss of skeletal muscle strength
- Risk for Loneliness related to changing role and decreasing functional status

Actual Diagnoses

- Caregiver Role Strain related to severity of illness, complexity of caregiving tasks
- Diversional Activity Deficit related to impaired mobility or impaired thought processes
- Fatigue related to compromised circulatory or respiratory system and/or effects of medications
- Grieving related to debilitating effects of chronic illness
- Hopelessness related to deteriorating physical condition
- Chronic Sorrow of parent, caregiver, or individual client related to chronic physical or mental disability of client
- Ineffective Therapeutic Regimen Management related to lack of community resources
- Impaired Physical Mobility related to pain, age, pathologic changes in joints, or neuromuscular impairment
- Powerlessness related to unpredictability of complex disease processes and complex treatments
- Ineffective Protection related to decreased immunity
- Activity Intolerance related to weakness, fatigue, or pain related to joint and muscle deterioration and subsequent disuse of joints
- Ineffective Role Performance related to chronic illness
- Functional Urinary Incontinence related to immobility or dementia
- Wandering related to cognitive impairment, disorientation, and sedation
- Bathing/Hygiene Self-Care Deficit related to impaired physical or cognitive functioning
- Dressing/Grooming Self-Care Deficit related to impaired physical or cognitive functioning
- Acute Confusion related to adverse effects of medication, infection, or dehydration

Selected Collaborative Problems

Often, abnormalities identified in the nursing assessment (including functional) will require a collaborative approach. Since the geriatric syndromes are usually caused by acute pathology, they almost always require referral and/or nurse-physician collaboration. After grouping the data, certain collaborative problems may become apparent. Remember that collaborative problems differ from nursing diagnoses in that nursing interventions cannot prevent them. However, these physiologic complications of medical conditions can be detected and monitored by the nurse. In addition, the nurse can use physician- and nurse-prescribed interventions to minimize the complications of the problems. In such situations, the nurse may also have to refer the client for further treatment of the problem. Following is a list of collaborative problems that may be identified when assessing the frail elderly client. These problems are worded as Risk for Complications (or RC), followed by the problem. It is important to remember, however, that any complication in the very old is likely to manifest as any one of the geriatric syndromes (GS).

Geriatric Syndromes: FALLS

- RC: Cardiac—syncope, orthostasis, dysrhythmias
- RC: Musculoskeletal—loss of strength, osteoporosis, osteoarthritis
- RC: Neurologic—dizziness, poor balance and gait, intracranial hemorrhage
- RC: Sensory—loss of vision
- RC: Infection

Geriatric Syndromes: Urinary Incontinence

- RC: Urinary obstruction—prostatic hypertrophy
- RC: Infection
- RC: Constipation, fecal impaction
- RC: Adverse medication effect

Geriatric Syndromes: Acute Mental Status Decline

- RC: Infection—pneumonia, urinary tract, sepsis
- RC: Adverse medication effect
- RC: Dehydration
- RC: Cardiovascular—heart failure, cerebrovascular accident (CVA)
- RC: Metabolic—hypothyroidism/hyperthyroidism, hypoglycemia
- RC: Depression

Geriatric Syndromes: Weakness, Fatigue, Anorexia, and Dyspnea

- RC: Cancer
- RC: Pain
- RC: Dysphagia
- RC: Adverse medication effect
- RC: Renal failure
- RC: Infection

CASE STUDY

You are doing the home health intake assessment on Mrs. Doris Miller, an 82-year-old Caucasian widow who has come to live with her daughter, Delores Ralston. Mrs. Miller fell in her own home three weeks ago and was hospitalized for repair and pinning of a fractured right femur.

Mrs. Miller is sitting in a chair and appears to be thin, pale, and distracted as you enter the room and introduce yourself. Mrs. Miller answers some of your questions appropriately, but frequently apologizes for her appearance and defers to her daughter to answer any questions with regard to her recent fall and hospitalization. She says in a very weak, raspy voice, "I don't know how I ended up here. I don't know what I'd do without Delores but if I could just walk and didn't hurt so bad everything would be O.K . . . I've always been able to take care of things. This just all seems like such of a fuss over nothing. She reaches up to wipe her eyes with a tissue that she is holding in her right hand with noticeably contracted fingers with swan-neck deformities and enlarged distal, interphalangeal joints.

Delores reports that Mrs. Miller can put just enough weight on her right leg to use a walker, but needs assistance with bathing, cooking, and dressing. She says that her mother is not eating very well and seems to be getting choked easily, especially when she is drinking, and that she complains frequently of a "dry mouth." Bedpads are used to manage a small amount of incontinence during the night. Delores is setting the alarm for 3:00 AM to assist her mother onto a bedside commode. Mrs. Miller has a history of Parkinson's, osteoarthritis, osteo-

porosis, and mitral valve disease. She has fallen numerous times, but this was the first time that she broke any bones with the fall. Her current medications are Sinemet 25/250 mg every day; warfarin 5 mg every day; MS Contin 15 mg every 12 hours; MS 10 mg oral solution (10 mg per 2.5 ml) every 8 hours prn breakthrough pain; levothyroxin 0.05 mg every a.m.; Miralax every other day as needed for constipation.

Your physical exam reveals a resting tremor of the hands, and several large bruises on her right shoulder, upper arm, and hip. She has slight ectropion and reddened eyes. You note crepitus and a grating, popping sound bilaterally when you assist her to raise her arms as well as increased resistance and rigidity. Mrs. Miller's blood pressure is 85/45 on the right and 108/64 on the left. Her heart rate is 92 and irregularly irregular. Lung sounds are clear but only heard in the upper lobes. Her height is reported at 5'0" and her weight prior to the fall and hospitalization was 89 lbs. Although her skin is pale, thin, and dry in most areas, it appears intact and well cared for. Incision line on right leg is dry, slightly red, but without swelling or drainage. However, some redness is noted on the elbows and sacrum, and the antecubital spaces are moist with some beginning maceration. Mrs. Miller has 1+ pitting pedal edema bilaterally.

References and Selected Readings

Administration on Aging. (2003). Statistics: A profile of older Americans. Retrieved May 20, 2004. Available at http://www.aoa.dhhs.gov

Amella, E. (2004). Presentation of illness in older adults. *American Journal of Nursing, 104* (10), 40–51.

Amella, E. (2001). Nutrition: Eating/meals for older adults. In Mezey, M., Fumoer, T., & Mariano, C. (eds.). *Best practices in care for older adults: Incorporating essential gerontologic content into baccalaureate nursing education and staff development* (3rd ed.). New York: New York University.

American Association for Geriatric Psychiatry. (2004). Geriatrics and mental health—The facts. Retrieved May 20, 2004. Available at http://www.aagpgpa.org/prof

Atchison, K. A. (1997). The general oral health assessment index. In G. D. Slade (ed.), *Measuring oral health and quality of life.* Chapel Hill: University of North Carolina, Dental Ecology.

Beers, M. H. (1997). Explicit criteria for determining inappropriate medication use by the elderly, An update. *Archives of Internal Medicine, 157,* 1521–1536.

Brink, T., Yesavage, J. A., Lum, O., Heersema, P., Adey, M., & Rose, T. (1992). Screening tests for a geriatric depression. *Clinical Gerontologist, 1*(1), 37–44.

Brown, J., Bedford, N., & White, S. (1999). *Gerontological protocols for nurse practitioners.* Philadelphia: Lippincott Williams & Wilkins.

Burke, M., & Walsh, M. (1997). *Gerontologic nursing: Holistic care of the older adult* (2nd ed.). St. Louis: Mosby.

Chichin, E., Fulmer, T., Mariano, C., & Mezey, T. (2001). Caregiving/mistreatment of older adults. In Mezey, M., Fulmer, T., & Mariano, C. (eds.). *Best practices in care for older adults: Incorporating essential gerontologic content into baccalaureate nursing education and staff development* (3rd ed.). New York: New York University.

Douzjian, M., Wilson, C., Shultz, M., Berger, J., Tapnio, J., & Blanton, V. (2002). A program to use pain control medication to reduce psychotropic drug use in residents with difficult behavior. *Nursing home medicine: The annals of long-term care,* 1–7. Retrieved May 20, 2004. Available at http://www.mmhe.com

Fitzpatrick, J., Fulmer, T., Wallace, M., & Flaherty, E. (eds.). (2000). *Geriatric nursing research digest.* New York: Springer.

Folstein, M., Folstein, S., & McHugh, P. (1975). Mini-Mental State: A practical method for grading the cognitive state of patients for the clinician. *Journal of Psychiatric Research, 12,* 189–198.

Francis, D., Fletcher, K., & Simon, L. (1998). The geriatric resource model of care. *Nursing Clinics of North America, 33*(3), 482–496.

Fulmer, T. (1991). The geriatric nurse specialist role: A new model. *Nursing Management, 22*(3), 91–93.

Hammerman, D (1999). Toward an understanding of frailty. *Annals of Internal Medicine, 130*(11), 945–950.

Herr, K. A., & Mobily, P. R. (1993). Comparison of selected pain assessment tools for use with the elderly. *Applied Nursing Research, 6*(1), 39–46.

Johnson, B. P. (2005). The elderly. In N. C. Frisch & L. E. Frisch (eds.). *Psychiatric mental health nursing* (3rd ed.). Albany, NY: Delmar Publishers.

Katz, S., Down, T. D., Cash, H. R., & Grotz, R. C. (1970). Progress in the development of the index of ADL. *Gerontologist, 10,* 20–30.

Kennedy-Malone, L., Fletcher, K., & Plank, L. (2000). *Management guidelines for gerontological nurse practitioners.* Philadelphia, PA: F. A. Davis.

Kresevic, D. M. (1997). New-onset urinary incontinence among hospitalized elders (Doctoral dissertation, Case Western Reserve University, 1997). (UMI No. 9810934).

Lawton, M. P. (1971). Functional assessment of elderly people. *Journal of the American Geriatrics Society, 9*(6), 465–481.

Lonergan, E. (Ed.). (1996). *Geriatrics.* Stanford, CT: Appleton and Lange.

McGann, E. (2000). Pulmonary changes in elders. In J. Fitzpatrick, T. Fulmer, M. Wallace & E. Flaherty (eds.), *Geriatric nursing research digest* (pp. 80–84). New York: Springer.

Mezey, M., Rauckhorst, L., & Stokes, S. (1993). *Health assessment of the older individual* (2nd ed.). New York: Springer.

Micelli, D. & Mezey, M. (2007). Critical thinking related to complex care of older adults, Geriatric Nursing Education Consortium, The John A. Hartford Foundation Institute for Geriatric Nursing.

Molony, S. (2002). Beers' criteria for potentially inappropriate medication use in the elderly. *Best practices in nursing care to older adults* (16). New York University: The Hartford Institute for Geriatric Nursing.

Palmer, M., Baumgarten, M., Langenberg, P., & Carson, J. L. (2002). Risk factors for hospital-acquired incontinence in elderly female hip fracture patients. *Journal of Gerontology, 10,* 672–677.

Parshall, M. (1999). Adult emergency visits for chronic cardiorespiratory disease: Does dyspnea matter? *Nursing Research, 48*(2), 62–70.

Podsinlo, D., & Richardson, S. (1991). The timed "Get Up and Go": A test of basic functional mobility for frail elderly persons. *Journal of the American Geriatric Society, 39,* 142–148.

Robinson, B. (1983). Validation of a Caregiver Strain Index. *Journal of Gerontology, 38,* 344–348.

Rubenstein, L. Z., Josephson, K. P., & Osterwell, D. (1996). Falls and fall prevention in the nursing home. *Clinics in Geriatric Medicine, 12*(4), 881–902.

Sullivan, T. (2002). Caregiver strain index (CSI). In S. Molony (Ed.), *Best practices in nursing care to older adults* (14). The Hartford Institute for Geriatric Nursing, New York University: The Hartford Institute for Geriatric Nursing.

Task Force on Aging Research Funding (2003). *Sustaining the commitment.* Retrieved May 20, 2004. Available at http://www.agingresearch.org

Tideiksaar, R. (1998). *Falls in older persons: Prevention and management.* Baltimore, MD: Health Professions Press.

Wallace, M., Richardson, B., & Seley, P. B. (2001). Pain/palliation of older adults. In Mezey, M., Fulmer, T., & Mariano, C. (eds.). *Best practices in care for older adults: Incorporating essential gerontologic content into baccalaureate nursing education and staff development* (3rd ed.). New York: New York University.

White, J. V., Ham, R. J., Lipschitz, D. A., Dwyer, J. T., & Wellman, N. S. (1991). Consensus of the nutrition screening initiative. Risk factors and indicators of poor nutritional status in older Americans. *Journal of the American Dietetics Society, 91,* 783–787.

Yesavage, J. A., & Brink, T. L. (1983). Development and validation of a geriatric depression screening scale: A preliminary report. *Journal of Psychiatric Research, 17,* 37–49.

Zembrzuski, C. (2001). *Clinical companion for assessment of the older adult.* Albany, NY: Delmar.

Websites

Administration on Aging
   http://www.aoa.gov
The John A. Hartford Foundation Institute for Geriatric Nursing
   http://hartfordign.org
Alzheimer's Association
   http://www.alz.org
American Geriatrics Society
   http://www.americangeriatrics.org
American Academy of Hospice and Palliative Medicine
   http://www.aahpm.org

33

Assessing Families

Structure and Function

Family assessment varies with the nurse's level of education in family nursing. It also varies with the type of family nursing care to be provided.

WHAT IS FAMILY ASSESSMENT?

The usual approach to family assessment taken by nurses who are not specialists in family nursing is to focus on the individual as client and the family as context for the client's illness and care. This type of family assessment focuses on determining strengths and problem areas within the family's structure and function that influence the family's ability to support the client.

A more advanced knowledge of family nursing is required to care for the family as client. Using this approach, the nurse views the family unit as a system and does not focus on any one family member. Instead the nurse works at all times simultaneously with a mental picture of the family system and the individuals in the system. The nurse caring for the family system can still provide care to the individual when necessary, but the primary assessment and interventions are directed toward the family as a dynamic system.

The information provided in this chapter is relevant to either approach, but omits expert family systems nursing concepts. To assess a family, the nurse must first determine who constitutes a family. The traditional definition of family was based on relationships of blood, marriage, or adoption. This definition has evolved over the years, and a number of different groups of people living together are now considered to be families (e.g., single-parent families, extended families, communes, gay and lesbian couples, multigenerational families). Therefore, at the turn into the 21st century, those involved in family nursing incorporated a broader definition of family, thought to be more relevant to the times. This definition is "The family is a social system composed of two or more persons who coexist within the context of some expectations of reciprocal affection, mutual responsibility, and temporal duration. The family is characterized by commitment, mutual decision making and shared goals" (Department of Family Nursing, Oregon Health Sciences University, 1985, quoted in Hanson & Boyd, 1996, p. 6).

Based on this definition, it is relatively simple for the nurse to determine who constitutes a family: *the family is whoever they say they are.* If there is disagreement within a family about who is a part of the family and who is not, the nurse should note this difference of opinion and determine that the family for the assessment consists of those people who interact the most frequently. Chapter 2 provides examples of different types of families.

WHY ASSESS FAMILIES?

Among the many reasons for nurses to understand the concepts of family assessment, three stand out as important to a nursing assessment text:

- An ill person's family is an essential part of the context in which the illness occurs.
- The family members, the ill person, and even the illness itself interact in such a way that no one component can be really separated from the rest.
- The statistics on family caregiving show that families are very much involved in providing care for an ill family member. (For an overview of the many people involved in caring for ill, chronically ill, or disabled family members in the United States, see Display 33-1.)

The dynamic interactions of the ill family member, the illness, and the other family members will become clear as the elements of family assessment are described throughout this chapter.

COMPONENTS OF FAMILY ASSESSMENT

In recent years, a variety of nursing models or frameworks have been developed as tools for assessing the family. Nurses have developed these models on the basis of family theories because none of the non-nursing fields has captured the necessary elements of the nursing of families. The framework used in this chapter for assessing the family is a modified combination of the Calgary Family Assessment Model (Wright & Leahey, 2005) and Friedman's (1998) Family Assessment Model. Regardless of which model or framework you use to assess the family, there are three essential components of family assessment especially prominent in all family assessment models:

- Structure
- Development
- Function

Environmental components, cultural-ethnic variations, and areas of family coping, family stress, and family communication are usually incorporated into these three essential components. However, some models of family assessment may address them separately.

DISPLAY 33-1	Family Caregiving Statistics*

Caregiving Statistics

If you're a caregiver, you are not alone. You've probably heard that before, but you may not know just how much company you have. A recent study by the National Alliance for Caregiving and AARP found that 44.4 million Americans age 18 or older are providing unpaid care to an adult. If we had to pay for this care, it would cost approximately $257 billion per year.

Overall

- The typical caregiver is a 46-year-old Baby Boomer woman with some college education who works and spends more than 20 hours per week caring for her mother who lives nearby.
- Female caregivers provide more hours of care and provide a higher level of care than male caregivers.
- Almost seven in ten (69%) caregivers say they help one person.
- The average length of caregiving is 4.3 years.
- Many caregivers fulfill multiple roles. Most caregivers are married or living with a partner (62%), and most have worked and managed caregiving responsibilities at the same time (74%).

Caregivers and Work

- Almost 60% of all caregivers either work or have worked while providing care.
  - 62 percent have had to make adjustments to their work life, such as reporting late to work or giving up work entirely.

- Male caregivers are more likely to be working full or part-time than female caregivers (66% vs. 55%)

Who Do Caregivers Care For?

- Most caregivers (89%) are helping relatives.
- Nearly 80% of care recipients are over fifty with the other 20% 18-49.
- Caregivers who help someone age 50 or older say the most common health problems the person they care for has are diabetes, cancer, and heart disease.
- One quarter of caregivers helping someone age 50 or older reports the person they care for is suffering from Alzheimer's, dementia, or other mental confusion.

Caregivers' Unmet Needs

- The most frequently reported unmet needs are finding time for myself (35%), managing emotional and physical stress (29%), and balancing work and family responsibilities (29%).
- About three in ten caregivers say they need help keeping the person they care for safe (30%) and finding easy activities to do with the person they care for (27%).
- One in five caregivers say they need help talking with doctors and other healthcare professionals (22%) or making end-of-life decisions (20%)

*Reprinted from Family Caregiving 101: Caregiving Statistics with permission of the National Family Caregivers Association, Kensington, MD, the nation's only organization for all family caregivers. 1 800 896 3650; www.thefamilycaregiver.org(2004).

Family Structure

Family structure has three elements: internal structure, external structure, and context. Some theorists focus on a structural–functional framework that, when applied to family assessment, examines the interaction between the family and its internal and external environment (Friedman, 1998). Other theorists separate the assessment of family structure from assessment of family function within the structural component. This chapter focuses on the interaction between the family structure and its internal and external environment.

Internal Structure

The internal structure of a family refers to the ordering of relationships within the confines of that family. It consists of all the details in the family that define the structure of the family. Elements of internal structure include

- Family composition
- Gender (and gender roles)
- Rank order
- Subsystems
- Boundaries
- Power structure

FAMILY COMPOSITION

Family composition can be illustrated by recording the family tree graphically as a genogram. A genogram helps the nurse to view the whole family as a unit. It shows names, relationships, and other information such as ages, marriages, divorces, adoptions, and health data. Behavior and health–illness patterns can be examined using the genogram because both of these patterns tend to repeat through the generations. Figure 33-1 illustrates the format and symbols used for a simple three-generation family genogram.

GENDER ROLES

A family member's gender often determines his or her role and behavior in the family. Beliefs about male and female roles and behaviors vary from one family to another. Also there may be female or male subsystems that share common interests or activities.

RANK ORDER

Rank order refers to the sibling rank of each family member. For instance, families treat the oldest child differently from the way they treat the youngest child. The rank order and gender of each family member in relation to other siblings' rank order and

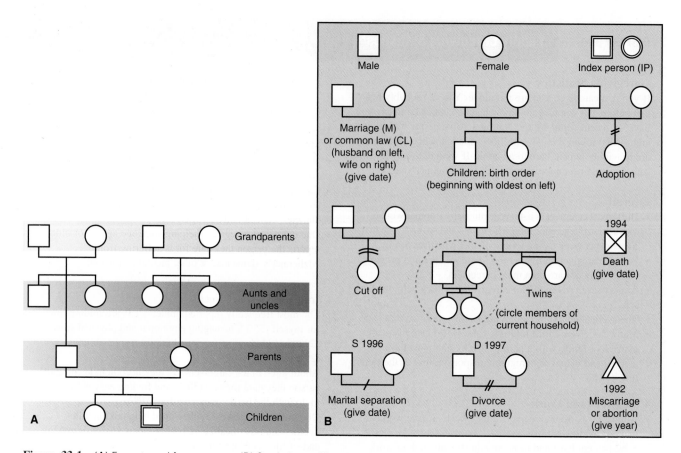

Figure 33-1 (A) Format used for genogram. (B) Symbols used in genogram.

gender make a difference in how the person will eventually relate to a spouse and children. For example, an older sister of a younger brother may bring certain expectations of how women relate to men into a marriage. If the older sister marries a man who is an older brother to a younger sister, there may be conflict or competition because each may expect to be the responsible leader.

SUBSYSTEMS

Each member of a family may belong to several subsystems. Subsystems may be related to gender, generational position (parents, grandparents, children), shared interests or activities (e.g., music, sports, hobbies), or to function (work at home, work away from home). Examples of subsystems are parent–child, spousal, sibling, grandmother–granddaughter, mother–daughter, and father–son. Subsystems in a family relate to one another according to rules and patterns, which are often not perceived by the family until pointed out by an outsider.

BOUNDARIES

Boundaries keep subsystems separate and distinct from other subsystems. They are maintained by rules that differentiate the particular subsystem's tasks from those of other subsystems. The most functional families have subsystems with clear boundaries; however, some connection between subsystems is maintained along with the boundaries. According to a theory by the family therapist Salvator Minuchin, the family and its subsystems may have problems with connectedness, so that boundaries are either too rigid or too diffuse. Disengaged

families have rigid boundaries, which leads to low levels of effective communication and support among family members. Enmeshed families have diffuse boundaries, which make it difficult for individuals to achieve individuation from the family.

POWER STRUCTURE

Power structure has to do with the influences each member has on the family processes and function. Some distribution of power is necessary to maintain order so the family can function. There is usually a power hierarchy, with the parents having more authority than the children. In the most functional families, parents have a sense of shared power and children gain increasing power as they mature and become more responsible.

A tool to help the nurse and family examine family structure and function within the structure is the Family Attachment Diagram. This is a diagram of the family members' interactions. It represents the reciprocal nature and quality of interactions. Figure 33-2 represents both a nuclear family with close and balanced relationships and a family with some conflicting, negatively attached relationships.

External Structure

External structure refers to those outside groups or things to which the family is connected. External structures may influence aspects of the internal structure of the family. Two elements of external structure include extended family and external systems.

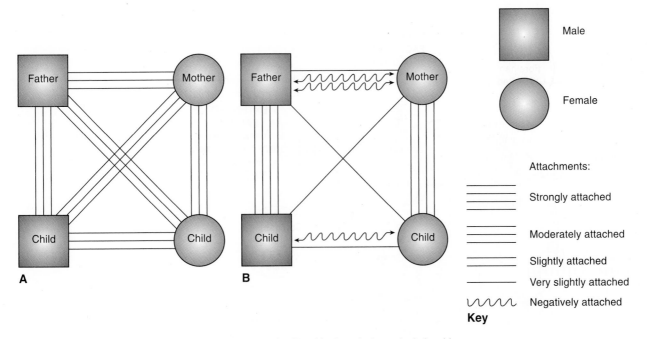

Figure 33-2 Family attachment diagram: **(A)** nuclear family with close, balanced relationship; **(B)** nuclear family with some conflicting, negatively attached relationships.

EXTENDED FAMILY

Extended family may consist of family members not residing in the home but with whom the family interacts frequently such as grandparents or an aunt and uncle who live only 5 minutes away. It also may include family members with whom the family interacts infrequently such as a first cousin who lives across the country and with whom the family communicates only through Christmas cards and a visit once every few years. However, the family feels confident that this cousin would be supportive in time of need. Another type of extended family is the "cut off" family member. An example would be a brother who left home 10 years ago and with whom there is no contact at all. This brother may still be considered extended family.

EXTERNAL SYSTEMS

External systems are those systems that are larger than the family and with which the family interacts. These systems include institutions, agencies, and significant people outside the family. Some specific examples of external systems include a family's health center, school, jobs, volunteer agency, church, recreational organizations, friends, neighbors, coworkers, and extended family (only those with whom interaction is frequent).

An ecomap can be used to assess the family members' interactions with the systems outside the family. The diagram, illustrated in Figure 33-3, is similar to the attachment diagram and shows the positive or conflicting nature of the family's relationships with outside groups or organizations.

Context

The context of a family refers to the interrelated conditions in which the family exists: it is the family's setting. Four elements make up the context of the family structure:

- Race-ethnicity
- Social class
- Religion
- Environment

Race or ethnicity may influence family structure and interactions. Assessment should include how much the family identifies with and adheres to traditional practices of a particular culture, whether the family's practices are similar to those of the neighborhood of residence, and whether the family has more than one ethnic or racial makeup.

The effects of *social class* and *religion* provide context for the family structure and lifestyle.

Environmental characteristics of the residence, neighborhood, and family and *neighborhood interactions* clarify the context for the family structure and interactions.

Family Development

Like individuals, families go through stages of growth and development. These stages of development are as important to the health and well-being of the family as they are to the individual. In fact, a static family structure is dysfunctional. Friedman (1998) developed theories about family life-cycle stages and associated tasks. Three of these stages—the traditional nuclear family, divorced family, and remarried family stages and tasks—are described by Wright and Leahey (2005) and are presented in Displays 33-2, 33-3, and 33-4.

Family Function

Friedman (1998) defined five basic family functions: affective, socialization and social placement, reproductive, economic, and health care. For purposes of this chapter's approach to family assessment, however, the components of family function are organized into four areas:

- *Instrumental:* Instrumental function is the ability of the family to carry out activities of daily living in normal circumstances and in the presence of a family member's illness.

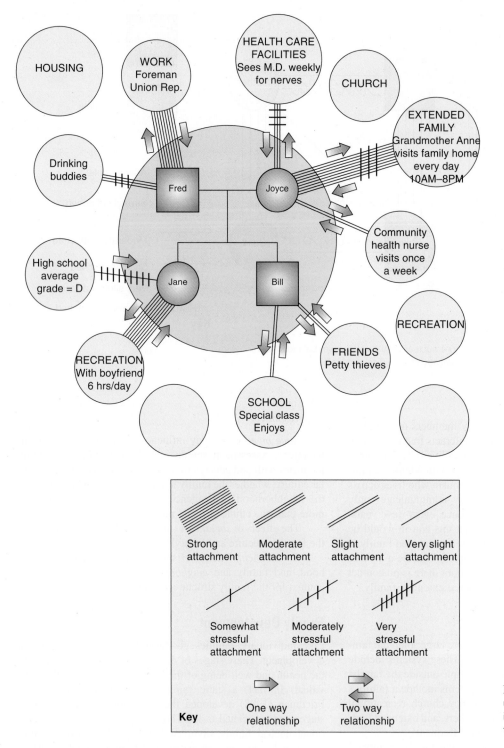

Figure 33-3 An ecomap is used to assess family members' interactions with systems outside the family.

- *Affective and socialization:* Affective function refers to the family's response to all members' needs for support, caring, closeness, intimacy, and the balance of needs for separateness and connectedness. Socialization function refers to the family's ability to bring about healthy socialization of children.
- *Expressive:* Expressive function refers to communication patterns used within the family. Members of well-functioning families are able to express a broad range of emotions; clearly express feelings and needs; encourage feedback; listen attentively to one another; treat one another with respect; avoid displacing, distorting, or masking verbal messages; avoid negative circular communication patterns; and use encouraging versus punishment methods to influence behavior.
- *Health care:* Assessment of health care function is useful for the nurse. It refers to family members' beliefs about a health problem; its etiology, treatment, and prognosis; and the role of professionals. Whether all family members agree or some members disagree with the beliefs helps the nurse to understand the family. The family's health promotion practices are also assessed.

DISPLAY 33-2 | **Two-Parent Nuclear Family Life Cycle**

Stage I—Beginning Families (stage of marriage)

Tasks

- Establishing a mutually satisfying marriage
- Relating harmoniously to the kin network
- Planning a family (decisions about parenthood)

Stage II—Childbearing Families (oldest child is infant through 30 months)

Tasks

- Setting up the young family as a stable unit (integrating new baby into family)
- Reconciling conflicting developmental tasks and needs of various family members
- Maintaining a satisfying marital relationship
- Expanding relationships with extended family by adding parenting and grandparenting roles

Stage III—Families with Preschool Children (2½ to 6 years)

Tasks

- Meeting family members' needs for adequate housing, space, privacy, and safety
- Socializing the children
- Integrating new child members while still meeting the needs of other children
- Maintaining healthy relationships within the family (marital and parent–child) and outside the family (extended family and community)

Stage IV—Families with School Children (6 to 13 years)

Tasks

- Socializing the children, including promoting school achievement and fostering of healthy peer relations of children
- Maintaining a satisfying marital relationship
- Meeting the physical health needs of family members

Stage V—Families with Teenagers (13 to 20 years)

Tasks

- Balancing of freedom with responsibility as teenagers mature and become increasingly autonomous
- Refocusing the marital relationship
- Communicating openly between parents and children

Stage VI—Launching Young Adults (from first to last child leaving home)

Tasks

- Expanding the family circle to include new family members acquired by marriage of children
- Continuing to renew and readjust in the marital relationship
- Assisting aging and ill parents of the husband or wife

Stage VII—Middle Aged Parents (empty nest through retirement)

Tasks

- Providing a health-promoting environment
- Sustaining satisfying and meaningful relationships with aging parents and adult children
- Strengthening the marital relationship

Stage VIII—Family in Retirement and Old Age (retirement to death of both spouses)

Tasks

- Maintaining a satisfying living arrangement
- Adjusting to a reduced income
- Maintaining marital relationships
- Adjusting to loss of spouse
- Maintaining intergenerational family ties
- Continuing to make sense out of one's existence (life review and integration)

Adapted from Friedman, M. (1998). *Family nursing: Theory and practice* (4th ed., pp. 113–138). Norwalk, CT: Appleton & Lange.

THEORETICAL CONCEPTS OF FAMILY FUNCTION

Some components of family function discussed previously are based on theoretical concepts found in systems theory, Bowen's family system theory, and communication theory. It is important for the nurse to have a good understanding of these concepts before performing an assessment of family function.

Systems Theory

Systems theory holds that a system is composed of subsystems interconnected to the whole system and to each other by means of an integrated and dynamic self-regulating feedback mechanism. Systems theory can be applied to any group with reciprocal

dynamic interaction. According to Boyd (1996), the major principles of systems theory as applied to family are

- Each system has its own characteristics.
- The whole is greater than the sum of the parts (rather than just the sum of the characteristics of individual parts of the system).
- All parts of the system depend on one another (even though each part has its own role within the system).
- There are mechanisms for exchange of information within the system (subsystems) and within the broader environment (suprasystem).

Wright and Leahey (2005) list the major concepts of systems theory that apply to families: A family is part of a larger suprasystem and is also composed of many subsystems

DISPLAY 33-3	The Divorce and Postdivorce Family Life Cycle

Divorce Stage One: Deciding to Divorce

Issues

Accepting one's own part in the failure of the marriage

Divorce Stage Two: Planning the Break-up of the System

Issues

Working cooperatively on problems of custody, visitation, and finances

Dealing with extended family about the divorce

Divorce Stage Three: Separation

Issues

Mourning loss of nuclear family

Restructuring marital and parent–child relationships and finances; adaptation to living apart

Realigning relationships with extended family; staying connected with spouse's extended family

Divorce Stage Four: Divorce

Issues

Mourning loss of intact family

Retrieving hopes, dreams, and expectations from the marriage

Staying connected with extended families

Postdivorce Stage: Single-parent (Custodial)

Issues

Making flexible visitation arrangements with ex-spouse and his or her family

Rebuilding own financial resources

Rebuilding own social network

Postdivorce Stage: Single-parent (Noncustodial)

Issues

Finding ways to continue effective parenting relationship with children

Maintaining financial responsibilities to ex-spouse and children

Rebuilding own social network

Postdivorce Stage: Single Parent (custodial)

Issues

Making flexible visitation arrangements

Rebuilding own financial resources

Rebuilding own social network

Adapted from Friedman, M. (1998). *Family nursing: Theory and practice* (4th ed., p. 140). Norwalk, CT: Appleton & Lange.

DISPLAY 33-4	The Remarried Family Formation

Stage One: Entering the New Relationship; Conceptualizing and Planning the New Marriage and Family

Issues

Recommitting to marriage and to forming a family

Developing openness in the new relationship

Planning financial and coparental relationships with ex-spouse

Planning to help children deal with fears, loyalty conflicts, and membership in two systems

Realigning relationships with extended family to include new spouse and children

Planning maintenance of connections for children with extended family of ex-spouse(s)

Stage Two: Remarriage and Family Reconstitution

Issues

Restructuring family boundaries to allow for inclusion of new spouse/step-parent

Realigning relationships and financial arrangements throughout subsystems

Making room for relationships of all children with custodial and noncustodial parents and grandparents

Sharing memories and histories to enhance step-family integration

Adapted from Friedman, M. (1998). *Family nursing: Theory and practice* (4th ed., p. 141). Norwalk, CT: Appleton & Lange.

(e.g., parent–child, sibling, marital); the family as a whole is greater than the sum of its parts; a change in one family member affects all family members; the family is able to create a balance between change and stability; and family members' behaviors are best understood from a view of circular rather than linear causality. For example, any behavior of family member A affects family member B, and B's behavior then affects A. Therefore, rather than an individual causing a family problem, the behavior pattern or system causes another behavior.

Bowen's Family System Theory

The family therapist Bowen (discussed in Shepard & Moriarty, 1996) developed several concepts that are widely used to assess family function. Bowen views the nuclear family as part of a multigenerational extended family with patterns of relating that tend to repeat over generations. When the pattern of projecting anxiety onto a child continues across generations, it is called the *multigenerational transmission process*. Bowen theorizes that familial emotional and interaction patterns are reflected in eight interwoven concepts. Two of these concepts—differentiation of self and triangles—are especially important to grasp for assessment of family function.

Differentiation of Self

Differentiation of self is assessed in relation to the boundaries of the subsystems in the structure of the family. This concept is based on a balance of emotional and intellectual levels of function. The emotional level, associated with lower brain centers, relates to feelings. The intellectual level, associated with the cerebral cortex, relates to cognition. How connected these levels, or systems, are affects the person's social functioning. The greater the balance between thinking and feeling, the higher the differentiation of self and the better the person is at managing anxiety.

Frisch and Kelley (1996) provide a summary of key elements of the concept of differentiation of self. The family with highly differentiated adult members is flexible in its interactions, seeks to support all members, understands each member as unique, and encourages members to develop differently from one another. Family roles are assigned on the basis of knowledge, skill, and interest.

The family with low levels of differentiation has adult members who demonstrate impulsive actions, who have difficulty delaying gratification, who cannot analyze a situation before reacting, and who cannot maintain intimate interpersonal relationships (similar to the developmental level of a 2-year-old child). Intense, short-term relationships are the norm, and emotionally based reactions can escalate into violence. Family roles are assigned on the basis of family tradition.

A moderately differentiated person is less dominated by emotions, but personal relationships are often emotion-dominated. Life is rule-bound, and thinking is usually dualistic (things and people are black and white, good or bad, smart or stupid). A situation cannot be perceived from any but a personal perspective. The person tends to "fuse" or become enmeshed with another in emotional relationships, losing himself in the efforts to please the other. Families with moderately differentiated members exhibit rigid patterns of interactions that are rule-bound and have defined roles and acceptable behaviors.

Triangles

Triangles are discussed in relation to subsystems of family structure. Shepard and Moriarty (1996) describe Bowen's triangle as a relational pattern or emotional configuration that exists among one or two family members and another person, object, or issue. Triangles exist in all families; who makes up a triangle can change depending on the situation. However, when two people avoid dealing with emotional closeness or an issue that produces anxiety, the two people may use a third person to evade the stress. For instance, a wife may pull in a child as a third person in the couple's relationship; the husband may distance himself from the conflict by deeper involvement in work. As the intensity of the relationship changes, the amount of interaction is usually balanced, so that as two members move closer, the third withdraws.

Communication Theory

Communication theory concerns the sending and receiving of both verbal and nonverbal messages. The focus is on how individuals interact with one another. According to Wright and Leahey (1994), the major concepts of communication theory applied to families are

1. All nonverbal communication is meaningful.
2. All communication has two major channels for transmission (verbal and nonverbal including body language, facial expression, voice tone, music, poetry, painting, and so forth).
3. A dyadic (two-person) relationship has varying degrees of symmetry and complementarity (both of which may be healthy depending on context).
4. All communication consists of two levels: content (what is said) and relationship (of those interacting).

Cybernetics

Cybernetics combines communication and general systems theory. Wright and Leahey (1994) state that the major concepts of cybernetics as applied to families are that families possess self-regulating abilities through the process of feedback, and feedback processes can occur simultaneously at different systems' levels within families.

Circular Communication

One example of a feedback system in communications is circular communication. Circular communication is a reciprocal communication between two people. Wright and Leahey (1994) note that most relationship issues have a pattern of circular communication. One person speaks and the other person interprets what is heard, then reacts and speaks on the basis of the interpretation, creating a circular feedback loop based on the individuals' perceptions and reactions.

Circular communication can be positive or negative. An example of negative circular communication is as follows: An angry wife criticizes her husband; the husband feels angry and withdraws; the wife becomes even angrier and criticizes more; the husband becomes angrier and withdraws further. Each person sees the problem as the other's, and each person's communication influences the other person's behavior. Positive and negative circular communication patterns are illustrated in Figure 33-4.

Family Assessment

Wright and Leahey (2005) assert that family knowledge can be obtained and applied even in very brief meetings with a family. They provide a guide to a 15-minute (or shorter) family interview. Key elements of the interview, which occurs only in the context of a therapeutic relationship, are manners, therapeutic conversation, family genogram (and ecomap as appropriate), therapeutic questions, and commendations. See Display 33-5 for a summary of the interview technique.

FAMILY INTERVIEW TECHNIQUES

The brief interview consists of several elements, which are described thoroughly by Wright and Leahey in the context of the Calgary Family Assessment Model and the Calgary Family Intervention Model. Essential points follow.

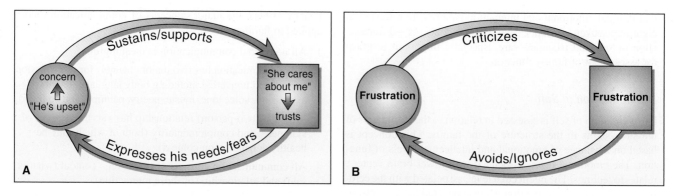

Figure 33-4 **(A)** Positive circular communication. **(B)** Negative circular communication.

DISPLAY 33-5	**Tips for Conducting the 15-Minute Family Interview**

- Introduce yourself and use good manners in interactions.
- Seek opportunities to involve family in care delivery and decision making.
- Use active listening, create family genograms (ecomaps), and ask key therapeutic questions to help family

members (and the nurse) better understand the family's needs and beliefs about themselves and the illness.
- Seek opportunities to commend individuals and the family.

Manners

The simple acts of good manners that invite a trusting relationship are

- Always call the client(s) by name.
- Introduce yourself by name.
- Examine your attitude and adjust responses to convey interest and acceptance.
- Explain your role for the time you will spend with the client/family.
- Explain any procedure before entering the room with equipment to perform the procedure.
- Keep appointments and promises to return.
- Be honest.

Therapeutic Conversation

Therapeutic conversation is purposeful and time-limited. The art of listening is paramount. The nurse *not only* makes information giving and client involvement in decision making an integral part of the care delivery process but also seeks opportunities to engage in purposeful conversations with families. Nurse–family therapeutic conversations can include such basic ideas as

- Invitations to accompany the client to the unit, clinic, or hospital
- Inclusion of family members in health care facility admission procedures
- Encouragement to ask questions during client orientation to a health care facility
- Acknowledgment of client and family's expertise in managing health problems by asking about routines at home
- Presentation of opportunities to practice how client will handle different interactions in the future such as telling

family members and others that they cannot eat certain foods
- Consultation with families and clients about their ideas for treatment and discharge (Wright & Leahey, 2000, p. 280)

Family Genograms and Ecomaps

The genogram (see Fig. 33-1) acts as a continuous visual reminder to caregivers to "think family." In addition, the ecomap (see Fig. 33-3) illustrates the family's interactions with outside systems.

Commendations

Offer at least one or two commendations during each meeting with the family. The individual or family can be commended on strengths, resources, or competencies observed or reported to the nurse. Commendations are observations of behavior. Look for patterns, not onetime occurrences to commend. Examples include "Your family shows much courage in living with your wife's cancer for 5 years"; "Your son is so gentle despite feeling so ill" (Wright & Leahey, 2000, p. 282). The commendations offer family members a new view of themselves. Wright and Leahey propose that many families experiencing illness, disability, or trauma have a "commendation-deficit disorder" (p. 282). Changing the view of themselves helps the family members to look differently at the health problem and more toward solutions.

ASSESSMENT PROCEDURE

As appropriate, incorporate some of the following interview components/techniques in your practice.

(text continues on page 805)

FAMILY ASSESSMENT

Assessment Procedure	Normal Findings	Abnormal Findings

Family Structure

Internal Family Structure

Assess family composition. Use a genogram and fill in as much information as possible. Ask the following questions:

- What is the family type (nuclear, three generation, single-parent)?
- Who does the family consider to be family?
- Has anyone recently moved in or out? Has anyone recently died?

Family identifies family type and members of the family. A new baby born into family or young adult moving out reflects normal life cycle tasks. Death is also a normal part of life, but it is not often viewed as a family strength.

A new baby or a young adult moving out may cause excessive stress for family. Death of a family member often causes a variety of different reactions including denial, extreme grief, depression, and even relief. Serious family problems may result when family members react to, and deal with, the death differently.

Determine gender roles in the family. Gender often determines an expected family role. Ask each family member the following question:

What are the expected behaviors for men in your family? For women?

> ➤ **Clinical Tip** • It is important to ask both the men and women what they perceive to be the roles of men and women in the family because they may perceive the roles differently.

Family members understand and agree on expected gender-related behaviors; expected behaviors are flexible.

Rigid, traditional gender-related behaviors reduce the family's flexibility for meeting family needs. One or more family members have different beliefs about expected behaviors for men and women, which can lead to family conflict.

Evaluate rank order. Spousal rank order often plays a significant role in family harmony. Ask spouses: What rank order did you have in your childhood family (e.g., older sister, youngest brother)? Using the family's answers and information you know concerning birth order, ask yourself:

Are spouses' birth rank orders likely to be complementary or competitive?

Complementary birth order of spouses can support each spouse's interaction with the other based on past experiences with siblings (e.g., older brother marries younger sister).

Competitive birth order of spouses may result in problems. For example, if an older brother marries an older sister, both may be used to being the responsible leader.

Assess subsystems. Ask the family questions about attachments within the family. For example, is there a mother–daughter relationship? How strong is it? Use a family attachment diagram to determine family subgroups. Assessment of the function of family subgroups is covered under assessment of family function.

Family subgroups are present and appear healthy.

Family subgroups are absent or appear excessively strong, excluding other family members. For instance, a strong female subgroup of mother and daughters may work to exclude the father/ husband from important family activities or decision-making. Or an overly strong spousal subsystem may impose an emotional distance between parents and children.

Assess family boundaries. Boundaries separate family subsystems. Ask the family questions about how the subsystems are fixed within the family. For example, is the mother–daughter subsystem totally separated from the father–son subsystem? Based on the family's answers, ask yourself the following questions:

Permeable boundaries are present.

Rigid or diffuse boundaries are present.

continued

FAMILY ASSESSMENT *Continued*

Assessment Procedure	Normal Findings	Abnormal Findings
Are there boundaries between subsystems?		
What types of boundaries are present? *Note:* Assessment of the function of family boundaries is covered under "Family Function."		
Evaluate the family power structure. Ask the family to rate the structure of the family on a scale with chaos (no leader) at one end, equality in the middle, and domination by one individual at the other end. If the family is dominated by one individual, ask the clients who that person is.	A power hierarchy with parents equally in control, but tending toward egalitarian and flexible power shifts, is considered normal. This type of structure demonstrates respect for all family members and encourages family development and effective functioning.	Chaotic or authoritarian power structures tend to prevent effective family functioning and individual development.
External Structure		
Assess the extended family. Ask "Are extended family members available to help support your immediate family?"	Extended family can provide emotional and other support to the family.	Lack of extended family or no contact with extended family results in no support for immediate family.
Assess external systems. Ask the family questions about relationships with external systems (e.g., agencies and people outside immediate family). Use an ecomap to record and view these relationships. Then ask yourself the following questions based on the ecomap:		
What relationship is there between the family and external systems?	Positive relationships with external systems are beneficial to the family.	Conflictual relationships with external systems add stress to the family.
Are external systems overinvolved or underinvolved with the family?	Balanced involvement with external systems adds to the health of the family.	Too little or too much involvement with external systems can prevent the family from effectively using resources to meet its needs. In addition, either overinvolvement or underinvolvement with external systems can add great stress to the immediate family.
Assess context. Ask questions that relate to ethnicity, social class, religion, and environment.	A family that has a strong ethnic identity and lives in a similar ethnic society will usually have plentiful support.	Racial or ethnic difference from the neighborhood or larger society can produce misunderstanding and negatively affect communications and interactions.
How does the family's race or ethnicity affect the family structure and function?		
How does the family's race or ethnicity affect interactions with neighbors?		
How does the family's race or ethnicity affect interactions with external systems?		

continued

Assessment Procedure	Normal Findings	Abnormal Findings
What social class is most representative of the family? Do social class factors affect the family's ability to meet its needs?	Cultural, social, and economic factors of the family's social class support the family's ability to meet its needs.	Cultural, social, and economic resources associated with social class may be inadequate to meet family needs.
Is religion important to the family?	Religion provides the family with supportive spiritual beliefs.	Religious controversies among family members may produce family conflict.
Are environmental characteristics of the residence and neighborhood adequate to meet family needs?	The residence and neighborhood are safe, and necessary resources are available.	The residence or neighborhood is not safe. Resources are not readily available.

Family Development: Life-Cycle Stages and Tasks

Ask the family questions about the family's life-cycle stage(s). Can the family meet the tasks of the current life-cycle stage(s) with which it is dealing?	The family has successfully met the tasks of previous life-cycle stages and can meet the tasks of its current life-cycle stage.	The family has not adequately met tasks of previous life-cycle stages and may be unable to meet tasks of the current stage.

Family Function

Assess instrumental function. Evaluate if the family can carry out routine activities of daily living.	The family has successfully met routine daily living needs of all family members.	The family cannot carry out one or more activities of daily living.
Does a family member's illness affect the family's ability to carry out activities of daily living?	The family can continue to carry out activities of daily living even with the added stress of an ill family member.	The added stress of caring for an ill family member prevents the family from adequately carrying out one or more activities of daily living.
Note affective and socialization function. Observe family interactions and ask questions to determine if family members provide mutual support and nurturance to one another.	Families that can meet psychological needs for support and nurturance of family members provide an opportunity for each individual adequately to self-differentiate and reach emotional maturity.	Families that cannot provide for psychological needs for support and nurturance make self-differentiation and emotional health of the members unlikely.
Are parenting practices appropriate for healthy socialization of the children?	Parenting practices based on respect, guidance, and encouragement (rather than punishment) encourage socialization.	Parenting practices based on control, coercion, and punishment discourage socialization. Chapter 9 discusses nursing assessment of families using violence.
What function do subgroups serve within the family?	Subgroups are flexible and assist the family to meet changing needs.	Rigid subgroups do not easily change to meet individual needs.
Are there alliances that produce triangles?	Flexible alliances and triangles form to maintain family functioning.	Rigid alliances and triangles are formed to balance negative forces and stress. They are a coping mechanism.
What function do boundaries serve within the family?	Permeable boundaries encourage emotional development and self-differentiation of family members.	Rigid or diffuse boundaries discourage emotional development and self-differentiation.

continued

FAMILY ASSESSMENT *Continued*

Assessment Procedure	Normal Findings	Abnormal Findings
Are family members enmeshed (overly involved with each other)? Disengaged (underinvolved with each other)?	Adequate involvement of family members without enmeshment or disengagement serves as support for family function and individual development.	Enmeshed or disengaged family members cannot adequately self-differentiate.
Evaluate expressive function. Ask the family and observe interactions to *assess emotional communication:* Do all family members express a broad range of both negative and positive emotion?	Open expression and acceptance of feelings and emotions within a family encourages positive family functioning.	Lack of acceptance of emotional expression or acceptance of emotional expression by only some family members tends to prevent effective family development and functioning.
Assess verbal communication: Are verbal messages clearly stated?	Clear verbal messages increase open communication.	Displaced, masked, or distorted messages obstruct open communication and may reflect underlying problems in family functioning.
Assess nonverbal communication: Do nonverbal communications match verbal content?	Clear and open communications have verbal and nonverbal elements that match.	Nonverbal communications that do not match verbal content suggest a lack of honesty or openness in the communication.
Assess circular communication: Is there an evident pattern of circular communication? If so, is it negative or positive?	Positive circular communication helps to build up the participants.	Negative circular communication reinforces interpersonal conflict and prevents an understanding of the intended message.
Assess the family's health care function. Ask the following questions: What do family members believe about the etiology, treatment, prognosis of the health problem? What do family members believe about the role of professionals, role of the family, and level of control the family has relative to the health problem? Are family members' beliefs in agreement or discord?	Agreement among family members reduces conflict.	Disagreement among family members produces conflict and draws on energy and emotional resources needed to handle the health problem.
What strengths does the family believe it has for coping with the health problem?	If the family perceives strengths, it will be more likely to cope effectively.	If the family does not perceive strengths, it will have difficulty coping with the health problem.
Are the family's health promotion practices supportive of family health?	A pattern of health promotion practices provides a basis for building in health care for a particular health problem.	A family that has little practice of health promotion behaviors will have difficulty incorporating health care practices for a particular problem into its routines.
Assess for multigenerational patterns. Look back over the assessment and determine if there are any multigenerational patterns evident in any categories.	Multigenerational patterns of positive behaviors are often seen in effectively functioning families.	Multigenerational patterns of ineffective or destructive behaviors make change more difficult.

VALIDATING AND DOCUMENTING FINDINGS

Validate the family assessment data that you have collected. This is necessary to verify that the data are reliable and accurate. Document the assessment data following the health care facility or agency policy.

Sample of Subjective and Objective Data

Family is composed of two parents, one grown child, and one grandmother—a three-generation family. The family also considers two other grown children and their spouses as immediate family. The second-oldest child was married recently and moved away, and the family views the event positively. Family members agree on expected gender-related behaviors, which are flexible. The wife is the youngest daughter of her family, and the husband is the oldest son of his family. Subgroups and triangles between family members are flexible. The boundaries between subgroups are permeable.

The two parents are equally in control, but the grown child and grandmother share equally in decisions that affect the family. The grandmother's other daughter and family live nearby and provide emotional and financial support in caring for her. The family is positively involved in the local church, the grown child has a group of supportive friends, the grandmother goes to the local senior center 3 days a week, and the parents enjoy being involved with the local garden club. Time spent with groups outside the family is balanced evenly with time spent with the immediate family.

The family lives in a safe home and in a neighborhood with people of similar ethnicity. The family's cultural, social, and economic factors support their ability to live well. The family is currently able to meet the tasks of its life cycle stage. The family has met routine activities of daily living needs of its members despite the fact that the grandmother needs care because of arthritis and macular degeneration. Family meets the psychological needs for support and nurturance of all family members. Family members feel free to express and accept feelings and emotions openly. The family, including the extended family, is in agreement about caring for the grandmother's health conditions and feels confident that they can meet her needs. Multigenerational patterns of positive behaviors are seen in this family.

Analysis of Data

After you have collected your assessment data, you will need to analyze the data, using diagnostic reasoning skills.

DIAGNOSTIC REASONING: POSSIBLE CONCLUSIONS

Listed below are some possible conclusions following assessment of the family.

Selected Nursing Diagnoses

After collecting subjective and objective data pertaining to the family, you will need to identify abnormal data and cluster the data to reveal any significant patterns or abnormalities. These data will then be used to make clinical judgments (nursing diagnoses: wellness, risk, or actual) about the status of the family. Following is a list of selected nursing diagnoses that you may identify when analyzing data for this part of the assessment.

Wellness Diagnoses

- Readiness for Enhanced Family Coping
- Health-Seeking Behaviors
- Readiness for Enhanced Spiritual Well-Being
- Readiness for Enhanced Parenting
- Readiness for Enhanced Home Maintenance
- Readiness for Enhanced Family Processes

Risk Diagnoses

- Risk for Caregiver Role Strain
- Risk for Impaired Parent/Infant/Child Attachment
- Risk for Impaired Parenting
- Risk for Compromised Family Coping
- Risk for Dysfunctional Family Processes
- Risk for Impaired Home Maintenance

Actual Diagnoses

- Caregiver Role Strain
- Compromised Family Coping
- Ineffective Family Coping: Disabling
- Dysfunctional Family Processes: Alcoholism
- Interrupted Family Processes
- Impaired Home Maintenance
- Ineffective Family Therapeutic Regimen Management
- Parental Role Conflict
- Impaired Parenting
- Impaired Social Interaction
- Social Isolation
- Spiritual Distress
- Ineffective Role Performance

Selected Collaborative Problems

After grouping the data, it may become apparent that certain collaborative problems emerge. Remember that collaborative problems differ from nursing diagnoses in that they cannot be prevented by nursing interventions. However, these physiologic complications of medical conditions can be detected and monitored by the nurse. In addition, the nurse can use physician- and nurse-prescribed interventions to minimize the complications of these problems. The nurse may also have to refer the client in such situations for further treatment of the problem. Following is a list of collaborative problems that may be identified when assessing the family. These problems are worded as Risk for Complications (or RC), followed by the problem.

- RC: Marital conflict
- RC: Child abuse
- RC: Spouse abuse

Medical Problems

After grouping the data, it may become apparent that the family has signs and symptoms that may require medical or mental health professional diagnosis and treatment. Referral to a primary care provider is necessary.

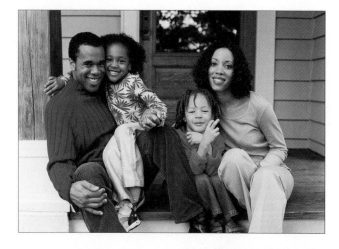

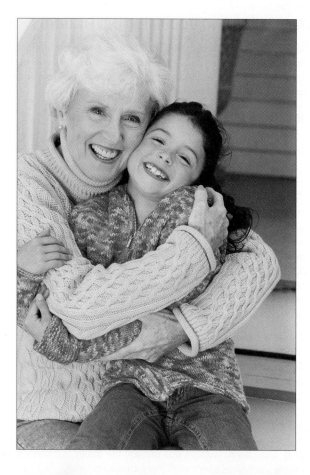

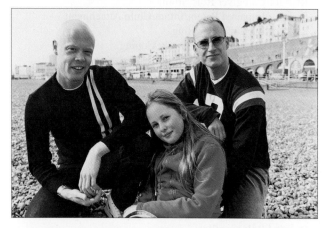

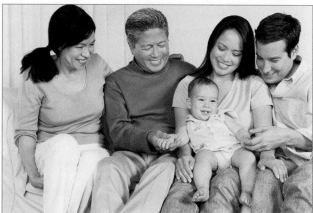

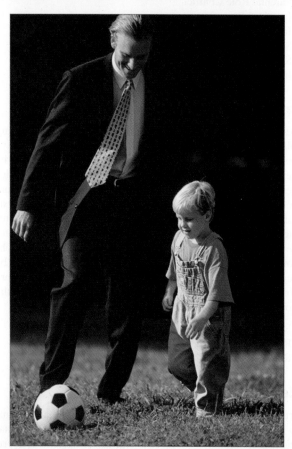

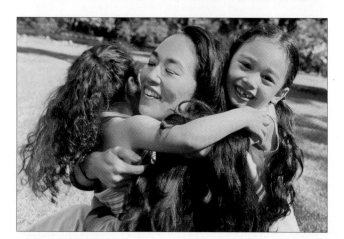

CASE STUDY

The case study presents assessment data for a specific family. It is followed by an analysis of the data to arrive at specific conclusions.

The Ross family has returned to the clinic for help with dealing with Dan's recent diagnosis and treatment for type 1 diabetes mellitus. Dan is a 17-year-old high school senior who is scheduled to leave for college in 6 months. He was diagnosed with type 1 diabetes mellitus 4 months ago. He is not following the diet–exercise–insulin protocol (prescribed 4 months ago). Dan has been seen by the physician and in the emergency room five times in the past 4 months for complications resulting from not following the protocol. The physician refers the Ross family to the nurse to help the family address the identified problem of Dan's refusal to follow the protocol. Because the diet and food preparation affect the whole family, sister Jenna attends the family session as well. Dan's file includes a genogram (Fig. 33-5).

Mr. and Mrs. Ross express concern and caring for Dan's well-being and request assistance with dealing with Dan's diagnosis and treatment. You ask how everyone feels about Dan's disease and treatment. Both the parents and Jenna appear tense when describing the effect of trying to deal with Dan's disease and his refusal to follow the protocol. Mr. and Mrs. Ross express frustration with inability to get Dan to follow the doctor's orders. Dan expresses frustration at having a disease and at being asked to follow a protocol that makes him different from his friends and unable to do the things that they do (e.g., diet, exercise, partying). Dan expresses frustration at having his parents tell him what to do. Jenna expresses frustration at Dan for upsetting the family, especially at mealtime, particularly in regard to what family members eat and how they interact. When you ask the family to tell you about Dan's disease and treatment, Dan and his parents describe a good understanding of the disease and reasons for the protocol.

The following concept map illustrates the diagnostic reasoning process.

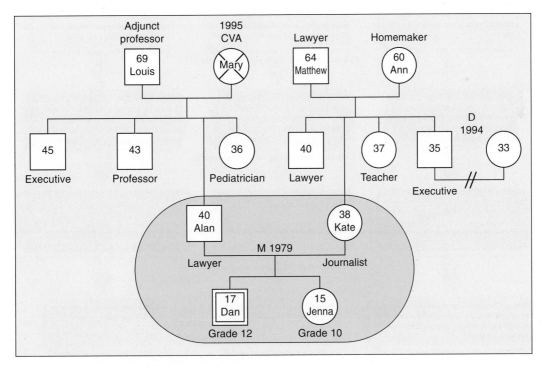

Figure 33-5 Genogram of the Ross family.

I) Identify abnormal findings and client strengths

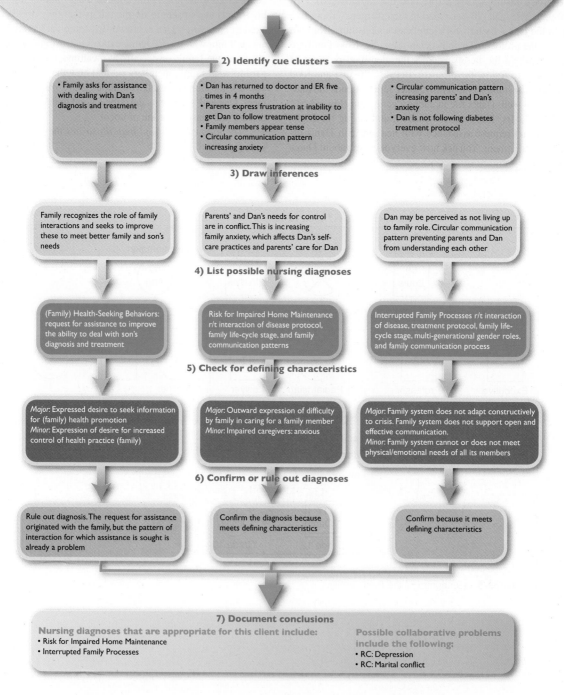

Subjective Data

- Dan refuses to follow prescribed diabetes protocol
- Parents express concern and caring for Dan's well-being and request assistance with dealing with Dan's diagnosis and treatment
- Parents express frustration with inability to get Dan to follow the doctor's orders
- Dan expresses frustration at having a disease and at a protocol that makes him different from his friends
- Dan expresses frustration at having his parents tell him what to do
- Jenna expresses frustration at Dan for upsetting the family, especially at mealtime

Objective Data

- Family members appear tense when describing the effect of trying to deal with Dan's disease and his refusal to follow the protocol
- Dan is a 17-year-old high school senior who is scheduled to leave for college in 6 months. He was diagnosed with type 1 diabetes mellitus 4 months ago
- Dan has been seen by the physician and in the emergency room five times in the past 4 months for complications resulting from not following the protocol
- Dan and his parents describe a good understanding of the disease and reasons for the protocol
- A circular pattern of communication has developed: Between the parents and between the father and Dan. Dan is not following the protocol, which increases the parents' anxiety and frustration. In addition, the parents' expressions of displeasure cause Dan's sense of loss of control, anxiety, and frustration to increase

2) Identify cue clusters

- Family asks for assistance with dealing with Dan's diagnosis and treatment

- Dan has returned to doctor and ER five times in 4 months
- Parents express frustration at inability to get Dan to follow treatment protocol
- Family members appear tense
- Circular communication pattern increasing anxiety

- Circular communication pattern increasing parents' and Dan's anxiety
- Dan is not following diabetes treatment protocol

3) Draw inferences

Family recognizes the role of family interactions and seeks to improve these to meet better family and son's needs

Parents' and Dan's needs for control are in conflict. This is increasing family anxiety, which affects Dan's self-care practices and parents' care for Dan

Dan may be perceived as not living up to family role. Circular communication pattern preventing parents and Dan from understanding each other

4) List possible nursing diagnoses

(Family) Health-Seeking Behaviors: request for assistance to improve the ability to deal with son's diagnosis and treatment

Risk for Impaired Home Maintenance r/t interaction of disease protocol, family life-cycle stage, and family communication patterns

Interrupted Family Processes r/t interaction of disease, treatment protocol, family life-cycle stage, multi-generational gender roles, and family communication process

5) Check for defining characteristics

Major: Expressed desire to seek information for (family) health promotion
Minor: Expression of desire for increased control of health practice (family)

Major: Outward expression of difficulty by family in caring for a family member
Minor: Impaired caregivers: anxious

Major: Family system does not adapt constructively to crisis. Family system does not support open and effective communication.
Minor: Family system cannot or does not meet physical/emotional needs of all its members

6) Confirm or rule out diagnoses

Rule out diagnosis. The request for assistance originated with the family, but the pattern of interaction for which assistance is sought is already a problem

Confirm the diagnosis because meets defining characteristics

Confirm because it meets defining characteristics

7) Document conclusions

Nursing diagnoses that are appropriate for this client include:
- Risk for Impaired Home Maintenance
- Interrupted Family Processes

Possible collaborative problems include the following:
- RC: Depression
- RC: Marital conflict

References and Selected Readings

Bomar, P. (2004). *Promoting health in families* (3rd ed.). Philadelphia: Saunders.

Boyd, S. (1996). Theoretical and research foundations of family nursing. In S. Hanson & S. Boyd (eds). *Family health care nursing* (pp. 41–53). Philadelphia: F. A. Davis.

Duvall, E. (1984). *Marriage and family development* (6th ed.). Philadelphia: J. B. Lippincott.

Friedman, M. (1998). *Family nursing: Theory and practice* (4th ed.). Norwalk, CT: Appleton & Lange.

Frisch, N., & Kelley, J. (1996). *Healing life's crises.* Albany, NY: Delmar.

Hanson, S., & Boyd, S. (1996). *Family health care nursing.* Philadelphia: F. A. Davis.

Lewis, M., Hepburn, K., Corcoran-Perry, S., Narayan, S., & Lally, R. M. (1999). Options, outcomes, values, likelihoods decision making guide for patients and their families. *Journal of Gerontological Nursing, 25*(12), 19–25.

Shepard, M., Moriarty, H. (1996). Family mental health nursing. In S. Hanson & S. Boyd (eds.). *Family health care nursing* (pp. 303–326). Philadelphia: F. A. Davis.

Wright, L., & Leahey, M. (2000). *Nurses and families: A guide to family assessment and intervention.* Philadelphia: F. A. Davis.

Wright, L., & Leahey, M. (2005). *Nurse and families: A guide to family assessment and intervention* (4th ed.). Philadelphia: F. A. Davis.

Wright, L., Watson, W., & Bell, J. (2000). Family nursing unit: Therapeutic approach. Available at http://www.ucalgary.ca/nu/

_____ (1996). *Beliefs: The heart of healing in families and illness.* New York: Basic Books.

Useful Website Resources

http://www.familynursingresources.com (Includes books, DVDs/videos)

34

Assessing Communities

WHAT IS COMMUNITY ASSESSMENT?

A thorough assessment of a community first requires an understanding of the concept of community. *Community* may be defined several ways depending on the conceptual view of the term. It may be defined from a sociologic perspective as "a collection of people in a place who interact with one another and whose common interests and goals give them a sense of belonging" (Stackhouse, 1998, p. 79). Another definition of *community* is an "open social system characterized by people in a place over time who have common goals" (Maurer & Smith, 2005, p. 341).

Classification of community, then, depends on the definition. For purposes of assessment, communities are classified according to either location or social relationship. The first classification is a geopolitical community in which people have a time-and-space relationship. Geopolitical communities may be determined by natural boundaries such as rivers, lakes, or mountain ranges. For example, the Mississippi River separates the states of Missouri and Illinois. Geopolitical boundaries also may be man-made: counties, cities, voting districts, or school districts. Another example of a geopolitical community is a census tract, which is determined by the government to organize demographic data collection.

Communities also may be classified by relationships among a group of people. These communities are usually centered on a specific goal or function. For example, a group such as Mothers Against Drunk Drivers (MADD) may center on eliciting support for a new ordinance regulating hours of bars and taverns. These types of communities can be organized to address a common interest or problem, such as a state student nurses' association or a support group for family and friends of Alzheimer's patients. Another example of this type of community would be those with similar religious or political beliefs. Any number of social communities may exist within the boundaries of a geopolitical community.

The purpose of community assessment is to determine the health-related concerns of its members, regardless of the type of the community. The nurse gets to know the community, its people, its history, and its culture through the assessment process. A thorough and accurate assessment provides the foundation for diagnosis and for planning appropriate nursing interventions.

MODELS OF COMMUNITY ASSESSMENT

A number of different models or frameworks have been used to provide the structure for assessing both geopolitical and social communities. The Partners in Caring Model served as the framework for a partnership between the University of Connecticut and the Visiting Nurse Association of Central Connecticut, Inc. as a partnership was developed to assist community agencies in meeting the challenge of providing care to clients who have declining resources. This cooperative program also provided nursing students with community-based clinical experiences (Bernal, Shellman, & Reid, 2004). The Mobilizing for Action through Planning and Partnerships (MAAP) model was used as the guide for a community-wide health assessment in Clarendon County in South Carolina. Data generated through this assessment identified gaps in services as well as service opportunities in the community (McClellan, 2005). The Bergen County Department of Health Services in New Jersey and Pace University's Lienhard School of Nursing together developed a "partnership model" to bring together both academia and practice. This model provided the health agency with support in assessment, assurance, and policy development. The Community Readiness Model was applied as a framework for the assessment of childhood obesity and the implementation of a program for its prevention and control (Findholt, 2007).

The Community as Partner model provides a comprehensive guide for data collection (Anderson & McFarlane, 2004). Central to the model are the people, or core, of the community. This component includes demographic information as well as information about the history, culture, and values and beliefs of the people. Also identified are eight subsystems that are affected by the people of the community and that directly contribute to the health status of the community. These include housing, fire and safety, health, education, economics, politics and government, communication, and recreation.

The Community as Partner model has been adapted for use in this chapter. The nursing assessment section (below) is a step-by-step assessment of the community; it has three categories: people, environment, and health. What to assess in each category and how to assess it are discussed. The nursing component is inherent throughout each category.

Community Assessment

Community assessment involves both subjective and objective data collection using a variety of methods. Subjective data collection includes perceptions of the community by the nurse as well as by members of the community. The nurse should spend time in the community to "get to know" the people and get a sense of their values and beliefs. Through the process of participant observation, the nurse hopes to become accepted as a member of the community. This method of data collection allows the nurse to participate in the daily life of the community, make observations, and obtain information about the structures and influences that affect the community. The nurse should ask key members or leaders of the community as well as "typical" residents to provide further information and insight about the community. Objective methods of data collection include using surveys and analyzing existing data such as census information, health records, and other public documents.

(text continues on page 821)

COMMUNITY ASSESSMENT

Assessment Procedure	Normal Findings	Abnormal Findings
Community History		
Study the history of the community. Look for this information at the local library or ask local residents. Use this information to gain insights into the health practices and belief systems of community members.	The community history should include initial development, any specific ethnic groups that may have settled there, past economic trends, and past population trends.	The history of some communities may include episodes that have had a disruptive influence on the people of the community such as relocation because of repeated flooding, a history of racial or ethnic problems, or the closing of a factory.
Demographic Information		
Age and Gender **Obtain age and gender information from census data.** Age is the most important risk factor for health-related problems. Gender may be another important risk factor.	A healthy/typical community has a distribution of individuals in various age ranges: younger than 5, 5 to 19, 30 to 34, 35 to 54, 55 to 64, and 65+ years as well as no significant difference between percentages of males and females.	Communities with a large percentage of elderly people or very young children generally have more health-related problems. Communities with a preponderance of women of child-bearing age may need to improve access to or expand family planning and prenatal services as well as well-baby programs.
Racial and Ethnic Groups **Study census figures and state and local population reports.** Use this information to learn about racial and ethnic groups that reside in the community.	The lack of significant numbers of racial or ethnic groups suggests that special screenings or programs to meet their needs may not be required.	A large percentage of ethnic or racial minorities may indicate that certain health concerns exist within these groups of individuals. For example, Native Americans often have a higher incidence of diabetes or alcohol-related health problems, and sickle cell anemia is prevalent among African Americans. Therefore, special screenings and programs to meet the needs of particular racial or ethnic groups become more important to these communities.
Vital Statistics **Obtain vital statistics data.** This data can be obtained from the National Center for Health Statistics, state and local agencies, and from hospital records. These include birth and death records as well as crude death rates (age and cause), specific death rates, and infant—maternal mortality. Morbidity (disease) data also	Expected birth, death, and morbidity data should generally reflect overall rates for the United States. See Displays 34-1, 34-2, 34-3, and 34-4 for age-related causes of mortality.	Higher-than-expected birth, death, and morbidity rates, especially age- and cause-specific rates, may indicate a lack of services or programs in critical areas. For example, higher-than-expected teen birth rates may be related to a lack of family planning services or education; high mortality rates associated

continued on page 813

DISPLAY 34-1   Causes of Neonatal Mortality—United States

1. Congenital malformations, deformations, and chromosomal abnormalities
2. Disorders related to short gestation and low birth weight, not classified elsewhere
3. Newborn affected by maternal complications of pregnancy
4. Newborn affected by complications of placenta, cord, and membranes
5. Respiratory distress of newborn
6. Bacterial sepsis of newborn

Source: Center for Disease Control. (September 30, 2005). *Monthly Morbidity and Weekly Reports 54*(38), 966.

DISPLAY 34-2   Causes of Infant Mortality—United States

1. Congenital malformation, deformations, and chromosomal abnormalities
2. Disorders related to short gestation/low birth weight
3. Sudden infant death syndrome
4. Newborn affected by maternal complications of pregnancy
5. Unintentional injuries
6. Newborn affected by complications of placenta, cord, and membranes

Source: National Center for Health Statistics. (2007). *Health, United States.* Available at www.cdc.gov/nchs/hus.htm

DISPLAY 34-3   Causes of Childhood Mortality—United States

Ages 1–4
1. Unintentional injuries
2. Congenital malformations, deformations, and chromosomal abnormalities
3. Malignant neoplasms
4. Homicide
5. Diseases of the heart

Ages 5–14
1. Unintentional injuries
2. Malignant neoplasms
3. Congenital malformations, deformations, and chromosomal abnormalities
4. Homicide
5. Suicide

Source: National Center for Health Statistics. (2007). *Health, United States.* Available at www.cdc.gov/nchs/hus.htm

DISPLAY 34-4   Causes of Teen and Adult Mortality—United States

Ages 15–24
1. Unintentional injuries
2. Homicide
3. Suicide
4. Malignant neoplasms
5. Diseases of the heart

Ages 45–64
1. Malignant neoplasms
2. Diseases of the heart
3. Unintentional injuries
4. Diabetes mellitus
5. Chronic lower respiratory disease

Ages 25–44
1. Unintentional injuries
2. Malignant neoplasms
3. Diseases of the heart
4. Suicide
5. Homicide

Ages 65 and Older
1. Diseases of the heart
2. Malignant neoplasms
3. Cerebrovascular diseases
4. Chronic lower respiratory diseases
5. Alzheimer's disease

Source: National Center for Health Statistics. (2007). *Health, United States.* Available at www.cdc.gov/nchs/hus.htm

Assessment Procedure	Normal Findings	Abnormal Findings

are important indicators of the health status of the community.

with motor vehicles, especially when alcohol is involved, indicate that alcohol awareness programs should be instituted; and greater-than-expected rates of tuberculosis or sexually transmitted infections indicate that primary and secondary prevention efforts should be increased.

Household Size, Marital Status, Mobility

Refer to the U.S. Census Bureau for the following information: Number of people per household, their marital status, and the stability of the population.

The Census Bureau identifies three major types of households: Married couple (Fig. 34-1), female householder (no husband present), and male householder (no female present). The nature and size of households in the United States have changed significantly in the last 50 years. Household size has decreased from 3.3 to 2.6 persons per household. The number of divorced people has quadrupled since 1970. According to the 2000 U.S. Census, married couples currently make up 51.7% of all households (down from 55% in 1990), and the number of unmarried partner households grew from 3.2 million in 1990 to 5.5 million in 2000. The number of female family households (no husband present) increased from 6.6% to 7.2% in 2000. Multigenerational family households make up 3.7% of all households. Americans also are a mobile population, moving for education, jobs, or retirement. A healthy community adjusts to these changes and organizes to meet the needs of the population.

Single parents (teenage mothers and fathers, in particular) are at greater risk for health problems, especially those related to role overload. This occurs because single parents often have to assume the role of the missing parent in addition to their own roles. Single mothers report a higher incidence of children's academic and behavioral problems than mothers in two-parent families. Unmarried people have a higher mortality rate than do married people. Elderly people living alone also are at higher risk for health problems. In addition, some immigrant groups, such as migrant farm families, are at higher risk. Communities that do not adapt to meet the needs of the mobile population compromise the continuity and quality of care for these people.

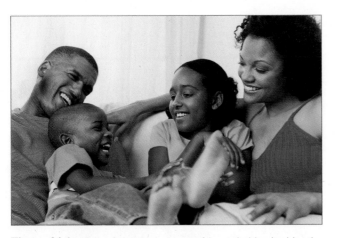

Figure 34-1 One of the three types of households cited by the Bureau of the Census is a married couple with children.

continued

COMMUNITY ASSESSMENT *Continued*

Assessment Procedure	Normal Findings	Abnormal Findings

Values and Religious Beliefs

Obtain data to determine values and religious beliefs of the community. These data can be obtained from the local Chamber of Commerce, community directories, surveys, and personal observation and interview. Each community's values are unique, rooted in tradition, and exist to meet the needs of the population (Fig. 34-2) (Anderson & McFarlane, 2004). Religious beliefs and culture are closely related to the community's values.

Healthy communities demonstrate an awareness and respect for different values and religions. There is a deliberate effort among various subgroups to communicate and to work together. Many communities form ministerial alliances, in which various denominations collaborate to meet the needs of the community. They may provide emergency shelters, operate soup kitchens or food pantries, and provide help for special populations. Certain religious beliefs directly affect health practices such as use of family planning services.

Some communities exhibit conflict among subgroups. Different values, beliefs, and practices are seen as a threat to one group's own values and beliefs. An unhealthy community may fail to recognize the existence of cultural or religious differences and believe that all members of the community should conform to one set of values. In such communities, anyone who does not fit the accepted norm is "suspect." Such an atmosphere does not enhance the overall health status of the community, which makes it difficult or even impossible for members to collaborate on problem solving.

Physical Environment

Geographic Boundaries

Identify geographic boundaries of the community. This information may be obtained from the library or local assessor's office.

Boundaries of a community should be clear, uncontested, and accepted by all members.

Boundaries may not always be clearly identified, and communities may not be able to resolve disputes without legal action. One community may seek to annex part of another because of access to certain resources, or a group or neighborhood may attempt to separate legally from the larger community because of ideologic differences, zoning regulations, or other issues. Disagreement about such issues may disrupt delivery of services.

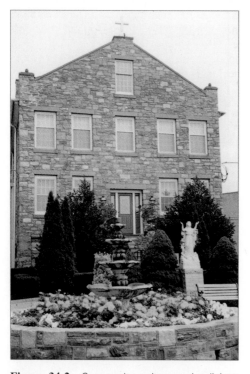

Figure 34-2 Community values and religious beliefs are unique and rooted in tradition.

continued

Assessment Procedure	Normal Findings	Abnormal Findings
Neighborhoods Identify the neighborhood(s) that comprise the area. Note characteristics. Neighborhoods have specific populations and boundaries and may vary a great deal in culture, leadership, and ties to the larger community. They may be composed of certain ethnic groups, economic classes, or age groups.	Neighborhoods should be cohesive with a sense of identity yet have strong ties to the larger community.	Some neighborhoods may seek to isolate themselves from the larger community or may be resistant to others who wish to move into the neighborhood. In such situations, conflicts often arise and mistrust may be widespread.
Housing **Obtain housing information from census documents, local housing authority, and local realtors.** A community should provide a variety of housing options.	A healthy community can provide enough safe, affordable housing to meet the needs of its members. It is estimated that of the 3.5 million people who experience homelessness each year, 1.35 million are children (National Law Center on Homelessness and Poverty, 2007).	A lack of adequate housing may be a serious problem in some communities. A shortage of safe, low-income housing contributes directly to the growing number of homeless individuals and families. Other communities may have a serious shortage of adequate rental property or special housing for the elderly or disabled. Inadequate housing contributes to various health problems related to safety, lead poisoning, and communicable diseases.
Climate and Terrain **Determine climate and geographic terrain of the area.** This information may be obtained from the local library, government agencies, and direct observation. Climate varies from region to region as does geographic terrain. Both have a direct effect on the health of the community.	Healthy communities have the resources to deal with whatever problems climate and terrain present. Such problems include extreme cold or heat, floods, fires, blizzards, tornadoes, and earthquakes. Certain health problems may be more prevalent in particular geographic areas (e.g., West Nile virus, Hanta virus). Safety programs, civil defense and disaster plans, and health education programs should be in place.	Communities inadequately prepared to deal with disasters or health problems related to climate or terrain do not adequately meet the needs of their members. This may result in a higher incidence of the following problems: heat exhaustion, deaths due to overexposure to cold, myocardial infarctions related to shoveling snow, skin cancers, infectious diseases, and deaths and injuries related to other natural disasters.

Health and Social Services

Hospitals, Clinics, Emergency Care, Private Practitioners **Determine the number of health care facilities and providers available to the community.** Information about health services can be obtained from the Chamber of Commerce, local professional organizations, telephone directories, and from personal interviews and observations.	A healthy community provides adequate primary health care services (Fig. 34-3). These services include private and non-profit facilities staffed with physicians, nurse practitioners, and nurses who provide medical/surgical, obstetric/gynecologic, pediatric, emergency, and various diagnostic and preventive services. Specialty services, such as neonatal intensive care, should be easily accessible to the community. In addition to physicians and nurses, the health care delivery system should include dentists,	Many communities (particularly rural ones) cannot provide needed services, especially in obstetric care. It is not unusual for a person to be 100 miles or more away from the nearest services. In addition, funding problems have caused many small rural hospitals to close, leaving residents miles away from any health care at all. Ambulance service also may be of concern for some communities. Accessibility may be limited because fewer health care providers are willing to accept some types of

continued

COMMUNITY ASSESSMENT *Continued*

Assessment Procedure	Normal Findings	Abnormal Findings
	physical therapists, and dietitians among others. Facilities and providers should accept third-party reimbursement including insurance, workers' compensation, Medicare, and Medicaid.	third-party reimbursement, especially Medicaid.
Public Health and Home Health Services **Obtain data concerning public health and home health services.** This information can be obtained from local directories, the Chamber of Commerce, and personal interviews. Local public health agencies have the responsibility for protecting the health of the general population. Program objectives are related to primary prevention and early diagnosis and are directed toward meeting health objectives of the federal program Healthy People 2010. Home health care is a fast growing component of the health care system as hospital stays become briefer while the need for skilled care remains.	Local public health services are usually delivered through county or city health departments. Wellness programs also may be offered through nonofficial agencies such as hospitals. Home health services may be provided through a number of different agencies such as a Visiting Nurses Association (VNA), official agencies, and free-standing proprietary agencies. Services provided include skilled nursing care, homemaker and home health aides, medical social services, nutritional consultation, and rehabilitation services (Fig. 34-4).	Many public health services are supported through local tax revenues. Therefore, small rural communities may not be able to provide the types of services needed, and limited access to these services may be another problem. Certain services may not be offered by home health agencies, and funding to cover visits for people who are not eligible for third-party reimbursement may be limited.
Social Service Agencies **Determine what level of social services is available in the community.** Information may be obtained through local directories, the Chamber of Commerce, or personal interviews.	A community should provide agency social services—both public and voluntary—for people of all ages. Official agencies include mental health facilities and children and family services such as Medicaid, Medicare, and Aid to Families with Dependent Children.	Access to social service agencies may be an obstacle in urban areas. In addition, funding may limit the number of programs and people these agencies serve. Availability of programs may be limited in rural areas. For example, homeless shelters and shelters for

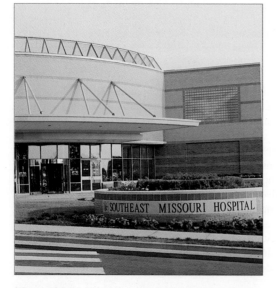

Figure 34-3 Healthy communities have access to adequate primary health care services.

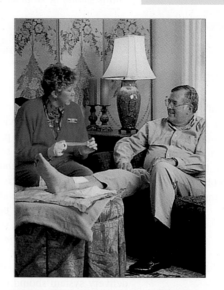

Figure 34-4 Healthy communities have adequate and available home health and skilled nursing care, among other services.

continued

Assessment Procedure	Normal Findings	Abnormal Findings
	Other agencies may be substance abuse treatment facilities, centers for abused women, hospices, and shelters for the homeless. Volunteer agencies (e.g., Meals on Wheels, Salvation Army) also offer community services (Fig. 34-5). Additional social programs may come from groups such as the YMCA and Parents Without Partners. Safe and certified child care facilities for children and the elderly should also be available.	abused women are nonexistent in many rural areas. Lack of transportation in rural areas may also make programs inaccessible. The cost of certain treatment programs can limit accessibility for those who are uninsured.
Long-Term Care Services **Determine if long-term care services are available in the community.** Long-term care services are those that meet the needs of elderly members, those with a chronic disabling illness, and those who have suffered disabilities due to accidents. Information can be obtained from local directories and the Chamber of Commerce.	A community should provide services for long-term care assistance in the home as well as extended care for those who can no longer function in their homes. For example, personal care assistance or a visiting nurse and skilled nursing and intermediate care facilities for those needing certain levels of nursing care should be available. Rehabilitation centers, boarding homes, continuing care, and retirement or assisted living centers are other types of long-term care facilities.	The capacity of available agencies may not meet the needs of a given community. Facilities that provide care for special concerns (e.g., Alzheimer's disease) may not be available in all communities. Facilities in urban areas may be inaccessible because of cost. Rural areas, in general, are likely to have inadequate long-term care resources. This is especially true in areas such as respite care and personal care assistance in the home.
Economics Gather community economic data. This data should include median household income, per capita income, percentage of households or individuals below the poverty level, percentage of people on public assistance, and unemployment statistics. In addition, collect data about local business and industry, types of occupations/jobs in which people are employed, and occupational health risks associated with certain occupations. Data can be collected from census records, Department of Labor, the Chamber of Commerce, and local and state unemployment offices.	Income has a direct relationship to the health of the residents of the community. The income of the members of the community determines its tax base and, therefore, the ability of the community to provide needed services (Clark, 2008) to its members. Businesses and other local employment opportunities are key factors in economic well-being. Businesses provide not only jobs but also goods and services such as groceries, pharmaceuticals, and clothing.	Economic instability in a community can lead to a number of health-related concerns. Poverty is associated with higher morbidity and mortality rates. High unemployment creates a stressful environment and a threat to the psychological well-being of the community. Occupationally related death and injuries cost the nation billions of dollars a year with lung diseases and musculoskeletal injuries being the most frequent causes.

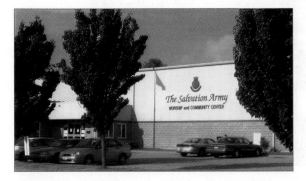

Figure 34-5 The Salvation Army is a voluntary agency that provides full-scale community services.

continued

COMMUNITY ASSESSMENT Continued

Assessment Procedure	Normal Findings	Abnormal Findings

Safety: Fire, Police, Environmental Protection

Gather information regarding fire, police, and environmental services in the community. This information can be obtained from local and regional police departments, fire departments, environmental agencies, and state health departments. Fire, police, and environmental services also are given the responsibility to protect the community from direct and indirect threats to its health and safety (Fig. 34-6). These services have both a direct and an indirect relationship to a community's well-being in knowing that it is safe from a variety of threats.

Police should be equipped with personnel, equipment, and facilities to protect the community. Education programs such as Drug Abuse Resistance Education (DARE); property and personal identification programs; support programs such as Neighborhood Watch; and animal control programs may also be run by the police department. Number of firemen, equipment, response time, and education programs contribute to adequate fire protection services. Environmental protection includes a wide range of programs such as water and air quality, solid and hazardous waste disposal, sewage treatment, food/restaurant inspection, and monitoring of public swimming pools, motels, and other public facilities.

Violent crimes, such as homicide, rape, robbery, and assault or increases in loss of life and property due to fires, may indicate that police and fire protection services are inadequate. This also contributes to a general sense of fear or uneasiness throughout the community and can lead to increased levels of stress and a loss of a sense of well-being. Poor environmental protection can result in repeated cases of illnesses, injuries, and even death. A number of health problems can be linked to the environment (e.g., waterborne illnesses and lead poisonings).

Transportation

Determine transportation options available in the community. Obtain information from local businesses through interviews, from county and state highway departments, and direct observation.

The most common means of transportation in most communities is the private automobile. Other sources of transportation locally, in addition to walking, are taxis, buses, subways, and trains. Long-distance transportation, in addition to the car, includes air, rail, and bus service. Roads, highways, and sidewalks should be kept in good repair, and communities should have adequate programs for snow and ice removal. Special transportation needs include school transportation and

Lack of a private automobile is a particular problem in rural areas where public means of transportation are often nonexistent. Personal safety or cost may make public transportation inaccessible for many in urban areas. Inability to access health care services because of transportation difficulties is a particular problem for the elderly and for mothers with young children (Fig. 34-7).

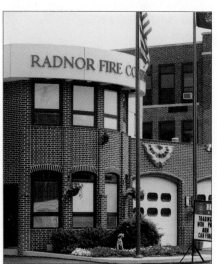

Figure 34-6 Adequate fire and police department protection are hallmarks of healthy communities.

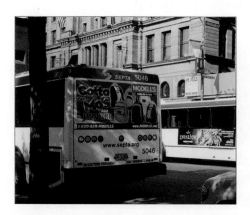

Figure 34-7 Access to transportation has a direct relationship to access to health care and other essential services.

continued

Assessment Procedure	Normal Findings	Abnormal Findings
	transportation for the elderly or disabled people.	

Education

Review levels of education, current school enrollment, and education resources in the community. Information may be obtained from census reports, local school districts, and state education agencies.

In general, the higher the community's education level, the healthier the community. Resources needed to meet community educational needs include preschool and early intervention programs, public or private elementary and secondary schools, and access to advanced education. Adequate supply of qualified educators, up-to-date facilities and equipment, and programs that meet the needs of those with special needs are keys to a successful education system (Fig. 34-8). Low absenteeism and higher-than-average scores on standardized achievement tests are indicators of effectiveness. Adult education, including GED classes, should be available. Additionally comprehensive school health programs directed by nurses, school meal programs, and after-school programs contribute to the health of a community. Public libraries are an important community supplement to the school system.

Funding for school systems is a growing problem for many communities, especially those in areas where the economy is weak. Many school districts are supported in part by property taxes. So in an area where the tax base is low and unemployment is a problem, schools may struggle to maintain even minimum standards. As a result, many districts must cut equipment purchases, special programs, and extracurricular activities such as music and athletics. School violence is a growing problem for many communities. Another indication of problems in the school system is a high dropout rate and a low graduation rate. Availability of post-high school colleges or technical programs may be limited in rural areas. Access may be limited because of a lack of financial resources. Libraries often depend on local taxes. So in times of economic difficulty, these facilities often face cutbacks.

Government and Politics

Review the government and political structures of the community. Information may be obtained from local government agencies, local political organizations, and local directories.

The government of a community and its leaders should be responsible and accessible to the community. Members should participate in the governance of the community as evidenced by voter

If the government is not responsive to the views of the citizens, members of the community will become increasingly apathetic. As a result, the formal power structure becomes ineffective in meeting

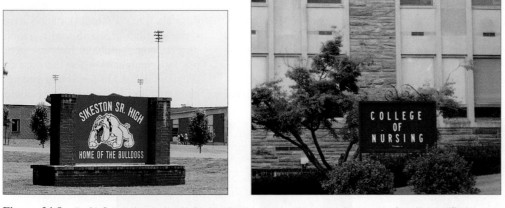

Figure 34-8 (Left) Secondary schools (high schools) need to be up-to-date and safe with qualified staff and programs that meet the needs of students and the community. (Right) Schools at a higher level (community colleges and universities) offer the community significant opportunities for learning and vocational fulfillment.

continued

COMMUNITY ASSESSMENT *Continued*

Assessment Procedure	Normal Findings	Abnormal Findings
Government agencies are often directly involved in planning and implementing programs that affect the health of the community. In addition, the political system is responsible for health-related legislation. It is important to assess both the formal and informal power structures in the community.	registration and percentage of registered voters who actually vote in elections. Open community meetings should be held to allow citizens a forum in which they may express their views. Political organizations should represent the differing views of the citizens; there should be an atmosphere of tolerance among the different groups.	the needs of the community. Low voter turnout and little representation of groups with different views and interests may be indicative of an unresponsive or unrepresentative government.

Communication

Assessment Procedure	Normal Findings	Abnormal Findings
Determine both the formal and informal means of communication in the community. Sources of information include the Chamber of Commerce, telephone book, and personal interviews and observations.	Open channels of communication are an important factor in maintaining the health of a community (Fig. 34-9). Larger communities usually have many types of formal communication sources including local television and radio stations, local cable access, and one or more daily newspapers. Smaller communities usually have access to fewer television and radio stations, and newspapers are typically published weekly. Mail delivery may also be limited. However, online services are usually available in all communities. Informal communications include word of mouth; newsletters; bulletin board notices at community centers, stores, businesses, and churches; and fliers distributed by mail or door-to-door.	Traditional means of communication may not be sufficient for some people in the community. Those who do not speak or understand English may not be able to obtain necessary information through either formal or informal means. Some people may not have access to telephone or other means of communication. Elderly people and others who are isolated also may be at a disadvantage.

Recreation

Assessment Procedure	Normal Findings	Abnormal Findings
Determine availability of community recreation and leisure programs for individuals and groups in all age ranges in the community. Information may be obtained from the Chamber of Commerce, park and recreation departments, churches, schools, businesses, and personal interview.	Schools in the area should have a regular program of physical education in which all students must participate. In addition, schools should provide equipment and programs for extracurricular activities, including both team and individual sports (e.g., tennis, softball), art, music, and foreign language programs, and other types of recreational programs. Churches may provide recreational programs, senior citizen dinners and outings, youth programs, church festivals,	Communities with a poor economic base or those with a large percentage of rural residents may not be able to provide adequate programs for recreation. Finding funds for building and maintaining recreational facilities is difficult: Lack of transportation may seriously limit access. Social isolation may become a problem for these people. In a community where there are no programs available for young people, gang activity and alcohol/drug abuse

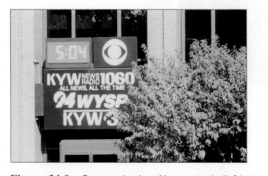
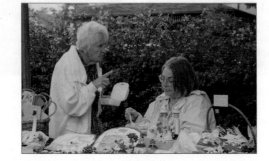

Figure 34-9 Communication: News travels (left) over the airways and (right) by word of mouth.

continued

Assessment Procedure	Normal Findings	Abnormal Findings

and special holiday activities. A comprehensive, community-based program is essential. Indoor or outdoor facilities (e.g., swimming pools, ball fields) should be available to all citizens, easily accessible, and kept in good repair. Organized activities for individuals and groups of all ages, genders, social status, and physical abilities should be available at minimal or no cost (Fig. 34-10).

may develop. In communities where activities such as water sports or snow sports are common, lack of programs related to safety issues could result in serious injury or even death.

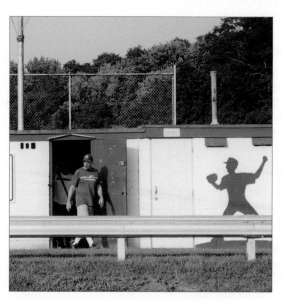
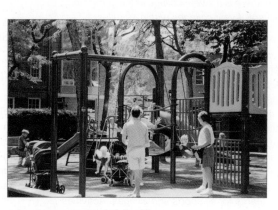

Figure 34-10   Recreational and leisure activities are directly related to a community's health status in that they connect people in the community and provide opportunities to socialize.

VALIDATING AND DOCUMENTING FINDINGS

Validate the community assessment data you have collected. This is necessary to verify that the data are reliable and accurate. Document the assessment data following the health care facility or agency policy.

Sample Documentation of Subjective and Objective Data

The community developed 100 years ago and has grown steadily in economic status and population over the years. There is an even age and gender population distribution. There is a large Hispanic population group in the community (20% Hispanic). Birth, death, and morbidity data reflect the overall rates for the United States. Most households consist of married couples with and without

children. Religious organizations are predominantly Methodist, Catholic, and Jewish; they work closely together to provide services to all community members. Boundaries are clear and uncontested, neighborhoods are cohesive but linked to larger community, and housing needs are met for all community members.

The geographic terrain is mountains and desert, and the climate is hot and dry. The community provides teaching about sun- and heat-related health problems. There is a community hospital that provides medical—surgical, obstetric—gynecologic, and emergency care. A large urban hospital with a trauma unit and specialized programs is 20 miles away, accessible by the community ambulance service. Other health services, such as physical therapy, nutrition consultation, dentistry, and ophthalmology, are available in the community. Most health care facilities accept third-party reimbursement. The public health service is well funded and home health agencies provide extensive services. Most social service needs of the community are through official, nonofficial, and voluntary health services. Some are located 20 miles away in the urban area, but a shuttle is provided for those requiring the services. Long-term care is available in the home and in four skilled nursing and rehabilitation facilities.

The median income of the community is slightly higher than the national average. A variety of local businesses adequately meet the needs of the community. The police, fire, and environmental agencies are adequately staffed and supplied with equipment to provide protection to the community. There is a bus system, a rail station, and a small airport; most people own at least one car. The public school system for the community is well funded; there is an RN school nurse at the elementary, middle, and high schools; therefore, many programs are available for the children and adolescents. In addition, there is a 2-year college in the community and there are several 4-year colleges within 40 miles.

The community government is representative of the views of the people, community meetings occur once a month, and most community members vote regularly. There are several local network affiliate television stations, a variety of radio stations, and a daily newspaper that focuses primarily on community news. The local public school system offers a variety of recreational programs, and the community churches offer activities for people of all ages. Many of the local companies (including the hospital) offer recreation and exercise facilities and sponsor community programs. The community itself offers an extensive recreation program. There are teams for all sports and all ages. Activities are also available at minimal cost to all members of the community. Several clubs and associations in the area offer unique recreational activities such as mountain climbing, a nature club, and a runners' club.

Analysis of Data

After collecting subjective and objective data pertaining to community assessment, identify abnormal findings and clients strengths. Then cluster the data to reveal any significant patterns or abnormalities. These data may then be used to make clinical judgments about the status of the community.

DIAGNOSTIC REASONING: POSSIBLE CONCLUSIONS

Listed are some possible conclusions after a community assessment.

Selected Nursing Diagnoses

After collecting subjective and objective data pertaining to the community, you will need to organize and group the data to reveal any significant patterns of abnormalities. These data will then be used to make clinical judgments (nursing diagnoses: wellness, risk, or actual) about the status of the client. Following is a listing of selected nursing diagnoses that you may identify when analyzing data for this part of the assessment.

Wellness Diagnoses

- Readiness for Enhanced Community Coping
- Health-Seeking Behaviors: initiation of comprehensive wellness program for elderly

Risk Diagnoses

- Risk for Other-Directed Violence related to insufficient police protection
- Risk for Impaired Community Processes related to subgroup of non-English–speaking people
- Risk for Trauma related to high-crime neighborhood

Actual Diagnoses

- Ineffective Community Therapeutic Regimen Management related to the presence of occupational health hazards
- Ineffective Community Therapeutic Regimen Management related to lack of substance abuse treatment programs
- Ineffective Community Coping related to increased unemployment
- Ineffective Community Coping related to inadequate resources for day care
- Fear related to rising incidence of crime
- Social isolation

Selected Collaborative Problems

After grouping the data, certain collaborative problems may emerge. Remember that collaborative problems differ from nursing diagnoses in that they cannot be prevented by nursing interventions. However, medical or other conditions can be detected and monitored by the nurse. In addition, the nurse can use physician- and nurse-prescribed interventions to minimize the complications of these problems. The nurse may also have to refer the client in such situations for further treatment of the problem. Following is a list of collaborative problems that may be identified when assessing the community. These problems are worded as Risk for Complications (or RC) followed by the problem.

- RC: Post-traumatic stress syndrome, community

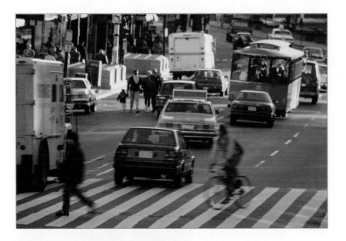

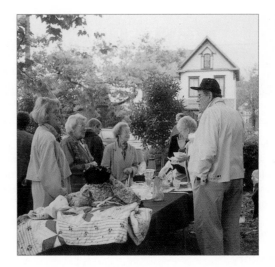

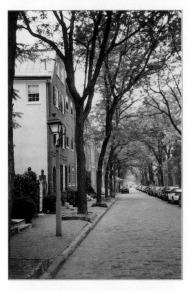

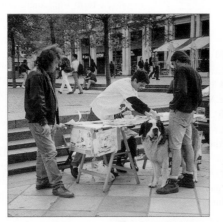

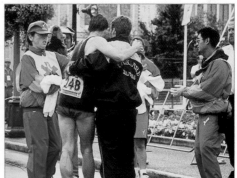

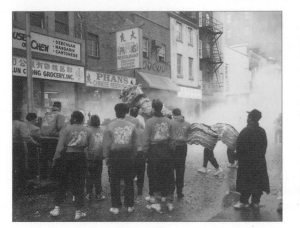

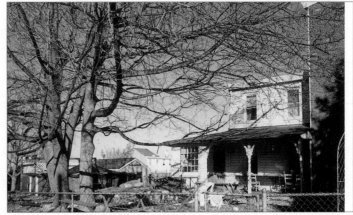

CASE STUDY

The case study demonstrates how to analyze spiritual assessment data for a specific client. The critical thinking exercises included in the study guide/lab manual and interactive product that complement this text also offer opportunities to analyze assessment data.

The following is an abbreviated case study of an assessment of a small town. In actual practice, a thorough assessment of a community would require more in-depth data collection than is described in this vignette. Such assessments may be quite lengthy, which is beyond the scope of this book.

The following concept map illustrates the diagnostic reasoning process.

History
Native American hunters and trappers first inhabited the area in and around Maple Grove. Later German immigrants settled in the region and the lumber/logging industry became the economic base of the community. The town derived its name from the large stands of hardwood trees, especially maples, that grew in the area.

Demographics
The total population for the town of Maple Grove as of the year 2000 was 2352, a decrease of 13.6% from the 1990 census. Of the total number of residents, 56% are female and 26.3% are 65 years of age or older. Racial distribution includes 94.5% white, 3% African American, 1.3% Hispanic, and 1.2% other. Most residents aged 15 years and older are married (65.4%), 10.1% are either separated or divorced, 12.3% are single, and 12.2% are widowed. The leading cause of death in Maple Grove is cardiovascular disease. The German immigrants who originally settled the area brought with them their Lutheran faith and over 80% still practice that religion. There is also a small Baptist congregation in Maple Grove as well as small Methodist and Catholic churches.

Physical Environment
Maple Grove is situated in a very rural area and is bordered on the north by national forest land. The Cache River runs along its western border and an interstate highway lies 2 miles from the city limits on the east. The southern edge of the town is surrounded by farmland. Average temperature in January is 31.2°F, and in June 87.3°F.

Health and Social Services
Maple Grove has no hospital; the nearest is 25 miles away and is an 85-bed, full-service facility. It is the only hospital in the county. A family practice physician and a nurse practitioner have an office in Maple Grove. The office is open 4 days a week. The county health department has a branch office in Maple Grove and offers immunizations, Special Supplemental Nutrition Program for Women, Infants and Children (WIC), sexually transmitted disease (STD) screening, family planning, and environmental services. A local Visiting Nurse Association (VNA) office offers home health services as well as hospice care. The nearest mental health center is approximately 25 miles away as are many other services including county government offices. There is a 50-bed skilled nursing facility in Maple Grove operating at full capacity.

Several residents have expressed their concern about this to the nurse. A committee has been formed to examine ways in which the capacity of the facility could be increased.

Economics
The median household income for Maple Grove is $32,245, which is lower than the national average, and the median per capita income is $17,320, also below the national average. Of the nearly 2,400 people living in Maple Grove, 15.1% live below the poverty level (the national average is 12.7%). The single largest employer in the community is a minimum-security state correctional facility. Other areas of employment include forestry-related occupations, farming, and local businesses such as automobile sales, farm implement sales, grocery, and the like. The unemployment rate is 7.8%, which is higher than the state average.

Safety
Maple Grove maintains a small local police force of five full-time officers, two part-time officers, and one dispatcher/office worker. The community also receives services from the county sheriff's office and the state police. Maple Grove has a fire department with seven part-time firemen and a small group of volunteer firemen. There are no trained emergency medical personnel working with the fire department. The equipment is slightly outdated but still functional. Environmental services are provided through the county health department. The crime rate is relatively low with the incidence of violent crime below the state average.

Transportation
There is no public transportation in Maple Grove except for a small taxi service (one taxicab) and a van supported by the area Agency on Aging, which provides transportation for senior citizens. There is an interstate bus service available on a limited basis. The nearest airport is 70 miles away.

Education
Maple Grove supports an elementary school and a high school with a total of approximately 450 students in kindergarten through twelfth grade. There is no school nurse available. School administrators expressed some concern about this. Although health-related problems are referred to the local health department, schools have difficulty getting the required screenings completed and school immunization records are not up to date. The school principals also are concerned that there is no one available to care for injuries or illness when they occur. The high school provides a limited number of extracurricular activities including boys' and girls' basketball, baseball, softball, and track. The closest junior college is 30 miles away, and the nearest university is 55 miles from Maple Grove. There is a small library open in the afternoons and on Saturday. The community

continued on page 825

residents are proud of their library because it is entirely funded through contributions. They often hold chili suppers, raffles, and other fundraising events to support it.

Politics and Government

Maple Grove has a mayor/city council form of government. The mayor was more than willing to meet with the nurse and invited her to attend the city council meeting on the first Monday of the month. Those members of the community with whom the nurse talked indicated that they felt comfortable with their elected officials and that they were free to voice concerns and opinions at any time. Both the Democratic and Republican parties are active in the town. The number of registered voters who voted in the last election was higher than the state average.

Communication

A radio station is located approximately 25 miles away, and the nearest television station is 50 miles from Maple Grove. The town has cable television service and a post office. A small local newspaper is published weekly.

Recreation

Maple Grove has a small city park equipped with playground equipment, three ball fields, and a picnic shelter. There are softball and baseball leagues for children ages 7 to 18 along with Boy Scout and Girl Scout troops. Other organized recreation activities, such as senior citizen programs, are offered through the churches.

1) Identify abnormal findings and client strengths

Subjective Data

- Expressed concern about insufficient number of long-term care beds
- Expressed concern regarding lack of school nurse
- Members feel comfortable with city government
- Difficulty in meeting requirements for school screenings
- Expressed concern that no one is available to care for injuries or illnesses that occur during school hours

Objective Data

- Maintain a community library through volunteer efforts
- Long-term care facility at full capacity
- Committee formed to increase capacity of long-term care facility
- No school nurse employed by district
- School immunization records not complete
- Median household and per capita income below national average
- Unemployment above state average
- Family practice physician and nurse practitioner available 4 days a week
- No emergency medical technicians available through the fire department

2) Identify cue clusters

- Citizens comfortable with government
- Organized effort to maintain community library
- Committee formed to increase long-term care bed capacity

- No school nurse
- Immunization records not up-to-date
- Physician and nurse practitioner available only 4 days/week
- No EMT with fire department

- Per capita and household income below average
- Unemployment rate above average

3) Draw inferences

Community has open system of communication and has the necessary resources to work together and solve problems

School health program inadequate. Physician and emergency care limited

Community may be facing economic crisis

4) List possible nursing diagnoses

Opportunity to Enhance Community Coping

Ineffective Management of Therapeutic Regimen, Community, r/t lack of school nurse and availability of emergency care

Risk for Ineffective Community Coping r/t low income and high unemployment

5) Check for defining characteristics

Major: Successful coping with previous crisis or problem
Minor: Positive communication
Active problem solving by community

Major: Verbalized difficulty in meeting health needs
Minor: None

Major: None
Minor: None

6) Confirm or rule out diagnoses

Confirm. Meets defining characteristics

Confirm, based on defining characteristics

Confirm. Monitor for changes in ability to meet own needs

7) Document conclusions

Nursing diagnoses that are appropriate for this client include:
- Opportunity to Enhance Community Coping
- Ineffective Management of Therapeutic Regimen, Community, r/t lack of school nurse
- Risk for Ineffective Community Coping r/t low income, high unemployment, and availability of emergency care

References and Selected Readings

Allender, J. A., & Spradley, B. W. (2005). *Community health nursing—promoting and protecting the public's health.* Philadelphia: Lippincott Williams & Wilkins.

Anderson, E., & McFarlane, J. (2004). *Community as partner.* Philadelphia: Lippincott Williams & Wilkins.

Aponte, J., & Nickitas, D. M. (2007). Community as client: Reaching an underserved urban community and meeting unmet primary health care needs. *Journal of Community Health Nursing, 24*(3), 177–190.

Bernal, H., Shellman, J., & Reid, K. (2004). Essential concepts in developing community-university partnerships. Carelink: The partners in caring model. *Public Health Nursing, 21*(1), 32–40.

Centers for Disease Control. (2005). Leading causes of neonatal and postneonatal deaths—United States. *Morbidity and Mortality Weekly Reports, 54*(38), 966.

Clark, M. J. (2008). *Community Health Nursing.* Upper Saddle River, NJ: Pearson/Prentice-Hall.

Cox, C. (2007). Finding community. *American Journal of Health Education, 38*(5), 301–303.

Findholt, N. (2007). Application of the Community Readiness Model for childhood obesity prevention. *Public Health Nursing, 24*(6), 565–70.

Fluhr, J. D., Oman, R. F., Allen, J. R., Lanphier, M. G., & McLeroy, K. R. (2004). A collaborative approach to program evaluation of community-based teen pregnancy prevention projects. *Health Promotion Practice, 5*(2), 127–137.

Huttlinger, K., Schaller-Ayers, J., & Lawson, T. (2004). Health care in Appalachia: A population-based approach. *Public Health Nursing, 21*(2), 103–110.

Livingood, W. C., Goldhagen, J., Bryant, T., Winterbauer, N., & Woodhouse, L. D. (2007). A community-centered model of the academic health department and implications for assessment. *Journal of Public Health Management and Practice, 13*(6), 662–669.

Maurer, F., & Smith, C. (2005). *Community/public health nursing practice.* St. Louis: Elsevier Saunders.

McClellan, C. S. (2005). Utilizing a national performance standards local public health assessment instrument in a community assessment process: The Clarendon County Turning Point Initiative. *Journal of Public Health Management Practice, 11*(5), 428–432.

National Center for Health Statistics. Health, United States, 2007 with Chartbook on Trends in the Health of Americans. Hyattsville, MD: 2007. Available at www.cdc.gov/nchs/hus.htm

National Law Center on Homelessness and Poverty. (January 2007). Homeless in the United States and the human right to housing. Available at www.nationalhomeless.org

Running, A., Martin, K., & Tolle, L. W. (2007). An innovative model for conducting a participatory community health assessment. *Journal of Community Health Nursing 24*(4), 203–213.

Schumacher, P. (2006). Responding to the changing needs of public health assessment in the information age: The evolution of a program. *Journal of Public Health Management and Practice, 12*(2), 109–112.

Truglio-Londrigan, M., & Macali, M. (2005). Partnership model for practice and education. *Journal of the New York State Nurses Association,* Spring/Summer, 20–23.

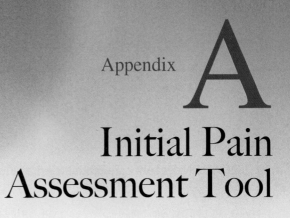

Appendix **A**

Initial Pain
Assessment Tool

Date _____

Patient's name _____ Age _____ Room _____

Diagnosis _____ Physician _____

Nurse _____

1. LOCATION: Patient or nurse marks drawing.

2. INTENSITY: Patient rates the pain. Scale used _____
   Present: _____
   Worst pain gets: _____
   Best pain gets: _____
   Acceptable level of pain: _____

3. QUALITY: (Use patient's own words, e.g., prick, ache, burn, throb, pull, sharp)
   _____

4. ONSET, DURATION, VARIATION, RHYTHMS: _____
   _____

5. MANNER OF EXPRESSING PAIN: _____
6. WHAT RELIEVES THE PAIN? _____
7. WHAT CAUSES OR INCREASES THE PAIN? _____
8. EFFECTS OF PAIN: (Note decreased function, decreased quality of life.)
   Accompanying symptoms (e.g., nausea) _____
   Sleep _____
   Appetite _____
   Physical activity _____
   Relationship with others (e.g., irritability) _____
   Emotions (e.g., anger, suicidal, crying) _____
   Concentration _____
   Other _____

9. OTHER COMMENTS: _____
   _____

10. PLAN: _____
   _____

McCaffery M, Pasero C: Pain: Clinical Manual, St. Louis, Mosby, ed.2, 1999

NANDA-Approved Nursing Diagnoses (2009–2011)

Activity Intolerance

Activity Intolerance, Risk for

Ineffective Activity Planning

Airway Clearance, Ineffective

Allergy Response, Latex

Allergy Response, Risk for Latex

Anxiety

Anxiety, Death

Aspiration, Risk for

Attachment, Risk for Impaired Parent/Child

Autonomic Dysreflexia

Autonomic Dysreflexia, Risk for

Behavior, Risk-Prone Health

Risk for Bleeding

Body Image, Disturbed

Body Temperature, Risk for Imbalanced

Bowel Incontinence

Breastfeeding, Effective

Breastfeeding, Ineffective

Breastfeeding, Interrupted

Breathing Pattern, Ineffective

Cardiac Output, Decreased

Caregiver Role Strain

Caregiver Role Strain, Risk for

Readiness for Enhanced Childbearing Process

Comfort, Readiness for Enhanced

Impaired Comfort

Communication, Impaired Verbal

Communication, Readiness for Enhanced

Conflict, Decisional

Conflict, Parental Role

Confusion, Acute

Confusion, Chronic

Confusion, Risk for Acute

Constipation

Constipation, Perceived

Constipation, Risk for

Contamination

Contamination, Risk for

Coping, Compromised Family

Coping, Defensive

Coping, Disabled Family

Coping, Ineffective

Coping, Ineffective Community

Coping, Readiness for Enhanced

Coping, Readiness for Enhanced Community

Coping, Readiness for Enhanced Family

Death Syndrome, Risk for Sudden Infant

Decision Making, Readiness for Enhanced

Denial, Ineffective

Dentition, Impaired

Development, Risk for Delayed

Diarrhea

Dignity, Risk for Compromised Human

Distress, Moral

Disuse Syndrome, Risk for

Diversional Activity, Deficient

Risk for Disturbed Maternal/Fetal Dyad

Risk for Electrolyte Imbalance

Energy Field, Disturbed

Environmental Interpretation Syndrome, Impaired

Failure to Thrive, Adult

Falls, Risk for

Family Processes, Dysfunctional: Alcoholism

Family Processes, Interrupted

Family Processes, Readiness for Enhanced

Fatigue

Fear

Fluid Balance, Readiness for Enhanced

Fluid Volume, Deficient

Fluid Volume, Excess

Fluid Volume, Risk for Deficient

Fluid Volume, Risk for Imbalanced

Gas Exchange, Impaired

Dysfunctional Gastrointestinal Motility

Risk for Dysfunctional Gastrointestinal Motility

Glucose, Risk for Unstable Blood

Grieving, Anticipatory

Grieving, Complicated

Grieving, Risk for Complicated

Growth and Development, Delayed

Growth, Risk for Disproportionate

Health Maintenance, Ineffective

Ineffective Self Health Maintenance

Home Maintenance, Impaired

Hope, Readiness for Enhanced

Hopelessness

Hyperthermia

Hypothermia

Identity, Disturbed Personal

Immunization Status, Readiness for Enhanced

Incontinence, Functional Urinary

Incontinence, Overflow Urinary

Incontinence, Reflex Urinary

Incontinence, Stress Urinary

Incontinence, Urge Urinary

Incontinence, Risk for Urge Urinary

Infant Behavior, Disorganized

Infant Behavior, Risk for Disorganized

Infant Behavior, Readiness for Enhanced Organized

Infant Feeding Pattern, Ineffective

Infection, Risk for

Injury, Risk for

Injury, Risk for Perioperative-Positioning

Insomnia

Intracranial Adaptive Capacity, Decreased

Knowledge, Deficient (Specify)

Knowledge, Readiness for Enhanced

Lifestyle, Sedentary

Liver Function, Risk for Impaired

Loneliness, Risk for

Memory, Impaired

Mobility, Impaired Bed

Mobility, Impaired Physical

Mobility, Impaired Wheelchair

Nausea

Neglect, Unilateral

Neonatal Jaundice

Noncompliance

Nutrition, Imbalanced: Less Than Body Requirements

Nutrition, Imbalanced: More Than Body Requirements

Nutrition, Readiness for Enhanced

Nutrition, Risk for Imbalanced: More Than Body Requirements

Oral Mucous Membrane, Impaired

Pain, Acute

Pain, Chronic

Parenting, Readiness for Enhanced

Parenting, Impaired

Parenting, Risk for Impaired

Peripheral Neurovascular Dysfunction, Risk for

Poisoning, Risk for

Post-Trauma Syndrome

Post-Trauma Syndrome, Risk for

Power, Readiness for Enhanced

Powerlessness

Powerlessness, Risk for

Protection, Ineffective

Rape-Trauma Syndrome

Readiness for Enhanced Relationship

Religiosity, Impaired

Religiosity, Readiness for Enhanced

Religiosity, Risk for Impaired

Relocation Stress Syndrome

Relocation Stress Syndrome, Risk for

Risk for Compromised Resilience

Readiness for Enhanced Resilience

Impaired Individual Resilience

Role Performance, Ineffective

Self-Care, Readiness for Enhanced

Self-Care Deficit, Bathing/Hygiene

Self-Care Deficit, Dressing/Grooming

Self-Care Deficit, Feeding

Self-Care Deficit, Toileting

Self-Concept, Readiness for Enhanced

Self-Esteem, Chronic Low

Self-Esteem, Situational Low

Self-Esteem, Risk for Situational Low

Readiness for Enhanced Self Health Management

Self-Mutilation

Self-Mutilation, Risk for

Self Neglect

Sensory Perception, Disturbed
   (Specify: Visual, Auditory, Kinesthetic,
   Gustatory, Tactile, Olfactory)

Sexual Dysfunction

Sexuality Pattern, Ineffective

Risk for Shock

Skin Integrity, Impaired

Skin Integrity, Risk for Impaired

Sleep Deprivation

Sleep Pattern, Disturbed

Sleep, Readiness for Enhanced

Social Interaction, Impaired

Social Isolation

Sorrow, Chronic

Spiritual Distress

Spiritual Distress, Risk for

Spiritual Well-Being, Readiness for Enhanced

Stress Overload

Suffocation, Risk for

Suicide, Risk for

Surgical Recovery, Delayed

Swallowing, Impaired

Therapeutic Regimen Management, Ineffective

Therapeutic Regimen Management, Ineffective Family

Therapeutic Regimen Management, Readiness
   for Enhanced

Thermoregulation, Ineffective

Tissue Integrity, Impaired

Tissue Perfusion, Ineffective Cardiac

Tissue Perfusion, Ineffective Peripheral

Transfer Ability, Impaired

Trauma, Risk for

Risk for Vascular Trauma

Urinary Elimination, Impaired

Urinary Elimination, Readiness for Enhanced

Urinary Retention

Ventilation, Impaired Spontaneous

Ventilatory Weaning Response, Dysfunctional

Violence, Risk for Other-Directed

Violence, Risk for Self-Directed

Walking, Impaired

Wandering

NANDA International. (2009). *Nursing diagnoses: Definitions and Classifications 2009–2011.* Philadelphia: NANDA.

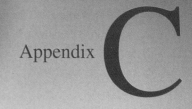
Selected Collaborative Problems*

RISK FOR COMPLICATION: CARDIAC/VASCULAR

RC: Decreased Cardiac Output

RC: Dysrhythmias

RC: Pulmonary Edema

RC: Deep Vein Thrombosis

RC: Hypovolemia

RC: Compartmental Syndrome

RC: Pulmonary Embolism

RISK FOR COMPLICATION: RESPIRATORY

RC: Hypoxemia

RC: Atelectasis, Pneumonia

RC: Tracheobronchial Constriction

RC: Pneumothorax

RISK FOR COMPLICATION: METABOLIC/IMMUNE/HEMATOPOIETIC

RC: Hypo/Hyperglycemia

RC: Negative Nitrogen Balance

RC: Electrolyte Imbalances

RC: Sepsis

RC: Acidosis (Metabolic, Respiratory)

RC: Alkalosis (Metabolic, Respiratory)

RC: Allergic Reaction

RC: Thrombocytopenia

RC: Opportunistic Infections

RC: Sickling Crisis

RISK FOR COMPLICATION: RENAL/URINARY

RC: Acute Urinary Retention

RC: Renal Insufficiency

RC: Renal Calculi

RISK FOR COMPLICATION: NEUROLOGIC/SENSORY

RC: Increased Intracranial Pressure

RC: Seizures

RC: Increased Intraocular Pressure

RC: Neuroleptic Malignant Syndrome

RC: Alcohol Withdrawal

RISK FOR COMPLICATION: GASTROINTESTINAL/HEPATIC/BILIARY

RC: Paralytic Ileus

RC: GI Bleeding

RC: Hepatic Dysfunction

RC: Hyperbilirubinemia

RISK FOR COMPLICATION: MUSCULAR/SKELETAL

RC: Pathologic Fractures

RC: Joint Dislocation

RISK FOR COMPLICATION: REPRODUCTIVE

RC: Prenatal Bleeding

RC: Preterm Labor

RC: Pregnancy-Associated Hypertension

RC: Fetal Distress

RC: Postpartum Hemorrhage

RISK FOR COMPLICATION: MEDICATION THERAPY ADVERSE EFFECTS

RC: Anticoagulant Therapy Adverse Effects

RC: Antianxiety Therapy Adverse Effects

RC: Adrenocorticosteroid Therapy Adverse Effects

RC: Antineoplastic Therapy Adverse Effects

RC: Anticonvulsant Therapy Adverse Effects

RC: Antidepressant Therapy Adverse Effects

RC: Antiarrhythmic Therapy Adverse Effects

RC: Antipsychotic Therapy Adverse Effects

RC: Antihypertensive Therapy Adverse Effects

RC: β-Adrenergic Blocker Therapy Adverse Effects

RC: Calcium Channel Blocker Therapy Adverse Effects

RC: Angiotensin-Converting Enzyme Inhibitor Therapy Adverse Effects

(Carpenito-Moyet, L. J. [2010]. *Nursing diagnosis: Application to clinical practice* [13th ed.]. Philadelphia: Lippincott Williams & Wilkins.)
*Frequently used collaborative problems are represented on this list. Other situations not listed here could qualify as collaborative problems.

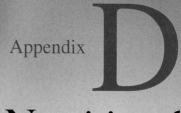

Mini-Nutritional Assessment (MNA)

Nestlé Nutrition INSTITUTE

Mini Nutritional Assessment
MNA®

Last name:	First name:	Sex:	Date:

Age:	Weight, kg:	Height, cm:	I.D. Number:

Complete the screen by filling in the boxes with the appropriate numbers.
Add the numbers for the screen. If score is 11 or less, continue with the assessment to gain a Malnutrition Indicator Score.

Screening

A Has food intake declined over the past 3 months due to loss of appetite, digestive problems, chewing or swallowing difficulties?
0 = severe loss of appetite
1 = moderate loss of appetite
2 = no loss of appetite ☐

B Weight loss during the last 3 months
0 = weight loss greater than 3 kg (6.6 lbs)
1 = does not know
2 = weight loss between 1 and 3 kg (2.2 and 6.6 lbs)
3 = no weight loss ☐

C Mobility
0 = bed or chair bound
1 = able to get out of bed/chair but does not go out
2 = goes out ☐

D Has suffered psychological stress or acute disease in the past 3 months
0 = yes   2 = no ☐

E Neuropsychological problems
0 = severe dementia or depression
1 = mild dementia
2 = no psychological problems ☐

F Body Mass Index (BMI) (weight in kg) / (height in m²)
0 = BMI less than 19
1 = BMI 19 to less than 21
2 = BMI 21 to less than 23
3 = BMI 23 or greater ☐

Screening score (subtotal max. 14 points) ☐ ☐
12 points or greater   Normal – not at risk – no need to complete assessment
11 points or below   Possible malnutrition – continue assessment

Assessment

G Lives independently (not in a nursing home or hospital)
0 = no   1 = yes ☐

H Takes more than 3 prescription drugs per day
0 = yes   1 = no ☐

I Pressure sores or skin ulcers
0 = yes   1 = no ☐

Ref. Vellas B, Villars H, Abellan G, et al. Overview of the MNA® - Its History and Challenges. J Nut Health Aging 2006;10:456-465.
Rubenstein LZ, Harker JO, Salva A, Guigoz Y, Vellas B. Screening for Undernutrition in Geriatric Practice: Developing the Short-Form Mini Nutritional Assessment (MNA-SF). J. Geront 2001;56A: M366-377.
Guigoz Y. The Mini-Nutritional Assessment (MNA®) Review of the Literature - What does it tell us? J Nutr Health Aging 2006; 10:466-487.

For more information : www.mna-elderly.com

J How many full meals does the patient eat daily?
0 = 1 meal
1 = 2 meals
2 = 3 meals ☐

K Selected consumption markers for protein intake
• At least one serving of dairy products (milk, cheese, yogurt) per day   yes ☐   no ☐
• Two or more servings of legumes or eggs per week   yes ☐   no ☐
• Meat, fish or poultry every day   yes ☐   no ☐
0.0 = if 0 or 1 yes
0.5 = if 2 yes
1.0 = if 3 yes ☐.☐

L Consumes two or more servings of fruits or vegetables per day?
0 = no   1 = yes ☐

M How much fluid (water, juice, coffee, tea, milk…) is consumed per day?
0.0 = less than 3 cups
0.5 = 3 to 5 cups
1.0 = more than 5 cups ☐.☐

N Mode of feeding
0 = unable to eat without assistance
1 = self-fed with some difficulty
2 = self-fed without any problem ☐

O Self view of nutritional status
0 = views self as being malnourished
1 = is uncertain of nutritional state
2 = views self as having no nutritional problem ☐

P In comparison with other people of the same age, how does the patient consider his/her health status?
0.0 = not as good
0.5 = does not know
1.0 = as good
2.0 = better ☐.☐

Q Mid-arm circumference (MAC) in cm
0.0 = MAC less than 21
0.5 = MAC 21 to 22
1.0 = MAC 22 or greater ☐.☐

R Calf circumference (CC) in cm
0 = CC less than 31   1 = CC 31 or greater ☐

Assessment (max. 16 points)	☐ ☐.☐
Screening score	☐ ☐
Total Assessment (max. 30 points)	☐ ☐.☐

Malnutrition Indicator Score

17 to 23.5 points   at risk of malnutrition ☐

Less than 17 points   malnourished ☐

Appendix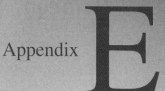

Testicular Self-Examination

Testicular self-examination (TSE) is to be performed once a month; it is neither difficult nor time consuming. A convenient time is often after a warm bath or shower when the scrotum is more relaxed.

1. Stand in front of a mirror and check for scrotal swelling.

2. Use both hands to palpate the testis; the normal testicle is smooth and uniform in consistency.

3. With the index and middle fingers under the testis and the thumb on top, roll the testis gently in a horizontal plane between the thumb and fingers (**A**).

4. Feel for any evidence of a small lump or abnormality.

5. Follow the same procedure and palpate upward along the testis (**B**).

6. Locate the epididymis (**C**), a cordlike structure on the top and back of the testicle that stores and transports sperm.

7. Repeat the examination for the other testis. It is normal to find that one testis is larger than the other.

8. If you find any evidence of a small, pealike lump, consult your physician. It may be due to an infection or a tumor growth.

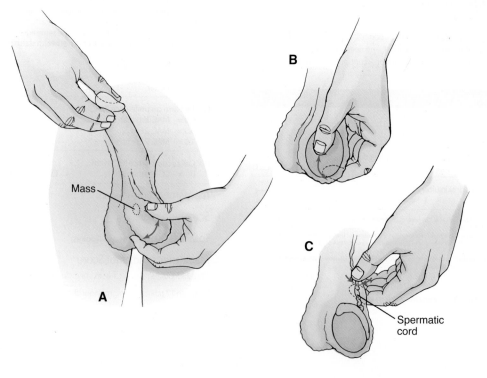

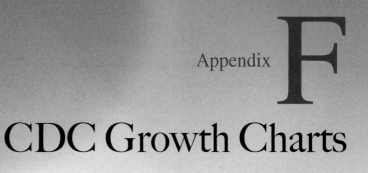

Appendix F

CDC Growth Charts

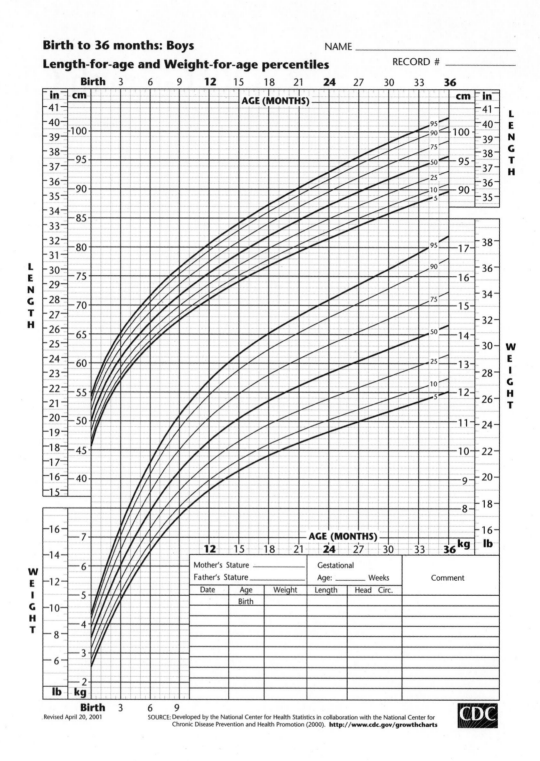

Birth to 36 months: Boys

Length-for-age and Weight-for-age percentiles

NAME _____

RECORD # _____

Revised April 20, 2001

SOURCE: Developed by the National Center for Health Statistics in collaboration with the National Center for Chronic Disease Prevention and Health Promotion (2000). **http://www.cdc.gov/growthcharts**

Birth to 36 months: Boys
Head circumference-for-age and
Weight-for-length percentiles

NAME _____

RECORD # _____

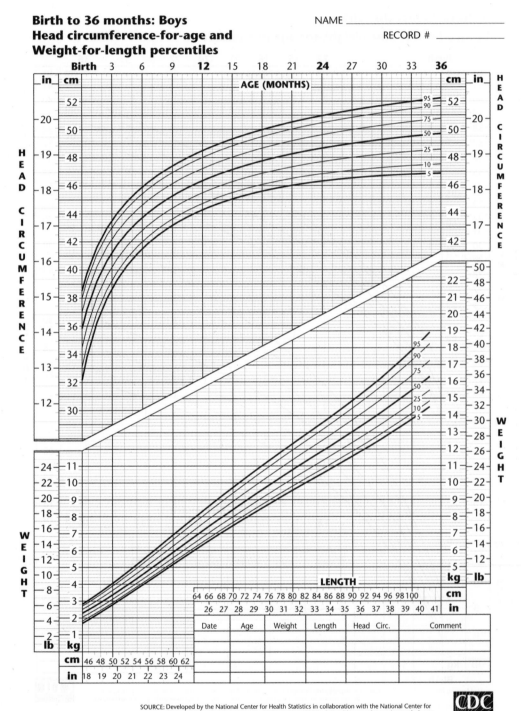

SOURCE: Developed by the National Center for Health Statistics in collaboration with the National Center for Chronic Disease Prevention and Health Promotion (2000). **http://www.cdc.gov/growthcharts**

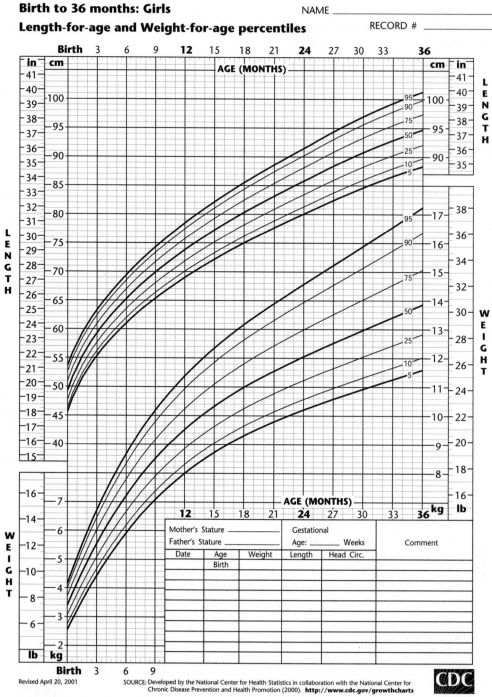

Birth to 36 months: Girls
Length-for-age and Weight-for-age percentiles

NAME _____

RECORD # _____

Revised April 20, 2001

SOURCE: Developed by the National Center for Health Statistics in collaboration with the National Center for Chronic Disease Prevention and Health Promotion (2000). http://www.cdc.gov/growthcharts

Birth to 36 months: Girls
Head circumference-for-age and
Weight-for-length percentiles

NAME _____

RECORD # _____

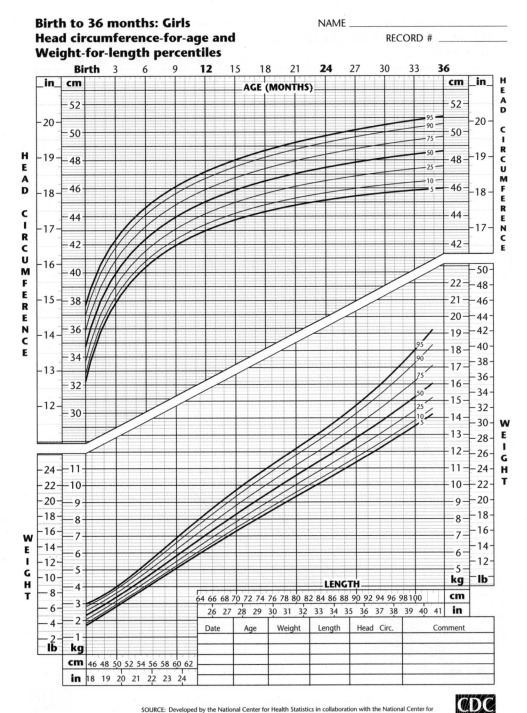

SOURCE: Developed by the National Center for Health Statistics in collaboration with the National Center for Chronic Disease Prevention and Health Promotion (2000). http://www.cdc.gov/growthcharts

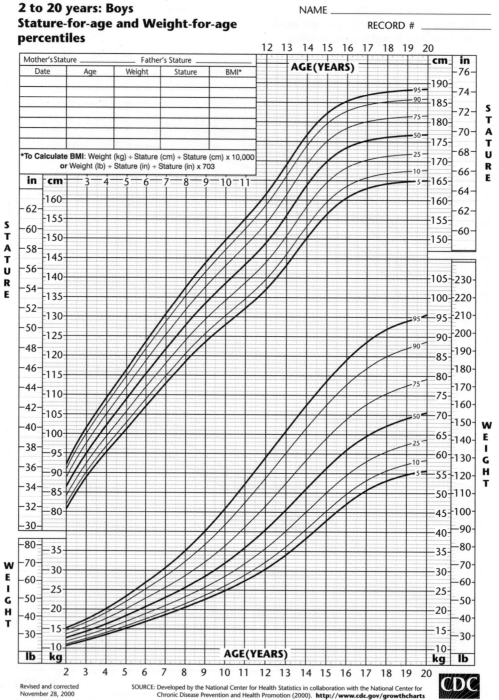

2 to 20 years: Boys
Stature-for-age and Weight-for-age percentiles

NAME _____

RECORD # _____

SOURCE: Developed by the National Center for Health Statistics in collaboration with the National Center for Chronic Disease Prevention and Health Promotion (2000). http://www.cdc.gov/growthcharts

2 to 20 years: Boys
Body mass index-for-age percentiles

NAME _____

RECORD # _____

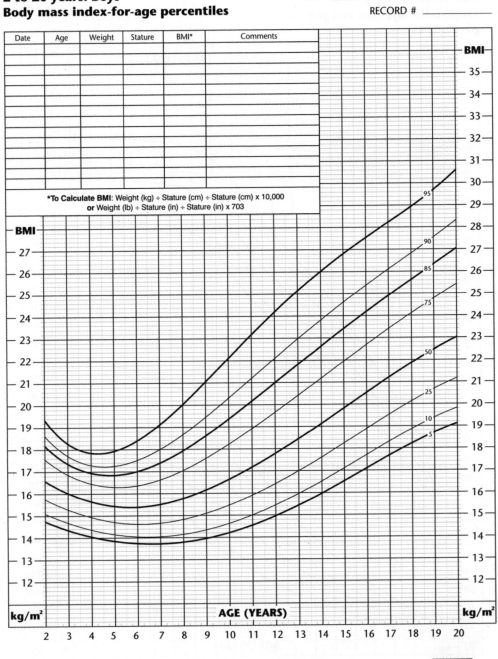

Date	Age	Weight	Stature	BMI*	Comments

*To Calculate BMI: Weight (kg) ÷ Stature (cm) ÷ Stature (cm) x 10,000
or Weight (lb) ÷ Stature (in) ÷ Stature (in) x 703

AGE (YEARS)

SOURCE: Developed by the National Center for Health Statistics in collaboration with the National Center for
Chronic Disease Prevention and Health Promotion (2000). **http://www.cdc.gov/growthcharts**

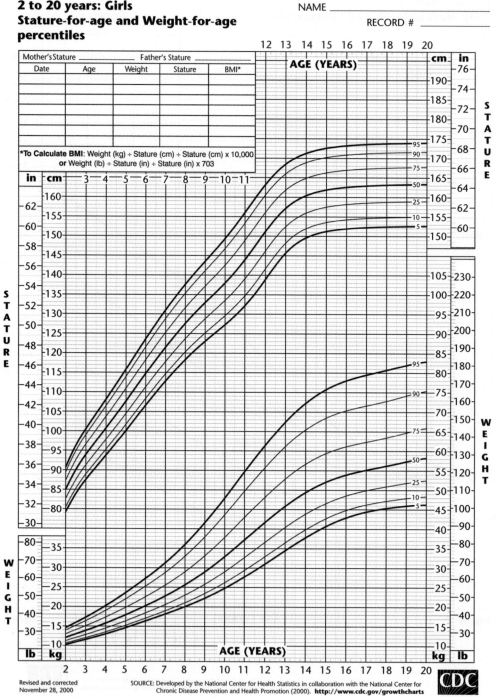

2 to 20 years: Girls
Stature-for-age and Weight-for-age percentiles

NAME _____

RECORD # _____

2 to 20 years: Girls
Body mass index-for-age percentiles

NAME _____

RECORD # _____

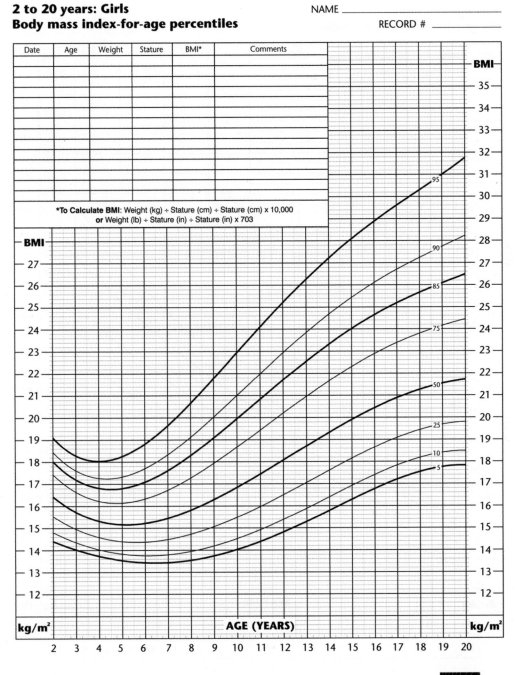

Date	Age	Weight	Stature	BMI*	Comments

*To Calculate BMI: Weight (kg) ÷ Stature (cm) ÷ Stature (cm) x 10,000
or Weight (lb) ÷ Stature (in) ÷ Stature (in) x 703

AGE (YEARS)

kg/m²

SOURCE: Developed by the National Center for Health Statistics in collaboration with the National Center for Chronic Disease Prevention and Health Promotion (2000). http://www.cdc.gov/growthcharts

2 to 5 years: Boys
Weight-for-stature percentiles

NAME _____

RECORD # _____

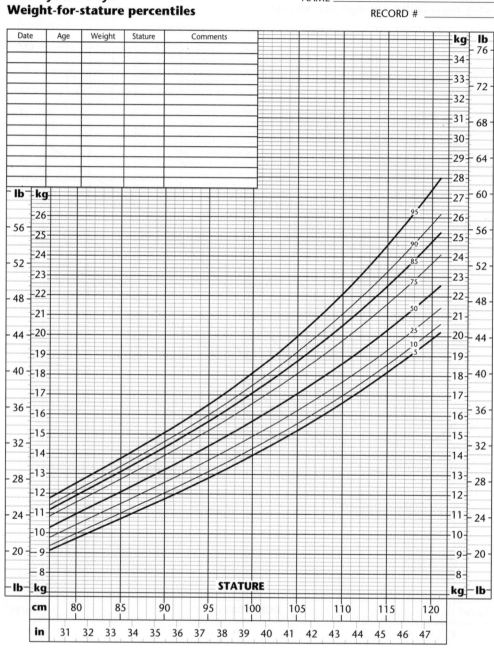

SOURCE: Developed by the National Center for Health Statistics in collaboration with the National Center for
Chronic Disease Prevention and Health Promotion (2000). **http://www.cdc.gov/growthcharts**

CDC

2 to 5 years: Girls
Weight-for-stature percentiles

NAME _____

RECORD # _____

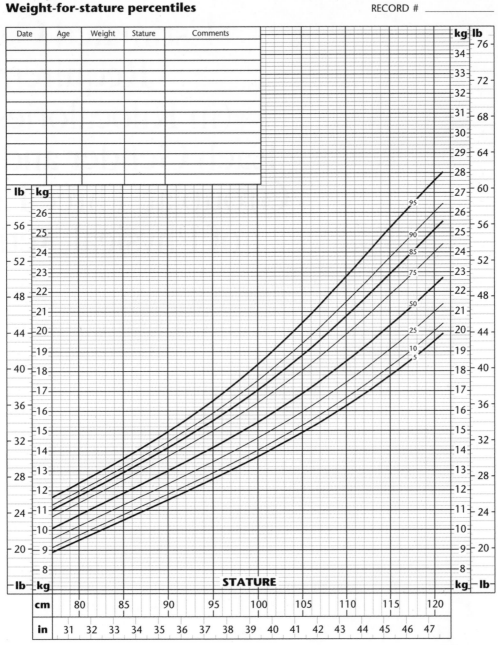

STATURE

SOURCE: Developed by the National Center for Health Statistics in collaboration with the National Center for Chronic Disease Prevention and Health Promotion (2000). http://www.cdc.gov/growthcharts

Appendix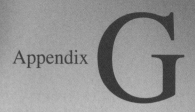

Estimated Calorie Requirements (in Kilocalories) for Each Gender and Age Group at Three Levels of Physical Activity[a]

Estimated amounts of calories needed to maintain energy balance for various gender and age groups at three different levels of physical activity. The estimates are rounded to the nearest 200 calories and were determined using the Institute of Medicine equation.

| Gender | Age (years) | Activity Level[b,c,d] | | |
		Sedentary[b]	Moderately Active[c]	Active[d]
Child	2–3	1,000	1,000–1,400[e]	1,000–1,400[e]
Female	4–8	1,200	1,400–1,600	1,400–1,800
	9–13	1,600	1,600–2,000	1,800–2,200
	14–18	1,800	2,000	2,400
	19–30	2,000	2,000–2,200	2,400
	31–50	1,800	2,000	2,200
	51+	1,600	1,800	2,000–2,200
Male	4–8	1,400	1,400–1,600	1,600–2,000
	9–13	1,800	1,800–2,200	2,000–2,600
	14–18	2,200	2,400–2,800	2,800–3,200
	19–30	2,400	2,600–2,800	3,000
	31–50	2,200	2,400–2,600	2,800–3,000
	51+	2,000	2,200–2,400	2,400–2,800

[a]These levels are based on Estimated Energy Requirements (EER) from the Institute of Medicine Dietary Reference Intakes macronutrients report, 2002, calculated by gender, age, and activity level for reference-sized individuals. "Reference size," as determined by IOM, is based on median height and weight for ages up to age 18 years of age and median height and weight for that height to give a BMI of 21.5 for adult females and 22.5 for adult males.

[b]Sedentary means a lifestyle that includes only the light physical activity associated with typical day-to-day life.

[c]Moderately active means a lifestyle that includes physical activity equivalent to walking about 1.5 to 3 miles per day at 3 to 4 miles per hour, in addition to the light physical activity associated with typical day-to-day life.

[d]Active means a lifestyle that includes physical activity equivalent to walking more than 3 miles per day at 3 to 4 miles per hour, in addition to the light physical activity associated with typical day-to-day life.

[e]The calorie ranges shown are to accommodate needs of different ages within the group. For children and adolescents, more calories are needed at older ages. For adults, fewer calories are needed at older ages.

Reprinted from *Dietary guidelines for Americans, 2005,* United States Departments of Agriculture and Health and Human Services.

Appendix **H**

The Dietary Approaches to Stop Hypertension (DASH) Eating Plan at 1,600-, 2,000-, 2,600-, and 3,100-Calorie Levels[a]

The DASH eating plan is based on 1,600, 2,000, 2,600 and 3,100 calories. The number of daily servings in a food group vary depending on caloric needs (see Table 9-3 to determine caloric needs). This chart can aid in planning menus and food selection in restaurants and grocery stores.

Food Groups	1,600 Calories	2,000 Calories	2,600 Calories	3,100 Calories	Serving Sizes	Examples and Notes	Significance of Each Food Group to the DASH Eating Plan
Grains[b]	6 servings	7–8 servings	10–11 servings	12–13 servings	1 slice bread, 1 oz dry cereal, ½ cup cooked rice, pasta, or cereal[c]	Whole wheat bread, English muffin, pita bread, bagel, cereals, grits, oatmeal, crackers, unsalted pretzels, and popcorn	Major sources of energy and fiber
Vegetables	3–4 servings	4–5 servings	5–6 servings	6 servings	1 cup raw leafy vegetable ½ cup cooked vegetable 6 oz vegetable juice	Tomatoes, potatoes, carrots, green peas, squash, broccoli, turnip greens, collards, kale, spinach, artichokes, green beans, lima beans, sweetpotatoes	Rich sources of potassium, magnesium, and fiber

continued

The Dietary Approaches to Stop Hypertension (DASH) Eating Plan at 1,600-, 2,000-, 2,600-, and 3,100-Calorie Levels[a] Continued

Food Groups	1,600 Calories	2,000 Calories	2,600 Calories	3,100 Calories	Serving Sizes	Examples and Notes	Significance of Each Food Group to the DASH Eating Plan
Fruits	4 servings	4–5 servings	5–6 servings	6 servings	6 oz fruit juice 1 medium fruit ¼ cup dried fruit ½ cup fresh, frozen, or canned fruit	Apricots, bananas, dates, grapes, oranges, orange juice, grapefruit, grapefruit juice, mangoes, melons, peaches, pineapples, prunes, raisins, strawberries, tangerines	Important sources of potassium, magnesium, and fiber
Low-fat or fat-free dairy foods	2–3 servings	2–3 servings	3 servings	3–4 servings	8 oz milk 1 cup yogurt 1½ oz cheese	Fat-free or low-fat milk, fat-free or low-fat buttermilk, fat-free or low-fat regular or frozen yogurt, low-fat and fat-free cheese	Major sources of calcium and protein
Meat, poultry, fish	1–2 servings	2 or less servings	2 servings	2–3 servings	3 oz cooked meats, poultry, or fish	Select only lean; trim away visible fats; broil, roast, or boil instead of frying; remove skin from poultry	Rich sources of protein and magnesium
Nuts, seeds, legumes	3–4 servings	4–5 servings	1 serving	1 serving	⅓ cup or 1½ oz nuts 2 Tbsp or ½ oz seeds ½ cup cooked dry beans or peas	Almonds, filberts, mixed nuts, peanuts, walnuts, sunflower seeds, kidney beans, lentils	Rich sources of energy, magnesium, potassium, protein, and fiber
Fat and oils[d]	2 servings/week	2–3 servings/week	3 servings	4 servings	1 tsp soft margarine 1 Tbsp low-fat mayonnaise 2 Tbsp light salad dressing	Soft margarine, low-fat mayonnaise, light salad dressing, vegetable oil (such as olive, corn, canola, or safflower)	DASH has 27 percent of calories as fat (low in saturated fat), including fat in or added to foods
Sweets	0 servings	5 servings/week	2 servings	2 servings	1 tsp vegetable oil 1 Tbsp sugar 1 Tbsp jelly or jam ½ oz jelly beans 8 oz lemonade	Maple syrup, sugar, jelly, jam, fruit-flavored gelatin, jelly beans, hard candy, fruit punch sorbet, ices	Sweets should be low in fat

[a]NIH publication No. 03-4082; Karanja NM et al. *JADA* 8:519–27, 1999.

[b]Whole grains are recommended for most servings to meet fiber recommendations.

[c]Equals ½–1¼ cups, depending on cereal type. Check the product's Nutrition Facts Label.

[d]Fat content changes serving counts for fats and oils: For example, 1 Tbsp of regular salad dressing equals 1 serving; 1 Tbsp of a low-fat dressing equals ½ serving; 1 Tbsp of a fat-free dressing equals 0 servings.

Reprinted from *Dietary Guidelines for Americans, 2005,* United States Departments of Agriculture and Health and Human Services.

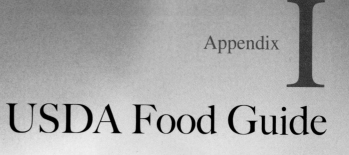

Appendix I

USDA Food Guide

The suggested amounts of food to consume from the basic food groups, subgroups, and oils to meet recommended nutrient intakes at 12 different calorie levels. Nutrient and energy contributions from each group are calculated according to the nutrient-dense forms of foods in each group (e.g., lean meats and fat-free milk). The table also shows the discretionary calorie allowance that can be accommodated within each calorie level, in addition to the suggested amounts of nutrient-dense forms of foods in each group.

Daily Amount of Food From Each Group (vegetable subgroup amounts are per week)

Calorie Level	1,000	1,200	1,400	1,600	1,800	2,000	2,200	2,400	2,600	2,800	3,000	3,200
Food Group[1]	Food group amounts shown in cup (c) or ounce-equivalents (oz-eq), with number of servings (srv) in parentheses when it differs from the other units. See note for quantity equivalents for foods in each group.[2] Oils are shown in grams (g).											
Fruits	1 c (2 srv)	1 c (2 srv)	1.5 c (3 srv)	1.5 c (3 srv)	1.5 c (3 srv)	2 c (4 srv)	2 c (4 srv)	2 c (4 srv)	2 c (4 srv)	2.5 c (5 srv)	2.5 c (5 srv)	2.5 c (5 srv)
Vegetables[3]	1 c (2 srv)	1.5 c (3 srv)	1.5 c (3 srv)	2 c (4 srv)	2.5 c (5 srv)	2.5 c (5 srv)	3 c (6 srv)	3 c (6 srv)	3.5 c (7 srv)	3.5 c (7 srv)	4 c (8 srv)	4 c (8 srv)
Dark green veg.	1 c/wk	1.5 c/wk	1.5 c/wk	2 c/wk	3 c/wk	3 c/wk	3 c/wk	3 c/wk	3 c/wk	3 c/wk	3 c/wk	3 c/wk
Orange veg.	.5 c/wk	1 c/wk	1 c/wk	1.5 c/wk	2 c/wk	2 c/wk	2 c/wk	2 c/wk	2.5 c/wk	2.5 c/wk	2.5 c/wk	2.5 c/wk
Legumes	.5 c/wk	1 c/wk	1 c/wk	2.5 c/wk	3 c/wk	3 c/wk	3 c/wk	3 c/wk	3.5 c/wk	3.5 c/wk	3.5 c/wk	3.5 c/wk
Starchy veg.	1.5 c/wk	2.5 c/wk	2.5 c/wk	2.5 c/wk	3 c/wk	3 c/wk	6 c/wk	6 c/wk	7 c/wk	7 c/wk	9 c/wk	9 c/wk
Other veg.	4 c/wk	4.5 c/wk	4.5 c/wk	5.5 c/wk	6.5 c/wk	6.5 c/wk	7 c/wk	7 c/wk	8.5 c/wk	8.5 c/wk	10 c/wk	10 c/wk
Grains[4]	3 oz-eq	4 oz-eq	5 oz-eq	5 oz-eq	6 oz-eq	6 oz-eq	7 oz-eq	8 oz-eq	9 oz-eq	10 oz-eq	10 oz-eq	10 oz-eq
Whole grains	1.5	2	2.5	3	3	3	3.5	4	4.5	5	5	5
Other grains	1.5	2	2.5	2	3	3	3.5	4	4.5	5	5	5
Lean meat and beans	2 oz-eq	3 oz-eq	4 oz-eq	5 oz-eq	5 oz-eq	5.5 oz-eq	6 oz-eq	6.5 oz-eq	6.5 oz-eq	7 oz-eq	7 oz-eq	7 oz-eq
Milk	2 c	2 c	2 c	3 c	3 c	3 c	3 c	3 c	3 c	3 c	3 c	3 c
Oils[5]	15 g	17 g	17 g	22 g	24 g	27 g	29 g	31 g	34 g	36 g	44 g	51 g
Discretionary calorie allowance[6]	165	171	171	132	195	267	290	362	410	426	512	648

[1]Food items included in each group and subgroup:

Fruits All fresh, frozen, canned, and dried fruits and fruit juices: for example, oranges and orange juice, apples and apple juice, bananas, grapes, melons, berries, raisins. In developing the food patterns, only fruits and juices with no added sugars or fats were used. *See note 6 on discretionary calories if products with added sugars or fats are consumed.*

Vegetables In developing the food patterns, only vegetables with no added fats or sugars were used. *See note 6 on discretionary calories if products with added fats or sugars are consumed.*
- **Dark green vegetables** All fresh, frozen, and canned dark green vegetables, cooked or raw: for example, broccoli; spinach; romaine; collard, turnip, and mustard greens.
- **Orange vegetables** All fresh, frozen, canned orange and deep yellow vegetables, cooked or raw: for example, carrots, sweetpotatoes, winter squash, and pumpkin.
- **Legumes (dry beans and peas)** All cooked dry beans and peas and soybean products: for example, pinto beans, kidney beans, lentils, chickpeas, tofu. (See comment under meat and beans group about counting legumes in the vegetable or the meat and beans group.)
- **Starchy vegetables** All fresh, frozen, and canned starchy vegetables: for example, white potatoes, corn, green peas.
- **Other vegetables** All fresh, frozen, and canned other vegetables, cooked or raw: for example, tomatoes, tomato juice, lettuce, green beans, onions.

Grains In developing the food patterns, only grains in low-fat and low-sugar forms were used. *See note 6 on discretionary calories if products that are higher in fat and/or added sugars are consumed.*
- **Whole grains** All whole-grain products and whole grains used as ingredients: for example, whole-wheat and rye breads, whole-grain cereals and crackers, oatmeal, and brown rice.
- **Other grains** All refined grain products and refined grains used as ingredients: for example, white breads, enriched grain cereals and crackers, enriched pasta, white rice.

USDA Food Guide Continued

Meat, poultry, fish, dry beans, eggs, and nuts (meat & beans)

All meat, poultry, fish, dry beans and peas, eggs, nuts, seeds. Most choices should be lean or low-fat. *See note 6 on discretionary calories if higher fat products are consumed.* Dry beans and peas and soybean products are considered part of this group as well as the vegetable group, but should be counted in one group only.

Milk, yogurt, and cheese (milk)

All milks, yogurts, frozen yogurts, dairy desserts, cheeses (except cream cheese), including lactose-free and lactose-reduced products. Most choices should be fat-free or low-fat. In developing the food patterns, only fat-free milk was used. *See note 6 on discretionary calories if low-fat, reduced-fat, or whole milk or milk products—or milk products that contain added sugars are consumed.* Calcium-fortified soy beverages are an option for those who want a non-dairy calcium source.

²Quantity equivalents for each food group:

Grains

The following each count as 1 ounce-equivalent (1 serving) of grains: ½ cup cooked rice, pasta, or cooked cereal; 1 ounce dry pasta or rice; 1 slice bread; 1 small muffin (1 oz); 1 cup ready-to-eat cereal flakes.

Fruits and vegetables

The following each count as 1 cup (2 servings) of fruits or vegetables: 1 cup cut-up raw or cooked fruit or vegetable, 1 cup fruit or vegetable juice, 2 cups leafy salad greens.

Meat and beans

The following each count as 1 ounce-equivalent: 1 ounce lean meat, poultry, or fish; 1 egg; ¼ cup cooked dry beans or tofu; 1 Tbsp peanut butter; ½ ounce nuts or seeds.

Milk

The following each count as 1 cup (1 serving) of milk: 1 cup milk or yogurt, 1½ ounces natural cheese such as Cheddar cheese or 2 ounces processed cheese. Discretionary calories must be counted for all choices, except fat-free milk.

³Explanation of vegetable subgroup amounts: Vegetable subgroup amounts are shown in this table as weekly amounts, because it would be difficult for consumers to select foods from each subgroup daily. A daily amount that is one-seventh of the weekly amount listed is used in calculations of nutrient and energy levels in each pattern.

⁴Explanation of grain subgroup amounts: The whole grain subgroup amounts shown in this table represent at least three 1-ounce servings and one-half of the total amount as whole grains for all calorie levels of 1,600 and above. This is the minimum suggested amount of whole grains to consume as part of the food patterns. More whole grains up to all of the grains recommended may be selected, with offsetting decreases in the amounts of other (enriched) grains. In patterns designed for younger children (1,000, 1,200, and 1,400 calories), one-half of the total amount of grains is shown as whole grains.

⁵Explanation of oils: Oils (including soft margarine with zero *trans* fat) shown in this table represent the amounts that are added to foods during processing, cooking, or at the table. Oils and soft margarines include vegetable oils and soft vegetable oil table spreads that have no *trans* fats. The amounts of oils listed in this table are not considered to be part of discretionary calories because they are a major source of the vitamin E and polyunsaturated fatty acids, including the essential fatty acids, in the food pattern. In contrast, solid fats are listed separately in the discretionary calorie table (appendix A-3). Oils, they are higher in saturated fatty acids and lower in vitamin E and polyunsaturated and monounsaturated fatty acids, including essential fatty acids. The amounts of each type of fat in the food intake pattern were based on 60% oils and/or soft margarines with no *trans* fats and 40% solid fat. The amounts in typical American diets are about 42% oils or soft margarines and about 58% solid fats.

⁶Explanation of discretionary calorie allowance: The discretionary calorie allowance is the remaining amount of calories in each food pattern after selecting the specified number of nutrient-dense forms of foods in each food group. The number of discretionary calories assumes that food items in each food group are selected in nutrient-dense forms (that is, forms that are fat-free or low-fat and that contain no added sugars). Solid fat and sugar calories always need to be counted as discretionary calories, as in the following examples:

• The fat in low-fat, reduced fat, or whole milk or milk products or cheese and the sugar and fat in chocolate milk, ice cream, pudding, etc.
• The fat in higher fat meats (e.g., ground beef with more than 5% fat by weight, poultry with skin, higher fat luncheon meats, sausages)
• The sugars added to fruits and fruit juices with added sugars or fruits canned in syrup
• The added fat and/or sugars in vegetables prepared with added fat or sugars
• The added fats and/or sugars in grain products containing higher levels of fats and/or sugars (e.g., sweetened cereals, higher fat crackers, pies and other pastries, cakes, cookies)

Total discretionary calories should be limited to the amounts shown in the table at each calorie level. The number of discretionary calories is lower in the 1,600-calorie pattern than in the 1,000-, 1,200-, and 1,400-calorie patterns. These lower calorie patterns are designed to meet the nutrient needs of children 2 to 8 years old. The nutrient goals for the 1,600-calorie pattern are set to meet the needs of adult women, which are higher and require that more calories be used in selections from the basic food groups. Additional information about discretionary calories, including an example of the division of these calories between solid fats and added sugars, is provided in appendix A-3.

Reprinted from *Dietary Guidelines for Americans, 2005*, United States Departments of Agriculture and Health and Human Services.

Appendix **J**

Canada's Food Guide

Health Canada · Santé Canada
Your health and safety... our priority.
Votre santé et votre sécurité... notre priorité.

Eating Well with Canada's Food Guide

Canada

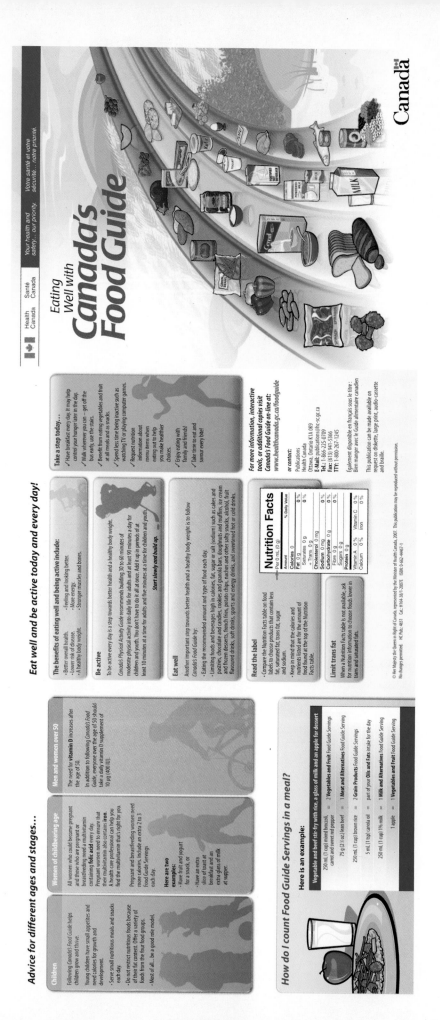

Advice for different ages and stages...

Children

Following *Canada's Food Guide* helps children grow and thrive.

Young children have small appetites and need calories for growth and development.

- Serve small nutritious meals and snacks each day.
- Do not restrict nutritious foods because of their fat content. Offer a variety of foods from the four food groups.
- Most of all... be a good role model.

Women of childbearing age

All women who could become pregnant and those who are pregnant or breastfeeding need a multivitamin containing **folic acid** every day.

Pregnant women need to ensure that their multivitamin also contains **iron**.

A health care professional can help you find the multivitamin that's right for you.

Pregnant and breastfeeding women need more calories. Include an extra 2 to 3 Food Guide Servings each day.

Here are two examples:
- Have fruit and yogurt for a snack, or
- Have an extra slice of toast at breakfast and an extra glass of milk at supper.

Men and women over 50

The need for **vitamin D** increases after the age of 50.

In addition to following *Canada's Food Guide*, everyone over the age of 50 should take a daily vitamin D supplement of 10 µg (400 IU).

How do I count Food Guide Servings in a meal?

Here is an example:

Vegetable and beef stir-fry with rice, a glass of milk and an apple for dessert

250 mL (1 cup) mixed broccoli, carrot and sweet red pepper	= 2 **Vegetables and Fruit** Food Guide Servings
75 g (2½ oz.) lean beef	= 1 **Meat and Alternatives** Food Guide Serving
250 mL (1 cup) brown rice	= 2 **Grain Products** Food Guide Servings
5 mL (1 tsp) canola oil	= part of your **Oils and Fats** intake for the day
250 mL (1 cup) 1% milk	= 1 **Milk and Alternatives** Food Guide Serving
1 apple	= 1 **Vegetables and Fruit** Food Guide Serving

Eat well and be active today and every day!

The benefits of eating well and being active include:

- Better overall health.
- Lower risk of disease.
- A healthy body weight.
- Feeling and looking better.
- More energy.
- Stronger muscles and bones.

Be active

To be active every day is a step towards better health and a healthy body weight.

Canada's Physical Activity Guide recommends building 30 to 60 minutes of moderate physical activity into daily life for adults and at least 90 minutes a day for children and youth. You don't have to do it all at once. Add it up in periods of at least 10 minutes at a time for adults and five minutes at a time for children and youth.

Start slowly and build up.

Eat well

Another important step towards better health and a healthy body weight is to follow *Canada's Food Guide* by:

- Eating the recommended amount and type of food each day.
- Limiting foods and beverages high in calories, fat, sugar or salt (sodium) such as cakes and pastries, chocolate and candies, cookies and granola bars, doughnuts and muffins, ice cream and frozen desserts, french fries, potato chips, nachos and other salty snacks, alcohol, fruit flavoured drinks, soft drinks, sports and energy drinks, and sweetened hot or cold drinks.

Read the label

- Compare the Nutrition Facts table on food labels to choose products that contain less fat, saturated fat, trans fat, sugar and sodium.
- Keep in mind that the calories and nutrients listed are for the amount of food found at the top of the Nutrition Facts table.

Limit trans fat

When a Nutrition Facts table is not available, ask for nutrition information to choose foods lower in trans and saturated fats.

Nutrition Facts
Per 0 mL (0 g)

Amount	% Daily Value
Calories 0	
Fat 0 g	0 %
Saturates 0 g	0 %
+ Trans 0 g	0 %
Cholesterol 0 mg	0 %
Sodium 0 mg	0 %
Carbohydrate 0 g	0 %
Fibre 0 g	0 %
Sugars 0 g	
Protein 0 g	
Vitamin A 0 %	Vitamin C 0 %
Calcium 0 %	Iron 0 %

Take a step today...

- Have breakfast every day. It may help control your hunger later in the day.
- Walk wherever you can — get off the bus early, use the stairs.
- Benefit from eating vegetables and fruit at all meals and as snacks.
- Spend less time being inactive such as watching TV or playing computer games.
- Request nutrition information about menu items when eating out to help you make healthier choices.
- Enjoy eating with family and friends!
- Take time to eat and savour every bite!

For more information, interactive tools, or additional copies visit *Canada's Food Guide* on-line at: www.healthcanada.gc.ca/foodguide

or contact:
Publications
Health Canada
Ottawa, Ontario K1A 0K9
E-Mail: publications@hc-sc.gc.ca
Tel.: 1-866-225-0709
Fax: (613) 941-5366
TTY: 1-800-267-1245

Également disponible en français sous le titre : Bien manger avec le Guide alimentaire canadien

This publication can be made available on request on diskette, large print, audio-cassette and braille.

Recommended Number of Food Guide Servings per Day

Age in Years	Children			Teens		Adults			
	2-3	4-8	9-13	14-18		19-50		51+	
Sex	Girls and Boys			Females	Males	Females	Males	Females	Males
Vegetables and Fruit	4	5	6	7	8	7-8	8-10	7	7
Grain Products	3	4	6	6	7	6-7	8	6	7
Milk and Alternatives	2	2	3-4	3-4	3-4	2	2	3	3
Meat and Alternatives	1	1	1-2	2	3	2	3	2	3

The chart above shows how many Food Guide Servings you need from each of the four food groups every day.

Having the amount and type of food recommended and following the tips in *Canada's Food Guide* will help:

- Meet your needs for vitamins, minerals and other nutrients.
- Reduce your risk of obesity, type 2 diabetes, heart disease, certain types of cancer and osteoporosis.
- Contribute to your overall health and vitality.

What is One Food Guide Serving?
Look at the examples below.

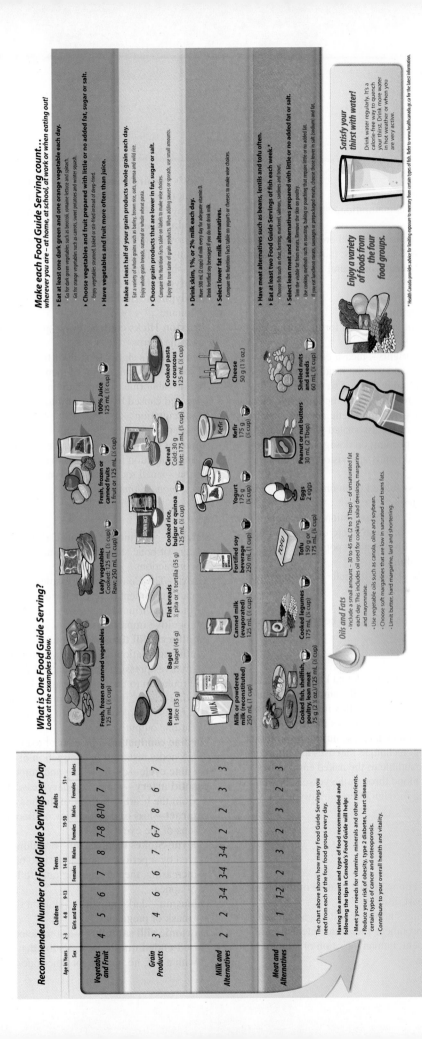

Vegetables and Fruit

Fresh, frozen or canned vegetables
125 mL (½ cup)

Leafy vegetables
Cooked: 125 mL (½ cup)
Raw: 250 mL (1 cup)

Fresh, frozen or canned fruits
1 fruit or 125 mL (½ cup)

100% Juice
125 mL (½ cup)

Grain Products

Bread
1 slice (35 g)

Bagel
½ bagel (45 g)

Flat breads
½ pita or ½ tortilla (35 g)

Cooked rice, bulgur or quinoa
125 mL (½ cup)

Cereal
Cold: 30 g
Hot: 175 mL (¾ cup)

Cooked pasta or couscous
125 mL (½ cup)

Milk and Alternatives

Milk or powdered milk (reconstituted)
250 mL (1 cup)

Canned milk (evaporated)
125 mL (½ cup)

Fortified soy beverage
250 mL (1 cup)

Yogurt
175 g (¾ cup)

Kefir
175 g (¾ cup)

Cheese
50 g (1 ½ oz.)

Meat and Alternatives

Cooked fish, shellfish, lean meat, poultry, lean meat
75 g (2 ½ oz.)/125 mL (½ cup)

Cooked legumes
175 mL (¾ cup)

Tofu
150 g or 175 mL (¾ cup)

Eggs
2 eggs

Peanut or nut butters
30 mL (2 Tbsp)

Shelled nuts and seeds
60 mL (¼ cup)

Make each Food Guide Serving count...
wherever you are – at home, at work or when eating out!

Vegetables and Fruit

▸ Eat at least one dark green and one orange vegetable each day.
- Go for dark green vegetables such as broccoli, romaine lettuce and spinach.
- Go for orange vegetables such as carrots, sweet potatoes and winter squash.
▸ **Choose vegetables and fruit prepared with little or no added fat, sugar or salt.**
- Enjoy vegetables steamed, baked or stir-fried instead of deep-fried.
▸ **Have vegetables and fruit more often than juice.**

Grain Products

▸ **Make at least half of your grain products whole grain each day.**
- Eat a variety of whole grains such as barley, brown rice, oats, quinoa and wild rice.
- Enjoy whole grain breads, oatmeal or whole wheat pasta.
▸ **Choose grain products that are lower in fat, sugar or salt.**
- Compare the Nutrition Facts table on labels to make wise choices.
- Enjoy the true taste of grain products. When adding sauces or spreads, use small amounts.

Milk and Alternatives

▸ **Drink skim, 1%, or 2% milk each day.**
- Have 500 mL (2 cups) of milk every day for adequate vitamin D.
- Drink fortified soy beverages if you do not drink milk.
▸ **Select lower fat milk alternatives.**
- Compare the Nutrition Facts table on yogurts or cheeses to make wiser choices.

Meat and Alternatives

▸ **Have meat alternatives such as beans, lentils and tofu often.**
▸ **Eat at least two Food Guide Servings of fish each week.***
- Choose fish such as char, herring, mackerel, salmon, sardines and trout.
▸ **Select lean meat and alternatives prepared with little or no added fat or salt.**
- Trim the visible fat from meats. Remove the skin on poultry.
- Use cooking methods such as roasting, baking or poaching that require little or no added fat.
- If you eat luncheon meats, sausages or prepackaged meats, choose those lower in salt (sodium) and fat.

Oils and Fats
- Include a small amount – 30 to 45 mL (2 to 3 Tbsp) – of unsaturated fat each day. This includes oil used for cooking, salad dressings, margarine and mayonnaise.
- Use vegetable oils such as canola, olive and soybean.
- Choose soft margarines that are low in saturated and trans fats.
- Limit butter, hard margarine, lard and shortening.

Enjoy a variety of foods from the four food groups.

Satisfy your thirst with water!
Drink water regularly. It's a calorie-free way to quench your thirst. Drink more water in hot weather or when you are very active.

* Health Canada provides advice for limiting exposure to mercury from certain types of fish. Refer to www.health.canada.gc.ca for the latest information.

Glossary

A

ADLs—activities of daily living

adrenarche—adrenocortical maturation, which occurs during puberty

adventitious breath sounds—abnormal breath sounds heard during auscultation of the lung fields; may include rales (crackles), rhonchi (wheezes), or pleural friction rubs

alopecia—hair loss

AMB—as manifested by

anorexia—loss of appetite for food

anthropometer—a type of caliper used for measuring elbow breadth and other body parts

anthropometric measurements—measurements of the human body (eg, height and weight, head circumference, waistline, percentage of body fat, and so forth)

anticholinergic effects—responses to anticholinergic medications, which inhibit the parasympathetic nervous system; in older adults, symptoms are associated with increased or decreased heart rate (depending on dosage), constipation, urinary retention, dilated pupils and vision problems, dry mouth, and drowsiness

anxiety—apprehensiveness related to an unknown source; occurs in different degrees

apical impulse—a normal visible pulsation in the area of the midclavicular line in the left fifth intercostal space; impulse can be seen in about half of the adult population

apnea—cessation of breathing

Argyll Robertson pupils—small, irregular pupils unresponsive to light

arthritis—inflammation of a joint

articulation—place of union or junction between two or more bones of the skeleton

atelectasis—collapse of a lung

atopic—allergic

atrial gallop—low-frequency heart sound known as S_4; occurs at the end of diastole when the atria contract and produced by vibrations from blood flowing rapidly into the ventricles after atrial contraction; S_4 has the rhythm of the word "Ten-nes-see" and may increase during inspiration

auscultation—assessment technique that uses a stethoscope to hear body sounds inaudible to the naked ear (eg, heart sounds, movement of blood through the vessels, bowel sounds, and air moving through the respiratory tract)

AV—atrioventricular

B

BCP—birth control pills

benign breast disease—nonmalignant disease of the breast, such as fibrocystic breast disease

biologic variation—changes in physical status as a result of genetics and/or environment and/or the interaction of genetics and environment; human variation of a biologic and physiologic nature

Biot's respiration—breathing pattern marked by several short breaths followed by long irregular periods of apnea; may be seen with IICP or head trauma

bipolar disorder—mood disorder categorized as a psychosis and characterized by emotional ups and downs ranging from extreme depression to extreme elation

BP—blood pressure

bradycardia—heart rate less than 60 beats per minute

bradypnea—slow breathing pattern less than 10 breaths per minute

Braxton Hicks contractions—painless, irregular contractions of the uterus

Brudzinski's sign—flexion of the hips and knees in response to neck flexion; a sign of meningeal inflammation

bruit—abnormal sound; blowing, swishing, or murmuring sound caused by turbulent blood flow; heard during auscultation

bruxism—grinding the teeth

Buerger's disease—obliterative vascular disease marked by inflammation in small and medium-sized blood vessels.

bursa—small sac filled with synovial fluid that lubricates and cushions a joint

C

calcium—chemical element (Ca^{++}) that is a major component of bone structure and a necessary element for muscle contractions

CAM—The Confusion Assessment Method (CAM) is a two part instrument to screen for overall cognitive impairment and to delirium or reversible confusion from other types of cognitive impairment.

capillary refill time—time it takes for reperfusion to occur after circulation has been stopped; test for capillary refill involves pressing on a fingernail firmly enough to stop circulation to the digit (signaled by blanching of the underlying tissue), releasing the pressure, and measuring the time it takes for color to return to the tissue; test is used to assess cardiac output

cardiac conduction—process of excitation initiated in the SA node, resulting in contraction of the heart muscle

cardiac cycle—cyclic filling and emptying of the heart

carotid artery—major coronary vessel that transports blood from the heart to the rest of the body

cataract—loss of transparency or cloudiness in the crystalline lens of the eye

Cheyne-Stokes respiration—breathing pattern characterized by a period of apnea of 10 to 60 seconds, followed by increasing, then decreasing rate, followed by another period of apnea

chloasma—darkening of the skin on the face, known as the "mask of pregnancy"

chorionic villi sampling—test to detect birth defects

closed-ended question—question that can be answered with a yes, no, maybe, or other one- or two-word answers;

typically used to clarify or specify information contributed in answers to open-ended questions; often begins with the words Are? Do? Did? Is? or Can?

clubbing—enlargement of fingertips and flattening of the angle between the fingernail and nailbed, as a result of heart and/or lung disease

CO—cardiac output

collaborative problems—physiologic complications that nurses monitor to detect their onset or changes in status (Carpenito, 2000)

colonoscopy—internal examination and visualization of the colon performed by a physician with a colonoscope, a fiber-optic endoscope with a miniature camera attachment

compulsion—repetitive act that the client must perform and over which he or she has no control

crepitus—a crackling sound/tactile sensation due to air under the skin; may also be heard in joints

critical thinking—complex thought process that has many definitions; in this textbook, critical thinking is best described as a thinking process used to arrive at a conclusion about information that is available; necessary when trying to reason or analyze what a client's diagnosis is or is not; investigational process or inquiry used to examine data in order to arrive at a conclusion

culture—as defined by Purnell and Paulanka, "the totality of socially transmitted behavioral patterns, arts, beliefs, values, customs, lifeways, and all other products of human work and thought characteristic of a population or people that guide their worldview and decision making"; all verbal and behavioral systems that transmit meaning

culture-bound syndrome—condition or state defined as an illness by a specific cultural group but not interpreted or perceived as an illness by other groups; may have a mental illness component or a spiritual cause

CVA—cerebrovascular accident, stroke

CVS—*see* chorionic villi sampling

cyanosis—bluish or gray coloring of the skin due to decreased amounts of hemoglobin in the blood suggesting reduced oxygenation

cystocele—herniation of the urinary bladder through the vaginal wall

D

delirium—potentially reversible alteration in mental status that has developed over a short time and is characterized by a change in level of alertness

delusion—false feelings of self that are unreal; may be symptoms of psychotic disorders, delirium, or dementia

dementia—diagnostic category that includes multiple physical disorders characterized by slowly deteriorating memory and alterations in abstract thinking, judgment and perception to the degree that the person's ability to perform everyday activities is affected

diastole—period when the heart relaxes and the ventricles fill with blood; in blood pressure measurements, the "bottom" value represents diastole

diastolic blood pressure—pressure between heartbeats (the pressure when the last sound is heard)

dimpling—indentation or retraction of subcutaneous tissue

direct percussion—direct tapping of a body part with one or two fingertips to elicit tenderness

documentation—committing findings in writing to the client's record

DRE—digital rectal examination

drug resistance—phenomenon that occurs when microorganisms develop a resistance to the effects of drug therapy, particularly antibiotic therapy

dyskinesia—incoordination marked by darting movements of the tongue and jerking movement of the arms and legs

dysphagia—difficulty swallowing solids or liquids

dystonia—abnormal muscle tone

E

ectopic pregnancy—pregnancy outside of the uterus; also called tubal pregnancy

ectropion—eversion of the lower eyelid

edema—accumulation of fluid in body tissues, which may cause swelling

ejection click—high-frequency heart sound auscultated just after S_1; produced by a diseased valve in mid-to-late systole

embryonic milk line—line formed during embryonic development; line starts in the axillary area, runs through the nipple, and extends down the abdomen on the outer side of the umbilicus down onto the upper, inner thigh; supernumerary breasts may occur along this line

entropion—inversion of the lower eyelid

epistaxis—nasal bleeding

erythema—redness due to capillary dilation

ethnicity—identification with a socially, culturally, and politically constructed group of people with common characteristics not shared by others with whom the group member come in contact

ethnocentrism—perception that our worldview is the only acceptable truth and that our beliefs, values, and sanctioned behaviors are superior to all others

exophthalmos—protruding eyes

extrapyramidal tract—descending pathway of the nervous system outside of the pyramidal tract and responsible for conducting impulses to the muscles for maintaining muscle tone and body control

exudate—any fluid that has exuded out of tissues (e.g., pus)

F

fasciculations—fine tremors

fibroadenoma—abnormal formation of tissue or tumor of the glandular epithelium-forming fibrous tissue

FOBT—fecal occult blood test; examination of a stool specimen to detect bleeding of unknown origin

fremitus—tactile vibration felt in neck and over the upper thorax from the transmission of vocal sounds from the airways to the surface of the chest wall

friction rub—auscultatory sound resulting from inflammation of the pericardial sac as with pericarditis

fundus—top of the uterus

G

GCS—Glasgow Coma Scale, an instrument for evaluating level of consciousness

geriatric syndrome—symptoms that are common harbingers of disease and disability in a frail elderly person

graphesthesia—ability to identify letters and numbers and drawing by touch and without sight

H

heart murmur—sounds made by turbulent blood flow through the valves of the heart

hemorrhoids—varicose veins in the rectum

hepatomegaly—enlargement of the liver

Homan's sign—aching or cramping pain in the calf felt with passive dorsiflexion of the foot; sign of thrombosis of deep veins in the calf

HR—heart rate

hyperemesis gravidarum—severe and lengthy nausea with pregnancy

I

ICS—intercostal space

illusion—false interpretation of actual stimuli

indirect percussion—also known as mediate percussion; most common percussion method in which tapping elicits a tone that varies with the density of underlying structures (eg, as density increases, the tone decreases)

induration—hardening

inframammary transverse ridge—firm compressed tissue that may be palpated below the mammary gland in the lower edges of the breasts especially in large breasts; normal variation and not a tumor

inspection—physical examination technique using the senses (vision, smell, and hearing) to observe the condition of various body parts, including normal and abnormal findings

intercostal spaces—spaces between the ribs; the first intercostal space is directly below the first rib, the second intercostal space is below the second rib, and so forth

J

jaundice—yellowness of the skin, eye whites, or mucous membranes due to a deposit of bile pigments related to excess bilirubin in the blood; often seen in clients with liver or gallbladder disease, hemolysis, and some anemias

joint—place where two or more bones meet, providing a variety of ranges of motion; a joint may be classified as fibrous, cartilaginous, or synovial

jugular veins—major neck vessels that transport blood from the head and neck to the heart

K

keratin—protein that is the chief component of skin, hair, and nails

Kernig's sign—pain and resistance to extension of the knee in response to flexion of the leg at the hip and the knee; bilateral pain and resistance are signs of meningeal irritation

Korsakoff's syndrome—psychosis induced by excessive alcohol use and characterized by disorientation, amnesia, hallucinations and confabulation

kyphosis—abnormally increased forward curvature of the upper spine

L

lanugo—fine, downy hairs that cover newborn's body

leading statement—statement made to elicit more information from the client; statements may begins with Explain, Describe, Tell, or Elaborate

lentigines—benign, spotty, brown skin discolorations, known as age spots or liver spots

lesion—abnormal change of tissue usually from injury or disease

leukoplakia—thick white patches of cells that adhere to oral tissues; condition is precancerous

ligament—strong dense band of fibrous connective tissue that joins the bones in synovial joints

linea nigra—dark line associated with pregnancy that extends from the umbilicus to the mons pubis

lordosis—exaggerated lumbar concavity often seen in pregnancy or obesity

M

macular degeneration—thinning or torn membrane in the center of the retina

mania—hyperexcitation; "manic" stage of manic–depressive disorder currently known as bipolar disorder

MCL—midclavicular line

melanin—pigment responsible for hair and skin color

menarche—first menstrual period

mucous plug—clump of mucus that seals the endocervical canal and prevents bacteria from ascending into the uterus

N

NANDA—North American Nursing Diagnosis Association

nonverbal communication—communication through body language including stance or posture, demeanor, facial expressions, and so forth

norms—learned behaviors that are perceived to be appropriate or inappropriate

NSR—normal sinus rhythm

nursing diagnosis—clinical judgment about individuals, family, or community responses to actual and potential health problems and life processes (North American Nursing Diagnosis Association, 2001–2002); provides the basis for selecting nursing interventions to achieve outcomes for which the nurse is accountable

nystagmus—rhythmic oscillation of the eyes

O

objective data—findings that are directly or indirectly observed through measurements; data can be physical characteristics (eg, skin color, rashes, posture), body functions (eg, heart rate, respiratory rate), appearance (eg, dress, hygiene), behavior (eg, mood, affect), measurements (eg, blood pressure, temperature, height, weight), or the results of laboratory testing (eg, platelet count, x-ray findings)

obsession—uncontrollable thought or thoughts that are unacceptable to client; characteristic of some neurotic disorders

OD—right eye (from the Latin *oculus dexter*)

open-ended question—question that cannot be answered with a yes, no, or maybe; usually requires a descriptive or explanatory answer; often begins with the words What? How? When? Where? or Who?

opening snap—extra heart sound occurring in early diastole and resulting from the opening of a stenotic or stiff mitral valve; often mistaken for a split S_2 or an S_3

orthopnea—difficulty breathing unless in a sitting or standing position; not uncommon in severe cardiac and pulmonary disease

orthostatic hypotension—drop in blood pressure when client arises from a sitting or lying position

OS—left eye (from the Latin *oculus sinister*)

osteoporosis—low bone density that occurs when bone-forming cells cannot keep pace with bone-destroying cells

OU—each eye (from the Latin *oculus uterque*)

P

PAD—peripheral artery disease

pallor—paleness, lack of color

palpation—examination technique in which the examiner uses the hands to touch and feel certain body characteristics, such as texture, temperature, mobility, shape, moisture, and motion

PAOD—peripheral arterial occlusive disease

paralytic strabismus—eyes deviate from normal position depending on the direction of gaze

parkinsonism—symptoms of Parkinson's disease that are secondary to another condition such as cerebral trauma, brain tumor, infection, or an adverse drug reaction

Parkinson's disease—chronic progressive degeneration of the brain's dopamine neuronal systems that is characterized by muscle rigidity, tremor, and slowed movements

PC—potential complication

percussion—tapping a body chamber with fingers to elicit the sounds from underlying organs and structures

perforator vein—vein that connects a superficial vein with a deep vein; also called communicator vein

PERRL—pupils equally reactive and responsive to light

pica—a craving for non-nutritional substances such as dirt or clay

pneumothorax—accumulation of air in the pleural space

point localization—ability to identify points touched on body without seeing the points touched

polyhydramnios—excessive amniotic fluid associated with multiple gestation or fetal abnormalities

postural hypotension—orthostatic hypotension characterized by dizziness or lightheadedness upon rising from a lying or sitting position

precordium—anterior surface of the body overlying the heart and great vessels

presbycusis—inability to hear high-frequency sounds or to discriminate a variety of simultaneous sounds caused by degeneration of the hair cells in the inner ear

presbyopia—farsightedness; person can see print and objects from farther away than considered normal

primary pain—original source of pain

proctosigmoidoscopy—internal examination and visualization of the sigmoid colon performed by a physician with a sigmoidoscope, a fiberoptic endoscope with miniature camera attachment

prodromal—precursor or early warning symptom of disease (eg, aura before a migraine headache or seizure)

proprioception—sensory faculties mediated by sensory nerves located in tissues such as the muscles and tendons

prostatic hyperplasia—enlargement of the prostate gland

pruritus—itching

PSA—prostate-specific antigen

pseudodementia—depressive symptoms that are commonly mistaken in the elderly for a dementia

pterygium—thickening of the bulbar conjunctiva that grows over the cornea and may interfere with vision

ptosis—drooping eyelids

ptyalism—excessive salivation

pulse amplitude—strength of the pulse

pyramidal tract—descending pathway of the nervous system; carries impulses that produce voluntary movements requiring skill and purpose

R

range of motion—natural distance and direction of movement of a joint

referral problem—problem that requires the attention or assistance of other health care professionals besides nurses

referred pain—pain perceived in an area that is not related to its original source (eg, gallbladder pain may radiate to the right shoulder and pancreatic pain may radiate to the back)

reinforcement technique—presentation of a stimulus so as to modify a response; increasing of a reflex response by causing the person to perform a physical or mental task while the reflex is being tested

retraction—indentation

r/t—related to

ruga—wrinkle, or fold, of skin or mucous membrane

S

SA—sinoatrial

satiety—fullness, satisfaction commonly associated with meals

scleroderma—degenerative disease characterized by fibrosis and vascular abnormalities in the skin and internal organs

scoliosis—lateral curvature of the spine with an increase in convexity on the side that is curved

SLUMS—Saint Louis University Mental Status (SLUMS) Examination Tool to determine mild cognitive impairment and dementia

splenomegaly—enlargement of the spleen

stereognosis—ability to identify an object by touch rather than sight

sternal retraction—pulling in of sternum during respiration in a physiologic attempt to take in more oxygen; seen in hypoxia or air hunger

STI—sexually transmitted infection; also called sexually transmitted disease

subjective data—descriptive rather than measurable information; symptoms, sensations, feelings, perceptions, desires, preferences, beliefs, ideas, values, and personal information contributed by a client or other person and verifiable only by the client or other person

supernumerary nipple—more than two nipples

SV—stroke volume; the volume of blood pumped with each contraction of the heart

synovitis—inflammation of the synovial membrane; synovial membrane surrounds the joint space and contains synovial fluid that lubricates the joint and enhances movement; characterized by painful movement of the joint

system—interacting whole formed of many parts

systole—cardiac phase during which the ventricles contract and eject blood into the pulmonary and circulatory systems

systolic blood pressure—pressure of the blood flow when the heart beats (the pressure when the first sound is heard).

T

tachycardia—heart rate exceeding 100 beats per minute

tachypnea—rapid, shallow breathing pattern exceeding 20 breaths per minute

temporal event—relating to a particular time of day or activity

tendon—strong fibrous cord of connective tissue continuous with the fibers of a muscle; tendon attaches muscle to bone or cartilage

TENS—transcutaneous electrical nerve stimulation; treatment modality associated with muscle pain, particularly low back pain

thelarche—time during puberty when breasts develop in females

thrill—palpable vibration over the precordium or an artery; usually the result of stenosis or partial occlusion

TIA—transient ischemic attack; minor stroke, sometimes called mini-stroke

TMJ syndrome—temporomandibular joint problems; limited range of motion, swelling, tenderness, pain, or crepitation in the jaw area

torus palatinus—bony protuberance on the hard palate where the intermaxillary transverse palatine sutures join

trigger factors—factors (eg, touch, pressure and/or chemical substances) that initiate or stimulate a response such as pain

turgor—normal skin tone, tension, and elasticity

U

uterine prolapse—protrusion of the cervix down through the vagina

UTI—urinary tract infection

V

validation—verification

values—learned beliefs about what is held to be good or bad

varicocele—varicose veins of the scrotum, which feels like a bag of worms upon palpation

venous hum—benign chest sound like roaring water caused by turbulence of blood in the jugular veins; common in children

ventricular gallop—another term for S_3, the third heart sound, which has low frequency and is often accentuated during inspiration; sound has rhythm of the word "Kentucky" and results from vibrations produced as blood hits the ventricular wall during filling

verbal communication—conversation with words, either spoken or written

viscera (solid, hollow)—internal organs; may consist of solid tissue (eg, liver) or be hollow to fill with fluids or other substances (eg, stomach or bladder)

visual field—what a person sees with one eye; field has four parts of quadrants—upper temporal, lower temporal, upper nasal, and lower nasal

vital signs—measurable signs of cardiopulmonary and thermoregulatory health status; signs include pulse rate, respiratory rate and character, blood pressure, and temperature. (*Note:* Some experts do not consider temperature a vital sign.)

voluntary guarding—person's willful attempt to protect body against pain by holding breath or tightening muscles

The following pieces of art were borrowed from **Lippincott Williams & Wilkins** sources:

Figures 6.2, 6.3, the photos in Abnormal Findings 13.1, and figures in Abnormal Findings 21.2 from Bickley, L.S. (2007). *Bates' Guide to Physical Examination and History Taking*, 9th edition.

Figures 13.1a, 14.1, 15.2, 15.3, 16.1, 20.2, 20.3, 21.1, 22.3, 23.2, 26.1, 26.2, 26.3, 27.1, 27.2, 27.6, 27.7, and the figures from displays 22.1, 26.1, and 26.2 from Cohen, B.J. and Taylor, J. (2009). *Memmler's Structure and Function of the Human Body*, 9th edition.

Figures 13.10, 13.11, and the figures in Abnormal Findings 14.1 from Hall, J.C. (2006). *Sauer's Manual of Skin Diseases*, 9th edition.

Figures 30.2, 30.5, 30.6, 30.7, 30.15, 31.1, 31.4, 31.5, 31.6, 31.10, and 31.11 from Klossner, N.J., and Hatfield, N. (2006). *Introductory Maternity and Pediatric Nursing*.

Figure 29.19 from Pillitteri, A. (2008). *Maternal and Child Health Nursing*, 5th edition.

Figures 8.2 and 8.3 from Porth, C.M. (2007). *Essentials of Pathophysiology*, 2nd edition.

Figures 22.14, 22.18, 22.19, 22.22, 22.29, 23.7, 24.5, and 26.18 from Rhoads, J. (2006). *Advanced Health Assessment and Diagnostic Reasoning*.

Figure 21.15 from Rubin, R. and Strayer, D.S. (2007). *Rubin's Pathology: Clinicopathologic Foundations of Medicine*, 5th edition.

Figure 8.1 from Taylor, C., Lillis, C., LeMone, P. (2006). *Fundamentals of Nursing*, 6th edition.

Note: Page numbers followed by f indicate figures; those followed by t indicate tables; and those followed by d indicate display material.